Surgical Oncology

LIST OF CONTRIBUTORS BY SPECIALTY

Surgery

Kranthi Achanta MD (Laparoscopic Surgery)
Charles M Balch MD (Surgical Oncology)
Nicole Baril MD (General Surgery)
George Berci MD (Laparoscopic Surgery)
Leslie H Blumgart MD (Hepatobiliary Surgery)
Cedric G Bremner MD, BCh, ChM (General Surgery)
John A Butler MD (Surgical Oncology)
Blake Cady MD (Surgical Oncology)
Linda S Callans MD (Surgical Oncology)
Mimi H Chiang PhD (Research)
Steven D Colquhoun MD (Transplant Surgery)
Caroline A Connelly PhD (Transplant Research)
Marvin L Corman MD (Colorectal Surgery)
John M Daly MD (Surgical Oncology)
Tom R DeMeester MD (Foregut Surgery)
Achilles A Demetriou MD, PhD (Transplant Surgery)
James E Duncan MD (General Surgery)
Rahila Essani MD (Laparoscopic Surgery)
Melanie H Friedlander MD (Laparoscopic Surgery)
Clark B Fuller MD (Thoracic Surgery)
Armando E Giuliano MD (Surgical Oncology)
Leo A Gordon MD (General Surgery)
Steven W Grant MD (Laparoscopic Surgery)
Seth P Harlow MD (Surgical Oncology)
Gila Hornreich MD (Gynecology)
James F Huth MD (Surgical Oncology)
Rosa F Hwang MD (General Surgery)
Ralph C Jones MD (Surgical Oncology)
Kim U Kahng MD (General Surgery)
Andreas M Kaiser MD (Laparoscopic Surgery)
Brian J Kaplan MD (Surgical Oncology)
Namir Katkhouda MD (Laparoscopic Surgery)
David N Krag MD (Surgical Oncology)
Walter Lawrence Jr MD (Surgical Oncology)
Alan T Lefor MD, MPH (Surgical Oncology)

Craig A Lipkin* MD (Transplant Surgery)
Megan McGarvey BA (Research)
Robert J McKenna Jr MD (Thoracic Surgery)
Leslie Memsic MD (Surgical Oncology)
Lawrence R Menendez MD (Orthopedic Oncology)
Leon Morgenstern MD (General Surgery)
Monica Morrow MD (Surgical Oncology)
Theodore X O'Connell MD (Surgical Oncology)
Mitchell C Posner MD (Surgical Oncology)
Joe B Putnam Jr MD (Thoracic Surgery)
Kenneth P Ramming MD (Surgical Oncology)
Howard A Reber MD (General Surgery)
John L Rombeau MD (Colorectal Surgery)
Daniel F Roses MD (Surgical Oncology)
Joel L Roslyn* MD (General Surgery)
Jack A Roth MD (Thoracic Surgery)
Gordon F Schwartz MD, MBA (Surgical Oncology)
Allan W Silberman MD, PhD (Surgical Oncology)
Howard Silberman MD (Surgical Oncology)
Melvin J Silverstein MD (Surgical Oncology)
Muthukumaran Sivanandham PhD (Research)
Kristin A Skinner MD (Surgical Oncology)
Vernon K Sondak MD (Surgical Oncology)
Bruce E Stabile MD (General Surgery)
Valerie L Staradub MD (Surgical Oncology)
Christos I Stavropoulos MD (General Surgery)
Paul H Sugarbaker MD (Surgical Oncology)
Karen E Todd MD (General Surgery)
Josephine Tsai MD (Colorectal Surgery)
Lawrence D Wagman MD (Surgical Oncology)
Marc K Wallack MD (Surgical Oncology)
Sharon Weber MD (Hepatobiliary Surgery)
Julie A Wolfe MD (General Surgery)
Sherry M Wren MD (General Surgery)

Medical Oncology/Hematology

M William Audeh MD
Robert W Decker MD
John F DiPersio MD, PhD
Dan Douer MD
Charles Forscher MD
John A Glaspy MD

Steven M Grunberg MD
Toshiyasu Hirama MD
Syma Iqbal MD
William H Isacoff MD
Valerie Israel DO
John J Kavanagh MD

Nancy E Kemeny MD
Hanna Khoury MD
H Phillip Koeffler MD
Edmund S Lee MD
Heinz-Josef Lenz MD
Franco M Muggia MD

Christy A Russell MD
Gregory Sarna MD
Darcy V Spicer MD
Seisho Takeuchi MD, PhD
Kunihiro Tsukasaki MD
Steven J Tucker MD

James R Waisman MD
Jeffrey S Weber MD, PhD
Edward M Wolin MD

Molecular Biology/ Medical Genetics[1]

Robin D Clark MD
Wolf-Karsten Hofmann PhD
Carl W Miller PhD
Malcolm C Pike PhD

Pathology

Sunanda J Chatterjee MD, PhD
Richard J Cote MD
Debra Hawes MD
Michael D Lagios MD
A Munro Neville MD, PhD, DSc
Clive R Taylor MD PhD

Radiation Oncology

Silvia C Formenti MD
Bernard S Lewinsky MD

Radiology

Marc L Friedman MD
Yuri Parisky MD

Surgical Oncology

Multidisciplinary approach to difficult problems

Edited by

HOWARD SILBERMAN MD
Department of Surgery,
University of Southern California,
Los Angeles, California, USA

ALLAN W SILBERMAN MD, PhD
Cedars-Sinai Comprehensive Cancer Center,
Los Angeles, California, USA

ARNOLD

A member of the Hodder Headline Group
LONDON   NEW YORK   NEW DELHI

First published in Great Britain in 2002 by
Arnold, a member of the Hodder Headline Group,
338 Euston Road, London NW1 3BH

http://www.arnoldpublishers.com

Distributed in the United States of America by
Oxford University Press Inc.,
198 Madison Avenue, New York, NY10016
Oxford is a registered trademark of Oxford University Press

British Library Cataloguing in Publication Data
A catalogue record for this book is available from the British Library

Library of Congress Cataloging-in-Publication Data
A catalog record for this book is available from the Library of
Congress

ISBN 0 340 76242 X (hb)

1 2 3 4 5 6 7 8 9 10

Commissioning Editor: Nick Dunton
Development Editor: Michael Lax
Production Editor: Rada Radojicic
Production Controller: Martin Kerans
Cover Design: Mouse Mat Design

Typeset in 10/12 pt Minion by Charon Tec Pvt. Ltd, Chennai, India
Printed and bound in Italy by Giunti

This book is dedicated to the memory of our beloved parents, Albert and Bertha Silberman, and to our wonderful Aunt Esther, who gave us the strength and encouragement to pursue careers in surgery. Also, enough cannot be said for the love and support from our family, Kathy and Samantha, who were always there when we needed them.

Contents

*Deceased.

---

*Deceased.

Contributors

Kranthi Achanta MD
Instructor in Surgery, Keck School of Medicine, University of Southern California, Los Angeles, California, USA

M William Audeh MD
Associate Clinical Professor of Medicine, University of California, Los Angeles, Clinical Co-Chief, Hematology/Oncology, Cedars-Sinai Medical Center, Los Angeles, California, USA

Charles M Balch MD
Departments of Surgery and Oncology, Johns Hopkins Medical Institutions, Baltimore, Maryland and Executive Vice President, American Society of Clinical Oncology, Alexandria, Virginia, USA

Nicole Baril MD
Instructor in Surgery, Keck School of Medicine, University of Southern California, Los Angeles, California, USA

George Berci MD
Clinical Professor of Surgery, Keck School of Medicine, University of Southern California,
Director, Endoscopic Research and Training, Cedars-Sinai Medical Center, Los Angeles, California, USA

Leslie H Blumgart MD
Enid A Haupt Chair in Surgery,
Chief, Hepatobiliary Service, Director, Hepatobiliary Disease Management Program,
Memorial Sloan-Kettering Cancer Center,
New York, USA

Cedric G Bremner MD, BCh, ChM
Professor of Clinical Surgery, Keck School of Medicine, University of Southern California, Los Angeles, California, USA

John A Butler MD
Associate Professor and Chief, Division of Oncological Surgery, College of Medicine, University of California, Irvine, Orange, California, USA

Blake Cady MD
Professor of Surgery, Brown University, Director, Breast Health Center at Women and Infants' Hospital, Providence, Rhode Island, USA

Linda S Callans MD
Assistant Professor of Surgery, University of Pennsylvania School of Medicine, Philadelphia, Pennsylvania, USA

Sunanda J Chatterjee MD, PhD
Research Associate, Department of Pathology, Keck School of Medicine, University of Southern California, Los Angeles, California, USA

Mimi H Chiang PhD
Research Assistant Professor of Surgery, Keck School of Medicine, University of Southern California, Los Angeles, California, USA

Robin D Clark MD
Clinical Associate Professor of Pediatrics, Head, Cancer Genetics Unit, Keck School of Medicine, University of Southern California, Los Angeles, California, USA

Steven D Colquhoun MD
Associate Professor of Surgery, University of California, Los Angeles, Program Director, Center for Liver Diseases and Transplantation, Cedars-Sinai Medical Center, Los Angeles, California, USA

Caroline A Connelly PhD
Adjunct Assistant Professor, Department of Surgery, University of California, Los Angeles, Research Scientist, Section of Transplantation Research, Cedars-Sinai Medical Center, Los Angeles, California, USA

Marvin L Corman MD
Professor of Surgery, Division of Colon and Rectal Surgery, Keck School of Medicine, University of Southern California, Los Angeles, California, USA

Richard J Cote MD
Professor of Pathology and Urology, Keck School of Medicine, University of Southern California, Los Angeles, California, USA

John M Daly MD
Lewis Atterbury Stimson Professor of Surgery and Chair, Department of Surgery, Weill Medical College of Cornell University, New York, USA

Robert W Decker MD
Clinical Associate Professor of Medicine, University of California at Los Angeles, Attending, Hematology/Oncology, Tower Hematology–Oncology Medical Group, Cedars-Sinai Medical Center, Los Angeles, California, USA

Tom R DeMeester MD
Professor and Chair, Department of Surgery, Jeffrey P Smith Chair in Surgery, Keck School of Medicine,

University of Southern California, Los Angeles, California, USA

Achilles A Demetriou MD, PhD
Esther and Mark Shulman Chair in Surgery and Transplantation Medicine, Chair, Department of Surgery, Cedars-Sinai Medical Center, Los Angeles, California, USA

John F DiPersio MD, PhD
Professor of Medicine, Pathology, and Pediatrics, Chief, Division of Bone Marrow Transplantation and Stem Cell Biology, Barnard Cancer Center, Washington University School of Medicine, Saint Louis, Missouri, USA

Dan Douer MD
Associate Professor of Medicine, Keck School of Medicine, University of Southern California, Director, Bone Marrow Transplantation Program, USC/Norris Comprehensive Cancer Center, Los Angeles, California, USA

James E Duncan MD, LT, MC, USNR
Resident in General Surgery, United States Naval Medical Center, Bethesda, Maryland, USA

Rahila Essani MD
Research Assistant, Department of Surgery, Keck School of Medicine, University of Southern California, Los Angeles, California, USA

Silvia C Formenti MD
Professor and Chair, Radiation Oncology, New York University School of Medicine, New York, USA

Charles Forscher MD
Assistant Clinical Professor of Medicine, University of California at Los Angeles, Attending, Hematology/Oncology, Cedars-Sinai Medical Center, Los Angeles, California, USA

Melanie H Friedlander MD
Instructor in Surgery, Keck School of Medicine, University of Southern California, Los Angeles, California, USA

Marc L Friedman MD
Director, Vascular and Interventional Radiology, Department of Imaging, Cedars-Sinai Medical Center, Los Angeles, California, USA

Clark B Fuller MD
Assistant Professor of Cardiothoracic Surgery, Keck School of Medicine, University of Southern California, Attending, Thoracic Surgery, Cedars-Sinai Medical Center, Los Angeles, California, USA

Armando E Giuliano MD
Chief of Surgical Oncology, Saint John's Hospital and Health Center, John Wayne Cancer Institute, Santa Monica, California, USA

John A Glaspy MD
Professor of Medicine, University of California at Los Angeles, Los Angeles, California, USA

Leo A Gordon MD
Attending, General Surgery, Department of Surgery, Cedars-Sinai Medical Center, Los Angeles, California, USA

Steven W Grant MD
Instructor in Surgery, Keck School of Medicine, University of Southern California, Los Angeles, California, USA

Steven M Grunberg MD
Professor of Medicine, University of Vermont College of Medicine, Burlington, Vermont, USA

Seth P Harlow MD
Assistant Professor of Surgery, Department of Surgery, University of Vermont College of Medicine, Burlington, Vermont, USA

Debra Hawes MD
Assistant Professor of Clinical Pathology, Keck School of Medicine, University of Southern California, Los Angeles, California, USA

Toshiyasu Hirama MD
Division of Hematology/Oncology, Cedars-Sinai Medical Center, Los Angeles, California, USA

Wolf-Karsten Hofmann PhD
Research Scholar, Division of Hematology/Oncology, Cedars-Sinai Medical Center, Los Angeles, California, USA

Gila Hornreich MD
Senior Physician, Division of Gynecologic Surgery and Oncology, Shaare Zedek Medical Center, Jerusalem, Israel

James F Huth MD
Professor and Chair, Division of Surgical Oncology, Occidental Chemical Chair in Cancer Research, University of Texas Southwestern Medical Center, Dallas, Texas, USA

Rosa F Hwang MD
Fellow in Surgical Oncology, University of Texas MD Anderson Cancer Center, Houston, Texas, USA

Syma Iqbal MD
Fellow in Medical Oncology, Keck School of Medicine, University of Southern California, Los Angeles, California, USA

William H Isacoff MD
Assistant Clinical Professor of Medicine, University of California, Los Angeles, California, USA

Valerie Israel DO
Assistant Professor of Medicine, Keck School of Medicine, University of Southern California, Los Angeles, California, USA

Ralph C Jones MD, LCDR, MC, USN
Chief of Surgical Oncology, United States Naval Medical Center, Bethesda, Maryland, USA

Kim U Kahng MD
Associate Professor and Vice Chair for Veterans' Affairs, Department of Surgery, Medical College of Wisconsin, Chief, Surgical Subspecialties, Zablocki Veterans' Administration Medical Center, Milwaukee, Wisconsin, USA

Andreas M Kaiser MD
Fellow in Colorectal Surgery, Keck School of Medicine, University of Southern California, Los Angeles, California, USA

Brian J Kaplan MD
Assistant Professor of Surgery, Medical College of Virginia, Richmond, Virginia, USA

Namir Katkhouda MD
Professor of Surgery, Keck School of Medicine, University of Southern California, Los Angeles, California, USA

John J Kavanagh MD
Professor of Medicine, Chief, Section of Gynecologic Medical Oncology, Department of Clinical Investigation, University of Texas MD Anderson Cancer Center, Houston, Texas, USA

Nancy E Kemeny MD
Professor of Medicine, Weill Medical College of Cornell University, Attending Physician, Gastrointestinal Oncology Service, Memorial Sloan-Kettering Cancer Center, New York, USA

Hanna Khoury MD
Assistant Professor of Medicine, Division of Bone Marrow Transplantation and Stem Cell Biology, Washington University School of Medicine, Saint Louis, Missouri, USA

H Phillip Koeffler MD
Professor of Medicine, University of California at Los Angeles, Mark Goodson Endowed Chair for Hematology/Oncology, Cedars-Sinai Medical Center, Los Angeles, California, USA

David N Krag MD
Associate Professor of Surgery, University of Vermont College of Medicine, Burlington, Vermont, USA

Michael D Lagios MD
Medical Director, Breast Cancer Consultation Service, Saint Mary's Medical Center, San Francisco, California, USA

Walter Lawrence Jr MD
Professor of Surgery, Emeritus, Director, Emeritus, Massey Cancer Center, Virginia Commonwealth University, Richmond, Virginia, USA

Edmund S Lee MD
Fellow in Medical Oncology, Keck School of Medicine, University of Southern California, Los Angeles, California, USA

Alan T Lefor MD, MPH
Associate Professor of Clinical Surgery, University of California at Los Angeles, Director, Division of Surgical Oncology, Cedars-Sinai Medical Center, Los Angeles, California, USA

Heinz-Josef Lenz MD
Associate Professor of Medicine, Division of Medical Oncology, Keck School of Medicine, University of Southern California, Los Angeles, California, USA

Bernard S Lewinsky MD
Western Tumor Medical Group, Sherman Oaks, California, USA

Craig A Lipkin* MD
Research Fellow, Division of Liver Transplant Surgery, Department of Surgery, Cedars-Sinai Medical Center, Los Angeles, California, USA

Megan McGarvey BA
Research Assistant, Department of Surgery, Keck School of Medicine, University of Southern California, Los Angeles, California, USA

Robert J McKenna Jr MD
Clinical Professor of Thoracic Surgery, University of California at Los Angeles, Clinical Chief, General Thoracic Surgery, Cedars-Sinai Medical Center, Los Angeles, California, USA

Leslie Memsic MD
Division of Surgical Oncology, Cedars-Sinai Medical Center, Los Angeles, California, USA

Lawrence R Menendez MD
Professor of Clinical Orthopedics, Keck School of Medicine, University of Southern California, Los Angeles, California, USA

Carl W Miller PhD
Division of Hematology/Oncology, Cedars-Sinai Medical Center, Los Angeles, California, USA

Leon Morgenstern MD
Emeritus Professor of Surgery, University of California at Los Angeles, Emeritus Director of Surgery, Cedars-Sinai Medical Center, Los Angeles, California, USA

Monica Morrow MD
Director, Cancer Program, American College of Surgeons, Professor of Surgery, Northwestern University Medical School, Director, Lynn Sage Comprehensive Breast Program, Northwestern Memorial Hospital, Chicago, Illinois, USA

Franco M Muggia MD
Anne Murnick and David H Cogan Professor of Oncology, New York University School of Medicine, New York, USA

A Munro Neville MD, PhD, DSc
Associate Director, Ludwig Institute for Cancer Research, Visiting Professor, Royal Postgraduate Medical School, London, England

Theodore X O'Connell MD
Chief of Surgical Oncology, Southern California Permanente Medical Group, Los Angeles, California, USA

Yuri Parisky MD
Associate Professor of Radiology, Keck School of Medicine, University of Southern California, Los Angeles, California, USA

---

*Deceased.

Malcolm C Pike PhD
Flora L Thornton Professor of Preventive Medicine, Keck School of Medicine, University of Southern California, Los Angeles, California, USA

Mitchell C Posner MD
Associate Professor of Surgery, University of Chicago Medical Center, Chicago, Illinois, USA

Joe B Putnam Jr MD
Associate Professor and Vice Chair, Department of Thoracic and Cardiovascular Surgery, University of Texas MD Anderson Cancer Center, Houston, Texas, USA

Kenneth P Ramming MD
Director, Cancer Center, Century City Hospital, Los Angeles, California, USA

Howard A Reber MD
Professor and Vice Chair, Department of Surgery, University of California, Los Angeles, California, USA

John L Rombeau MD
Professor of Surgery, University of Pennsylvania School of Medicine, Philadelphia, Pennsylvania, USA

Daniel F Roses MD
Jules Leonard Whitehill Professor of Surgery, New York University Medical Center, New York, USA

Joel L Roslyn* MD
Alma Dea Professor and Chair, Allegheny University of the Health Sciences, Department of Surgery, Medical College of Pennsylvania – Hahnemann School of Medicine, Philadelphia, Pennsylvania, USA

Jack A Roth MD
Professor and Chair, Department of Thoracic and Cardiovascular Surgery, Bud S Johnson Clinical Chair of Tumor Biology, Director, WM Keck Center for Cancer Gene Therapy, University of Texas MD Anderson Cancer Center, Houston, Texas, USA

Christy A Russell MD
Associate Professor of Medicine, Keck School of Medicine, University of Southern California, Los Angeles, California, USA

Gregory Sarna MD
Clinical Professor of Medicine, University of California, Los Angeles, Attending, Hematology/Oncology, Cedars-Sinai Medical Center, Research Director, Cedars-Sinai Comprehensive Cancer Center, Los Angeles, California, USA

Gordon F Schwartz MD, MBA
Professor of Surgery, Jefferson Medical College, Philadelphia, Pennsylvania, USA

Allan W Silberman MD, PhD
Clinical Chief, Division of Surgical Oncology, Cedars-Sinai Medical Center, Los Angeles, California, USA

Howard Silberman MD
Professor of Surgery, Keck School of Medicine, University of Southern California, Los Angeles, California, USA

Melvin J Silverstein MD
Professor of Surgery, Henrietta C Lee Chair in Breast Cancer Research, Keck School of Medicine, University of Southern California, Director, Harold E and Henrietta C Lee Breast Center, USC/Norris Comprehensive Cancer Center, Los Angeles, California, USA

Muthukumaran Sivanandham PhD
Director, Surgical Research Laboratory, Department of Surgery, Saint Vincent Hospital and Medical Center, New York, USA

Kristin A Skinner MD
Assistant Professor of Surgery, Keck School of Medicine, University of Southern California, Los Angeles, California, USA

Vernon K Sondak MD
Associate Professor of Surgery, University of Michigan Medical School, Ann Arbor, Michigan, USA

Darcy V Spicer MD
Associate Professor of Clinical Medicine, Keck School of Medicine, University of Southern California, Los Angeles, California, USA

Bruce E Stabile MD
Professor of Surgery and Chair, Department of Surgery, Harbor–UCLA Medical Center, Torrance, California, USA

Valerie L Staradub MD
Assistant Professor of Surgery, Northwestern University Medical School, Chicago, Illinois, USA

Christos I Stavropoulos MD
Department of Surgery, Saint Vincent Hospital and Medical Center, New York, USA

Paul H Sugarbaker MD
The Washington Cancer Center, Washington Hospital Center, Washington, DC, USA

Seisho Takeuchi MD, PhD
Division of Hematology/Oncology, Cedars-Sinai Medical Center, Los Angeles, California, USA

Clive R Taylor MD, PhD
Professor and Chair, Department of Pathology, Keck School of Medicine, University of Southern California, Los Angeles, California, USA

Karen E Todd MD
Department of Surgery, University of California, Los Angeles, California, USA

Josephine Tsai MD
Resident in Colorectal Surgery, Keck School of Medicine, University of Southern California, Los Angeles, California, USA

Kunihiro Tsukasaki MD, PhD
Division of Hematology/Oncology, Cedars-Sinai Medical Center, Los Angeles, California, USA

*Deceased.

Steven J Tucker MD
Compassionate Oncology Medical Group, Los Angeles, California, USA

Lawrence D Wagman MD
Chair, Division of Surgery, City of Hope National Medical Center, Duarte, California, USA

James R Waisman MD
Associate Professor of Clinical Medicine, Keck School of Medicine, University of Southern California, Los Angeles, California, USA

Marc K Wallack MD
Professor and Chair, Department of Surgery, Saint Vincent Hospital and Medical Center, New York Medical College, New York, USA

Jeffrey S Weber MD, PhD
Associate Professor of Medicine, Keck School of Medicine, University of Southern California, Los Angeles, California, USA

Sharon Weber MD
Hepatobiliary Fellow, Department of Surgery, Memorial Sloan-Kettering Cancer Center, New York, New York, USA

Julie A Wolfe MD
Resident in Surgery, University of Michigan Medical School, Ann Arbor, Michigan, USA

Edward M Wolin MD
Attending, Hematology/Oncology and Stem-Cell Transplantation, Associate Medical Director, Cedars-Sinai Comprehensive Cancer Center, Los Angeles, California, USA

Sherry M Wren MD
Assistant Professor of Surgery, Stanford University School of Medicine, Chief of General Surgery, Palo Alto Veterans Administration Medical Center, Palo Alto, California, USA

Foreword

Not too long ago the management of patients with particular types of neoplasms was routinely assigned to surgery, radiation therapy or medical oncology, and then further divided into various anatomically oriented specialties. Fortunately, this pigeonholing is rapidly becoming obsolete. Sophisticated imaging technology, newer cytotoxic and antiangiogenesis drugs, antibody or vaccine immunotherapy, molecular-based laboratory assessments, and minimally invasive surgical techniques have brought us to a multidisciplinary approach to neoplastic disease. Thus, while surgery is still the most frequently used cancer therapy, it is most often curative when combined with nonsurgical interventions.

Today's surgical oncologists, medical oncologists, radiologists, nuclear medicine physicians, and pathologists are positioning themselves along a highly interactive treatment continuum. On this continuum, preoperative chemotherapy and radiation therapy may be used to minimize the extent and increase the efficacy of surgical resection; alternatively, cytoreductive surgery may be undertaken to reduce tumor volume and thereby improve the response to systemic chemotherapy or immunotherapy. A multimodal approach has made conservative surgery possible in breast carcinoma, bone and soft tissue sarcoma, prostate cancer, head and neck cancer, and other neoplasms, improving not only the duration but also the quality of life.

This text edited by brothers Drs. Howard and Allan Silberman is a most timely acknowledgement of the team approach to oncology. Most of its chapters are specialty-independent treatment scenarios for breast cancer, melanoma, esophageal cancer, and common gastrointestinal cancers. These chapters are accompanied by treatment algorithms, surgical diagrams, and carefully chosen tabular displays. Balancing these specific chapters are background chapters that overview the metastatic process and the molecular basis of cancer. Another unique aspect of the book is its inclusion of expert commentary at the end of each chapter, which serves as a complement, supplement, critique, and/or overview. This gives the reader added perspective, as do the selected abstracts at the end of each chapter. These abstracts were chosen by the editors and generally represent the most recently published studies for the oncology problem under discussion.

This text's comprehensive nature and practical, problem-solving approach make it useful for general surgeons and surgical residents, as well as for practicing surgical, medical, and radiation oncologists. Because surgery is increasingly combined with other treatment modalities, the team approach is essential. This text reminds us of our obligation to provide comprehensive multidisciplinary treatment that is defined not by the patient or by the type of neoplasm, but by the need to integrate the most recent advances in striving for a cure for each patient's cancer.

Donald L Morton, MD
Medical Director and Surgeon-in-Chief,
John Wayne Cancer Institute,
Santa Monica, California

Preface

The management of solid tumors has undergone dramatic evolution in the last century. The earlier approach to cure called for ever-more radical surgical extirpation in accordance with the Halstedian concept that cancer spreads primarily by contiguous extension throughout the body. Advances in cancer biology, pathology, and imaging sciences have led to more limited, conservative surgery with perioperative adjunctive therapies designed to address micrometastatic deposits now known to exist frequently, even at the earliest stages of clinically evident disease. Such occult systemic disease undoubtedly explains the treatment failures commonly observed after apparently successful surgical resection alone.

Thus, to provide optimal oncologic care in the twenty-first century, the surgeon must not only be technically adroit, but must also be well versed in the biology of cancer and have a thorough understanding of the range of therapies that other oncologic disciplines can offer patients in order to enhance outcome. The advantages of a multidisciplinary approach in the evaluation and treatment of patients with solid tumors have become increasingly clear over the last two decades. It is our view that neoadjuvant and/or adjuvant therapy are worthy of consideration in many, even the majority, of our patients at the present time, and we expect that such adjunctive treatment will be an essential component of therapy in virtually all patients with solid malignancies as research yields more potent pharmacologic and biologic agents.

We have not attempted to provide a comprehensive textbook of surgical oncology, but, instead, we present a multidisciplinary analysis of the common solid malignancies, highlighting the controversial issues in clinical judgment surrounding each problem. In addition, gene therapy, bone marrow and stem cell transplantation, and other non-surgical therapies are discussed, as well as some of the newer surgical techniques, such as sentinel lymph node analysis and therapeutic laparoscopy. A chapter on organ transplantation for malignant disease and malignant disease as a result of transplantation is also included.

Clinical judgments which must be rendered prior to the availability of conclusive scientific evidence often differ among even the most experienced physicians. We believe that, to understand such controversial issues, other viewpoints are often necessary to highlight and emphasize the problem. Thus, each of our primary chapters is followed by a commentary by another expert in the field to offer a contrasting opinion or to discuss a tangential issue which may not be discussed by the primary author. In addition, following each chapter and commentary, we have selected several abstracts from the recently published literature which also relate to the issues involved and allow us to provide the most current information possible in a book.

Finally, we wish to acknowledge associates whose assistance was invaluable as we worked through the conceptual development of this book, the recruitment of contributors, and the editing of the many manuscripts comprising this work. Dick Hebert, our editorial assistant and experienced writer in his own right, so competently managed the innumerable details of organizing the book and communicating with our many contributing authors and our editors at Arnold that we were able to complete this volume while still maintaining our usual clinical activities. Nick Dunton, at Arnold, rescued our fledgling project during a period of instability in the publishing industry, and he, with Michael Lax, supported our novel approach in which we use commentaries and current abstracts from the recent literature to facilitate the currency of the scientific material. We also express our thanks to Rada Radojicic, Production Editor at Arnold, and we must make special note of the extraordinary attention to detail provided by our Copy-editor, Jane Smith, who contributed so much to the accuracy of the final printed product.

Howard Silberman
Allan W Silberman
Los Angeles, California

Web-site

A web-site to accompany this book can be found at www.silberman-oncology.com. This fully interactive site has the following features:

- full bibliographic details of the book
- contents and introductory material
- expanded contributor list (including photographs, mini-biographies and links through to Institution web-sites)
- a sample chapter
- all current Abstracts from the book in searchable format with linking through to the PubMed version of the full article
- new abstracts will be added regularly to keep the book's content up to date

- a template for users to submit their own Commentaries on chapters. These would be subject to peer-review and, if acceptable, would be posted on the site and count as an on-line 'publication'
- links section – hot-links out to other sites of interest.

Please take the time to visit the site. We hope you will find the content of interest and that you will submit content to help build this into a valuable resource center for all clinicians working in Surgical Oncology.

Howard Silberman
Allan W Silberman
Los Angeles, California

Principles of molecular biology for cancer surgeons

ROSA F HWANG, NICOLE BARIL, MEGAN MCGARVEY, MIMI H CHIANG,
SILVIA C FORMENTI, AND KRISTIN A SKINNER

The past two decades have brought an explosion in our understanding of the molecular biology of cancer. From the mid-1970s, when it became accepted that cancer developed as a result of genetic mutations, we have identified and characterized many of the genes responsible for cancer formation. Malignant transformation is a complex process, involving not only cell proliferation and escape from normal regulation, but also alterations in gene expression, and in cell/matrix interactions, leading to invasion of surrounding tissues, angiogenesis, and metastasis formation. This chapter provides a brief overview of the current understanding of the molecular basis of oncogenesis, as well as of the potential clinical applications of these advances.

OVERVIEW OF THE MOLECULAR BIOLOGY OF CANCER

In order to understand the biology of cancer, it is necessary first to understand the biology of normal cellular processes. The normal cell undergoes a cycle of growth and division, called the cell cycle, that is a tightly controlled process. Control of cellular proliferation involves a cascade of events connecting extracellular signals to intranuclear responses. Angiogenesis and cell/matrix interactions are critical events in the pathogenesis of cancer. Alterations in oncogenes and tumor suppressor genes are involved in all of these processes.

Cell-cycle control

Replicating somatic cells progress through a defined process prior to cell division: an initial growth phase in the absence of DNA replication (G1), a period of DNA replication (S), a growth phase following DNA synthesis

(G2), and finally mitosis (M). At the completion of mitosis, a decision is made regarding whether the daughter cell is destined to replicate, entering G1, or whether it is to remain growth arrested, entering a phase termed G0 (Figure 1.1). The cell cycle is largely regulated by a special class of protein kinases, called cyclin-dependent kinases (cdks). These kinases are active only when complexed with unstable regulatory elements, called cyclins, that fluctuate in abundance during the cell cycle.[1] Progression through G1 is regulated by cyclin D in complex with cdk4 or cdk6. Progression through S-phase is regulated by cyclin E or cyclin A in complex with cdk2. Progression through M is regulated by cyclins A or B in complex with cdk1.[2] The activation of the cdks is controlled at multiple levels. Synthesis of the activating cyclins is regulated at the transcriptional level. Cyclin–cdk complexes are subject to both activating and inactivating phosphorylations. The cdks are further regulated by binding to specific cdk inhibitors (e.g., p15, p16, p21, p27) and other proteins such as sic1, an S-phase cdk inhibitor. Finally, the activating cyclins are periodically destroyed through proteolysis. At the G1–S transition, G1 cyclins undergo proteolysis, and sic1 is destroyed. During mitosis, the M-cdks are destroyed by the anaphase-promoting complex (An-PC).[3]

Each step in the cell cycle is tightly regulated, and progression is dependent on the completion of events in the previous step. At the completion of mitosis, most cells enter a resting state, termed G0. When the cell receives signals to proliferate (growth factors, nutritional signals, etc.) cyclin D is produced, which complexes with and activates cdk4 and cdk6. These active kinases then phosphorylate and inactivate pRB, the gene product of the retinoblastoma tumor suppressor gene. Inactivation of pRB leads to the activation of E2F, a transcription factor which then activates transcription of many genes that are required for DNA synthesis and chromosome duplication. Further,

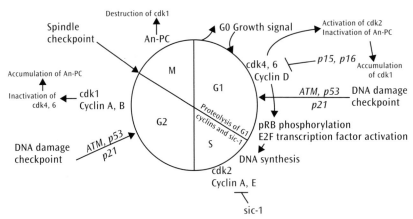

Figure 1.1 *Cell-cycle control. Cells rest in G0 unless stimulated by a growth signal, at which time they enter G1 growth phase via activation of cyclin D. Cyclin D, in turn, activates the G1 cyclin-dependent kinases (cdks), cdk4 and cdk6. Inhibitors of the G1 cdks include p15, p16, and p21. G1 cdks activate the S-phase cdk, cdk2, and inactivate the anaphase promoting complex (An-PC), allowing accumulation of cdk1. ATM, p53, and p21 mediate the DNA damage checkpoint in G1 and G2. If this checkpoint is successfully negotiated, the G1 cdks phosphorylate the retinoblastoma protein (pRB), leading to activation of the E2F transcription factor and induction of the proteins required for DNA synthesis. At the G1/S interface, the G1 cyclins and sic-1, an inhibitor of S-phase cdks, are inactivated, allowing progression of S-phase. After DNA synthesis and chromosome duplication are complete, the cell enters another growth phase, G2, during which the mitotic cdk, cdk1, is activated, leading to inactivation of the G1 cdks, and allowing accumulation of An-PC. At the G2/M interface, the spindle checkpoint ensures proper spindle formation and segregation of the chromosomes before mitosis begins. Completion of mitosis is mediated by An-PC. Accumulation of An-PC leads to inactivation of mitotic cdks. At the completion of mitosis, the cells enter the resting state, G0, unless stimulated by further growth signals.*

accumulation of the G1-cdks leads to the activation of the S-phase cdks and the inactivation of An-PC, which regulates the completion of mitosis. The inactivation of An-PC allows M-phase cdks to accumulate. Finally, proteins synthesized during G1 allow assembly of pre-replication complexes (Pre-RCs) at DNA origins of replication, rendering the DNA competent for replication. S-phase cdks trigger replication from origins with complete Pre-RCs, and inhibit the formation of new Pre-RCs. M-phase cdks also inhibit the formation of new Pre-RCs. Therefore, DNA replication is possible immediately after G1, the only time when Pre-RCs are formed. Activation of specific cdks in late G2 is required for progression into mitosis. M-phase cdks lead to chromosome alignment and spindle formation, as well as the inactivation of G1 cyclins. Once the spindle forms and the chromosomes are correctly aligned, An-PC is formed. An-PC causes segregation of the sister chromatids and the completion of mitosis. It also triggers the proteolysis of mitotic cdks, so that accumulation of G1 cyclins is possible and further cell division is not possible until another round of DNA synthesis has occurred.

There are two known checkpoints that ensure that the process of DNA replication and cell division are completed with the necessary fidelity to ensure the production of two identical daughter cells.[4] The first checkpoint is the DNA damage checkpoint. This is a mechanism that detects DNA damage and generates a signal that arrests cells in G1, slows down S-phase, or arrests cells in G2, and induces transcription of DNA repair genes. In this

way, damaged DNA is repaired before a round of cell division is allowed to proceed. If cells are not able to repair the DNA damage, they are then subject to apoptosis, or programmed cell death. The signal that activates this pathway is DNA damage. The sensor is thought to be a protein encoded by the *RAD9* gene, which activates the ataxia-telangiectasia mutated (*ATM*) gene, which is a member of the phosphinoside kinase superfamily. *ATM* then activates the *TP53* tumor suppressor gene which, in turn, activates the p21 cdk inhibitor, blocking cell-cycle progression, and activates the DNA repair genes or triggers apoptosis. This checkpoint ensures that DNA damage is repaired before replication occurs, so that each daughter cell receives an accurate copy of genomic DNA.

The second checkpoint is the spindle assembly checkpoint. This checkpoint is a mechanism that assures proper segregation of chromosomes at mitosis. Proper segregation requires assembly of a bipolar spindle, attachment of kinetochores of the sister chromatids to fibers from opposite poles of the spindle, and arrival of the chromosomes at the metaphase plate. If these events do not occur properly, anaphase is prevented. This mechanism ensures that each daughter cell receives a single copy of each chromosome at anaphase.

In summary, it is clear that, in normal cells, the cell cycle is tightly regulated so that each step must be completed before the subsequent steps are initiated. DNA can only be replicated once per cell cycle. Chromosomes can only segregate after they have correctly aligned. Checkpoints are in place to ensure that each daughter cell is an accurate copy of the parental cell. In cancer cells, these regulatory processes become altered. Oncogenic processes primarily target particular regulators of G1 phase progression. During G1, cells respond to extracellular signals either by advancing toward division or by withdrawing from the cell cycle and entering G0.[5]

Control of cellular proliferation

Most somatic cells reside in G0 until they receive a signal to proliferate, at which time they re-enter G1 and progress through the cell cycle. Proliferation signals include exposure to growth factors, electrolyte imbalances, and loss of contact inhibition. These signals originate in the extracellular domain and are transduced, through complex networks of molecules, to nuclear signals that alter gene expression, leading to cell growth and proliferation. A detailed description of these signal transduction pathways is beyond the scope of this chapter, but a generalized overview of the process is provided.

The cell membrane is a fluid structure with protein channels and receptors embedded in it. Most of these receptors are ligand specific, binding ligand with their extracellular domain and initiating signals with their intracellular domain. The signal is then carried to the nucleus through a series of second messenger molecules that typically act to alter the phosphorylation state of other molecules, resulting in activation of other messengers. The ultimate result is the activation of transcription factors, which turn on the expression of the 'immediate-early response genes,' which are required for cell proliferation. These genes, in turn, activate other genes and processes, ultimately leading to cell growth, DNA synthesis, and cell division (Figure 1.2).[6,7]

Angiogenesis and cell–matrix interactions

Angiogenesis refers to the process of formation of new capillary blood vessels from pre-existing capillaries and venules. Angiogenesis is critical for normal growth and development. In healthy adults, it is a tightly regulated process, normally occurring during the female menstrual cycle, placenta formation, and as a part of the inflammatory process and wound healing. Several disease states are associated with aberrant angiogenesis, including diabetic retinopathy, chronic inflammatory diseases, ischemic vascular disease, and cancer.[8]

The theory that angiogenesis is required for tumor growth, invasion, and metastasis was first proposed in 1971 by Judah Folkman, who suggested that tumors lie in a dormant state, unable to grow beyond a few millimeters in size in the absence of neovascularization.[9] Folkman postulated that tumors secrete angiogenic factors, initiating angiogenesis and leading to the vascularization of the tumor. In the process, tumor cells gain the ability to invade surrounding tissue and gain access to the vasculature,

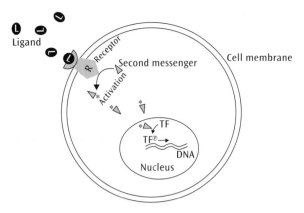

Figure 1.2 *A simplified illustration of the control of cellular proliferation. Proliferation is initiated when a growth signal, or ligand (●), binds to its receptor ( ) on the cell membrane. Ligand–receptor binding leads to activation (*) of a second messenger system (△). The activated second messenger carries the signal to the nucleus (sometimes through other mediators), where the signal is translated into the activation of transcription factors (TF), typically through phosphorylation (Ⓟ). These transcription factors can then bind DNA, leading to expression of genes required for proliferation.*

leading to metastasis formation. Over the past two decades, a large body of evidence has accumulated to support this theory and to elucidate the mechanism of angiogenesis. Multiple factors that either stimulate or inhibit angiogenesis have been identified (Table 1.1). The equilibrium between angiogenic factors and inhibitors of angiogenesis is responsible for the tight regulation of angiogenesis in normal tissues.

Prior to the acquisition of the angiogenic phenotype, tumors are in a dormant state in which the rate of cell proliferation equals the rate of apoptosis, so that the absolute cell number remains stable.[10] Angiogenesis leads to a decrease in the apoptotic rate, allowing tumor growth. Tumor-associated angiogenesis is initiated when the tumors develop the ability to shift the local equilibrium between the positive and negative regulators in favor of angiogenesis.

Tumor cells can overexpress angiogenic factors themselves, or they can cause release of angiogenic factors from the extracellular matrix or from host cells such as macrophages or other inflammatory cells. Recent studies have suggested that the tumor suppressor gene *VHL* (responsible for the von Hippel–Lindau syndrome) functions to suppress vascular endothelial growth factor (VEGF), a potent angiogenic factor. Loss of function of the *VHL* gene, then, would lead to increased expression of VEGF and thus to angiogenesis.[10]

Similarly, inhibitors of angiogenesis in the local environment may be down-regulated. Recent studies have shown that the loss of function of the tumor suppressor gene *TP53* leads to down-regulation of thrombospondin, a potent inhibitor of angiogenesis. The end result is an

Table 1.1 *Mediators of angiogenesis*

Stimulators	Inhibitors
Growth factors	Enzymes and related factors
Acidic fibroblast growth factor (aFGF)	Angiogenin-specific ribonuclease inhibitors
Basic fibroblast growth factor (bFGF)	Herbimycin A
Epidermal growth factor (EGF)	Laminin peptides
Interleukin-8	Methotrexate
Interleukin-1α	Platelet factor 4
Placental growth factor (PlGF)	Thallidomide
Platelet-derived endothelial growth factor	TIMPs (metalloprotease inhibitors)
Proliferin	Matrix degradation inhibitors
Transforming growth factor-α (TGF-α)	β-aminopropionitrile
Transforming growth factor-β (TGF-β)	Proline analogs
Tumor necrosis factor-α (TNF-α)	Retinoids
Vascular endothelial growth factor (VEGF)	
Non-growth factors	
Adenosine diphosphate	
Angiogenin	
Angiotensin II	
Ceruloplasmin	
Copper	
Heparin	
Lactate	
Nicotinamide	
Plasminogen activator	
Prostaglandins E1, E2	

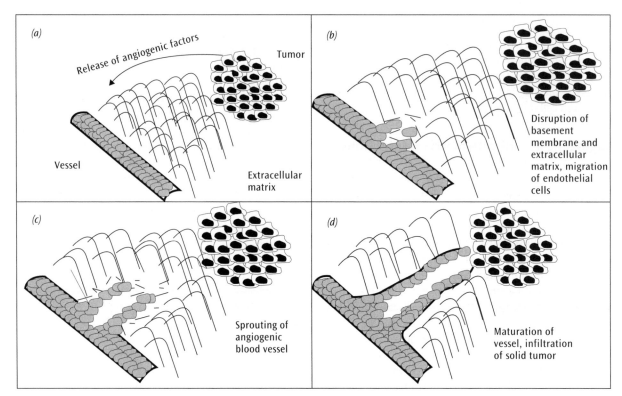

Figure 1.3 *Angiogenesis. (a) Tumor-associated angiogenesis begins when tumor cells, or the surrounding stroma, release angiogenic factors. (b) The angiogenic factors induce collagenase and matrix metalloproteinases that lead to the digestion of the vascular basement membrane and the extracellular matrix. The angiogenic factors also provide a chemotactic signal for vascular endothelial cells, leading to endothelial migration. (c) Further extracellular matrix destruction and cell migration culminate in the sprouting of angiogenic vessels. (d) Finally, the angiogenic vessels infiltrate the solid tumor and mature.*

increase in the local concentration of angiogenic factors, relative to the concentration of angiogenic inhibitors. The angiogenic factors, then, induce the expression and secretion of enzymes by tumor cells, endothelial cells, and stromal cells, such as collagenase and the matrix metalloproteinases, that break down the extracellular matrix and vascular basement membrane. Breakdown of the extracellular matrix allows migration of both tumor cells and endothelial cells. Furthermore, angiogenic factors provide a chemotactic signal for the endothelial cells, promoting migration, proliferation, lumen formation, and finally vessel maturation (Figure 1.3).[11] Immature capillaries have a fragmented basement membrane and are leaky, making them more penetrable to tumor cells, thus facilitating metastasis.[12] The importance of angiogenesis in tumor progression is supported by the findings that increased circulating levels of angiogenic factors or matrix metalloproteinases and the microvessel density within tumors all are predictive of poor prognosis.[10]

Oncogenes

Experiments extending back over the past 50 years have provided evidence that cancer is a genetic disease. Chemical carcinogens were shown to damage DNA and, in fact, their carcinogenic potential was correlated to their ability to mutate genes. This led to the belief that cancer cells carried mutant genes which were altered forms of normal cellular genes. The first cancer-causing gene (oncogene) was described in the mid-1970s as a gene carried by the Rous sarcoma virus, an animal RNA tumor virus, or retrovirus. Stehelin *et al.* showed in 1976 that the transforming gene of this retrovirus was, in fact, derived from a normal cellular gene.[12a] This gene, named *src*, when activated by overexpression by the virus, was capable of transforming the infected cells, leading to tumor formation. Over the next decade, many other viral oncogenes were identified, along with their cellular homologues. Subsequently, it has been shown that these cellular oncogenes are activated by mutations or genetic rearrangements in many human tumors.[13] Because many genetic alterations occur in tumor cells as a result of transformation rather than as a cause of it, an oncogene is strictly defined as a gene that, when introduced into a cell, causes transformation or tumor formation. Over the past two decades, approximately 50 oncogenes have been identified. Understanding the functions of these genes in normal cells has given us a greater understanding of the normal regulation of cell growth and differentiation.

In general, cellular oncogenes are all genes that are involved in cellular proliferation, and can be classified into several groups (Table 1.2).[14] Oncogenes in the first group encode growth factors. When aberrantly expressed, these oncogene products will stimulate cell growth through the normal mechanisms of the parent growth factor. Examples include the *sis* oncogene (platelet-derived growth factor, PDGF), *int-1* (unknown growth factor), *int-2* (fibroblast growth factor (FGF)-related), and *hst* (FGF-related). Oncogenes in the second group encode proteins that resemble growth factor receptors. Growth factor receptors are activated by binding of their specific ligand. The activated receptor then phosphorylates second messengers, leading to transmission of a signal to the nucleus and ultimately to alterations in gene expression, which lead to cellular proliferation. The oncogenes are constitutively activated forms of these receptors, which continuously signal the cell to proliferate. Oncogenes in the third group encode members of the signal transduction pathways within the cell. Normally, members of these pathways require activation by the previous step in the pathway. However, when overexpressed or aberrantly expressed, these oncogenes provide continuous stimulation, leading to cellular proliferation. The final group is the nuclear transcription factors. These genes are normally regulated by the signal transduction pathways and regulate expression of proliferation-associated genes. When overexpressed or aberrantly expressed, they lead to unbridled proliferation. Oncogenes, then, are positive regulators of proliferation, and gain of function of oncogenes leads to tumor formation.

Tumor suppressor genes

The first experimental evidence for tumor suppressor genes came nearly 30 years ago, when tumor cells were fused with normal cells and the resulting hybrid cells were found to have lost the potential to form tumors.[15–17] It was noted that the tumorigenic potential was regained if specific chromosomes derived from the normal parental cell were subsequently lost from the hybrid cell. Further, these same specific normal chromosomes were able to suppress the tumorigenic phenotype when introduced into tumor cells, and therefore must carry 'tumor suppressing' genes.

Unlike oncogenes, a tumor suppressor gene is a gene whose loss of function confers a malignant phenotype. It acts in a recessive fashion, in that both copies of the gene must be inactivated, through mutation, deletion, loss of heterozygosity, or transcriptional silencing, for the effect to be seen. Finally, returning a functional allele to a cell line deficient for a tumor suppressor gene will reverse the tumorigenic phenotype in test animals.[17]

The first tumor suppressor genes were identified through the study of human familial cancer syndromes. By studying family pedigrees, carriers could be identified and chromosomal analysis performed. In a proportion of these individuals, consistent areas of chromosomal loss could be identified, localizing potential tumor suppressor genes to particular regions of a chromosome. As more and more detailed genetic linkage analyses are undertaken, the specific gene can be identified.[18] In this manner,

Table 1.2 *Oncogenes*

Growth factor type	Receptor type	Signal transducer type	Transcription factor type
hst (fibroblast growth factor related)	c-erb-B2 (HER-2/neu) (receptor like)	abl (cytoplasmic/nuclear protein tyrosine kinase)	ets (sequence-specific DNA-binding protein)
int-1 (?)	erb-B (truncated epidermal growth factor)	fgr (membrane-associated protein tyrosine kinase)	fos (component of AP-1 transcription factor)
int-2 (fibroblast growth factor related)	fms (mutant CSF-1 receptor)	fps/fcs (cytoplasmic protein tyrosine kinase)	jun (sequence-specific DNA-binding protein)
sis (platelet-derived growth factor β-chain)	kit (truncated stem cell receptor-like protein)	fgr (membrane-associated protein tyrosine kinase)	myb (sequence-specific DNA-binding protein)
	met (soluble truncated receptor-like protein)	lck (membrane-associated protein tyrosine kinase)	L-myc (sequence-specific DNA-binding protein)
	ret (truncated receptor-like protein)	src (membrane-associated protein tyrosine kinase)	N-myc (sequence-specific DNA-binding protein)
	ros (receptor-like protein)	yes (membrane-associated protein tyrosine kinase)	myc (sequence-specific DNA-binding protein)
	trk (soluble truncated receptor-like protein)	H-ras (membrane-associated G-protein)	erbA (dominant negative mutant of thyroxine receptor)
		k-ras (membrane-associated G-protein)	rel (dominant negative mutant of NF-B-related protein)
		N-ras (membrane-associated G-protein)	evi-1 (transcription factor?)
		gip (mutant-activated form of Gi)	ski (transcription factor?)
		gsp (mutant-activated form of Gs)	vuv (transcription factor?)
		B-raf (protein-serine kinase)	
		cot (protein-serine kinase)	
		pim-1 (protein-serine kinase)	
		raf/mil (protein-serine kinase)	
		mos (cytostatic factor)	
		crk (SH2/SH3-containing protein)	

the first tumor suppressor gene, the retinoblastoma gene (*Rb*), was identified and cloned in 1987.[19] Subsequently, many other tumor suppressor genes have been identified and their functions are beginning to be elucidated (Table 1.3). In general, the function of the product of tumor suppressor genes is to control cellular proliferation. For many of the tumor suppressor genes, the exact mechanisms of action are not well understood, but the *Rb* and *TP53* pathways constitute the two main cell-cycle regulatory pathways and are quite elegant in their control.

The retinoblastoma pathway

The retinoblastoma gene encodes a 105 kDa protein, pRb, that is unphosphorylated in the G0/G1 phase of the cell cycle. The unphosphorylated form is capable of binding to and inhibiting the activity of the E2F transcription factor. E2F is required for the transcription of genes required for proliferation, DNA synthesis and replication; therefore, if pRb binds to E2F, the cell is unable to proliferate. In late G1, pRb is phosphorylated by cdk4 or cdk6, releasing E2F, allowing transcriptional activation of cell-cycle-promoting genes. Mutant pRb is incapable of binding E2F and so the process becomes deregulated. The cdk inhibitor *p16/INK-4a* inhibits the activity of cdk4 and cdk6 and so can inhibit the phosphorylation of pRb and prevent the release of E2F, maintaining G1 arrest.[20,21] Thus, both tumor suppressor genes *Rb* and *p16* function in this same pathway, giving a double layer of control.

The *TP53* pathway

Alterations in *TP53* are the most common genetic change documented in human malignancies, with over half of all cancers carrying mutations in *TP53*. *TP53* is a tumor suppressor gene that is induced in the presence of DNA damage and encodes a protein, p53, that acts as a transcription factor, activating genes that, in turn, transcriptionally regulate genes important for G1 arrest and DNA repair. p53 can also act to trigger apoptosis in the face of DNA damage. In this way, up-regulation of p53 will lead to G1 arrest, allowing the cell adequate time for DNA repair. If DNA repair fails, p53 then eliminates cells with the damaged DNA by inducing programmed cell death.[21] The end result is that mutations are prevented from accumulating and the fidelity of the genome is preserved through successive rounds of the cell cycle. The oncogene mdm2, overexpressed in 30–40% of sarcomas, encodes a protein that binds to and degrades p53, inhibiting its effects. The *p19/ARF* tumor suppresser gene encodes a protein that specifically binds to the mdm2 protein and leads to its degradation, blocking its inhibition of *p53*.[22,23] This is another example of two tumor suppresser genes functioning in the same regulatory pathway.

The story gets even more complex when you consider *p16/INK-4a* and *p19/ARF*. These are not really two distinct tumor suppressor genes because they are, in fact, encoded by the same piece of DNA. To date, they are the only known example of two completely distinct proteins (they have no amino-acid homology) being encoded by the same DNA, having distinct first exons (exon1α for *p16* and 1β for *p19*) and sharing exons 2 and 3, but using alternate reading frames.[24] Thus, there is one gene encoding two distinct tumor-suppressing proteins that function in the two major cell-cycle regulatory pathways.

In conclusion, normal cells are regulated at many levels. There are both extracellular and intracellular signals that control cellular proliferation, cell-cycle control, angiogenesis, and cell/matrix interactions. The expressions of oncogenes and tumor suppressor genes are involved in many of these functions. Mutations in any of these regulatory pathways can lead to unbridled growth and malignant degeneration.

APPLICATIONS OF MOLECULAR BIOLOGY TO CANCER TREATMENT

Molecular markers of tumor progression

Perhaps the most common use of molecular biology in the day-to-day practice of surgical oncology is that of biologic markers to diagnose cancer, predict prognosis, or detect recurrence. To use biologic markers effectively it is necessary to understand their significance and which markers are appropriate in which tumors.

Breast cancer

In planning the treatment of a patient with breast cancer, certain molecular biologic characteristics of the primary tumor carry prognostic significance. Whereas originally there was thought to be a striking difference in outcome for estrogen receptor (ER)-positive versus ER-negative tumors, follow-up studies have shown a more modest separation in survival.[25,26] Some authors feel that ER expression may be an indication of growth rate and not metastatic potential.[27] Expression of the progesterone receptor (PR) depends on ER function and, thus, evaluation of the PR status is another indicator of outcome based on biologic behavior. It has been well established that the ER and PR tissue content can predict the response to hormonal therapy, and thus is used to guide the use of adjuvant systemic therapy (Table 1.4).[28]

Numerous other tumor markers for breast cancer have been described. These include expression of the DF3 antigen, a high molecular weight mucin, and of the estrogen-related protein pS-2. Both markers are associated with a favorable clinical outcome.[29,30] Other studies have implicated that overexpression of certain enzymes, such as cathepsin-D or urokinase-plasminogen activator, or an adhesion molecule such as the laminin receptor, may positively or negatively associate with a metastatic phenotype.[31–33] These markers are not widely used clinically.

Table 1.3 *Tumor suppressor genes*

Gene	Proposed function	Associated cancer or disorder	Syndrome
APC	Regulation of β-catenin, signal transduction	Colon cancer, colon polyps, gastric and duodenal tumors, desmoid tumors (Gardner's syndrome)	Familial polyposis coli
ATM	DNA repair, induction of TP53	Lymphoma, cerebellar ataxia, immunodeficiency, breast cancer in heterozygotes	Ataxia-telangiaectasia
BLM	? DNA helicase	Solid tumors, immunodeficiency, small stature	Bloom's syndrome
BRCA1	Interact with RAD51, repair of double-stranded DNA breaks	Breast cancer, ovarian cancer	Familial breast cancer 1
BRCA2	? Interact with RAD51, repair of double-stranded DNA breaks?	Breast cancer, male breast cancer, pancreatic cancer?, others	Familial breast cancer 2
CDK4	Cyclin-dependent kinase	Melanoma	Familial melanoma
?DCC	Cell surface receptor similar to NCAM	Colon cancer	?
E-cadherin	Intracellular signaling	Gastric cancer	?
EXT1, EXT2, EXT3	?	Exostoses, chondrosarcoma	Multiple exostoses
FACC	? DNA repair	Acute myelogenous leukemia, pancytopenia, skeletal abnormalities	Fanconi's anemia
MEN1	?	Pancreatic islet cell tumors	Multiple endocrine neoplasia type 1
MET	Receptor for HGF	Renal cancers, ?others	Hereditary papillary renal cancer
MLH1, MSH1, PMS1, PMS2	DNA mismatch repair	Colon cancer, endometrial, ovarian, hepatobiliary, genitourinary	Hereditary non-polyposis colorectal cancer
NF1	GTPase-activating protein for p21 ras proteins	Neurofibromas, neurofibromosarcoma, brain tumors	Neurofibromatosis type 1
NF2	Links membrane proteins to cytoskeleton	Acoustic neuromas, meningiomas, gliomas, ependymomas	Neurofibromatosis type 2
P15	Cyclin-dependent kinase inhibitor	Hematologic malignancies	?
P16/INK-4A	Cyclin-dependent kinase inhibitor	Melanoma, pancreatic cancer, other	Familial melanoma
P19/ARF	Binds and degrades mdm2	?	?
P57/KIP2	Cell-cycle regulator	Wilms' tumor	Wiedmann–Beckwith syndrome
PTCH	Receptor for hedgehog signaling molecule	Basal cell carcinoma	Nevoid basal cell carcinoma syndrome
PTEN	Phosphatase with similarity to tensin	Breast cancer, follicular thyroid cancer, intestinal hamartomas, skin lesions	Cowden's disease
RB1	Cell-cycle and transcriptional regulator through E2F binding	Retinoblastoma, osteosarcoma, small-cell lung cancer, many others	Familial retinoblastoma
RET	Receptor tyrosine kinase for GDNF	Medullary thyroid cancer, pheochromocytoma, parathyroid hyperplasia, mucosal hamartomas	Multiple endocrine neoplasia type 2, familial medullary thyroid cancer
TP53	Transcription factor, response to stress and DNA damage, apoptosis	Sarcomas, breast cancers, brain tumors, leukemia, many others	Li–Fraumeni syndrome
VHL	Regulates transcriptional elongation by RNA polymerase III	Renal cell carcinoma, pheochromocytoma, retinal angiomas, hemangioblastomas	Von Hippel–Lindau syndrome
WT1	Transcriptional repressor	Wilms' tumor	Wilms' tumor
XPA, XPB, XPD	DNA repair helicases, nucleotide excision repair	Skin cancer, pigmentation abnormalities, hypogonadism	Xeroderma pigmentosum

Table 1.4 *Response to endocrine therapy by steroid receptor content*

Hormone receptor content		Response to endocrine therapy (%)
Estrogen receptor	Progesterone receptor	
Negative	Negative	9
Positive	Negative	32
Negative	Positive	42
Positive	Positive	68

Another marker shown to have prognostic significance in breast cancer is the detection of abnormalities in oncogenes. Amplification of the *HER-2/neu* proto-oncogene has been reported to be associated with a poorer clinical outcome in node-positive breast cancer patients. However, the results in node-negative patients have been less striking.[34–37] Two recent studies have suggested that overexpression of *HER-2/neu* might be associated with relative resistance to adjuvant chemotherapy with cyclophosphamide, methotrexate, and 5-fluorouracil (5-FU), and thus patients whose tumors have normal levels of the protein are more likely to benefit from adjuvant cytoxan, methotrexate, 5-FU (CMF) protocol chemotherapy.[38,39] However, in another study, patients with *HER-2/neu* overexpression were more likely to benefit from higher doses of cytoxan, doxorubicin (Adriamycin), 5-FU (CAF) chemotherapy, whereas patients with normal *HER-2/neu* expression had similar benefit from either low or high doses.[40] Obviously, these conclusions remain speculative and await confirmation in a large, prospective trial. *HER-2/neu* overexpression has also been demonstrated to impart a relative resistance to hormonal therapy, with less response to tamoxifen in ER-positive patients who also overexpress *HER-2/neu*.[41] Currently, *HER-2/neu* status is being used as part of the randomization schema in several multi-institutional adjuvant trials, and an antibody to the *HER-2/neu* protein, herceptin, has been developed for use as an adjuvant to chemotherapy.

The protein product of the tumor suppressor gene *TP53* has a very short half-life. Mutations of the *TP53* gene reduce or eliminate the product's tumor-suppressing function, and also seem to protect it from degradation, thus allowing its detection.[42] Detection of p53 protein in tumor tissue is associated with mutations at the genetic level. Recent studies have suggested that detection of p53 in primary breast cancers is associated with a worse prognosis, but these early findings must be placed in an appropriate clinical context.[43] This marker is not yet widely used.

Another potential use of biologic markers is to follow patients once the primary tumor has been removed. Because the natural history of breast cancer is heterogeneous, and the risk of relapse is present even 20 to 30 years after initial therapy, the use of circulating tumor markers to detect such relapses early is advantageous.[44]

Such circulating serum markers include carcinoembryonic antigen (CEA), tissue polypeptide antigen (TPA), gross cystic disease protein (GCDP), and a family of related mucin-like high molecular weight glycoproteins that includes CA 15-3, CA 27.29, CA 549, breast cancer mucin, mammary serum antigen and mucinous carcinoma antigen. Of these, CEA, CA 27.29, and CA 15-3 have been shown to become elevated prior to the development of symptoms or the detection of metastatic carcinoma by physical or radiographic findings.[45–48] In general, approximately 40–50% of patients who will develop metastases will have a preceding rise in CEA, CA 27.29, or CA 15-3, with lead times ranging from 3 to 18 months. However, the clinical utility of tumor markers in predicting relapse has not been proven, and the treatment of asymptomatic patients has not been shown to improve palliation,[49,50] and thus routine screening at this time is considered investigational. CA 27.29 has been shown to be more sensitive and specific than either CEA or CA 15-3 in detecting recurrence in stage II and stage III breast cancer patients,[48] and this is the main marker in wide clinical use at this time.

Both CEA and CA 15-3 are elevated because changes in serum levels of CEA and CA 15-3 are indicative of clinical course, these markers have been used to monitor patients with advanced disease. Approximately 80% of patients with metastatic breast cancer will have elevated serum levels of CA 15-3, and thus it can be used as an adjunct for follow-up.[51,52] There is often an initial rise in the levels of CEA and CA 15-3 early in the course of effective hormonal or chemotherapy treatment, but this is then followed by a fall to or below baseline level, creating a 'spike' effect, which should not be interpreted as progression of disease.[53]

Lung cancer

Serum tumor markers play a less specific role in lung cancer than in other solid malignancies, not because of an inability to reflect tumor status, but rather because of a lack of effective therapeutic interventions. Currently available tumor markers for lung cancer are not suitable for the screening of asymptomatic patients. Cytopathologic examinations have a better diagnostic yield and, thus, tumor markers are useful screening tools only in those patients whose debilitated status precludes more invasive tissue diagnosis. The main utility of serum biomarkers has been for the monitoring of disease status or progression to therapy. The use of tumor markers is unreliable for predicting staging in lung cancer due to overlap of levels in the different stages.[54]

For small-cell lung cancer (SCLC), the best tumor marker available is neuron-specific enolase (NSE). NSE can be used to differentiate between SCLC and lymphoma, both Hodgkin's and non-Hodgkin's.[55] NSE levels may be useful to monitor patients for SCLC recurrence, but they have not been shown to differentiate between a complete and partial remission. Therefore, a rising NSE level mandates further diagnostic work-up.[56]

CEA has also been used as a marker for SCLC; however, it is not specific, as it may be elevated in benign pulmonary conditions such as chronic obstructive pulmonary disease and tuberculosis. CEA has been shown to be more elevated in SCLC patients with more extensive disease than in those with limited tumor involvement. Also, survival was significantly shorter for patients with marked CEA elevations, although this may just be an indication of bulky disease rather than an independent prognostic factor.[57] CEA levels may possess some benefit for evaluating the response to chemotherapy, as one study showed a strong relation between a change in the CEA level and response.[58] However, other studies have not demonstrated such a clear-cut correlation.[59,60]

For non-small-cell lung cancer (NSCLC), the best marker is cytokeratin 19 fragment 21-1 (CYFRA 21-1).[61] This marker provides prognostic information for overall survival as patients with pretreatment elevated levels had a significantly shorter survival than those with normal levels in several studies.[62,63] An elevated CYFRA 21-1 level should drop to the normal range after curative resection, and may thus be used to monitor recurrence.[64,65] A few studies have evaluated the prognostic value of CEA in resectable, early-stage NSCLC; one study did find a correlation between an elevated preoperative CEA and a higher likelihood of recurrence.[66] CA 125 may also be a useful marker for predicting stage, resectability, and survival in NSCLC patients.[67,68]

For squamous cell carcinoma (SCC), the SCC antigen level should drop to baseline after curative resection, and thus a rising level indicates early tumor relapse.[69] The SCC antigen level is not affected by smoking, which eliminates the interference that is seen with CEA. In one study, 32% of patients with SCC who had a normal CEA level were found to have an elevated SCC antigen level. Both CEA and SCC antigen were found to adversely affect prognosis in patients with SCC.[70] CYFRA 21-1 is also a useful marker for SCC. There has been shown to be a correlation between the CYFRA 21-1 level and the patient's clinical response to chemotherapy in patients with inoperable SCC.[71]

Tissue polypeptide antigen is elevated in a variety of human malignancies, including lung cancer. One report showed a good correlation between the TPA level and clinical stage, and an elevated TPA level was associated with decreased survival independent of stage.[72,73] Another study revealed that TPA was more sensitive than CEA, and that elevated levels of TPA preceded the clinical recognition of recurrence or progression.[74]

Gastric cancer

CA 72-4 is found in a variety of human malignancies of epithelial origin, including NSCLC, breast, ovarian, pancreas, esophageal, and gastric cancers. It is rarely expressed in benign tissue lesions, and only appears in normal adult human tissue in the secretory endometrium. Several studies have shown that serum levels of CA 72-4 are elevated in patients with gastrointestinal adenocarcinoma, and that it has clinical relevance in the follow-up of carcinoma patients.[75] CA 72-4 levels correlate with the presence of lymph node or serosal involvement in gastric cancer.[76] Because the level of CA 72-4 will drop following curative resection, a subsequent rise is useful as a marker of recurrence, or a persistent elevation as an indication of incomplete resection.

CEA has also been used to monitor patients with gastric cancer, but it has a low sensitivity, and thus is not advocated as a first-choice tumor marker.[77,78] The serum CEA level appears to correlate with the tumor stage. Whereas approximately 40–60% of gastric tumors overall will be CEA positive over the course of disease, only 10–20% of patients with stage I and II gastric cancers will have an elevated CEA level, compared to 30% of those with stage III cancers.[79–82] Although an elevated CEA level is a predictor of unresectable disease, a normal level does not predict curability reliably. A complete resection should be associated with a return of an elevated CEA to normal, and failure to reach a normal level indicates either incomplete resection or early recurrence.[83] Similarly, a postoperative new elevation of CEA suggests recurrence.

Alfa-fetoprotein (AFP) may also be elevated in gastric cancer, with approximately 30% of patients having an elevated level and as many as 40% of patients with liver metastases showing elevations.[84] The elevations of CEA and AFP are non-overlapping in gastric cancer. CA 19-9 has also been shown to be elevated in gastric cancer. The level will return to normal following curative resection, thus allowing it to be used for recurrence detection.

Colorectal cancer

There is no tumor marker available for screening for colon cancer. CEA has been shown to be ineffective for screening, even in high-risk patients such as those with ulcerative colitis, adenomatous familial polyposis, or hereditary non-polyposis colon cancer syndrome.[85] CEA has been shown to be elevated in 65% of patients with stage D colon cancer, but significant elevations are less common among patients with potentially curable disease.[86,87] Preoperative CEA levels have been shown to have a prognostic value independent of tumor stage.[88] Elevated preoperative CEA levels should return to normal following resection; failure to do so is associated with a high risk of recurrence.[89] Some patients continue to maintain a marginally elevated level despite no evidence of recurrent disease; thus, although highly predictive of relapse, an elevated postoperative CEA is not absolute.[82] Several studies have evaluated the utility of CEA monitoring in postoperative patients; approximately half of the patients who might benefit from a second resection are identified by routine CEA testing.[82] In summary, CEA has no role in the screening of patients for colorectal cancer, but has a definite benefit in the assessment of preoperative and postoperative prognosis. There is limited benefit to the use of CEA for monitoring for recurrence or to assess the potential for second-look surgery or response to therapy.[82]

Pancreatic cancer

Pancreatic adenocarcinoma is fatal in over 95% of cases, and the only curative intervention is early surgery. CA 19-9 has been the main tumor marker for pancreatic cancer, although it is not specific. High CA 19-9 levels can differentiate pancreatic cancer from chronic pancreatitis, but not from other malignancies.[90] The serum levels appear to correlate with the extent of disease, with higher levels indicating more advanced tumors.[91,92] The presence of biliary disease or cholangitis can yield falsely elevated CA 19-9 levels. The level of CA 19-9 should return to normal following curative resection, and failure to do so is a poor prognostic indicator. Similarly, a subsequent rise in the marker following normalization indicates recurrence; in fact, the level may rise prior to clinical presentation.[82] There has not been a clear delineation between CA 19-9 levels and response to chemotherapy, in part due to limitations of the currently available treatments for the disease.

CEA may be associated with pancreatic cancer in 20–40% of patients, but it is much less specific and sensitive than CA 19-9.[92] Some authors have found that a low CEA level is associated with a better prognosis.[93] However, other studies have found no difference in prognosis when patients are controlled for stage.[94]

Hepatocellular carcinoma

Alfa-fetoprotein is the major tumor marker associated with hepatocellular carcinoma, and may even be used for screening in the high-risk population. Approximately 20–35% of tumors are not associated with an elevated AFP level.[95,96] In general, the degree of AFP elevation relates to tumor size. Currently, a screening combination of ultrasound and AFP determination is recommended for patients with hepatitis B or C and cirrhosis or chronic active hepatitis.[97] The level of AFP will fall following resection or chemoembolization, and a subsequent rise indicates recurrence.[80]

Ovarian cancer

Serum CA 125 levels are elevated in 80–90% of women with epithelial ovarian cancer. The expression is highest in serous, mixed and unclassified adenocarcinomas and lowest in mucinous types.[98] CA 125 does not have a high enough sensitivity to be used for screening, as up to 50% of patients with early disease will have a normal level,

as well as a low specificity, with benign conditions such as pelvic inflammatory disease producing elevations.[98] It may be used to differentiate between benign and malignant disease in women presenting with a pelvic mass, with a sensitivity of 78% and a specificity of 93%.[98] The degree of elevation appears to relate to the extent of disease.[99] It appears that CA 125 levels preoperatively do not have independent prognostic significance.[98,100] The presence of a persistently elevated level postoperatively might reflect the presence of residual or recurrent disease, and has been used as an indicator for a second-look operation. Some reports indicate that a change in CA 125 level during chemotherapy induction is associated with improved survival.[101]

Prostate cancer

The prostate-specific antigen (PSA) has greatly increased the diagnosis of prostate cancer, and there is growing evidence that PSA-diagnosed tumors are more likely to be organ confined and thus curable.[102] PSA is produced by both normal and malignant prostate tissue, and is thus prostate specific, not prostate cancer specific. The elevation of PSA in benign prostatic hypertrophy is usually mild, in contrast to the more striking elevations seen in prostatitis.[103] Clinical digital rectal examination has little effect on the PSA level, but greater manipulation, as might occur with prostatic massage, biopsy, and transurethral resection, will cause a striking elevation.[104] PSA appears to predict the success of radiotherapy as primary treatment.[105,106] It should rapidly decline following radical prostatectomy, and thus can be used as a marker for either incomplete resection or recurrence. Patients with a rising PSA level may have occult metastatic disease and thus must be evaluated fully. Decline of PSA levels is more latent after radiotherapy than with operative resection. In addition, the PSA level will decrease following androgen ablation, and thus a rising level indicates likely relapse.[107]

Molecular determinants of response to chemotherapy

Tumor specimens obtained before treatment can be analysed for potential markers that predict the response to available chemotherapy agents. Examples are mediators of drug-specific resistance mechanisms or protein products of genes involved in cell-cycle and apoptotic pathways. Biological profiles of the primary tumor can be prospectively acquired for each patient studied. Associations of the markers tested with the extent of clinical or pathological response of the primary tumor can be explored to generate hypotheses to explain mechanisms of tumor resistance to the tested regimen.[108,109] A clinical setting that allows for the testing of a single agent at a time is ideal for studying molecular determinants of response.

A good example is that of colorectal cancers, for 5-FU was for many years the only active drug for these tumors. Moreover, because only approximately 20–30% of patients responded to 5-FU, research directed at identifying markers of response/resistance became quite compelling. Thymidylate synthase (TS), the target enzyme of 5-FU, became a useful tool to predict response to this drug. Leichman et al. demonstrated a strong correlation between levels of TS gene expression and clinical response in recurrent/metastatic colorectal tumors treated with 5-FU.[110] Other markers, such as dihydropyrimidine dehydrogenase (DPD) and thymidine phosphorylase, have been found to complement TS in the identification of potential responders to fluoropyrimidines.[111,112] Probably the main limitation of the work done on colorectal tumors was the fact that the measurement of the effect was made by clinical assessment of response, which is often imprecise.

In 1993, the University of Southern California Interdisciplinary Breast Cancer Group started a series of clinical studies in locally advanced breast cancer. Pretreatment tumor core biopsies were obtained to prospectively study potential predictors for pathological response (at mastectomy) to first-line continuous infusion FU and radiation. Whereas 30/35 achieved objective clinical responses, only 12/35 patients achieved a pathological response to treatment. Noticeably, original p53 status measured at immunohistochemistry was significantly associated with pathological response ($p < 0.010$).[108] Because most patients with mutated p53 failed to respond, the second pilot study involved taxanes during radiation therapy, due to their presumed activity in p53-mutated tumors: this study is ongoing and preliminary data from the first 14 patients suggest that low expression of specific β-tubulin isoforms at reverse transcriptase–polymerase chain reaction (RT–PCR) may predict pathological response.[109]

Many other groups have focused on breast cancer: generally, biological markers have been evaluated in a retrospective fashion by examining the original paraffin blocks of tumors from patients whose outcome is known. Markers of apoptosis and resistance to chemotherapy were studied by Linn et al., who conducted immunohistochemical determination of p53 and p-glycoprotein (pGP) expression in 20 operable and 30 inoperable locally advanced breast cancer (LABC) patients. By using double immunostaining techniques, they demonstrated frequent concomitant expression of p53 and pGP ($p = 0.003$). Among patients with LABC, the combination of p53 and pGP overexpression was the strongest prognostic factor for shorter survival at multivariate analysis ($p = 0.004$).[113] Other studies have supported the role of pGP expression as an intermediate endpoint of drug response.[114,115] In-vitro studies have shown that the mutant TP53 gene product is capable of stimulating the MDR1 promoter gene, while wild TP53 gene product can exert a direct or indirect repressive action on MDR1 gene transcription;[116] these findings could account for the observed chemoresistance among breast cancer with TP53 mutations.[117,118] However, in another immunohistochemical study of LABC, Linn et al. found no correlation amongst pGP, multidrug resistance-associated protein (MRP), lung resistance protein (LRP), p53, and Ki-67, and pathological response to primary chemotherapy. Interestingly, the resistant clones found in the surgical specimen generally had a low proliferation rate.[117,119]

The effect of primary chemotherapy on tumor cell kinetics has also been investigated. Studies have measured the initial tritiated thymidine labeling index (TLI) in LABC. The technique provides an indirect estimate of the proportion of cancer cells in S-phase, when cells are capable of incorporating tritium-labeled thymidine. Generally, patients with low TLI in the diagnostic specimen fare better than those with high TLI.[120,121] However, Gardin et al. found that patients with high TLI tumors had better response to 5-FU, adriamycin, and cyclophosphamide (FAC) chemotherapy. Moreover, persistent high TLI after primary FAC was associated with the highest response rate and disease-free survival (DFS).[122] Other investigators have focused on the study of mitotic figure count and specific proliferation markers such as Ki-67, MIB-1, proliferating cell nuclear antigen (PCNA): MIB-1 positivity and mitotic figure count were associated with DFS in a study of 135 breast cancers ($p < 0.0005$ and $p < 0.0003$, respectively).[123] Brifford and co-workers conducted an interesting study of sequential fine-needle aspirations in 27 patients with T3, N0-1 breast cancers.[124] All patients had tumor fine needle aspiration biopsy (FNA) before and after the first cycle of a protocol of three cycles of preoperative adriamycin, vincristine cyclophosphamide, methotrexate, 5-FU (AVCMF). For each set of specimens, flow-cytometric DNA and S-phase analysis were compared to image analysis. The data were then correlated to the clinical response: 12 patients achieved measurable objective response, and 15 had no tumor regression. Each of the eight patients with non-diploid tumors and a pretreatment high percentage of cells in S and G2–M phases achieved objective tumor regression ($p < 0.001$). The investigators suggested that this technique should be used to prospectively select patients with responsive tumors to this regimen.[124]

The Southwestern Oncology Group conducted a study of sequential FNA in LABC patients treated with high physiological doses of estradiol to increase the number of cycling cancer cells in an attempt to increase chemotherapeutic efficacy. Flow cytometry was used to measure S-phase fraction and proliferative index (PI). Despite noticing an increase of S-phase fraction and PI after estradiol treatment, no major effect on the response to adriamycin-based chemotherapy was detected.[125]

The paradigm of treatment of primary chemotherapy or chemoradiation has generated in-vivo pathological data of the effects of these modalities. The non-neoplastic stromal component of breast tissue chemotherapy induces fibrosis and hyalinization, while cytoplasmic vacuolization is the most common finding among residual tumor cells.[126]

In patients undergoing pathological response to treatment, no residual tumor cells or only a few microscopic foci of invasive breast cancer cells are usually found in the context of a characteristic pattern of fibrous tissue with a cellular component of lymphocytes, iron-loaded macrophages, and hysticocytes with foamy cytoplasm. Honkoop *et al.* reported a pattern of reduced mitotic index and microvessel density after chemotherapy in general, without an association with pathological response.[127] Paulsen *et al.* reported a similar lack of association between microvessel density and clinical response to doxorubicin monochemotherapy in 63 patients with LABC.[128] More studies on the pathological verification of pretreatment and post-treatment angiogenesis markers are warranted.

Angiogenesis inhibitors

Angiogenesis is a critical event in tumor growth and metastasis. Agents that interrupt one or more steps of the neovascularization process promise to lead to novel therapies for cancer and related diseases. The principal approach of anti-angiogenic therapy is to inhibit the proliferation and migration of endothelial cells. This section reviews the current status of anti-angiogenic therapy.

There are three main strategies upon which anti-angiogenic therapies are based.[129] First, because anti-angiogenic therapies target only tumor-induced vascular endothelial cell growth, they have much lower toxicities compared to the presently used cytotoxic chemotherapy. Endothelial cells engaged in active tumor angiogenesis have a much shorter turnover rate than do normal adult endothelial cells (4 days compared to hundreds of days). Therefore, endothelial cells undergo little genetic mutation compared to cancer cells, reducing the risk of developing drug resistance.[130] Second, endothelial cells release growth factors in a paracrine manner that have a direct influence on tumor growth. Two such examples are insulin-like growth factors (IGFs) 1 and 2 and basic fibroblast growth factor (bFGF), which have been shown to promote tumor cell growth and migration.[131] Therefore, through inhibiting endothelial proliferation, it may be possible to inhibit tumor cell growth.[129] Finally, by preventing peripheral capillary formation, it may be possible to prevent metastasis of cancer brought about by tumor cells escaping into the bloodstream through leaky neovasculature. Currently, a number of anti-angiogenic agents have been identified and shown to have antitumor effects in preclinical models.

Agents in preclinical trials and/or early-phase clinical trials

SU5416

SU5416 therapy aims at controlling tumor growth by inhibiting the VEGF signaling cascade. *In vitro*, SU5416 shows inhibition of ligand-induced autophosphorylation of Flk-1, the signal partner of VEGF receptor heterodimer (Flk-1 and Flt-1).[132] As a result, SU5416 inhibits endothelial cell proliferation and migration. In preclinical evaluation, SU5416 showed inhibition of acquired immunodeficiency syndrome (AIDS)-related Kaposi's sarcoma (KS), a highly vascularized tumor, both *in vitro* and *in vivo*.[133] The dose-limiting toxicity of SU5416 in dogs and rats was hepatocellular injury.[132] Toxicities of SU5416 in patients include fatigue, change in voice, pain at injection site, and allergic reaction. SU5416 for the treatment of KS and other human tumors is moving into phase II trials.[133]

IM-862

IM-862 is a dipeptide, identified from the soluble fractions of the thymus.[133] It has been shown to have antitumor activity without toxicity to the tumor cells, thus leading to evaluation of a potential anti-angiogenic role. Although this compound has been shown to have no direct effect on endothelial cell growth or migration, it has been shown in chicken allantoid membrane (CAM) assays to inhibit angiogenesis.[133] Murine tumor models bearing human xenografts have been shown to have an IM-862 dose-dependent tumor growth inhibition.[133] A phase I/II trial in KS was done using a fixed dose amount of the peptide. A third of the patients in the study responded with noticeable tumor reduction, including patients who had failed prior cytotoxic chemotherapy.[133] A double-blind, randomized trial will begin shortly. Trials in other human cancers, including breast, prostate, and melanoma, are either in progress or in development.

Tecogalan

Tecogalan is a 29-kDa sulfated polysaccharide peptidoglycan derived from the *Arthrobacter* species AT-25. It has shown inhibition of proliferation and migration of endothelial cells. Phase I trials have shown that tecogalan's anti-angiogenic activity is enhanced when it is administered in conjunction with either cortisone acetate or tetrahydro S.[131] In addition, when administered with tamoxifen, endothelial cell proliferation inhibition is enhanced.[134] A phase I trial of tecogalan in AIDS–KS patients showed tumor size reduction and tumor-associated edema improvement, but no durable responses were seen.[133] Toxicities included fever, chills, and rigor during the first few hours of infusion. The dose-limiting toxicity was anti-coagulation, manifested by an increased activated partial thromboplastin time (APTT).[131]

TNP-470

An analog of fumagillin, TNP-470 is a secreted antibiotic product of the fungus *Aspergillus fumigatus*. TNP-470 is a more potent, less toxic anti-angiogenic compound than the previously tested fumagillan.[135] It was given to 38 AIDS–KS patients in a phase I clinical trial: 18% of the patients showed a response lasting for a median of 11 weeks, with a range of 3 to 26+ weeks.[133] *In-vitro* studies show inhibition of proliferation and migration of endothelial cells. Further studies showed *in-vitro* capillary tube formation inhibition at concentrations that were cytostatic not cytotoxic.[131] TNP-470 is currently in phase II trials.

Angiostatin

An 812 amino acid protein, angiostatin is an endogenous inhibitor of the angiogenic response. First shown in 1994 to suppress micrometastatic growth from Lewis lung carcinoma in mice, angiostatin is thought to have potent anti-angiogenic activity.[136] Angiostatin was first isolated by O'Reilly *et al.* from the urine of tumor-bearing mice.[136a] It is a 38-kDa subunit of a precursor protein, plasminogen.[136] *In-vitro* proliferation assays show angiostatin to inhibit endothelial cell growth yet have no effect on the growth of other cell types such as fibroblast, epithelium, or myoblast. Angiostatin has also been shown to reduce the growth of several tumor types in murine tumor models.[136]

Endostatin

Endostatin was also isolated by Folkman's group. A 20-kDa protein portion of collagen XVIII, it is a more potent inhibitor of angiogenesis.[137] Endostatin was administered to mice carrying a significant tumor burden equivalent to a 1.5-lb human tumor. It induced regression of tumors in murine models without the evolution of resistance.[137] At the present time, the group is moving toward human testing.

Agents in late-phase trials and/or in clinical use

Thalidomide

Thalidomide, originally used as a sedative, has recently been shown to inhibit angiogenesis. *In-vitro* assays of the thalidomide drug itself did not show inhibition of endothelial cell growth, nor did *in-vivo* studies, using chorioallantoic membrane (CAM) assays, show anti-angiogenic activity.[131] It has subsequently been shown that the hepatically generated epoxide metabolite carries anti-angiogenic activity. Later discoveries have shown that thalidomide blocks tumor necrosis factor-alpha (TNF-α) production, and inhibits basement membrane formation and intercellular adhesion molecules.[133] Substantial toxicities were reported and include neutropenia, rash, fever, myositis, and depression. Other clinical trials using thalidomide as anti-angiogenic therapy involve breast cancer, prostrate cancer, and primary brain tumors.[131]

Marimastat

Marimastat has been shown to inhibit the growth and metastatic spread of tumors through its ability to inhibit matrix metalloproteases (MMP) and is orally bioavailable.[129] Phase III trials of marimastat have shown that 50% of the patients in the trial had dose-related reductions in the expression of cancer-associated serum tumor markers such as CA 19-9, PSA and CA 125.[131] Commonly reported toxicities include fibrosis and inflammation of the knee and ankle joints and some muscle necrosis. Overall, maximum bioactivity and long-term tolerability were achieved through lower dosage (10 mg twice daily).[129]

Interleukin-12

Interleukin-12 (Il-12) is a cytokine that possesses potent anti-angiogenic activity through its induction of interferon-γ (IFN-γ). IFN-γ induces human IFN-inducible protein 10 (IP-10), which is the actual inhibitor of angiogenesis.[131] Currently, AIDS–KS phase III trials are underway.

In conclusion, anti-angiogenic therapy may be very promising in the development of novel anticancer treatment. At this point, a more detailed understanding of tumor-induced angiogenesis is needed in order to understand the full ramifications of anti-angiogenic therapy. Most studies indicate that, in order for anti-angiogenic tumor therapy to be successful, long-term administration is required. It is unknown at this time what, if any, long-term side-effects of anti-angiogenic therapy there will be. Additionally, anti-angiogenic therapy is costly. To be suitable for long-term chronic uses, agents should possess little toxicity, be easily administered, and be available at reasonable cost. Obviously, further studies are needed to define the potential and role of this new class of therapeutic agents in the treatment of cancer.

Gene therapy

All cancers involve some type of genetic dysfunction, although the specific gene or genes involved may not have been identified. The aberrant gene may be a genetic accident, present at birth and resulting in the development of a cancer. Alternatively, the cancer may be the consequence of environmental factors, such as chemicals, radiation, or viruses, activating a proto-oncogene or inactivating a tumor suppressor gene. As more details of the molecular behavior of cancers are discovered, more potential exists for genetic engineering in the treatment of human cancers. Thus, the recent developments in gene transfer techniques may lead to novel therapies for patients with cancer.

The first clinical trial involving gene transfer in humans occurred in 1989 with the insertion of a neomycin-resistant marker gene into tumor-infiltrating lymphocytes from melanoma patients. This study demonstrated that an exogenous gene could be transferred safely into human patients and subsequently detected in their cells.[138] In September 1990, gene therapy was first attempted in humans to treat adenosine deaminase (ADA) deficiency. When the ADA gene was transferred into the peripheral T lymphocytes of patients with ADA deficiency, cellular and humoral immunity was restored.[139]

Since these initial steps, there have been over 200 clinical trials involving genes, the majority of which are for human cancers.[140] Despite major improvements recently in conventional cancer therapies involving surgery, radiation, or chemotherapy, many of the current treatments ultimately fail to result in a cure. Surgical resection is the primary treatment for many forms of cancer. However, a single residual tumor cell left behind can theoretically generate the development of recurrence and metastases; it is the growth of metastases that is most difficult to control and often results in patient death. Radiation and chemotherapy are limited by their toxic effects on normal cells and are unable to target tumor cells specifically. Gene therapy, therefore, is an important new therapeutic approach that potentially can treat cancers in an effective as well as a selective manner.

Techniques of gene transfer

Although various methods exist for delivering genes to target tissues, no ideal vector has yet been developed. The best vector for gene transfer would be safe to the host, easily produced in high quantities, efficient at transferring the gene of interest, and result in long-lasting effects. The earliest vehicles for gene delivery were viral vectors, because a natural part of the viral life cycle is to infect host cells and transfer their genetic material. These viral-dependent approaches probably remain the most efficient methods of gene delivery. However, issues of safety and possible host inflammatory responses led to the development of other non-viral-dependent strategies.

Viral vectors

The first gene therapy trials utilized retroviral vectors, and they are currently still the most commonly used gene transfer method in human trials.[140] Retroviruses contain genomes composed of RNA, which is reverse-transcribed into DNA during viral replication. Interestingly, they are the same viruses that were found to cause tumors in chickens, leading to the discovery of the first oncogenes nearly 30 years ago. To make the vector safe for use in humans, the retrovirus is rendered replication incompetent by deleting the genes necessary for viral replication (gag, pol, and env) and replacing them with the gene of interest. Once the retroviral vector infects the target cell, it integrates its genome into that of the host and continues replication of the gene of interest, which is then expressed by the cell.[141] Because the viral DNA becomes stably integrated with the host genome, expression of the transferred gene can be long term. However, one disadvantage of retroviral vectors is their reliance on cell proliferation for gene transfer, because replication of the retrovirus requires DNA synthesis and integration into the host genome. As a result, transduction efficiency is typically around 10–20% in vitro and even less in vivo. Furthermore, current methods of retroviral vector production are unable to produce high concentrations of viral supernatant and the titer is usually 10^5–10^6 cfu/ml. To achieve adequate titers for in-vivo use, the retroviral supernatant must be concentrated in a labor-intensive process. Finally, the possibility exists that replication-competent virus may be produced

through recombination events, although this likelihood is remote with newer modifications of the retroviral vector and screening assays.[142,143]

In contrast to the low transduction efficiency of retroviral vectors, adenoviruses are able to achieve very high levels of transduction because they can efficiently infect non-dividing cells. Adenoviral vectors can also be prepared as high-titer supernatants (10^{10} pfu/ml). Thus, adenoviruses have been useful in many in-vivo experiments including systems using non-proliferating cells such as hepatocytes, cardiac muscle, smooth muscle, and endothelial cells. Despite these advantages, adenoviruses are limited by the inflammatory response generated by the host immune response to viral antigens expressed along with the therapeutic gene.[145] In addition, the adenoviral genome is not integrated into, and replicated along with, the host genome. This property, together with the host immune response against adenoviral proteins, results in a more limited duration of transgene expression in the host compared to retroviral vectors. New generations of adenoviral vectors lacking specific gene regions (E1, E3, and E4) are unable to replicate independently and may be less immunogenic to the host.[146]

Adeno-associated virus (AAV) contains a small DNA genome that requires a helper virus such as adenovirus or herpes virus in order to replicate.[146] Without a helper virus, AAV cannot replicate, but becomes integrated into the host genome in a site-specific manner, preferentially to a small region on human chromosome 19. AAV vectors are able to integrate into non-dividing cells, although the mechanism is not fully understood. The small size of the AAV genome makes it amenable to purification processes; however, the transgene insert size is also limited to approximately 4.5 kb.

The herpes simplex virus (HSV) is a large DNA virus that is able to infect neuronal cells (its natural target) and almost every other mammalian cell. HSV may remain in a latent state after infection of a target cell and be activated to undergo lysis by various stimuli. For use as a method of gene transfer, the pathogenic regions of the HSV genome can be deleted, resulting in long-term expression of only the transgene. The advantages of HSV for gene delivery include the large size of its genome (150 kb), which allows large amounts of foreign DNA to be inserted, and the relative ease of production of high-titer supernatants.[147] The toxicity of HSV, however, limits its clinical role in gene therapy trials. Certain lytic viral genes that are present in current HSV vectors cause host-cell toxicity and death.

Another viral approach to gene transfer utilizes vaccinia virus, which is a member of the poxvirus family and contains a large DNA genome. Vaccinia viruses have been mostly used in immunization protocols.[144,148,149] The large size of the vaccinia genome allows for a 25-kb capacity for the gene insert. Vaccinia is also able to infect a broad range of host cells, and construction of recombinant vaccinia virus is relatively simple.[150] However, vaccinia viral vectors continue to have problems with cytopathic effects on infected cells *in vivo*,[150] although recent development of non-replicating vectors may abrogate the viral toxic effects.[151]

Non-viral vectors

Several types of non-viral vectors have been developed to avoid the various disadvantages associated with viral vectors. For example, many of the viral-based vectors have toxic effects, often relating to the host inflammatory response to viral antigens. Viral vectors also may have the potential for recombination, resulting in replication of the virus or even development of malignancy. In addition, construction of recombinant viral vectors in sufficient quantities is often tedious and labor intensive. The non-viral approaches summarized here may circumvent these problems, but, in general, are less efficient in gene transfer and have a shorter duration of gene expression than viral methods.

Liposomes have been engineered for gene delivery by mixing positively charged lipids with negatively charged DNA. After addition of the synthetic liposomes to target cells, non-specific fusion of the liposome with the cell membrane occurs, releasing the DNA into the cytoplasm.[152] Gene transfer efficiency can be quite variable with the various compositions of liposomes under investigation, although up to 90% gene transfer has been reported.[153] To improve the efficacy of liposome entry into the target cell, liposomes have been complexed with viral proteins as well as with target cell-specific antibodies to create 'virosomes' and 'immunoliposomes'.[153,154] The clinical applicability of liposome-mediated gene transfer is still limited by the transient nature of gene expression, which is probably due to host immune responses against the foreign gene as well as to loss of the plasmid containing the foreign gene from the liposome or to down-regulation of the plasmid promoter. When liposomes carrying a marker gene were injected into the tail vein of mice, gene expression was present at 24 h, but gradually declined by 20–150-fold by 3 weeks.[155]

Gene delivery can also be achieved by simply directly injecting the gene of interest into target tissue. The exact mechanism of incorporation of the DNA into cells is not fully understood, but appears to involve endocytic or electrical processes resulting in internalization of the DNA into myofiber cells.[156] Specific tissues seem to be more capable of expressing directly injected DNA: muscle, subcutaneous tissue, liver, and thyroid follicular cells.[157–159] A non-linear structure of the injected DNA is also important for uptake into target cells. A newly developed device, the Accell gene gun, is able to deliver DNA, coated with gold particles, at high velocities with a burst of helium gas into the target tissue. The transfection procedure takes 5 s and genes are able to be delivered through 30–50 cell layers into subcutaneous tumors.[160]

Direct gene transfer usually results in only transient gene expression; however, a biologic effect has been shown in several animal models. Delivery of human IL-6 in four to five applications into fibrosarcomas in mice resulted in reduction of tumor growth and significant serum levels of the cytokine.[161]

A variation of direct gene injection uses engineered skeletal muscle cells to express the gene of interest. Skeletal myoblasts are harvested and transduced with a retroviral vector carrying the gene of interest. When the transduced myoblasts are injected into the host skeletal muscle, they are able to produce and secrete the foreign protein locally as well as systemically. Gene expression has been shown to persist for 2 years at high levels.[162] Myoblast-mediated gene transfer has been utilized for expression of proteins such as human growth hormone, coagulation factor IX, and erythropoietin.

Applications to cancer treatment

Immunotherapy

Three main strategies have been proposed using gene therapy techniques to stimulate the immune response to treat tumors:

1 enhancement of the immunogenicity of the tumor by a cancer vaccine;
2 blocking mechanisms by which tumors evade immunological destruction;
3 increasing antitumor activity of immune cells.

Because tumor cells are poor immunogens despite having certain tumor-associated antigens (TAA), all of these approaches attempt to enhance the natural immune response to tumors.

Immunization protocols have used vectors carrying various antigens such as major histocompatibility complex (MHC), CEAs, and virus antigens to provoke an antitumor response in the host.[163–165] A plasmid carrying the human CEA cDNA was shown to elicit humoral and cellular immune responses that were CEA-specific *in vivo*. In addition, the plasmid was able to function as a vaccine and protect against syngeneic colon carcinoma cells that expressed CEA.[164]

Genes encoding accessory proteins in the immune response have been incorporated in tumor vaccines. The B7 family of molecules is expressed on the surface of antigen-presenting cells and is required as a costimulation factor to activate T lymphocytes by interaction with the CD28 and CTLA-4 molecules on the lymphocytes. When the B7 gene was transfected into tumor cells in animals, tumor regression was observed and, furthermore, subsequent injections of tumor cells were rejected.[166,167] In a human clinical trial for melanoma, liposomes containing the *HLA-B7* gene were directly injected into subcutaneous melanoma nodules. In four of five patients, the injected nodules regressed. In one patient, the regression was seen in the injected nodule as well as in distant metastases.[168]

Another strategy of tumor vaccines involves the transfer of cytokine genes into tumor cells to create a paracrine effect from the cytokines at the tumor site, but without systemic toxicity. It is hoped that if tumor cells can be engineered to secrete a cytokine, cytotoxic T lymphocytes (CTLs) will be activated and sensitized. When injected into a patient, these tumor-specific T cells may be able to destroy remaining tumor cells. Clinical studies are underway utilizing the transfer of several cytokines, such as IL-2, IL-4, IL-7, TNF-α, IFN-γ, and granulocyte–macrophage colony-stimulating factor. IL-2 has been the focus of many investigators. This cytokine is secreted by activated T helper (CD4+) cells and, in turn, activates CTL (CD8+) cells to result in cell killing. Cancer patients, however, may have defective T helper cells and be unable to activate the CTL response. Transduction of tumor cells with the IL-2 gene would produce a local secretion of IL-2 at the tumor site to directly activate tumor-specific CTLs. IL-2 may also activate natural killer (NK) cells and lymphokine-activated killer cells (LAK). Preclinical studies have demonstrated that, when tumor cells are transduced with IL-2 and re-injected into animals, specific antitumor activity is seen, along with a systemic response. The immune response against autologous tumor is enhanced and protects against re-challenge with tumor cells.[165,169]

Some tumors have the ability to evade immunological detection and destruction by the production of certain cytokines. For example, glioblastoma multiforme and breast cancers secrete IGF-1, although the mechanism by which IGF-1 protects the tumor cells is not clear.[170] When tumor cells were transfected with IGF-1 and implanted into animals, the tumors were rejected by the host immune system.[171]

To mount an effective immune response against tumor cells, tumor-infiltrating lymphocytes (TILs) can be isolated from a surgically excised tumor and stimulated to proliferate *in vitro* in the presence of IL-2. These TILs have been shown to travel to tumor sites *in vivo*[172] and, thus, could be used to deliver cytokines to tumor sites. In an intracerebral murine tumor model, TILs transduced with the IL-2 gene were able to reduce B16F10 lung metastasis, with prolonged survival time in the animals.[173] TILs carrying the neomycin resistance marker gene (NeoR) were detected by PCR analysis in tumor deposits up to 64 days after infusion and in the systemic circulation at 189 days.[174]

Suicide genes

With the suicide strategy of gene therapy, a gene encoding an enzyme is transferred into tumor cells, which activates a non-toxic prodrug to produce a toxic agent, resulting in death of the transduced tumor cell. In the best-known system, the herpes simplex virus thymidine kinase (*HSV-tk*) gene is transduced into tumor cells. When the tumor cell is exposed to the prodrug ganciclovir, thymidine kinase phosphorylates the molecule, producing an intermediate that interferes with DNA synthesis and leads to cell death.[175] Theoretically, cytotoxic effects could be directed specifically to tumor cells transduced with the

HSV-tk gene without systemic toxicity. Culver *et al.* injected murine fibroblast cells producing the HSV-tk retroviral vector directly into brain tumors in rats. After systemic treatment with ganciclovir, significant tumor regression was observed without surrounding toxicity.[176] Other investigators have transduced the gene encoding cytosine deaminase (CD) into tumor cells, allowing the metabolism of the non-toxic prodrug 5-fluorocytosine to the toxic metabolite 5-FU.[177] In the first clinical trial using suicide gene therapy, a positive response was seen in five of the eight patients with glioblastoma multiforme treated with a retroviral HSV-tk vector.[178] Preclinical studies in a nude mouse model of metastatic pancreas cancer have also demonstrated that intraperitoneal administration of retroviral HSV-tk vector followed by injections of ganciclovir significantly inhibited the growth of primary pancreas tumors as well as metastatic peritoneal tumor deposits.[179] An important mechanism in the HSV-tk system is the bystander effect, by which neighboring untransduced cells are killed by ganciclovir treatment when transduced tk+ cells are killed. This is thought to be mediated by the transfer of the toxic phosphorylated ganciclovir metabolite from transduced tumor cells through gap junctions in cell membranes to adjacent untransduced cells.[180,181] Because current techniques of gene transfer often have low transduction efficiency, a strong bystander effect is essential for successful tumor killing. Tumor-cell killing was observed even when only 10% of cells were transduced with the *HSV-tk* gene.[180] The delivery of the *HSV-tk* gene, and thus cell killing, can be targeted to specific tumor cells by the use of tumor-specific promoters. For instance, when the CEA promoter was linked to the *HSV-tk* gene in a plasmid and transfected into lung cancer cells, only CEA-positive cells were killed in response to ganciclovir treatment. Similarly, viral vectors containing the AFP promoter have been effective against hepatocellular carcinomas and the c-*eRbB*-2 promoter for pancreatic and breast cancers.[182,183]

Modulation of oncogenes and tumor suppressor genes

In order to inhibit tumor growth at its molecular origin, one approach in cancer gene therapy is either to ablate the function of an oncogene or to enhance the function of tumor suppressor genes. The goal of these strategies is to restore the normal mechanisms for growth control and differentiation.

To block oncogene function, investigators have used triplex formation of double-stranded DNA oligonucleotides in order to prevent transcription. Binding of these specific oligonucleotides changes the conformation of the DNA helix, preventing further transcription. The cyclin D1 proto-oncogene is involved in the regulation of cell growth and is often amplified in breast, esophageal, hepatocellular, and head/neck carcinomas. Kim *et al.* designed a triplex-forming oligonucleotide targeted to the promoter region for the human cyclin D1 proto-oncogene. This molecule was able to bind to the cyclin D1 promoter and inhibit transcription in HeLa cells.[184] Antisense oligonucleotides to oncogenes also inhibit gene expression, although the exact mechanism is not clear. They are thought to induce the arrest of translation by either binding to the oncogene mRNA or inducing RNase H to cleave the RNA. Several oncogenes have been effectively inhibited by antisense oligonucleotides, for example c-abl, c-fos, c-myc, c-src and ras.[185] A retroviral vector containing the antisense sequence to human cyclin G1 was shown to inhibit the proliferation of human osteosarcoma cells in vitro.[186] Anti-oncogene ribozymes are RNA molecules with catalytic activity, like protein enzymes that are able to bind and cleave specific target RNA sequences in oncogenes, preventing translation of the gene into a protein product. Anti-ras ribozymes have been designed to cleave the H-ras mRNA in human bladder carcinoma EJ cells, resulting in growth suppression in vitro. When EJ cells were transduced ex vivo with an adenoviral vector bearing the H-ras ribozyme and injected subcutaneously into nude mice, tumorigenicity was abrogated in the animals, in contrast to mice injected with empty control vectors, which grew large tumor nodules in 28 days.[187] Other strategies using gene transfer to abolish activated oncogenes include: dominant negative mutants, which produce mutant proteins that inhibit the wild-type function of endogenous proteins[188] (e.g. H-ras), and single-chain antibodies against oncogenes such as erbB2 that have been shown effectively to reverse the malignant phenotype of cells.[189]

Many cancers are thought to arise from either mutations or deletions in tumor suppressor genes. Thus, replacement of the defective tumor suppressor gene with the wild-type gene may restore the regulatory controls necessary for normal cell growth. To be effective, however, this approach relies first on the identification of the defective gene responsible for cancer. Moreover, the wild-type version of the gene must be delivered into a sufficient number of cells to exert a tumor-suppressive effect. Finally, cancers probably do not arise from a single defect in a single gene, but involve multiple genetic abnormalities.

Several tumor suppressor genes have been identified and found to be mutated in various forms of human cancers, including the Rb retinoblastoma susceptibility gene and the TP53 tumor suppressor gene. The Rb gene functions to inhibit the cell cycle at the G1 phase checkpoint. When the gene is inactivated by phosphorylation, this control point in the cycle is lost and the cell is able to proceed through DNA replication and mitosis. The inactivated form of Rb gene has been found in retinoblastomas as well as in adult tumors such as breast, prostate, bladder, and SCLCs.[190] When the normal Rb gene was transferred into retinoblastoma or osteosarcoma cells with inactivated Rb genes, cell growth and tumorigenicity in nude mice were reduced.[191]

The TP53 tumor suppressor gene is induced when DNA is damaged in cells, releasing a cascade of events that ultimately results in arrest of the cell cycle at the G1–S checkpoint, apoptosis, and cell death.[192] Mutations in the TP53 gene are found in over 50% of human cancers and have been shown to be correlated with a poor prognosis.[193,194] Transfer of the wild-type TP53 gene by viral vectors has been shown to inhibit tumor growth in human lung cancer, head and neck cancer, and prostate cancer.[195–197] Intraperitoneal injections of a retroviral vector containing the human wild-type TP53 gene resulted in significant inhibition of growth of primary pancreas tumors in nude mice as well as of peritoneal metastases.[198] Treatment with the retroviral TP53 vector induced apoptosis in the transduced pancreas tumor cells and increased expression of WAF1/p21 protein, a downstream mediator of TP53. Because transduction efficiency is very low in vivo, the tumor inhibition observed in these studies was probably mediated by a bystander effect in which untransduced cells are also affected by the function of the TP53 in neighboring transduced cells. Although the mechanism is not clear, Xu and colleagues postulated that an inhibition of angiogenesis might be involved in the TP53 bystander effect because TP53 has been found to induce thrombospondin.[199]

Improving the response to chemotherapy and radiotherapy

The wild-type TP53 gene also seems to play a role in the sensitivity of tumors to chemotherapy. Lowe et al. demonstrated that fibroblasts were sensitized to undergo apoptosis after treatment with ionizing radiation, 5-FU, etoposide, and adriamycin only when the TP53 tumor suppressor gene was intact.[200] When exposed to DNA-damaging stimuli, a cell carrying the wild-type TP53 will be arrested in the cell cycle at G1 and will have time for DNA repair. If repair were not possible, TP53 would trigger apoptosis. The presence of a mutant TP53 gene has been shown to be correlated with resistance to chemotherapy and radiation, and patients have a poorer prognosis.[201–203] When human NSCLC cells with a deletion of TP53 were transduced with an adenoviral vector containing the wild-type TP53 gene, their sensitivity to cisplatin was significantly increased. Injection of the TP53 vector into subcutaneous tumors in nude mice, followed by intraperitoneal delivery of cisplatin, resulted in apoptosis and destruction of the tumors.[204]

Transduction of bone marrow cells with the multidrug resistance (MDR) gene may be a novel approach to improve the response to chemotherapy by protecting the host bone marrow against toxic effects and increasing the dose limit of a chemotherapy agent. The MDR gene encodes for a transmembrane channel that actively pumps cytotoxic agents out of cells, increasing resistance to drugs such as taxol, adriamycin, vincristine, and actinomycin D. Mouse bone marrow cells transduced with the MDR gene were implanted into animals and were able to be selected for after treatment with paclitaxel.[205] In a clinical trial for the treatment of breast cancer, patients' bone marrow stem cells will be transduced with the *MDR* gene to determine whether myelosuppression from paclitaxel can be reduced.[206]

Future directions

Remarkable advances have been made in the field of gene therapy since the initial human clinical trial was initiated in September 1990 for a patient with adenosine deaminase deficiency. The various types of gene-delivery vectors have expanded to include numerous viral as well as non-viral approaches. The possible applications for gene therapy technology have broadened and the number of clinical protocols is now over 200.[140] Significant obstacles will need to be overcome, however, if gene therapy for cancers is to be clinically successful. Currently, most vectors are unable to achieve 100% transduction of cells. To effectively cure a cancer, all tumor cells would need to be killed, because, theoretically, only a single remaining cell could give rise to a tumor. The bystander effect that has been described for some systems, such as the HSV-tk retroviral approach, seems to be able to overcome this deficiency to result in overall tumor killing. Safety concerns must always be an important consideration when developing new gene therapy techniques. Finally, to be effective in the clinical setting, all gene therapy strategies must have the ability to target the specific tissue of interest without harming surrounding tissues.

Continued efforts in basic science research will be essential to identify the molecular processes giving rise to cancers in order for gene therapy to be clinically successful. Surgeons have been important figures in the development of gene therapy since the very beginning when a surgeon initiated the first gene transfer trial in 1990.[207] The participation of surgeons is invaluable in the emerging field of gene therapy because surgeons are able to provide fresh human tissue specimens for investigation and, moreover, with their direct contact with human disease, surgeons have a unique position in the understanding of pathologic processes. Though many surgeons may feel molecular biology is impenetrable and irrelevant, an understanding of the fundamentals of gene therapy technology will be useful for this emerging field.

CONCLUSIONS

The molecular biology of cancer is a complex field that has exploded over the past two decades. With the increasing understanding of the origin of the disease, we are also beginning to have a better understanding of how to prevent and to treat cancer. The next two decades will bring further advances in the area of cancer prevention, early detection, molecular biology, molecular medicine, gene therapy for cancer, and tailoring chemotherapy using biologic markers, all of which will probably make cancer a curable disease.

REFERENCES

1. Nasmyth K. Viewpoint: putting the cell cycle in order. Science 1996; 274:1643–6.
2. Edgar BA, Lehner CF. Developmental control of cell cycle regulators: a fly's perspective. Science 1996; 274:1646–52.
3. King RW, Deshaies RJ, Peters J-M, Kirschner MW. How proteolysis drives the cell cycle. Science 1996; 274:1652–9.
4. Elledge SJ. Cell cycle checkpoints: preventing an identity crisis. Science 1996; 274:1664–72.
5. Scherr CJ. Cancer cell cycles. Science 1996; 274:1672–7.
6. Hunter T. Oncoprotein networks. Cell 1998; 88:333–46.
7. Review M. Oncogenes: 20 years later. Genes Dev 1995; 9:1289–301.
8. Bischoff J. Perspective series: cell adhesion in vascular biology. Cell Adhes Angiogen 1997; 99(3):373–6.
9. Folkman J. Tumor angiogenesis: therapeutic implications. N Engl J Med 1971; 285:1182–6.
10. Pluda J. Tumor-associated angiogenesis: mechanisms, clinical implications, and therapeutic strategies. Semin Oncol 1997; 24(2):203–18.
11. Risau W. Mechanism of angiogenesis. Nature 1997; 386:671–4.
12. Gastl G, Hermann T, Steurer M, *et al.* Angiogenesis as a target for tumor treatment. Oncology 1997; 54:177–84.
12a. Stehelin D, Varmus HE, Bishop JM, Vogy PK. DNA related to the transforming gene(s) of avian sarcoma virus is present in normal avian DNA. Nature 1976; 260:170–3.
13. Weinberg RA. Oncogenes and tumor suppressor genes. CA Cancer J Clin 1994; 44:160–70.
14. Yamamoto T. Molecular basis of cancer: oncogenes and tumor suppressor genes. Microbiol Immunol 1993; 37(1):11–22.
15. Weinberg RA. Tumor suppressor genes. Science 1991; 254:1138–45.
16. Marshall C. Tumor suppressor genes. Cell 1991; 64:313–28.
17. Levine J. The tumor suppressor genes. Annu Rev Biochem 1993; 62:623–51.
18. Fearon ER. Human cancer syndromes: clues to the origin and nature of cancer. Science 1997; 278:1043–50.
19. Lee W-H, Bookstein R, Hong F, *et al.* Human retinoblastoma susceptibility gene: cloning, identification, and sequence. Science 1987; 235:1394–9.

20. Sager R. Tumor suppressor genes in the cell cycle. Curr Opin Cell Biol 1992; 4:155–60.

21. Hoppe-Seyler F, Butz K. Tumor suppressor genes in molecular medicine. Clin Invest 1994; 72:619–30.

22. Zhang Y, Xiong Y, Yarbrough W. ARF promotes MDM2 degradation and stabilizes p53: ARF-INK4a locus deletion impairs both the Rb and p53 tumor suppression pathways. Cell 1998; 92:725–34.

23. Pomerantz J, Schrerer-Agus N, Liegeois N, et al. The Ink4a tumor suppressor gene product, p19^Arf, interacts with MDM2 and neutralizes MDM2's inhibition of p53. Cell 1998; 92:713–23.

24. Quelle DE, Zindy F, Ashmun R, Scherr CJ. Alternative reading frames of the Ink4a tumor suppressor gene encode two unrelated proteins capable of inducing cell cycle arrest. Cell 1995; 83:993–1000.

25. Elledge R, McGuire W, Osborne C. Prognostic factors in breast cancer. Semin Oncol 1992; 19:244–53.

26. Andry G, Sciu S, Pratola D, et al. Relation between estrogen receptor concentration and clinical and histological factors: their relative prognostic importance after radical mastectomy for primary breast cancer. Eur J Cancer 1989; 25:319–29.

27. Hayes D. Tumor markers for breast cancer: clinical utilities and future prospects. Hematol Oncol Clin North Am 1994; 8(3):485–506.

28. Osborne C. Receptors. Philadelphia, Lippincott, 1991.

29. Foekins J, Rio M, Sequin P, et al. Prediction of relapse and survival in breast cancer patients by pS2 protein status. Cancer Res 1990; 50:3832–7.

30. Hayes D, Mesa-Tejada R, Papsidero L, et al. Prediction of prognosis in primary breast cancer by detection of a high molecular weight mucin-like antigen using monoclonal antibodies DF3, F36/22 and CU18: a Cancer and Leukemia Group B Study. J Clin Oncol 1991; 9:1–10.

31. Duffy M, O'Grady P, Devaney D, et al. Tissue plasminogen activator, a new prognostic marker in breast cancer. Cancer Res 1988; 48:1348–9.

32. Marques L, Franco E, Torloni H, et al. Independent prognostic value of laminin receptor expression in breast cancer survival. Cancer Res 1990; 50:1479–83.

33. Tandon A, Clark G, Chamness G, et al. Cathepsin D and prognosis in breast cancer. N Engl J Med 1990; 322:297–302.

34. Borg A, Tandon A, Sigurdsson H, et al. HER-2/neu amplification predicts poor survival in node-positive breast cancer. Cancer Res 1990; 50:4332–7.

35. Slamon D, Clark G, Wong S, et al. Human breast cancer: correlation of relapse and survival with amplification of the HER-2/neu oncogene. Science 1987; 235:177–82.

36. Tandon A, Clark G, Chamness G, et al. HER-2/neu oncogene protein and prognosis in breast cancer. J Clin Oncol 1989; 7:1120–8.

37. Toikkanen S, Helin H, Isola J, Joensu H. Prognostic significance of HER-2 oncoprotein expression in breast cancer: a 30 year follow-up. J Clin Oncol 1992; 10:1044–8.

38. Gusterson B, Gelber R, Goldhirsch A, et al. Prognostic importance of c-erbB-2 expression in breast cancer. J Clin Oncol 1992; 10:1049–56.

39. Allred D, Clark G, Tandon A, et al. HER-2/neu in node-negative breast cancer: prognostic significance of overexpression influenced by the presence of in situ carcinoma. J Clin Oncol 1992; 10:599–605.

40. Muss H, Thor A, Berry D, et al. c-erbB-2 expression and S-phase activity predict response to adjuvant therapy in women with node positive early breast cancer. N Engl J Med 1994; 330(18):1260–6.

41. Wright C, Nicholson S, Angus B, et al. Relationship between c-erbB-2 protein product expression and response to endocrine therapy in advanced breast cancer. Br J Cancer 1992; 65:118–21.

42. Allred D, Clark G, Elledge R, et al. Association of p53 protein expression with tumor cell proliferation rate and clinical outcome in node-negative breast cancer. J Natl Cancer Inst 1993; 85:200–6.

43. Thor A, Yandell D. Prognostic significance of p53 overexpression in node-negative breast carcinoma: preliminary studies suggest cautious optimism. J Natl Cancer Inst 1993; 85:176–7.

44. Rosen P, Groshen W, Saigo P, et al. A long term follow-up study of survival in stage 1 (TIN0M0) and stage 2 (TINIM0) breast carcinoma. J Clin Oncol 1989; 7:355–66.

45. Colomer R, Ruibal A, Genoballa J, et al. Circulating CA 15-3 levels in the post surgical follow-up of breast cancer patients and in nonmalignant diseases. Breast Cancer Res Treat 1989; 13:123–33.

46. Kallioniemi O, Oksa H, Aaran R, et al. Serum CA 15-3 assay in the diagnosis and follow-up of breast cancer. Br J Cancer 1988; 58:213–15.

47. Safi F, Lohler I, Rottinger E, et al. Comparison of CA 15-3 and CEA in diagnosis and monitoring of breast cancer. Int J Biol Markers 1989; 4:207–14.

48. Chan D, Beveridge R, Muss H, et al. Use of Truquant BR radioimmunoassay for early detection of breast cancer recurrence in patients with stage II and III disease. J Clin Oncol 1997; 15(6):2322–8.

49. Stierer M, Rosen H. Influence of early diagnosis on prognosis of recurrent breast cancer. Cancer 1989; 64:1128–31.

50. Hayes D, Kaplan W. Evaluation of patients following primary therapy. Philadelphia, JB Lippincott, 1991.

51. Hayes D, Tondini C, Kufe D. Clinical applications of CA 15-3. Totowa, NJ, Humana Press, 1992.

52. Hayes D, Zurawski VJ, Kufe D. Comparison of circulating CA 15-3 and carcinoembryonic antigen levels in patients with breast cancer. J Clin Oncol 1986; 41:1542–50.

53. Hayes D, Kiang D, Korzun A, et al. CA 15-3 and CEA spikes during chemotherapy for metastatic breast cancer. Proc Am Soc Clin Oncol 1988; 7:38a.

54. Ebert W, Leichtweis B, Schaphler B, Muley T. The new tumour marker CYFRA is superior to SCC antigen and CEA in the primary diagnosis of lung cancer. Tumordiagn Ther 1993; 3:91–9.

55. Hansen M. Serum tumor markers in lung cancer. Comments and critique. Eur J Cancer 1993; 29A:483–4.

56. Cooper E, Splinter T, Brown D, et al. Evaluation of radio-immunoassay for neuro-specific enolase in small cell lung cancer. Br J Cancer 1985; 52:333–8.

57. Laberge F, Fritsche H, Umsawasdi T, et al. Use of carcinoembryonic antigen in small cell lung cancer. Cancer 1987; 59:2047–52.

58. Sculier J, Field R, Evans W, et al. Carcinoembryonic antigen: a useful prognostic marker in small cell lung cancer. J Clin Oncol 1985; 3:1349–54.

59. Krischke W, Niederle N, Schutte J, et al. Is there any clinical relevance of serial determinations of serum carcinoembryonic antigen in small cell lung cancer patients? Cancer 1988; 62:1348–54.

60. Lokich J. Plasma CEA levels in small cell lung cancer. Correlation with stage, distribution of metastases, and survival. Cancer 1982; 50:2154–6.

61. Steiber P, Dienemann H, Hasholzener U, et al. Comparison of CYFRA 21-1, TPA and TPS in lung cancer, urinary bladder cancer and benign disease. Int J Biol Markers 1994; 9:82–8.

62. Ebert W, Bodenmuller H, Holzel W. CYFRA 21-1 – medical decision making and analytical standardization and requirements. Scand J Clin Lab Invest 1995; 55(Suppl. 221):72–80.

63. Pujol J-L, Grenier J, Daures J-P, et al. Serum fragment of cytokeratin subunit 19 measured by CYFRA 21-1. Immunoradiometric assay as a marker of lung cancer. Cancer Res 1993; 53:61–6.

64. Ebert W, Muley T, Drings P. Does the assessment of serum markers in patients with lung cancer aid in the clinical decision making process? Anticancer Res 1996; 16:2161–8.

65. Ebert W, Dienemann H, Fateh-Moghadam A, et al. Cytokeratin 19 fragment CYFRA 21-1 compared with carcinoembryonic antigen, squamous cell carcinoma antigen and neuron-specific enolase in lung cancer: results of an International Multicentre Study. Eur J Clin Chem Clin Biochem 1994; 32(3):189–99.

66. Gail M, Eagan R, Feld R, et al. Prognostic factors in patients with resected stage I NSCLC: a report from the Lung Cancer Study Group. Cancer 1984; 54:1802–13.

67. Diez M, Cerdan F, Ortega M, et al. Evaluation of serum CA-125 as a tumor marker in non-small cell lung cancer. Cancer 1991; 67:150–4.

68. Kimura Y, Fujii T, Hamamoto K, et al. Serum CA-125 is a good prognostic indicator in lung cancer. Br J Cancer 1990; 62:676–8.

69. Ebert W, Leichweis B, Bulzebruck I, Drings P. The role of Imx SCC assays in the detection and prognosis of primary squamous carcinoma of the lung. Diagn Oncol 1992; 2:203–10.

70. Strauss G, Skarin A. Use of tumor markers in lung cancer. Hematol Oncol Clin North Am 1994; 8(3):507–32.

71. Van der Gaast A, Schoenmakers C, Kok T, et al. Evaluation of a new tumor marker in patients with non small cell lung cancer: CYFRA 21-1. Br J Cancer 1994; 69:525–8.

72. Buccheri G, Ferrigno D. Prognostic value of the tissue polypeptide antigen in lung cancer. Chest 1992; 92:101–87.

73. Buccheri G, Ferrigno D. Usefulness of tissue polypeptide antigen in staging, monitoring, and prognosis of lung cancer. Chest 1988; 93:565–70.

74. Buccheri G, Ferrigno D, Sartoris A, et al. Tumor markers in bronchogenic carcinoma: superiority of tissue polypeptide antigen to carcinoembryonic antigen and carbohydrate antigenic determinant 19-9. Cancer 1987; 60:42–50.

75. Spila A, Roseli M, Cosimelli M, et al. Clinical utility of CA 72-4 serum marker in the staging and immediate post surgical management of gastric cancer patients. Anticancer Res 1996; 16:2241–8.

76. Byrne D, Browning MC, Cuschieri A. Ca 72-4: a new tumour marker for gastric cancer. Br J Surg 1990; 77:1010–13.

77. Koga T, Kano T, Souda K, et al. The clinical usefulness of preoperative CEA determination in gastric cancer. Jpn J Surg 1987; 17:342–7.

78. Hamazoe R, Maeta M, Matsui T, et al. CA 72-4 compared with carcinoembryonic antigen as a tumor marker for gastric cancer. Eur J Cancer 1992; 28A:1351–4.

79. Maehara Y, Sugimachi K, Akagi M, et al. Serum carcinoembryonic antigen level increases correlate with tumor progression in patients with differentiated gastric carcinoma following noncurative resection. Cancer Res 1990; 50(13):3952–5.

80. Posner M, Mayer R. The use of serologic tumor markers in gastrointestinal malignancies. Hematol Oncol Clin North Am 1994; 8(3):533–53.

81. Shimizu N, Wakatsuki T, Murakami A, et al. Carcinoembryonic antigen in gastric cancer patients. Oncology 1987; 44:240–4.

82. Steele G, Ellenberg D, Ramming K, et al. CEA monitoring among patients in multi-institutional adjuvant GI therapy protocols. Ann Surg 1982; 196:162–9.

83. Tomoda H, Furusawa M, Ohmachi S, et al. Carcinoembryonic antigen in the management of gastric cancer patients. Jpn J Clin Oncol 1981; 11:69–73.

84. Ravry M, McIntire R, Moertel C, et al. Brief communication: carcinoembryonic antigen and alpha-fetoprotein in the diagnosis of gastric and

colonic cancer: a comparative clinical evaluation. J Natl Cancer Inst 1974; 52:1019–24.

85. Fletcher R. Carcinoembryonic antigen. Ann Intern Med 1986; 104:66–73.

86. Goslin R, Steele G, McIntyre J, et al. The use of preoperative plasma CEA levels for the stratification of patients after curative resection of colorectal cancers. Ann Surg 1990; 192:747–51.

87. Wolmark N, Fisher B, Wieand S, et al. The prognostic significance of preoperative carcinoembryonic antigen levels in colorectal cancer. Ann Surg 1984; 199:375–82.

88. Moertel C, O'Fallon J, Go V, et al. The preoperative carcinoembryonic antigen test in the diagnosis, staging and prognosis of colorectal cancer. Cancer 1986; 58:603–10.

89. Wanebo JH, Stearns M, Schwartz M. Use of CEA as an indicator of early recurrence and as a guide to a selected second-look procedure in patients with colorectal cancer. Ann Surg 1978; 188:481–93.

90. Gullo L. CA 19-9: the Italian experience. Pancreas 1994; 9:717–19.

91. Glenn J, Steinberg W, Kurtzman S, et al. Evaluation of the utility of radioimmunoassay for serum CA 19-9 levels in patients before and after the treatment of carcinoma of the pancreas. J Clin Oncol 1988; 6:462–8.

92. Pleskow D, Berger H, Gyves J, et al. Evaluation of serologic marker, CA 19-9, in the diagnosis of pancreatic cancer. Ann Intern Med 1989; 110:704–9.

93. Yasue M, Sakamoto J, Teramukai S, et al. Prognostic values of preoperative CEA and CA 19-9 levels in pancreatic cancer. Pancreas 1994; 9:735–40.

94. Lundin J, Roberts P, Kuusela P, et al. The prognostic value of preoperative serum levels of CA 19-9 and CEA in patients with pancreatic cancer. Br J Cancer 1994; 69:515–19.

95. Taketa K. Alpha-fetoprotein: reevaluation in hepatology. Hepatology 1990; 12:1420–32.

96. Tsukuma H, Hiyama T, Tanaka S, et al. Risk factors for hepatocellular carcinoma among patients with chronic liver disease. N Engl J Med 1993; 328:1797–801.

97. Di Biscegile A, Rustgi V, Hoffnagle J, et al. Hepatocellular carcinoma. Ann Intern Med 1988; 108:390–401.

98. Ozols R. Gynecologic oncology. Norwell, MA, Kluwer, 1998.

99. Makar A, Kristensen G, Kaern J, et al. Prognostic value of pre- and postoperative serum CA-125 levels in ovarian cancer: new aspects and multivariate analysis. Obstet Gynecol 1992; 79:1002–10.

100. Makar A. Prognostic studies in cancer of the ovary and fallopian tube, with emphasis on the CA 125 antigen and c-erbB-2 oncogene. PhD, Norway, University of Oslo.

101. Rustin G, Gennings J, Nelstrop A. Use of CA 125 levels to predict survival of patients with ovarian cancer. J Clin Oncol 1989; 7:1667–71.

102. Catalona W, Smith D, Ratliff T, et al. Detection of organ confined prostate cancer is increased through prostate-specific antigen-based screening. JAMA 1993; 270:948–54.

103. Neal D, Clejan S, Sarma D, Moon T. Prostate specific antigen and prostatitis I. Effect of prostatitis on serum PSA in the human and non-human primate. Prostate 1992; 20:105–11.

104. Oesterling J, Rice D, Glenski W, Bergstrahl E. Effect of cystoscopy, prostate biopsy, and transurethral resection of prostate on serum prostate-specific antigen concentration. Urology 1993; 42:276–82.

105. Zagars G. Prostate-specific antigen as a prognostic factor for prostate cancer treated by external beam radiotherapy. Int J Radiat Oncol Biol Phys 1992; 23:47–53.

106. Pisansky T, Cha S, Earle J, et al. Prostate-specific antigen as a pretherapy prognostic factor in patients treated with radiation therapy for clinically localized prostate cancer. J Clin Oncol 1993; 11:2158–66.

107. Dupont A, Cusan L, Gomez J, et al. Prostate specific antigen and prostatic acid phosphatase for monitoring therapy of carcinoma of the prostate. J Urol 1991; 146:1064–8.

108. Formenti S, Dunnington G, Uzieli B, et al. Original p53 status predicts for pathological response in locally advanced breast cancer patients treated pre-operatively with continuous infusion 5-fluorouracil and radiation therapy. Int J Radiat Oncol Biol Phys 1997; 39(5):1059–68.

109. Formenti S, Danenberg K, Danenberg P. Primary paclitaxel in breast cancer: is β-tubulin a predictor for pathological response? Proc First Eur Breast Cancer Symp 1998; 1:543.

110. Leichman C, Lenz H, Leichman L, et al. Quantitation of intratumoral thymadylate synthase expression predicts for disseminated colorectal cancer response and resistance to protracted-infusion fluorouracil and weekly leucovorin. J Clin Oncol 1997; 15:3223–9.

111. Metzger R, Danenberg K, Leichman C, et al. High basal level gene expression of thymidine phosphorylase (platelet-derived endothelial cell growth factor) in colorectal tumors is associated with nonresponse to 5-fluorouracil. Clin Cancer Res 1998; 4(10):2371–6.

112. Danenberg K, Salonga D, Park J, et al. Dihydropyrimidine dehydrogenase (DPD) and thymidylate synthase (TS) gene expression identify a high percentage of colorectal tumors responding to 5-fluorouracil (5-FU). Proc Annual Meeting Am Soc Clin Oncol 1998; 17:A992.

113. Linn S, Honkoop A, Hoekman K, et al. p53 and P-glycoprotein are often co-expressed and are

associated with poor prognosis in breast cancer. Br J Cancer 1996; 74:63–8.

114. Chung H, Rha S, Kim J, et al. P-glycoprotein: the intermediate end point of drug response to induction chemotherapy in locally advanced breast cancer. Breast Cancer Res Treat 1997; 42:65–72.

115. Veneroni S, Zaffaroni N, Daidone M, et al. Expression of P-glycoprotein and in vitro or in vivo resistance to doxorubicin and cisplatin in breast and ovarian cancer. Eur J Cancer 1994; 30A(7):1002–7.

116. Chin K, Ueda K, Pastan I, et al. Modulation of activity of the promoter of the human MDRI gene by Ras and p53. Science 1992; 255:459–62.

117. Buser K, Joncourt F, Altermatt H, et al. Breast cancer: pretreatment drug resistance parameters (GSH system, ATPase, P-glycoprotein) in tumor tissue and their correlation with clinical and prognostic characteristics. Ann Oncol 1997; 8(4):335–41.

118. Lowe S, Ruley H, Jacks T, Housman D. p53 dependent apoptosis modulates the cytoxicity of anticancer agents. Cell 1993; 74:957–67.

119. Linn S, Pinedo H, Van Ark-Otte J, et al. Expression of drug resistance proteins in breast cancer, in relation to chemotherapy. Int J Cancer 1997; 71:787–95.

120. Tubiana M, Pejovic M, Chavaudra N, et al. The long-term prognostic significance of the thymidine index in breast cancer. Int J Cancer 1984; 33:441–5.

121. Silvestrini R, Daidone M, Valagussa P, et al. Cell kinetics as a prognostic marker in locally advanced breast cancer. Cancer Treat Rep 1987; 71:375–9.

122. Gardin G, Alama A, Rosso R, et al. Relationship of variations in tumor cell kinetics induced by primary chemotherapy to tumor regression and prognosis in locally advanced breast cancer. Breast Cancer Res Treat 1994; 32:311–18.

123. Keshgegian A, Cnaan A. Proliferation markers in breast carcinoma. Mitotic figure count, S-phase fraction, proliferating cell nuclear antigen, Ki-67 and MIB-1. Am J Clin Pathol 1995; 104:42–9.

124. Brifford M, Spyratos F, Hacene K, et al. Evaluation of breast carcinoma chemosensitivity by flow cytometric DNA analysis and computer assisted image analysis. Cytometry 1992; 13:250–8.

125. Fabian C, Kimler B, Mckittrick R, et al. Recruitment with high physiological doses of estradiol preceding chemotherapy: flow cytometric and therapeutic results in women with locally advanced breast cancer. A Southwest Oncology Group Study. Cancer Res 1994; 54:5357–62.

126. Aktepe F, Kapucuoglu N, Pak I. The effects of chemotherapy on breast cancer tissue in locally advanced breast cancer. Histopathology 1996; 29:63–7.

127. Honkoop A, Pinedo H, De Jong J, et al. Effects of chemotherapy on pathologic and biologic characteristics of locally advanced breast cancer. Am J Clin Pathol 1997; 107:211–18.

128. Paulsen T, Aas T, Borrensen A, et al. Angiogenesis does not predict clinical response to doxorubicin monotherapy in patients with locally advanced breast cancer (Letter). Int J Cancer 1997; 74:138–40.

129. Twardowski P, Gradishar WJ. Clinical trials of antiangiogenic agents. Curr Opin Oncol 1997; 9:584–9.

130. Boehm T, Folkman J, Browder T, O'Reilly MS. Antiangiogenic therapy of experimental cancer does not induce acquired drug resistance. Nature 1997; 390:404–7.

131. Pluda JM. Tumor-associated angiogenesis: mechanisms, clinical implications, and therapeutic strategies. Semin Oncol 1997; 24(2):203–18.

132. Rosen LS, Kabbinavar F, Rosen P, et al. Phase I trial of SU5416, a novel angiogenesis inhibitor in patients with advanced malignancies. Proc Annual Meeting Am Soc Clin Oncol 1998; 17:218a.

133. McGarvey ME, Tupule A, Cai J, et al. Emerging treatments for epidemic (AIDS-related) Kaposi's sarcoma. Curr Opin Oncol 1998; 10:413–21.

134. Tanaka NG, Sakamoto N, Korenaga H, et al. The combination of a bacterial polysaccharide and tamoxifen inhibits angiogenesis and tumour growth. Int J Radiat Biol 1991; 60:79–83.

135. Dezube BJ, Roenn JHV, Holden-Wiltse J, et al. Fumagillin analog in the treatment of Kaposi's sarcoma: a Phase I AIDS Trial Group Study. J Clin Oncol 1998; 16(4):1444–9.

136. Colville-Nash PR, Wiloughby DA. Growth factors in angiogenesis: current interest and therapeutic potential. Mol Med Today 1997; 3:14–23.

136a. O'Reilly MS, Holmgren L, Shing Y, et al. Angiostatin: a novel angiogenesis inhibitor that mediates the suppression of metastases by a Lewis lung carcinoma. Cold Spring Harbor Symp Quant Biol 1994; 59:471–82.

137. O'Reilly MS, Boehm T, Shing Y, et al. Endostatin: an endogenous inhibitor of angiogenesis and tumor growth. Cell 1997; 88:277–85.

138. Rosenberg S, Aebersold P, Cornetta K, et al. Gene transfer into humans – immunotherapy of patients with advanced melanoma, using tumor infiltrating lymphocytes modified by retroviral gene transduction. N Engl J Med 1990; 323:570–8.

139. Blaese R, Culver K, Miller A, et al. T lymphocyte-directed gene therapy for ADA-SCID: initial trial results after 4 years. Science 1995; 270:475–80.

140. Human gene marker/therapy clinical protocols. Hum Gene Ther 1998; 9:935–76.

141. Boris-Lawrie K, Temin H. The retroviral vector. Replication cycle and safety considerations for retrovirus-mediated gene therapy. Ann NY Acad Sci 1994; 716:59–70.

142. Miller A, Buttimore C. Redesign of retrovirus packaging cell lines to avoid recombination leading

to helper virus production. Mol Cell Biol 1986; 6:2895–902.

143. Cornetta K, Morgan R, Anderson W. Safety issues related to retroviral-mediated gene transfer in humans. Hum Gene Ther 1991; 2:5–20.

144. Cole D. Phase I study of recombinant CEA vaccine with post vaccination CEA peptide challenge. Hum Gene Ther 1997; 8:1138.

145. Yang Y, Numes F, Berencsi K, et al. Cellular immunity to viral antigens limits El-deleted adenoviruses for gene therapy. Proc Natl Acad Sci USA 1994; 91:4407–11.

146. Berns K, Giraud C. Adenovirus and adeno-associated virus as vectors for gene therapy. Ann NY Acad Sci 1995; 772:95–104.

147. Glorioso J, DeLuca N, Fink D. Development and application of herpes simplex virus vectors for human gene therapy. Annu Rev Microbiol 1995; 49:675–710.

148. Rosenberg S. Phase I trial in patients with metastatic melanoma of immunization with a recombinant fowlpox virus encoding the GP-100 melanoma antigen. Hum Gene Ther 1997; 8:1974–5.

149. Conry R. Phase IB trial of intratumoral injection of a recombinant canarypox virus encoding the human interleukin-12 gene (ALVAC-hIL-12) in patients with surgically incurable melanoma. Hum Gene Ther 1998; 9:913.

150. Moss B. Genetically engineered poxviruses for recombinant gene expression, vaccination, and safety. Proc Natl Acad Sci USA 1996; 93:11341–8.

151. Tsung K, Yim J, Marti W, et al. Gene expression and cytopathic effect of vaccinia virus inactivated by psoralen and long-wave UV light. J Virol 1996; 70:165–71.

152. Felger P, Tsai Y, Sukhu L, et al. Improved cationic lipid formulations for in vivo gene therapy. Ann NY Acad Sci 1995; 772:126–39.

153. Ledley F. Non-viral gene therapy: the promise of genes as pharmaceutical products. Hum Gene Ther 1995; 6:1129–44.

154. Trubetskoy V, Torchilin V, Kennel S, Huang L. Cationic liposomes enhance targeted delivery and expression of exogenous DNA mediated by N-terminal modified poly (L-lysine)-antibody conjugate in mouse lung endothelial cells. Biochim Biophys Acta 1992; 1131:311–33.

155. Liu Y, Liggitt D, Zhong W, et al. Cationic liposome-mediated intravenous gene delivery. J Biol Chem 1995; 270:24864–70.

156. Manthorpe M, Cornefert-Jensen F, Hartikka J, et al. Gene therapy by intramuscular injection of plasmid DNA: studies on firefly luciferase gene expression in mice. Hum Gene Ther 1993; 4:419–31.

157. Raz E, Carson D, Parker S, et al. Intradermal gene immunization: the possible role of DNA uptake in the induction of cellular immunity to viruses. Proc Natl Acad Sci USA 1994; 91:9519–23.

158. Hickman M, Malone R, Lehmann K, et al. Gene expression following direct injection of DNA into liver. Hum Gene Ther 1994; 5:1477–83.

159. Sikes M, O'Malley BJ, Finegold M, Ledley F. In vivo gene transfer into rabbit thyroid follicular cells by direct DNA injection. Hum Gene Ther 1994; 5:837–44.

160. Yang N, Sun W. Gene gun and other non-viral approaches for cancer gene therapy. Nat Med 1995; 1:481–3.

161. Sun W, Burkholder J, Sun J, et al. In vivo cytokine gene transfer by gene gun reduces tumor growth in mice. Proc Natl Acad Sci USA 1995; 92:2889–93.

162. Blau H, Springer M. Muscle-mediated gene therapy. N Engl J Med 1995; 333:1554–6.

163. Zweibel J, Su N, MacPherson A, et al. The gene therapy of cancer: transgenic immunotherapy. Semin Hematol 1993; 30:119–29.

164. Conry R, LoBuglio A, Loechel F, et al. A carcinoembryonic antigen polynucleotide vaccine has in vivo antitumor activity. Gene Ther 1995; 2:59–65.

165. Pardoll D. Immunotherapy with cytokine gene-transduced tumor cells: the next wave in gene therapy for cancer. Curr Opin Oncol 1992; 4:1124–9.

166. LaMotte R, Rubin M, Barr E, et al. Therapeutic effectiveness of the immunity elicited by P815 tumor cells engineered to express the B7-2 costimulatory molecule. Cancer Immunol Immunother 1996; 42:161–9.

167. Dunussi-Joannopoulos K, Weinstein H, Nickerson P, et al. Irradiated B7-1 transduced primary acute myelogenous leukemia (AML) cells can be used as therapeutic vaccines in murine AML. Blood 1996; 87:2938–46.

168. Nabel G, Nabel E, Yang Z, et al. Direct gene transfer with DNA liposome complexes in melanoma: expression, biologic activity and lack of toxicity in humans. Proc Natl Acad Sci USA 1993; 90:11307–11.

169. Yu M. Advances in cancer gene therapy. McGill J Medicine 1996; 2:93–106.

170. Yee D, Paik S, Lebovic G, et al. Analysis of IGF-1 expression in malignancy – evidence for a paracrine role in human breast cancer. Mol Endocrinol 1989; 3:509–17.

171. Trojan J, Johnson T, Rudin S. Treatment and prevention of rat glioblastoma by immunogenic C6 cells expressing antisense insulin-like growth factor 1 RNA. Science 1993; 259:94–7.

172. Hwu P, Rosenberg S. The use of gene-modified tumor-infiltrating lymphocytes for cancer therapy. Ann NY Acad Sci 1994; 716:188–99.

173. Nakamura Y, Wakimoto H, Abe J, et al. Adoptive immunotherapy with murine tumor-specific

T lymphocytes engineered to secrete interleukin 2. Cancer Res 1994; 54:5757–60.

174. Rosenberg S, Anderson W, Blaese M, *et al*. The development of gene therapy for the treatment of cancer. Ann Surg 1993; 218:455–64.

175. Moolten F. Tumor chemosensitivity conferred by inserted herpes thymidine kinase genes: paradigm for a prospective cancer control strategy. Cancer Res 1986; 46:5276–81.

176. Culver K, Ram Z, Walbridge S, *et al*. In vivo gene transfer with retroviral vector producer cells for treatment of experimental brain tumors. Science 1992; 256:1550–2.

177. Mullen C, Kilstrup M, Blaese R. Transfer of the bacterial gene for cytosine deaminase to mammalian cells confers lethal sensitivity to 5-fluorocytosine: a negative selection system. Proc Natl Acad Sci USA 1992; 89:33–7.

178. Ram Z, Culver K, Walbridge S, *et al*. Toxicity studies of retroviral-mediated gene transfer for the treatment of brain tumors. Neurosurgery 1993; 79:400–7.

179. Yang L, Hwang R, Pandit L, *et al*. Gene therapy of metastatic pancreas cancer with intraperitoneal injections of concentrated retroviral herpes simplex thymidine kinase vector supernatant and ganciclovir. Ann Surg 1996; 224:405–17.

180. Freeman S, Abboud C, Whartenby K, *et al*. The 'bystander effect' tumor regression when a fraction of the tumor mass is genetically modified. Cancer Res 1993; 53:5274–83.

181. Colombo B, Benedetti S, Ottolenghi S, *et al*. The 'bystander' effect: association of U-87 cell death with ganciclovir-mediated apoptosis of nearby cells and lack of effect in athymic mice. Hum Gene Ther 1995; 6:763–72.

182. Walther W, Stein U. Cell type specific and inducible promoters for vectors in gene therapy as an approach for cell targeting. J Mol Med 1996; 74:379–92.

183. Sikora K, Harris J, Hurst H, *et al*. Therapeutic strategies using c-erb B-2 promoter-controlled drug activation. Ann NY Acad Sci 1994; 716:115–24.

184. Kim H, Miller D. A novel triplex-forming oligonucleotide targeted to human cyclin D1 (bcl-1, proto-oncogene) promoter inhibits transcription in Hela cells. Biochemistry 1998; 37:2666–72.

185. Zhang W. Antisense oncogene and tumor suppressor gene therapy of cancer. J Mol Med 1996; 74:191–204.

186. Skotzko M, Wu L, Anderson W, *et al*. Retroviral vector-mediated gene transfer of antisense cyclin G1 (CYCG1) inhibits proliferation of human osteogenic sarcoma cells. Cancer Res 1995; 55:5493–8.

187. Kashani-Sabet M, Funato T, Tone T, *et al*. Reversal of the malignant phenotype by an anti-ras ribozyme. Antisense Res Dev 1992; 2:3–15.

188. Ogiso Y, Sakai N, Watari H, *et al*. Suppression of various human tumor cell lines by a dominant negative H-ras mutant. Gene Ther 1994; 1:332–7.

189. Beerli R, Wels W, Hynes N. Intracellular expression of single chain antibodies reverts erbB-2 transformation. J Biol Chem 1994; 269:23931–6.

190. Wiman K. The retinoblastoma gene: role in cell-cycle control and cell differentiation. FASEB J 1993; 7:841–5.

191. Huang H, Yee J, Shew J, *et al*. Suppression of the neoplastic phenotype by replacement of the *RB* gene in human cancer cells. Science 1988; 242:1563–6.

192. Hartwell L, Kastan M. Cell cycle control and cancer. Science 1994; 266:1821–8.

193. Vogelstein B. Cancer. A deadly inheritance. Nature 1990; 348:681–2.

194. Quinlan D, Davidson A, Summers C, *et al*. Accumulation of p53 protein correlates with a poor prognosis in human lung cancer. Cancer Res 1992; 52:4828–31.

195. Cai D, Mukhopadhyay T, Liu Y, *et al*. A stable expression of the wild-type p53 gene in human lung cancer cells after retrovirus-mediated gene transfer. Hum Gene Ther 1993; 4:617–24.

196. Liu T, Zhang W, Taylor D, *et al*. Growth suppression of human head and neck cancer cells by the introduction of a wild-type p53 gene via a recombinant adenovirus. Cancer Res 1994; 54:3662–7.

197. Eastman J, Hall S, Sehgal I, *et al*. In vivo gene therapy with p53 or p21 adenovirus for prostate cancer. Cancer Res 1995; 55:5151–5.

198. Hwang R, Gordon E, Anderson W, Parekh D. Gene therapy of primary and metastatic pancreas cancer with intraperitoneal retroviral vector bearing wild type p53 gene. Surgery 1998; 124(2):143–50.

199. Xu M, Kumar D, Srinivas S, *et al*. Parenteral gene therapy with p53 inhibits human breast tumors in vivo through a bystander mechanism without evidence of toxicity. Hum Gene Ther 1997; 8:177–85.

200. Lowe S, Ruley H, Jacks T, Housman D. p53-dependent apoptosis modulates the cytotoxicity of anticancer agents. Cell 1993; 74:957–67.

201. Davidoff A, Herndon J, Glover N, *et al*. Relation between p53 overexpression and established prognostic factors in breast cancer. Surgery 1991; 110:259–64.

202. Horio Y, Takahashi T, Kuroishi T, *et al*. Prognostic significance of p53 mutations and 3p deletions in primary resected non-small cell lung cancer. Cancer Res 1993; 53:1–4.

203. Sun X, Carstensen J, Zhang H, *et al*. Prognostic significance of cytoplasmic p53 oncoprotein in colorectal adenocarcinoma. Lancet 1992; 340:1369–73.

204. Fujiwara T, Grimm E, Mukhopadhyay T, *et al*. Induction of chemosensitivity in human lung cancer

cells in vivo by adenovirus-mediated transfer of the wild-type p53 gene. Cancer Res 1994; 54: 2287–91.

205. Sorrentino B, Brandt S, Bodine D, *et al.* Retroviral transfer of the human MDRI gene permits selection of drug-resistant bone marrow cells in vivo. Science 1992; 257:99–103.

206. Bank A. A phase-I study of gene therapy for breast cancer. Hum Gene Ther 1994; 5:102–6.

207. Rosenberg S, Aebersold P, Cornetta K, *et al.* Gene transfer into humans: immunotherapy of patients with advanced melanoma using tumor infiltrating lymphocytes modified by retroviral gene transduction. N Engl J Med 1990; 323:570–8.

Commentary

WOLF-KARSTEN HOFMANN, CARL W MILLER, SEISHO TAKEUCHI, TOSHIYASU HIRAMA, KUNIHIRO TSUKASAKI, AND H PHILLIP KOEFFLER

TECHNIQUES: THE ENGINE OF MEDICAL ADVANCES

Our understanding of cancer and its diagnosis is dependent on advances in technology. For the first part of the 1900s, we relied on light microscopy and special vital stains to diagnose cancer. Subsequent advances included the development of antibodies against cell surface and intracellular products, which helped to phenotype the cancer cell and determine what proteins were aberrantly expressed in these cells. Over the last 20–30 years, we have focused our attention on the chromosomes and genes of cancer cells, as a result of advancements in cytogenetics and molecular biological techniques.

Cancer cytogenetics has played a significant role in clinical care and basic sciences. In 1960, the discovery of the first consistent chromosomal abnormality in a human cancer was the Philadelphia chromosome in chronic myelocytic leukemia. Since then, improved cell culture, chromosome banding, and molecular cytogenetic methodologies, such as fluorescence *in situ* hybridization (FISH), have resulted in progress in cancer genetics. Cytogenetics is helpful for diagnosis and essential for making therapeutic decisions for many malignancies, especially for hematological ones. Also, cancer cytogenetics has provided a guide to identify the genes apparently responsible for multistep carcinogenesis, such as oncogenes and tumor suppressor genes. Chromosomal analyses are useful for the identification of karyotypic aberrations and imbalances, but they are less reliable for chromosomal amplifications. FISH allows the rapid, accurate ability to look for specific chromosomal changes. The relatively new technique of comparative genomic hybridization (CGH) can rapidly detect DNA copy-number variations across the whole genome, using differentially labeled test and reference genomic DNAs co-hybridized to normal chromosome. CGH is more reliable than cytogenetics for the recognition of potentially amplified regions.

The very recent technique of DNA microarray analysis can detect the expression of genes in a cell. The genes that are to be examined are arrayed or spotted, often on a glass surface, which is also called a 'chip.' Many of these genes have been isolated as a result of the genome project, which has identified and sequenced many of the human genes. The genes are represented on the chip either as oligonucleotides or as segments of the complementary copy of the RNA of the gene. RNA from the tumor is changed into a fluorescent probe and hybridized to the chip. A special fluorescence detector determines which genes are expressed and the intensity of expression. This allows for a genome-wide analysis of gene expression, which affords the opportunity to genotype the tumor, and identifies genetic pathways that are aberrant. These can then become targets to identify therapeutic agents that can correct the abnormal pathway.

These advances in methodology will ultimately identify specific genetic abnormalities that are associated with each person's cancer. Furthermore, therapy will be tailored for the specific genetic defect. In addition, individuals can undergo genetic testing to determine which cancers they are susceptible to develop.

NORMAL CELL-CYCLE CONTROL AND ALTERATIONS OF THE CELL-CYCLE MACHINERY IN CANCER

Central to many or most cancers is aberrant expression of one or several protein components that drive the cell cycle. Abnormalities of these proteins allow either rapid or unbridled cell division. Therefore, understanding the cell cycle is critical to understanding many of the genetic alterations that can occur in cancer. Cell division is governed by the concerted action of cyclin-dependent kinases (cdks), and their regulatory subunits, cyclins (Figure 1). The cells are at rest during G0. A critical point when a cell is going to decide to divide is the G1/S junction.

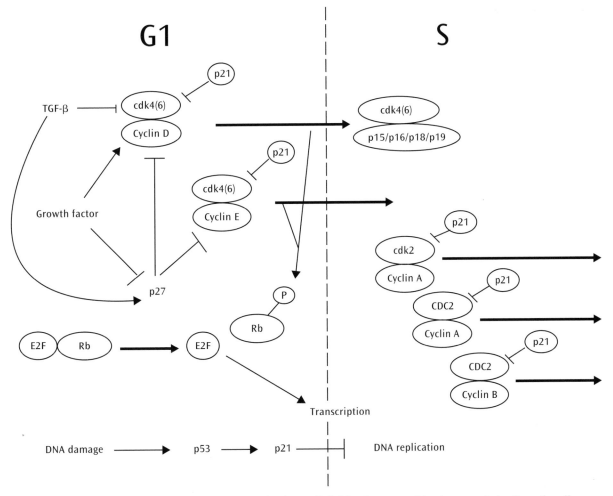

Figure 1 *Normal cell-cycle control at the G1 to S checkpoint. Cell division is governed by the concerted action of cyclin-dependent kinases (cdks) and their regulatory subunit, cyclins. Abbreviations: CDC2, cell division cycle 2; TGF-β, transforming growth factor β; E2F, E2F transcription factor; Rb, retinoblastoma protein.*

Cyclin D and cyclin E and their associated cdks have a critical function to progress through this checkpoint.[1] Cyclin D is associated with either cdk4 or cdk6, and is induced by growth factors, which means that cyclins are one of the links between extracellular signals and regulation of the cell cycle.[2] Cyclin E is associated with cdk2. Both the cyclin D/cdk4 and cdk6 and cyclin E/cdk2 kinase complexes are necessary for the G1/S transition. These G1–cdks phosphorylate the retinoblastoma protein (pRB). The growth-inhibitory effect of pRB occurs in its underphosphorylated form, at which time it binds to a family of cellular transcription factors known as E2F.[3] The phosphorylation of pRB allows E2F to become a transcriptional activator. Many genes important for DNA synthesis and cell proliferation have an E2F-binding site in their promoter, and these are induced to be expressed at the G1/S boundary by E2F after Rb is phosphorylated.

Dysregulation of the cell-cycle machinery can lead to uncontrolled cell division, which may be a key event in the development of cancer. Table 1 lists associations between aberrations of the cell cycle and the development of cancer. The cyclin-dependent kinase inhibitors (cdki) known as p16[INK4A] and p15[INK4B] are the most frequently altered cell-cycle-related proteins in cancer (Table 2).

TUMOR SUPPRESSOR GENES IDENTIFIED BY DETECTION OF LOSS OF HETEROZYGOSITY AND MUTATIONAL ANALYSIS

Inactivation of tumor suppressor genes is a crucial event in oncogenesis, which can be identified by assays for loss of heterozygosity (LOH). The rationale for LOH is that one allele of a tumor suppressor gene sustains a mutation and then the normal remaining allele is lost through a variety of possible means, such as deletion or recombination. If a polymorphic marker is in the region of this tumor suppressor gene, LOH will occur with loss of the normal allele. A powerful way to analyse for such loci is by polymerase chain reaction (PCR) using microsatellite markers, which anneal to polymorphic DNA loci that

Table 1 *Alterations of the components of cell cycle machinery in cancers*

Protein	Chromosome	Changes in cancer
Cyclin D1	11q13	Overexpression associated with many cancers
Cyclin D2	12p13	Overexpression associated with a colorectal cancer line
Cyclin E	19q12	Overexpression associated with several types of cancers
Cyclin A	4(q25-q31)	Overexpressed in breast cancers
Cyclin B1	5(q13-qter)	Overexpressed in breast cancers
Cyclin C	6q21	Hemizygously deleted in some ALLs
CDC2	10	Overexpressed in breast cancers
cdk4	12q13	Amplified in brain tumors and sarcoma and glioma cell lines
p21WAF1/Cip1	6p21	Very rare
p27Kip1	12p13	Decreased protein level in some cancers, sometimes associated with poor prognosis
p57Kip2	11p15.5	Very rare
p16^{INK4A}	9p21	Deletions and, less frequently, mutations associated with many cancers
p15^{INK4B}	9p21	Deletions associated with many cancers
p18^{INK4C}	1p32	Very rare
p19^{INK4D}	19p13	Very rare

Abbreviations: CDC2, cell division cycle 2; cdk4, cyclin-dependent kinase 4; WAF1, wild-type p53-activated fragment 1; Cip1, cdk-interacting protein 1; INK4A–INK4D, inhibitor of kinase 4A–4D; ALL, acute lymphoblastic leukemia.

Table 2 *Alterations of the p15^{INK4B} and p16^{INK4A} genes in cancers*

Neoplasm	p15^{INK4B} (%)	p16^{INK4A} (%)
Cervical	Rare	Rare
Ovarian	Rare	Rare
Endometrial	Rare	Rare
Testicular	Rare	Rare
Breast	Rare	Rare
NSC lung	9	12
Osteosarcoma	Rare	Rare
Sarcomas	Rare	9
AML	Rare	7
Lymphomas	Rare	Rare
Myeloma	14	14
ATL	18	26
B-ALL	10	15
T-ALL	64	77
Pancreas	82	Not reported
Melanoma	28	18

Abbreviations: AML, acute myelogeneous leukemia; ATL, adult T-cell leukemia; ALL, acute lymphoblastic leukemia; NSC, non-small cell.

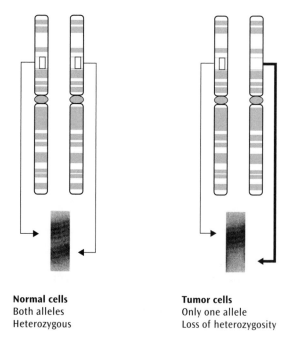

Normal cells
Both alleles
Heterozygous

Tumor cells
Only one allele
Loss of heterozygosity

Figure 2 *Schematic representation of loss of heterozygosity. Pairwise analysis of genomic DNA from tumor cells as well as from normal cells from the same individual.* Left. *In the normal cells, both polymorphic alleles are detected by polymerase chain reaction using primers for the microsatellite marker D1S450 from chromosome 1.* Right. *In the tumor cells, one allele is missing (bold arrow).*

contain a repeated nucleotide sequence (2–6 bp repeats). The most common microsatellite in the human genome is the $(CA)_n$ repeat. These can be found on average once every 30–60 kb and are generally polymorphic for $n > 10$.

Traditionally, determination of LOH uses electrophoretic microsatellite analysis of normal versus tumor DNA pairs by PCR amplification of each of the respective microsatellite alleles. Gel-based microsatellite analysis of LOH requires that a marker is informative (heterozygous) in the normal sample, and that genomic DNA from normal and tumor tissue is available for comparison. As shown in Figure 2, the PCR amplification of the microsatellite marker D1S450 from chromosome 1 results in products from both polymorphic alleles in the normal tissue, whereas in the tumor cells from the same patient only one allele could be detected. The bold arrow indicates the loss of the second allele in the tumor sample representing LOH for this locus.

Table 3 *Chromosomal regions that probably contain a mutated tumor suppressor gene, and the frequency of loss of heterozygosity (LOH) at these regions in several tumors*

Cancer	Chromosomal locus	Frequency of LOH (%)	Reference
Lung	3p	71–91	4
Lung	1p34	–	5
Non-small-cell lung	8p	39	6
Breast	3p24–25	–	7
Breast	8p22	52	8
Colorectal	8p	48	9
Colorectal	18q21	20	10
	5q21–22	26	
Medullary thyroid	1p	42	11
	17p	24	
	22q	31	
Ovarian	6q27	–	12
Squamous cell (head/neck)	7q31	53	13
Acute lymphoblastic leukemia	9p21	57	14
Acute myeloid leukemia	7q	27	15
Adult T-cell leukemia	6q	41	16
Chronic myeloid leukemia	1p36	47	17
Myelodysplastic syndrome	5q	40	18
	7q	45	
	1p	36	
	1q	35	

p, short chromosomal arm; q, long chromosomal arm.

Table 3 shows a summary of chromosomal loci that are frequently affected by LOH in several types of tumors. Furthermore, these sites of LOH, like cemetery gravestones, mark the location of a tumor suppressor gene whose mutation may be of importance in tumor pathogenesis. Also, LOH analysis of a tumor can help to evaluate its prognosis and perhaps its sensitivity to therapy.

Having determined a site of LOH in a tumor, the investigator attempts to identify candidate genes in the region that may represent the tumor suppressor gene that is mutated in that cancer. Knowledge of which tumor suppressor genes are mutated can help the physician to determine the prognosis and/or therapy for the patient. Analysis of single-point mutations can be done by several different methods, which can be broadly grouped into gel-based and advanced technologies.[19] The traditional methods are single strand conformation polymorphism (SSCP, see below) and heteroduplex analysis (HA). The resolution of nucleotide heteroduplex strands from homoduplex strands can be accomplished by several methods, such as denaturing gradient gel electrophoresis, temperature gradient gel electrophoresis, constant denaturant gel electrophoresis, and base excision sequence scanning. Furthermore, direct DNA sequencing is able to detect single-point mutations, but usually this technique is used for the analysis of a small number of samples, and it is not applicable for the screening of patient material.

During the last few years, a number of 'high-tech' methods have been developed to interrogate DNA samples for mutations, such as microarray analysis, mass spectrometry, and high performance liquid chromatography (HPLC)-based DNA fragment analysis. In the future, automated DNA array technology will be capable of the simultaneous mutational analysis of thousands of genes. However, until more reliable, efficient and cost-effective high-throughput methods become accessible, current available methods will rely upon more primitive means for screening for mutations of genes.

The polymerase chain reaction–single strand conformation polymorphism (PCR–SSCP) technique detects small deletions, insertions, and point mutations in genes. Mutations alter the mobility of single-strand DNA by changing its conformation in non-denaturing gels. PCR primers are designed and synthesized so that they can initiate amplification spanning the sequences of a gene where a mutation is expected. As a control, the same region of the DNA of a normal sample is also amplified. After amplification, the radioactive labeled (^{32}P-dCTP) products are subjected to non-denaturing polyacrylamide gel electrophoresis. The conformational change caused by the presence of a mutation is detected as a mobility difference, a shifted band. Figure 3 shows that a mutation can cause a change in the conformation of DNA resulting in a change in its rate of migration during electrophoresis in a gel. In sample number 4, an aberrantly shifted band from the DNA of bone marrow cells from a patient with preleukemia – also known as myelodysplastic syndrome (MDS) – was detected. Direct sequencing of this genomic DNA sample found a point mutation changing a cytosine to guanosine, resulting in the amino acid change of alanine to glycine.

This technique allows a large number of clinical samples of DNA to be screened effectively for mutations. One pitfall of the PCR–SSCP technique is that novel migrating bands require direct nucleotide sequencing or cloning of the PCR product and sequencing of the nucleotides in order to determine if the new band represents a mutation versus a polymorphism.

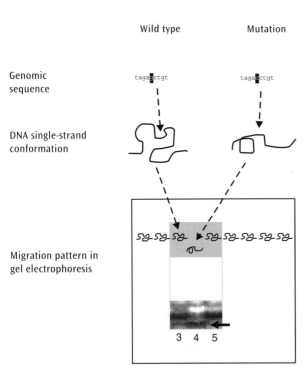

Figure 3 *Mutation analysis by polymerase chain reaction–single strand conformation polymorphism. The point mutation (g to c) results in a conformational change of the single-strand DNA. After electrophoresis, the DNA from the mutated cells shows a different migration pattern compared with that from the wild-type cells. The bold arrow indicates the shifted band.*

The *p53* tumor suppressor gene

This gene is frequently altered in many types of cancer. A familial predisposition to develop multiple tumors, known as the Li–Fraumeni syndrome, is usually due to inheritance of a mutant *p53* gene on chromosome 17.[20,21] Mice without *p53*, while viable at birth, develop tumors later in life.[22] These examples strongly imply that aberrant *p53* plays a very specific role in the development of cancer. The *p53* tumor suppressor is often described as a guardian of the genome, stalling cell division in order for the cell to repair the DNA or inducing apoptosis in cells with severely damaged DNA.[23,24] *p53* is critical in other circumstances, such as metabolic and temperature stress, and aberrant growth signals.[25,26] These pathways are central to guarding against oncogenesis; tolerance of damaged DNA and growth in the absence of growth factors are characteristic of cancer cells (Figure 4).

Several steps in the activation of *p53* after gamma-ray irradiation have recently been elucidated (Figure 4). Double-stranded DNA breaks induced by irradiation activate a kinase known as *ATM*.[27] *ATM* is mutated in a familial syndrome with neurological and cancer symptoms known as ataxia-telangectasia (AT), hence the name AT mutated (*ATM*).[27] Activated *ATM* phosphorylates a kinase called *CHK2* (also known as Cds1).[28,29] *CHK2* is a DNA damage kinase, originally discovered in yeast, which is mutated in some Li–Fraumeni cancer syndrome families.[30] The N-terminal region of the *p53* protein is phosphorylated by activated *CHK2*,[31–33] which blocks a binding site for murine double minute 2 (*MDM2*).[34] The *MDM2* protein targets *p53* for degradation by the ubiquitination pathway.[35–37] Thus, phosphorylation by *CHK2* stabilizes the *p53* protein. The *MDM2* gene is frequently amplified in liposarcomas.[38,39] The double-stranded DNA break pathway is an excellent illustration of how *p53* can be activated. Especially notable, mutations inactivating *ATM*, *CHK2* or *p53*, or amplification of *MDM2* contribute to oncogenesis.

Stabilized *p53* binds specific DNA sequences, resulting in activation of transcription of the cdk p21[WAF1], as well

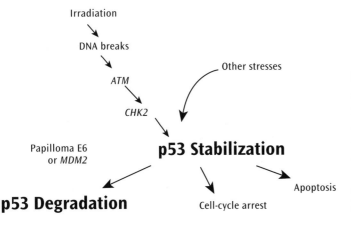

Figure 4 *The* p53 *pathways. The* p53 *activity is modulated by stabilization, induced by cellular stress. For example, at* left, *irradiation induces DNA breaks, which activates* ATM, *which turns on* CHK2, *which phosphorylates* p53, *making it become stable. Degradation of* p53 *takes place through the ubiquination pathway, initiated by the cellular protein* MDM2 *or viral proteins such as papilloma virus E6.*

as other proteins.[40,41] Increased expression of p21 leads to inhibition of cdks acting at cell-cycle checkpoints (see Figure 1).[40,41] Cells blocked at G1 are prevented from beginning new DNA synthesis; cells in G2 are prevented from going through mitosis. These pauses allow cellular repair to proceed. If damage is too great, *p53* accumulates in the absence of transcription, producing cell death by apoptosis.[42,43] However, p21 mutation and inactivation are not a feature of cancer.[44] Perhaps, apoptosis induced by *p53* has primacy in controlling cancer cells.

In human tumors, *p53* is inactivated by several mechanisms, including direct alterations of the *p53* gene, abnormalities affecting the *p53* activation pathways, and targeting of *p53* by viral-inactivating and host-inactivating proteins (Table 4). Physical alterations of the *p53* gene can occur by deletions of all or parts of it or by nucleotide changes resulting in coding alterations.[45,46] These alterations are usually missense mutations, yielding an aberrant *p53*, which can be inactive or even interfere with normal *p53* function.[45,46] Nucleotide changes causing premature termination, such as frameshift and nonsense mutations, are also common.[45,46] The nucleotide structure of *p53* gene alterations bares witness to the mutagenic assault implicated in the cancer. For example, G to T mutations are especially common in smoking-related cancers such as small-cell lung cancers.[47] By contrast, spontaneous mutations such as are found in osteosarcoma are predominantly C to T mutations caused by deamination of methylated cytosine residues.[47] Others, such as the occurrence of G to T mutations in cervical

cancer, suggest an as yet unidentified mutagenic process.[48] Mutations of *p53* are collected into a public database that has become a valuable resource for studying mutagenesis in human cancer and the effects of mutation on *p53* function.[49] Mutations of *p53* protein are concentrated in the central domain of the molecule.[45] The pattern of protein alterations observed in different types of cancer reflects the mutagenic process in a given tumor. For unknown reasons, different types of cancer have distinct frequencies of *p53* mutation (Table 5).[50,51]

Specific viral proteins evolved to inactivate *p53*, as *p53* also apparently acts to limit the effects of viral infection. The presence of a 53 kDa host protein binding to simian virus 40 (SV40) T-antigen protein originally led to the discovery of *p53*.[52,53] In human cancers, the targeting of *p53* for degradation by papilloma E6 protein is a striking example of this phenomenon.[54] The viral proteins that interact with *p53* are typically oncogenic.[54] Expression of these proteins alone can contribute to the neoplastic conversion of cells. Targeting SV40 T-antigen to specific murine tissues results in tumors in the target tissue.[55] Viral proteins known to interact with *p53* include SV40 T-antigen, papilloma virus E6, adenovirus E2B, and Epstein–Barr virus EBNA5.[56]

Tumors have been identified that modulate *p53* by exploiting host proteins that regulate the *p53* pathway. As mentioned above, overexpression of *MDM2* can decrease the stability of *p53* leading to degradation and inactivation of the protein.[38,39] Also, *p53* activity can be abrogated by the targeting of the upstream *p53* activation pathway including *CHK2* and *ATM*.[27,30] In addition, poorly understood cellular processes sequester abundant wild-type *p53* in the cytoplasm in some neuroblastomas and inflammatory breast cancers.[57] Transcriptional and apoptotic processes of *p53* are thus blocked.[57]

Stabilization and accumulation of *p53* lead to cell-cycle arrest and eventually to cell death. These properties are abolished or weakened by mutation of *p53*. Reintroduction of wild-type *p53* into tumor cells harboring a mutant *p53* is a therapeutic approach.[58] Certain anti-*p53* antibodies or *p53* peptides, if they enter the cell, may normalize mutant *p53* or cause mobilization of

Table 4 *Mechanisms of* p53 *inactivation*

Mechanism	Examples
Mutation	G to T transversions in smoking-related cancers
	C to T transitions characteristic of spontaneous mutations
	Rearrangements in osteosarcoma
Viral antigens	SV40, BKV and JCV T-antigen
	Papillomavirus E6
	Adenovirus E2F
	Epstein–Barr virus EBNA5
Sequestration	Cytoplasmic p53 in neuroblastoma and inflammatory breast cancer
Degradation	Papilloma virus E6 mediates p53 degradation
	Overexpression of *MDM2* in liposarcoma leads to p53 degradation
Upstream	Inactivation of *ATM* and *CHK2*, which act upstream of *p53*, leads to functional inactivation

Table 5 *Frequency of* p53 *mutation in diverse tumors*

Cancer type	Mutant *p53* (%)
Small-cell lung	80
Bladder	60
Colorectal	60
Osteosarcoma	50
Prostate	25
Non-small-cell lung	25
Neuroblastoma	5
Childhood acute lymphoblastic leukemia	1
Testicular	0

cytoplasmically sequestered *p53* to the nucleus.[59–61] In either case, only cells containing the wild type-like *p53* will undergo cell cycle arrest or apoptosis. One of the practical barriers to *p53* gene and protein therapy is the efficient delivery of the *p53* vector, peptides or antibody to a significant portion of the tumor cells.

Another approach is to take advantage of weaknesses inherent in cells without wild-type *p53*. Chemotherapy may work in part through the inability of cells having a mutant *p53* to recover from assaults by agents designed to damage DNA.[61] In addition, cells lacking *p53* are more sensitive to destruction by defective viruses. This characteristic has been exploited with some success using a defective version of an adenovirus known as ONYX-051.[62] One advantage of these approaches is that they target the whole *p53* response pathway and thus should work regardless of how the pathway is damaged.

In summary, knowledge of the functional and structural integrity of *p53* in a cancer may define prognosis and may suggest a course of treatment. Improved delivery systems and understanding of the *p53* pathway will probably lead to exciting approaches to cancer treatment.

HYPERMETHYLATION OF TUMOR SUPPRESSOR GENES

Numerous studies have shown that DNA methylation of the promoter of genes can inhibit their transcription. Most genes have binding sites for transcription factors in their promoters, and these genes synthesize more RNA product when the transcription factors bind to these regions (Figure 5a).[63] If the CpG nucleotides are methylated, transcription factors can no longer bind to the promoter region of the target gene, leading to silencing of

transcription (Figure 5b). Therefore, tumor suppressor genes can be inactivated by hypermethylation of promoter sequences. This is an alternative means for the inactivation of tumor suppressor genes in addition to point mutations or gene deletions. The following tumor suppressor genes are frequently inactivated through promoter CpG methylation: *p16^{INK4A}*, *p15^{INK4B}*, *VHL*, *hMLH1*.[64] A number of techniques to detect DNA hypermethylation have been developed. A recent, powerful approach is the bisulfate reaction. Using this technique, all unmethylated cytosines are converted to uracils, while 5-methylcytosines remain unaltered. Thus, the sequence of the treated DNA will differ if the DNA was originally methylated versus unmethylated. PCR products can be analysed by sequencing of the DNA (Figure 6).[65]

MISMATCH REPAIR DEFICIENCY AND CANCER

In cells with normal mismatch repair function, DNA mutations are repaired by proteins coded by the family of mismatch repair genes including *hMSH2*, *hMSH3*, *hMSH6*, and *hMLH1* (Figure 7a). However, cells without mismatch repairs accumulate mutations during their cell division, and eventually a cancerous mutation may occur (Figure 7b).

Microsatellites are short tracts of cytosine and adenosine nucleotide – $(C-A)_n$ – repeats which exist throughout the genome. Microsatellite instability (MSI) represents either an expansion or reduction of these sequences. This abnormality was initially reported in hereditary nonpolyposis colorectal cancer.[66] MSI appears to reflect multiple replication errors because of defective mismatch repair genes, including *hMSH2*, *hMLH1*, *hPMS1*, and *hPMS2* (Figure 8).[67] MSI has been reported in many kinds

(a) Normal active transcription of tumor suppressor genes

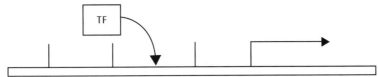

(b) Silencing of transcription by methylation

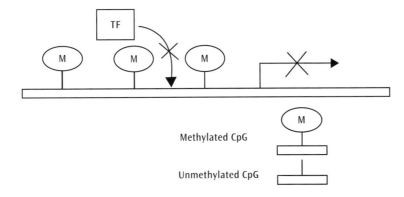

Methylated CpG

Unmethylated CpG

Figure 5 *Inactivation of tumor suppressor genes by promoter methylation. If the CpG nucleotides are methylated (M), transcription factors (TF) can no longer bind to the promoter region of the target gene, leading to silencing of transcription.*

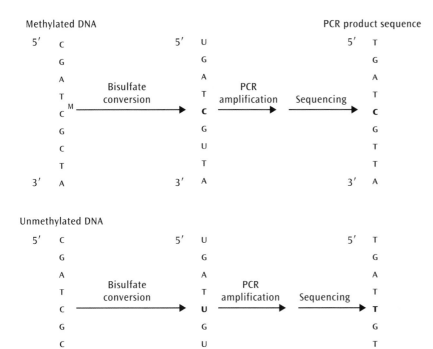

Figure 6 *Technique to detect hypermethylation. By bisulfate conversion, all unmethylated cytosines are converted to uracils, while 5-methylcytosines remain unaltered. Thus, the sequence of the treated DNA will differ depending on whether the DNA was originally methylated or unmethylated. Polymerase chain reaction products can be analysed by sequencing of DNA.*

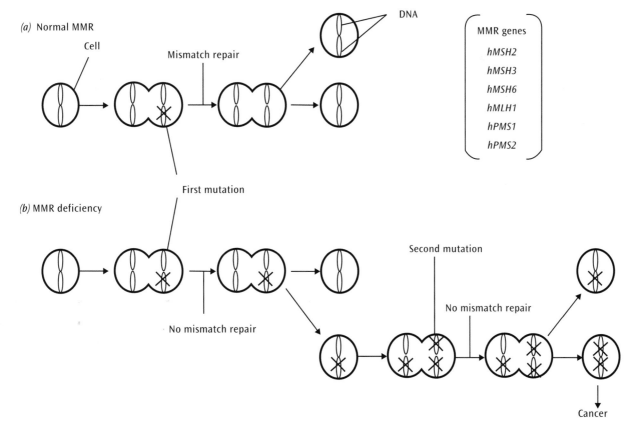

Figure 7 *Mismatch repair deficiency and development of cancer. (a) In cells with normal mismatch repair function, DNA mutations are repaired by proteins coded from mismatch repair genes. (b) However, in cells without mismatch repair, mutations accumulate in the course of cell division, and eventually a cancerous mutation occurs. MMR, mismatch repair.*

Microsatellite instability

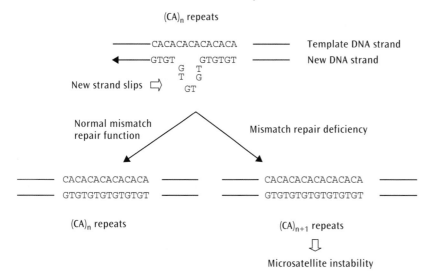

Figure 8 *Microsatellite instability. Increase in the number of microsatellite repeats occurs when the new strand slips down one repeat in its binding to the old template strand. If mismatch repair does not function correctly, this extra microsatellite cannot be removed and is reflected as microsatellite instability.*

of solid tumors, including sporadic colorectal, gastric, pancreatic, endometrial, prostatic, and renal cell carcinomas, as well as small-cell lung cancers.

LOSS OF IMPRINTING

Genomic imprinting plays a critical role in the repression of transcription of genes and it is important for the control of cell growth and development. Imprinting is the phenomenon by which individual alleles of certain genes are expressed differentially according to their parental origin. To date, approximately 25 imprinted genes have been identified; most of them are situated within a 500-kb region of chromosome 11p15. This region includes growth promoter genes such as insulin-like growth factor 2 (*IGF2*) and tumor suppressor genes such as *H19*, *p57^{KIP2}* (a member of the p21 cdkis), or *wt-1* (Wilms' tumor suppressor gene).

The *IGF2* has been confirmed to be involved directly in the regulation of cell growth. It is one of the most important genes that is imprinted in normal human embryonal tissue, resulting in mono-allelic expression of paternal *IGF2*. The expression of both alleles of *IGF2*, also known as loss of imprinting (LOI), was initially described in embryonal tumors of childhood, but other solid tumors and hematological malignancies have also been reported to have LOI (Table 6). LOI of *IGF2* is particularly frequent in tumors with a high proliferative rate (invasive breast cancer, acute myeloid leukemia), indicating the importance of bi-allelic expression of this gene for enhanced cell growth. Furthermore, animal models have shown that overexpression of *IGF2* promotes tumor growth of intestinal adenomas in mice.

The imprinting status can be investigated by PCR with specific primers for *IGF2*. *IGF2* is polymorphic for

Table 6 *Frequency of loss of imprinting (LOI) of the* IGF2 *gene in several tumors*

Cancer	Frequency of LOI (%)	Reference
Wilms' tumor	60–90	68
Glioma	57	69
Gastric	53	70
Colorectal	44	71
Renal cell	50	72
Head and neck squamous cell	38	73
Invasive breast	100	74
Ovarian	25	75
Acute myeloid leukemia	100	76
Chronic myeloid leukemia	100	77

the binding site of the restriction enzyme Apa 1. The PCR product amplified from the genomic DNA (both alleles of *IGF2* are targeted by the primers) is subjected to the restriction enzyme Apa 1, which cuts only the PCR product amplified from the genotype B. Electrophoresis can discriminate between the genotype AA (292 bp band) or BB (231 bp band). If the individual is heterozygous for *IGF2*, each of the bands at 292 bp and 231 bp is visible (AB). The distribution of the genotypes in Caucasians is as follows: 20% AA, 40% BB, 40% AB. Figure 9 shows the PCR products of all three genotypes amplified from genomic DNA after cutting with Apa 1.

Allelic specific expression can be determined by analysing RNA from those individuals showing heterozygosity for *IGF2* (genotype AB) using reverse transcriptase PCR. If the gene is physiologically imprinted, only amplification of the paternal allele of *IGF2* will occur, resulting in one band of 292 bp. The detection of two

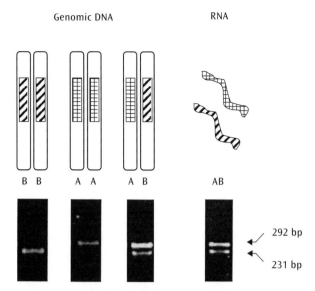

Genomic DNA   RNA

B B   A A   A B   AB

292 bp

231 bp

Figure 9 *Loss of imprinting of the* IGF2 *gene.* Left. *Genomic DNA was amplified by polymerase chain reaction (PCR) using specific primers for* IGF2. *The PCR products were cut by the restriction enzyme Apa 1, resulting in fragments of 292 bp for allele A and 231 bp for allele B. Results from all three genotypes are shown.* Right. *Reverse transcriptase PCR was performed from RNA from the same individual, which showed the genotype AB. After cutting with Apa 1, two different amplification products are separated by gel electrophoresis. The appearance of both bands reflects the expression of both alleles, showing the loss of imprinting in this sample.*

amplification products from the RNA reflects a loss of imprinting of *IGF2*, implying that both alleles of this gene are expressed in this population of cells (Figure 9). The LOI of *IGF2* may lead to overexpression of this growth factor, which may stimulate the proliferation of these transformed cells.

SUMMARY

Cancer can be analogized to rapid evolution at the cellular level; the genetic alterations will become established if each provides growth advantage to the transformed cell over its normal counterpart. By understanding these genetic alterations, we can begin fully to categorize each cancer, leading to an accurate diagnosis and full understanding of the prognosis. Identifying aberrant cellular pathways will allow us to tailor therapy that specifically attacks the particular abnormality with minimal toxicity to normal cells. New techniques drive innovation and discovery in medicine. We now have incredibly powerful molecular biology techniques and bio-informatics to revolutionize our approach to cancer.

ACKNOWLEDGMENTS

This work was supported by US Defense and NIH grants as well as by the CaPCure Foundation, Lymphoma Foundation of America, Parker Hughes Trust, C. and H. Koeffler Fund, Horn Trust, and the Aron Eschman Fund. H.P.K. is the holder of the Mark Goodson Endowed Chair for Hematology/Oncology and is a member of the Jonsson Cancer Center.

REFERENCES

1. Hirama T, Koeffler HP. Role of the cyclin-dependent kinase inhibitors in the development of cancer. Blood 1995; 86(3):841–54.
2. Sherr CJ. Mammalian G1 cyclins [Review]. Cell 1993; 73(6):1059–65.
3. Nevins JR. E2F: a link between the Rb tumor suppressor protein and viral oncoproteins. Science 1992; 258(5081):424–9.
4. Wistuba II, Behrens C, Virmani AK, *et al.* High resolution chromosome 3p allelotyping of human lung cancer and preneoplastic/preinvasive bronchial epithelium reveals multiple, discontinuous sites of 3p allele loss and three regions of frequent breakpoints. Cancer Res 2000; 60(7):1949–60.
5. Mendoza C, Sato H, Hiyama K, *et al.* Allelotype and loss of heterozygosity around the *L-myc* gene locus in primary lung cancers. Lung Cancer 2000; 28(2):117–25.
6. Lerebours F, Olschwang S, Thuille B, *et al.* Fine deletion mapping of chromosome 8p in non-small-cell lung carcinoma. Int J Cancer 1999; 81(6):854–8.
7. Matsumoto S, Minobe K, Utada Y, *et al.* Loss of heterozygosity at 3p24–p25 as a prognostic factor in breast cancer. Cancer Lett 2000; 152(1):63–9.
8. Utada Y, Haga S, Kajiwara T, *et al.* Allelic loss at the 8p22 region as a prognostic factor in large and estrogen receptor negative breast carcinomas. Cancer 2000; 88(6):1410–16.
9. Lerebours F, Olschwang S, Thuille B, *et al.* Deletion mapping of the tumor suppressor locus involved in colorectal cancer on chromosome band 8p21. Genes Chromosomes Cancer 1999; 25(2):147–53.
10. Sturlan S, Kapitanovic S, Kovacevic D, *et al.* Loss of heterozygosity of APC and DCC tumor suppressor genes in human sporadic colon cancer. J Mol Med 1999; 77(3):316–21.
11. Khosla S, Patel VM, Hay ID, *et al.* Loss of heterozygosity suggests multiple genetic alterations in pheochromocytomas and medullary thyroid carcinomas. J Clin Invest 1991; 87(5):1691–9.
12. Saito S, Sirahama S, Matsushima M, *et al.* Definition of a commonly deleted region in ovarian cancers to a 300-kb segment of chromosome 6q27. Cancer Res 1996; 56(24):5586–9.

13. Zenklusen JC, Thompson JC, Klein-Szanto AJ, Conti CJ. Frequent loss of heterozygosity in human primary squamous cell and colon carcinomas at 7q31.1: evidence for a broad range tumor suppressor gene. Cancer Res 1995; 55(6):1347–50.

14. Takeuchi S, Seriu T, Tasaka T, et al. Microsatellite instability and other molecular abnormalities in childhood acute lymphoblastic leukaemia. Br J Haematol 1997; 98(1):134–9.

15. Koike M, Tasaka T, Spira S, Tsuruoka N, Koeffler HP. Allelotyping of acute myelogenous leukemia: loss of heterozygosity at 7q31.1 (D7S486) and q33-34 (D7S498, D7S505). Leuk Res 1999; 23(3): 307–10.

16. Hatta Y, Yamada Y, Tomonaga M, Miyoshi I, Said JW, Koeffler HP. Detailed deletion mapping of the long arm of chromosome 6 in adult T-cell leukemia. Blood 1999; 93(2):613–16.

17. Mori N, Morosetti R, Spira S, et al. Chromosome band 1p36 contains a putative tumor suppressor gene important in the evolution of chronic myelocytic leukemia. Blood 1998; 92(9):3405–9.

18. Xie D, Hofmann WK, Mori N, Miller CW, Hoelzer D, Koeffler HP. Allelotype analysis of the myelodysplastic syndrome. Leukemia 2000; 14(5):805–10.

19. Gupta KC. Deviations from the norm: systems for mutation detection reveal hidden potentials. The Scientist 1999; 13(15):25–30.

20. Li FP, Strong LC, Fraumeni JF Jr, et al. Germ line p53 mutations in a familial syndrome of breast cancer, sarcomas, and other neoplasms. Science 1990; 250:1233–8.

21. Srivastava S, Zou ZQ, Pirollo K, Blattner W, Chang EH. Germ-line transmission of a mutated p53 gene in a cancer-prone family with Li–Fraumeni syndrome. Nature 1990; 348:747–9.

22. Donehower LA, Harvey M, Stagle BL, et al. Mice deficient for p53 are developmentally normal but susceptible to spontaneous tumours. Nature 1992; 356:215–21.

23. Dasika GK, Lin SC, Zhao S, Sung P, Tomkinson A, Lee EY. DNA damage-induced cell cycle checkpoints and DNA strand break repair in development and tumorigenesis. Oncogene 1999; 18(55):7883–99.

24. Kastan MB, Onyekwere O, Sidransky D, Vogelstein B, Craig RW. Participation of p53 protein in the cellular response to DNA damage. Cancer Res 1991; 51:6304–11.

25. Goto A, Shomori K, Ohkumo T, Tanaka F, Sato K, Ito H. Hyperthermia-induced apoptosis occurs both in a p53 gene-dependent and -independent manner in three human gastric carcinoma cell lines. Oncol Rep 1999; 6(2):335–9.

26. Lotem J, Sachs L. Hematopoietic cells from mice deficient in wild-type p53 are more resistant to induction of apoptosis by some agents. Blood 1993; 82(4):1092–6.

27. Lavin MF, Khanna KK. ATM: the protein encoded by the gene mutated in the radiosensitive syndrome ataxia-telangiectasia. Int J Radiat Biol 1999; 75(10):1201–14.

28. Matsuoka S, Huang M, Elledge SJ. Linkage of ATM to cell cycle regulation by the Chk2 protein kinase. Science 1998; 282(5395):1893–7.

29. Brown AL, Lee CH, Schwarz JK, Mitiku N, Piwnica-Worms H, Chung JH. A human Cds1-related kinase that functions downstream of ATM protein in the cellular response to DNA damage. Proc Natl Acad Sci USA 1999; 96(7):3745–50.

30. Bell DW, Varley JM, Szydlo TE, et al. Heterozygous germ line hCHK2 mutations in Li–Fraumeni syndrome. Science 1999; 286(5449):2528–31.

31. Hirao A, Kong YY, Matsuoka S, et al. DNA damage-induced activation of p53 by the checkpoint kinase Chk2. Science 2000; 287(5459):1824–7.

32. Shieh SY, Ahn J, Tamai K, Taya Y, Prives C. The human homologs of checkpoint kinases Chk1 and Cds1 (Chk2) phosphorylate p53 at multiple DNA damage-inducible sites. Genes Dev 2000; 14(3):289–300.

33. Chehab NH, Malikzay A, Appel M, Halazonetis TD. Chk2/hCds1 functions as a DNA damage checkpoint in G(1) by stabilizing p53. Genes Dev 2000; 14(3):278–88.

34. Chehab NH, Malikzay A, Stavridi ES, Halazonetis TD. Phosphorylation of Ser-20 mediates stabilization of human p53 in response to DNA damage. Proc Natl Acad Sci USA 1999; 96(24):13777–82.

35. Honda R, Tanaka H, Yasuda H. Oncoprotein MDM2 is a ubiquitin ligase E3 for tumor suppressor p53. FEBS Lett 1997; 420(1):25–7.

36. Haupt Y, Maya R, Kazaz A, Oren M. MDM2 promotes the rapid degradation of p53. Nature 1997; 387:296–9.

37. Kubbutat MH, Jones SN, Vousden KH. Regulation of p53 stability by MDM2. Nature 1997; 387:299–303.

38. Momand J, Zambetti GP, Olson DC, George D, Levine AJ. The MDM2 oncogene product forms a complex with the p53 protein and inhibits p53-mediated transactivation. Cell 1992; 69:1237–45.

39. Oliner JD, Kinzler KW, Meltzer PS, George DL, Vogelstein B. Amplification of a gene encoding a p53-associated protein in human sarcomas. Nature 1992; 358:80–3.

40. Bunz F, Dutriaux A, Lengauer C, et al. Requirement for p53 and p21 to sustain G2 arrest after DNA damage. Science 1998; 282:1497–501.

41. El-Deiry WS, Tokino T, Velculescu VE, et al. WAF1, a potential mediator of p53 tumor suppression. Cell 1993; 75:817–25.

42. Caelles C, Helmberg A, Karin M. p53-dependent apoptosis in the absence of transcriptional activation of p53-target genes. Nature 1994; 370:220–3.

43. Bates S, Vousden KH. p53 in signaling checkpoint arrest or apoptosis. Curr Opin Genet Devel 1996; 6(1):12–18.

44. Shiohara M, El-Deiry WS, Wada M, et al. Absence of WAF1 mutations in a variety of human malignancies. Blood 1994; 84:3781–4.

45. Walker DR, Bond JP, Tarone RE, et al. Evolutionary conservation and somatic mutation hotspot maps of

p53: correlation with p53 protein structural and functional features. Oncogene 1999; 18(1):211–18.

46. Hainaut P, Hollstein M. p53 and human cancer: the first ten thousand mutations. Adv Cancer Res 2000; 77:81–137.

47. Miller CW, Simon KJ, Aslo A, et al. p53 mutation in human lung tumors. Cancer Res 1992; 52:1695–8.

48. Park DJ, Wilczynski SP, Paquette RL, Miller CW, Koeffler HP. p53 mutations in HPV-negative cervical carcinoma. Oncogene 1994; 9:205–10.

49. Hernandez-Boussard T, Rodriguez-Tome P, Montesano R, Hainaut P. IARC p53 mutation database: a relational database to compile and analyze p53 mutations in human tumors and cell lines. International Agency for Research on Cancer. Hum Mutat 1999; 14(1):1–8.

50. Wang XW, Harris CC. p53 tumor-suppressor gene: clues to molecular carcinogenesis. J Cell Physiol 1997; 173(2):247–55.

51. Miller C, Koeffler HP. p53 mutations in human cancer. Leukemia 1993; 2:S18–21.

52. Lane DP, Crawford LV. T antigen is bound to a host protein in SV40-transformed cells. Nature 1979; 278:261–3.

53. Linzer DI, Levine AJ. Characterization of a 54K dalton cellular SV40 tumor antigen present in SV40-transformed cells and uninfected embryonal carcinoma cells. Cell 1979; 17:43–52.

54. Scheffner M, Werness BA, Huibregtse JM, Levine AJ, Howley PM. The E6 oncoprotein encoded by human papillomavirus types 16 and 18 promotes the degradation of p53. Cell 1990; 63:1129–36.

55. Furth PA. SV40 rodent tumour models as paradigms of human disease: transgenic mouse models. Devel Biol Standard 1998; 94:281–7.

56. Neil JC, Cameron ER, Baxter EW. p53 and tumour viruses: catching the guardian off-guard. Trends Microbiol 1997; 5(3):115–20.

57. Moll UM, Ostermeyer AG, Haladay R, Winkfield B, Frazier M, Zambetti G. Cytoplasmic sequestration of wild-type p53 protein impairs the G1 checkpoint after DNA damage. Mol Cell Biol 1996; 16(3):1126–37.

58. Roth JA, Nguyen D, Lawrence DD, et al. Retrovirus-mediated wild-type p53 gene transfer to tumors of patients with lung cancer. Nat Med 1996; 9:985–91.

59. Selivanova G, Kawasaki T, Ryabchenko L, Wiman KG. Reactivation of mutant p53: a new strategy for cancer therapy. Semin Cancer Biol 1998; 8(5):369–78.

60. Ostermeyer AG, Runko E, Winkfield B, Ahn B, Moll UM. Cytoplasmically sequestered wild-type p53 protein in neuroblastoma is relocated to the nucleus by a C-terminal peptide. Proc Natl Acad Sci USA 1996; 93(26):15190–4.

61. Fan S, Smith ML, Rivet DJ II, et al. Disruption of p53 function sensitizes breast cancer MCF-7 cells to cisplatin and pentoxifylline. Cancer Res 1995; 55:1649–54.

62. Heise C, Sampson-Johannes A, Williams A, McCormick F, Von Hoff DD, Kirn DH. ONYX-015, an E1B gene-attenuated adenovirus, causes tumor-specific cytolysis and antitumoral efficacy that can be augmented by standard chemotherapeutic agents. Nat Med 1997; 3(6):639–45.

63. Singal R, Ginder GD. DNA methylation. Blood 1999; 93(12):4059–70.

64. Tasaka T, Asou H, Munker R, et al. Methylation of the p16INK4A gene in multiple myeloma. Br J Haematol 1998; 101:558–64.

65. Herman JG, Graff JR, Myöhänen S, et al. Methylation-specific PCR: a novel PCR assay for methylation status of CpG islands. Proc Natl Acad Sci USA 1996; 93:9821–6.

66. Loeb LA. Microsatellite instability: marker of a mutator phenotype in cancer. Cancer Res 1994; 54:5059–63.

67. Fishel R, Lescoe MK, Roa MRS, et al. The human mutator gene homolog MSH2 and its association with hereditary nonpolyposis colon cancer. Cell 1993; 75:1027–38.

68. Steenman MJ, Rainier S, Dobry CJ, Grundy P, Horon IL, Feinberg AP. Loss of imprinting of IGF2 is linked to reduced expression and abnormal methylation of H19 in Wilms' tumour. Nat Genet 1994;7(3):433–9.

69. Uyeno S, Aoki Y, Nata M, et al. IGF2 but not H19 shows loss of imprinting in human glioma. Cancer Res 1996; 56(23):5356–9.

70. Wu MS, Wang HP, Lin CC, et al. Loss of imprinting and overexpression of IGF2 gene in gastric adenocarcinoma. Cancer Lett 1997; 120(1):9–14.

71. Cui H, Horon IL, Ohlsson R, Hamilton SR, Feinberg AP. Loss of imprinting in normal tissue of colorectal cancer patients with microsatellite instability. Nat Med 1998; 4(11):1276–80.

72. Oda H, Kume H, Shimizu Y, Inoue T, Ishikawa T. Loss of imprinting of IGF2 in renal-cell carcinomas. Int J Cancer 1998; 75(3):343–6.

73. el-Naggar AK, Lai S, Tucker SA, et al. Frequent loss of imprinting at the IGF2 and H19 genes in head and neck squamous carcinoma. Oncogene 1999; 18(50):7063–9.

74. Pedersen IS, Dervan PA, Broderick D, et al. Frequent loss of imprinting of PEG1/MEST in invasive breast cancer. Cancer Res 1999; 59(21):5449–51.

75. Chen CL, Ip SM, Cheng D, Wong LC, Ngan HY. Loss of imprinting of the IGF-II and H19 genes in epithelial ovarian cancer. Clin Cancer Res 2000; 6(2):474–9.

76. Wu HK, Weksberg R, Minden MD, Squire JA. Loss of imprinting of human insulin-like growth factor II gene, IGF2, in acute myeloid leukemia. Biochem Biophys Res Commun 1997; 231(2):466–72.

77. Randhawa GS, Cui H, Barletta JA, et al. Loss of imprinting in disease progression in chronic myelogenous leukemia. Blood 1998; 91(9):3144–7.

Editors' selected abstracts

Markers of DNA repair and susceptibility to cancer in humans: an epidemiologic review.

Berwick M, Vineis P.

Department of Epidemiology and Biostatistics, Memorial Sloan-Kettering Cancer Center, New York, NY, USA.

Journal of the National Cancer Institute 92(11):874–97, 2000, June 7.

DNA repair is a system of defenses designed to protect the integrity of the genome. Deficiencies in this system probably lead to the development of cancer. The epidemiology of DNA repair capacity and of its effect on cancer susceptibility in humans is, therefore, an important area of investigation. We have summarized all of the published epidemiologic studies on DNA repair in human cancer through 1998 ($n = 64$) that addressed the association of cancer susceptibility with a putative defect in DNA repair capacity. We have considered study design, subject characteristics, potential biases, confounding variables, and sources of technical variability. Assays of DNA repair capacity used, to date, can be broadly grouped into five categories: (1) tests based on DNA damage induced with chemicals or physical agents, such as the mutagen sensitivity assay, the G(2)-radiation assay, induced micronuclei, and the Comet assay; (2) indirect tests of DNA repair, such as unscheduled DNA synthesis; (3) tests based on more direct measures of repair kinetics, such as the host cell reactivation assay; (4) measures of genetic variation associated with DNA repair; and (5) combinations of more than one category of assay. The use of such tests in human populations yielded positive and consistent associations between DNA repair capacity and cancer occurrence (with odds ratios in the range of 1.4–75.3, with the majority of values between 2 and 10). However, the studies that we have reviewed have limitations, including small sample size, 'convenience' controls, the use of cells different from the target organ, and the use of mutagens that do not occur in the natural environment. The evolving ability to study polymorphisms in DNA repair genes may contribute to new understandings about the mechanisms of DNA repair and the way in which DNA repair capacity affects the development of cancer.

Microsatellite instability in colorectal-cancer patients with suspected genetic predisposition.

Calistri D, Presciuttini S, Buonsanti G, Radice P, Gazzoli I, Pensotti V, Sala P, Eboli M, Andreola S, Russo A, Pierotti M, Bertario L, Ranzani GN.

Dipartimento di Genetica e Microbiologia, University of Pavia, Italy.

International Journal of Cancer 89(1):87–91, 2000, January 20.

Hereditary non-polyposis colorectal cancer (HNPCC) is a dominantly inherited syndrome linked to DNA-mismatch-repair (MMR) gene defects, which also account for microsatellite instability (MSI) in tumour tissues. Diagnosis is based mainly on family history, according to widely accepted criteria (Amsterdam Criteria: AC). The aim of this work was to assess MSI in colorectal-cancer patients with suspected genetic predisposition, and to verify whether MSI represents a tool to manage MMR gene (hMSH2 and hMLH1) mutation analysis. We investigated 13 microsatellites (including the 5 NCI/ICG-HNPCC markers) in 45 patients with suspected hereditary predisposition (including 16 subjects from HNPCC families fulfilling the AC). We found MSI-H (high frequency of instability, i.e., in ≥ 30% of the markers) in 85% of the HNPCC patients and in 16% of the non-HNPCC subjects. The 5 NCI/ICG-HNPCC microsatellites proved to be the most effective in detecting MSI, being mononucleotide repeats, the most unstable markers. We investigated the association between hMSH2 and hMLH1 gene mutations and MSI. Our results indicate that AC are highly predictive both of tumour instability and of MMR-gene mutations. Therefore, as the most likely mutation carriers, HNPCC subjects might be directly analyzed for gene mutations, while to test for MSI in selected non-HNPCC patients and to further investigate MMR genes in MSI-H cases, appears to be a cost-effective way to identify subjects, other than those from kindred fulfilling AC, who might benefit from genetic testing.

p53 gene mutation, microsatellite instability and adjuvant chemotherapy: impact on survival of 388 patients with Dukes' C colon carcinoma.

Elsaleh H, Powell B, Soontrapornchai P, Joseph D, Goria F, Spry N, Iacopetta B.

Department of Surgery, University of Western Australia, Nedlands, Australia.

Oncology 58(1):52–9, 2000.

Two common genetic alterations in colon carcinoma, p53 mutation and microsatellite instability (MSI), were investigated to determine their prognostic importance for cancer-specific survival and response to adjuvant chemotherapy in patients with Dukes' C colon cancer. The p53 tumour suppressor gene encodes for a nuclear phosphoprotein involved in cellular response to DNA damage, while MSI is a characteristic feature of tumours with defective DNA mismatch repair. The cellular response mechanisms to DNA-damaging agents in tumours with mutant p53 or MSI may as a consequence differ, and this might translate into different outcomes following adjuvant chemotherapy. A consecutive series of 388 Dukes' C colon carcinomas with 5-year median follow-up was analysed for p53 mutation and for MSI (in proximal/transverse carcinomas only) using polymerase chain reaction single-strand conformation polymorphism. The incidence of p53 mutation was 28% in all carcinomas while that of MSI in proximal/transverse carcinomas was 19%. One hundred and thirty-three patients (34%) received adjuvant chemotherapy (5-fluorouracil/levamisole) with curative intent. The presence of p53 mutation did not predict for survival in either the treated or untreated groups. The presence of MSI in the proximal/transverse colon carcinoma group was associated with significantly better 5-year survival: 58 versus 32% ($p = 0.015$, log rank test). This was largely due to better survival observed in the MSI subgroup that received adjuvant chemotherapy ($p = 0.017$, log rank test). Further work in prospective, randomised clinical trials investigating the effects of adjuvant therapy should consider incorporating MSI status in order to determine whether this is an independent predictive factor for survival and/or response to adjuvant chemotherapy.

Angiogenesis and cancer metastasis.

Fidler IJ.

Department of Cancer Biology, The University of Texas, M.D. Anderson Cancer Center, Houston, TX, USA.

Cancer Journal from Scientific American 6(Suppl. 2): S134–41, 2000, April.

The growth and spread of neoplasms depend on the establishment of an adequate blood supply, that is, angiogenesis. The onset of angiogenesis involves a change in the local equilibrium between proangiogenic and antiangiogenic regulators that are produced by tumor cells, surrounding stromal cells, and infiltrating leukocytes. In most normal tissues, factors that inhibit angiogenesis predominate, whereas in rapidly dividing tissues, the balance of angiogenic molecules favors stimulation of the process. A potent inhibitor of angiogenesis is interferon-alpha or -beta, shown to down-regulate transcription and protein production of basic fibroblast growth factor, collagenase type IV, and interleukin-8. The daily systemic administration of low (but not high) dose of interferon-alpha can produce significant inhibition of angiogenesis and, hence, regression of human tumors implanted orthotopically in nude mice. The recent elucidation of the interaction among proangiogenic molecules during physiological processes and the apparent disruption of this balance in neoplasia should allow the design of potent antiangiogenic therapies against primary cancers and metastases.

Chromosomal breakage-fusion-bridge events cause genetic intratumor heterogeneity.

Gisselsson D, Pettersson L, Hoglund M, Heidenblad M, Gorunova L, Wiegant J, Mertens F, Dal Cin P, Mitelman F, Mandahl N.

Department of Clinical Genetics, University Hospital, SE-221 85 Lund, Sweden.

Proceedings of the National Academy of Sciences of the United States of America 97(10):5357–62, 2000, May 9.

It has long been known that rearrangements of chromosomes through breakage-fusion-bridge (BFB) cycles may cause variability of phenotypic and genetic traits within a cell population. Because intercellular heterogeneity is often found in neoplastic tissues, we investigated the occurrence of BFB events in human solid tumors. Evidence of frequent BFB events was found in malignancies that showed unspecific chromosome aberrations, including ring chromosomes, dicentric chromosomes, and telomeric associations, as well as extensive intratumor heterogeneity in the pattern of structural changes but not in tumors with tumor-specific aberrations and low variability. Fluorescence in situ hybridization analysis demonstrated that chromosomes participating in anaphase bridge formation were involved in a significantly higher number of structural

aberrations than other chromosomes. Tumors with BFB events showed a decreased elimination rate of unstable chromosome aberrations after irradiation compared with normal cells and other tumor cells. This result suggests that a combination of mitotically unstable chromosomes and an elevated tolerance to chromosomal damage leads to constant genomic reorganization in many malignancies, thereby providing a flexible genetic system for clonal evolution and progression.

Angiogenesis: potentials for pharmacologic intervention in the treatment of cancer, cardiovascular diseases, and chronic inflammation.

Griffioen AW, Molema G.

Tumor Angiogenesis Laboratory, Department of Internal Medicine, University Hospital Maastricht, Maastricht, The Netherlands.

Pharmacological Reviews 52(2):237–68, 2000, June.

Angiogenesis, or the formation of new blood vessels out of pre-existing capillaries, is a sequence of events that is fundamental to many physiologic and pathologic processes such as cancer, ischemic diseases, and chronic inflammation. With the identification of several proangiogenic molecules such as the vascular endothelial cell growth factor, the fibroblast growth factors, and the angiopoietins, and the recent description of specific inhibitors of angiogenesis such as platelet factor-4, angiostatin, endostatin, and vasostatin, it is recognized that therapeutic interference with vasculature formation offers a tool for clinical applications in various pathologies. Whereas inhibition of angiogenesis can prevent diseases with excessive vessel growth such as cancer, diabetes retinopathy, and arthritis, stimulation of angiogenesis would be beneficial in the treatment of diseases such as coronary artery disease and critical limb ischemia in diabetes. In this review we highlight the current knowledge on angiogenesis regulation and report on the recent findings in angiogenesis research and clinical studies. We also discuss the potentials, limitations, and challenges within this field of research, in light of the development of new therapeutic strategies for diseases in which angiogenesis plays an important role.

DNA microsatellite instability and mismatch repair protein loss in adenomas presenting in hereditary non-polyposis colorectal cancer.

Iino H, Simms L, Young J, Arnold J, Winship IM, Webb SI, Furlong KL, Leggett B, Jass JR.

First Department of Surgery, Yamanashi Medical University, Yamanashi, Japan.

Gut 47(1):37–42, 2000, July.

Background and aim: Hereditary non-polyposis colorectal cancer (HNPCC), as its name implies, is associated with few adenomas, and the early evolution of colorectal neoplasia is poorly understood. In this study our aim was to clarify the genetic profiles of benign polyps in subjects with HNPCC using a combined molecular and immunohistochemical approach. *Methods:* Thirty adenomas and 17 hyperplastic polyps were obtained from 24 affected HNPCC subjects. DNA was extracted from paraffin embedded tissue by microdissection and analysed for the presence of microsatellite instability (MSI) and mutations in five genes known to be targets in mismatch repair deficiency (TGFbetaRII, IGF2R, BAX, hMSH3, and hMSH6). Serial sections were stained by immunohistochemistry for hMLH1 and hMSH2. *Results:* Twenty four (80%) of 30 adenomas showed MSI. Of MSI positive adenomas, 66.7% showed MSI at more than 40% of markers – high level of MSI (MSI-H). Two of 17 hyperplastic polyps revealed MSI at one marker – low level of MSI (MSI-L). A significant association was found between MSI-H and high grade dysplasia in adenomas ($p = 0.004$). Eight of nine adenomas with mutations of coding sequences revealed high grade dysplasia and all nine were MSI-H. Four of the nine ranged in size from 2 to 5 mm. The presence of the hMSH6 mutation was significantly correlated with high levels of MSI (80% of markers) ($p < 0.02$). Twenty four adenomas gave evaluable results with immunohistochemistry. One of six (17%) microsatellite stable, six of seven (86%) MSI-L, and 11 of 11 (100%) MSI-H adenomas showed loss of either hMLH1 or hMSH2. *Conclusions:* Most adenomas in subjects with a definite diagnosis of HNPCC show MSI (80%). The finding of MSI-L is usually associated with loss of expression of hMLH1 or hMSH2, unlike the situation in MSI-L sporadic colorectal cancer. The transition from MSI-L to MSI-H correlated with the finding of high grade dysplasia and mutation of coding sequences and may be driven by mutation of secondary mutators such as hMSH3 and hMSH6. Advanced genetic changes may be present in adenomas of minute size.

Sequence of molecular genetic events in colorectal tumorigenesis.

Laurent-Puig P, Blons H, Cugnenc PH.

Laboratoire de Toxicologie Moleculaire, INSERM U490, Paris, France.

European Journal of Cancer Prevention 8(Suppl. 1): S39–47, 1999, December.

Intensive screening for genetic alteration in colorectal cancer led to the identification of two types of colorectal tumours that are distinct by their carcinogenesis processes. The first group, named LOH (for loss of heterozygosity) positive, is characterized by hyperploidy and allelic losses involving preferentially chromosome 18q and chromosome 17p. More than two-thirds of colorectal cancers belong to this group. The second group, called multiple microsatellite loci (MSI)-positive cancers, is characterized by genetic instability at microsatellite loci. Although colorectal cancer cells are characterized by specific microsatellite alterations, the same four different signalling pathways, WNT/Wingless pathway, K-ras pathway, transforming growth factor (TGF) beta pathway and p53 pathway, could be implicated in tumour progression. The WNT/Wingless pathway could be altered in two different ways according to whether the cancer cells belong to the group of LOH-positive or MSI-positive tumours. LOH-positive tumours activate the WNT/Wingless signalling pathway through an adenomatous polyposis coli (APC) mutation, whereas the MSI-positive tumours activate this pathway through a beta-catenin stabilizing mutation. Beta-catenin and APC mutations were observed as early as

the adenomatous stage of colorectal neoplasia. In TGFbeta pathways LOH-positive tumours inactivated SMAD2 (similar to mother against decapentaplegic drosophilia) or SMAD4, whereas in MSI-positive tumours the TGFbeta type II receptor is frequently deleted. Alteration of these genes correlated closely with the progression of the adenoma to cancer. In the p53 pathway LOH-positive tumours showed frequent p53 mutation, whereas MSI-positive tumours demonstrated BAX (BCL-2-associated X protein)-inactivating mutation. These alterations contribute to the adenoma–carcinoma transition.

Aneuploidy vs. gene mutation hypothesis of cancer: recent study claims mutation but is found to support aneuploidy.

Li R, Sonik A, Stindl R, Rasnick D, Duesberg P.

Department of Molecular and Cell Biology, Stanley Hall, University of California, Berkeley, CA, USA.

Proceedings of the National Academy of Sciences of the United States of America 97(7):3236–41, 2000, March 28.

For nearly a century, cancer has been blamed on somatic mutation. But it is still unclear whether this mutation is aneuploidy, an abnormal balance of chromosomes, or gene mutation. Despite enormous efforts, the currently popular gene mutation hypothesis has failed to identify cancer-specific mutations with transforming function and cannot explain why cancer occurs only many months to decades after mutation by carcinogens and why solid cancers are aneuploid, although conventional mutation does not depend on karyotype alteration. A recent high-profile publication now claims to have solved these discrepancies with a set of three synthetic mutant genes that 'suffices to convert normal human cells into tumorigenic cells.' However, we show here that even this study failed to explain why it took more than '60 population doublings' from the introduction of the first of these genes, a derivative of the tumor antigen of simian virus 40 tumor virus, to generate tumor cells, why the tumor cells were clonal although gene transfer was polyclonal, and above all, why the tumor cells were aneuploid. If aneuploidy is assumed to be the somatic mutation that causes cancer, all these results can be explained. The aneuploidy hypothesis predicts the long latent periods and the clonality on the basis of the following two-stage mechanism: stage one, a carcinogen (or mutant gene) generates aneuploidy; stage two, aneuploidy destabilizes the karyotype and thus initiates an autocatalytic karyotype evolution generating preneoplastic and eventually neoplastic karyotypes. Because the odds are very low that an abnormal karyotype will surpass the viability of a normal diploid cell, the evolution of a neoplastic cell species is slow and thus clonal, which is comparable to conventional evolution of new species.

Environmental and heritable factors in the causation of cancer – analyses of cohorts of twins from Sweden, Denmark, and Finland.

Lichtenstein P, Holm NV, Verkasalo PK, Iliadou A, Kaprio J, Koskenvuo M, Pukkala E, Skytthe A, Hemminki K.

Department of Medical Epidemiology, Karolinska Institute, Stockholm, Sweden.

New England Journal of Medicine 343(2):78–85, 2000, July 13.

Background: The contribution of hereditary factors to the causation of sporadic cancer is unclear. Studies of twins make it possible to estimate the overall contribution of inherited genes to the development of malignant diseases. *Methods:* We combined data on 44 788 pairs of twins listed in the Swedish, Danish, and Finnish twin registries in order to assess the risks of cancer at 28 anatomical sites for the twins of persons with cancer. Statistical modeling was used to estimate the relative importance of heritable and environmental factors in causing cancer at 11 of those sites. *Results:* At least one cancer occurred in 10 803 persons among 9512 pairs of twins. An increased risk was found among the twins of affected persons for stomach, colorectal, lung, breast, and prostate cancer. Statistically significant effects of heritable factors were observed for prostate cancer (42 percent; 95 percent confidence interval, 29 to 50 percent), colorectal cancer (35 percent; 95 percent confidence interval, 10 to 48 percent), and breast cancer (27 percent; 95 percent confidence interval, 4 to 41 percent). *Conclusions:* Inherited genetic factors make a minor contribution to susceptibility to most types of neoplasms. This finding indicates that the environment has the principal role in causing sporadic cancer. The relatively large effect of heritability in cancer at a few sites suggests major gaps in our knowledge of the genetics of cancer.

The causes of cancer: implications for prevention and treatment.

Madhukar BV, Trosko JE.

Department of Pediatrics and Human Development, College of Human Medicine, Michigan State University, East Lansing, MI, USA.

Indian Journal of Pediatrics 64(2):131–41, 1997, March–April.

The final clinical manifestation of cancer is a result of complex series of changes in a single cell. This review summarizes some of the new concepts and hypotheses that explain the evolution of cancers. The emphasis is on cancer as a disease of the stem cells within a tissue that undergo initiation as a result of mutational insult to one or more genes that are critical for cell growth. During the second stage (promotion stage) the initiated cells acquire proliferative capacity due to epigenetic changes, i.e., altered expression of genes whose products play a central role in signal transduction. This requires continued exposure to agents and events causing such changes. This stage is, therefore, reversible and the various components of this stage are central targets for the development of mechanism based anti-cancer drugs. During the stage of progression, the neoplastic lesions acquire additional genetic alterations and become clinically manifestable malignant neoplasms. At the biochemical and molecular level, neoplastic transformation involves aberrations in the expression and regulation of oncogenes, tumor suppression genes, transcription factors and components of the cell signal transduction cascades. The understanding of the various cellular biochemical and molecular events that metamorphose a normal cell

into a cancer cell is central to the development of rational new drugs that are targeted against the various components. Such drugs in combination with the conventional chemotherapeutic agents that are currently used, provide a more effective control of cancer without the risk of toxic side effects.

Role of telomerase in normal and cancer cells.

Meyerson M.

Department of Adult Oncology, Dana-Farber Cancer Institute, Boston, MA, USA.

Journal of Clinical Oncology 18(13):2626–34, 2000, July.

Shortening of the telomeric DNA at chromosome ends is postulated to limit the lifespan of human cells. In contrast, activation of telomerase, the enzyme that synthesizes telomeric DNA, is proposed to be an essential step in cancer cell immortalization and cancer progression. This review discusses the structure and function of telomeres and telomerase, the role of telomerase in cell immortalization, and the effects of telomerase inactivation on normal and cancer cells. Moreover, data on the experimental use of telomerase assays for cancer detection and diagnosis are reviewed. Finally, the review considers the evidence regarding whether telomerase inhibitors could be used to treat human cancers.

Molecular biology of pancreatic cancer; oncogenes, tumour suppressor genes, growth factors, and their receptors from a clinical perspective.

Sakorafas GH, Tsiotou AG, Tsiotos GG.

Department of Surgery, 251 Hellenic Air Force (HAF) Hospital, Messogion and Katehaki, Athens, Greece.

Cancer Treatment Reviews 26(1):29–52, 2000, February.

Pancreatic cancer represents the fourth leading cause of cancer death in men and the fifth in women. Prognosis remains dismal, mainly because the diagnosis is made late in the clinical course of the disease. The need to improve the diagnosis, detection, and treatment of pancreatic cancer is great. It is in this type of cancer, in which the mortality is so great and the clinical detection so difficult that the recent advances of molecular biology may have a significant impact. Genetic alterations can be detected at different levels. These alterations include oncogene mutations (most commonly, K-ras mutations, which occur in 75% to more than 95% of pancreatic cancer tissues), tumour suppressor gene alterations (mainly, p53, p16, DCC, etc.), over-expression of growth factors (such as EGF, TGF alpha, TGF beta 1–3, aFGF, bTGF, etc.) and their receptors (i.e., EGF receptor, TGF beta receptor I–III, etc.). Insights into the molecular genetics of pancreatic carcinogenesis are beginning to form a genetic model for pancreatic cancer and its precursors. These improvements in our understanding of the molecular biology of pancreatic cancer are not simply of research interest, but may have clinical implications, such as risk assessment, early diagnosis, treatment, and prognosis evaluation. [References: 315.]

Molecular approach in human tumor investigation: oncogenes, tumor suppressor genes and DNA tumor polyomaviruses.

Scarpa A, Tognon M.

Institute of Anatomical Pathology, School of Medicine, University of Verona, Verona, Italy.

International Journal of Molecular Medicine 1(6):1011–23, 1998, June.

Molecular analyses are useful for diagnosis, prognosis and follow-up of the patients, as well as for addressing therapeutic choices. Most of the molecular methods are based on the analysis of nucleic acids. The DNA and RNA methodologies of routine applicability include Southern and Northern hybridizations and polymerase chain reaction (PCR) techniques. Southern blot hybridization recognizes major DNA rearrangements, and detection of oncogenic viral sequences present in high copy number, whereas PCR-based methods allow the detection of gross chromosomal modifications, fine gene alterations and low amount of tumor virus footprints. PCR techniques also allow the analysis of the partially degraded nucleic acids from formalin-fixed paraffin-embedded tissues. We present an overview of the use of molecular techniques for the analysis, diagnosis, prognosis and follow-up of neoplastic diseases, using examples from our experience in both leukemias and solid tumors.

Targeting vascular endothelial growth factor (VEGF) for anti-tumor therapy, by anti-VEGF neutralizing monoclonal antibodies or by VEGF receptor tyrosine-kinase inhibitors.

Schlaeppi JM, Wood JM.

Core Technology, Novartis Pharmaceuticals, Novartis Limited, Basle, Switzerland.

Cancer and Metastasis Reviews 18(4):473–81, 1999.

Vascular endothelial growth factor/vascular permeability factor (VEGF/VPF) is an important mediator of tumor-induced angiogenesis and represents a potential target for innovative anticancer therapy. In several animal models, neutralizing anti-VEGF/VPF antibodies have shown encouraging inhibitory effects on solid tumor growth, ascites formation and metastatic dissemination. Targeting the VEGF signaling pathway by means of VEGF receptor tyrosine-kinase inhibitors has shown similar efficacy in animal tumor models. Several of these anti-VEGF therapies are currently being tested in clinical trials in cancer patients. The profiles and effects of the neutralizing anti-VEGF/VPF antibodies and the VEGF receptor tyrosine-kinase inhibitors in animal models are reviewed and the risks and benefits of VEGF blockade by one or the other treatments are discussed.

COX-2 is expressed in human pulmonary, colonic, and mammary tumors.

Soslow RA, Dannenberg AJ, Rush D, Woerner BM, Khan KN, Masferrer J, Koki AT.

Department of Pathology, New York Presbyterian Hospital–Weill Medical College of Cornell University, New York, NY, USA.

Cancer 89(12):2637–45, 2000, December 15.

Background: The cyclooxygenase (COX) enzyme catalyzes the formation of prostaglandins, which can affect cell proliferation and alter the response of the immune system to malignant cells. The inducible form of COX, COX-2, has been shown to be important in carcinogenesis. *Methods:* The authors studied COX-1 and -2 expression in 20 tumors of the lung, colon, and breast (60 total) by using commercially available monoclonal and polyclonal antibodies on formalin fixed, paraffin embedded tissue. Our evaluation also included seven carcinoma-associated colonic adenomas and 10 mammary ductal carcinomas in situ (DCIS). Quantitation of immunoreactivity was accomplished using an immunohistochemical scoring system that approximates the use of image analysis-based systems. *Results:* Ninety percent of lung tumors (squamous cell carcinomas and adenocarcinomas), 71% of colon adenocarcinomas and 56% of breast tumors (DCIS and infiltrating ductal and lobular carcinomas) expressed COX-2 at a moderate to strong level, which was significantly different from the negligible expression in distant nonneoplastic epithelium (controls; $p < 0.0001$). Poorly differentiated histologic features were correlated with low COX-2 expression overall, especially in colon carcinomas. Among breast carcinomas, DCIS was more likely to express COX-2 than invasive carcinomas. Adenomatous colonic epithelium showed moderate COX-2 expression, as did adjacent nonneoplastic epithelium. COX-1 immunoreactivity was essentially weak to moderate in all tissues evaluated. *Conclusions:* COX-2 expression is upregulated in well and moderately differentiated carcinomas of the lung, colon, and breast whereas COX-1 appears to be constitutively expressed at low levels. A possible COX-2 paracrine effect is suggested by moderate immunoreactivity in adjacent nonneoplastic epithelium.

The p53 tumor suppressor gene: from molecular biology to clinical investigation.

Soussi T.

Institut Curie, Laboratoire de Genotoxicologie des Tumeurs, Paris, France.

Annals of the New York Academy of Sciences 910:121–37; discussion 137–9, 2000, June.

The tumor suppressor p53 is a phosphoprotein barely detectable in the nucleus of normal cells. Upon cellular stress, particularly that induced by DNA damage, p53 can arrest cell cycle progression, thus allowing the DNA to be repaired; or it can lead to apoptosis. These functions are achieved, in part, by the transactivational properties of p53, which activate a series of genes involved in cell cycle regulation. In cancer cells bearing a mutant p53, this protein is no longer able to control cell proliferation, resulting in inefficient DNA repair and the emergence of genetically unstable cells. The most common changes of p53 in human cancers are point missense mutations within the coding sequences of the gene. Such mutations are found in all major histogenetic groups, including cancers of the colon (60%), stomach (60%), breast (20%), lung (70%), brain (40%), and esophagus (60%). It is estimated that p53 mutations are the most frequent genetic event in human cancers, accounting for more than 50% of cases. One of the most striking features of the inactive mutant p53 protein is its increased stability (half-life of several hours, compared to 20 min for wild-type p53) and its accumulation in the nucleus of neoplastic cells. Therefore, positive immunostaining is indicative of abnormalities of the p53 gene and its product. Several studies have shown that p53 mutations are associated with short survival in colorectal cancer, but the use of p53 as a tumoral marker is still a matter of debate.

Role of telomerase in cell senescence and oncogenesis.

Urquidi V, Tarin D, Goodison S.

Cancer Center, University of California, San Diego School of Medicine, La Jolla, CA, USA.

Annual Review of Medicine 51:65–79, 2000.

The ends of linear chromosomes are capped by specialized nucleoprotein structures termed telomeres. Telomeres comprise tracts of noncoding hexanucleotide repeat sequences that, in combination with specific proteins, protect against degradation, rearrangement, and chromosomal fusion events. Due to the polarity of conventional DNA synthesis, a net loss of telomeric sequences occurs at each cell division. It has been proposed that this cumulative telomeric erosion is a limiting factor in replicative capacity and elicits a signal for the onset of cellular senescence. To proliferate beyond the senescent checkpoint, cells must restore telomere length. This can be achieved by telomerase, an enzyme with reverse-transcriptase activity. This enzyme is absent in differentiated somatic tissues, but telomerase reactivation has been detected in most tumors. Much investigative effort is focusing on telomere dynamics with a view to possible manipulation of cellular proliferative potential. In this article, we review the role of telomeres and telomerase in senescence and tumor progression, and we discuss the potential use of telomerase in diagnosis and treatment.

2

Bone marrow transplantation in the management of solid tumors

DAN DOUER

INTRODUCTION

The delivery of systemic anticancer therapy is limited by dose-related toxicity to the function of the bone marrow to produce blood cells. Dose intensification of most chemotherapy drugs or whole-body irradiation will gradually lead to a more profound and prolonged neutropenia and thrombocytopenia with more serious infections and bleeding complications. Eventually, high doses of a single cycle of most anticancer drugs or radiation of sufficient intensity would lead to irreversible bone marrow failure. However, because many types of cancer cannot be cured by standard doses of chemotherapy, attempts are made to intensify chemotherapy or radiation approaches by providing measures that rescue the hematopoietic system. The underlying concept of this approach is that marrow-ablative doses of chemotherapy and/or radiation that may otherwise be lethal can be administered safely provided that hematopoietic precursor cells are subsequently transplanted into the patient. Hematopoietic precursors are responsible for restoring blood-cell production, and they can be collected from the bone marrow, from the peripheral blood, or from cord blood. They can be obtained from a histocompatible donor, usually a human leukocyte antigen (HLA)-identical sibling or an HLA-matched, unrelated donor. This approach is termed bone marrow or blood stem allogeneic transplantation. Its applicability is limited by the need for a suitable donor and the problems of graft rejection and graft versus host disease. An alternative is to use the patient's own hematopoietic precursors, obtained from the bone marrow or from the peripheral blood prior to administration of high-dose therapy. This is referred to as autologous bone marrow or peripheral blood progenitor cell transplantation or autotransplantation. This chapter discusses the biology and the technique of bone marrow and peripheral blood autotransplantation and reviews the results of this approach in patients with solid tumors.

DOSE INTENSITY

Data from experimental animal tumors indicate that higher doses of anticancer drugs could have correspondingly greater antitumor effects.[1–3] In several human tumors, an improved response was observed with more intensive treatment[4–6] within a drug dose range that produces minimal marrow toxicity. A dose–response effect was also shown in randomized studies with certain solid tumors, including breast,[7] testicular,[8] and ovarian[9] cancers, as well as with acute leukemia.[10] In these studies, the drug dose in the higher dose arm produced a better outcome. Transplantation of hematopoietic precursor allows further dose escalation of chemotherapy agents and total-body radiation, regardless of bone marrow toxicity. The dose intensification cannot be increased indefinitely because unacceptable non-hematological toxicities would eventually develop, and therefore transplantation of hematopoietic precursors provides a 'window' of high doses that can be tested in clinical trials. This strategy has been shown to be successful, for example, in patients with intermediate or high-grade lymphoma who relapse after initial chemotherapy, and are incurable with the use of further conventional salvage chemotherapy regimens. However, if still responsive at the time of salvage treatment, the use of high-dose therapy and autotransplantation can result in 40–50% long-term disease-free survival.[11–13]

HEMATOPOIETIC PRECURSOR CELLS

Hematopoietic precursors are the cells responsible for bone marrow repopulation after marrow or peripheral blood transplantation. The most primitive hematopoietic precursor cells are termed pluripotent stem cells, which are bone marrow cells with the capacity for both self-renewal and differentiation that will ultimately develop into functional multilineage blood cells. These stem cells produce progenitor cells that are slightly more mature and have minimal self-renewal capability but proliferate and differentiate along several cell lineages or are committed to a specific cell lineage. The concentration of stem cells and progenitor cells in the bone marrow is very low and these cells cannot be identified morphologically. The stem cells can be assayed in lethally irradiated mice in terms of their ability for long-term hematopoietic reconstitution, but in humans the true self-renewing pluripotent hematopoietic stem cell cannot be measured reliably. The hematopoietic progenitors can be assayed by a semisolid culture that estimates the concentration of committed granulocyte–macrophage progenitors by counting the number of colonies they form. The progenitor cells measured are thus called colony-forming units (CFUs). This assay is not well standardized, is time consuming, and the results vary between centers depending on the culture conditions. A second assay for progenitor cells uses monoclonal antibodies against the CD34 antigen. Cells expressing surface CD34 include almost all of the committed and pluripotent progenitors, as well as very primitive B and T lymphocyte precursors. One percent to 4% of the normal human bone marrow and a very small fraction of the peripheral blood cells are CD34+ cells. Flow-cytometric measurement of CD34+ cells in harvested bone marrow or peripheral blood is the most frequently used method for assessing the quality of the transplanted cells (see below). A more immature subpopulation of CD34+ cells has been identified as those expressing the thy-1 antigen but not CD38, HLA-DR, or any of the linear-specific antigens; the true pluripotent stem cell fraction probably resides within this subpopulation.

To a certain degree, the dose of chemotherapy can be intensified using hematopoietic growth factors, without transplantation of hematopoietic precursors. Granulocyte colony stimulating factor (G-CSF) or granulocyte–monocyte colony stimulating factor (GM-CSF) given as a daily subcutaneous injection after intensified treatment can shorten the duration and degree of neutropenia, and the recently discovered thrombopoietin molecule may also reduce the problems of thrombocytopenia. However, these drugs require the presence of hematopoietic progenitor cells as targets for their activity and, therefore, the dose of chemotherapy can only be increased by twofold to threefold. More intense treatment, causing irreversible damage to the hematopoietic precursor cell, will require a source of hematopoietic cells for transplantation.

Autologous bone marrow cells

Hematopoietic precursor cells can be collected without loss of functional integrity to the bone marrow and then cryopreserved, thawed, and re-infused. Autologous bone marrow cells are collected under general or epidural anesthesia by multiple needle aspirations from both posterior iliac crest bones in sterile conditions in the operating room. This approach requires a single collection of approximately 1–1.5 L of bone marrow, with an approximate loss of 2 units of red blood cells. Complications from the procedure such as local infections and bleeding are extremely rare and the local pain usually lasts for 2–3 days.

Autologous peripheral blood progenitor cells

Under normal circumstances, hematopoietic precursor cells are resident within the bone marrow and will home to the marrow if infused intravenously. The bone marrow has therefore served as the major source for autologous stem cells for transplantation in patients with cancer. However, in-vitro assays have demonstrated that pluripotent and committed progenitor cells circulate in the peripheral blood. Parabiotic experiments in mice, dogs, and baboons, in which the blood circulation of a lethally irradiated animal was joined with the circulation of a non-irradiated animal, have shown the restoration of hematopoietic function in the irradiated animals.[14–16] Peripheral blood cells collected by leukapheresis restore hematopoietic function when re-infused after lethal doses of chemotherapy or total-body irradiation in animals[16] and humans.[17–19] Over the past decade, transplantation of peripheral blood progenitor cells (PBPCs) has emerged as the most common method for autologous hematopoietic rescue after high-dose chemotherapy.[20,21]

There are a number of advantages in using autologous PBPCs as opposed to bone marrow:

1 PBPCs can be collected without the need for general anesthesia or the discomfort associated with multiple bone marrow aspirations from the iliac crest.
2 PBPCs can be harvested from patients who have undergone prior radiation to the pelvic area.
3 Bone marrow that appears histologically normal can still be contaminated by occult tumor cells, as demonstrated when sensitive immunological or histochemical methods are used.[22,23]

The potential advantage of progenitor cells collected from the peripheral blood is that they may contain fewer or no occult malignant cells. However, apart from all of these factors, the most significant value of PBPCs appears to be the more rapid recovery of neutrophils and platelets after autologous PBPC autotransplantation compared to bone marrow transplantation.[21] This advantage can be obtained only if the PBPCs are collected after prior exposure of the patient to chemotherapy or hematopoietic growth factors, or both, a process called mobilization.[24–27] Re-infusion of PBPCs mobilized in this way results in a shorter time to engraftment, less need for transfusions, a decrease in the number of days on antibiotics, and a decreased period of hospitalization when compared to patients receiving autologous bone marrow transplantation.[28–33]

However, PBPCs usually require several collections, whereas bone marrow is collected only once. PBPC collections can also be associated with central venous catheter-related infections and thrombotic episodes. In addition, patients with excessive prior exposure to chemotherapy or those with histologically proven cancer in the marrow may not manifest the same progenitor cell expansion following mobilization,[34] and the advantage of rapid recovery may be lost. Further, occult tumor cells can also circulate in the blood. PBPC harvests have been found to contain lymphoma, neuroblastoma, or breast cancer cells when sensitive molecular or immunohistochemical assays were employed.[35–37] Even if the blood did contain a smaller percentage of tumor cells than the bone marrow, the higher number of cells collected by leukapheresis may result in a higher absolute number of tumor cells than might be obtained from a single bone marrow harvest.

Allogeneic transplantation

Transplantation of hematopoietic stem cells from a suitable HLA-matched related or unrelated donor is not done in solid tumors except in rare experimental cases, but is mostly used in acute leukemia or chronic myelogenous leukemia. This procedure is also associated with more complications than autologous transplantation and a higher mortality rate due to graft versus host disease and infections.

In recent years, peripheral blood progenitor cells have also started to be used in allogeneic transplantation. This requires the administration of G-CSF to normal donors to mobilize the progenitor cells and then one or two leukapheresis procedures. This approach was studied carefully, because the blood contains a higher number of T-cells than the bone marrow and there is a potentially higher risk of chronic graft versus host disease.[38]

Umbilical cord blood

The cord blood contains a large concentration of colony forming cells and CD34+ cells, which are usually discarded.

These cells can be collected and frozen and provide an opportunity to create a bank of hematopoietic cells of diverse HLA subtypes intended for allogeneic transplantation to ethnically diverse heterogeneous population.[39]

Biology of hematopoietic reconstitution

Little is known of the biology of autologous marrow graft recovery. Sustained hematopoiesis requires a population of multipotential stem cells that are capable of self-renewal and differentiation to the various cell lineages. More mature progenitor cells, even though capable of proliferation and multipotential differentiation, have a more limited self-renewal capacity. It is unknown whether cryopreserved marrow contains viable true stem cells for long-term engraftment, or whether the autograft only provides temporary replenishment of committed progenitor cells. In this case, endogenous stem cells that have survived the most intense pretransplant conditioning may eventually recover and repopulate the marrow. There have also been some concerns that peripheral blood may not contain the appropriate repopulating stem cells necessary for long-term engraftment. It is also unknown if stem cells circulating in the blood differ from their corresponding bone marrow progenitors. For example, mobilized peripheral blood stem cells may have altered expression of adhesion molecules, with impaired stroma binding that could reduce the repopulating capability.[40] The accelerated blood cell production after the transplantation of mobilized PBPCs probably reflects the presence of a high number of relatively mature and lineage-restricted progenitors, which proliferate and differentiate very early after transplantation. These cells are probably present in sufficient numbers to produce the early release of neutrophils and platelets without necessarily contributing to long-term engraftment. Although long-term recovery has already been demonstrated in patients undergoing PBPC transplantation, this is not necessarily proof of prolonged or sustained engraftment. The early repopulation could later be superseded by permanent hematopoiesis from endogenous stem cells or from stem cells present in the grafted bone marrow if autologous bone marrow transplantation was also performed. Recent clinical gene transfer trials have indicated that bone marrow cells or peripheral blood mobilized PBPCs marked by a retroviral vector can contribute to long-term hematopoietic engraftment of multiple lineages.[41,42]

CELL COLLECTION AND PROCESSING

Cells harvested from the bone marrow are passed in the operating room through 200–500-μ filters to remove small clots and bony particles to yield single-cell suspensions, and are then transferred to the bone marrow transplantation laboratory for processing. Hematopoietic reconstitution of autologous cells from bone marrow can be routinely achieved with bone marrow cells that contain more than 1×10^8 nucleated cells/kg, which includes approximately 1×10^4 CFU-GM/kg or 10^6 CD34+ cells/kg. The number of progenitor cells varies between patients and the minimal requirement in the bone marrow autograft is not accurately established.

PBPCs are collected by leukapheresis with cell separators that are programmed to collect the mononuclear cell population that includes the progenitor cells. Leukapheresis is not done in steady state, but requires a mobilization procedure. It has been known for several years[20,21] that, as blood counts recover to normal after chemotherapy, there is an increase in the circulating myeloid progenitors in the blood. Subsequently, it was shown that injections of hematopoietic growth factors, such as GM-CSF or G-CSF, can also increase the number of circulating progenitor cells. These cytokines also augment the increase of progenitor cells after a cycle of chemotherapy. PBPCs are collected after the progenitor cells are mobilized by pretreating the patient with G-CSF or GM-CSF, with or without a cycle of chemotherapy.

When a cytosine such as G-CSF or GM-CSF is used alone for mobilization, it is given for 4–6 days, followed by several days of leukapheresis. Mobilizing chemotherapy can consist of either a cycle of chemotherapy designed for the particular patient's cancer or a single high dose of cyclophosphamide in a range of 3–6 g/m². G-CSF or GM-CSF is started after chemotherapy is completed, to enhance hematopoietic recovery as well as to increase the yield of circulating progenitor cells, and is continued until all leukapheresis procedures have been completed. The optimal time to begin leukapheresis after chemotherapy/cytosine mobilization is not accurately established, but it is usually done when the white blood cell counts begin to increase above 1000/mm³ because it is felt that at this time there is an outburst of progenitor cells into the circulation. A more accurate, but less commonly used, method is to time the beginning of the leukapheresis procedure to coincide with an increase in CD34+ cells in the circulation.

The number of CD34+ cells in the PBPC collection is considered to be the best predictor of neutrophil and platelet engraftment rate after high-dose therapy. The collections continue until at least 2.5×10^6 CD34+ cells per kg are harvested.[21] Studies in which PBPCs were used alone have shown that, when the infused number of CD34+ cells exceeds 2.5×10^6/kg, nearly all patients have prompt recovery of neutrophils and platelets.[21,24] However, the minimum number of CD34+ cells that is necessary for recovery has not yet been established. Delays in neutrophil and especially platelet recovery are more frequent in patients in whom lower numbers of CD34+ cells are administered.[21] Another factor that predicts success in mobilizing stem cells is the number of previous treatments that the patient has received. Patients without extensive prior treatment are likely to have good yields.[43] There is a negative impact of previous therapy on determining the success of mobilization and the subsequent recovery of the neutrophil and platelet counts following autologous transplantation.[29,44,45]

Cell cryopreservation

Because autologous cells, from the bone marrow or the blood, are collected days to years before they are returned to the recipient, it is necessary to preserve the normal hematopoietic precursor cell function. Marrow cells can be preserved at 4 °C for up to several days without substantial loss of stem cell function. Preservation for longer periods requires freezing and storage at low temperatures. The cells suspended in plasma are mixed with a cellular cryoprotectant, usually dimethylsulfoxide (DMSO), at a final concentration of approximately 5%. The cells are then cooled at a controlled rate of -1 °C to -2 °C per min to approximately -80 °C. Shortly after cooling has begun (at -6 °C to -12 °C), the cells enter a transition phase, during which the fusion heat is released and will cause the temperature to rise and remain elevated for several minutes. This temperature change adversely affects progenitor cell survival. To reduce the length of the transition phase, the sample is temporarily supercooled by programmable, controlled-rate freezing devices. Once the sample is cooled to -80 °C, the cells are transferred to the vapor or liquid phase of liquid nitrogen and stored at -156 °C to -196 °C until transfused to the patient. An alternative method, using a cryoprotectant mixture of DMSO and hydroxyethyl starch, does not require the controlled-rate device because placing samples in a -80 °C temperature will cause a gradual decrease in the temperature at a rate of approximately -3 °C.

It may be preferable to store the cells at lower volumes to reduce the amount of DMSO that the patient will receive, which can be achieved by increasing the concentration of cells in the suspension. Cryopreservation at cell concentrations of approximately 400×10^6 nucleated cells per mL has been shown to have no significant effect on viability, CD34+ cell number, CFU growth, or engraftment.[46] A typical bone marrow collection containing $2-3 \times 10^8$ nucleated cells per kg can be stored in high cell concentrations at a volume of 50 mL. A more recent approach to reduce the volume is to enrich the harvest with CD34+ cells by eliminating those cells that are not responsible for marrow reconstitution, using anti-CD34 antibodies and magnetic beads.[47]

Thawing and re-infusion

The cryopreserved cells are thawed at the bedside and infused intravenously, through the central venous catheter, 24–72 h after completion of chemotherapy or radiation. Precise timing depends on the clearance rates of the drugs used to condition the patient. Because DMSO is toxic to cells in liquid state, each bag of cells is thawed rapidly in a 37 °C waterbath and infused in less than 5 min. The entire procedure usually requires 2–3 h, during which time the patient is closely monitored for symptoms and signs of fluid overload. There may be a disagreeable odor of the DMSO, which may also cause increased blood pressure and bradycardia during the re-infusion.[48] A recent study has shown that a few patients may develop electrocardiographic heart block, although this was of no clinical consequence.[49] Patients may develop fever during the infusion, and hemoglobin that is released from hemolysing red cells may cause hemoglobinuria in the first 24 h. Hemoglobinuria is less common in PBPC re-infusion because fewer red cells are collected by leukapheresis.

ENGRAFTMENT

The intensive drug and radiation conditioning is followed by a rapid decline in white cell, platelet, and red cell counts. During this period, the patient is at high risk for infection and bleeding, and close follow-up and intensive supportive measures are essential. In most instances, patients are hospitalized in rooms with positive airflow pressure equipped with HEPA filters and are cared for by a specially trained nursing staff, skilled in providing the unique needs of patients with bone marrow function failure. Platelets are transfused when the patients have severe thrombocytopenia or bleeding. All blood cell products are irradiated to prevent potentially fatal graft versus host disease. The most serious complications from severe neutropenia are infections, and patients are often treated prophylactically with oral quinalone antibiotics and fluconazol and, when febrile, by broad-spectrum intravenous antibiotics. The infections are usually those that are seen in patients with severe and profound neutropenia, including Gram-positive or Gram-negative bacteremia. In most patients, an infection presents as fever without physical, radiological signs. Patients with prolonged severe neutropenia can develop fungal infections such as *Candida* bacteremia or lung aspergillosis. A variety of empiric systemic antibiotic approaches for the treatment of fever in neutropenic patients have been developed over the years and have resulted in a significant reduction of infection-related complications. The early use of amphotericin-B when fungal infection is clinically suspected is also important. Patients also receive a hematopoietic growth factor such as GM-CSF or G-CSF, which can shorten the duration of neutropenia. On average, it takes 9–12 days for the neutrophil count to increase above the 500/mm^3 and approximately 12–15 days for platelets to increase above 50 000/mm^3. The engraftment may be slower when bone marrow is purged to reduce contamination by tumor cells. Also, PBPC transplantation low in CD34+

cells or cells obtained from patients with prolonged or intensive prior chemotherapy is associated with delayed engraftment.

Because of the increased experience with autologous transplantation and the shorter duration of bone marrow failure, several centers have developed programs to care for patients in an outpatient setting. Patients are seen daily at the hospital by the transplant team and receive the necessary treatment before being sent to a nearby hotel for an overnight stay. Patients are required to have a caregiver who is a family member or close friend and who can monitor the patient for 24 h. The patient and the caregiver remain in direct telephone contact with the transplant center in case any questions or symptoms arise, and the patient is admitted as an inpatient when the clinical condition indicates. This outpatient approach for autotransplantation is feasible and safe, and is not associated with more infections, morbidity, or mortality.[50] In addition to reducing the costs of transplantation, an outpatient program provides patients with other choices of care. However, the critical element of care, in both the inpatient and the outpatient settings, is the availability of a nursing team skilled in recognizing the potential complications that may occur in a patient undergoing intensive chemotherapy, such as infections, bleeding, fluid overload, and various non-hematological toxicities. For example, early recognition and immediate treatment of fever during the severe neutropenic period are essential in preventing serious complications and mortality. Therefore, autotransplantation should be performed in centers that have the ability to provide this particular level of nursing on a continuous basis.

NON-HEMATOLOGICAL TOXICITIES

High doses of drugs and radiation can damage tissues other than the bone marrow, which usually occurs early after transplantation. Problems developing after several months are more likely to be related to tumor recurrence. In most instances, non-marrow toxicities of high-dose therapy are mild to moderate, but severe complications may contribute to post-transplantation mortality. Mortality from autologous transplantation is less than 5% and in many centers less than 2%, and is usually from non-hematological complications.

The most common non-hematological organ to be adversely affected is the gastrointestinal tract. Almost all patients develop nausea or vomiting while receiving the intensive chemotherapy regimen, which can be ameliorated by selective serotonin 5-HT3 receptor blockers such as ondansetron or granisetron. Patients may continue to have these symptoms after completing the chemotherapy, which is probably due to damage by the intensive regimen to the stomach mucosa, and ondansetron and granisetron are less effective. Diarrhea is also common, but it is usually not severe, and somatitis, which may be severe, interferes with the oral intake of food or fluids. In addition, most patients have a poor appetite, which can last for several weeks after the high-dose regimens, and therefore may lose a considerable amount of weight. Hyperalimentation is used in several centers, but there is no evidence that it enhances recovery and, therefore, except for a very severe drop in weight, it is probably not indicated.

Pulmonary toxicity is occasionally related to bacterial, fungal, or viral infectious etiologies. However, several forms of non-infectious pulmonary toxicity can occur after autotransplantation, which can cause morbidity and even lead to death.[51,52] During the first days of engraftment, usually while white cell counts are rising, patients may develop a pulmonary syndrome characterized by non-productive cough, dyspnea, fever, hypoxia, interstitial pulmonary infiltrates, and respiratory distress. No infectious cause can be identified in these cases and the condition can deteriorate rapidly to pulmonary failure and death.[53–55] High doses of steroids are very effective and should be started at the earliest signs of this complication.[56] Clinicians should be aware of this complication and should start steroid treatment even if an infectious cause has not yet been completely ruled out. In the meantime, empiric antibiotics can be given or bronchoscopy performed. The cause of this pulmonary syndrome is unknown, but it has been attributed to the production of cytokines during the engraftment, or possibly to neutrophil influx into the lung, or to damage to the pulmonary cells by chemotherapy. Another pulmonary complication that can occur later after engraftment is pulmonary interstitial fibrosis, which is considered to be a toxic effect of the high doses of chemotherapy or radiation therapy and can cause serious respiratory failure with hypoxia. Fortunately, this complication is uncommon and is more likely to develop in patients who have received prior chest radiation and/or when patients have lower diffusion capacities. Although investigators have not been able to identify a relationship with any individual component of the treatment, pulmonary toxicity has been related to high-dose BCNU.[52]

A serious liver toxicity of high-dose chemotherapy and bone marrow transplantation is veno occlusive disease (VOD) of the liver.[57,58] It is characterized by edema, thrombosis, and fibrosis of the terminal hepatic venules and small sublobular veins. The resulting obstruction of blood flow leads to liver enlargement, ascites, hepatic cellular necrosis, and, in the most severe cases, encephalopathy. VOD usually reappears within 8–25 days after the high-dose regimen. The clinical features are: jaundice, hepatomegaly, right upper quadrant pain, ascites, and unexplained weight gain with no other identifiable cause for liver disease. The definitive diagnosis can be made by liver biopsy, although this is often not possible because of thrombocytopenia. The cause of venous edema and obstruction has not been clearly defined, but it has been postulated that injury to the subendothelium of the hepatic venules by cytokines activates the coagulation system and consequently generates thrombus. The reported incidence of VOD varies significantly amongst studies, ranging between 5% and 50%, which is probably dependent on the criteria used to identify this condition. Pretransplant hepatitis is the most important predictor of subsequent VOD in patients receiving a high-dose chemotherapy regimen.

Cardiac toxicity after bone marrow transplantation can occur in 4% of patients, with life-threatening cardiac complications occurring in less than 2% of all patients,[59] including arrhythmia, congestive heart failure, and pericardial effusion. Cyclophosphamide administered as part of the high-dose regimens is the agent most frequently associated with cardiac toxicity, although it has also been described following regimens that do not include this drug. Cardiac toxicity was reported to occur significantly more often in patients with pretransplant reduced lower left ventricular ejection fraction. However, major toxicity has also been reported in patients with normal results in cardiologic prescreening. In one study,[59] the risk of developing major cardiac toxicity was only 5% in patients with reduced ejection fraction, compared with 1% in patients with normal ejection fraction. During the first hours after re-infusion of the cryopreserved cells, patients may develop mild hypertension and bradycardia and, in rare cases, also heart block. However, in a recent study,[49] bradycardia and heart block were shown to be of little clinical significance and may be related to the DMSO-containing cells in the autologous graft.

TUMOR RESPONSE

As a general rule, the more active an agent is against a specific disease, the more likely it is that a clinical benefit can be detected with increasing dose. There is no standard drug or radiation schedule that is useful for all patients, but most trials use complex multimodality regimens of combination chemotherapy with or without radiation. The drugs selected usually have marrow toxicity as their major limiting factor to dose escalation. The high sensitivity of hematological malignancies to conventional doses of chemotherapy makes them more suitable diseases for exploring high-dose therapy; in these diseases, autotransplantation frequently led to durable responses and some patients were cured. In a recent European randomized trial, patients with acute myelogenous leukemia in first remission undergoing autologous bone marrow transplantation had a lower relapse rate compared to patients receiving less intensive chemotherapy.[60] In another study, patients with intermediate or high-grade non-Hodgkin's lymphoma responding to salvage chemotherapy after first relapse were randomized to receive high-dose chemotherapy and autologous bone marrow transplantation or additional standard-dose chemotherapy.[13] This study, which did not use peripheral blood stem cells, showed that the 5-year disease-free survival was 46% and the overall survival was 53% in the transplant arm, compared to 12% and 32%, respectively, in the control arm. In other non-randomized trials, patients with incurable relapsed non-Hodgkin's lymphoma could achieve long-term disease-free survival with autotransplantation.[11,12,61–63] In solid tumors, autologous transplantation could be more problematic, because of the limited number of available cytotoxic agents that are effective at conventional doses. Although several empiric combinations of chemotherapy were able to induce a higher response rate than standard dose of chemotherapy in patients with a variety of solid tumors, in most cases the responding patients relapsed without an overall survival benefit.

Another general concept in autotransplantation is that a better outcome can be achieved when it is performed while the tumor burden is lowest, after the patient responds to chemotherapy and preferably when no tumor is clinically detected. In several studies, solid tumors in complete remission or near-complete remission responded better to autotransplantation than patients transplanted with apparent disease.[64,65] Although no randomized trials have been done to prove this concept, autotransplantation in patients with minimal tumor burden who are still responding to salvage chemotherapy seems to be an approach that is more likely to yield more durable clinical responses. To a large extent, autologous transplantation has been studied in patients with solid tumors who have metastatic disease.[64] It is likely that survival would be improved by treating patients at the time of minimal tumor burden, and adjuvant autotransplantation may be the optimal approach. The reduced mortality and the lower morbidity of autotransplantation now allow for a wider exploration of this approach in patients who have no clinical evidence of disease.

The mechanism of relapse after high-dose chemotherapy and autotransplantation is unknown. In solid tumors and lymphoma, relapse often occurs at sites of original disease, indicating that the treatment was insufficient to overcome tumor-cell resistance. It is also possible that occult tumor cells may survive in the cryopreserved autograft and, when re-infused, may contribute to relapse. Whether the bone marrow or blood-derived cells differ in this respect is unknown. This is important, because, if elimination of residual cancer cells from the re-infused cells is essential to the success of high-dose therapy, methods of tumor-cell purging or positive stem-cell selection need to be developed. On the other hand, if the cause of relapse is not related to transplantable occult tumor cells, then improving the pretransplant regimen may be more important than purging. Data from current clinical trials comparing the frequency of relapses in the absence or presence of contaminating tumor cells are still inconclusive. Tumors such as lymphoma, breast cancer, or small-cell lung cancer are often associated with bone marrow involvement.

However, even in patients in remission or in whom the disease is localized, occult tumor cells can be found. Although, in theory, the peripheral blood is expected to contain fewer tumor cells than the bone marrow, occult circulating tumor cells have been detected in the peripheral blood stem cell harvests of patients with breast cancer,[35,66] neuroblastoma,[67] and lymphoma.[37,38,68] Some studies suggest that, in breast cancer or lymphoma, tumor cells occur less frequently in PBPC products than in bone marrow autografts.[35,66] However, in a recent study with breast and lung cancer patients,[69] mobilization of stem cells by chemotherapy and G-CSF also resulted in mobilization of tumor cells in the blood. The mere presence of tumor cells in the bone marrow or PBPCs does not necessarily imply that they can regrow after transplantation. In lymphoma, indirect evidence has suggested that the presence of lymphoma cells in bone marrow autograft contributes to relapse.[70] In another study, the relapse rate after PBPCs in patients with lymphoma was lower than with bone marrow.[71] More direct evidence can be obtained by gene marking techniques.[72,73] In leukemia and neuroblastoma patients, aliquots of remission bone marrow were first marked *ex vivo* with a retroviral vector containing a marker gene. These cells were then re-infused into the patient following high-dose chemotherapy. In a few patients, tumor cells obtained from relapsed tissue containing the marker gene were found, thus confirming the contribution of re-infused tumor cells to disease recurrence. There are no such data in cases of breast cancer or solid tumors.

In acute myeloid leukemia, several investigators purged the autologous bone marrow by *ex-vivo* chemotherapy manipulation before re-infusion, but, so far, no advantage has been demonstrated of this approach over transplantation of unpurged bone marrow. In fact, in these patients, purging the marrow with chemotherapy drugs resulted in delayed engraftment and more transplant-related complications due to prolonged marrow failure. In other studies, *ex-vivo* purging was performed using antibodies directed against antigens on the surface of tumor cells. Alternatively, it is possible to perform a positive selection of normal hematopoietic precursors by isolating CD34+ cells from peripheral blood and bone marrow harvests instead of a negative selection of the tumor cells. Solid tumors and multiple myeloma cells have been shown not to express the CD34 antigen, and selection of CD34+ cells resulted in a marked reduction of contaminated tumor cells in the autograft.[74] Transplantation of CD34+ bone marrow cells or PBPCs resulted in good engraftment, similar to that of unselected cells, but whether the re-infusion of cells containing fewer tumor cells will result in fewer relapses is still unclear.[47]

Different tumors pose different problems when autotransplantation is considered. Regimens active in one tumor may not be as effective in others. Tumors may differ in their response to standard-dose therapy, bone marrow involvement, organ damage, and age distribution, which may affect the eligibility for transplantation or overall outcome. The next section reviews the current results of autotransplantation in various solid tumors.

BREAST CANCER

Breast cancer is a tumor that is sensitive to chemotherapy, and several studies have shown a correlation between dose intensity and outcome when the treatment doses remained within the conventional dose range.[7,75,76] Breast cancer is the most common cancer in women and is second only to lung cancer as the leading cause of cancer-related deaths. It is also the most common solid tumor to be treated by autologous transplantation and is becoming the most frequent indication for this approach. The Autologous Blood and Marrow Transplant Registry of North America (ABMTR) registered 23 057 autotransplantations performed between 1989 and 1995. The most common indication was breast cancer, with 33% of the autotransplants, and then non-Hodgkin's lymphoma, with 25%. Because of recent studies described below the number of autotransplantations in breast cancer has significantly dropped.

In breast cancer, autologous transplantation is considered for metastatic disease or for patients with stage II/III as part of the overall primary treatment plan. Initially, autologous transplantation was performed in women with metastatic disease refractory to standard-dose chemotherapy. Although high-dose chemotherapy produced tumor responses and, in some cases, even complete responses, it failed to translate into longer survival.[77,78] Autologous transplantation is therefore not recommended for patients with refractory metastatic disease and the focus has shifted to studying this approach earlier in the course of the disease. In an early phase II trial, Peters et al. treated 22 patients who had not received prior chemotherapy for metastatic disease with high doses of cyclophosphamide, cisplatin, and BCNU.[79] Fifty-four percent of the patients attained a complete response, with an overall response of 73%. This study demonstrated that a single course of high-dose chemotherapy can induce a higher rate of complete responses than conventional doses. Nevertheless, the survival of the patients did not improve, as only 14% remained in complete remission beyond 16 months. Since this landmark study, most studies have focused on improving the duration of the response by initial cytoreduction using salvage standard-dose chemotherapy followed by high-dose chemotherapy. Several of these studies reported an overall response rate of 60–90%, with complete responses of 25–40% after the high-dose phase.[80–83] Although most patients relapsed and ultimately developed resistant disease, a minority of the women, in the range of 13–25%, have experienced prolonged progression-free survival. In two studies reported from the Dana Farber Cancer Institute

(DFCI), 62 patients received standard-dose chemotherapy cytoreduction followed by a single cycle of high doses of cyclophosphamide, thiotepa, and carboplatin. The 5-year progression-free survival was 21%, with a median observation of 50 months.[33,65,80]

Not all patients have the same chance of benefiting from standard-dose chemotherapy followed by a high-dose regimen, and several prognostic factors have been recognized for patients with metastatic disease.[84] The ABMTR analysed 1058 patients with metastatic breast cancer transplanted between 1989 and 1994.[85] The most commonly used high-dose regimens contained cyclophosphamide and thiotepa with or without carboplatin. The survival rate after 2 years was 41% and the progression-free survival was 17%, which are comparable to the results from the single institutions. A better outcome was seen, however, in patients with bone metastasis, complete response prior to transplantation, longer duration from diagnosis to metastasis, and estrogen-receptor-positive disease. The importance of achieving a complete response in predicting a longer duration of the response was emphasized by the DFCI study. In this study, patients who attained a complete remission to induction therapy had a 5-year progression-free survival of 31% as compared to 21% for the whole group.[65] In fact, even those with a reduction in tumor bulk of more than 90% but less than complete remission failed to do better than those with partial remission. In a multivariant analysis performed in that study, the most significant predictors for progression-free survival in addition to attainment of complete remission were a single metastatic site and a long interval from primary diagnosis to onset of metastatic disease. Overall, these results appear to be better than those of metastatic breast cancer treated by standard-dose chemotherapy, which are generally considered to be less than 1 year of median response duration and a median survival that is usually between 1 and 2 years. However, these studies do not clarify whether the improved results can be attributed to the high-dose chemotherapy or to a selection of a subset of patients who would have faired well even without auto-transplantation.[86] The first phase III study suggesting an advantage to the high-dose approach was reported from South Africa.[87] Ninety patients who were previously untreated for metastatic disease were randomized to receive either two cycles of high doses of cyclophosphamide, mitoxantrone, and etoposide with autologous transplantation, or six to eight cycles of conventional doses of cyclophosphamide, mitoxantrone, and vincristine. This study did not use standard-dose induction chemotherapy prior to the high-dose regimen. The overall response and complete response rates were 95% and 51% for the high-dose regimen compared to 51% and 4%, respectively, in the standard-dose group. The median response duration was 52 weeks in the high-dose group, which was higher than the 34 weeks for the standard-dose group. The median survival was 90 weeks versus 45 weeks, respectively. There was no mortality from toxicity in this study. The credibility of the study has recently been strongly questioned because another randomized trial reported by the same author in primary breast cancer was found to be fraudulent (see below).

At the 1999 meeting of the American Society of Clinical Oncology the results of two randomized trials in metastatic breast cancer were presented. The largest trial was initiated in 1990 by the Philadelphia Bone Marrow Transplant Group (PBTG).[88] In 1995, the Eastern Cooperative Group (ECOG) assumed coordination of the trial as it became the only nationwide randomized trial. The Southwestern Oncology Group (SWOG) also joined the study. According to the study design, patients first received standard induction chemotherapy with four to six cycles of cyclophosphamide, adriamycin, and 5-fluorouracil (CAF) with cyclophosphamide, methotrexate, and 5-fluorouracil (CMF). Those patients responding to this treatment and willing to proceed were randomized either to receive high-dose chemotherapy (with cyclophosphamide, thiotepa, or carboplatin) or to continue with conventional-dose maintenance treatment. Five hundred and fifty-three women were enrolled in the trial, but only 199 patients were randomized, of whom 184 were analysed (110 patients to the transplant arm, 89 to conventional chemotherapy maintenance). The remainder of the original group either did not achieve a complete or partial response or did not agree to be randomized. After a median follow-up of 37 months, the results showed no difference in the overall survival, regardless of complete or partial response to induction therapy (Table 2.1). This study shows that the use of high-dose chemotherapy and autologous hematopoietic rescue is not justified in metastatic breast cancer patients, even if they respond to chemotherapy.

A smaller randomized trial was initiated in 1992 in France, in which 61 women with metastatic breast cancer responding to standard-dose chemotherapy were randomized either to high-dose chemotherapy with mitoxantrone, cyclophosphamide, and melphalan, or to conventional maintenance chemotherapy.[89] After 5 years of follow-up, there were no statistically significant differences in the progression-free survival or overall survival between the groups (Table 2.2). Interestingly, the relapse for patients on the higher-dose chemotherapy arm was delayed, which could offer a better quality of life without chemotherapy for more time.

The conclusion from these trials is that, as autologous transplantations are currently done, they do not provide any significant benefits over standard chemotherapy in patients who have relapsed and who respond to standard-dose chemotherapy.

Primary breast cancer

It is possible that the effect of high-dose chemotherapy in metastatic disease is limited by the disease bulk despite cytoreduction by chemotherapy. Therefore, autotransplantation is being applied in the adjuvant setting in patients with newly diagnosed stage II/III disease, in particular those who are at higher risk for relapse despite standard-dose adjuvant chemotherapy. These patients, before developing metastatic disease, are more likely to have minimal disease burden. Furthermore, because autotransplantation is performed early in the course of the disease, the likelihood of the tumor cells acquiring drug resistance is lower. In addition, because the prior chemotherapy that these patients had received is minimal, they have less residual damage to the hematopoietic system and other organs and therefore the toxicity of autotransplantation is expected to be low. Indeed, in our own experience, the recovery rate of blood counts after autologous PBPC transplantation is the fastest in primary breast compared to other disease categories.

Table 2.1 *Randomized trials in metastatic breast cancer*

	Number of patients	Complete remission (%)	3-year survival (%)	Median survival (months)	Median time to progress (months)
High dose	110	42	32	24	9.6
Maintenance	89	49	38	26	9.0

The 'Philadelphia' Intergroup and ECOG Trial.[88]

Table 2.2 *Randomized trial in metastatic breast cancer*

	Number of patients	Complete remission (%)	Relapse at 5 years (%)	5-year survival (%)	Median PFS (months)
High dose	32	42	91	30	27
Maintenance	29	49	91	19	16
					$p = 0.08$

The 'French' study, reported from ASCO meeting 1999.[89]
PFS, progression-free survival.

Despite the improvement in standard-dose adjuvant chemotherapy, disease-free survival continues to be disappointing in patients with four or more involved axillary lymph nodes. The 5-year relapse-free survival in several major centers for patients with four to nine positive nodes was reported as 37–76%, and for ten or more positive nodes was 21–47%.[90–94] Because prospective randomized trials showed a dose–response relationship with outcome for patients with primary breast cancer,[7] it was felt that consolidating the adjuvant chemotherapy with high-dose chemotherapy followed by autotransplantation may reduce the recurrence rate.

Peters et al.[95] studied 102 patients who had stage II/III primary breast cancer with ten or more positive nodes who were treated after surgery with four cycles of standard-dose adjuvant chemotherapy followed by a high dose of cyclophosphamide, cisplatin, and BCNU. The 5-year event-free survival was 72%. These patients were compared to historical controls treated by the same salvage chemotherapy without high-dose therapy who had an event-free survival of only 25%. Although the therapy-related mortality was high (12%), the study was performed between 1989 and 1991, before hematopoietic growth factors and PBPCs were introduced.

The Milan group also treated breast cancer patients with ten or more positive axillary lymph nodes with a short, high-dose regimen consisting of sequential administration of three chemotherapy courses ending with PBPC transplantation.[96] In 67 patients, the relapse-free survival at 5 years was 56% and only one patient died from toxicity. In two historical control groups using standard-dose chemotherapy alone, the relapse-free survival was only 41% and 33%. Both studies point to the same direction: high-dose chemotherapy used after adjuvant chemotherapy reduces the recurrence rate in women with primary breast cancer who are at high risk of relapse.

In the 1999 meeting of the American Society of Clinical Oncology, preliminary results of three randomized trials were presented (Table 2.3). The largest trial was conducted by Cancer and Leukemia Group B (CALGB).[97] Enrollment opened in January 1992 and remained open until May 1998. Eight hundred and seventy-four women with primary breast cancer with ten or more axillary lymph nodes were enrolled and received four cycles of standard-dose CAF chemotherapy; 784 were randomized either to high-dose BCNU, cyclophosphamide, and cisplatinum followed by hematopoietic stem cell rescue, or to a lower intermediate dose of the same drugs with G-CSF support. All patients received tamoxifen for 5 years. At a median follow-up of 3 years, there were no statistically significant differences between the two arms in overall survival and event-free survival. These data are only preliminary because of the short follow-up. It is possible that, with a longer follow-up, a difference between the arms will emerge. In addition, in 29 patients (7.4%), treatment-related deaths occurred among 394 patients randomized to the high-dose therapy, but not among those on the intermediate-dose arm. Currently, in centers experienced with autotransplantation, the mortality rate with high-dose therapy in primary event cancer is 1% or less. It is possible that with lower mortality rates in the transplant arm the overall results would have been better.

The largest study outside the USA was conducted by the Scandinavian Breast Cancer Study Group,[98] which treated 525 patients who were assumed to have a greater than 70% chance of relapse within 5 years with standard therapy. This study was conducted between 1994 and 1998. Patients were randomized to receive nine courses of BFU, epirubicin, and cyclophosphamide (FEC) supported by G-CSF, or three cycles of FEC followed by high-dose therapy consisting of cyclophosphamide, thiotepa, and carboplatin followed by FEC mobilized peripheral blood progenitor cells. All patients in both arms received locoregional radiotherapy and tamoxifen for 5 years. This study has a short follow-up period, with a median of 23.7 months. The overall survival was not different between the groups (80% and 88% in the standard versus the high-dose arm). Two patients died from treatment complications in the high-dose arm and seven patients developed acute myelogenic leukemia and myelodysplasia. Despite the large number of patients enrolled, the follow-up is still too short to draw firm conclusions. Another report of a randomized trial was presented at a plenary session of the 1999 ASCO meeting by Bezoada from South Africa. This author claimed benefit from high-dose therapy,[99] but the results were found to be fraudulent. The report was retracted after an independent review discovered that the data were falsified.

To summarize, so far there has been no clear advantage to high-dose therapy in primary breast cancer in terms of reducing the high-risk for relapse. The studies have shown that high-dose chemotherapy can be safely

Table 2.3 *Primary breast randomized CALGB trial*

	Number of patients	Overall survival (%)	Event-free survival (%)	Relapse number	Treatment-related deaths (%)
High dose	394	78	68	74	7.4
Maintenance	389	86	64	107	0

Reported from ASCO Meeting 1999.[97]

administered to these patients. However, this conclusion can be taken only as preliminary due to the following factors: the follow-up is too short, and the Southwest Oncology Group (SWOG) is still following a large group of patients in a randomized trial in which patients in the transplant arm received high-dose cyclophosphamide plus thiotepa, the results of which have not yet been published. Another national randomized trial is being conducted in patients with four to nine positive nodes after early studies showed that this approach is feasible.[100]

One potential problem in transplanting patients with breast cancer is the concern regarding relapse of the disease from the re-infusion of occult breast cancer cells in the autograft. Occult micrometastases are found in the bone marrow of patients with stage II disease as well as of patients with metastatic disease and, theoretically, these could be re-infused back into the patient and re-establish the growth of the tumor. Because in metastatic disease relapse after high-dose chemotherapy occurs predominantly at sites of previous bulky disease, it was felt that the relapse occurs mainly as a result of failure of the high-dose regimen. It is still unclear if the use of PBPCs, which may contain fewer occult tumor cells than bone marrow cells, or the use of CD34 selected cells, which have fewer occult tumor cells, will reduce the relapse rate.

OVARIAN CANCER

High-dose chemotherapy and autologous transplantation are applicable for ovarian cancer for several reasons:

1 Ovarian cancer is a tumor with considerable chemosensitivity.
2 Patients who fail the initial therapy with standard doses have a very poor outcome: patients with advanced ovarian cancer have a 5-year survival rate of 21%.
3 There is evidence for the importance of dose intensification in the treatment of ovarian cancer within the standard dose range.[96–102] A retrospective study demonstrated a correlation between increasing the dose of cisplatin and both the response rate and overall survival.[101,102] The best response and overall survival rates from intensified doses were seen mostly with patients with optimally debulked disease.[103–107]
4 The bone marrow is rarely involved and therefore, in contrast to breast cancer, the potential for re-infusion of occult ovarian cancer cells is considered to be of less importance.

Despite the appropriateness of this disease for autotransplantation, the results of the clinical trials so far are inconclusive. In the ABMTR, 2% of autotransplantation cases were reported in patients with ovarian cancer. Most of the published reports consist of small groups of patients, treated after various numbers of prior chemotherapy cycles with a variety of regimens,

and separate analysis of each study is not productive.[108–112] In general, patients who are refractory to standard-dose chemotherapy may still respond to the high-dose regimen, but the response is usually of short duration. A review from 1994 of more than 200 patients collected from the small studies showed a response rate after high-dose chemotherapy and transplantation of 70–82%.[113] Most patients had advanced disease and, despite the high doses, no survival advantage was seen.

Stiff et al. surveyed 100 ovarian cancer patients with relapsed or refractory disease (almost all with bulky disease) who had autologous transplantation.[114] The overall response rate was 85%, with a complete response rate of 43%. However, patients who were still sensitive to cisplatin had a complete response of 73%, whereas those who were chemoresistant had a complete response of 34%. Unfortunately, only 14% of the patients remained disease free at 1 year.

Murakami et al. reported 42 patients who underwent primary cytoreductive surgery but with no prior chemotherapy before entering the study.[112] The patients received two cycles of high-dose cyclophosphamide, doxorubicin, and cisplatin. In the 22 patients without residual disease, the 5-year survival was 78%, whereas for those with macroscopic residual disease it was 26%. Overall, both studies[112,114] indicate that low tumor bulk and maintaining the sensitivity to standard-dose chemotherapy are important predictive factors for the effectiveness of high-dose therapy.

Another report evaluated 53 patients, most of whom did not have bulky, residual disease.[115] The 5-year overall survival was 60% and disease-free survival was 25%, which is comparable to 20% and 30% in patients receiving standard-dose chemotherapy.[116] Therefore, current trials are focusing on patients who are responding to initial chemotherapy with minimal residual disease after second-look surgery. In this group of patients, it would be possible to demonstrate whether high-dose chemotherapy is able to prolong survival. The ability to collect and store a very large number of hematopoietic progenitor cells from the peripheral blood by several collections has also allowed investigators to administer more than one cycle of high-dose chemotherapy.[117] This provides the opportunity to test the effect of multiple high-dose cycles with short intervals rather than one single high-dose cycle. So far, early study results indicate that even multiple courses of high-dose chemotherapy do not appear to overcome resistance in advanced bulky disease.[118] The introduction of paclitaxel in the treatment of ovarian cancer requires reconsideration of high-dose chemotherapy because of the survival advantage with this drug.[119]

A phase III trial is now being conducted by the Gynecological Oncology Group (GOG), which is randomizing patients with minimal disease to standard chemotherapy with paclitaxel and cisplatin or to high-dose chemotherapy with cyclophosphamide, mitoxantrone, and cisplatin with bone marrow or peripheral blood stem cell transplantation.

GERM-CELL CANCER

Testis cancer is one of the most chemosensitive solid tumors, approximately 70% of patients who present with advanced disease being cured by a combination of bleomyocin, etoposide, and cisplatin.[120] However, salvage chemotherapy for patients who relapse or fail to respond completely can achieve a complete remission in only 50%, and the disease-free survival is only 10–25%.[121–123] In these patients, high-dose chemotherapy followed by autotransplantation is offered in an attempt to improve the results. In 1992, Nichols *et al.* reported an ECOG trial using high-dose carboplatin and etoposide followed by autologous transplantation in 38 patients with recurrent or resistant germ-cell tumor.[124] The protocol did not include an attempt at debulking before high-dose chemotherapy. Of 38 evaluated patients, 17 (45%) had a response, with 9 (24%) showing a complete response. Five patients remained disease free for over 1 year. The results were poor because 13% died from treatment-related complications which today would probably have been much less common. This trial in a very poor prognosis group of patients indicated the curative potential of high-dose carboplatin and etoposide, even in highly refractory germ-cell cancer. Siegert *et al.* studied, in a larger group of patients, the effect of adding high-dose cyclophosphamide to the carboplatin and etoposide regimen.[123] This population of patients also had recurrent or refractory disease, but a better prognosis than the cohort reported by Nichols *et al.* because 37% were transplanted in complete remission. After high-dose chemotherapy, 51% were in complete remission and the event-free survival at 2 years for this group was 35%. This study also showed a correlation between tumor sensitivity and survival. The event-free survival was 4% for patients who were refractory to chemotherapy and 50% for those with sensitive disease. Other studies using similar drug regimens reported similar results.[125–129] These studies established the principle that a few patients with refractory germ-cell cancer can be cured by high-dose therapy, with a higher number of patients being cured when the disease is still chemosensitive. Similar to the developments seen in breast cancer, the focus has shifted to using this approach in patients who are receiving initial treatment but are at high risk of relapse. These include patients who are slow responders to initial therapy or have prolonged tumor marker half-life on conventional-dose chemotherapy. In two studies by Motzer,[130,131] high-risk, relapsed patients received high-dose chemotherapy and autotransplantation in the early stage after initial response to standard dose. The 3-year disease-free survival was 45%, compared to 25% in a similar group of historical patient from the same institution receiving standard-dose

chemotherapy. A randomized trial is now ongoing to examine the validity of these data.

SMALL-CELL LUNG CANCER

Lung cancer is the leading cause of cancer-related mortality in the USA. Nevertheless, only few patients were considered as candidates for autologous transplantation and most of them had small-cell lung cancer. Autologous transplantation, however, may be of considerable importance in the treatment of small-cell lung cancer because this tumor is known to have significant sensitivity to chemotherapy but very rarely are patients cured.[132] The almost universal relapse after complete response to chemotherapy is attributed to a small population of tumor cells that are resistant to chemotherapy and persist after the standard doses of therapy. The rationale for high-dose chemotherapy is to overcome this resistance and eradicate these persisting cells. Initial studies have clearly shown that only patients with limited disease would benefit from this approach, whereas patients with extensive disease uniformly relapse after autotransplantation.[67] With this subset of patients with limited disease, early studies have shown that approximately 10% of patients remained disease free 2–3 years after autotransplantation.[67]

The only randomized trial in small-cell lung cancer comparing high-dose chemotherapy intensification versus conventional-dose therapy was reported by Humblet, with disappointing results.[133] One hundred and one patients received five cycles of standard-dose chemotherapy. The 44 patients who responded were randomized to receive either one cycle of conventional-dose chemotherapy or one cycle of high-dose cyclophosphamide, BCNU, and etoposide followed by autotransplantation. No chest radiotherapy was given. Although high-dose chemotherapy resulted in a higher complete remission rate, there was no statistically significant difference between the study arms in the overall survival. However, the failure to show a survival benefit in this randomized trial could have been caused by two factors:

1 the treatment-related death was higher in the high-dose arm and therefore the disease-free survival did not translate into better overall survival;
2 most relapses after high-dose chemotherapy, which was given without radiotherapy, were inside of the primary tumor region.

Several studies have shown that the addition of chest radiotherapy to conventional-dose chemotherapy can improve the survival rates of limited disease compared to chemotherapy alone.[134–136]

Elias *et al.* treated patients with limited disease who responded to first-line conventional chemotherapy, who were younger than 60 years, with adequate lung function and good performance status, with high-dose chemotherapy, autologous transplantation and then chest radiotherapy.[137] The survival at 2 years was 50%, which is higher than that reported in this disease after standard-dose therapy. In small-cell lung cancer, most patients are smokers and therefore cardiopulmonary toxicity related to the high-dose chemotherapy may be of special importance when considering a high-dose chemotherapy with radiation therapy that involves the heart and lungs. So far, dose intensification and high-dose therapy with auto-transplantation have not shown the benefits to be better than those of a standard cisplatin/etoposide regimen.[138] In small-cell lung cancer, it is possible that new agents, which would modify the underlying biology of the disease, could, in the future, improve the outcome of this disease instead of chemotherapy dose intensification.[138]

OTHER SOLID TUMORS

In other tumors which are less sensitive to conventional-dose chemotherapy, high-dose chemotherapy has not yet demonstrated any advantage. One such tumor that was studied is metastatic melanoma, which is considered to be very resistant to standard-dose chemotherapy. Meisenberg *et al.* reported preliminary data using high-dose chemotherapy and autologous transplantation for melanoma patients in the adjuvant setting.[139] Following primary resection, patients with more than four regional lymph nodes involved with metastasis were randomized to treatment with a high-dose chemotherapy regimen versus observation. Eighteen of the 20 patients randomized to observation have relapsed, as opposed to 15 of the 19 patients who received high-dose chemotherapy. With other tumors that are essentially resistant to chemotherapy, such as gastrointestinal or pancreatic tumors, there is no evidence that dose intensification and autotransplantation are of benefit.

ACKNOWLEDGMENTS

The author wishes to acknowledge Gus Miranda and Brandy Wong for their assistance in preparing the manuscript.

REFERENCES

1. Bruce WR, Meeker BE, Valeriote FA. Comparison of the sensitivity of normal hematopoietic and transplanted lymphoma colony-forming cells to chemotherapeutic agents administered in vivo. J Natl Cancer Inst 1966; 37:233–45.
2. Skipper HE, Schobel FM Jr, Wilcox WS. Experimental evaluation of potential anticancer agents. XIII. On the criteria and kinetics associated with 'curability' of experimental leukemia. Cancer Chemother Rep 1964; 35:1–111.
3. Frei E III, Teicher BA, Holden SA, *et al.* Preclinical studies and clinical correlation of the effect of alkylating dose. Cancer Res 1988; 48:6417–23.
4. Ziegler JL. Treatment results of 54 American patients with Burkitt's lymphoma are similar to the African experience. N Engl J Med 1977; 297:75–80.
5. Cohen MH, Creaven PJ, Fossieck BE Jr, *et al.* Intensive chemotherapy of small cell bronchogenic carcinoma. Cancer Treat Rep 1977; 61:349–54.
6. Einhorn LH, Donohue J. Cis-diamminedichloro-platinum, vinblastine, and bleomycin combination chemotherapy in disseminated testicular cancer. Ann Intern Med 1977; 87:293–8.
7. Wood W, Budman D, Korzun A, *et al.* Dose and dose intensity of adjuvant chemotherapy for stage II, node-positive breast carcinoma. N Engl J Med 1994; 330:1253–9.
8. Sampson MK, Rivkin SE, Jones SE, *et al.* Dose–response and dose–survival advantage for high versus low-dose cisplatin combined with vinblastine and bleomycin in disseminated testicular cancer: a Southwest Oncology Group study. Cancer 1984; 53:1029.
9. Kaye SB, Lewis CR, Paul J, *et al.* Randomized study of two doses of cisplatin with cyclophosphamide in epithelial ovarian cancer. Lancet 1992; 340:329–33.
10. Mayer RJ, Davis RB, Schiffer CA, *et al.* Intensive postremission chemotherapy in adults with acute myeloid leukemia. N Engl J Med 1994; 331:896–903.
11. Freedman AS, Takvorian T, Anderson KC, *et al.* Autologous bone marrow transplantation in B-cell non-Hodgkin's lymphoma: very low treatment-related mortality in 100 patients in sensitive relapse. J Clin Oncol 1990; 8(5):784–91.
12. Freedman AS, Takvorian T, Neuberg D, *et al.* Autologous bone marrow transplantation in poor-prognosis intermediate-grade and high-grade B-cell non-Hodgkin's lymphoma in first remission: a pilot study. J Clin Oncol 1993; 11:931–6.
13. Philip T, Guglielmi C, Hagenbeek A, *et al.* Autologous bone marrow transplantation as compared with salvage chemotherapy in relapses of chemotherapy-sensitive non-Hodgkin's lymphoma. N Engl J Med 1995; 333:1540–5.
14. Brecher G, Cronkite EP. Post-radiation parabiosis and survival in rats. Proc Soc Exp Biol Med 1951; 77:292–4.
15. Epstein RB, Graham TC, Buckner CD. Allogeneic marrow engraftment by cross circulation in lethally irradiated dogs. Blood 1966; 28:692–707.
16. Storb R, Graham TC, Epstein RB, *et al.* Demonstration of hematopoietic stem cells in the peripheral blood of baboons by cross circulation. Blood 1977; 50:537.
17. Abrams RA, Glaubiger D, Appelbaum FR, Deisseroth AB. Result of attempted hematopoietic

reconstitution using isologous, peripheral blood mononuclear cells: a case report. Blood 1980; 56:516–20.

18. Kessinger A, Armitage JO, Landmark JD, et al. Reconstitution of human hematopoietic function with autologous cryopreserved circulating stem cells. Exp Hematol 1986; 14:192.

19. Korbling M, Dorken B, Ho AD, et al. Autologous transplantation of blood-derived hemopoietic stem cells after myeloablative therapy in a patient with Burkitts' lymphoma. Blood 1986; 67:529.

20. Lee JH, Klein HG. Collection and use of circulating hematopoietic progenitor cells. Hematol/Oncol Clin N Am 1995; 9:1–22.

21. Cooper DL. Peripheral blood stem cell transplantation. In *Principles and practice of oncology update,* Number 12. New York, Lippincott, Williams & Wilkins, 1994.

22. Cote RJ, Rosen PP, Hakes TB, et al. Monoclonal antibodies detect occult breast carcinoma metastases in the bone marrow of patients with early stage disease. Am J Surg Pathol 1988; 12:333–40.

23. Sharp JG, Joshi SS, Armitage JO, et al. Significance of detection of occult non-Hodgkin's lymphoma in histologically uninvolved bone marrow by a culture technique. Blood 1992; 79:1074–80.

24. Socinski MA, Cannistra SA, Elias A, et al. Granulocyte–macrophage colony-stimulating factor expands the circulating haemopoietic progenitor cell compartments in man. Lancet 1988; 1:1194–8.

25. Gianni AM, Bregni M, Siena S, et al. Rapid and complete hemopoietic reconstitution following combined transplantation of autologous blood and bone marrow cells. A changing role for high dose chemo-radiotherapy? Hematol Oncol 1989; 7:139–48.

26. Sheridan WP, Begley CG, Juttner CA, et al. Effect of peripheral-blood progenitor cells mobilized by filgrastim (G-CSF) on platelet recovery after high-dose chemotherapy. Lancet 1992; 339:640–4.

27. Peters WP, Rosner G, Ross M, et al. Comparative effects of granulocyte–macrophage colony-stimulating factor (GM-CSF) and granulocyte colony-stimulating factor (G-CSF) on priming peripheral blood progenitor cells for use with autologous bone marrow after high-dose chemotherapy. Blood 1993; 81:1709–19.

28. Chao NJ, Schriber JR, Grimes K, et al. Granulocyte colony stimulating factor 'mobilized' peripheral blood progenitor cells accelerate granulocyte and platelet recovery after high-dose chemotherapy. Blood 1993; 81:2031–5.

29. Hass R, Mohle R, Fruhauf S, et al. Patients' characteristics associated with successful mobilizing and autografting of peripheral blood progenitor cells in malignant lymphomas. Blood 1994; 83:3787–94.

30. Bensinger W, Singer J, Appelbaum F, et al. Autologous transplantation with peripheral-blood mononuclear cells collected after administration of recombinant granulocyte stimulating factor. Blood 1993; 81:3158–63.

31. Bishop MR, Anderson JR, Jackson JD, et al. High-dose therapy and peripheral blood progenitor cell transplantation: effects of recombinant human granulocyte–macrophage colony-stimulating factor on the autograft. Blood 1994; 83:610–16.

32. To LB, Shepard KM, Haylock DN, et al. Single high doses of cyclophosphamide enable the collection of high numbers of hemopoietic stem cells from the peripheral blood. Exp Hematol 1990; 18:442–7.

33. Elias AD, Ayash L, Anderson K, et al. Mobilization of peripheral blood progenitor cells by chemotherapy and GM-CSF for hematologic support after high-dose intensification for breast cancer. Blood 1992; 79:3036–44.

34. Dreger P, Kloss M, Petersen B, et al. Autologous progenitor cell transplantation: prior exposure to stem cell-toxic drugs determines yield and engraftment of peripheral blood cell but not of bone marrow grafts. Blood 1995; 86:3970–98.

35. Ross AA, Cooper BW, Lazarus HM, et al. Detection and viability of tumor cells in peripheral blood stem cell collections from breast cancer patients using immunocytochemical and clonogenic assay techniques. Blood 1993; 82:2605–10.

36. Moss TJ, Cairo M, Santana VM, et al. Clonogenicity of circulating neuroblastoma cells: implications regarding peripheral blood stem cell transplantation. Blood 1994; 83:3085–9.

37. Gribben JG, Neuberg D, Barber M, et al. Detection of residual lymphoma cells by polymerase chain reaction in peripheral blood is significantly less predictive for relapse than detection in bone marrow. Blood 1994; 83:3800.

38. Bensinger WI, Clift RA, Anasetti C, et al. Transplantation of allogeneic peripheral blood stem cells mobilized by recombinant human granulocyte colony stimulating factor. Stem Cells 1996; 14:90–105.

39. Wagner JE, Kernan NA, Steinbuch M, Broxmeyer HE, Gluckman E. Allogeneic sibling umbilical-cord-blood transplantation in children with malignant and non-malignant disease. Lancet 1995; 346:214–19.

40. Papayannopoulou T, Nakamoto B. Peripherization of hematopoietic progenitors in primates treated with anti-VLA4 integrin. Proc Natl Acad Sci 1993; 90:9374–8.

41. Brenner MK, Rill DR, Holladay MS, et al. Gene marking to determine whether autologous marrow infusion restores long-term haemopoiesis in cancer patients. Lancet 1993; 342:1134–7.

42. Dunbar CE, Cottler-Fox M, O'Shaughnessy JA, et al. Retrovirally marked CD34-enriched peripheral blood and bone marrow cells contribute to long-term engraftment after autologous transplantation. Blood 1995; 85:3048–57.

43. Pettengell R, Morgenstern GR, Woll PJ, et al. Peripheral-blood progenitor-cell transplantation in

lymphoma and leukemia using a single apheresis. Blood 1993; 82:3770–7.

44. Kotasek D, Shepard KM, Sage RE, *et al.* Factors affecting blood stem cell collections following high-dose cyclophosphamide mobilization in lymphoma, myeloma, and solid tumors. Bone Marrow Transplant 1992; 9:11.

45. Bolwell BJ, Fishleder A, Andresen SW, *et al.* G-CSF primed peripheral blood progenitor cells in autologous bone marrow transplantation: parameters affecting bone marrow engraftment. Bone Marrow Transplant 1993; 12:609.

46. Rowley SD, Bensinger WI, Gooley TA, Buckner CD. Effect of cell concentration on bone marrow and peripheral blood stem cell cryopreservation. Blood 1994; 83:2731–6.

47. Shpall EJ, Jones RB, Bearman SI, *et al.* Transplantation of enriched CD34-positive autologous marrow into breast cancer patients following high-dose chemotherapy: influence of CD34-positive peripheral-blood progenitor and growth factors on engraftment. J Clin Oncol 1994; 12:28.

48. Davis JM, Rowley SD, Braine HG, Piantadosi S, Santos GW. Clinical toxicity of cryopreserved bone marrow graft infusion. Blood 1990; 75:781–6.

49. Keung YK, Lau S, Elkayam U, Chen SC, Douer D. Cardiac-arrhythmia after infusion of cryopreserved stem-cells. Bone Marrow Transplant 1994; 14:363–7.

50. Meisenberg BR, Miller WE, McMillan R, *et al.* Outpatient high-dose chemotherapy with autologous stem-cell rescue for hematologic and nonhematologic malignancies. J Clin Oncol 1997; 15:11–17.

51. Crilley P, Topolsky D, Styler MJ, *et al.* Extramedullary toxicity of a conditioning regimen containing busulphan, cyclophosphamide and etoposide in 84 patients undergoing autologous and allogeneic bone marrow transplantation. Bone Marrow Transplant 1995; 15:361–5.

52. Valteau D, Hartmann O, Benhamou E, *et al.* Nonbacterial nonfungal interstitial pneumonitis following autologous bone marrow transplantation in children treated with high-dose chemotherapy without total-body irradiation. Transplantation 1988; 45:737–40.

53. Robbins RA, Linder J, Stahl MG, *et al.* Diffuse alveolar hemorrhage in autologous bone marrow transplant recipients. Am J Med 1989; 87:511–18.

54. Seiden MV, Elias A, Ayash L, *et al.* Pulmonary toxicity associated with high dose chemotherapy in the treatment of solid tumors with autologous marrow transplant: an analysis of four chemotherapy regimens. Bone Marrow Transplant 1992; 10:57–63.

55. Lee CK, Gingrich RD, Hohl RJ. A distinctive clinical syndrome accompanying the engraftment process in autologous bone marrow transplantation (ABMT). Blood 1994; 84:490a.

56. Chao NJ, Duncan SR, Long GD, Horning SJ, Blume KG. Corticosteroid therapy for diffuse alveolar hemorrhage in autologous bone marrow transplant recipients. Ann Intern Med 1991; 114:145–6.

57. McDonald GB, Sharma P, Matthews DE, Shulman HW, Thomas ED. Venoocclusive disease of the liver after bone marrow transplantation: diagnosis, incidence, and predisposing factors. Heptatology 1984; 4:116–22.

58. McDonald GB, Hinds MS, Fisher LD, *et al.* Veno-occlusive disease of the liver and multiorgan failure after bone marrow transplantation: a cohort study of 355 patients. Ann Intern Med 1993; 118:255–67.

59. Hertenstein B, Stefanic M, Schmeiser T, *et al.* Cardiac toxicity of bone marrow transplantation: predictive value of cardiologic evaluation before transplantation. J Clin Oncol 1994; 12:998–1004.

60. Zittoun RA, Mandelli F, Willemze R, *et al.* Autologous or allogeneic bone marrow transplantation compared with intensive chemotherapy in acute myelogenous leukemia. European Organization for Research and Treatment of Cancer (EORTC) and GIMEMA. N Engl J Med 1995; 332:217–23.

61. Takvorian T, Canellos GP, Ritz J, *et al.* Prolonged disease-free survival after autologous bone marrow transplantation in patients with non-Hodgkin's lymphoma with a poor prognosis. N Engl J Med 1987; 316:1499–505.

62. Nademanee A, Sniecinski I, Schmidt GM, *et al.* High-dose therapy followed by autologous peripheral-blood stem-cell transplantation for patients with Hodgkin's disease and non-Hodgkin's lymphoma using unprimed and granulocyte colony-stimulating factor-mobilized peripheral-blood stem cells. J Clin Oncol 1994; 12:2176–86.

63. Gribben JG, Goldstone AH, Linch DC, *et al.* Effectiveness of high-dose combination chemotherapy and autologous bone marrow transplantation for patients with non-Hodgkin's lymphomas who are still responsive to conventional-dose therapy. J Clin Oncol 1989; 7:1621–9.

64. Shpall EJ, Stemmer SM, Bearman SI, Jones RB. Role of autotransplantation in treatment of other solid tumors. Hematol/Oncol Clin N Am 1993; 7:663–86.

65. Ayash LJ, Wheeler C, Fairclough D, *et al.* Prognostic factors for prolonged progression-free survival with high-dose chemotherapy with autologous stem-cell support for advanced breast cancer. J Clin Oncol 1995; 13:2043–9.

66. Douer D, Chaiwun B, Glaspy J, Watkins K, Vesco R, Cote R. Analysis of peripheral blood progenitor cell (PBPC) harvests for occult breast cancer micrometastasis using a sensitive immuno-histochemical method. Proc Am Soc Clin Oncol 1993; 12:62a.

67. Moss TJ, Sanders DJ, Lasky LC, *et al.* Contamination of peripheral blood stem cell harvests by circulating neuroblastoma cells. Blood 1990; 76:1879–83.

68. Sharp JG, Kessinger A, Vaughan WP, *et al*. Detection and clinical significance of minimal tumor cell contamination of peripheral stem cell harvests. Int J Cell Cloning 1992; 10(Suppl. 1):92–4.

69. Brugger W, Bross KJ, Glatt M, *et al*. Mobilization of tumor cells and hematopoietic progenitor cells into peripheral blood of patients with solid tumors. Blood 1994; 83:636–40.

70. Gribben JG, Freedman AS, Neuberg D, *et al*. Immunologic purging of marrow assessed by PCR before autologous bone marrow transplantation for B-cell lymphoma. N Engl J Med 1991; 325:1525–33.

71. Vose JM, Anderson JR, Kessinger A, *et al*. High-dose chemotherapy and autologous hematopoietic stem-cell transplantation for aggressive non-Hodgkin's lymphoma. J Clin Oncol 1993; 11:1846–51.

72. Rill DR, Santana VM, Roberts M, *et al*. Direct demonstration that autologous bone marrow transplantation for solid tumors can return a multiplicity of tumorigenic cells. Blood 1994; 84:380–3.

73. Brenner MK, Rill DR, Moen RC, *et al*. Gene-marking to trace origin of relapse after autologous bone marrow transplantation. Lancet 1993; 341:85–6.

74. Berenson RJ. Transplantation of CD34+ hematopoietic precursors: clinical rationale. Transplant Proc 1992; 24:3032–4.

75. Hryniuk W, Bush H. The importance of dose intensity in chemotherapy of metastatic breast cancer. J Clin Oncol 1984; 2:1281–8.

76. Tannock I, Boyd N, DeBoer G, *et al*. A randomized trial of two dose levels of cyclophosphamide, methotrexate, fluorouracil chemotherapy for patients with metastatic breast cancer. J Clin Oncol 1988; 6:1377–87.

77. Kaminer LS, Williams SF, Beschorner J, *et al*. High-dose chemotherapy with autologous hematopoietic stem cell support in the treatment of refractory stage IV breast carcinoma. Bone Marrow Transplant 1989; 4:359–62.

78. Peters WP, Eder JP, Henner ED, *et al*. High-dose combination alkylating agents with autologous bone marrow support: a phase I trial. J Clin Oncol 1986; 4:646–54.

79. Peters WP, Shpall EJ, Jones RB, *et al*. High-dose combination alkylating agents with bone marrow support as initial treatment for metastatic breast cancer. J Clin Oncol 1988; 6:1368–76.

80. Antman K, Ayash L, Elias A, *et al*. A phase II study of high-dose cyclophosphamide, thiotepa, and carboplatin with autologous marrow support in women with measurable advanced breast cancer responding to standard-dose therapy. J Clin Oncol 1992; 10:102–10.

81. Williams SF, Gilewski T, Mick R, *et al*. High-dose consolidation therapy with autologous stem-cell rescue in stage IV breast cancer: follow-up report. J Clin Oncol 1992; 10:1743–7.

82. Kennedy MJ, Beveridge RA, Rowley SD, *et al*. High-dose chemotherapy with reinfusion of purged autologous bone marrow following dose-intense induction as initial therapy for metastatic breast cancer. J Natl Cancer Inst 1991; 82:920–6.

83. Dunphy FR, Spitzer G, Buzdar AU, *et al*. Treatment of estrogen receptor-negative or hormonally refractory breast cancer with double high-dose chemotherapy intensification and bone marrow support. J Clin Oncol 1990; 8:1207–16.

84. Dunphy FR, Spitzer G, Rossiter-Fornoff JE, *et al*. Factors predicting for long-term survival in metastatic breast cancer treated with high-dose chemotherapy and bone marrow support. Cancer 1994; 73:2157.

85. Rowlings PA, Antman KS, Horowitz MM, *et al*. Prognostic factors in autotransplants for metastatic breast cancer. Blood 1995; 86(Suppl. 1):618a.

86. Kennedy JM. High-dose chemotherapy of breast cancer: is the question answered? J Clin Oncol 1995; 13:2477–9.

87. Bezwoda WR, Seymour L, Dansey RD. High-dose chemotherapy with hematopoietic rescue as primary treatment for metastatic breast cancer: a randomized trial. J Clin Oncol 1995; 13:2483–9.

88. Stadtmauer EA, O'Neill A, Goldstein LJ, *et al*. Conventional-dose chemotherapy compared with high-dose chemotherapy plus autologous hematopoietic stem-cell transplantation for metastatic breast cancer. N Engl J Med 2000; 342: 1069–76.

89. Lotz JP, Cure H, Janvier M, *et al*. and the PEGASE Group. High-dose chemotherapy (HD-CT) with hematopoietic stem cells transplantation (HSCT) for metastatic breast cancer (MBC): results of the French protocol PEGASE 04. J Clin Oncol 1999; 18:43a.

90. Early Breast Cancer Trialist's Collaborative Group. Systemic treatment of early breast cancer by hormonal, cytotoxic, or immune therapy. Lancet 1992; 339:1–15, 71–85.

91. Moon TE, Jones SE, Bonadonna G, *et al*. Development and use of a natural history data base of breast cancer studies. Am J Clin Oncol 1987; 10:396–403.

92. Jones SE, Moon PE, Bonadonna G, *et al*. Comparison of different trials of adjuvant chemotherapy in stage II breast cancer using a natural history data base. Am J Clin Oncol 1987; 10:387–95.

93. Buzzoni R, Bonadonna G, Valagussa P, *et al*. Adjuvant chemotherapy with doxorubicin plus cyclosphosphamide, methotrexate and fluorouracil in the treatment of resectable breast cancer with

more than three positive nodes. J Clin Oncol 1991; 9:2134–40.

94. Bonadonna G, Zambetti M, Valagussa P. Sequential or alternating doxorubicin and CMF regimens in breast cancer with more than three positive nodes. Ten-year results. JAMA 1995; 273:542–7.

95. Peters WP, Ross M, Vredenburgh JJ, *et al.* High-dose chemotherapy and autologous bone marrow support as consolidation after standard-dose adjuvant therapy for high-risk primary breast cancer. Pro Am Soc Clin Oncol 1995; 14:90a.

96. Gianni AM, Siena S, Bregni M, *et al.* 5-year results of high dose sequential (HDS) adjuvant chemotherapy in breast cancer with ≥10 positive nodes. J Clin Oncol 1955; 14:90.

97. Peters WP, Rosner G, Vredenburgh J, *et al.* for CALGB, SWOG, and NCICJ. A prospective, randomized comparison of two doses of combination alkylating agents (AA) as consolidation after CAF in high-risk primary breast cancer involving ten or more axillary lymph nodes (LN): preliminary results of CALGB 9082/SWOG9114/NCIC MA-13. Clin Oncol 1999; 18:1a.

98. The Scandinavian Breast Cancer Study Group 9401. Results from a randomized adjuvant breast cancer study with high dose chemotherapy with CTCb supported by autologous bone marrow stem cells versus dose escalated and tailored FEC therapy. J Clin Oncol 1999; 18:1a.

99. Bezwoda WR. Randomised, controlled trial of high dose chemotherapy (HD-CNVp) vs standard dose (CAF) chemotherapy for high risk, surgically treated, primary breast cancer. J Clin Oncol 1999; 18:2a.

100. Bearman SI, Overmoyer BA, Bolwell BG, *et al.* High dose chemotherapy with autologous peripheral blood progenitor cells for primary breast cancer in patients with 4–9 involved axillary lymph nodes: a feasibility study. Pro Am Soc Clin Oncol 1996; 15:333a.

101. Levin L, Hryniuk WM. Dose intensity analysis of chemotherapy regimens in ovarian carcinoma. J Clin Oncol 1987; 5:756–67.

102. Levine L, Simon R, Hryniuk W. Importance of multiagent chemotherapy regimens in ovarian carcinoma: dose-intensity analysis. J Natl Cancer Inst 1993; 85:1732–42.

103. Kaye SB, Lewis CR, Paul J, *et al.* Randomized study of two doses of cisplatin and cyclophosphamide in epithelial ovarian cancer. Lancet 1992; 340:329–33.

104. Ngan HYS, Choo YC, Cheung M, *et al.* A randomized study of high-dose versus low-dose cisplatinum combined with cyclophosphamide in the treatment of advanced ovarian cancer. Chemotherapy 1989; 35:221–7.

105. Ehrlich CE, Einhorn L, Stehman FB, *et al.* Treatment of advanced epithelial ovarian cancer using

cisplatin, adriamycin, and cytoxan: the Indiana University experience. Clin Obstet Gynecol 1983; 10:325–35.

106. Colombo N, Pittelli MR, Parma G, *et al.* Cisplatin dose intensity in advanced ovarian cancer: a randomized study of dose-intense versus standard-dose cisplatin monochemotherapy. Proc Am Soc Clin Oncol 1993; 12:255.

107. Conte PF, Bruzzone M, Gadducci A, *et al.* High doses versus standard doses of cisplatin in combination with epidoxorubicin and cyclosphosphamide in advanced ovarian cancer patients with bulky residual disease: a randomized trial. Proc Am Soc Clin Oncol 1993; 12:273.

108. Mulder POM, Willemse PHB, Aalders JG, *et al.* High-dose chemotherapy with autologous bone marrow transplantation in patients with refractory ovarian cancer. Eur J Cancer Clin Oncol 1989; 25:645–9.

109. Viens P, Maraninchi D, Legros M, *et al.* High dose melphalan and autologous marrow rescue in advanced epithelial ovarian carcinomas: a retrospective analysis of 35 patients treated in France. Bone Marrow Transplant 1990; 5:227–33.

110. Shpall EJ, Pearson-Clarke D, Soper JT, *et al.* High-dose alkylating agent chemotherapy with autologous bone marrow support in patients with stage III/IV epithelial ovarian cancer. Gynecol Oncol 1990; 38:386–91.

111. Broun ER, Belinson JL, Berek JS, *et al.* Salvage therapy for recurrent and refractory ovarian cancer with high-dose chemotherapy and autologous bone marrow support: a Gynecologic Oncology Group pilot study. Gynecol Oncol 1994; 54:142–6.

112. Murakami M, Shinozuka T, Kuroshima Y, Tokuda Y, Tajima T. High-dose chemotherapy with autologous bone marrow transplantation for the treatment of malignant ovarian tumors. Semin Oncol 1994; 21:29–32.

113. Shpall EJ, Jones RB, Berman SL, *et al.* Future strategies for the treatment of advanced epithelial ovarian cancer using high-dose chemotherapy and autologous bone marrow support. Gynecol Oncol 1994; 54:357–61.

114. Stiff PJ, Bayer R, Kerger C, *et al.* High dose chemotherapy with autologous transplantation for persistent/relapsed ovarian cancer. A multivariant analysis of survival of 100 consecutively treated patients. J Clin Oncol 1997; 15:1309–17.

115. Legros M, Dauplat J, Fleury J, *et al.* High-dose chemotherapy with hematopoietic rescue in patients with stage III to IV ovarian cancer: long-term results. J Clin Oncol 1997; 15:1302–8.

116. Thigpen JT. Dose-intensity in ovarian carcinoma: hold, enough? J Clin Oncol 1997; 15:1291–3.

117. Shea TC, Mason JR, Storniolo AM, *et al.* Sequential cycles of high-dose carboplatin administered with

recombinant human granulocyte-macrophage colony-stimulating factor and repeated infusions of autologous peripheral blood progenitor cells: a novel and effective method for delivering multiple courses of dose-intensive therapy. J Clin Oncol 1992; 10:464–73.

118. Herrin VE, Thigpen JT. High-dose chemotherapy in ovarian carcinoma. Semin Oncol 1999; 26: 99–105.

119. McGuire WP, Hoskins WJ, Brady MF, *et al.* Cyclophosphamide and cisplatinum compared with paclitaxel and cisplatin in patients with stage III and stage IV ovarian cancer. N Engl J Med 1996; 334:1–6.

120. Williams S, Birch R, Einhorn LH, *et al.* Treatment of disseminated germ cell tumors with cisplatin, bleomycin and either vinblastine or etoposide. N Engl J Med 1987; 316:1435–40.

121. Harstrick A, Schmoll HJ, Wilke H, *et al.* Cisplatin, etoposide, and ifosfamide salvage therapy for refractory or relapsing germ cell cancer. J Clin Oncol 1991; 9:1549–55.

122. Loehrer PJ, Einhorn LH, Williams SD. VP-16 plus ifosfamide plus cisplatin as salvage therapy in refractory germ cell cancer. J Clin Oncol 1986; 4:528–36.

123. Siegert W, Beyer J, Strohscheer I, *et al.* High-dose treatment with carboplatin, etoposide, and ifosfamide followed by autologous stem-cell transplantation in relapsed or refractory germ cell cancer: a phase I/II study. J Clin Oncol 1994; 12:1223–31.

124. Nichols CR, Andersen J, Lazarus HM, *et al.* High-dose carboplatin and etoposide with autologous bone marrow transplantation in refractory germ cell cancer: an Eastern Cooperative Oncology Group protocol. J Clin Oncol 1992; 10:558–63.

125. Lotz JP, Andre T, Donsimoni R, *et al.* High dose chemotherapy with ifosfamide, carboplatin and etoposide combined with autologous bone marrow transplantation for the treatment of poor risk germ cell tumors and metastatic trophoblastic disease in adults. Cancer 1995; 75:874–88.

126. Broun ER, Nichols CR, Kneebone P, *et al.* Long-term outcome of patients with relapsed and refractory germ cell tumors treated with high-dose chemotherapy and autologous bone marrow rescue. Ann Intern Med 1992; 117:124–8.

127. Barnett MJ, Coppin CML, Murray N, *et al.* High-dose chemotherapy and autologous bone marrow transplantation for patients with poor prognosis non-seminomatous germ cell tumours. Br J Cancer 1993; 68:594.

128. Chevreau C, Droz JP, Pico JL, *et al.* Early intensified chemotherapy with autologous bone marrow transplantation in first line treatment of poor risk non-seminomatous germ cell tumours. Eur Urol 1993; 23:213–18.

129. Droz JP, Kramar A, Pico JL. Prediction of long-term response after high-dose chemotherapy with autologous bone marrow transplantation in the salvage treatment of non-seminomatous germ cell tumours. Eur J Cancer 1993; 29A(6): 818–21.

130. Motzer RJ, Mazumdar M, Bajorin DF, Bosl GJ, Lyn P, Vlamis V. High-dose carboplatin, etoposide, and cyclophosphamide with autologous bone marrow transplantation in first-line therapy for patients with poor-risk germ cell tumors. J Clin Oncol 1997; 15:2546–52.

131. Motzer RJ, Mazumdar M, Gulati SC, *et al.* Phase II trial of high-dose carboplatin and etoposide with autologous bone marrow transplantation in first-line therapy for patients with poor-risk germ cell tumors. J Natl Cancer Inst 1993; 85:1828–35.

132. Seifter EJ, Ihde DC. Therapy of small cell lung cancer: a perspective on two decades of clinical research. Semin Oncol 1988; 15:278–99.

133. Humblet Y, Symann M, Bosly A, *et al.* Late intensification chemotherapy with autologous bone marrow transplantation in selected small-cell carcinoma of the lung: a randomized study. J Clin Oncol 1987; 5:1864–73.

134. Perry MC, Eaton WL, Propert KJ, *et al.* Chemotherapy with or without radiation therapy in limited small-cell carcinoma of the lung. N Engl J Med 1987; 316:912–18.

135. Bunn PA, Lichter AS, Makuch RW, *et al.* Chemotherapy alone or chemotherapy with chest radiation therapy in limited stage small cell lung cancer. Ann Intern Med 1987; 106:655–62.

136. Kies MS, Mira JG, Crowley JJ, *et al.* Multimodal therapy for limited small-cell lung cancer: a randomized study of induction combination chemotherapy with or without thoracic radiation in complete responders; and with wide-field versus reduced-field radiation in partial responders: a Southwest Oncology Group study. J Clin Oncol 1987; 5:592–600.

137. Elias AD, Ayash L, Frei E III, *et al.* Intensive combined modality therapy for limited stage small cell lung cancer. J Natl Cancer Inst 1993; 85:559–66.

138. Johnson DH, Carbone DP. Increased dose-intensity in small cell lung cancer: a failed strategy? J Clin Oncol 1999; 17:2297–9.

139. Meisenberg B, Ross M, Jones R, *et al.* Adjuvant high-dose combination alkylating agent chemotherapy (HDCAA) with autologous bone marrow support (ABMS) in multi-node positive melanoma. Proc Am Soc Clin Oncol 1992; 11:345.

Commentary

HANNA KHOURY AND JOHN F DIPERSIO

Despite years of research, the importance of the chemotherapy drug dose in the management of various non-hematologic malignancies remains unresolved. The concept that dose might be correlated with outcome is based on laboratory models in which delivery of the highest possible doses of chemotherapy leads to maximum tumor cell killing.[1] Additionally, chemoresistance, commonly observed after initial tumor response, can often be overcome, in the laboratory, by using fivefold to tenfold higher doses of chemotherapy.[2] Clinically, some correlation between chemotherapy dose and response has long been recognized,[3] but before modern hematopoietic support strategies, systematic analysis of dose–response relationships has proven problematic. Dose quantified per unit time, and expressed in drug dose administered per square meter per week, was accepted as a method for quantifying dose–response relationships in patients treated with chemotherapy.[4] This method, far from being perfect, served as a basis for several randomized trials in which dose intensity was the most important variable analysed. Disappointingly, the results of these studies were mixed, with only few trials showing increased response rate for regimens with greater dose intensity. However, these increments in chemotherapy dose were modest and thus produced, at best, only modest effects on survival.[5] The limiting toxicity of higher chemotherapy doses being myelosuppression for many, if not all, cytotoxic agents, hematopoietic stem cells have been used to ensure prompt marrow recovery after supralethal doses of chemotherapy and radiotherapy. Advances in supportive care and the widespread availability of technologies to harvest, store, and re-infuse hematopoietic stem cells have provided the impetus for this approach and allowed the systematic testing of high-dose chemotherapy (HDC) in the management of various cancers. Initial experience was limited to patients with advanced disease; but the observation that patients with small metastatic tumor volume and sensitivity to salvage chemotherapy have the highest chance of response and the longest disease-free survival led to the application of HDC to earlier disease stages. The rationale for using HDC early, as adjuvant therapy for patients at high risk for relapse, was based on the hypothesis that, for a chemoresponsive malignancy, effective therapy whose limiting toxicity is marrow failure, administered early in the course of the disease when tumor burden and drug resistance are minimal, followed by a rescue with a source of progenitor cells that are free of tumor cells, may be a curative treatment modality. As outlined in the excellent review by Douer, initial phase I–II studies using HDC and hematopoietic stem cell transplantation (HSCT) have indeed been encouraging,

for both early and advanced disease stages. However, these high hopes have yet to be realized in the setting of randomized clinical trials. In contrast to ongoing randomized trials for germ-cell tumors and ovarian cancer, results of randomized trials for breast cancer are now available.[6–11]

For women with metastatic breast carcinoma, data from two randomized trials[6,7] suggest that it is unlikely that a single course of HDC with alkylating agents will result in superior disease-free and overall survival when compared to conventional-dose chemotherapy. These results are in sharp contrast with data published by Bezwoda et al.,[8] thus raising the question of how to interpret discordant results obtained from randomized trials (see endnote). One can speculate that the use of HDC upfront, the inclusion of high-dose anthracycline in the preparative regimen, or the use of a combination of alkylating agents in tandem may account for these apparent differences. At the present time, neither historical controls nor the completed large Philadelphia Intergroup randomized trial[6] support the use of HDC and HSCT on a routine basis for patients with metastatic breast cancer. However, a potential beneficial role for patients who achieve a complete remission with salvage chemotherapy may still be possible. Unfortunately, this question remains open, as the power of the available randomized trials is inadequate to provide meaningful information. Such information would be of great importance, and may answer a common criticism that relates to patient selection in HDC trials.

Preliminary results of randomized adjuvant trials[9–11] seem to indicate that a high cumulative total dose of chemotherapy may be equivalent to one cycle of myeloablative HDC and HSCT. Indeed, the CALGB trial[10] does not compare HDC to conventional 'standard'-dose adjuvant chemotherapy, but rather to 'intermediate'-dose combined alkylating agents therapy. It is also of particular interest that the outcome for patients enrolled in this trial and who were not transplanted appears better than in any previously reported randomized trial within the CALGB for this patient population. Better patient selection, more effective therapy, consolidation with combined intermediate-dose alkylating agents, locoregional radiation therapy, and hormonal therapy may all have played a role in contributing to this improved outcome. Similarly to the CALGB trial, the Scandinavian Breast Cancer Study Group[11] randomized high-risk breast cancer patients to receive nine courses of individually tailored 5-FU, epirubicin, and cyclophosphamide (FEC), or three courses of intermediate-dose FEC followed by HDC and HSCT. The tailored regimen was used in an attempt to compensate for the significant interindividual variation in drug clearance rates, and was determined based on the hematologic toxicity profile. This study did not address the relative effectiveness of transplant versus conventional therapy as the planned cumulative doses for the tailored therapy arm actually exceeded those for the HDC arm. This trial rather questions the optimal way of delivering chemotherapy, i.e., one cycle of high-dose chemotherapy versus six cycles of intensified, intermediate-dose chemotherapy with a higher cumulative chemotherapy dose.

While the results of the ongoing or recently completed large randomized trials from Europe and the USA comparing HDC with conventional therapy in solid tumors mature and become available, newer strategies are being actively investigated in an attempt to improve the outcome of HDC. These include methods to overcome tumor resistance, methods for purging hematopoietic stem cells of malignant cells, and the addition post-transplant of an effective, non-toxic anticancer treatment.

One approach to overcome *cancer cell resistance* might involve, as in the South African trials,[8–9] the upfront use of tandem transplants. Another might include strategies to harness the immune response to eliminate minimal residual disease. Numerous pilot studies are currently ongoing in this regard. They can be regrouped into three large categories:

1 non-specific strategies attempting to induce an autologous[12] or an allogeneic[13] graft versus tumor effect;
2 approaches using targeted humoral immunity with monoclonal antibodies (e.g., monoclonal antibodies directed to the breast cancer growth factor receptor, HER2/*neu*);
3 attempts to improve antigen presentation by using various vaccination strategies (e.g., vaccination against antigens commonly expressed in adenocarcinomas such as *muc-1*).

The precise value of *graft purging* is difficult to assess in most disease settings, especially in breast cancer. Several methods of purging have been reported and include the use of chemotherapy,[14] CD-34+ selection,[15] purging with monoclonal antibodies,[16] and *ex-vivo* expansion of stem cells.[17] Most of the evaluations of purging strategies have focused thus far on safety and engraftment issues, and none has been tested in randomized clinical trials. Nevertheless, therapeutic results for tumor purging so far do not appear meaningfully different from those of studies in which purging has not been performed.

Finally, the *addition post-transplant of an effective therapy* as recently demonstrated in a randomized trial of 13-cis-retinoic acid (RA) in patients with high-risk neuroblastoma is an interesting avenue to explore.[18] Based on the observation that 13-cis-RA can induce differentiation and growth arrest of neuroblastoma cell lines *in vitro*, the trial was designed to determine if 13-cis-RA can prevent recurrences from minimal residual disease after intensive therapy. In this study, 539 patients with high-risk neuroblastoma were randomized, after induction chemotherapy, either to myeloablative chemoradiotherapy supported by purged autologous HSCT or to intense non-myeloablative chemotherapy. Both study arms were then randomized upon completion of their assigned treatment to 13-cis-RA (160 mg/m^2/d $\times$ 2 weeks/month $\times$ 6 months) or no further therapy. 13-cis-RA was well tolerated, and the study clearly demonstrated a significant improvement of the 3-year disease-free survival with autologous transplantation and the post-transplant addition of 13-cis-RA (55% versus 39%).

It has become clear from initial trials investigating the role of chemoradiotherapy dose escalation that high-dose therapy alone does not eradicate the malignancy in many patients. Additionally, the benefit of a potential lower relapse rate in patients receiving higher doses of chemoradiotherapy was offset by increased transplant-related toxic deaths.[19] Initially, the hematopoietic stem cells have been regarded as a supportive care modality for restoring hematopoiesis, and this is indeed the case for autologous HSCT. Nevertheless, in the allogeneic transplant setting, an antitumor potential of allogeneic leukocytes has been recognized and well documented. Indirect evidence supporting the existence of a 'graft-versus-tumor' reaction associated with allogeneic HSCT has been observed in patients with hematologic malignancies. These include the following observations:

1 Abrupt withdrawal of immunosuppression or a flare of acute graft-versus-host disease (GVHD) can re-establish complete remission in some patients with relapsed leukemia.[20]
2 The risk of leukemic relapse is higher in recipients of syngeneic marrow grafts compared to recipients of allogeneic grafts.[21]
3 GVHD after allogeneic HSCT may be protective against relapse.[22]
4 T-cell depletion of an allogeneic graft results in an increased relapse rate, especially in patients with chronic myeloid leukemia.[23]

Based on these observations, newer methods for performing allogeneic transplantation have emerged. Conditioning regimens 'de-escalating' the intensity of chemotherapy and/or radiation therapy were designed and developed, not with the aim of eradicating the malignancy, but to provide sufficient myelosuppression to allow the engraftment of allogeneic stem cells and to permit development of a graft-versus-tumor effect. These relatively non-toxic conditioning regimens have produced less morbidity and allowed older and more medically infirm patients, who cannot tolerate conventional high-dose preparative regimens, to be transplanted. This approach may prove beneficial in diseases where graft-versus-malignancy exists and is effective. Initial studies focused on indolent hematologic malignancies for which the success of this strategy requires the development of an effective graft-versus-tumor effect before the underlying disease can progress.[24] These studies have shown the feasibility of this approach, and a number of patients have experienced clinical, and occasionally molecular, remissions of their underlying malignancies. This new concept has opened the door for a wider application of adoptive allogeneic cell-mediated immunotherapy in a number of clinical indications such as solid tumors. Ongoing trials assessing the potential role of allogeneic HSCT using a non-myeloablative conditioning in renal cell carcinoma[25,26] and malignant melanoma[26] are promising, but thus far too preliminary to provide meaningful conclusions. An important and unresolved issue following non-myeloablative allogeneic transplantation is the optimal immunosuppressive therapy. As acute GVHD does occur and remains a significant hurdle to successful transplantation after non-myeloablative regimens, efforts have focused on effective strategies to separate GVHD from the graft-versus-tumor effect. Such strategies are critical for the success of this treatment approach and are being actively investigated.

In conclusion, the role of HDC and autologous HSCT in the management of solid tumors is far from being well defined and remains an active area of continued study in cancer therapy. Fortunately, the recent completion of several large, randomized trials from Europe and the USA comparing HDC with conventional therapy in solid tumors promises that more definitive information will emerge over the next few years. The immune graft-versus-malignancy effect responsible for part of the benefit observed after allogeneic HSCT is a promising new modality in cancer treatment. The reduction of the acute toxicities with the non-myeloablative conditioning regimens may allow a broader application for such regimens and provide an effective, less hazardous anticancer therapy mediated by the immune system.

ENDNOTE

These results should be viewed in the light of recent information suggesting that data from a randomized trial of HDC for locally advanced breast cancer by Bezwoda[9] may have been contaminated. Therefore, the validity and conclusions of the present study[8] may also be compromised.

REFERENCES

1. Hill RP, Stanley JA. The response of hypoxic B16 melanoma cells to in vivo treatment with chemotherapeutic agents. Cancer Res 1975; 35:1147–53.

2. Schabel FM, Griswold DP, Corbett TH, *et al*. Increasing the therapeutic response rate to anticancer drugs by applying the basic principles of pharmacology. Cancer 1984; 50:1160–7.

3. Frei III E, Canellos GP. Dose, a critical factor in cancer chemotherapy. Am J Med 1980; 69:585–94.

4. Hryniuk WM, Bush H. The importance of dose intensity in chemotherapy of metastatic breast cancer. J Clin Oncol 1984; 2:1281–7.

5. Henderson IC, Hayes DF, Gelman R. Dose-response in the treatment of breast cancer: a critical review. J Clin Oncol 1988; 6:1501–15.

6. Stadtmauer EA, O'Neill A, Golstein LJ, *et al*. Phase III randomized trial of high-dose chemotherapy and stem cell support shows no difference in overall survival or severe toxicity compared to maintenance chemotherapy with CMF for women with metastatic breast cancer who are responding to conventional induction chemotherapy: the Philadelphia Intergroup Study 'PBT-1'. Proc Am Soc Clin Oncol 1999; 18:1a.

7. Lotz J-P, Cure H, Janvier M, *et al*. High dose chemotherapy with hematopoietic stem cells transplantation for metastatic breast cancer: results of the French protocol PEGASE 04. Proc Am Soc Clin Oncol 1999; 18:43a.

8. Bezwoda WR, Seymour L, Dansey RD. High-dose chemotherapy with hematopoietic rescue as primary treatment for metastatic breast cancer: a randomized trial. J Clin Oncol 1995; 13:2483.

9. Bezwoda WR. Randomized controlled trial of high dose chemotherapy (HD-CNVp) versus standard dose (CAF) chemotherapy for high risk surgically treated primary breast cancer. Proc Am Soc Clin Oncol 1999; 18:2a.

10. Peters W, Rosner G, Vredenburgh J, *et al*. A prospective randomized comparison of two doses of combination alkylating agents as consolidation after CAF in high-risk primary breast cancer involving ten or more axillary lymph nodes: preliminary results of CALGB 9082/SWOG 9114/NCIC MA-13. Proc Am Soc Clin Oncol 1999; 18:1a.

11. The Scandinavian Breast Cancer Study Group 9401. Results from a randomized adjuvant breast cancer study with high-dose chemotherapy with CTCb supported by autologous bone marrow stem cells versus dose escalated and tailored FEC therapy. Proc Am Soc Clin Oncol 1999; 18:2a.

12. Kennedy MJ, Vogelsang GB, Jones RJ, *et al*. Phase I trial of interferon gamma to potentiate cyclosporine-induced graft-versus-host disease in women undergoing autologous bone marrow transplantation for breast cancer. J Clin Oncol 1994; 12:249–57.

13. Eibl B, Schwaighofer H, Nachbaur D, *et al*. Evidence for a graft-versus-tumor effect in a patient treated with marrow ablative chemotherapy and allogeneic bone marrow transplantation for breast cancer. Blood 1996; 88:1501–8.

14. Shpall EJ, Jones RB, Bast RC. 4-Hydroperoxycyclo-phosphamide purging of breast cancer from the mononuclear cell fraction of bone marrow in patients receiving high-dose chemotherapy and autologous

marrow support: a phase I trial. J Clin Oncol 1991; 9:85–93.

15. Franklin WA, Shpall EJ, Archer P, *et al*. Immunocyto-chemical detection of breast cancer cells in marrow and peripheral blood of patients undergoing high-dose chemotherapy with autologous stem cell support. Breast Cancer Res Treat 1996; 41:1–13.

16. Anderson I, Shpall EJ, Leslie D, *et al*. Elimination of malignant clonogenic breast cancer cells from human bone marrow. Cancer Res 1989; 49:4659–64.

17. Williams SF, Lee WJ, Bender JG, *et al*. Selection and expansion of peripheral blood CD 34+ cells in autologous stem cell transplantation for breast cancer. Blood 1996; 87:1687–91.

18. Matthay KK, Villablanca JG, Seeger RC, *et al*. Treatment of high-risk neuroblastoma with intensive chemotherapy, radiotherapy, autologous bone marrow transplantation, and 13-cis-retinoic acid. Children's Cancer Group. N Engl J Med 1999; 341(16):1165–73.

19. Clift R, Buckner D, Appelbaum FR, *et al*. Allogeneic marrow transplantation in patients with chronic myeloid leukemia in the chronic phase: a randomized trial of two irradiation regimens. Blood 1991; 77:1660–5.

20. Odom L, August C, Githens J, *et al*. Remission of relapsed leukemia during a graft versus-host reaction: a graft-versus-leukemia reaction in man? Lancet 1978; 2:537–40.

21. Gale PR, Horowitz M, Ash R, *et al*. Identical-twin bone marrow transplants for leukemia. Ann Intern Med 1994; 120:646–52.

22. Weiden P, Sullivan K, Flournoy N, *et al*. Anti-leukemic effect of chronic graft-versus-host disease: contribution to improved survival after allogeneic marrow transplantation. N Engl J Med 1981; 304:1529–33.

23. Apperley J, Mauro F, Goldman J, *et al*. Bone marrow transplantation for chronic myeloid leukemia in first chronic phase: importance of a graft-versus-leukemia effect. Br J Haematol 1988; 69:239–45.

24. Khouri IF, Keating M, Korbling M, *et al*. Transplant-lite: induction of graft-versus-malignancy using fludarabine-based non-myeloablative chemotherapy and allogeneic blood progenitor-cell transplantation as treatment of lymphoid malignancies. J Clin Oncol 1998; 16:2817–24.

25. Childs R, Contentin N, Clave E, *et al*. Sustained regression of metastatic renal cell carcinoma following non-myeloablative allogeneic peripheral blood stem cell transplantation: a new application of allogeneic immunotherapy. Blood 1999; 94:710a.

26. Porter DL, Connors JM, Van Deerlin VM, *et al*. Graft-versus-tumor induction with donor leukocyte infusions as primary therapy for patients with malignancies. J Clin Oncol 1999; 17:1234–43.

Editors' selected abstracts

Typhlitis complicating autologous blood stem cell transplantation for breast cancer.

Boggio L, Pooley R, Roth SI, Winter JN.

Department of Medicine, Division of Hematology/Oncology, The Robert H Lurie Comprehensive Cancer Center, Northwestern University Medical School, Chicago, IL, USA.

Bone Marrow Transplantation 25(3):321–6, 2000, February.

Three cases of typhlitis occurring during autologous blood stem cell transplantation (ABSCT) for metastatic breast cancer are described. Typhlitis is a rare complication of neutropenia and has uncommonly been reported in the autologous transplant setting. Although it has been most commonly described in children with leukemia, typhlitis has increasingly been reported in adult leukemias and in association with neutropenia secondary to chemotherapy for a number of solid tumors. Only five previous cases of typhlitis in the setting of ABSCT have been described. Whereas diarrhea and fever are common toxicities associated with high-dose chemotherapy, it is likely that many cases of typhlitis go unrecognized.

Importance of radiation therapy for breast cancer patients treated with high-dose chemotherapy and stem cell transplant.

Buchholz TA, Tucker SL, Moore RA, McNeese MD, Strom EA, Jhingran A, Hortobagyi GN, Singletary SE, Champlin RE.

Department of Radiation Oncology, The University of Texas M.D. Anderson Cancer Center, Houston, TX, USA.

International Journal of Radiation Oncology, Biology, Physics 46(2):337–43, 2000, January 15.

Purpose: To determine local–regional failure rates in breast cancer patients treated with surgery and high-dose chemotherapy with stem cell transplant and to relate local–regional failure to the use and timing of radiation treatment. *Methods and materials:* We retrospectively reviewed the records of 165 breast cancer patients treated on institutional protocols with surgery and high-dose chemotherapy with stem cell transplant. All patients had either Stage III disease, 10 or more positive axillary lymph nodes, or 4 or more positive axillary lymph nodes following neoadjuvant chemotherapy. Twelve patients had inflammatory breast cancer. Thirteen patients treated with breast preservation and 5 patients who died from toxicity within 30 days of transplant were excluded from the analyses of local–regional recurrences. In the remaining 147 patients, 108 were treated with adjuvant radiation and 39 were not. The disease stage distribution for these two groups was comparable. The median follow-up for surviving patients was 35 months. *Results:* The 3- and 5-year actuarial disease-free survival (DFS) for the entire group was 60% and 51%, respectively. The 5-year rates of freedom from isolated local–regional recurrence were 95% in the patients treated with adjuvant radiation and 86% in the patients who did not receive radiation ($p = 0.014$, log rank comparison). The 5-year rates of any local–regional recurrence as a first event (isolated recurrences plus those with simultaneous local–regional and distant recurrences) were 92% versus 82%, respectively for patients whose treatment did and did not include radiation ($p = 0.038$). We could not demonstrate a correlation of the timing of radiation with the risk of local–regional recurrence. *Conclusions:* These data indicate that high-dose chemotherapy does not negate the importance of radiation in optimizing local–regional control in patients with high-risk breast cancer. Given the results of recent randomized trials studying postmastectomy radiation, which show that improving local–regional control improves overall survival (OS), we believe that all breast cancer patients with high-risk primary breast cancer who are treated with high-dose chemotherapy with stem cell transplant should receive radiation as a component of their treatment.

Mobilization of peripheral-blood stem cells by concurrent administration of daniplestim and granulocyte colony-stimulating factor in patients with breast cancer or lymphoma.

DiPersio JF, Schuster MW, Abboud CN, Winter JN, Santos VR, Collins DM, Sherman JW, Baum CM.

Division of Bone Marrow Transplantation and Stem Cell Biology, Washington University School of Medicine, St Louis, MO, USA.

Journal of Clinical Oncology 18(14):2762–71, 2000, July.

Purpose: To evaluate the safety and hematopoietic activity of daniplestim administered concurrently with granulocyte colony-stimulating factor (G-CSF) for peripheral-blood stem-cell (PBSC) mobilization. *Patients and methods:* In the initial dose-escalation phase, 25 patients with adenocarcinoma of the breast (AB; 13 patients) or lymphoma (12 patients) were given daniplestim at doses ranging from 0.1 to 3.75 microgram/kg/d plus G-CSF 10 microgram/kg/d. In the randomized phase, 52 patients with AB (27 patients) or lymphoma (25 patients) were randomized within disease categories to the daniplestim dose chosen in the dose-escalation phase plus G-CSF 10 microgram/kg/d (D + G) or placebo plus G-CSF 10 microgram/kg/d (P + G) for up to 7 days. *Results:* A daniplestim dose of 2.5 microgram/kg/d was chosen for further study because it was hematopoietically active and had an acceptable side-effect profile. In the randomized phase, in patients with AB, D + G was associated with a higher probability ($p = 0.0696$) of collecting $\geq 2.5 \times 10^6$ CD34(+) cells/kg and significantly higher circulating CD34(+) cell counts ($p = 0.0498$) on days 6 through 9 after the initiation of dosing. The target level was more likely to be reached with additional leukaphereses in the patients given D + G. Patients given P + G did not benefit from additional leukaphereses beyond the first procedure. The type of mobilization did show a trend toward a shorter duration of neutropenia in the D + G group. The adverse events with D + G consisted largely of mild to moderate flu-like symptoms, including headache and fever, and occurred more frequently than with P + G. *Conclusion:* Daniplestim administered at 2.5 microgram/kg/d is tolerable and active when combined with G-CSF, and the combination may prove more effective than G-CSF alone in promoting the collection of adequate numbers of CD34(+) cells for PBSC infusion in patients with AB.

Delphi-panel analysis of appropriateness of high-dose chemotherapy and blood cell or bone marrow autotransplants in women with breast cancer.

Gale RP, Park RE, Dubois R, Bitran JD, Buzdar A, Hortobagyi G, Jones SE, Lazar GS, Spitzer G, Swain SM, Vaughn CB, Vogel CE, Martino S.

Salick Health Care, Inc., Los Angeles, CA, USA.

Clinical Transplantation 14(1):32–41, 2000, February.

Background: There is controversy whether high-dose chemotherapy and a blood cell or bone marrow autotransplant is a better treatment than conventional-dose chemotherapy for women with local/regional or metastatic breast cancer. Subject selection and time-to-treatment biases make definitive comparison impossible. Recent results of randomized trials are contradictory. *Objective:* Determine appropriateness of high-dose chemotherapy and a blood cell or bone marrow autotransplant in women with breast cancer. *Panelists:* Nine breast cancer experts from diverse geographic sites and practice settings. *Evidence:* Boolean MEDLINE searches of 'breast cancer' and 'chemotherapy' and/or 'blood cell' or 'bone marrow transplants'. *Process:* We used a modified Delphi-panel group judgement process. Clinical variables were permuted to define 2058 clinical settings. Each panelist rated appropriateness of high-dose therapy and an autotransplant versus conventional therapy on a 9-point ordinal scale (1: most inappropriate, 9: most appropriate). An appropriateness index was developed based on median rating and amount of disagreement. The relationship of appropriateness indices to the permuted clinical variables was considered by analysis of variance and recursive partitioning. *Conclusions:* In women with local/regional breast cancer autotransplants were rated: (1) appropriate in those with ≥ 10 cancer-involved lymph nodes; (2) uncertain in those with 4–9 cancer-involved nodes; and (3) inappropriate in women with ≤ 3 cancer-involved lymph nodes. In women with metastatic breast cancer autotransplants were rated: (1) appropriate in those with metastases to 'favorable' sites (skin, lymph node, pleura) and a complete or partial response to chemotherapy; (2) uncertain in women with metastases to 'unfavorable' sites (lung, liver, or central nervous system) and a complete response to chemotherapy or those with bone metastases and a complete or partial response or stable disease after chemotherapy; and (3) inappropriate in other settings.

Clinical outcome of breast and ovarian cancer patients treated with high-dose chemotherapy, autologous stem cell rescue and THERATOPE STn-KLH cancer vaccine.

Holmberg LA, Oparin DV, Gooley T, Lilleby K, Bensinger W, Reddish MA, MacLean GD, Longenecker BM, Sandmaier BM.

Clinical Research Division, Fred Hutchinson Cancer Research Center, Seattle, WA, USA.

Bone Marrow Transplant 25(12):1233–41, 2000, June.

The purpose of this study was to evaluate the toxicity and potential efficacy of administering the THERATOPE STn-KLH cancer vaccine to ovarian and breast cancer patients after an autologous stem cell transplant. Forty patients (11 high-risk stage II/III breast cancer, 22 stage IV breast cancer, and seven stage III/IV ovarian cancer patients) were treated with high-dose chemotherapy followed by autologous/syngeneic stem cell rescue and vaccination with THERATOPE STn-KLH (Sialyl-Tn-KLH with Detox-B Stable Emulsion). Each patient was scheduled to receive a total of five vaccinations beginning on days 30–151 after stem cell infusion. The vaccine was well tolerated. Induration and erythema at the site of injection were the most common side-effects. When one compares the outcome of patients vaccinated with 66 breast and ovarian cancer patients who were not, following risk-adjustment analysis, vaccinated patients appeared more likely to survive ($p = 0.07$) and less likely to relapse ($p = 0.10$). Vaccinated patients with the greatest specific lytic activity against STn + OVCAR tumor cells relative to nonspecific killing of Daudi cells tended to remain in remission longer than patients who displayed less specific immune activity ($p = 0.057$). We conclude that the THERATOPE STn-KLH cancer vaccine is well tolerated in breast and ovarian cancer patients after autologous transplant and, while not statistically significant, the trends in data support the concept that THERATOPE vaccine may decrease the risk for relapse and death and thus warrants further study.

Randomized trial of high-dose chemotherapy and blood cell autografts for high-risk primary breast carcinoma.

Hortobagyi GN, Buzdar AU, Theriault RL, Valero V, Frye D, Booser DJ, Holmes FA, Giralt S, Khouri I, Andersson B, Gajewski JL, Rondon G, Smith TL, Singletary SE, Ames FC, Sneige N, Strom EA, McNeese MD, Deisseroth AB, Champlin RE.

Department of Breast Medical Oncology, The University of Texas M.D. Anderson Cancer Center, Houston, TX, USA.

Journal of the National Cancer Institute 92(3):225–33, 2000, February 2.

Background: Uncontrolled studies have reported encouraging outcomes for patients with high-risk primary breast cancer treated with high-dose chemotherapy and autologous hematopoietic stem cell support. We conducted a prospective randomized trial to compare standard-dose chemotherapy with the same therapy followed by high-dose chemotherapy. *Patients and methods:* Patients with 10 or more positive axillary lymph nodes after primary breast surgery or patients with four or more positive lymph nodes after four cycles of primary (neoadjuvant) chemotherapy were eligible. All patients were to receive eight cycles of 5-fluorouracil, doxorubicin (adriamycin), and cyclophosphamide (FAC). Patients were stratified by stage and randomly assigned to receive two cycles of high-dose cyclophosphamide, etoposide, and cisplatin with autologous hematopoietic stem cell support or no additional chemotherapy. Tamoxifen was planned for postmenopausal patients with estrogen receptor-positive tumors and chest wall radiotherapy was planned for all. All *p* values are from two-sided tests. *Results:* Seventy-eight patients (48 after primary surgery and 30 after primary chemotherapy) were registered. Thirty-nine patients were randomly assigned to FAC and 39 to FAC followed by high-dose chemotherapy. After a median follow-up of 6.5 years, there have been 41 relapses. In intention-to-treat analyses, estimated 3-year relapse-free survival rates were 62% and 48% for FAC and FAC/high-dose chemotherapy, respectively ($p = 0.35$), and 3-year survival rates were 77% and 58%, respectively ($p = 0.23$). Overall, there was greater and more frequent morbidity associated with high-dose chemotherapy than with FAC; there was one septic death associated with high-dose chemotherapy. *Conclusions:* No relapse-free or overall survival advantage was associated with the use of high-dose chemotherapy, and morbidity was increased with its use. Thus, high-dose chemotherapy is not indicated outside a clinical trial.

Evaluation of the predictive value of Her-2/neu overexpression and p53 mutations in high-risk primary breast cancer patients treated with high-dose chemotherapy and autologous stem-cell transplantation.

Nieto Y, Cagnoni PJ, Nawaz S, Shpall EJ, Yerushalmi R, Cook B, Russell P, McDermit J, Murphy J, Bearman SI, Jones RB.

University of Colorado Bone Marrow Transplant Program and Departments of Pathology and Biostatistics, University of Colorado, Denver, CO, USA.

Journal of Clinical Oncology 18(10):2070–80, 2000, May.

Purpose: To ascertain the predictive value of Her-2/neu overexpression and p53 mutations, assessed by immunohistochemistry, in high-risk primary breast cancer (HRPBC) treated with high-dose chemotherapy (HDCT). *Patients and methods:* We obtained paraffin-embedded tumor blocks from 146 HRPBC patients previously enrolled at our program onto clinical trials of HDCT for four to nine involved axillary lymph nodes, ≥10 involved axillary nodes, or inflammatory carcinoma. All patients received the same HDCT regimen, with cyclophosphamide, cisplatin, and carmustine (STAMP-I), followed by autologous stem-cell transplantation. Median follow-up was 42 months (range, 5 to 90 months). The same pathologist, blinded to clinical outcome, reviewed all immunostained slides. *Results:* Positive results for Her-2/neu and p53 were found in 44.5% and 34% of the patients, respectively. Positivity for Her-2/neu was significantly associated with increased risk of relapse and death. No correlation was found between p53 mutations and relapse-free survival (RFS) or overall survival (OS). Multivariate analyses included Her-2/neu overexpression and the following variables previously identified as independent predictors of outcome in this population: tumor size, nodal ratio (number of involved nodes/number of dissected nodes), and hormone receptor status. All four variables had independent value. *Conclusion:* Her-2/neu overexpression is an independent negative predictor of RFS and OS in HRPBC treated with HDCT. Its inclusion in our previously described predictive model increases the predictive capacity of this model for the low-risk subgroup. In contrast, p53 mutations lack predictive value in this setting.

High-dose chemotherapy with stem cell support for solid tumors in adults.

Rodenhuis S, de Vries EG.

Het Nederlands Kankerinstituut/Antoni van Leeuwenhoek Ziekenhuis, afd. Medische Oncologie, Amsterdam, The Netherlands.

Nederlands Tijdschrift voor Geneeskunde 143(14):731–8, 1999, April 3.

High-dose chemotherapy for advanced solid malignancies has been the subject of many clinical studies. The replacement of autologous bone marrow transplantation by peripheral blood haematopoietic progenitor cell transplantation and other advances in supportive care have led to a considerable reduction of therapy-related mortality and morbidity. In certain rare disorders, such as germ cell tumours or paediatric sarcomas in adults, high-dose therapy is currently considered the therapeutic standard. It is likely that a subgroup of patients with high-risk or disseminated breast cancer can also benefit in terms of survival from this treatment modality, but final proof from randomized studies remains to be generated. On theoretical grounds, high-dose chemotherapy could also be effective in small cell lung cancer and ovarian cancer, and randomized studies to answer this question are in progress. Many investigators concur that high-dose chemotherapy often leads to dramatic cytoreduction in solid tumours, but only rarely achieves cure. Novel therapeutic modalities are required to control the residual microscopic disease.

Conventional-dose chemotherapy compared with high-dose chemotherapy plus autologous hematopoietic stem-cell transplantation for metastatic breast cancer.

Stadtmauer EA, O'Neill A, Goldstein LJ, Crilley PA, Mangan KF, Ingle JN, Brodsky I, Martino S, Lazarus HM, Erban JK, Sickles C, Glick JH.

From the University of Pennsylvania Cancer Center, Philadelphia, PA (E.A.S., C.S., J.H.G.); Dana-Farber Cancer Institute, Boston, MA (A.O.); Fox Chase Cancer Center, Philadelphia, PA (L.J.G.); Hahnemann University, Philadelphia, PA (P.A.C., I.B.); Temple University, Philadelphia, PA (K.F.M.); Mayo Clinic, Rochester, MN (J.N.I.); John Wayne Cancer Institute, Santa Monica, CA (S.M.); University Hospitals of Cleveland, Cleveland, OH (H.M.L.); and Tufts–New England Medical Center, Boston, MA (J.K.E.), USA.

New England Journal of Medicine 342:1069–76, 2000, April 13.

Background: We conducted a randomized trial in which we compared high-dose chemotherapy plus hematopoietic stem-cell rescue with a prolonged course of monthly conventional-dose chemotherapy in women with metastatic breast cancer. *Methods:* Women 18 to 60 years of age who had metastatic breast cancer received four to six cycles of standard combination chemotherapy. Patients who had a complete or partial response to induction chemotherapy were then randomly assigned to receive either a single course of high doses of carboplatin, thiotepa, and cyclophosphamide plus transplantation of autologous hematopoietic stem cells or up to 24 cycles of cyclophosphamide, methotrexate, and fluorouracil in conventional doses. The primary end point was survival. *Results:* The median follow-up was 37 months. Of 553 patients who enrolled in the study, 58 had a complete response to induction chemotherapy and 252 had a partial response. Of these, 110 patients were assigned to receive high-dose chemotherapy plus hematopoietic stem cells and 89 were assigned to receive conventional-dose chemotherapy. In an intention-to-treat analysis, we found no significant difference in survival overall at three years between the two treatment groups (32 percent in the transplantation group and 38 percent in the conventional-chemotherapy group). There was no significant difference between the two treatments in the median time to progression of the disease (9.6 months for high-dose chemotherapy plus hematopoietic stem cells and 9.0 months for conventional-dose chemotherapy). *Conclusions:* As compared with maintenance chemotherapy in conventional doses, high-dose chemotherapy plus autologous stem-cell transplantation soon after the induction of a complete or partial remission with conventional-dose chemotherapy does not improve survival in women with metastatic breast cancer.

3

Occult metastases

SUNANDA J CHATTERJEE, DEBRA HAWES, CLIVE R TAYLOR, A MUNRO NEVILLE, AND RICHARD J COTE

INTRODUCTION

The goal of diagnostic surgical oncology is twofold: to arrive at the specific diagnosis (benign or malignant and cell of origin) and to stage the tumor. These are the two important parameters that determine the rational treatment of any type of tumor. Using pathological criteria in conjunction with clinical parameters, the pathologist and the clinician attempt to determine the outcome for a patient. Staging criteria are used to evaluate almost any type of solid tumor and are important not only in predicting prognosis, but also in selecting appropriate therapy.

Specific staging criteria for most tumors of epithelial origin (carcinomas) include the presence or absence of invasion through basement membrane, invasion to surrounding structures, and the presence of metastases; these criteria vary for each type of tumor. Although staging can provide estimates of outcome for populations of patients who have tumors with similar characteristics, stage cannot determine the outcome for an individual patient. For example, in the case of breast cancer, the single most important prognostic parameter is the presence or absence of metastases to the axillary lymph nodes. However, a proportion of patients with no evidence of nodal involvement will experience recurrence. Conversely, not all patients who have metastases in the axillary lymph nodes develop recurrent disease. In other words, it is not possible to determine which individual will relapse based on current clinical and pathological staging parameters alone.

The most important factor affecting the outcome for patients with invasive cancers is whether the tumor has spread, either regionally (to regional lymph nodes) or systemically. However, a proportion of patients with no evidence of systemic dissemination will develop recurrent disease after primary therapy. Clearly, these patients had occult systemic spread of disease that was undetectable by methods routinely employed (careful pathological, clinical, biochemical, and radiological evaluation). In addition, the success of adjuvant therapy is assumed to stem from its ability to eradicate occult metastases before they become clinically evident.[1] Therefore, methods for the detection of occult metastases in patients with the earliest stage of cancer, i.e., prior to the detection of metastases by any other clinical or pathological analysis, have received a great deal of attention. This chapter focuses on the detection and significance of occult metastatic cells in the bone marrow and lymph nodes of patients with various types of tumors.

METHODS USED FOR THE DETECTION OF OCCULT METASTASES

Immunohistochemistry

Following pioneering studies at the Ludwig Institute and Royal Marsden Hospital in London, England,[2] a number of groups have used immunohistochemical procedures to identify occult metastatic cancer cells in the bone marrow and lymph nodes of patients with cancer. Whereas many of the initial studies focused on breast cancer,[2–6] tumors from other organs, such as colon,[7–9] prostate,[10–14] and lung,[15–19] are now under investigation. Immunohistochemical methods are based on the ability of monoclonal antibodies to distinguish between cells of different histogenesis (i.e., epithelial cancer cells versus the hematopoietic and stromal cells of the bone marrow and lymph nodes). The results indicate that it is possible to identify occult metastatic cancer cells in lymph nodes and bone marrow prior to their detection by any other method, and that the presence of these cells may be an important risk factor for disease recurrence.

The most widely used monoclonal antibodies to detect occult metastatic cells are antibodies to epithelial-specific antigens. These antibodies do not react with normal hematopoietic or stromal cells present in the bone marrow or lymph nodes. None of the antibodies used in any study is specific for cancer; all react with normal and malignant epithelial cells. They are useful because they can identify an extrinsic population of epithelial cells in bone marrow or lymph nodes, where there are normally no epithelial elements. The reported sensitivity of the immunohistochemical method ranges from the detection of one epithelial cell in 10 000 [3] to that of two to five epithelial cells in a million hematopoietic cells.[3,6,20]

Molecular methods

Recently, molecular methods have been used to detect occult metastatic cells. The method usually employed is reverse transcriptase–polymerase chain reaction (RT–PCR), which differentiates gene expression between epithelial and lymphoid cells to identify epithelial cancer cells. RT–PCR entails the isolation and reverse transcription of epithelial-specific messenger RNA to complementary DNA (cDNA) and, thereafter, involves PCR-based amplification of the cDNA template between specific primers. This results in a several thousand-fold amplification of the signal, and makes the method theoretically extremely sensitive. The drawbacks of the method include the chance of a low level of epithelial gene expression from lymphoid cells that could result in high background, and the inability to employ morphologic criteria to confirm the presence of metastatic cells; this has been the case in our studies. However, RT–PCR has been successfully used for the detection of occult metastases to the bone marrow in melanoma and carcinoma of the prostate and colon.

Flow cytometry

A flow-cytometric assay has recently been developed to detect rare cancer cells in bone marrow and blood.[21] The method is reported to be extremely sensitive, with an ability to detect one positive cell in ten million blood cells in a model system; this is in contrast to all other reports on the sensitivity of flow cytometry.[22] One major disadvantage of most flow-cytometric systems is the inability to morphologically characterize the cells constituting the 'positive' events. However, by employing sophisticated cell-sorting technologies, in which the extrinsic cell population can be captured for subsequent morphologic evaluation, the rate of detection might be improved.

With this overview, the following sections describe the significance of detecting occult metastatic cells in bone marrow and lymph nodes from patients with various cancers.

DETECTION OF OCCULT METASTASES IN THE BONE MARROW

Bone marrow is a frequent site of distant metastasis in a variety of cancers, such as carcinoma of the breast and prostate. Epithelial cancer cells detected in the bone marrow do not necessarily have the potential to form metastatic lesions at the sample site; rather, they may merely be cells in transit. In this regard, we have found that extrinsic cells could be identified in the bone marrow of patients with metastatic disease, even when aspirates were taken from sites distant from the areas of clinically detectable tumor involvement.[23] Moreover, tumors that do not usually metastasize to the bone marrow, such as colon cancer, can be detected in the bone marrow aspirates in patients with early-stage disease.[24]

Peripheral blood would clearly be the most convenient sample site for studies to detect occult metastatic cells. Unfortunately, the yield of occult metastatic cells from peripheral blood is extremely low. Redding et al.[2] found that 28.2% of patients with breast cancer showed extrinsic cancer cells in their bone marrow, but only 2.7% of these patients had detectable cells in their peripheral blood. It is not clear why tumor cells are detected less commonly in peripheral blood than in bone marrow. The bone marrow vasculature consists of a unique sinusoidal system that may simply act as a filter that traps or concentrates malignant cells. The marrow environment may provide a more favorable support system for tumor cell proliferation than does blood. One may also speculate that cancer cells that are released into the systemic circulation represent a small subpopulation of cells with altered expression of cell adhesion molecules. Whatever the reason, bone marrow offers the best opportunity to detect cancer cells that have been released into the blood. Therefore, the majority of studies to detect occult metastatic cells in the systemic circulation have investigated bone marrow as a site of spread.

Detection of occult metastases in the bone marrow in patients with breast cancer

The majority of patients with newly diagnosed breast cancer have operable disease, and these patients are considered potentially curable. However, 35–40% of these patients, including up to 24% of patients with no evidence of metastasis at the time of diagnosis, develop recurrent disease after primary therapy. The most reliable prognostic parameters (lymph node status and tumor size) cannot predict which particular individual will progress. As a result, several groups have recommended adjuvant treatment for patients with lymph node-negative disease. While this is controversial (because the majority of node-negative patients will be clinically cured without adjuvant therapy), it is in this group of patients who have minimal occult metastases that adjuvant therapy should be most successful. It would be of great value, therefore, to be able to discriminate further and identify those patients with early-stage disease who are most likely to show recurrence. Detection of occult metastatic cells in these patients could be extremely beneficial in determining prognosis and in making treatment decisions.

Bone marrow is the single most common site of breast cancer metastasis, and up to 80% of patients with recurrent tumors will develop bony metastases at some point during the evolution of their disease;[25] it is also the most frequent initial site of clinically detectable breast cancer metastasis.[26] Tumor cells are estimated to be present in the bone marrow of 20–45% of patients with primary operable breast cancer,[2,5,23,27–29] and in 20–70% of patients with metastatic breast cancer.[30] As with most cancers, the most widely used method to detect occult metastatic cells is immunohistochemistry.

Immunohistochemical methods for detecting occult bone marrow metastases

Antibodies

A variety of antibodies have been used to detect metastatic breast cancer cells in the bone marrow. It is important to emphasize that the distinguishing feature of these antibodies is that they are epithelial specific, and do not react with bone marrow elements. The antibodies used in all the studies fall into two general classes (Table 3.1): (i) those reactive with cell surface antigens, and (ii) those reactive with cytostructural antigens.

Among antibodies to cell-surface molecules, those to epithelial membrane antigen (EMA) have been most widely used; these have been reported to react with plasma cells,[31] which could result in false-positive staining in bone marrow preparations. In addition, surface antigens tend to be unstable with certain types of fixation and handling; this can make their detection less reliable. As a result, several groups have used antibodies directed against cytoplasmic structural antigens, particularly low molecular weight cytokeratin intermediate filament proteins, to detect extrinsic cells in the bone marrow.[4,23,24] These antigens are usually well expressed by epithelial cells and are generally stable in a wide variety of fixatives.

Because of antigenic heterogeneity in all tissues (including malignant neoplasms), none of the antigens being detected is expressed in all of the cells in any given lesion. In order to minimize this problem and to ensure identification of the maximum number of extrinsic epithelial cells, we have used cocktails of antibodies that include antibodies to cell surface and cytokeratin intermediate filament antigens. The specificities of the antibodies used in all of the studies have been well characterized; they are all specific for epithelial cells and react with virtually all breast carcinomas. In addition, the antibodies used in our own studies have been tested on bone marrow samples from over 200 individuals, including normal individuals and those undergoing staging for lymphoma and leukemia.[20] No reactivity has been observed with normal or neoplastic hematopoietic cells. This feature is critical, because the assay is based on the differential antigenic expression of epithelial versus bone marrow mononuclear cells.

Bone marrow aspiration and cell separation

In general, bone marrow aspirates collected at the time of surgery are used to concentrate contaminating epithelial cells. Dearnaley et al.[32] found that the yield of positive cells improved when aspirates from multiple sites were obtained. Redding et al.[2] obtained bone marrow samples from eight sites (two sternal, one anterior iliac, two posterior iliac, and two sacral) for each patient. In our own studies, aspirations were collected from both anterior iliac crests and the sternum.

We have shown that separation of cells on a Ficoll-Hypaque density gradient results in a marked concentration of extrinsic epithelial cells. This method is superior to collection of the buffy coat layer followed by red-cell lysis for selectively concentrating epithelial cells in the bone marrow.[20] Most published studies have used the Ficoll-Hypaque density gradient to concentrate epithelial cells.

These methods should provide significant advantages over routinely sampled, formalin-fixed, paraffin-embedded bone marrow aspirates in bone biopsy samples. A large number of cells can be examined by using smears of cells that have a significantly concentrated population of the cells of interest. Also, the fixation used is less disruptive to the antigens than paraffin processing and decalcification, thus minimizing the risk of epitope loss, particularly in the case of cell-surface antigens.

Immunohistochemistry

Visualization of antigen-positive cells has been performed using light microscopy either manually or by

Table 3.1 *Antibodies used to detect breast cancer occult metastases*

Type of antigen	Specific antigen	References
Cell-surface antigens	EMA	Redding et al. (1983)[2]
		Mansi et al. (1987)[29]
	MBr 1	Porro et al. (1988)[30]
	17-1A	Schlimok et al. (1987)[24]
	T16, C26	Cote et al. (1988)[23]
Cytostructural antigens	Cytokeratin intermediate filament (e.g., AE-1, CAM 5.2)	Cote et al. (1988)[23]
		Schlimok et al. (1987)[24]
		Ellis et al. (1989)[4]

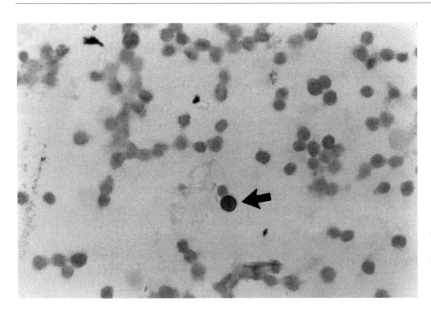

Figure 3.1 *Immunohistochemical staining with monoclonal antibodies to cytokeratin (AE1 and CAM5.2), showing a single cancer cell in the bone marrow of a patient with breast cancer.*

automated methods, or indirect immunofluorescence methods. Light microscopic visualization utilizes the immunoperoxidase and immunoalkaline phosphatase systems to develop color in the positive cells. These methods give good results (Figure 3.1),[2,20,24] and have certain advantages over immunofluorescence techniques. Not only do they provide a permanent record, but they also allow better cytologic evaluation of the cells.

Sensitivity

The sensitivity of methods used to detect extrinsic cells in the bone marrow is an important issue. In patients with early-stage cancers, the concentration of such extrinsic cells is presumably quite low; these cells cannot be detected by routine imaging procedures, biochemical determinations, or even cytologic examination of the bone marrow. The limits of detection of our methods have been studied using a model system in which the breast cancer cell lines MCF-7 and MDA-MB-468 were diluted in bone marrow cells of normal donors.[3,5,20] These studies demonstrate that, by using the methods described (immunofluorescence, immunoalkaline phosphatase, or immunoperoxidase), as few as two to five extrinsic epithelial cells can be detected in a background of one million bone marrow mononuclear cells.[3,6,20]

Automated detection of occult metastases

Although immunohistochemical methods are extremely sensitive, manual microscopic screening of rare positive (i.e., antigen-expressing) tumor cells is labor intensive, time consuming, and requires much expertise. Automated slide screening may facilitate the routine use of immunohistochemical methods to detect occult metastases. Attempts have already been undertaken along this line, with encouraging results.[10,33–35]

We have compared an automated method[34,35] to our standard, clinically validated manual methods for detecting rare tumor cells in bone marrow and blood. The automated system displayed a useful level of sensitivity, as evidenced by comparing the detection rates of automated versus manual screening. Evaluation of the sensitivity, accuracy, and reproducibility of the automated system was based on a comparison between results obtained by manual and automated screening methods. Two groups of specimens were used for this comparative study: a model system consisting of a cell line and clinical cases of lung carcinoma.

In the model cell line system, the breast cancer cell line MDA-MB-468 (MDA) was serially diluted in peripheral blood mononuclear cells (PBMCs) or the Raji (B-cell) line from original concentrations of 1–1000 MDA cells/10^6 PBMCs or Raji cells. In order to test the accuracy of cell selection by the automated system, all slides in the model system were analysed by the system as well as being manually reviewed by two investigators (blinded to MDA dilution) using a conventional microscope. At the lowest concentration (1 MDA cell/10^6 PBMCs), a single cancer cell was detected on two of three slides using both manual and automated screening.

In the clinical cases of lung carcinoma, bone marrow from patients with stage I–III non-small-cell lung cancer was used. The bone marrow samples were obtained from the sections of rib removed routinely at the time of surgery.[18] These bone marrow samples were curetted into heparinized media and placed in an insulated container at room temperature. Storage of bone marrow aspirates was possible for 24–48 h without significant adverse effects on epithelial cell antigenicity.[20] The results of these studies have shown that the sensitivity of the automated system is virtually identical to that of manual methods. The application of the automated system in the detection of occult metastases may provide a powerful tool for the assessment of lung cancer. However, at present automated image analysis is not reliable enough to be used for routine screening for occult metastases.

Molecular methods for detecting occult metastases in the bone marrow

Whereas immunohistochemical methods are effective in identifying occult metastases in the bone marrow of patients with operable breast cancer, these methods are laborious and require considerable technical expertise to perform and interpret. Efforts are now underway to develop molecular techniques based on the PCR to detect occult cancer metastases. These methods are theoretically more sensitive and provide the possibility of automation. Keratin 18 or 19 mRNA that is expressed in epithelial cells has been the most frequent target for amplification to detect cancer occult metastases. Datta et al.[36] used the keratin 19 transcript to identify cancer cells in the bone marrow and peripheral blood of breast cancer patients. It is known that a pseudogene for keratin 19 exists which shares a very high homology with the mature mRNA from the keratin 19 gene. Contamination of DNA in the RNA sample used for reverse transcription can result in amplification of the pseudogene, giving rise to specific 'background' bands in the negative controls (known negative bone marrow and blood; Figure 3.2).[14] Furthermore, non-epithelial cells may have a low level of expression of epithelial transcripts, leading to background staining. To circumvent this problem, we have attempted to amplify transcripts from epithelial and breast cell-specific genes, such as GCDFP-15, MUC-1, and GA733-2, to detect small numbers of breast cancer cells among cells of lymphoid origin. We observed specific amplification from lymphoid cells, such as peripheral

blood and bone marrow from patients with lymphoma, and the Raji B-cell line. Thus, these epithelial-associated and breast-associated transcripts are expressed at low levels in lymphoid cells present in bone marrow and blood. In another recent study,[37] we evaluated the specificity of carcinoembryonic antigen (CEA), cytokeratin 19 (CK 19), cytokeratin 20 (CK 20), gastrointestinal tumor-associated antigen 733.2 (GA 733.2), and mucin-1 (MUC-1) in the blood of healthy donors and lymph nodes from patients without cancer by RT–PCR (Figure 3.3).[37] CK 20 was the only mRNA marker not detected in lymph nodes or blood from patients without cancer. This will clearly limit the application of PCR techniques for the detection of breast cancer occult metastases, at least for the foreseeable future. For the present, immunohistochemical assays remain the method of choice for the detection of bone marrow occult metastatic cells in breast cancer.

Rate of detection of bone marrow occult metastases in patients with early-stage breast cancer

Because immunohistochemistry is the most widely used (and, currently, the most reliable) method for the detection of occult metastases in the bone marrow in breast cancer patients, we have summarized the results from several groups performing immunohistochemical assays using monoclonal antibodies (Table 3.2).

The percentage of patients with early-stage breast cancer in whom extrinsic cells were detected in the bone marrow ranges from 16% to 38%. The possible reasons for some of the variations observed include:

1 use of single antibodies to detect extrinsic cells in some of the studies,
2 differences in patient populations, although all the results were from patients with early-stage disease,

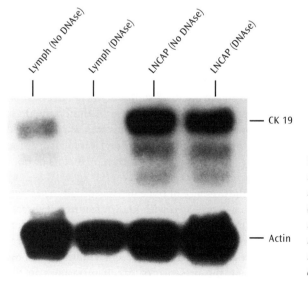

Figure 3.2 Upper panel. *Southern blot of DNAse-treated and non-DNAse-treated LNCAP prostate cancer cell line and lymphocyte specimens (lymph) amplified with cytokeratin 19 (CK 19) primers using RT–PCR. An amplified product is seen in LNCAP and non-DNAse-treated samples, but no signal is seen in the DNAse-treated lymphocyte sample. (Courtesy of Dr D. Wood, Louisville, KY.) Lower panel. RT–PCR showing amplification of actin mRNA in all samples evaluated.*

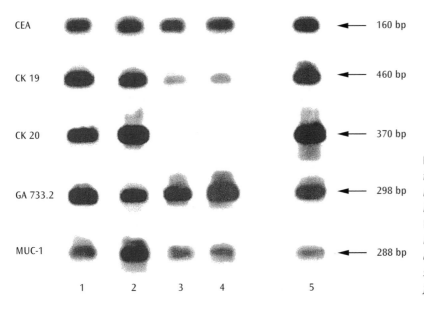

CEA ← 160 bp

CK 19 ← 460 bp

CK 20 ← 370 bp

GA 733.2 ← 298 bp

MUC-1 ← 288 bp

1   2   3   4   5

Figure 3.3 *Representative examples of the expression of specific mRNA markers in healthy donor lymphocytes by RT–PCR and Southern blot assay. Lane 1: breast cancer cell line; lane 2: breast tumor biopsy; lanes 3–5: healthy donor lymphocytes. (For abbreviations, see text.) Reprinted with permission from reference 37.*

Table 3.2 *Detection of bone marrow occult metastases (BMOM) in patients with early-stage breast cancer*

Number of patients in the study	Number of patients with BMOM (%)	References
110	31 (28)	Redding *et al.* (1983)[2]
307	81 (26)	Mansi *et al.* (1987)[29]
155	28 (18)	Schlimok *et al.* (1987)[24]
51	18 (35)	Cote *et al.* (1988)[23]
159	25 (16)	Porro *et al.* (1988)[30]
211	79 (37)	Diel *et al.* (1992)[40]
116	35 (30)	Pantel *et al.* (1993)[17]
197	62 (31)	Menard *et al.* (1994)[38]
Total 1306	359 (27)	

3 differences in the antibody reactivity with breast cancer cells,

4 the presence of antigenic heterogeneity.

However, what is evident and striking is that occult metastases in the bone marrow were detected in all of the studies. Furthermore, it is becoming apparent that the rate of detection of occult metastases in the bone marrow in patients with operable breast cancer is approximately 30% when appropriate antibodies are used. Finally, bone marrow occult metastases can be detected in a proportion of patients with no evidence of metastatic spread beyond the axilla.

Detection of occult metastases in the bone marrow in patients with early-stage breast cancer: clinical significance

Bone marrow occult metastases have been correlated with known predictors of prognosis in several studies. In our studies,[5] extrinsic cells were detected in 27% of node-negative patients and in 41% of node-positive patients. On average, the lymph node-negative group had fewer extrinsic cells than the lymph-node positive group, suggesting a trend toward a greater metastatic tumor burden in patients with lymph node metastases.

The presence of occult metastases in the bone marrow has been correlated with pathologic tumor, node, metastasis (TNM) stage in breast cancer. In our study, 23% of stage I, 38% of stage II, and 50% of stage III patients had extrinsic cells in the bone marrow.[23] Several other investigators have obtained similar results (Table 3.3). In the original study from the Ludwig Institute,[2] the presence of bone marrow occult metastases was correlated with the tumor stage ($p = 0.05$) and vascular invasion ($p < 0.01$), both of which are known predictors of poor prognosis.

While the presence of bone marrow occult metastases appears to be correlated with known features of disease progression, the ultimate utility of this test will be determined by whether bone marrow occult metastases predict breast cancer recurrence. Several studies now show that, in fact, the presence of occult metastases in the

Table 3.3 *Detection of bone marrow occult metastases (BMOM) in breast cancer: correlation with lymph node (LN) status*

Percentage of patients with BMOM (number)		References
LN−	LN+	
27 (6/22)	41 (12/29)	Cote *et al.* (1988)[23]
17 (17/101)	14 (8/58)	Porro *et al.* (1988)[30]
7 (1/14)	43 (10/23)	Dearnaley *et al.* (1991)[39]
19 (32/170)	32 (49/153)	Mansi *et al.* (1991)[41]
30 (40/133)	58 (74/127)	Diel *et al.* (1992)[40]
31 (112/360)	55 (203/367)	Diel *et al.* (1996)[42]
Total 26 (208/800)	47 (356/757)	

Table 3.4 *Prognostic significance of bone marrow occult metastases (BMOM) in breast cancer: correlation with clinical outcome*

Percentage of patients with recurrence (number)		Comments, *p* value	References
BMOM+	BMOM−		
31 (8/26)	85 (11/13)	$p < 0.05$	Dearnaley *et al.* (1991)[39]
25 (64/261)	48 (43/89)	$p < 0.005$	Mansi *et al.* (1991)[41]
16 (5/31)	39 (7/18)	BMOM associated with early recurrence, $p < 0.04$	Cote *et al.* (1991)[5]
3 (4/130)	27 (22/81)	BMOM associated with shorter relapse-free survival, $p = 0.0001$	Diel *et al.* (1992)[40]
Total 18 (81/448)	41 (83/201)		

bone marrow identifies a population of patients at high risk for recurrence (Table 3.4). Our own studies[5] have revealed that the presence of occult metastases in the bone marrow significantly predicts recurrence; the 2-year recurrence rate for patients with no evidence of bone marrow occult metastases was 3%, compared with 33% for patients with detectable bone marrow occult metastases ($p < 0.04$; Figure 3.4). In a study with long-term follow-up (median 9.5 years), Dearnaley *et al.*[39] found that 11 of 13 (85%) patients with bone marrow occult metastases developed recurrence, compared with 8 of 26 (31%) patients with no evidence of occult metastases in the bone marrow, regardless of the lymph node status ($p < 0.05$). This study demonstrates that, over the long term, the presence of occult metastases in the bone marrow may identify a subset of patients who are all at high risk for recurrence. Diel *et al.*[40] followed up 211 patients over a mean period of 24 months. Among 81 patients with occult metastases in the bone marrow, there was recurrence in 22 (27%), but only in 4/130 (3%) patients without occult bone marrow metastases. In addition, the relapse-free survival was highly significantly related to the presence of tumor cells in the bone marrow ($p = 0.0001$). Mansi *et al.*[41] have followed a large number of patients (350) for an extended period (median 76 months) and have demonstrated that,

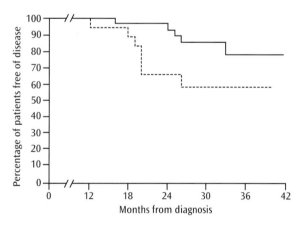

Figure 3.4 *Kaplan Meier curve showing the disease-free interval of patients with breast cancer according to the presence or absence of bone marrow occult metastases. Patients with detectable tumor cells in the bone marrow (----) had significantly shorter time to recurrence than patients without occult metastases (—), p < 0.04. Reprinted with permission from reference 5.*

regardless of lymph node status, nearly one-half of patients with bone marrow occult metastases experienced recurrence (43 of 89, 48%), compared with 64 of 261 (25%) of patients with no evidence of occult metastases in the bone marrow ($p < 0.005$). Finally, Diel and associates[42] studied 727 patients with primary operable breast cancer. They were able to detect tumor cells in the bone marrow of 203 of 367 (55%) lymph node-positive patients and of 112 of 360 (31%) lymph node-negative patients. They found that the occult bone marrow metastases were associated with larger tumor size ($p < 0.001$), lymph node involvement ($p = 0.001$), and higher tumor grade ($p = 0.002$). After a median follow-up of 36 months, patients with cancer cells in their bone marrow had reduced disease-free survival times and reduced overall survival (both p values < 0.001). They also found that the presence of occult metastases in bone marrow was an independent prognostic indicator for both dis-tant disease-free survival and overall survival that was superior to axillary lymph node status, tumor stage, and tumor grade. This large study provides definitive evidence that the detection of occult metastases in the bone marrow by immunohistochemical methods is prognostically important. The presence of bone marrow occult metastases predicts a higher risk for recurrence in bone as well as in other distant sites. Of particular importance in all of these findings is the fact that the presence of bone marrow occult metastases identifies patients with node-negative disease who are at a higher risk for recurrence; this subset of patients can therefore be the target of more aggressive adjuvant therapy.

In fact, several studies have now shown that the bone marrow status can be combined with other prognostic factors, such as axillary lymph node status. This allows groups of patients to be stratified[5,17,39,41,42] as follows:

1 those with very low recurrence rates (lymph node negative, bone marrow negative),
2 those with moderate rates of recurrence (lymph node negative, bone marrow positive, and lymph node positive, bone marrow negative),
3 those with high recurrence rates (lymph node positive, bone marrow positive)[5,40–42] (Figure 3.5).

Detection of bone marrow occult metastases: effect of tumor burden

Another interesting finding from our studies[5] in the detection of occult metastases in the bone marrow is that the number of carcinoma cells detected in the bone marrow (the bone marrow tumor burden) was significantly associated with disease recurrence. In our study, the bone marrow aspirates were processed so that the concentration of bone marrow elements was equal for each patient. Consequently, the number of extrinsic cells counted for each case could be compared among patients; the number of extrinsic cells identified in the bone marrow was considered to be reflective of the peripheral tumor burden in each patient. Among patients with occult bone

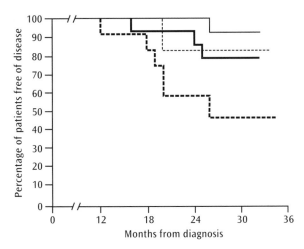

Figure 3.5 *Disease-free interval of patients with breast cancer according to bone marrow status and axillary lymph node status. Patients who were lymph node positive, bone marrow positive (----, thick line) had a significantly shorter time to recurrence than patients who were lymph node negative, bone marrow negative (—, thin line), $p < 0.04$. Patients who were lymph node negative, bone marrow positive (----, thin line) and lymph node positive, bone marrow negative (—, thick line) had intermediate time to recurrence. Reprinted with permission from reference 5.*

Table 3.5 *Effect of bone marrow tumor burden on recurrence[5]*

Variable (n)	Estimated 2-year recurrence rate	p value
Patients with:		
0 ≤ 10 cells (36)	6	< 0.006
≥ 10 cells (13)	46	

marrow metastases, those who did not show recurrence had, on average, fewer extrinsic cells in their marrow than those who did show recurrence (15 versus 43 cells, respectively). In addition, the estimated 2-year recurrence rate for patients with ten or more cells (46%) was significantly higher than that for patients with fewer than 10 cells (6%, $p < 0.006$; Table 3.5). Further, the number of extrinsic cells detected in the bone marrow was an independent predictor of prognosis.

Occult metastatic cells: biologic properties

While correlation of occult metastases in the bone marrow with survival data indicates that the presence of occult metastatic cells is clinically significant, the biological capability of such cells to proliferate has also been demonstrated. Pantel *et al.*[17] showed that, among patients with localized breast cancer, the occult metastatic cells from 48/71 (68%) patients also expressed proliferation-associated antigens (Erb B2). Also, in all of the patients (23/23) with metastatic breast cancer, the occult metastatic cells expressed Erb B2. Such expression of proliferation-associated antigens by disseminated tumor cells may indicate both that viable tumor cells are still present and that these individuals are at particular risk of later clinical relapse.

Detection of occult bone marrow metastases in patients with advanced breast carcinoma

Another situation in which detecting occult bone marrow metastases could be of importance is in advanced-stage breast cancer patients who will receive autologous bone marrow transplantation therapy. It is logical to assume that tumor cells in the bone marrow may be re-infused along with the stem cells during such therapy. Whether or not they are a cause of subsequent relapse is not clearly understood. In patients with hematopoietic tumors who have received bone marrow transplantation, disease relapse is thought to result from both re-infusion of tumor cells and regrowth of tumor not killed by systemic treatment. However, in the case of solid tumors, such as breast cancer, the cause of relapse following autologous bone marrow transplantation remains to be determined. Clearly, re-infusion of contaminating tumor cells and regrowth of existent tumor may both play a role. Tumor cells in the bone marrow may be either the cause of relapse or simply a manifestation of tumor deposits outside of bone and, thus, a measure of systemic tumor burden; patients with increased systemic tumor burden may also be at an increased risk for treatment failure. In any event, the presence of bone marrow occult metastases may place patients who will receive autologous bone marrow transplantation at an increased risk for treatment failure and relapse. Several studies examining patients with neuroblastoma and lymphoma suggest that peripheral blood progenitor cell samples may contain fewer tumor cells than bone marrow.[43–45] We have shown that the frequency of detecting breast cancer cells in a peripheral blood progenitor cell harvest from patients with localized or metastatic breast cancer is low, even when the bone marrow demonstrates overt or occult disease. Whereas this suggests that bone marrow might be a more suitable site for detecting occult metastases in early-stage breast cancer, it also suggests that peripheral blood may be a more suitable source of progenitor cells for hematopoietic support following high-dose chemotherapy. Peripheral blood has certain other advantages over bone marrow for autologous stem-cell transplantation therapy, including convenience and a faster hematopoeitic recovery. Thus, during the past few years, autologous peripheral blood progenitor cell transplantation therapy has been used increasingly in patients with solid tumors, as well as in those with hematologic malignancies.

Detection of occult metastases in the bone marrow in patients with lung cancer

Although lung cancer is the third most common form of cancer, it is the leading cause of cancer deaths in both men and women in the USA. Once a tumor has developed, surgery (either alone or in combination with adjuvant therapy) represents the only potentially curative modality of treatment.[46] Of the four major histologic types of lung cancer (squamous, adenocarcinoma, large cell, small cell), only small-cell carcinoma is generally considered refractory to surgical therapy. However, small-cell carcinoma accounts for only 22% of lung tumors overall;[47] thus, 78% of lung cancers would be potentially curable by surgery if detected early enough. Approximately 50% of all patients with lung cancer are candidates for, and will undergo, definitive surgical resection.[46]

The use of the TNM staging system and the staging map of the mediastinal lymph nodes[48] have been very helpful in establishing treatment plans and prognosis for resectable lung cancer.[49–53] For non-small-cell lung cancer, accurate staging of disease has greater prognostic significance than cell type. Patients with T1N0M0 (stage I) lung cancer treated with surgical resection have an anticipated 5-year survival rate of 60–85%.[49,53–55] For larger carcinomas such as T2N0M0 (stage I), patients have a 50–60% 5-year survival rate. However, survival rates decrease dramatically with increasing stage of disease, particularly in relation to the presence of metastases in regional lymph nodes. In the case of stage III lung cancer, survival rates as low as 5% have been reported for patients with stage IIIb disease, despite the absence of clinically detectable systemic metastases at the time of surgery.[46]

The ability to detect the earliest spread of lung cancer would identify several important groups of patients, including those with low-stage (stage I) disease who have evidence of occult tumor metastases and who may, therefore, benefit from adjuvant systemic treatment. In addition, among patients with locally advanced (stage III) disease, who are generally not considered to be surgical candidates, a subset of patients without occult metastases may be identified who may benefit from more aggressive local (surgical) control of their tumor.

Significance of occult bone marrow metastases in patients with lung cancer

Detection of occult bone marrow metastases in patients with non-small-cell lung cancer

The earliest study, by Frew et al.,[15] did not show any advantage of using immunohistochemistry to detect occult metastases in the bone marrow in non-small-cell lung cancer over routine histopathologic examination. Bone marrow occult metastases in one case of squamous cell carcinoma that was detected by immunohistochemistry were also detected by conventionally stained smears. This is in marked contrast to studies in patients with breast cancer, and to larger, more definitive, studies of patients with non-small-cell lung cancer. Pantel *et al.*[17] observed that bone marrow occult metastases could be detected in up to 22% (18 of 82) cases of operable non-small-cell lung cancer (Table 3.6). These investigators demonstrated that the detection of bone marrow occult metastases is significantly associated with the size and histological grade of the primary carcinoma. However, the association with metastatic involvement of regional lymph nodes as determined with routine histological staining was weaker. This supports the view that hematogenous spread of lung cancer cells may be an event that is distinct from regional spread of tumor (to lymph nodes).

We have shown that occult bone marrow metastases can be detected in a substantial proportion of patients with lung cancer who show no clinical evidence of systemic metastasis, including patients with the earliest stage of disease (stage I).[18] The rate of detection of occult bone marrow metastases was associated with stage of disease; 29% of patients with stage I or II and 46% of patients with stage III disease had detectable bone marrow occult metastases.

Pantel *et al.*[17] observed that the presence of occult bone marrow metastases in patients with non-small-cell lung cancer was significantly associated with the development of metastatic disease (Table 3.7). Disease recurrence was seen in 10/15 (67%) cases with bone marrow occult metastases, and in only 15/41 (37%) cases with no detectable bone marrow occult metastases. The presence of occult metastases in the bone marrow was most highly associated with skeletal metastases, but not with the local outgrowth of residual tumor cells. In our own study,[18] we

showed that the presence of occult bone marrow metastases was significantly associated with higher recurrence rates and a shorter time to recurrence for patients with primary localized (stage I–III) non-small-cell lung cancer. The median time to recurrence for patients with no detectable bone marrow occult metastases was 35.1 months, compared to 7.3 months for patients with bone marrow occult metastases, ($p = 0.0009$; Figure 3.6). Furthermore, for patients with stage I or II disease, the presence of occult bone marrow metastases was significantly associated with a high rate of recurrence ($p = 0.0004$; Figure 3.7). Similar results were seen in comparisons of bone marrow status to overall survival

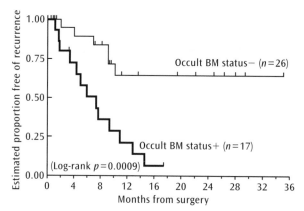

Figure 3.6 *Recurrence-free interval for patients with stage I to III lung cancer according to bone marrow (BM) status. Patients with detectable tumor cells in the bone marrow (thick line) had significantly shorter time to recurrence than patients with no bone marrow occult metastases detected (thin line), p = 0.0009. Reprinted with permission from reference 18.*

Table 3.6 *Detection of bone marrow occult metastases (BMOM) in lung cancer*

Tumor type	References	Antibody	Number of patients in study	Number of patients with BMOM (%)
Non-small-cell lung cancer	Pantel *et al.* (1993)[17]	CK 18	82	18 (22)
	Cote *et al.* (1995)[18]	CK	43	17 (40)
Small-cell lung cancer	Leonard *et al.* (1990)[16]	EMA, CK	12	8 (67)

Table 3.7 *Prognostic significance of bone marrow occult metastases (BMOM) in lung cancer*

Tumor type	References	Percentage of patients with recurrence (number)		p value, other findings
		BMOM−	BMOM+	
Non-small-cell lung cancer	Pantel *et al.* (1993)[17]	37 (15/41)	67 (10/15)	BMOM associated with skeletal metastases
	Cote *et al.* (1995)[18]	23 (6/26)	76 (13/17)	$p = 0.0004$, BMOM associated with shorter recurrence-free survival
Small-cell lung cancer	Leonard *et al.* (1990)[16]	75 (3/4)	88 (7/8)	

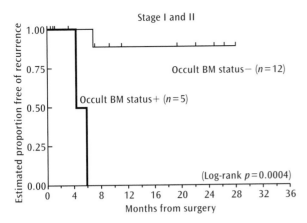

Figure 3.7 *Recurrence-free interval for patients with early-stage lung cancer (stage I, II) according to bone marrow (BM) status. Patients with bone marrow occult metastases detected (thick line) had significantly shorter time to recurrence than patients with no detectable bone marrow occult metastases (thin line), p = 0.0004. Reprinted with permission from reference 18.*

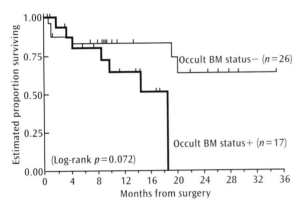

Figure 3.8 *Survival of patients with stage I to III lung cancer according to bone marrow (BM) status. Patients with bone marrow occult metastases detected (thick line) died sooner, on average, than patients with no bone marrow occult metastases detected (thin line). This did not reach statistical significance (p = 0.07). Reprinted with permission from reference 18.*

(Figure 3.8). Although the presence of occult bone marrow metastases was related to stage of disease, it was independent of stage in predicting recurrence.

In another study, Pantel *et al.*[19] demonstrated that occult metastases in the bone marrow could be detected in 83/139 (60%) patients with non-small-cell lung cancer without evidence of distant metastases. The presence of occult metastases in the bone marrow was a significant and independent predictor for a later clinical recurrence in node-negative patients ($p = 0.004$), with recurrence seen in 19/54 (35%) patients without detectable occult metastases versus 9/12 (75%) patients with occult metastases. Furthermore, for patients with node-negative disease (pT1–3pN0M0), those who showed more than one

cell per 4×10^5 bone marrow cells were significantly more likely to suffer relapse.

Ohgami *et al.*[56] compared 39 patients with stage I–III non-small-cell lung cancer who underwent curative resection using immunohistochemistry with monoclonal antibody to CK 18 to detect tumor cells in the bone marrow. They also performed immunostaining of p53 protein in the corresponding primary tumors. CK 18-positive cells were detected in 15 of the 39 (38%) patients and overexpression of p53 was associated with positivity of the tumor cells in the bone marrow. Also, patients with CK 18-positive cells in the bone marrow demonstrated a significantly earlier recurrence than patients without detectable occult metastases in the bone marrow.

The presence of occult bone marrow metastases thus appears to be a clinically important and independent predictor of recurrence and survival in patients with non-small-cell lung carcinoma.

Detection of occult metastases in the bone marrow in patients with small-cell lung cancer

Small-cell lung cancer remains a therapeutic challenge to surgeons, radiotherapists, and medical oncologists. It has a high propensity for metastasis, both to regional lymph nodes and to distant sites. Because of this, primary surgical therapy (even in combination with chemotherapy and radiation therapy) is not considered a viable therapeutic option. The clinical remission obtained by combination chemotherapy is only temporary; successive relapses become increasingly resistant to further therapy. Although small-cell lung cancer is a radiosensitive tumor, only combination chemotherapy has shown a major impact upon survival. In order to identify patients who may benefit most from adjuvant therapy, studies to detect occult metastases have been undertaken.

Initial studies by Frew *et al.*[15] failed to detect any occult metastases by immunohistochemistry that were not identified by routine histology in the bone marrow of patients with primary small-cell lung cancer. However, Leonard *et al.*[16] showed that occult bone marrow metastases could be detected in 8/12 (67%) cases of small-cell lung cancer (see Table 3.6). Moreover, recurrences were observed in 7/8 (88%) of patients with detectable occult bone marrow metastases, and in 3/4 (75%) of patients with no detectable bone marrow occult metastases (see Table 3.7). In a more recent study by Pasini *et al.*,[57] 108 bone marrow samples were taken from 60 patients with small-cell lung cancer and stained with mAb MluC1 using the immunohistochemical method. They were able to detect positive cells in 23 patients (38%). In 16 of these patients, there were more than ten positive cells or clumps of cells in aspirates (14 patients) or a positive bone marrow biopsy (two patients). This group of patients had a poorer median survival (5.5 versus 11 months, $p = 0.01$) than those with negative bone marrow samples or fewer than ten positive cells in the aspirates.

The role of detection of occult metastases in the bone marrow in patients with lung cancer

In early-stage non-small-cell lung cancer (stage I, II), the presence of occult bone marrow metastases may define patients who are at a higher risk for recurrence and death (who will presumably benefit most from adjuvant chemotherapy), and may provide more rational grounds for making treatment decisions. For patients with locally advanced (stage III) disease, the role of surgery can be controversial. However, by identifying those stage III patients at lowest risk of recurrence, it may be possible to determine which patients will benefit most from local (surgical) control of tumor. Finally, in patients with small-cell carcinoma, this technology may identify those who may benefit from a primary surgical approach (those patients with no evidence of occult metastases in the bone marrow). Thus, the study of occult bone marrow metastases in patients with small-cell lung cancer may substantially alter the possible therapeutic options. The detection of these occult metastases appears to be an important new prognostic factor in lung cancer that can greatly affect the selection of patients who may benefit most from adjuvant therapy, and the selection of patients with advanced disease who may benefit from surgery.[55] Therefore, the detection of occult metastases in the bone marrow not only has prognostic significance, it may also provide useful information to determine therapeutic options. This approach provides a great improvement in staging accuracy, and hence allows for the formulation of truly homogeneous treatment groups in future clinical trials.

Detection of occult metastases in the bone marrow in patients with colorectal cancer

Colorectal carcinoma is one of the most common malignancies in the Western world, and still shows an increasing incidence. Despite advances in early detection, the 5-year survival rate of patients with resectable tumors is only about 50%.[58] Therefore, identification of the subset of patients in whom the primary tumor has metastasized would have considerable significance.

Several investigators have examined the clinical significance of detecting occult metastatic cells in the bone marrow of patients with colorectal cancer, even though colorectal cancer rarely involves the skeleton as the metastatic site. These studies have demonstrated the presence of occult bone marrow metastases in substantial proportions of patients with colorectal cancer (Table 3.8).[7–9,59–61] Schlimok et al.[7] found that cytokeratin-positive cells (epithelial cells) were present in 27% (42 of 156) of cases with Duke's stage A–D colorectal cancer. The presence of occult metastases in the bone marrow was correlated with histologic evidence of lymph node metastases. Consistent with the clinical observation that rectal cancers metastasize more frequently to the bone than do colon cancers, these investigators found that patients with rectal cancer had a higher incidence of cytokeratin-positive cells in their bone marrow. Of note is the consistency with which the investigators could detect occult metastatic cells in repeated bone marrow aspirations from patients undergoing adjuvant therapy. In addition, using double-labeling techniques, they also found that 20–50% of the occult metastatic cells expressed proliferation-associated antigens (i.e., the cells were probably capable of proliferating). Finally, as the ultimate evidence of the clinical significance of detecting occult bone marrow metastases in colorectal cancer, it was found that patients with occult bone marrow metastases had shorter recurrence-free intervals than those without ($p = 0.0084$),[8] and that detection of occult bone marrow metastases was an independent indicator of disease relapse ($p = 0.0035$). Recurrence rates for patients with occult bone marrow metastases were higher than those for patients without occult metastases (Table 3.9).

Subsequent to these studies, other investigators have found occult metastatic cells in the bone marrow of patients with colorectal cancer (see Table 3.8). Silly et al.[9] also observed that increased numbers of occult metastatic cells are an indicator of poor prognosis in colorectal cancer. Similarly, Braun and Pantel[61] found individual keratin-positive cells in the bone marrow of approximately 30% of patients with colon cancer. Additionally, they were able to show that the presence of occult metastases in the bone marrow of these patients was a

Table 3.8 *Detection of bone marrow occult metastases (BMOM) in colorectal cancer*

Number of patients in study	Number of patients with BMOM (%)	References
156 (stage A–D)	42 (27)	Schlimok et al. (1990)[7]
7 (M0)	5 (71)	Silly et al. (1992)[9]
12 (M1)	1 (8)	
195 (M0)	53 (27)	Pantel et al. (1993)[17]
82 (M1)	32 (39)	
11 (stage I)	3 (27)	Juhl et al. (1994)[60]
31 (stage II, III)	7 (23)	
12 (stage IV)	4 (33)	

Table 3.9 *Prognostic significance of bone marrow occult metastases (BMOM) in colorectal cancer*

Percentage of patients with recurrence (number)			References
BMOM−	BMOM+	*p* value	
32 (19/60)	68 (17/25)	0.002	Schlimok *et al.* (1990)[7]
30 (18/60)	57 (16/28)	BMOM is associated with shorter disease-free survival, *p* = 0.008	Lindemann *et al.* (1992)[8]

strong independent indicator of subsequent disease relapse.[61]

There has been speculation about the discrepancy between clinically rare bony metastasis and the frequently detected occult bone marrow metastases in colon cancer. According to Paget's original concept,[62] Schlimok *et al.*[7] suggested that although the 'seed' (the tumor itself) is capable of proliferating and developing into metastatic deposits, the 'soil', or the microenvironment (in this case the bone marrow), also determines whether the tumor cells will proliferate. Although overt metastases may not develop in the skeleton, the disseminative capability of metastatic cells from an individual tumor is demonstrated by their presence in the bone marrow.

Attempts have been made to develop molecular methods to detect occult metastatic cells in the bone marrow from patients with colorectal cancer. Although cytokeratin mRNA transcripts have not proved to be helpful in this context (due to the presence of pseudogenes), Gerhard *et al.*[63] have successfully used CEA to detect a small number of metastatic colon cancer cells in the bone marrow by RT–PCR. The method is based on the fact that the majority of colorectal cancers express CEA, whereas bone marrow cells do not. The method is reported to be highly sensitive; it can detect one cancer cell in $2-5 \times 10^7$ bone marrow cells. These investigators could detect CEA mRNA in 67% (10 of 15) cases with abdominal cancers. In addition, some of the cases that were negative by immunohistochemistry were positive by RT–PCR. One major concern is the confirmation that CEA mRNA transcripts are not normally present in bone marrow; if CEA transcripts are found in normal bone marrow, then the detection of CEA mRNA may not signify the presence of tumor. Pending this confirmation and clinical correlation between the detection of occult bone marrow metastases by RT–PCR and the outcome, immunohistochemistry remains the most reliable method to detect bone marrow occult metastatic cells in colorectal cancer.

Detection of occult metastases in patients with prostate cancer

Carcinoma of the prostate is the most common malignancy and the second leading cause of cancer-related death in men in the USA. Unfortunately, only 30% of patients with prostate cancer have potentially curable disease at presentation.[64] A 15-year disease-free survival of 36% has been reported in patients after radical prostatectomy with negative pelvic lymph nodes. Thus, two-thirds of patients with lymph node-negative disease will fail after radical prostatectomy; 15% will have local recurrence, and 50% will fail with distant metastases.[65]

The most frequent site of distant metastasis is the axial skeleton. Of those patients who develop bony metastases, approximately 50% die of their disease within 5 years.[66] Patients with apparently localized prostate cancer who relapse following radical prostatectomy are presumed to have undetected occult metastatic dissemination at initial presentation. The ability to identify this group of patients could modify therapy aimed at local control of disease, and might form the basis for the administration of adjuvant therapy early in the disease process.

Detection of bone marrow metastases by radionuclide bone scan in patients with apparently localized prostate cancer ranges between 8% and 33%.[66] Conventional microscopic examination of bone marrow aspirates in this group of patients has been of limited utility in the past.[67–69] Using an immunohistochemical method that identifies epithelial cells, Mansi *et al.*[70] demonstrated that 13% of patients with operable (stage A–C) prostate cancer had occult metastatic cells in the bone marrow, whereas 73% of cases with confirmed metastatic disease had detectable occult metastatic cells in the bone marrow (Table 3.10). Oberneder *et al.*[12] were able to detect CK 18-positive cells in the bone marrow samples of 33% of patients with stage N0M0 prostate cancer; the incidence of occult metastatic cells showed a significant correlation with established risk factors, such as local tumor extent, distant metastases, and tumor differentiation. In our own study,[13] we used a panel of monoclonal antibodies that recognize epithelial cell-specific membrane and cytoskeletal antigens in an immunofluorescence assay. We found that 22% cases with localized disease and 36% of cases with metastatic prostate cancer, including 100% of patients with bony metastases, had antigen-positive cells in the bone marrow. The serum prostate-specific antigen (PSA) level, a parameter used widely to detect residual/recurrent disease, appeared to correlate with the presence of occult metastases. In addition, the number of antigen-positive cells detected appears to correlate with the stage of disease.[13]

Efforts are underway to use molecular methods to detect circulating occult metastatic cells in patients with

Table 3.10 *Detection of bone marrow occult metastases (BMOM) in prostate cancer*

Percentage of patients with BMOM (%)		References
Localized	Metastatic	
13 (2/15)	73 (11/15)	Mansi *et al.* (1988)[10]
22 (2/9)	36 (4/11)	Bretton *et al.* (1994)[13]
20 (1/5)	100 (2/2)	Wood *et al.* (1994)[14] (RT–PCR)
38 (25/65)	78 (14/18)	Katz *et al.* (1994)[72] (RT–PCR)

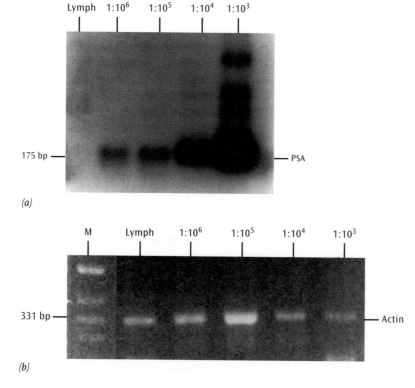

(a)

(b)

Figure 3.9 *(a) Southern blot of LNCAP prostate cancer cell line dilutions amplified with PSA primers using RT–PCR. An amplified product is seen in all dilutions, but no signal is present in the lymphocyte (lymph) sample. (b) Ethidium bromide-stained gel showing an amplified product for actin in all the specimens evaluated in 3.9(a). M refers to metastatic prostate cancer cell. (Courtesy Dr D. Wood, Louisville, KY.)*

prostate cancer, where it is particularly advantageous to use RT–PCR because antigens such as PSA and prostate-specific membrane antigen (PSMA) are considered to be specific to prostate tissue; any positive result is expected to be from circulating prostate cancer cells (unlike CK 19, the pseudogene for which can be amplified from non-epithelial cells giving rise to false-positive results). Moreno *et al.*[11] demonstrated that 4/12 (33%) patients with stage D1–3 prostate cancer tested positive for PSA mRNA by RT–PCR. Wood *et al.*[14] evaluated the sensitivity and specificity of immunohistochemistry and PCR amplification of PSA mRNA to detect prostate cancer cells in bone marrow samples. Using serial dilutions of the prostate cancer cell line LNCAP in lymphocytes, they demonstrated that both techniques were specific and highly sensitive; PCR was more sensitive at highest dilutions (10^5 and 10^6, $p = 0.003$; Figure 3.9). In addition, 2/2 patients with known metastatic prostate cancer, and 1/5 patients with clinically localized tumor had occult metastatic cells detectable by both immunohistochemistry and RT–PCR. In another study, Wood *et al.* detected PSA mRNA by RT–PCR in 29/55 (53%) patients with prostate cancer, including 5/7 patients with lymph node metastases and 5/5 patients with bony metastases.[71] Among 43 patients with clinically localized prostate cancer, 19 (44%) had detectable PSA mRNA amplification. Out of 24 patients who had PSA mRNA amplification by RT–PCR, immunohistochemistry demonstrated prostate cancer cells in only 19 (44%), suggesting that RT–PCR may be more sensitive than immunohistochemistry in detecting occult metastases. Katz *et al.*[72] reported that 25 of 65 (38%) patients with clinically localized disease (T1–2b) were positive for PSA by RT–PCR from blood specimens obtained prior to surgery. In addition, there was a correlation between positivity on this assay and the presence of capsular penetration, a known predictor of poor prognosis. Israeli *et al.*[73] used the sensitive nested RT–PCR method to detect PSA and PSMA mRNA in bone marrow samples. Although the primers for both PSA and PSMA yielded similar sensitivities in the model system (serial dilutions of LNCAP cells in the breast cancer cell line MCF-7), PSMA primers detected occult bone marrow metastases in 48/77 (62%) patients with prostate cancer, whereas PSA primers detected occult metastases in only 7/77 (9%). This represents a remarkable inconsistency with other reports.

Although the use of RT–PCR technology for the detection of prostate cancer occult metastases appears promising, it has certain theoretical disadvantages over immunohistochemical methods. The primary one is that the positive events cannot be morphologically evaluated to confirm that they are consistent with malignant epithelial cells. Further, there is a possibility that mRNA transcripts of PSA may enter into the circulation; thus, detection of these transcripts may not always be associated with the presence of tumor cells. This may account for the high detection rate of PSA mRNA in the blood of patients with apparently localized disease; the detection rate is far higher than the expected recurrence rate. Finally, non-prostate cells may produce PSA. This has, in fact, been clearly demonstrated; PSA can be expressed even by female mammary epithelium.[74] Using nested-primer RT–PCR, Smith *et al.*[74] demonstrated PSA mRNA in epithelial and leukemia cell lines, as well as in blood. The low level of expression of PSA mRNA in blood cells may interfere with PCR methods to detect prostate cancer occult metastases.

In general, from 13% to 38% of patients with apparently localized prostate cancer have been shown to have detectable occult metastatic cells in the bone marrow using a variety of technologies. The best criterion regarding the malignant nature of the occult metastatic cells is whether or not they were present in patients who ultimately developed recurrent disease. This has been demonstrated in the case of breast cancer; the presence of bone marrow occult metastases identifies a population of patients at increased risk of recurrence.[3–5] Whether or not this is the case with prostate cancer remains to be determined through more extensive studies and clinical follow-up. If the presence of occult bone marrow metastases proves to be clinically significant, this will have to be considered in recommendations for therapy, particularly in the case of patients with apparently localized prostate cancer who are at present candidates for radical surgery.

Detection of occult metastases in the bone marrow in patients with neuroblastoma

Neuroblastoma is the most common extracranial solid tumor in childhood.[75] Although the prognosis of this malignancy has improved with advances in medical management, the overall 5-year survival rate is currently only 55%. Prognostic markers currently employed are stage, age, serum ferritin level, histopathologic features, tumor DNA content, and tumor N-*myc* gene copy number.[76–79] Evaluation of bone marrow by standard cytologic analysis is a routine and important component of clinical staging. Morphological distinction between

tumor cells and primitive lymphoblasts can be difficult; immunohistochemical methods have therefore been employed to detect circulating malignant cells.

Moss *et al.*[80] studied the bone marrow specimens of 197 patients with newly diagnosed neuroblastoma using monoclonal antibodies specific to neuroblastoma cells; 131 (66%) of these cases had occult bone marrow metastases detectable by immunohistochemistry (Table 3.11). Among patients with only localized or regional disease (stage I, II, III), 35% (23/65) were shown to have occult bone marrow metastases. Tumor content predicted clinical outcome in relation to the age of the patient; progression-free survival in patients with stage I, II, and III disease diagnosed after the age of 1 year was lower in those with occult bone marrow metastases than in those without such occult metastases ($p = 0.006$). In addition, in patients with stage IV disease diagnosed at an age of less than 1 year, bone marrow tumor load was associated with poorer progression-free survival.

Naito *et al.*[81] used RT–PCR to detect tyrosine hydroxylase mRNA from neuroblastoma cells diluted in bone marrow cells (Table 3.11). They achieved a sensitivity of detection of one neuroblastoma cell per 10 000 normal bone marrow cells. This detection was specific; none of the control bone marrow samples had detectable amplification. Subsequently, Mattano *et al.*[82] used RT–PCR to detect the neuronal gene *PGP 9.5* in neuroblastoma cells. These investigators report a sensitivity of detecting one neuroblastoma cell in ten million blood mononuclear cells. They also showed a higher rate of detection of occult metastatic cells in patient samples by RT–PCR than by immunohistochemistry. While Moss *et al.*[80] showed a prognostic significance of detecting occult bone marrow metastases by immunohistochemistry, a detailed clinical evaluation of the significance of detecting these occult metastases by RT–PCR remains to be done.

Detection of occult metastases in the bone marrow in patients with other cancers

The presence of occult bone marrow metastases or circulating tumor cells has been studied for a variety of solid tumors. These are listed in Table 3.11.[83–85]

With improvements in techniques, it may be possible to standardize the detection of occult metastases. Studies of larger groups of patients with long-term follow-up will enable detailed analyzes of the clinical significance of occult bone marrow metastases in different cancers. When the presence of occult bone marrow metastases is combined with other prognostic parameters, patients with high and low risk of recurrence can be identified. In future, it may be possible to predict the outcome for an individual patient when known predictors of prognosis (such as grade and stage) are considered in conjunction with newer prognostic factors, such as the status of

Table 3.11 *Detection of bone marrow occult metastases (BMOM) in other cancers*

Tumor	Method	Target gene/antigen	Percentage of patients with BMOM (number)	Comment	References
Neuroblastoma	IHC	Neuroblastoma-specific antigens	66 (131/197)	BMOM can predict clinical outcome in relation to age	Moss *et al.* (1991)[45]
	RT–PCR	Tyrosine hydroxylase	NA	NA	Naito *et al.* (1991)[81]
	RT–PCR	PGP 9.5	44 (8/18)	RT–PCR is more sensitive than IHC	Mattano *et al.* (1992)[82]
Uveal melanoma	RT–PCR	Tyrosinase	50 (3/6)		Tobal *et al.* (1993)[83]
Ovarian cancer	IHC	Cytokeratin	24 (12/50)		Cain *et al.* (1990)[84]
Pancreatic cancer	IHC	CEA, mucin	58 (15/26)		Juhl *et al.* (1994)[60]
Gastric cancer	IHC	CEA, mucin	25 (9/36)		Juhl *et al.* (1994)[60]
Cervical cancer	RT–PCR	HPV E6/E7	91 (10/11)		Czegledy *et al.* (1995)[85]

IHC, immunohistochemistry; RT–PCR, reverse transcriptase–polymerase chain reaction; CEA, carcinoembryonic antigen; HPV, human papillomavirus; NA, not applicable.

oncogenes and tumor suppressor genes, and the evidence of occult metastasis.

DETECTION OF OCCULT METASTASES IN THE LYMPH NODES

Despite the explosion of knowledge of the biology of cancer, the single most important prognostic factor for most solid tumors is the presence of histologically detectable regional lymph node metastases: patients with tumors that have not metastasized to the regional lymph nodes tend to do far better than patients with lymph node metastases. A significant proportion of node-negative patients will, however, develop distant metastasis. As we have seen, systemic dissemination may take place by routes other than lymphatic spread; the presence of bone marrow occult metastases in node-negative patients demonstrates this. Nevertheless, a proportion of node-negative patients without evidence of bone marrow metastases will experience recurrence. It has now become clear that another possible site for occult tumor spread in histologically node-negative patients is the regional lymph nodes.

Routine histopathological examination of lymph nodes is in reality only a lymph node sampling; in fact, Gusterson and Ott[86] have calculated that a pathologist has only a 1% chance of identifying a metastatic focus of cancer of a diameter of three cells in cross-section occupying a lymph node. It has also been clearly shown that re-examination of lymph node sections initially considered negative for tumor after routine histopathologic screening frequently shows metastatic deposits, demonstrating that even when tumor cells are present in the section, they can be missed.[87] It is evident that routine processing and histologic examination of regional lymph nodes are inadequate to detect the presence of tumor in all cases.

As with bone marrow occult metastases, most studies have involved the detection of regional (axillary) lymph node occult metastases in patients with breast cancer.[87–94] These studies can be classified into two major categories:

1 Detection of metastasis after more intensive histological examination of the lymph node, including analysis of multiple serial sections.
2 Studies that use immunohistochemistry to take advantage of the differential expression of antigens between normal lymph node constituents and epithelial carcinoma cells in order to detect occult tumor in lymph nodes. In fact, this is the same principle as that used for detecting occult tumor in bone marrow.

Attempts have also been made to use molecular techniques to detect lymph node occult metastatic cells. While studies concerning occult lymph node metastases are most advanced for breast cancer, there is now a growing body of literature on the detection and clinical significance of occult lymph node metastases in other tumors, such as colon, lung, and prostate carcinoma, and melanoma (discussed in the following sections).

Detection of occult metastases in the lymph nodes of patients with breast cancer

As mentioned above, a significant proportion of patients with node-negative breast cancer will develop distant metastases. Disease recurrence in these patients is strongly associated with the presence of bone marrow occult metastases. However, a subset of node-negative patients without evidence of bone marrow occult metastases will also experience recurrence. It has now become clear that another possible site for occult tumor spread in node-negative breast cancer patients is the axillary lymph nodes.[94–107]

Detection of occult lymph node metastases by histological review

Studies undertaken to detect occult lymph node metastases by routine histologic methods have generally been performed by cutting serial sections from all paraffin blocks containing lymph nodes, followed by routine staining and microscopic review.[98,101] However, several studies have simply re-reviewed the original histologic slides. All of these studies have demonstrated that deposits of tumor can be detected using these methods. Between 7% and 33% of previously node-negative cases convert to node-positive after review (Table 3.12). As reviewed by Neville et al.,[105] the mean conversion rate is approximately 13%.

Detection of occult lymph node metastases by immunohistochemistry

Several investigators have used various antibodies in order to detect occult lymph node metastases in patients with breast cancer using immunohistochemical methods.

In general, most studies have used antibodies specific for low molecular weight intermediate filament proteins to distinguish the epithelial tumor deposits from normal node elements. Other studies have used antimucin antibodies raised against human mammary carcinoma cells.[104] In our own studies, we have used a cocktail of two antikeratin antibodies, AE1 and Cam5.2 (which, in combination, recognize CK 18 and CK 19, the predominant intermediate filament proteins in simple epithelial cells). Although antibodies to cytokeratins have been reported to react with dendritic reticulum cells (with the possibility of producing false-positive results), this has not been a significant problem in our own experiments. Furthermore, as with the bone marrow examination previously described, the morphologic evaluation of the 'positive' cells is critical; cells that do not possess the morphologic characteristics of malignant epithelial cells are not considered to be tumor cells in our studies.

Unlike routine histological evaluation for the detection of occult metastases in which multiple sections from each block are studied, most of the studies employing

Table 3.12 *Detection of axillary lymph node occult metastases in patients with histologically node-negative breast cancer*

Histologic methods

Saphir and Amromin (1948)[88]	30 cases, 33% conversion rate
Pickren (1961)[89]	51 cases, 22% conversion rate
Fisher et al. (1978)[90]	78 cases, 24% conversion rate
Wilkinson et al. (1982)[91]	525 cases, 17% conversion rate
International (Ludwig) Breast Cancer Study Group (1990)[92]	921 cases, 9% conversion rate; lymph node occult metastases are prognostically significant
deMascarel et al. (1992)[93]	1680 cases, 7% conversion rate; lymph node occult metastases are prognostically important

Immunohistochemical methods

Wells et al. (1984)[94]	45 cases, 15% conversion rate
Bussolati et al. (1986)[95]	50 cases, 24% conversion rate
Byrne et al. (1987)[96]	40 cases, 10% conversion rate
Trojani et al. (1987)[97]	150 cases, 14% conversion rate; lymph node occult metastases are prognostically important
Apostolikas et al. (1989)[98]	50 cases, 14% conversion rate
Sedmak et al. (1989)[99]	45 cases, 20% conversion rate; lymph node occult metastases are prognostically significant
Cote et al. (1992)[100]	251 cases, 24% conversion rate; lymph node occult metastases are prognostically significant
Neville et al. (1991)[105]	285 cases, 16% conversion rate; lymph node occult metastases are prognostically significant
Elson et al. (1993)[102]	97 cases, 20% conversion rate
Nasser et al. (1993)[103]	159 cases, 14% conversion rate
Hainsworth et al. (1993)[104]	343 cases, 12% conversion rate; lymph node occult metastases are prognostically significant
Cote et al. (1999)[111]	736 cases, 20% conversion rate; prognostically important in post menopausal women

immunohistochemical techniques have tested only a single section. When a single section is studied, the percentage of patients who convert from node negative to node positive ranges from 14% to 30%, with a mean conversion rate of 16%, as reviewed by Neville[87,105] (Table 3.12).

Detection of occult lymph node metastases by RT–PCR

Attempts are being made to detect occult lymph node metastases by molecular techniques such as RT–PCR. As in the case of immunohistochemistry, epithelial-specific gene expression is used to distinguish between epithelial (cancer) cells and lymphoid cells. However, as with the results found in the case of occult bone marrow metastases, false-positive results can be obtained when cytokeratin mRNA is used to detect cancer cells. Schoenfeld et al.[106] used RT–PCR to detect keratin 19 mRNA from breast cancer cells metastatic to the lymph nodes. While they could detect keratin 19 mRNA from all histologically involved lymph nodes and a proportion of lymph nodes showing no evidence of metastasis by immunohistochemistry, all normal lymph nodes also showed the keratin 19 PCR product when the number of cycles was increased to make the method more sensitive. On the matter of using PCR as a method of detection of occult lymph node metastases, Schoenfeld[106] states, '… the sensitivity is limited by the specificity of the tumor marker.'

Other investigators[107,108] have used MUC-1 mRNA expression to detect breast cancer cells among lymphoid cells. MUC-1, the core protein of polymorphic epithelial mucin, is known to be expressed in most breast cancers.[109] Noguchi et al.[107] used serial dilutions of the breast cancer cell line MCF7 in lymph node cells and could detect as few as one MCF7 cell in a million lymph node cells; they also showed that RT–PCR was more sensitive than immunohistochemistry using antibodies to MUC-1 antigen. However, in our own studies (unpublished), we observed that MUC-1 gene expression is not restricted to epithelial cells alone; by RT–PCR, MUC-1 mRNA was also detected in lymphoid cells from bone marrow. CK 20 protein is not expressed by the majority of breast carcinomas, yet we have shown that CK 20 mRNA can be detected in the majority of breast cancers.[37] Other markers, such as CK 7 and gross cystic disease fluid protein (GCDFP), are currently under investigation as possible markers for the detection of occult metastases in breast cancer patients. Regardless of the marker chosen, clinical correlation with survival and recurrence data and comparisons with well-established immunohistochemical protocols for the detection of occult metastases need to be performed before RT–PCR becomes a routinely used method for the detection of occult lymph node metastases.

While it may, at some point, be possible to detect occult metastases in the lymph nodes of patients with breast cancer using PCR methods, this procedure continues to have major drawbacks compared with immunohistochemistry. The lymph nodes used must be fresh (or fresh frozen), and all lymph nodes in their entirety must be disaggregated to undergo RNA extraction (as we have shown that metastases in node-negative cases usually occurs to only one lymph node). Therefore, these lymph nodes will be totally unavailable for histologic review, and the method will test for both histologic and occult positives.

Clinical significance of occult lymph node metastases in patients with breast cancer

Although virtually all studies have demonstrated that lymph node metastases can be overlooked, there is a surprising disagreement about the prognostic importance of these occult tumor deposits. Many of the studies using routine histologic review of sections have found that the presence of occult lymph node metastases does not influence the recurrence rates in a statistically significant way;[89–91] several studies using immunohistochemical techniques have reported similar findings.[95,96,102,110] In order to begin to understand this, a few basic observations need to be made. Many earlier studies have involved fewer than 100 patients; in fact, some have involved even fewer than 50 patients. Cote and Groshen have demonstrated that, even if the finding of occult lymph node metastases is prognostically important, there is no possibility that studies of the clinical impact of occult lymph node metastases involving few patients will provide statistically significant data (personal communication). In fact, Fisher et al.[90] were the first to point this out clearly: 'it has been mathematically estimated that differences in survival of 10 percent, if indeed they occur between the two groups [true lymph node negative versus occult lymph node positive], would require a study of approximately 1400 cases.' Therefore, studies involving a few patients are not suitable to address the issue of the prognostic significance of occult lymph node metastases. This dilemma is well illustrated by a study done by Byrne et al.[96] using immunohistochemical methods to detect occult lymph node metastases. This group studied 40 patients and found a 10% incidence of occult lymph node metastases; patients with occult metastases had a 5-year recurrence rate of 75% and a 5-year survival rate of 50%, compared with 5-year recurrence and survival rates of 25% and 86%, respectively, for patients without evidence of occult lymph node metastases. However, these authors concluded that the detection of occult lymph node metastases is of no clinical value, because the differences were not statistically significant.

Fortunately, investigators from the Ludwig Institute and International Breast Cancer Study Group have performed a definitive study of the importance of occult lymph node metastases in patients with node-negative breast cancer.[92] They examined serial sections of 921 node-negative breast cancer patients by routine histological methods. Nine percent of these patients were found to have occult lymph node metastases; these patients had a poorer disease-free ($p = 0.003$) and overall survival ($p = 0.002$) after 5 years' median follow-up, compared with patients whose nodes remained negative after serial sectioning.[92] Six-year median follow-up data give even more conclusive evidence of the prognostic significance of occult lymph node metastases.[101] Another large-scale study was performed by deMascarel et al.,[93] with a median follow-up of 7 years. These investigators studied the lymph nodes from 1121 patients with primary operable breast cancer, by serial macroscopic sectioning; they found single occult lymph node metastases in 120 patients. A significant difference in recurrence ($p = 0.005$) and survival ($p = 0.04$) was found between node-negative patients and those with single occult metastases. However, in multivariate analysis using the Cox model, occult metastases were not a predicting factor. Several studies using immunohistochemical methods have also shown the prognostic significance of occult lymph node metastases[97,99,104] (see Table 3.12). We studied 251 patients with breast cancer and histologically negative lymph nodes for the presence of occult metastases using immunohistochemistry;[100] occult lymph node metastases were detected in 60 patients (24%). Preliminary analysis has shown that patients with occult lymph node metastases are at increased risk for recurrence (5-year recurrence rate of lymph node occult metastases positive versus negative: 27% versus 37%, $p = 0.02$). In a more recent study, we examined the lymph nodes from 736 patients with breast cancer who were involved in Trial V of the International (Ludwig) Breast Cancer Study for the presence of metastases. Occult metastases were detected by immunohistochemistry in 148 (20%) of the 736 patients. These occult metastases were associated with significantly poor disease-free and overall survival in postmenopausal patients but not in premenopausal patients. Immunohistochemically detected occult lymph node metastases remained an independent and highly significant predictor of recurrence, even after control for tumor grade, tumor size, estrogen-receptor status, vascular invasion, and treatment ($p = 0.007$).[111]

While there is ample evidence showing that occult lymph node metastases can be detected in a substantial proportion of node-negative patients and that the presence of such deposits is probably prognostically significant, the best method for detecting these deposits is not yet clear. Re-examination of multiple serial sections is laborious, time consuming, and expensive. Immunohistochemical assays, on the other hand, are more sensitive and certainly less laborious. Definitive comparative analyses are now ongoing;[100] results from these studies suggest that immunohistochemical methods may be superior to histologic re-examination of lymph node serial sections.

Lung cancer

Although lung cancer is the leading cause of cancer-related death in both men and women, surprisingly few studies have been done on the significance of lymph node occult metastases. Chen et al.[112] used the polyclonal antikeratin antibody to demonstrate that keratin-positive cells could be detected in the regional lymph nodes of 38/60 (63%) cases with node-negative non-small-cell lung cancer (Table 3.13). The median survival of patients with occult metastases was shorter than that of patients whose nodes contained no tumor, although this finding did not reach the level of statistical significance.

Passlick et al.[113] used the monoclonal antibody Ber-Ep4 against two glycoproteins of 34 and 49 kDa present on the surface and cytoplasm of epithelial cells[114–116] to study the regional lymph nodes of 72 patients with node-negative non-small-cell lung cancer. They found that 11/72 (15%) of patients demonstrated positively staining cells in the lymph nodes (Table 3.13). The detection of occult metastatic cells was positively correlated with a shorter disease-free survival, whereas no correlation was obtained with grade, size of tumor, or the presence of occult bone marrow metastases (Table 3.14). A strong predictive value of nodal occult metastatic cells was demonstrated; tumor relapses in patients with occult metastases occurred approximately 5.3 times more frequently than they did in patients without occult metastases ($p = 0.005$).

Izbicki et al.[114] looked at 73 non-small-cell lung cancer patients with node-negative disease by routine hematoxylin and eosin staining and found, using monoclonal antibody BerEp4 by immunohistochemical techniques, that 20 (27%) had occult nodal metastases.

The rate of detection of nodal occult metastases differed markedly among these three studies.[112–114] This discrepancy may reflect methodological differences and different patient populations.

Table 3.13 *Detection of lymph node occult metastases (LNOM) in node-negative lung cancer*

Antibody	Number of patients in study	Number of patients with LNOM (%)	References
Polyclonal antikeratin	60	38 (63)	Chen *et al.* (1993)[112]
Monoclonal BerEp4 (antiglycoprotein)	72	11 (15)	Passlick *et al.* (1994)[113]
Monoclonal BerEp4	73	20 (27)	Izbicki *et al.* (1996)[114]

Table 3.14 *Prognostic significance of lymph node occult metastases (LNOM) in node-negative lung cancer*

Percentage of patients with recurrence (number)		Other findings	Reference
LNOM−	LNOM+		
14 (8/56)	50 (5/10)	LNOM is correlated with shorter disease-free survival, $p = 0.005$	Passlick et al. (1994)[113]

Table 3.15 *Detection of lymph node occult metastases (LNOM) in colorectal cancer*

Number of patients in study	Number of patients with LNOM (%)	Antibodies	Prognostic significance	References
46	12 (26)	CEA, CK	Not significant	Cutait et al. (1991)[122]
22	8 (36)	CK	Not done	Haboubi et al. (1992)[123]
77	19 (25)	CK	Not significant	Jeffers et al. (1994)[124]
50	14 (28)	CK	LNOM is correlated with poor survival, $p = 0.0013$	Greenson et al. (1994)[125]
45	17 (38)	CK	Not significant	Florentine et al. (1996)[126]
26	14 (54)	CEA	$p = 0.02$	Liefers et al. (1998)[127]

CEA, carcinoembryonic antigen; CK, cytokeratin.

Colorectal cancer

Colorectal cancer is one of the most common malignancies in the Western world. Several factors have been related to prognosis in colorectal cancer, but Dukes' staging is considered the most important in clinical practice.[117–123] Dukes' staging is based on histopathologic studies performed with the classic hematoxylin and eosin staining technique. A central point in staging is the involvement of the regional lymph nodes with metastatic tumor cells. Considering that approximately 25% of patients with Dukes' stage B carcinoma (i.e., no histologic evidence of lymph node metastases) die within 5 years, it is obvious that, in these patients, microscopic dissemination of their tumor had occurred at the time of initial diagnosis. Therefore, detection of these microscopic tumor deposits that are undetectable by routine histopathology may be of great relevance in diagnosing tumors that are no longer localized.

Immunohistochemical detection of occult metastatic cells in patients with localized disease (Dukes' B) has been demonstrated by several investigators (Table 3.15). Although most of the studies showed that a substantial proportion of patients with localized colorectal cancer demonstrate occult metastases in the regional lymph nodes, not all studies show the prognostic significance of finding these occult metastases. Cutait et al.[122] and Jeffers et al.[124] did not find a correlation between the presence of occult metastases and long-term survival. Greenson et al.,[125] however, showed that the presence of cytokeratin-positive cells within the lymph nodes correlated with a significantly poorer prognosis. We studied[126] the lymph nodes from 45 patients with stage II colon cancer for the presence of occult metastatic cells, using monoclonal antibodies to cytokeratin. Occult metastatic cells were detected in 46 lymph nodes from 17/45 (38%) patients, varying from 1 to 300 cells per lymph node. Recurrence was seen in 8/17 (47%) patients with lymph node occult metastases, whereas it occurred in only 8/28 (29%) patients without lymph node occult metastases.

Molecular methods have also been used to identify occult metastases in colorectal cancer patients. Liefers et al.[127] have analysed the lymph nodes from 26 patients with stage II colorectal cancer using CEA-specific nested RT–PCR. They were able to detect CEA positivity in the sample of 14 of 26 patients (54%). In addition, they found a significant difference in the 5-year survival rate between the two groups of patients. The 5-year survival rates were 50% in the node-positive group and 91% in the node-negative group ($p = 0.02$). This study assumed that CEA positivity is cancer specific. This assumption is in contrast to data from other studies that show that CEA is expressed in normal epithelial and non-epithelial tissues.[37,128] Larger prospective studies are required to confirm the prognostic significance of detecting occult metastases and to evaluate the appropriateness of adjuvant chemotherapy in patients whose disease is upstaged by immunohistochemical staining.

Prostate cancer

As previously indicated, a subset of patients with prostate cancer who undergo radical prostatectomy will suffer recurrence, even in the absence of clinically or pathologically detectable regional or systemic metastases.

The thought of developing a method to reliably determine the risk of developing advanced disease by a simple peripheral blood test is seductive. Because PSA has long been thought to be specific for prostate – an idea now seriously in doubt – and the longstanding clinical use of serum PSA levels in the follow-up of patients with cancer of the prostate has been shown to be of value in determining disease progression, methods to increase the sensitivity of PSA detection in the blood have been developed. Most promising has been the use of RT–PCR on peripheral blood samples to determine the presence of PSA. However, there are indications from some groups that the RT–PCR methods to detect PSA may be *too* sensitive. Henke and associates[129] studied 34 subjects, 10 of whom were healthy women, 12 were either healthy men or men with benign prostatic hypertrophy, and 12 had cancer of the prostate. PSA was detected in all groups, including in the women and men with no disease or benign hypertrophy. Henke *et al.* therefore concluded that the expression of PSA was not tumor specific.[129]

The highest recurrence and progression rates in patients with regionally confined disease occur among those with pathological stage C (pT3N0) tumors, that is, tumors with no histologic evidence of lymph node metastases.[130] Recurrence in these cases is presumably due to occult spread of tumor. The detection of regional or systemic spread of tumor at its earliest stages might therefore identify patients at the greatest risk for recurrence and progression of disease.

Although the most frequent site of distant metastasis in prostate cancer is the axial skeleton, the initial site of dissemination is the regional (pelvic) lymph nodes. In fact, the presence of lymph node metastases is the most important pathologic predictor for progression and recurrence in patients undergoing radical prostatectomy. Pathological analyses using routine histochemical methods can detect lymph node metastases in 10–15% of patients undergoing surgery for clinical stages A to C (T1–T3).[130] The extent of pelvic lymph node involvement has been shown to correlate with disease progression and death, with increasing rates of each with single,

multiple, and gross nodal involvement.[21,131–135] Thus, the detection of regional lymph node metastases is crucial to predict the outcome in patients with prostate cancer.

Initial studies[131,132] performed to detect pelvic lymph node occult metastases in prostate cancer patients involved small and heterogeneous populations of patients with prostate cancer (clinical and pathological stages A through D). These studies concluded that occult lymph node metastases are found in a small percentage of patients (approximately 3%) with prostate cancer and suggested that the immunohistochemical detection of occult lymph node metastases is neither cost effective nor practical (Table 3.16). To define more completely the incidence of lymph node occult metastases in prostate cancer, we performed a larger study involving a pathologically homogeneous group of patients with operable prostate cancer at high risk for recurrence (stage pT3N0); i.e., tumors with extracapsular spread but no histologic evidence of lymph node metastases.[136] As in the previous two studies, we used monoclonal antibodies to cytokeratin (Figure 3.10) and PSA to detect and confirm the presence of metastatic cells of prostatic origin in the regional (pelvic) lymph nodes. Occult lymph node metastases were detected in 15/95 (16%) cases. The presence of occult lymph node metastases was associated with known clinical and pathological predictors of disease progression; occult lymph node metastases were more frequent in patients with high primary Gleason grade tumors and in tumors with seminal vesicle involvement ($p = 0.03$). Preliminary analysis of this group indicates that the presence of occult lymph node metastases may be an important predictor of recurrence and survival in stage C prostate cancer.[137] Although the 5-year recurrence rate for patients with occult lymph node metastases (47%) was greater than that for patients without occult lymph node metastases (32%), this difference did not reach statistical significance due to the small sample size. However, patients with occult lymph node metastases had a significantly worse survival (80% and 67% at 5 and 10 years) compared to patients without occult lymph node metastases (95% and 88% at 5 and 10 years, $p = 0.025$). In addition, among 59 patients with Gleason scores 7–10, the detection of occult lymph node

Table 3.16 *Detection of lymph node occult metastases (LNOM) in prostate cancer*

Number of patients in study	Number of patients with LNOM (%)	Other findings	References
23 (stage A, B)	0 (0)	LNOM are infrequent	Gomella *et al.* (1993)[131]
9 (stage C)	1 (11)		
11 (stage D)	1 (9)		
32 (localized)	1 (3)	LNOM are infrequent	Moul *et al.* (1994)[132]
95 (stage C)	15 (16)	LNOM are associated with known predictors of prognosis, i.e., high Gleason grade and seminal vesicle invasion, $p = 0.03$	Freeman *et al.* (1996)[137]

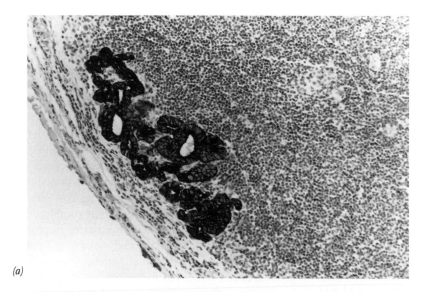

(a)

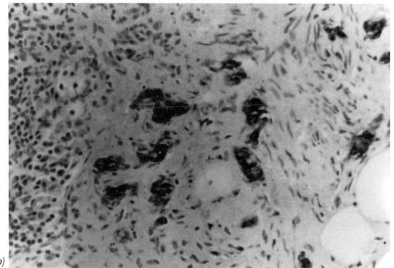

(b)

Figure 3.10 *Regional lymph node from a patient with prostate cancer stained immunohistochemically with (a) anticytokeratin monoclonal antibodies (AE1 and CAM 5.2), showing occult metastases with gland formation by tumor in the subcapsular sinus, and (b) anti-PSA antibody showing prostatic occult metastatic cells. Reprinted with permission from reference 14.*

metastases was significantly associated with increased risk of recurrence ($p = 0.0015$) and with increased risk of death ($p = 0.014$).

Molecular methods (RT–PCR) have been used to detect PSA mRNA in lymph nodes to identify those with occult metastatic involvement. The method appears to be very sensitive, detecting as few as one positive cell in a million peripheral blood mononuclear cells.[138] However, RT–PCR has certain inherent drawbacks. As mentioned above, PSA has been shown to be expressed by non-prostate cells. In addition, in order to use this method to detect occult metastatic cells from lymph nodes, the entire lymph node (which has to be fresh or immediately snap frozen) has to be disaggregated to isolate the mRNA. We have shown that usually only a single lymph node is involved with occult metastases. Therefore, all lymph nodes must be disrupted to detect tumor cells by PCR. Thus, the lymph nodes will not be available for any type of routine morphologic evaluation. In contrast, immunohistochemical methods, in which a single or a few sections from each block containing lymph nodes are

studied, allow routine pathological evaluation and morphological assessment of the occult metastases. However, PCR techniques may have certain advantages, including technical ease of performance and interpretation, and the possibility of increased sensitivity and automation. The relative advantage of immunohistochemistry versus PCR techniques in the detection of occult lymph node metastases remains to be evaluated.

Malignant melanoma

The prognosis for patients with melanoma is influenced by the presence of malignant involvement of regional lymph nodes; the survival rate is significantly decreased when the lymph nodes are involved. Prophylactic regional lymph node dissection is recommended for patients with intermediate-thickness melanomas (0.76–4 mm);[139] the absence of malignant cells in the regional lymph nodes indicates a good prognosis. However, 33% of patients reported to have lymph nodes free of metastases will

Table 3.17 *Detection of lymph node occult metastases (LNOM) in malignant melanoma*

Number of patients in study	Number of patients with LNOM (%)	Method	References
100	14 (14)	IHC (S-100)	Cochran et al. (1988)[141]
62	15 (24)	IHC on LN cultures	Heller et al. (1993)[142]
29	19 (66)	RT–PCR (tyrosinase)	Wang et al. (1994)[143]

IHC, immunohistochemistry; RT–PCR, reverse transcriptase–polymerase chain reaction; LN, lymph node.

Table 3.18 *Prognostic significance of lymph node occult metastases (LNOM) in malignant melanoma*

Percentage of patients who died of disease (number)		Reference
LNOM−	LNOM+	
21 (18/86)	43 (6/14)	Cochran et al. (1988)[141]

die of recurrent disease within 5 years.[140] Clearly, these patients had occult systemic spread of disease that was undetectable by the methods routinely employed. The presence of lymph node metastases is an important criterion in determining the appropriate adjuvant therapy. Because of the prognostic and therapeutic implications, it is important to identify occult lymph node metastases in patients with melanoma.

Cochran et al.[141] studied the lymph nodes from 100 patients with clinical stage I cutaneous melanoma for the presence of microscopic deposits of tumor. Occult lymph node metastases were detected in 14/100 (14%) patients by immunohistochemistry using antibodies to S-100 protein (Table 3.17). The incidence of occult metastases was correlated with known predictors of prognosis (deeply invasive, micrometrically thick tumors). In addition, the presence of occult lymph node metastases was associated with a poorer survival: 6/14 (43%) patients with occult lymph node metastases died of their disease, compared to only 18/86 (21%) without occult metastases (Table 3.18).

An interesting study was done by Heller et al.,[142] in which the investigators isolated lymph nodes from standard dissection and placed a portion of the lymph node in culture, to grow possible occult metastatic cells (see Table 3.17). These cells were confirmed to be melanoma cells by cytology and immunohistochemistry. Lymph nodes cultures from 15/62 (24%) patients with stage I or II melanomas had occult metastases. In a 24-month follow-up, disease recurrence was observed only in patients with culture-positive lymph nodes. In addition, patients with lymph nodes positive by both histology and culture had the highest recurrence rate, whereas no recurrence was observed in the histologically positive, culture-negative population. This study demonstrated that occult metastatic cells in lymph nodes are prognostically significant, and that they have a capability to form metastatic deposits.

Recently, Wang et al.[143] used RT–PCR to detect tyrosinase mRNA to identify metastatic cells in the lymph nodes from patients with stage I and II melanoma. Out of 29 patients, 19 (66%) were positive for tyrosinase (see Table 3.17). These included all of the 11 cases that were detected by pathology. However, until larger studies are performed showing the prognostic importance of detecting occult lymph node metastases by RT–PCR, the significance of finding these occult metastases cannot be validated.

SUMMARY AND FUTURE PROSPECTS

The concept of occult metastases has existed for over four decades. Over the years, investigators have attempted to improve techniques for detecting occult metastatic cells, and to attribute clinical significance to the detection of such occult metastases. While the majority of the work has been done in breast cancer, an increasing body of literature exists on occult metastases' detection in other cancers.

Occult metastases in the bone marrow have been shown to be prognostically significant in a variety of malignancies, e.g., breast, lung, and colorectal cancer, and neuroblastoma. On the other hand, there has been a surprising disagreement about the prognostic importance of occult lymph node metastases, especially in breast cancer, although, increasingly, more studies are now showing a clinical significance of detecting such occult metastases. Similarly, in colorectal cancer, the prognostic significance of occult lymph node metastases has not been shown conclusively. In lung cancer, prostate cancer, and melanoma, detection of occult lymph node metastases has been shown to be prognostically important.

The presence of occult metastases (in the lymph nodes and/or bone marrow) may not only define patients who are at higher risk for recurrence and death at worse prognosis, but may also identify biologically distinct mechanisms of tumor spread (e.g., lymphatic versus vascular dissemination). The use of techniques to detect occult metastases may also allow us to identify biologically important populations of cells, i.e., those cells constituting the earliest metastatic population of tumor cells. Thus, techniques that identify occult metastases may be valuable in furthering our understanding of the events regulating tumor dissemination.

Although molecular methods such as RT–PCR have an advantage of potential automation and increased sensitivity, the most widely used methods remain immunohistochemistry in the detection of occult metastases in the bone marrow, and serial sectioning and immunohistochemistry in the detection of occult lymph node metastases. With improvements in screening methods and standardization of the immunohistochemical procedures, it might become possible to apply this technology in the clinical management of patients.

A new concept that is emerging in the staging of cancers is the TNnMm classification, where the traditional T (tumor), N (node), and M (metastasis) may be complemented by n and m (nodal and systemic occult metastases). With larger studies on the prognostic significance of occult metastases, in either bone marrow or lymph nodes, this staging may be applied clinically, and the estimates of outcome for populations of patients may be narrowed down to those for subpopulations of patients (i.e., those with or without occult metastases). Similarly, in future, treatment decisions may be based on the detection of occult metastases.

ACKNOWLEDGMENTS

The authors thank Dr David P. Wood for his generous contribution of data on the detection of occult metastases in prostate cancer; Dr John Glaspy for his collaboration in the bone marrow occult metastases studies; Dr Benjaporn Chaiwun for her valuable work on immunohistochemical detection of occult metastases; Dr Shan Rong Shi for his overall contribution to the immunohistochemical techniques; Dr John Freeman for his work on lymph node occult metastases in prostate cancer; and Ms Christina Yang for technical assistance.

REFERENCES

1. Schabel FM. Rationale for adjuvant chemotherapy. Cancer 1977; 39:2875–82.
2. Redding WH, Monaghan P, Imrie SF, et al. Detection of micrometastases in patients with primary breast cancer. Lancet 1983; 2:1271–4.
3. Osborne MP, Asina S, Wong GY, et al. Immunofluorescent monoclonal antibody detection of breast cancer in bone marrow: sensitivity in a model system. Cancer Res 1989; 49:2510–13.
4. Ellis G, Fergusson M, Yamanaka E, et al. Monoclonal antibodies for detection of occult carcinoma cells in bone marrow of breast cancer patients. Cancer 1989; 63:2509–14.
5. Cote RJ, Rosen PP, Lesser ML, et al. Prediction of early relapse in patients with operable breast cancer by detection of occult bone marrow metastases. J Clin Oncol 1991; 9:1749–56.
6. Osborne MP, Wong GY, Asina S, et al. Sensitivity of immunocytochemical detection of breast cancer cells in human bone marrow. Cancer Res 1991; 51:2706–9.
7. Schlimok G, Funke I, Bock B, Schweiberer B, Witte J, Riethmuller G. Epithelial tumor cells in bone marrow of patients with colorectal cancer: immunocytochemical detection, phenotypic characterization, and prognostic significance. J Clin Oncol 1990; 8:831–7.
8. Lindemann F, Schlimok G, Dirschedl P, Witte J, Riethmuller G. Prognostic significance of micrometastatic tumor cells in bone marrow of colorectal cancer patients. Lancet 1992; 340:685–9.
9. Silly H, Samonigg H, Stoger H, Brezinschek HP, Wilders-Truschnig M. Micrometastatic tumor cells in bone marrow in colorectal carcinoma. Lancet 1992; 340:1288.
10. Mansi JL, Mesker WE, McDonnel T, et al. Automated screening for micrometastases in bone marrow smears. J Immunol Methods 1988; 112:105–11.
11. Moreno JG, Croce CM, Fischer R, et al. Detection of hematogenous micrometastases in patients with prostate cancer. Cancer Res 1992; 52:6110–12.
12. Oberneder R, Riesenberg R, Kriegmair M, et al. Immunocytochemical detection and phenotypic characterization of micrometastatic tumour cells in bone marrow of patients with prostate cancer. Urol Res 1994; 22:3–8.
13. Bretton PR, Melamed MR, Fair WR, Cote RJ. Detection of occult micrometastases in the bone marrow of patients with prostate carcinoma. Prostate 1994; 25:108–14.
14. Wood DP, Banks ER, Humphreys S, Rangnekar VM. Sensitivity of immunohistochemistry and polymerase chain reaction in detecting prostate cancer cells in the bone marrow. J Histochem Cytochem 1994; 42:505–11.
15. Frew AJ, Ralfkaier N, Ghosh AK, Gatter KC, Mason DY. Immunohistochemistry in the detection of bone marrow micrometastases in patients with primary lung cancer. Br J Cancer 1986; 53:555–6.
16. Leonard RCF, Duncan LW, Hay FG. Immunocytological detection of residual marrow disease at clinical remission predicts metastatic relapse in small cell lung cancer. Cancer Res 1990; 50:6545–8.
17. Pantel K, Izbicki JR, Angsrwurm M, et al. Immunocytological detection of bone marrow micrometastasis in operable non-small cell lung cancer. Cancer Res 1993; 53:1027–31.
18. Cote RJ, Beattie EJ, Chaiwun B, et al. Detection of occult bone marrow metastases in patients with operable lung carcinoma. Ann Surg 1995; 222:415–25.
19. Pantel K, Izbicki J, Passlick B, et al. Frequency and prognostic significance of isolated tumour cells in bone marrow of patients with non-small cell lung cancer without overt metastases. Lancet 1996; 347:649–53.

20. Chaiwun B, Saad AD, Chen S-C, *et al.* Immunohistochemical detection of occult carcinoma in bone marrow and blood. Diagn Oncol 1992; 2:267–76.

21. Gross HJ, Verwer B, Houck D, Hoffman RA, Recktenwald D. Model study detecting breast cancer cells in peripheral blood mononuclear cells at frequencies as low as 10^{-7}. Proc Natl Acad Sci USA 1995; 92:537–41.

22. Leslie DS, Johnston WW, Daly L, *et al.* Detection of breast carcinoma cells in human bone marrow using fluorescence-activated cell sorting and conventional cytology. Am J Clin Pathol 1990; 94:8–13.

23. Cote RJ, Rosen PP, Hakes TB, *et al.* Monoclonal antibodies detect occult breast carcinoma metastases in bone marrow of patients with early stage disease. Am J Surg Pathol 1988; 12:333–40.

24. Schlimok G, Funke I, Holzman B, *et al.* Micrometastatic cancer cells in bone marrow: in vitro detection with anticytokeratin and in vivo with anti-17-1A monoclonal antibody. Proc Natl Acad Sci USA 1987; 84:8672.

25. Theriult RL, Hortobagyi GN. Bone metastases in breast cancer. Anticancer Drugs 1992; 3:455–62.

26. Body JJ. Metastatic bone disease: clinical and therapeutic aspects. Bone 1992; 13(Suppl.):857–62.

27. Berger U, Bettelheim R, Mansi JL, et *al.* The relationship between micrometastases in the bone marrow, histopathologic features in the primary tumor in breast cancer and prognosis. Am J Clin Pathol 1988; 90:1–6.

28. Osborne MP, Rosen, PP. Detection and management of bone marrow micrometastases in breast cancer. Oncology (Huntingt) 1994; 8(8):25–31.

29. Mansi JL, Berger U, Easton D, *et al.* Micrometastases in bone marrow in patients with primary breast cancer: evaluation as an early predictor of bone metastases. BMJ 1987; 295:1093–6.

30. Porro G, Menard S, Tagliabue E, *et al.* Monoclonal antibody detection of carcinoma cells in bone marrow biopsy specimens from breast cancer patients. Cancer 1988; 61:2407–11.

31. Boo K, Cheng S. A morphological and immuno-histochemical study of plasma cell proliferative lesions. Malasian J Pathol 1992; 14:45–8.

32. Dearnaley DP, Sloan JP, Imrie S, *et al.* Detection of isolated mammary carcinoma cells in marrow of patients with primary breast cancer. J R Soc Med 1983; 76:359–64.

33. Mesker WE, Marja JM, Oud PS, *et al.* Detection of immunocytochemically stained rare events using image analysis. Cytometry 1994; 17(3):209–15.

34. Makarewicz K, MsDuffie L, Shi S-R, *et al.* Immunohistochemical detection of occult micrometastases using an automated intelligent microscopy system [abstract]. In Proceedings of the 88th Annual Meeting of the American Association for Cancer Research, 1997, April 14, San Diego, CA. Abstract 1805, 1997; p.38.

35. Cote RJ, Shi S-R, Beattie EJ, *et al.* Automated detection of occult bone marrow micrometastases in patients with operable lung carcinoma [abstract]. In Proceedings of the American Society of Clinical Oncology 33rd Annual Meeting; 1997, May 17–19; Denver, CO. Abstract 1645, 1997; p.458a.

36. Datta YH, Adams PT, Drobyski WR, *et al.* Sensitive detection of occult breast cancer by reverse-transcriptase polymerase chain reaction. J Clin Oncol 1994; 12:475–82.

37. Bostick PJ, Chatterjee S, Chi DD, *et al.* Limitations of specific reverse-transcriptase polymerase chain reaction markers in the detection of metastases in the lymph nodes and blood of breast cancer patients. J Clin Oncol 1998; 16(8):2632–40.

38. Menard S, Squicciarini P, Luini A, *et al.* Immunodetection of bone marrow micrometastases in breast carcinoma patients and its correlation with tumour prognostic features. Br J Cancer 1994; 69:1126–9.

39. Dearnaley DP, Ormerod MG, Sloane JP. Micrometastases in breast cancer: long-term follow-up of the first patient cohort. Eur J Cancer 1991; 27:236–9.

40. Diel IJ, Kaufman M, Goerner R, *et al.* Detection of tumor cells in bone marrow of patients with primary breast cancer: a prognostic factor for distant metastases. J Clin Oncol 1992; 10:1534–9.

41. Mansi JL, Easton U, Berger JC, *et al.* Bone marrow micrometastases in primary breast cancer: prognostic significance after six years' follow-up. Eur J Cancer 1991; 27:1552–5.

42. Diel IJ, Kaufmann M, Costa SD, *et al.* Micrometastatic breast cancer cells in bone marrow at primary surgery: prognostic value in comparison with nodal status. J Natl Cancer Instit 1996; 88(22):1652–8.

43. Henry JM, Sykes PJ, Brisco MJ, To LB, Juttner CA, Morley AA. Comparison of myeloma cell contamination of bone marrow and peripheral blood stem cell harvests. Br J Haematol 1996; 92:614–19.

44. Kessinger A, Armitage JO, Smith DM, *et al.* High-dose therapy and autologous peripheral blood stem cell transplantation for patients with lymphoma. Blood 1989; 74:1260–5.

45. Moss TJ, Reynolds CP, Sather SN, *et al.* Prognostic value of immunohistochemical detection of bone marrow metastases in neuroblastoma. N Engl J Med 1991; 324:219–26.

46. Minna JD, Pass H, Glatstein EJ, Ihde DC. Cancer of the lung. In Devita VT, Hellman S, Rosenberg SA, eds. *Cancer, principles and practice of oncology.* Philadelphia, JB Lippincott, 1989, 591–705.

47. Rosenow EC, Carr DT. Bronchogenic carcinoma. CA Cancer J Clin 1979; 29:233–46.

48. Beahrs OH, Henson DE, Hutter RVP, Myers MH, eds. *American Joint Committee in Cancer manual for staging cancer*, 3rd edn. Philadelphia, JB Lippincott, 1988.

49. Martini N, Beattie EJ. Results of surgical treatment in stage I lung cancer. J Thorac Cardiovasc Surg 1977; 74:499–506.

50. Martini N, Flehinger BJ, Nagasaki F, *et al*. Prognostic significance of N1 disease in carcinoma of the lung. J Thorac Cardiovasc Surg 1983; 86:646–53.

51. Martini N, Flehinger BJ, Zaman MB, Beattie EJ Jr. Results of resection in non-oat cell carcinoma of lung with mediastinal metastases. Ann Surg 1983; 198:386–97.

52. Melamed MR, Flehinger BJ, Zaman MB, *et al*. Screening for early lung cancer: results of the Memorial Sloane Kettering in New York. Chest 1984; 86:44–53.

53. Mountain CF, Hermes KE. Management implications of surgical staging studies. Prog Cancer Res Ther 1979; 11:233–42.

54. Williams DE, Pairolero PC, Davis CS, *et al*. Survival of patients surgically treated for stage I lung cancer. J Thorac Cardiovasc Surg 1981; 82:70–6.

55. Nohl-Oser HC. The long-term survival of patients with lung cancer treated surgically after selection by mediastinoscopy. Thorac Cardiovasc Surg 1980; 28(3):158–61.

56. Ohgami A, Tetsuya M, Kenji S, *et al*. Micrometastatic tumor cells in the bone marrow of patients with non-small cell lung cancer. Ann Thorac Surg 1997; 64:363–7.

57. Pasini F, Pelosi G, Verlato G, *et al*. Positive immunostaining with MLuC1 of bone marrow aspirate predicts poor outcome in patients with small-cell lung cancer. Ann Oncol 1998; 9:181–5.

58. Mentges B, Bruckner R. Das Kolonkarzinom: Prognostische Faktoren. Dtsch Med Wschr 1986; 111:1790–3.

59. Pantel K, Schlimok G, Braun S, *et al*. Differential expression of proliferation-associated molecules in individual micrometastatic carcinoma cells. J Natl Cancer Inst 1993; 85:1419–23.

60. Juhl H, Stritzel M, Wroblewski A, *et al*. Immunocytochemical detection of micrometastatic cells: comparative evaluation of findings in the peritoneal cavity and the bone marrow of gastric, colorectal and pancreatic cancer patients. Int J Cancer 1994; 57:330–5.

61. Braun S, Pantel K. Immunodiagnosis and immunotherapy of isolated tumor cells disseminated to bone marrow of patients with colorectal cancer. Tumori 1995; 81(Suppl.):78–83.

62. Paget S. The distribution of secondary growths in cancer of the breast. Lancet 1989; 1:571–3.

63. Gerhard M, Juhl H, Kalthoff H, Schreiber HW, Wegener C, Neumaier M. Specific detection of carcinoembryonic antigen-expressing tumor cells in bone marrow aspirates by polymerase chain reaction. J Clin Oncol 1994; 12:725–9.

64. Catalona WJ, Scott WW. Carcinoma of the prostate: a review. J Urol 1978; 119:1–8.

65. Schellhammer PF. Radical prostatectomy: patterns and survival in 67 patients. Urology 1988; 31:191–7.

66. Pollen JJ. Bone scanning in prostate cancer. Urology 1981; 17(Suppl.):31–2.

67. Clifton JA, Phillip RJ, Ludovic E, Fowler WM. Bone marrow and carcinoma of the prostate. Am J Med Sci 1952; 224:121–30.

68. Mehan DJ, Broun GO Jr, Hoover B, Storey G. Bone marrow findings in carcinoma of the prostate. J Urol 1966; 95:241–4.

69. Nelson CMK, Boatman DL, Flocks RH. Bone marrow examination in carcinoma of the prostate. J Urol 1973; 109:667–70.

70. Mansi JL, Berger U, Wilson P, Shearer R, Coombes RC. Detection of tumor cells in bone marrow of patients with prostatic carcinoma by immunocytochemical techniques. J Urol 1988; 139:545–8.

71. Wood DP Jr, Banks ER, Humphreys S, *et al*. Identification of bone marrow micrometastases in patients with prostate cancer. Cancer 1994; 74:2533–40.

72. Katz AE, Olsson CA, Raffo AJ, *et al*. Molecular staging of prostate cancer with the use of an enhanced reverse-transcriptase polymerase chain reaction assay. Urology 1994; 43:765–75.

73. Israeli RS, Miller WH, Su SL, *et al*. Sensitive nested reverse transcriptase polymerase chain reaction detection of circulating prostatic tumor cells: comparison of prostate-specific membrane antigen and prostate-specific antigen based assays. Cancer Res 1994; 54:6306–10.

74. Smith MR, Biggar S, Hussain M. Prostate-specific antigen messenger RNA is expressed in non-prostate cells: implications for detection of micrometastases. Cancer Res 1995; 55:2640–4.

75. Crist WM, Kun LE. Common solid tumors of childhood. N Engl J Med 1991; 324:461–71.

76. Silber JH, Evans AE, Fridman M. Models to predict outcome from childhood neuroblastoma: the role of serum ferritin and tumor histology. Cancer Res 1991; 51:1426–33.

77. Brodeur GM, Fong C. Molecular biology and genetics of human neuroblastoma. Cancer Genet Cytogenet 1989; 41:153–74.

78. Fong C, Dracopoli NC, White PS. Loss of heterozygosity for the short arm of chromosome 1 in human neuroblastomas: correlation with N-*myc* amplification. Proc Natl Acad Sci USA 1989; 86:3753–7.

79. Taylor SR, Blatt J, Costantino JP. Flow cytometric DNA analysis of neuroblastoma and ganglioneuroma. Cancer 1988; 62:749–54.

80. Moss TJ, Sanders DG, Lasky LC, Bostrom B. Contamination of peripheral blood stem cell harvests by circulating neuroblastoma cells. Blood 1990; 76:1879–83.

81. Naito H, Kuzumaki N, Uchino J, et al. Detection of tyrosine hydroxylase mRNA and minimal neuroblastoma cells by reverse transcriptase polymerase chain reaction. Eur J Cancer 1991; 27:762–5.

82. Mattano LA Jr, Moss TJ, Emerson SG. Sensitive detection of rare circulating neuroblastoma cells by reverse transcriptase polymerase chain reaction. Cancer Res 1992; 52:4701–5.

83. Tobal K, Sherman LS, Foss AJE, Lightman SL. Detection of melanocytes from uveal melanoma in peripheral blood using polymerase chain reaction. Invest Ophthalmol Vis Sci 1993; 34:2622–5.

84. Cain JM, Ellis GA, Collins C, et al. Bone marrow involvement in epithelial ovarian cancer by immunohistochemical assessment. Gynaecol Oncol 1990; 38:442–5.

85. Czegledy J, Iosif C, Hansson BG, et al. Can a test for E6/E7 transcripts of human papillomavirus type 16 serve as a diagnostic tool for the detection of micrometastases in cervical cancer? Int J Cancer 1995; 64:211–15.

86. Gusterson BA, Ott R. Occult axillary lymph node micrometastases in breast cancer. Lancet 1990; 336:434–5.

87. Neville AM. Breast cancer micrometastases in lymph nodes and bone marrow are prognostically important. Ann Oncol 1989; 2:13–14.

88. Saphir O, Amromin GD. Obscure axillary lymph node metastases in carcinoma of the breast. Cancer 1948; 1:238–41.

89. Pickren JW. Significance of occult metastases. A study of breast cancer. Cancer 1961; 14:1266–71.

90. Fisher ER, Saminoss S, Lee CH, et al. Detection and significance of occult axillary node metastases in patients with invasive breast cancer. Cancer 1978; 42:2025–31.

91. Wilkinson EJ, Hause LL, Hoffman RG, et al. Occult axillary lymph node metastases in invasive breast carcinoma: characteristics of the primary tumor and the significance of metastases. Pathol Ann 1982; 17:67–91.

92. International (Ludwig) Breast Cancer Study Group. Prognostic importance of occult lymph node micrometastases from breast cancers. Lancet 1990; 335:1565–8.

93. deMascarel I, Bonichon F, Coindre JM, Trojani M. Prognostic significance of breast cancer axillary lymph node micrometastases assessed by two special techniques: reevaluation with longer follow-up. Br J Cancer 1992; 66:523–7.

94. Wells CA, Heryet A, Brochier J, et al. The immunohistochemical detection of axillary micrometastases in breast cancer. Br J Cancer 1984; 50:193–7.

95. Bussolati G, Gugliotta P, Morra Z, et al. The immunohistochemical detection of lymph node micrometastases from infiltrating lobular carcinoma of the breast. Br J Cancer 1986; 54:631–6.

96. Byrne J, Waldron R, McAvinchey D, et al. The use of monoclonal antibodies for the histopathological detection of mammary axillary micrometastases. Eur J Surg Oncol 1987; 13:409–11.

97. Trojani L, Mascarel I, Bonichon F, et al. Micrometastases to axillary lymph nodes from carcinoma of the breast: detection by immunohistochemistry and prognostic significance. Br J Cancer 1987; 55:303–6.

98. Apostolikas N, Petraki C, Agnantis NJ. The reliability of histologically negative axillary lymph nodes in breast cancer. Pathol Res Pract 1989; 184:35–8.

99. Sedmak DD, Meineke TA, Knechtges DS, et al. Prognostic significance of cytokeratin-positive breast cancer metastases. Mod Pathol 1989; 2:516–20.

100. Cote RJ, Chaiwun B, Qu J, et al. Prognostic importance of occult lymph node metastases in patients with breast cancer. Proc Am Assoc Cancer Res 1992; 33:202.

101. Neville AM, Price KN, Gelber RD, et al. Axillary node micrometastases and breast cancer. Lancet 1991; 337:1110.

102. Elson CE, Kufe D, Johnston WW. Immunohistochemical detection and significance of axillary lymph node micrometastases in breast cancer – a study of 97 cases. Ann Quant Cytol Histol 1993; 15(3):171–8.

103. Nasser IA, Lee AKC, Bosari S, Saganich R, Heatley G, Silverman ML. Occult axillary lymph node metastases in 'node-negative' breast cancer. Hum Pathol 1993; 24:950–7.

104. Hainsworth PJ, Tjandra JJ, Stillwell RG, et al. Detection and significance of occult metastases in node-negative breast cancer. Br J Surg 1993; 80:459–63.

105. Neville AM. Prognostic factors and primary breast cancer. Diag Oncol 1991; 1:53–63.

106. Schoenfeld A, Luqmani Y, Smith D, et al. Detection of breast cancer micrometastases in axillary lymph nodes by using polymerase chain reaction. Cancer Res 1994; 54:2986–90.

107. Noguchi S, Aihara T, Nakamori S, et al. The detection of breast cancer micrometastases in axillary lymph nodes by means of reverse transcriptase–polymerase chain reaction. Cancer 1994; 74:1595–600.

108. Noguchi S, Aihara T, Motomura K, Inaji H, Imaoka S, Koyama H. Detection of breast cancer micrometastases in axillary lymph nodes by means of reverse transcriptase–polymerase chain reaction. Comparison between MUC1 mRNA and keratin 19

mRNA amplification. Am J Surg Pathol 1996; 148:649–56.

109. Ho SB, Niehans GA, Lyftogt C, *et al.* Heterogeneity of mucin gene expression in normal and neoplastic tissues. Cancer Res 1993; 53:641–51.

110. Cote RJ, Taylor CR. Tumors of the breast. In Taylor C, Cote RC, eds. *Immunomicroscopy: a diagnostic tool for the surgical pathologist.* Philadelphia, 1994, WB Saunders, 200–36.

111. Cote RJ, Peterson HF, Chaiwun B, *et al.* Role of immunohistochemical detection of lymph-node metastases in management of breast cancer. Lancet 1999; 354(9182):896–900.

112. Chen ZL, Perez S, Holmes EC, *et al.* Frequency and distribution of occult micrometastases in lymph nodes of patients with non-small-cell lung cancer. J Natl Cancer Inst 1993; 85:493–8.

113. Passlick B, Izbicki JR, Kubuschak B, *et al.* Immunohistochemical assessment of individual tumor cells in lymph nodes of patients with non-small-cell lung cancer. J Clin Oncol 1994; 12:1827–32.

114. Izbicki JR, Passlick B, Hosch SB, *et al.* Mode of spread in the early phase of lymphatic metastasis in non-small cell lung cancer: significance of nodal micrometastasis. J Thorac Cardiovasc Surg 1996; 112(3):623–30.

115. Momburg F, Moldenhauer G, Hammerling GJ, *et al.* Immunohistochemical study of the expression of a Mr 34,000 human epithelium-specific surface glycoprotein in normal and malignant tissues. Cancer Res 1987; 47:2883–91.

116. Latza U, Niedobitek G, Schwarting R, *et al.* Ber-EP4: new monoclonal antibody which distinguishes epithelia from mesothelia. J Clin Pathol 1990; 43:213–19.

117. Phillips RK, Hittinger R, Blesovsky L, Fry JS, Fielding LP. Large bowel cancer: surgical pathology and its relationship to survival. Br J Surg 1984; 71:604–10.

118. Chapuis PH, Deut OF, Fisher R, *et al.* A multivariate analysis of clinical and pathological variables in prognosis after resection of large bowel cancer. Br J Surg 1985; 72:698–702.

119. Steinberg SM, Barkin JS, Kaplan RS, Stablein DM. Prognostic indicators of colon tumors. The Gastrointestinal Tumour Study Group experience. Cancer 1986; 57:1866–70.

120. Jass JR, Atkin WS, Cuzick J, *et al.* The grading of rectal cancer: historical perspectives and a multivariate analysis of 447 cases. Histopathology 1986; 10:437–59.

121. Dukes CE. Discussion on major surgery in carcinoma of the rectum with or without colostomy, excluding the anal canal and including the rectosigmoid. Proc R Soc Med 1957; 50:1031.

122. Cutait R, Alves VAF, Lopez LC, *et al.* Restaging of colorectal cancer based on the identification of lymph node micrometastases through immunoperoxidase staining of CEA and cytokeratins. Dis Colon Rectum 1991; 34:917–22.

123. Haboubi NY, Clark P, Kaftan SM, Schonfield PF. The importance of combining xylene clearance and immunohistochemistry in the accurate staging of colorectal carcinoma. J R Soc Med 1992; 85:386–8.

124. Jeffers MD, O'Dowd GM, Mulcahy H, Stagg M, O'Donoghue DP, Toner M. The prognostic significance of immunohistochemically detected lymph node micrometastases in colorectal cancer. J Pathol 1994; 172:183–7.

125. Greenson JK, Isenhart CE, Rice R, *et al.* Identification of occult micrometastases in pericolic lymph nodes of Duke's B colorectal cancer patients using monoclonal antibodies against cytokeratins and CC49. Cancer 1994; 73:563–9.

126. Florentine B, Ettekal B, Leichman CG, *et al.* Prognostic importance of occult lymph node metastases detected by cytokeratin immunohistochemical techniques in stage II colon cancer. Proceedings of ASCO, Abstract, 1996.

127. Liefers G-J, Cleton-Jensen A-M, van de Velde CJH, *et al.* Micrometastases and survival in stage II colorectal cancer. N Engl J Med 1998; 339(4):223–8.

128. Zippelius P, Kufer P, Honold G, *et al.* Limitations of reverse-transcriptase polymerase chain reaction analysis for detection of micrometastatic epithelial cancer cells in bone marrow. J Clin Oncol 1997; 15:2701–8.

129. Henke W, Jung M, Jung K, *et al.* Increased analytical sensitivity of RT-PCR of PSA mRNA decreases diagnostic specificity of detection of prostatic cells in blood. Int J Cancer 1997; 70:54–6.

130. Freeman JA, Lieskovsky G, Cook DW, *et al.* Radical retropubic prostatectomy and post-operative radiation for pathologic stage C (PCN0) prostate cancer from 1976–1989: intermediate findings. J Urol 1993; 149:1029–34.

131. Gomella LG, White JL, McCue PA, Byrne DS, Mulholland SG. Screening for occult nodal metastasis in localized carcinoma of the prostate. J Urol 1993; 149:776–8.

132. Moul JW, Lewis DJ, Ross AA, Kahn DG, Ho CH, McLeod DG. Immunohistologic detection of prostate cancer pelvic lymph node micrometastases: correlation to pre-operative serum prostate-specific antigen. Urology 1994; 43:68–73.

133. Prout GR Jr, Heaney JA, Griffith PP, Daly JJ, Shipley WU. Nodal involvement as a prognostic indicator in patients with prostatic carcinoma. J Urol 1980; 124:226–31.

134. Gervasi LA, Mata J, Easley JD, *et al.* Prognostic significance of lymph nodal metastases in prostate cancer. J Urol 1989; 142:332–6.

135. Smith JA, Middleton RG. Implications of volume on nodal metastases in patients with adenocarcinoma of the prostate. J Urol 1985; 133:617–19.

136. Freeman JA, Esrig D, Grossfeld GD, *et al*. Incidence of occult lymph node metastases in pathological stage C (pT2N0) prostate cancer. J Urol 1995; 154:474–8.

137. Freeman JA, Chapel Hill NC, Esrig D, *et al*. Occult lymph node metastases correlate with recurrence and survival in pathologic stage C (pT3N0) prostate cancer. J Urol 1996;155.

138. Deguchi T, Doi T, Ehara H, *et al*. Detection of micrometastatic prostate cancer cells in lymph nodes by reverse transcriptase–polymerase chain reaction. Cancer Res 1993; 53:5350–4.

139. Reintgen DS, Cox EB, McCarty KS, Seigler HF. Efficacy of elective node dissections in patients with intermediate thickness melanoma. Ann Surg 1983; 198:379–85.

140. Cancer statistics 1990. CA Cancer J Clinic 1990; Jan/Feb:40.

141. Cochran AJ, Wen DR, Morton DL. Occult tumor cells in the lymph nodes of patients with pathological stage I malignant melanoma. Am J Surg Pathol 1988; 12:612–18.

142. Heller R, King B, Backey P, Cruse W, Reintgen D. Identification of submicroscopic lymph node metastases in patients with malignant melanoma. Semin Surg Oncol 1993; 9:285–9.

143. Wang X, Heller R, VanVoorhis N, *et al*. Detection of submicroscopic lymph node metastases with polymerase chain reaction in patients with malignant melanoma. Ann Surg 1994; 220:768–74.

Commentary

MICHAEL D LAGIOS

Over the last 50 years, prognostication for a patient with cancer has evolved from rudimentary evaluations of size and stage made by gross pathologic examination to include an entire suite of sophisticated techniques designed to detect increasingly more minute evidence of metastatic disease. Chatterjee and his colleagues provide an encyclopedic review of the existing and emerging technologies designed to detect micrometastatic deposits in bone marrow and regional lymph nodes, either as a morphologically definable group of cells or merely as mRNA sequences detectable by polymerase chain reaction (PCR) technology. These endeavors are designed to detect either intact cells or specific mRNA sequences which are foreign to either marrow or regional lymph nodes, with the expectation that they will reflect a subset of patients, regardless of conventional stage, who are at greater risk for dissemination and progression of disease. The technological advances described, e.g., an automated, computerized screening system that can identify potential micrometastases by immunohistochemistry and reserve images for subsequent visual confirmation, might greatly reduce the time and expense involved in the application of such methods to a clinical setting.

Before oncologists peruse this very useful and clearly written summary, they should be aware of the vagaries in the conventional pathologic assessment of regional lymph nodes, the most commonly utilized sample screened for metastases, and alluded to by the authors. Pathology practice varies greatly in the degree to which lymph nodes removed during a staging procedure for carcinoma are sampled. In the recent past, some practices sampled only grossly involved lymph nodes and would stop sampling at ten nodes. More recently, and occasionally to this day, grossly uninvolved lymph nodes were bisected and half submitted for evaluation and the remainder discarded. Currently, common practice for breast cancer is to bisect lymph nodes and submit both halves, but only to sample larger grossly uninvolved or 'fatty' nodes. The sentinel lymph node procedure has markedly increased scrutiny of the sentinel lymph node(s), but practice is hardly uniform. Some practices continue only to bisect the node without levels, others make an attempt to slice the node into thinner segments before embedding and then obtain levels. The number of levels and the use of immunohistochemistry to identify micrometastases are quite variable. Thus, even for sentinel nodes removed for breast cancer, the specific pathologic methodology employed by a particular laboratory may result in a marked variation in the yield, particularly for micrometastases. These differences in yield are exemplified in the authors' data and in recent work by Dowlatshahi *et al*.[1] in which serial levels of a sentinel lymph node at 0.25-mm intervals stained by immunohistochemistry produced a yield of 52% for conventionally lymph node-negative T1a,b (1–10 mm) invasive breast cancer – a yield approximately six times that of conventional hematoxylin and eosin identifiable metastases for such carcinomas.

Such extraordinarily high yields have only a tenuous relationship to outcome. For T1a,b carcinomas detected mammographically, only 10% would be expected to have identifiable metastases by conventional means. The 90% of breast carcinomas in this subset would be expected to have a 95% 10-year disease-free survival.

In a similar disjunct with outcome, several recent studies that employed sentinel lymph node technology for mastectomies with pure ductal carcinoma *in situ* (DCIS) have revealed immunohistochemistry-identifiable micrometastatic rates of 6–8%, and yet the expected disease-free survival for patients with DCIS treated by mastectomy is 99% at 15 years of follow-up.

These discordant findings should inject some degree of caution into the use of the information gathered by these new technologies. All existing outcome data are based on conventional lymph node examination, however flawed and variable that may be. This fact has been lost on many colleagues who equate a grossly identifiable 3-mm metastasis to a single cluster of three immunohistochemistry-positive cells in a sentinel node.

Carter et al.[2] have recently described artifactual mechanisms capable of displacing benign as well as non-invasive neoplastic breast epithelium into lymphatics and resulting in 'micrometastatic' deposits in lymph nodes. Neither type of epithelium is capable of metastatic growth, but both scenarios can result in serious clinical misinterpretation, resulting in adjuvant chemotherapy. Although immunohistochemistry-identifiable micrometastases should exhibit a cytology and pattern consistent with the invasive primary, this is often difficult to establish because such deposits are so frequently detected as single cells. For example, tubular carcinomas generally metastasize as small tubular glands, not single cells or small solid cell masses of 8–15 cells. As the authors note, the inability to identify morphologically the purported micrometastasis is one of the serious limitations with PCR technology.

The evaluation of outcome data for the presence of occult micrometastases must be corrected for the T stage. Although significant differences in outcome have been demonstrated for immunohistochemistry-positive micrometastases in conventionally negative regional lymph nodes and bone marrow, much of this difference is likely to reflect the impact of larger carcinomas. As an example, the recent work of Braun et al.[3] corroborates the authors' previous conclusions regarding the significance of immunohistochemistry-identifiable bone marrow micrometastases, confirming the presence of such cells in bone marrow aspirates as an independent prognostic factor for distant disease-free survival, and cause specific survival equivalent to a node-positive status. Braun et al. demonstrated a relative risk of death of a positive bone marrow among node-negative patients of 13.26, and among node-positive patients of 3.32. However, these data reflect the inherently poorer prognosis associated with the 34% of patients with T2, T3, and T4 carcinomas, which contributed 53% of all micrometastases in that study. Most positive bone marrows contained a scant median number of these cells (93%); only 7% contained cell clusters. One of the authors,[4] in a previous publication, noted that breast cancer outcome for axillary immunohistochemistry micrometastases in particular may be dependent on the number of identifiable cells. Patients whose occult immunohistochemistry micrometastases numbered 100 or fewer cells had only a 6% difference in disease-free survival at 10 years, whereas more than 100 cells resulted in a 37% reduction relative to node-negative patients.

Disconcerting are the 23% of pT1a and 35% of pT1b patients who exhibited immunohistochemistry-bone marrow micrometastases despite expected disease-free survivals of 98% and 95% at N0 stage at 10 years. Remarkably, 22% (11/51) of T1a,b,N0, grade I or II, estrogen receptor-positive carcinomas exhibited immunohistochemistry-positive bone marrows, yet Tabar et al.[5] and Joensuu et al.[6] have showed cause-specific survivals of 97% at 16 years and 93% at 25 years of follow-up for this or comparable subsets. Given the large frequency of immunohistochemistry-positive bone marrows in this subset, and the recent work of the authors and of Dowlatsahi et al.,[1] which demonstrate frequencies of immunohistochemistry-positive axillary lymph nodes in 52% of T1a,bN0 carcinomas, a large percentage of such patients might be classified as both immunohistochemistry lymph node and marrow positive and at high risk. Would adjuvant chemotherapy be appropriate for these patients? Do scant immunohistochemistry-positive single cells in bone marrow have a significance similar to that of comparably scant immunohistochemistry-positive occult metastases in axillary lymph nodes in premenopausal patients?[4]

The techniques reviewed by the authors hold great promise for a more rational use of adjuvant chemotherapy. Future randomized trials may better define the level of advantage expected for those patients who do benefit, and identify those who will not benefit.

REFERENCES

1. Dowlatshahi K, Fan M, Bloom KJ, et al. Occult metastases in the sentinel lymph nodes of patients with early stage breast carcinoma: a preliminary study. Cancer 1999; 86:990–6.
2. Carter BA, Jensen RA, Simpson JF, Page DL. Benign transport of breast epithelium into axillary lymph nodes after biopsy. Am J Clin Pathol 2000; 113:259–65.
3. Braun S, Pantel K, Muller P, et al. Cytokeratin-positive cells in the bone marrow and survival of patients with stage I, II or III breast cancer. N Engl J Med 2000; 342:525–33.
4. Cote RJ, Peterson HF, Chalwun B, et al. Role of immunohistochemical detection of lymph node metastases in management of breast cancer. Lancet 1999; 354:896–900.
5. Tabar L, Duffy S, Vitak B, et al. The natural history of breast carcinoma. What have we learned from screening? Cancer 1999; 86:449–62.
6. Joensuu H, Pylkkanen L, Tolkkanen S. Late mortality from pT1 N0 M0 breast carcinoma. Cancer 1999; 85:2183–9.

Editors' selected abstracts

Evidence for colorectal cancer micrometastases using reverse transcriptase–polymerase chain reaction analysis of *MUC2* in lymph nodes.

Bernini A, Spencer M, Frizelle S, Madoff RD, Willmott LD, McCormick SR, Niehans GA, Ho SB, Kratzke RA.

Department of Surgery, Minneapolis VA Medical Center and the University of Minnesota Medical School, Minneapolis, MN, USA.

Cancer Detection & Prevention 24(1):72–9, 2000.

Poor survival in patients following resection for early stage colorectal cancer is thought to be due in part to the presence of occult micrometastases at the time of surgery. The *MUC2* mucin gene is highly expressed in the colon and associated colorectal tumors and may be a candidate marker for colorectal cancer micrometastases. We have used RT–PCR to detect expression of *MUC2* mRNA transcripts in order to identify possible lymph node micrometastases in node negative (Stage I and II, or Dukes A and B) colorectal cancer patients. A total of 396 nodes (histologic stage N0) from 34 colon and nine rectal cancers were studied by RT–PCR analysis with nested primers for *MUC2* (an average of 7.6 nodes per case). In the primary tumors, 42/43 (98.1%) were positive for *MUC2* by RT–PCR. Evidence of the presence of *MUC2* was demonstrated in nodes from 0 of 10 (0%) patients with Tis or T1, one of six (16.7%) from T2, 10 of 25 (40%) from T3, and one of two (50%) from T4 tumors. *MUC2* RT–PCR was negative in six nodes from three patients with non-malignant colon disease and positive in histologically positive lymph nodes from six of six (100%) Stage III colon cancers. In this study, using RT–PCR to detect the presence of *MUC2* transcripts, we have found preliminary evidence for possible micrometastatic disease in approximately a third of histologically negative N0 colorectal cancer patients. The increased presence of *MUC2* expression also correlated with more advanced T stage. We conclude that *MUC2* RT–PCR may be a sensitive and specific marker for occult micrometastases. This technique has the potential to identify a group of colorectal cancer patients at risk for early cancer recurrence.

Lack of effect of adjuvant chemotherapy on the elimination of single dormant tumor cells in bone marrow of high-risk breast cancer patients.

Braun S, Kentenich C, Janni W, Hepp F, de Waal J, Willgeroth F, Sommer H, Pantel K.

I. Frauenklinik der Ludwig-Maximilians-Universitat, Munich, Germany.

Journal of Clinical Oncology 18(1):80–6, 2000, January.

Purpose: There is an urgent need for markers that can predict the efficacy of adjuvant chemotherapy in patients with solid tumors. This study was designed to evaluate whether monitoring of micrometastases in bone marrow can predict the response to systemic chemotherapy in breast cancer. *Patients and methods:* Bone marrow aspirates of 59 newly diagnosed breast cancer patients with either inflammatory ($n = 23$) or advanced ($>$ four nodes involved) disease ($n = 36$) were examined immunocytochemically with the monoclonal anticytokeratin (CK) antibody A45-B/B3 (murine immunoglobulin G(1); Micromet, Munich, Germany) before and after chemotherapy with taxanes and anthracyclines. *Results:* Of 59 patients, 29 (49.2%) and 26 (44.1%) presented with CK-positive tumor cells in bone marrow before and after chemotherapy, respectively. After chemotherapy, less than half of the previously CK-positive patients (14 of 29 patients; 48.3%) had a CK-negative bone marrow finding, and 11 (36.7%) of 30 previously CK-negative patients were CK-positive. At a median follow-up of 19 months (range, 6 to 39 months), Kaplan–Meier analysis of 55 assessable patients revealed a significantly reduced overall survival ($p = 0.011$; log-rank test) if CK-positive cells were detected after chemotherapy. In multivariate analysis, the presence of CK-positive tumor cells in bone marrow after chemotherapy was an independent predictor for reduced overall survival (relative risk = 5.0; $p = 0.016$). *Conclusion:* The cytotoxic agents currently used for chemotherapy in high-risk breast cancer patients do not completely eliminate CK-positive tumor cells in bone marrow. The presence of these tumor cells after chemotherapy is associated with poor prognosis. Thus, bone marrow monitoring might help predict the response to systemic chemotherapy.

Cytokeratin-positive cells in the bone marrow and survival of patients with stage I, II, or III breast cancer.

Braun S, Pantel K, Muller P, Janni W, Hepp F, Kentenich CR, Gastroph S, Wischnik A, Dimpfl T, Kindermann G, Riethmuller G, Schlimok G.

I. Frauenklinik, Klinikum Innenstadt, Ludwig Maximilians University, Munich, Germany.

New England Journal of Medicine 342(8):525–33, 2000, February 24.

Background: Cytokeratins are specific markers of epithelial cancer cells in bone marrow. We assessed the influence of cytokeratin-positive micrometastases in the bone marrow on the prognosis of women with breast cancer. *Methods:* We obtained bone marrow aspirates from both upper iliac crests of 552 patients with stage I, II, or III breast cancer who underwent complete resection of the tumor and 191 patients with nonmalignant disease. The specimens were stained with the monoclonal antibody A45-B/B3, which binds to an antigen on cytokeratins. The median follow-up was 38 months (range, 10 to 70). The primary end point was survival. *Results:* Cytokeratin-positive cells were detected in the bone marrow specimens of 2 of the 191 control patients with nonmalignant conditions (1 percent) and 199 of the 552 patients with breast cancer (36 percent). The presence of occult metastatic cells in bone marrow was unrelated to the presence or absence of lymph-node metastasis ($p = 0.13$). After four years of follow-up, the presence of micrometastases in bone marrow was associated with the occurrence of clinically overt distant metastasis and death from cancer-related causes ($p < 0.001$), but not with locoregional relapse ($p = 0.77$). Of 199 patients with occult metastatic cells, 49 died of cancer, whereas of 353 patients without such cells, 22 died of cancer-related causes ($p < 0.001$). Among the 301 women without lymph-node metastases, 14 of the 100 with bone marrow micrometastases died of cancer-related causes, as did 2 of the 201 without bone marrow micrometastases ($p < 0.001$). The presence of occult metastatic cells in bone marrow, as compared with their absence, was an independent prognostic indicator of the risk of death from cancer (relative risk, 4.17; 95 percent confidence interval, 2.51 to 6.94; $p < 0.001$), after adjustment for the use of systemic adjuvant chemotherapy. *Conclusions:* The presence of occult cytokeratin-positive metastatic cells in bone marrow increases the risk of relapse in patients with stage I, II, or III breast cancer.

Detection of circulating tumor cells and micrometastases in stage II, III, and IV breast cancer patients utilizing cytology and immunocytochemistry.

Fetsch PA, Cowan KH, Weng DE, Freifield A, Filie AC, Abati A.

Cytopathology Section, National Cancer Institute, National Institutes of Health, Bethesda, MD, USA.

Diagnostic Cytopathology 22(5):323–8, 2000, May.

Evaluation for circulating tumor cells and bone marrow micrometastases has generated considerable interest due to a potential association with disease recurrence and poor prognosis. In this study, we examined bone marrow and apheresis samples from Stage II, III, and IV patients (n 120) enrolled in various clinical breast cancer trials at the National Institutes of Health/National Cancer Institute. For each patient sample, two Diff–Quik-stained cytospins were reviewed for morphology, and approximately 1×10^6 cells were analyzed for the expression of cytokeratins using an avidin-biotin immunoperoxidase method. Keratin-positive malignant cells appearing as single cells or in small clusters were detected in bone marrow samples from Stage IV patients only (9/68, 13%) and detected in apheresis samples from both Stage III and IV patients (13/245, 5%). These findings indicate that the combination of cytomorphology with immunocytochemistry can be utilized for the investigation of circulating tumor cells and bone marrow micrometastases, and that positive results appear to correlate with high tumor stage/burden.

Molecular detection of micrometastases and circulating tumor cells in melanoma prostatic and breast carcinomas.

Ghossein RA, Carusone L, Bhattacharya S.

Department of Pathology, Memorial Sloan-Kettering Cancer Center, New York, NY, USA.

In Vivo 14(1):237–50, 2000, January–February.

The molecular detection of circulating tumor cells (CTC) and micrometastases may help develop new prognostic markers in patients with solid tumors. In the last 10 years, numerous groups have attempted the detection of occult tumor cells in solid malignancies using the highly sensitive reverse transcriptase polymerase chain reaction (RT PCR) technique. These assays were in the vast majority directed against tissue specific markers. In most studies on prostatic carcinoma, RT PCR was able to specifically detect prostatic tissue specific markers in the peripheral blood (PB), bone marrow (BM) and lymph nodes of patients with localized and metastatic disease. Melanoma related transcripts were detected by RT PCR in the PB, BM and lymph nodes of patients with localized and advanced tumors. In most studies, melanoma related markers were shown to be specific except when assayed in lymph nodes. RT PCR positivity rates were highly variable between studies. Despite these discrepancies, many authors have shown a statistically significant correlation between RT PCR positivity and a poorer outcome in both melanoma and prostatic carcinoma. In breast carcinoma, all markers that have been extensively tested were shown to be non-specific. Because of the many limitations of RT PCR (e.g. false positives), many groups are developing new approaches for the detection of occult tumor cells. One of these techniques involves immunobead isolation of CTC and micrometastases prior to down stream analysis. The tumor rich magnetic fraction can be subjected to RT PCR, immunocytochemistry and flow cytometry. In conclusion, the molecular detection of occult tumor cells in solid tumors seems very promising and the techniques used for this purpose are in continuous evolution. Large prospective and interlaboratory variability studies are necessary to determine the accuracy and prognostic value of these assays.

Prognostic significance of an increased number of micrometastatic tumor cells in the bone marrow of patients with first recurrence of breast carcinoma.

Janni W, Gastroph S, Hepp F, Kentenich C, Rjosk D, Schindlbeck C, Dimpfl T, Sommer H, Braun S.

I. Frauenklinik, Klinikum Innenstadt, Ludwig-Maximilians-Universtiitaet, Munich, Germany.

Cancer 88(10):2252–9, 2000, May 15.

Background: Using cytokeratin (CK) as a histogenetic marker of epithelial tumor cells in the bone marrow of patients with primary breast carcinoma, a subgroup of patients with decreased survival can be identified. This study was designed to evaluate the frequency and prognostic relevance of such cells in patients with recurrent breast carcinoma. *Methods:* Bone marrow aspirates from 65 patients were analyzed immunocytochemically for the presence of CK positive cells. A quantitative immunoassay with monoclonal anti-CK antibody A45-B/B3 was used and 2×10^6 bone marrow cells per patient were evaluated. For prognostic evaluation the authors calculated a cutoff value of micrometastatic tumor cells by analogy to classification and regression tree (CART) analysis. Patients were monitored prospectively for a median of 37 months (range, 11–63 months). *Results:* Bone marrow micrometastases were present in 5 of 32 patients (16%) with locoregional recurrence and in 24 of 33 patients (73%) with distant recurrence. The bone marrow status yielded no prognostic indication for patients with locoregional recurrence. In contrast, a cutoff value of 2.5 tumor cells per 1 million bone marrow cells analyzed (2.5×10^6 tumor cells) correlated with a significantly different prognosis for women with distant disease. Patients with metastatic disease and a micrometastatic tumor load of $>2.5 \times 10^6$ tumor cells survived for a mean of 6 months (95% confidence interval [95% CI], 2.0–9.1) compared with 17 months (95% CI, 11.6–22.0) for patients with $\leqslant 2.5 \times 10^6$ tumor cells ($p < 0.0001$). Multivariate analysis, allowing for hormone receptor status, disease free interval prior to recurrence, manifestation site of metastases, age, and micrometastases in bone marrow, revealed that bone marrow involvement was an independent risk factor, with a hazard ratio of 7.4 (95% CI, 1.6–13.3) for disease-related death. *Conclusions:* An increased number of micrometastases identified in the bone marrow of patients with metastatic breast carcinoma represents an independent prognostic factor that may influence future therapeutic strategies for patients with metastatic breast carcinoma.

The prognostic dilemma of nodal micrometastases in breast carcinoma.

Leong AS.

Hunter Area Pathology Services, University of Newcastle, Newcastle, UK.

Gan to Kagaku Ryoho [*Japanese Journal of Cancer & Chemotherapy*], 27 Suppl. 2:315–20, 2000, May.

The presence of axillary lymph node metastasis in patients with breast cancer is a major prognostic factor and also determines the use of adjuvant chemotherapy. Micrometastasis has been arbitrarily defined as deposits of <2 mm dimension. Earlier studies of micrometastases failed to demonstrate prognostic relevance. However, when larger numbers of patients were followed up for longer periods, micrometastasis was shown to be a significantly poor prognostic parameter, with patients having a survival rate similar to those with macrometastasis or nodal disease. There are no compelling reasons to retain the term 'micrometastasis' in the light of these findings and our understanding of tumor biology. Routine histological examination of axillary lymph nodes is a notoriously inaccurate method for the detection of metastases. When serial or multilevel sectioning and/or immunohistochemical staining for cytokeratin were employed, detection rates increased by as much as 33%. Reverse transcriptase–polymerase chain reaction and Southern blotting for CK 19 may be a more accurate method of examination. However, there are inherent technical problems associated with this method, and the recent finding of a pseudogene with great homology to CK 19 in normal peripheral blood nucleated cells further emphasises the need for caution in this approach. It is not cost-effective to employ serial sectioning and immunohistochemistry when examining the axillary contents. However, the introduction of sentinel-node biopsy may allow detailed examination of the single node most likely to harbour a metastatic tumor.

Epithelial cells in bone marrow of oesophageal cancer patients: a significant prognostic factor in multivariate analysis.

Thorban S, Rosenberg R, Busch R, Roder RJ.

Department of Surgery, Technische Universitat Munchen, Germany.

British Journal of Cancer 83(1):35–9, 2000, July.

The detection of epithelial cells in bone marrow, blood or lymph nodes indicates a disseminatory potential of solid tumours. 225 patients with squamous cell carcinoma of the oesophagus were prospectively studied. Prior to any therapy, cytokeratin-positive (CK) cells in bone marrow were immunocytochemically detected in 75 patients with the monoclonal anti-epithelial-cell antibody A45-B/B3 and correlated with established histopathologic and patient-specific prognosis factors. The prognosis factors were assessed by multivariate analysis. Twenty-nine of 75 (38.7%) patients with oesophageal cancer showed CK-positive cells in bone marrow. The analyses of the mean and median overall survival time showed a significant difference between patients with and without epithelial cells in bone marrow ($p < 0.001$). Multivariate analysis in the total patient population and in patients with curative resection of the primary tumour confirmed the curative resection rate and the bone marrow status as the strongest independent prognostic factors, besides the T-category. The detection of epithelial cells in bone marrow of oesophageal cancer patients is a substantial prognostic factor proved by multivariate analysis and is helpful for exact preoperative staging, as well as monitoring of neoadjuvant therapy.

Detection of hematogenic tumor cell dissemination in patients undergoing resection of liver metastases of colorectal cancer.

Weitz J, Koch M, Kienle P, Schrodel A, Willeke F, Benner A, Lehnert T, Herfarth C, von Knebel Doeberitz M.

Division for Molecular Diagnostics and Therapy and the Division for Surgical Oncology, the Department of Surgery, University of Heidelberg, and the Central Unit Biostatistics, German Cancer Research Center, Heidelberg, Germany.

Annals of Surgery 232(1):66–72, 2000, July.

Objective: To determine the extent of pre- and intraoperative hematogenic tumor cell dissemination in patients undergoing liver resection for metastatic colorectal cancer. *Summary background data:* For patients with hepatic metastases of colorectal cancer, liver resection is the only potentially curative therapy. However, 38% to 53% of patients develop extrahepatic tumor recurrence, probably caused by tumor cells disseminated before or during surgery not detected by current staging systems. *Methods:* Blood samples harvested before, during, and after surgery from 41 patients and bone marrow samples from 30 patients undergoing resection of liver metastases of colorectal cancer were analyzed for disseminated tumor cells using cytokeratin 20 reverse transcriptase-polymerase chain reaction. *Results:* Tumor cells were detected in the blood samples of 26 of the 41 patients (63.4%) and in the bone marrow samples of 8 of the 30 patients (26.7%). Tumor cells were detected significantly more often during surgery than before or after surgery. Intraoperative tumor cell dissemination was detected in 41.7% of patients undergoing resection of two or more liver segments but only 14.3% of patients undergoing resection of one liver segment. Compared with resection of primary colorectal cancer, major liver resection carries an increased risk for intraoperative tumor cell dissemination. *Conclusions:* Detection of disseminated tumor cells in patients undergoing liver resection for metastases of colorectal cancer using cytokeratin 20 reverse transcriptase-polymerase chain reaction might help to identify patients at high risk for tumor recurrence who may benefit from adjuvant therapy. Major liver resection of metastases leads to frequent intraoperative tumor cell shedding, possibly preventable by alternative surgical strategies.

4

Laparoscopy in oncology: historical perspectives

GEORGE BERCI

INTRODUCTION

Around the turn of the twentieth century, Jacobeus in Sweden drew attention to a new procedure that he called peritoneoscopy.[1] His first patient was a female with ascites, who was suspected to have an intra-abdominal malignancy. Under local anesthesia, Jacobeus introduced a cystoscope into the abdomen and, after evacuating fluid, discovered liver metastases.

For the next few years, he collected a large number of cases in which this procedure was successful in finding a primary or secondary intra-abdominal lesion. Hans Kalk, however, was the real pioneer of laparoscopy. This German gastroenterologist designed a telescope with an electric globe. He advocated a second trocar approach to obtain visually guided liver biopsies. Ten years later, with Bruhl, he published a monograph in which he reported 2000 laparoscopies and liver biopsies without mortality. His procedures were performed under local anesthesia, with sedation. Room air was used as an insufflating agent.[2]

In 1934, Ruddock published a series of laparoscopic cases, also without mortality.[3] It was the gynecologists who took the lead with this technology.[4] They initially used it for diagnostics and then for therapeutic purposes. As this was progressing, advances in image transmission developed.[5] Because of the decreased light absorption of these new images, they were brighter, with a larger viewing angle and better image quality. With the advent of miniaturized television (charge couple device cameras), the projected image was magnified on the monitor and could easily be visualized from an optimal viewing distance.[6-8] Movements utilizing an assistant were coordinated, and videotape documentation resulted.

Several surgeons tried to popularize diagnostic laparoscopy,[9] but this technique did not occupy a central role in general surgery until the advent of laparoscopic cholecystectomy in the late 1980s. This procedure led to an explosion of interest in operative laparoscopy in the general surgical and oncologic community. Surgeons learned that the direct visualization of intra-abdominal organs was an extremely valuable diagnostic and therapeutic tool.[10] It permitted a safe target biopsy of suspicious lesions within the abdomen. As general surgeons were trained and educated to interpret visual findings, it became easy to target lesions.

Laparoscopy afforded the general surgeon an excellent close-up view of a small stab wound or buttonhole incision. Although some areas of the abdomen remained difficult to see, i.e., the dome of the liver, most could be evaluated and biopsied. The popularity of laparoscopy led surgeons to realize that diagnostic laparoscopy could decrease the number of laparotomies for non-resectable malignant lesions. It is this fact that has led to an increasing interest among oncologic surgeons as they seek to stage and treat oncology patients.[11-13]

Computerized tomography (CT) scanning is performed in many cases of suspected malignancy of the liver. If the lesion is larger than 1 cm, it will usually be seen on CT. Smaller lesions are difficult to see on CT, as parietal implants are difficult to see radiologically or sonographically. If a patient presents with a definite lesion on CT, a CT-directed biopsy may be performed. Often, these biopsies are non-diagnostic, even after several attempts; inadequate cell samples are the usual cause. A well-trained cytologist may be unable to make a diagnosis on a CT-guided biopsy. It is in this situation that laparoscopy has definite advantages.

Instrumentation

Every standard laparoscopic cholecystectomy set can be used for diagnostic laparoscopy in the oncologic setting. The operator has to check only whether the following instruments are present:

biopsy cup-forceps

hook-punch biopsy forceps

flat-punch forceps

aspiration cannula to remove fluid

an insulated suction coagulation device for hemostasis.

Documentation

In the majority of operating theaters where laparoscopic cholecystectomy is performed, a videotape recorder and a printer for color photos are standard. In previous years, many surgeons routinely videotaped all procedures performed through the laparoscope. Because this procedure (which was unique in 1990) is now a matter of routine, standard videotaping is not usually performed. Video documentation may be helpful to the pathologist, as well as for documentation of lesions that require radiation treatment. The teaching aspects of such documentation are obvious.

Anesthesia

The type of anesthesia is dependent on the patient's general condition, underlying diseases, and the surgeon's experience. Diagnostic laparoscopy may be performed under local anesthesia with sedation if an anesthesiologist is present. High-pressure pneumoperitoneum may be avoided. One of the appealing aspects of diagnostic laparoscopy under local anesthesia is that it can be performed safely in the high-risk patient.

Indications

Operative laparoscopy in the oncologic setting affords the surgical oncologist a direct method of identifying intra-abdominal disease. It can bypass many time-consuming and low-yield investigative studies.

Liver disease

Both lobes of the liver can be well visualized using laparoscopy. Asymmetry of appearance between lobes may give an indication of intraparenchymal disease. Dilated veins in the omentum or parietal peritoneum may signify portal hypertension. The laparoscopic surgeon can perform a liver biopsy in a safer manner than can be done in the standard blind percutaneous fashion. Bleeding or oozing may be controlled by compression or by coagulation. The biopsy site can be more accurately selected.

Suspected liver tumors

Cirrhotic patients have a higher incidence of hepatocellular carcinomas. Sometimes, these tumors originate from a normal-appearing liver. The value of laparoscopy in these patients hinges on the fact that smaller lesions may be missed by CT, and multicentricity may be detected laparoscopically.

Suspected metastases

If the clinical picture indicates dissemination of a primary lesion, laparoscopy can help to define this problem. Laparoscopically targeted biopsies yield larger tissue samples for the pathologist.

Palpable mass

Intra-abdominal masses that are palpable on physical examination may be specifically defined laparoscopically; they may be discovered to be extrahepatic. Retroperitoneal tumors protruding into the abdominal cavity may be better defined. Given the risk of venous bleeding with percutaneous biopsy, laparoscopy affords a safer method of biopsy in the patient with venous compression secondary to malignant disease.

Ascites of unknown origin

Radiologic examinations are impaired when large fluid volumes are present in the abdomen. Laparoscopy affords many benefits for the patient who has ascites of unknown origin. When performing laparoscopy in this setting, it is helpful to place the pneumoperitoneum needle parallel to the abdominal wall after insertion. This avoids creating bubbles in the ascitic fluid that may interfere with visibility. In the patient with dilated periumbilical veins, alternative sites of needle and trocar placement should be considered. During laparoscopy in the patient with ascites, usually a few milliliters of ascitic fluid are withdrawn to indicate that the needle is in the proper place. Trocars are placed after installation of the pneumoperitoneum. Unfortunately, ascites does not provide a 'protective cushion.' A small pneumoperitoneum is still required. The veress pneumoperitoneum needle after penetration of the abdominal wall should be kept parallel with the abdominal wall to avoid creation of a bubble in the ascitic fluid. Because the intestines are gas filled, they float on top of the ascitic fluid, presenting the risk of enteric perforation. Once the telescope has been successfully introduced above the fluid level of ascites, another small incision may be made for additional trocar placement. The patient is placed in a reverse Trendelenburg position, and the ascitic fluid is removed by suction. It is possible to evacuate several liters of fluid at this time. Anesthetic management is key to insuring the hemodynamic stability of the patient. Once the ascitic fluid has been removed, the liver and other viscera may be visualized. The cirrhotic liver may be seen. The undersurface of the liver may be examined by using additional instruments. Metastatic lesions may be discovered in the parietal peritoneum, falciform ligament, or even on the serosa of the intestine or stomach. It is suggested that trocar sites in patients with ascites be closed with fascial sutures and subcutaneous sutures to the skin. Laparoscopy in the patient with ascites of unknown origin will usually reveal the diagnosis within a short period of time.

Staging

One of the major issues in laparoscopy in oncology is the value of this procedure in staging the patient. Carcinoma of the pancreas is a good example. In approximately one-third of cases, there is peritoneal involvement at the time of diagnosis. At this stage, CT scan or ultrasound is not sensitive enough to detect small nodules on the parietal peritoneum or the diaphragm.[14] It is helpful to perform laparoscopy prior to any major oncologic procedure. If the patient is brought to surgery for resection prior to laparotomy, laparoscopy should be performed. This approach to pancreatic cancer can save the patient a full laparotomy as well as prolonged hospitalization.

Lymphogranulomatous disease

Non-Hodgkin's lymphoma, with its widespread appearance, can easily be seen and biopsied. In Hodgkin's disease, multiple liver biopsies can be performed on both lobes. This affords a larger sample for the pathologist. Larger lymph nodes presenting in the mesentery may also be biopsied. The assessment of splenic involvement in Hodgkin's disease is controversial.[15]

CONTRAINDICATIONS

Mechanical or paralytic ileus

There is widening experience of laparoscopy in the patient with bowel obstruction or ileus. The greatest danger is perforation of dilated intestinal loops; laparoscopy in this situation depends on the expertise of the surgeon and the severity of the ileus or obstruction.

Blood dyscrasias and coagulopathies

Hematologic abnormalities should be assessed and corrected prior to laparoscopy. There are large variations in the extent and severity of such coagulopathies, and each case should be individually evaluated. Special attention should be paid to aspirin intake and other platelet inhibitors.

Obesity

The obese patient presents several technical problems to the oncologic laparoscopist. It may be difficult to obtain pneumoperitoneum using the closed technique, and the technique may be changed to open laparoscopy, using a Hasson trocar. It is essential that longer instruments be available in the truly morbidly obese patient.

Cardiorespiratory disease

As with any surgical procedure, severe cardiac disease or recent myocardial infarction may prevent the performance of this laparoscopy. Compensated disease is usually not an absolute contraindication if the patient has been properly evaluated and is meticulously monitored. Severe chronic obstructive pulmonary disease should also be evaluated prior to the procedure.

Previous abdominal surgery

In the patient with previous abdominal surgery, it is essential that the puncture site be carefully selected and tested prior to the installation of the pneumoperitoneum. A precise history of the patient's previous surgery is important in assessing the extent of intra-abdominal adhesions.

TECHNIQUE

The technique of operative laparoscopy has been described elsewhere.[16] However, several points regarding the oncologic patient are worth mentioning. In sick or cachectic patients, the grade of CO_2 installation should be slow (1–1.5 L/min). Such patients may develop hemodynamic changes if there is a sudden interference with venous return or a vasovagal reflex due to sudden tension on the diaphragm. In cases of hypertension or other problems occurring during pneumoperitoneum, the surgeon should stop the pneumoperitoneum and deflate the abdomen. The same evacuation of pneumoperitoneum should occur if the trocar has been placed and a problem is identified by the anesthesiologist. Usually, the problem disappears, and the pneumoperitoneum may be attempted again at a slower rate. The usual pressure for such laparoscopies is in the 15–17 mmHg range. Operative laparoscopy is done in the supine position. If ascites is present or a better view of the liver is required, the reverse Trendelenburg position may facilitate observation. After the laparoscopy is completed, the abdominal cavity should be examined for bleeding as well as for evidence of organ injury. Trocar sites are usually infiltrated with local anesthesia to decrease postoperative pain and should be meticulously closed with a few subcutaneous stitches to avoid leakage.

The non-operated abdomen

In the non-operated abdomen, the pneumoperitoneum is usually instilled subumbilically. Needle aspiration is performed. The saline drop test is also performed to assure free flow at the tip of the needle. If a palpable mass is present in the midline, the needle may be placed in any number of lateral positions.

The operated abdomen

In the patient with previous surgery, alternate installation sites and trocar placement must be chosen. The left lower quadrant or right lower quadrant may be used in the patient who has had a previous upper midline incision or right subcostal incision. Needle and trocar placements are guided by the nature of the previous surgery, the patient's history, and the position of the scar. In case of difficulties the open (Hassan) technique should be considered. As with the placement of the pneumoperitoneum, any hemodynamic changes during trocar placement should lead to desufflation and intraoperative consultation with the anesthesiologist. Sudden hypotension should lead to a consideration of major vascular injury, with immediate abdominal exploration.

GENERAL ASPECTS

The laparoscope is prepared with an attached television camera. It is advisable to 'white balance' the camera, focus it, and have the lens prewarmed in warm saline. After the trocar is inserted and advanced, the laparoscope is slowly inserted under continuous observation. It is helpful to insert the laparoscope parallel to the abdominal wall. When evaluating the oncologic patient, it is useful to observe the falciform ligament: is it in the middle, or is it displaced by a mass? The parietal peritoneum is then examined as well as the architecture of the venous system. Once initial assessment is completed, an accessory trocar is placed. A finger indentation or transillumination facilitates the safe placement of these additional trocars. A probe is then used to move the omentum, examine the lobes of the liver, and 'palpate' the liver. The tactile sensation resulting from this probe may indicate the consistency of liver lesions. The probe is then used to examine the left lobe of the liver and to elevate it in order to inspect its undersurface. It is essential that, prior to biopsying any lesion, it is palpated to differentiate a solid from a cystic lesion. The color of the liver is noted, as is the appearance of its edge and surface. The parietal peritoneum is then observed. Small, whitish lesions, if present, are biopsied. Normally the spleen is not seen, as it is usually covered by omentum, but it may be observed if it is significantly enlarged. Rotating the table will facilitate visualization of the intra-abdominal organs. The operator may palpate the inferior surface of the stomach, examine the intestinal loops, the omentum, and the mesentery of the large and small bowel. Protruding lymph nodes may be noted at the root of the mesentery, which may be dissected and biopsied. If fluid is noted in the gutters, it may be evacuated and sent for cytologic examination. The gallbladder usually appears thin walled and bluish. In cases of jaundice with the presence of a collapsed gallbladder, a tumor of the bile duct may be suspected. A distended gallbladder which cannot be compressed may lead to a consideration of distal obstruction of the common bile duct. A cirrhotic liver may display typical scarring, regenerative nodules, and a solid–hard impression on palpation. Very large nodules accompanied by fibrosis may be indicative of postnecrotic cirrhosis.

COMPLICATIONS

The use of laparoscopy in the evaluation of the oncologic patient affords a relatively low-risk technique of assessment and staging. However, complications may occur. Bleeding from the abdominal wall can usually be treated by compression or direct suture ligation. Enterotomies of the intestine require exploration and repair. A routine part of laparoscopy should be careful observation of the abdominal cavity, looking particularly for the presence of blood or enteric contents. A variety of hemodynamic changes can occur during laparoscopy; these are usually treated by evacuation of the pneumoperitoneum.

Most patients recover uneventfully after laparoscopic evaluation for oncologic disease. Therefore, any complaint of pain or signs of hypotension should be evaluated.

POSTOPERATIVE OBSERVATION

Operative laparoscopy may safely be performed in the outpatient setting. For patients who have had extensive biopsies, it may be advisable to admit them for an overnight stay. An intravenous line is left in place, and oral fluid is begun. As with any operative procedure, early identification and treatment of complications will lessen the overall morbidity and mortality of these procedures.

CONCLUSIONS

Since the advent of laparoscopic cholecystectomy, there has been an explosion of interest in the use of laparoscopy in evaluating many types of patients. The abilities to evaluate the abdominal contents, to biopsy targeted lesions safely, and to document the extent of disease represent significant benefits for the oncologic patient. This technique should be a central part of the surgical–oncologic armamentarium.

REFERENCES

1. Jacobeus HC. Kurze Ubersicht über meine Erfahrungen mit der Laparoskopie. Münch med Wschr 1911; 58:2017–19.

2. Kalk H, Bruhl W. *Leitfaden der Laparoskopie.* Stuttgart, Thieme, 1951.

3. Ruddock JC. Peritoneoscopy. West J Surg Obstet Gynec 1934; 42:392–4.

4. Semm K. Die laparoskopie in der Gynekologie. J Geburtshilfe Frauenheilkd 1967; 27:1029.

5. Hopkins HH. Physics of the fiberoptic endoscope. In Berci G, ed. *Endoscopy.* New York, Appleton-Century-Crofts, 1976, 27–64.

6. Berci G, Davids J. Endoscopy and television. BMJ 1962; 1:1610.

7. Berci G, Schulman AG, Morgenstern L, *et al.* TV choledochoscopy. Surg Gynecol Obstet 1985; 160:176.

8. Berci G, Brooks PG, Paz-Partlow M. TV-laparoscopy: a new dimension in visualization and documentation of pelvic pathology. J Reprod Med 1986; 31:585–8.

9. Berci G, Cuschieri A. *Practical laparoscopy.* London: Baillère Tindall, 1986.

10. Cuschieri A, Berci G. *Laparoscopic biliary surgery,* 2nd edn. Philadelphia: Lippincott, 1992.

11. Berci G. Laparoscopy for oncology. In Moussa A, *et al.* eds. *Comprehensive textbook of oncology.* Baltimore, Williams and Wilkins, 1991, 210–19.

12. Cuschieri A. Value of laparoscopy in hepatobiliary disease. Ann R Coll Surg Engl 1975; 57:33–8.

13. Cuschieri A, Hall AW, Clark J. Value of laparoscopy in the diagnosis and management of pancreatic cancer. Gut 1978; 19:672–7.

14. Warshaw AL, Tepper JE, Shipley WU. Laparoscopy in the staging and planning of therapy for pancreatic cancer. Am J Surg 1986; 158:76–80.

15. Lightdale CJ. Clinical application of laparoscopy in patients with malignant neoplasms. Gastrointest Endosc 1982; 28:99–102.

16. Cuschieri A, Berci G. Technique of laparoscopic cholecystectomy. In Cuschieri A, Berci G, eds, with contributions by Paz-Bartlow M, Nathanson LK, Sackier J. *Laparoscopic biliary surgery,* 2nd edn. London: Blackwell Scientific Publications, 1992, 69–101.

Commentary

LEO A GORDON

Istuc est sapere, non quod aute pedes modo est.
Videre, sed etiam illa, quae futura sunt, Prospicere.

To be wise is to not see merely that which lies before your feet, but to foresee even those things which are in the womb of futurity.

Terentius (195–159 BC)

Dr Berci's illustrious endoscopic career provides a fitting bookend for an evaluation of laparoscopic applications to surgical oncology. He is the 'Father of Laparoscopy,' who has had the good fortune to see his 'child' grow to influential maturity and to dominate the surgical landscape for the last decade.

His contributions and lucid texts are the benchmark for anyone's observations on laparoscopy and its applications. I am personally honored to have been asked to comment on his chapter.

Laparoscopy provides several benefits for the oncologic patient. As techniques have been refined, the gulf between open exploration and laparoscopic exploration has been narrowed. Better cameras, better instruments, and widening experience all provide the surgeon with the ability to truly 'explore' the abdomen. Laparotomy for 'exploration' is becoming less common. The tactile sensations of open surgery, the assessment of erosion and growth into contiguous organs, and the technical data gained from laparoscopy have established criteria of unresectability. The advancing techniques of laparoscopic ultrasound have aided this immensely.

The surgical laparoscopist stands at the flashpoint of two advancing technologies – laparoscopy and non-invasive assessment of solid organs. At the time of this writing, these two modalities are converging and 'cross-pollinating,' to use a term of the surgical theorists. What we are seeing is less-invasive approaches generating more significant data. A tumor that is 'moveable' by older criteria can now be anatomically defined by refined sonographic techniques. Tissue planes, areas of extension, and relations to major vessels can now be delineated with more precision than by tactile assessment. Smaller and smaller laparoscopes are being fitted to better and better imaging systems.

The advent of mass scanning has special significance to the oncologic laparoscopist. In the near future, surgeons will be evaluating asymptomatic masses detected years before conventional symptoms. The time-honored 'chief complaint' of 'pain in the left side of my abdomen' will be replaced by the new chief complaint: 'Doctor, my body scan showed a 0.25-cm lesion in the tail of my pancreas.' This complaint will be a challenge for surgeon and oncologist alike: the surgical laparoscopist.

Several areas of laparoscopic surgical oncology have been examined in recent years: pancreatic cancer, gastric cancer, colon cancer, and lymphoproliferative disorders.

PANCREATIC CANCER

A dismal outlook and pervasive nihilistic attitude permeate the thinking of the working surgeon. In all but the most rarefied corners of academia, there is a reluctance to embark on resectional therapy for pancreatic cancer.

There has been an ongoing focus on the pancreas as newer imaging techniques have been refined. Helical CT scanning has been found to be sensitive and accurate for predicting unresectability.[1] Magnetic resonance (MR) has been compared with Endoscopic retrograde cholangiopancreatography (ERCP) in malignant biliary obstruction.[2] Because of its ability to detect vascular involvement, MR was found to have an advantage over ERCP. Building on these advances in imaging, the surgical laparoscopist has taken the next step: combining the non-invasive aspects of laparoscopy with these refined imaging techniques.

Laparoscopy for pancreatic cancer can help the patient by maximizing outpatient time. Many centers employ laparoscopy as the first step in assessing the newly discovered pancreatic lesion. As an adjunct to a planned laparotomy, the early detection of 'criteria of unresectability' greatly abbreviate hospital stays and allow definitive diagnosis of extrapancreatic tumor spread. There is morbidity and mortality associated with exploratory laparotomy for pancreatic cancer. The surgical goal is to maximize clinical information with the least morbidity.

Demonstrating an unusual and humanistic respect for the individual, medical economists have referred to this disease as a 'cost-loser.' In these times of scrutiny of medical costs, expenses engendered in the work-up and treatment of pancreatic cancer have been analysed.[3] Attempts at streamlining this diagnostic work-up have estimated that such measures can save approximately $6 million from the healthcare costs.

Exploratory laparoscopy offers several advantages to the patient with pancreatic cancer. This technique can document metastatic spread of tumor, obviating the need for laparotomy. Tumors can be clipped to map radiation therapy.

Laparoscopy is enhanced with the use of intraoperative endoscopic ultrasound. Minnard and associates at Sloan–Kettering found the greatest contribution of laparoscopic ultrasound in patients with equivocal laparoscopic findings. Twelve of the 13 patients with equivocal laparoscopic findings were found to have had vascular involvement when ultrasound was added. In their series, laparoscopic ultrasound combined with laparoscopy was 100% sensitive, 98% specific, and 98% accurate.[4]

Coupling fine-needle aspiration with laparoscopic ultrasound usually yields a tissue diagnosis.[5] This technique allows the differentiation between benign and malignant masses.

The sonographic criteria of unresectability for laparoscopic cases are similar to the criteria for open cases: metastases, mesocolic involvement, nodal involvement, and major vascular tumor encasement.

Several technical advances are underway to make the laparoscopic assessment of pancreatic tumors more specific. High-frequency/high-resolution transducers of smaller size are being developed. Laparoscopic instrumentation is being refined to provide tactile feedback – the cornerstone of anatomically responsible operative surgery. The actuations of many of the laparoscopic instruments are also being refined to provide the ultimate tool – an extension of the surgeon's hands. Couple these advances with the advent of 'minilaparoscopy,' using laparoscopes as small as 2 mm, and one can see the future of laparoscopy for pancreatic cancer.

Although some have relegated laparoscopic resectional therapy for pancreatic cancer to surgeons' 'fish stories,' this is an area of interest. I am reminded of the early days of laparoscopic cholecystectomy when surgeons would look into an operating room, see a distended gallbladder on the screen, shake their heads, and walk away. As fewer than 20% of pancreatic cancers are resectable, it makes sense to see if some of the operative techniques can be adapted to palliative procedures. The most feasible procedure is the laparoscopic gastroenterostomy (LGE), which builds on the increasing experience with laparoscopic colon surgery. It employs existing linear laparoscopic staples to perform a gastric bypass for outlet obstruction.[6] Some investigators noted no difference in the morbidity and mortality when comparing open versus laparoscopic gastro-jejunostomy.[7] Few patients will require this procedure, because they seldom present with gastric outlet obstruction.

Some surgeons advocate laparoscopic cholecystoenterostomy. Two issues must be kept in mind:

1 endoscopic biliary stenting is relatively effective,
2 cholecystoenterostomy requires a high level of advanced laparoscopic skill.

As with open cholecystoenterostomy, the malignant obstruction must be below the insertion of the cystic duct.[8] This occurs in roughly 20% of malignant obstructions.

Pancreatic cancer lends itself to laparoscopic assessment. This disease stands at the convergence of smaller laparoscopes, improved imaging techniques, and refined criteria of unresectability.

GASTRIC CANCER

We stand in a transition zone of surgical expertise. The classically trained, 'open' surgical anatomists are being replaced by newer graduates schooled in laparoscopic techniques. Just as the blood-letters and cauterizers of old looked suspiciously at the surgeons who dared to open body cavities, so do many surgeons today look suspiciously at resectional laparoscopic techniques for malignancies.

Gastric surgery, once the font of general surgical experience, is performed today mainly for malignancy. Laparoscopists have focused on gastric surgery with the two-'s' approach: stage the patient in an attempt to spare the patient.

Most patients with gastric cancer present at an advanced stage of the disease. More than one-third have unsuspected metastatic disease at the time of laparotomy. Laparoscopy has the advantage of sparing these patients laparotomy. It also has the advantage of detecting small metastatic deposits which are too small to be detected by preoperative imaging techniques. Laparoscopy combined with laparoscopic abdominal lavage leading to cytology may add even more sensitivity to laparoscopic assessment.[9]

Laparoscopic resectional therapy has its greatest application in early gastric lesions. Most of the reports have come from Japan, where gastric screening protocols have been in place for many years.[10] Resectional therapy has – as do most laparoscopic procedures – the advantages of less postoperative pain, a shorter stay in hospital, and a faster recovery. Endoscopic tumor staining and intraoperative endoscopy have been used to facilitate judgment regarding margins during laparoscopic gastrectomy.[11]

Several investigators describe 'laparoscopic palpation,' which is a unique term. It hints at the increasing experience of laparoscopists in striving to equal the open surgical mode. The goal is to transfer the tactile sense of open surgery to the laparoscopic setting. Laparoscopic resectional gastrectomy appears to be best suited for smaller, early lesions that are node negative.

COLON CANCER

There is much controversy, debate, seminar preparation, retreats, panel discussions, diatribes, and jeremiads in surgery today regarding laparoscopic colon resection. Much of the controversy could be resolved by adhering to semantically proper surgical terms. One must define the extent of the laparoscopic activity to assess a laparoscopic operation. Personal observations of laparoscopic colon surgery range from a thrilling assessment of the line of Toldt to laparoscopically assisted colectomy, to total intracorporeal laparoscopic colectomy. One need only look at the extent of 'axillary dissection' as evidenced by pathology reports for breast cancer to understand the need for better and more accurate definition of laparoscopic surgical activity.

The main issues to be resolved at this point in the development of laparoscopic colon surgery are:

1 *The effect of pneumoperitoneum on the spreading of colon cancer tumor cells.* Chen's work suggests the spread of tumor cells through the portal vein to the liver in the rat model.[12] Further work[13] implicates pneumoperitoneum as a cause of tumor dissemination and port-site metastases. The survival rates and patterns of spread are being analysed in an attempt to find out the long-term implications of pneumoperitoneum.

2 *The extent of resection by laparoscopic techniques.* The extent of resection has been the traditional benchmark for adequacy of resection. What are the survival implications of narrower margins? Can laparoscopic techniques reproduce the open setting? Is the extent of lymphadenectomy important and what is the influence of that lymphadenectomy on survival? These questions remain to be answered.

3 *The safety of the procedure.* What are the effects of capnoperitoneum on an aging population? What is the patient cost of the ever-present 'learning curve?' Do the complications of laparoscopy offset the complications of open surgery? As these issues are resolved, the relative safety of laparoscopic colon resection will be defined.

4 *The benefits of the procedure.* Laparoscopic colectomy generally results in a shorter hospital stay, earlier return of intestinal function, and earlier mobilization. Whether or not these benefits are 'statistically significant' must be put into the context of the patient population to see if they are 'logically significant.' By that I mean, what is the logic of employing a new procedure for 'earlier return to full activity' if the 'activity' is that of a sedentary retiree? I mean no disrespect to retirees, hoping to become one myself. However, short of full population mobilization in a war-time setting, the real benefit of 'earlier mobilization' must be examined.

5 *Port-site metastases as a complication of the procedure.* Every new technology has a surgically significant complication. I am reminded of the vascular surgeon who was unemployed until the new angiographer came to town. Such is the case with port-site metastases. The influences of positive intra-abdominal pressure, trocar tumor contamination, and body wall manipulation are being studied.[14] This issue is yet to be resolved as the studies present conflicting data.

Colon surgery is in transition as these issues are studied and resolved. An interesting medical–social scenario is playing out in the operating theaters of the USA as increasingly demanding technology faces decreasing remuneration.

LYMPHOPROLIFERATIVE DISORDERS

Few surgeons have ever felt the typical sense of surgical satisfaction after an open staging laparotomy for lymphoproliferative disease. Many of the patients are young. The open procedure of node biopsy, splenectomy, and liver biopsy has a defineable morbidity and mortality, and such staging procedures are often negative for intraabdominal disease. The thrill of a negative pathology report never totally obliterated the pain or scar arising from such procedures.

For this reason, the laparoscopic eye was turned to lymph node biopsy and splenectomy. For the surgical laparoscopist, the splenic embryology has done us a few favors: the organ is approachable, disposable, has a uniform blood supply, and has well-defined anatomic planes. All of these issues converge to make laparoscopic splenectomy and node biopsy appealing.

At the time of writing, it is clear that laparoscopic splenectomy for idiopathic thrombocytopenia purpura and staging for Hodgkin's disease represent an advance over the open technique. Many of these patients are young. The laparoscopic procedure allows return to work or to school much sooner than with the open technique. There is some evidence that one of the benefits of this approach may be the earlier institution of chemotherapy.[15]

CONCLUSION

As with any new operative procedure, laparoscopy in the field of surgical oncology has generated more questions than answers. This reflects the history of laparoscopic cholecystectomy, perhaps the single greatest surgical innovation of the last 20 years. The issues for the surgical laparoscopist, however, are broader, and therefore will require longer study.

Currently, laparoscopic surgery for oncologic problems appears to be most efficacious for clinical staging. Resectional therapy is evolving. As instrumentation becomes more refined and as a new generation of surgeons becomes more experienced, resectional therapy, based on evolving oncologic criteria, will have wider appeal. Should laparoscopic surgery for oncologic problems prove a failure, it is comforting to know that we have a 100-year track record of open surgery to fall back on.

REFERENCES

1. Furukawa H, Kosuge T, Mukai K, *et al.* Helical computed tomography in the diagnosis of portal vein invasion by pancreatic head carcinoma: usefulness for selecting surgical procedures and predicting the outcome. Arch Surg 1998; 133:61–5.
2. Georgopoulos SK, Schwartz LH, Jarnagin WR, *et al.* Comparison of magnetic resonance and endoscopic retrograde cholangiopancreatography in malignant pancreaticobiliary obstruction. Arch Surg 1999; 134:1002–7.
3. Alvarez C, Livingston EH, Ashley SW, Schwarz M, Reber HA. Cost–benefit analysis of the work-up for pancreatic cancer. Am J Surg 1993; 165:53–8; discussion 58–60.
4. Minnard EA, Conlon KC, Hoos A, Dougherty EC, Hann LE, Brennan MF. Laparoscopic ultrasound enhances standard laparoscopy in the staging of pancreatic cancer. Ann Surg 1998; 228:182–7.
5. Suits J, Frazee R, Erickson RA. Endoscopic ultrasound and fine needle aspiration for the evaluation of pancreatic masses. Arch Surg 1999; 134:639–42; discussion 642–3.
6. Casaccia M, Diviacco P, Molinello P, Danovaro L, Casaccia M. Laparoscopic gastrojejunostomy in the palliation of pancreatic cancer: reflections on the preliminary results. Surg Laparosc Endosc 1998; 8:331–4.
7. Bergamaschi R, Marvik R, Thoresen JE, Ystgaard B, Johnsen G, Myrvold HE. Open versus laparoscopic gastrojejunostomy for palliation in advanced pancreatic cancer. Surg Laparosc Endosc 1998; 8:92–6.
8. Park A, Schwartz R, Tandan V, Anvari M. Laparoscopic pancreatic surgery. Am J Surg 1999; 177:158–63.
9. Ribeiro U Jr, Garna-Rodrigues JJ, Bitelman B, *et al.* Value of peritoneal lavage cytology during laparoscopic staging of patients with gastric carcinoma. Surg Laparosc Endosc 1998; 8:132–5.
10. Shiraishi N, Adachi Y, Kitano S, Bondoh T, Katsuta T, Morimoto A. Indication for and outcome of laparoscopy-assisted Billroth I gastrectomy. Br J Surg 1999; 86:541–4.
11. Seshadri PA, Mamazza J, Poulin EC, Schlachta CM. Technique for laparoscopic gastric surgery. Surg Laparosc Endosc 1999; 9:248–52.
12. Chen WS, Lin W, Kou YR, Kuo HS, Hsu H, Yang WK. Possible effect of pneumoperitoneum on the spreading of colon cancer tumor cells. Dis Colon Rectum 1997; 40:791–7.
13. Chew DK, Borromeo JR, Kimmelstiel FM. Peritoneal mucinous carcinomatosis after laparoscopic-assisted anterior resection for early rectal cancer: report of a case. Dis Colon Rectum 1999; 42:424–6.
14. Gutt CN, Riemer V, Kim ZG, Jacobi CA, Paolucci V, Lorenz M. Impact of laparoscopic colonic resection on tumour growth and spread in an experimental model. Br J Surg 1999; 86:1180–4.
15. Berman RS, Yahanda AM, Mansfield PF, *et al.* Laparoscopic splenectomy in patients with hematologic malignancies. Am J Surg 1999; 178:530–6.

5

Laparoscopic surgery for cancer

ALAN T LEFOR

INTRODUCTION

Laparoscopy has become an important tool in the diagnosis and treatment of many diseases throughout the world over the past 10 years. However, it has been available for nearly 100 years, used mostly by gynecologists, hepatologists, and a few pioneer general surgeons. One of the major reasons for its new popularity is the availability of high-quality images on video monitors, making it easy for a team of surgeons to work together, each with the same view. In addition, the development of long-handled tools which function through ports has rapidly and widely expanded the scope of laparoscopic surgery as we enter the new millennium. Whereas laparoscopy is applied widely to a large number of surgical conditions, and has become the standard surgical approach for cholecystectomy since its introduction to the USA in 1988, its application to patients with cancer remains less well defined. In fact, at the present time, there are no specific indications for the use of laparoscopy in patients with malignancies. Naturally, this remains subject to immediate change as techniques become further refined.

There are two principles that guide the use of laparoscopy in the care of the cancer patient:

1 Similar to the conduct of any procedure, the procedure should not be performed simply because it can be done laparoscopically.
2 When laparoscopy is used in the care of the cancer patient for diagnosis, staging, treatment, or palliation, the laparoscopic conduct of the operation should compromise neither the nature of the procedure nor the amount or source of the tissue obtained.

Surgeons have been involved in the diagnosis, staging, treatment, and palliation of malignancies for centuries. Laparoscopy is assuming a role in each of these areas.

1 It has a role in establishing the *diagnosis* of cancer in some situations, allowing biopsy of intraperitoneal and retroperitoneal masses and lymph nodes, biopsy of visceral lesions, as well as the examination of abdominal contents with ultrasound probes.
2 It is useful in the *staging* of established malignancies such as pancreatic cancer, Hodgkin's lymphoma, and esophageal cancer.
3 It also has a role in the surgical *treatment* of a variety of malignancies, including gastric carcinoma, pancreatic cancer, renal tumors, adrenal tumors, colon cancer, and gynecologic tumors. It may be the appropriate approach for the definitive therapy of these lesions, or may be a way to provide a palliative procedure such as a cholecystojejunostomy in a patient with unresectable carcinoma of the pancreas.
4 It can play an important role in the *palliative care* of the cancer patient as a way of performing procedures such as feeding-tube placement or intestinal stoma creation with decreased hospitalization and recovery time.

PORT-SITE METASTASES

In the early years of modern laparoscopic surgery (*ca.* 1990), there were many attempts to duplicate the success observed with laparoscopic cholecystectomy in other anatomic sites, such as appendectomy, hernia repair, and colon resection. The technical ability to conduct these procedures was readily available, and so many surgeons 'pushed the envelope' of laparoscopic surgery. Soon after the laparoscopic treatment of malignancies began throughout the world, there appeared a number of reports of 'port-site metastases', that is, tumor recurrence at the sites of trocar placement in the postoperative period.[1–4] There was a large number of such anecdotal reports, which subjectively seemed far more common than wound recurrences after open colon resection. The true extent of the problem was difficult to determine. In a large series of open colon resections, Hughes *et al.* reported 11/1603 (0.7%) wound recurrences of tumor.[5] Several investigators began to look for port-site recurrences in a prospective manner. Ramos *et al.* reported

3/208 (1%) recurrences in a series of laparoscopic colon cancer resections.[6] Of these three patients, two had widespread disease.

A retrospective study of 372 patients who underwent laparoscopic colon resection for malignancy was conducted by Fleshman and colleagues.[7] This study had a relatively short follow-up, with a mean of just 23 months. The incidence of port-site metastases was 1.1%, which is similar to published data for open surgical resection of colon cancer. This study also demonstrated 3-year survival that was similar, stage for stage, to open colon resection data. In a large prospective study of 533 patients with a variety of intra-abdominal malignancies who underwent laparoscopic investigation, port-site recurrences were identified in just four patients (0.8%).[8] These investigators looked at the extent of disease as well, identifying port-site recurrences in 3/71 (4%) patients with advanced disease, compared with just 1/462 (0.2%) without advanced disease ($p < 0.003$), further supporting the concept that this phenomenon may be an indicator of advanced disease.

A number of investigators have attempted to explain this phenomenon using clinical studies and laboratory models of port-site recurrences, looking specifically at the effects of the insufflation gases. In a clinical study of 15 patients with malignancies, the insufflation gas effluent was directed through saline.[9] The saline was concentrated, suspended, put on a slide, and stained with Papanicolau stain. Malignant cells were found in specimens from only two patients, both of whom had carcinomatosis. These authors concluded that tumor cell aerosolization is unlikely to contribute to port-site metastases. In a study of effluent carbon dioxide, another group reported very low levels of tumor cells in the gas, but they did find large numbers of tumor cells on trocars and instruments that were used.[10] They suggest that port-site metastases might be reduced with the avoidance of mechanical contamination.

Other investigators have looked at the influence of tissue trauma on the formation of port-site metastases. In an animal experiment, tissue trauma was induced at the port sites, and a significantly greater amount of tumor grew there after insufflation than at port sites without induced trauma.[11] These investigators also identified the leakage of insufflating gas as a contributing factor. Other investigators have also looked at the influence of tissue

Table 5.1 *Possible causes of tumor cell dissemination in laparoscopic surgery for cancer*

Possible cause	Intervention to potentially minimize this cause
Dispersion of cells by carbon dioxide gas	Avoid sudden loss of pneumoperitoneum
Tumor spillage from manipulation and instrumentation	Avoid excessive manipulation of the tumor
Tumor spillage at extraction site	Protected tumor extraction (plastic bag)
Immunosuppressive effect of pneumoperitoneum	Irrigation of abdomen with tumoricidal solutions[16]

Table 5.2 *Experimental studies of laparoscopy and tumor dissemination*

Reference	Model	Results
Bessler *et al.* (1994)[14]	Murine tumor injected in dorsal skin; animals then underwent pneumoperitoneum, laparotomy, or no operation	Tumors were larger in laparotomy group than in pneumoperitoneum group
Jones *et al.* (1995)[135]	Human colon cancer cells injected into peritoneum of hamsters; animals then underwent laparotomy or pneumoperitoneum	Animals undergoing pneumoperitoneum had increased tumor recurrence in abdominal wall compared to laparotomy group
Jacobi *et al.* (1995)[136]	Colon carcinoma in rat model; animals were inoculated with tumor, then underwent laparotomy versus laparoscopy with air versus CO_2 versus no insufflation	Intraperitoneal tumor growth higher in laparotomy and air laparoscopy groups
Mutter *et al.* (1999)[13]	Intrapancreatic inoculation of carcinoma, then laparotomy versus laparoscopy, $\pm$ tumor manipulation	No differences without tumor manipulation; less tumor growth with manipulation in laparoscopy group
Allendorf *et al.* (1995)[15]	Mice had dermal tumor injection then insufflation, laparotomy, or anesthesia only	Laparotomy caused greater tumor growth
Bouvy *et al.* (1996)[137]	Intraperitoneal tumor administration in rats, then laparotomy, laparoscopy, or gasless laparoscopy	Tumor growth greatest in laparotomy group
Ikramuddin *et al.* (1998)[9]	Effluent CO_2 was bubbled through saline in 35 patients, and the cells collected and stained	Malignant cells were identified in just two patients, both of whom had carcinomatosis

injury, and found that peritoneal injury enhances peritoneal implantation of tumor cells.[12] A number of investigators have used laboratory models to compare laparotomy and laparoscopy. In the absence of tumor manipulation, there was no difference in intraperitoneal tumor growth and spread between laparotomy and laparoscopy in a rat model.[13] The possibility of immune mediation has been investigated by one group.[14,15] These investigators found that tumors were established and grew more readily and larger after laparotomy than after insufflation. In one of their studies, altered levels of tumor necrosis factor (TNF) were found, suggesting an association.[15] The relative immunosuppression of laparotomy may play a role.

There have been a number of explanations put forward to explain the phenomenon of port-site metastases. These are outlined briefly in Table 5.1. The potential causes of this problem suggest that technical modifications of the procedure may minimize the likelihood of the problem occurring. It is clear that early data suggest that the incidence of port-site recurrences after laparoscopic tumor resection is similar to the wound recurrence rate after open resections for colon cancer. Further clinical and experimental studies are in progress to determine the true extent of this problem, some of which are summarized in Table 5.2. Laparoscopic resection of malignancies off-protocol should be undertaken 'with circumspection' until the true incidence of the problem is known as a result of prospective randomized trials.[17]

LAPAROSCOPY IN THE DIAGNOSIS OF MALIGNANCY

Biopsy of masses

Masses identified on preoperative imaging studies are often amenable to laparoscopic biopsy. Laparoscopic 'fishing expeditions' may be less fruitful than such endeavors performed using conventional open techniques because of the perceived lack of tactile sensation. Some recent studies have evaluated the tactile sensation afforded by laparoscopic instruments and have found it to be almost comparable with open palpation.[18] The combined use of laparoscopy with laparoscopic intracorporeal ultrasound (LICU) may greatly improve the diagnostic yield of laparoscopic investigations. Whatever method is used, the surgeon must take great care to avoid losing the specimen; a retrieval bag may be useful for certain specimens. The techniques available for the biopsy of masses under laparoscopic control include:[19]

- Percutaneous insertion of a Tru-cut® biopsy needle with direct puncture of the mass: this is easily performed under the direct vision afforded by the laparoscope.

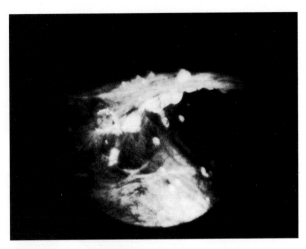

Figure 5.1 *Laparoscopic evaluation of the abdomen can sometimes reveal unexpected widespread metastatic disease, as shown here. These lesions are easily biopsied with cup forceps. Reprinted with permission from reference 20.*

- Wedge biopsy using electrocautery: this method should be used cautiously to avoid thermal destruction of the specimen.
- Cup forceps biopsy: careful use of these forceps allows the removal of adequate tissue for histopathologic examination while avoiding destruction of the specimen. This technique is extremely useful for the biopsy of small lesions such as those present on peritoneal surfaces (Figure 5.1).[20]

Liver biopsy and evaluation of liver tumors

Laparoscopy is extremely useful in the evaluation of liver lesions. It may be helpful in patients with liver lesions diagnosed by imaging studies, or in those with unknown hepatic lesions. Laparoscopic investigation of hepatic lesions can include inspection, palpation (with a probe), intraoperative ultrasound (discussed below), and directed biopsy.[21] Lesions that are located on the thin edge of the liver may be easily biopsied using two applications of the linear stapler, avoiding destruction of the tissue as shown in Figure 5.2.[22] This method is also useful in obtaining blind liver biopsies requiring larger specimens than those available with a Tru-cut® needle.

Lymph node biopsy

With careful dissection, laparoscopic access to most lymph node areas can be obtained. Specifically, mesenteric, portal, iliac, pelvic, periaortic, and celiac lymph nodes can be biopsied. In cases where specific lymph nodes are identified preoperatively with imaging studies, it may be helpful to mark the area of dissection with clips, to use intraoperative radiographs as a guide, and to assure that

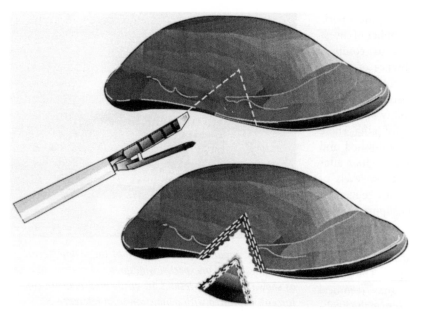

Figure 5.2 *The linear stapler can be used to obtain a wedge biopsy of the liver by firing twice at approximately 90-degree angles. The resulting specimen is of adequate size and lacks burn artifact caused by the use of the electrocautery to obtain the specimen. Reprinted with permission from reference 22.*

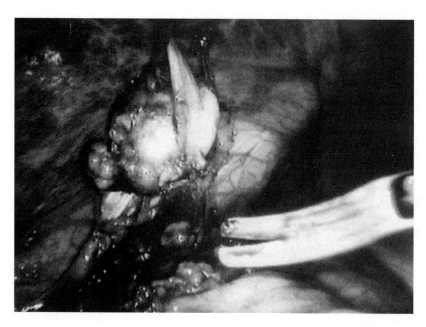

Figure 5.3 *A 70-year-old woman presented with fevers and non-specific abdominal pain. The work-up revealed a negative physical examination, with an enlarged celiac lymph node seen on CT scan. The celiac node was identified laparoscopically and excised. Histopathologic evaluation revealed non-Hodgkin's lymphoma. Reprinted with permission from reference 23.*

the desired area has been evaluated. Portal lymph nodes are fairly straightforward to approach. Mesenteric lymph nodes, when not pathologically enlarged, may be elusive. Iliac lymph nodes are approached by dissection around the vessels. Periaortic and pericaval lymph nodes require mobilization of the colon, which may require some practice but is not difficult to perform. The case of a 70-year-old woman illustrates the value of laparoscopy in the diagnosis of malignancy.[23] The woman presented with malaise and non-specific complaints, and underwent a computerized tomography (CT) scan of the abdomen. An enlarged periaortic node was identified; this was biopsied laparoscopically and the patient was discharged on the same day (Figure 5.3). Non-Hodgkin's lymphoma was diagnosed and therapy begun.

Laparoscopic intracorporeal ultrasound (LICU)

One of the most important recent developments in the laparoscopic evaluation of malignancies is the laparoscopic ultrasound probe.[24] Intraoperative ultrasound was first described in 1958 and, with advancements in the technology, has had significant impact on the intraoperative management of a number of complex problems.[25] The essential equipment consists of a probe and a scanner connected by a cable. The laparoscopic application of these devices is limited by the size and location of the access ports used. The direct contact of the probe to the liver affords superior resolution compared to that obtained with transabdominal ultrasound imaging.

A wide variety of probes is becoming available for laparoscopic examinations, including flexible or rigid tips, and linear or circular arrays.

The ability to examine the biliary tree with LICU has been described.[26] This report establishes the accuracy of this technique compared to cholangiography in determining common duct size and presence of choledocholithiasis. The use of LICU in 176 patients was reported.[27] In this series, 145 patients underwent laparoscopic cholecystectomy, and 31 patients underwent staging laparoscopy with examination of the liver. From these preliminary studies it appears that LICU has potential in the intraoperative evaluation of patients with malignancies. It is also clear that the value of this procedure is limited by operator skill. Therefore, it is important to gain experience with this technique whenever possible.

It is quite clear that the use of LICU is complementary to laparoscopy alone, particularly in the evaluation of hepatic lesions. In a study of 50 patients with potentially resectable liver tumors, laparoscopy alone demonstrated factors that rendered the patient unresectable in 23 cases (46%).[28] Of the remaining patients, LICU identified nine as unresectable. Patients in this study who underwent combined laparoscopic/LICU staging ultimately had a 93% resectability rate, compared with a 58% resectability rate among an historical group who did not have laparoscopic staging. In another study of 420 patients with a wide range of upper gastrointestinal malignancies, laparoscopy/LICU staging precluded laparotomy in 20% of patients deemed resectable by preoperative imaging studies, with an overall sensitivity of 70%.[29] The results of these studies and others demonstrate that the effective use of laparoscopy for tumor diagnosis requires the use of LICU as a complementary technique to evaluate the true extent of disease.

Laparoscopic techniques have the potential to improve patient care in the diagnosis of a variety of malignancies. These techniques include the biopsy of intra-abdominal masses, liver biopsy, and LICU. In some cases, several different techniques must be used in combination to maximize patient benefit. There are few, if any, prospective trials of laparoscopy in the diagnosis of malignancy. It seems unlikely that such trials will be feasible, or necessary. The application of this technology will depend on the judgment of the surgeon in the care of the individual patient.

LAPAROSCOPY IN THE STAGING OF MALIGNANCY

Laparoscopy is extremely accurate for the identification of peritoneal disease, which is often missed by standard, non-invasive imaging studies such as CT scanning, ultrasonography, and magnetic resonance imaging.[30] Lesions that are only a few millimeters in size can be biopsied with extreme accuracy. Liver and peritoneal disease is often found in patients with negative CT scans,

supporting the use of laparoscopy to identify these lesions.[30] A representative laparoscopic view of such lesions is shown in Figure 5.1.

A series of 162 patients with a variety of malignancies, including 98 patients with hepatic lesions and 64 patients with non-hepatic intra-abdominal malignancy, underwent laparoscopic staging.[31] All of these patients were felt to be resectable for cure, based on a number of preoperative imaging studies. Biopsies were performed in 37% of cases. In 36% of cases, laparoscopy yielded information that prevented unnecessary laparotomy because of the identification of lesions that were unresectable. Conversely, 12% of patients who had laparoscopic findings suggesting resectability were found at laparotomy to be unresectable. Sites missed included positive lymph nodes, hepatic vein involvement, and missed peritoneal metastases. This study supports the use of laparoscopy to prevent unnecessary laparotomy in those patients who will not benefit from resection.

Intra-abdominal malignancies commonly present with ascites, which is exudative in nature. Paracentesis is carried out initially. Laparoscopic examination is not necessary if cytologic examination demonstrates malignancy. However, if the cytology is negative for malignancy, then laparoscopy offers an excellent way to make a diagnosis. Preoperative CT scanning may help direct the exploration. Patients with CT scans that suggest ovarian disease are brought to open laparotomy because this is necessary in cases of ovarian cancer for definitive staging.

Laparoscopy is facilitated in patients with tense ascites by repeated paracentesis begun 24 h before surgery.[32] In a series of 47 patients with ascites, laparoscopy revealed carcinomatosis in 22, ovarian cancer in 11, three patients each with mesothelioma, hepatoma, or hepatic myelofibrosis, two patients with pancreatic cancer, and one patient with each of the following: squamous cancer, chronic lymphocytic leukemia, breast cancer, and lymphoma.[32] The accuracy of laparoscopy in the evaluation of malignant disease presenting as ascites has been reported in one series as 100%.[32]

Pancreatic tumors

Laparoscopy has been used in the staging of patients with carcinoma of the pancreas for some time. In fact, the first report of laparoscopy in the USA was the evaluation of a patient with carcinoma of the pancreas.[33] The goal of laparoscopy in the staging of patients with carcinoma of the pancreas is to avoid laparotomy in those patients deemed resectable by preoperative imaging studies. An early report describes the experience with 23 patients having pancreatic cancer.[34] This study was carried out before the widespread use of abdominal CT scan and the advent of quality optics for laparoscopy. The report emphasized the utility of biopsy under direct vision.

The ability of laparoscopy to detect metastatic disease not otherwise identified has been reported by others.[35] The use of laparoscopy and laparoscopic ultrasonography has been described in the evaluation of 40 consecutive patients felt to have a resectable pancreatic lesion.[36] Resectability was confirmed in 12 patients with negative laparoscopic examinations, for a sensitivity of 100%. Occult metastatic disease was identified in 14 patients, including liver lesions ($n = 10$), peritoneal surfaces ($n = 8$), and hilar lymphadenopathy ($n = 2$). Laparoscopy failed to demonstrate metastatic disease in three patients. As for predicting resectability, laparoscopy alone failed to identify the 12 patients with locoregional tumor unresectability, with an overall specificity of only 50%. However, the combined use of laparoscopy and laparoscopic ultrasonography resulted in a sensitivity of 92%, a specificity of 88%, and an accuracy of 89%.

More recently, several investigators have suggested that laparoscopy be used in a highly selective manner in patients with carcinoma of the pancreas, rather than as a standard staging modality.[37,38] Of 398 patients who underwent laparotomy for pancreatic or periampullary carcinoma at one center, 172 underwent resection, 150 had a palliative bypass, and 76 underwent exploratory laparotomy only.[38] Local signs of unresectability, identifiable only at laparotomy, were found in 47, leaving 29 patients (7%) who did not require palliation and whose signs of unresectability could have been determined by laparoscopy. These authors conclude that laparoscopy (with or without LICU) should be used selectively in patients considered probably unresectable who do not require a palliative surgical procedure. The laparoscopic conduct of palliative bypass procedures in patients with carcinoma of the pancreas may make laparoscopy somewhat more applicable than these data imply, however. In a retrospective study of 148 patients with pancreatic cancer, survival of patients with clinically resectable pancreatic cancer that was deemed unresectable at laparotomy was evaluated to determine the utility of staging laparotomy.[37] The importance of staging laparoscopy is enhanced if one believes that endoscopic stenting is the best palliation. These authors conclude that extensive laparoscopic evaluation is not necessary, because they contend that operative palliation is superior to endoscopic palliation. Staging laparoscopy is useful only to identify those patients with liver or peritoneal metastases who have an expected survival of about 6 months, and for whom endoscopic palliation is sufficient.

Liver tumors

The accurate evaluation of the liver is a critical component of tumor staging for many malignancies of interest to the surgeon, because the presence of metastatic disease in the liver often obviates the need for major resections. Radiologic imaging alone is imperfect, and several studies have demonstrated the scope of the problem. In one series, 63 of 150 (42%) patients with colorectal carcinoma were found to have unresectable hepatic disease at laparotomy after an imaging evaluation demonstrated resectable lesions.[39] In another series of 132 patients referred to the National Cancer Institute for liver tumor resection, 107 had negative staging evaluations and were brought to laparotomy. Extrahepatic disease was identified in 28 of these 107 (26%) patients.[40] These studies demonstrate one of the major potential benefits of laparoscopic staging: the ability to exclude from laparotomy those patients with unresectable lesions in a way that minimizes postoperative pain and hospitalization.

In a study of 29 patients with hepatic malignancies (12 with hepatoma and 17 with metastatic disease), laparoscopy was undertaken prior to laparotomy to evaluate the resectability of the lesions.[41] Laparoscopy alone demonstrated unresectability in 14 of the 29 (48%) patients evaluated. Unsuspected cirrhosis was identified in four, and unresectable or extrahepatic lesions were found in ten. Not surprisingly, these investigators found that patients who underwent laparoscopy had shorter hospital stays than historical controls who underwent laparotomy that identified unresectable disease, and concluded that laparoscopy should precede laparotomy for planned resection of hepatic malignancies.

In a study of 30 patients undergoing planned hepatic resection and 32 patients undergoing resection of a gastrointestinal primary malignancy, intraoperative ultrasonography was compared with CT angioportography.[42] Of the 30 patients planned to undergo hepatic resection, the procedure was changed or guided by the ultrasonographic result in 20 cases (67%). Of the 32 patients undergoing resection of their primary tumor, five (16%) had the stage of their disease altered by the results of intraoperative ultrasonography.

Having demonstrated the value of laparoscopy and intraoperative ultrasonography, combining the two procedures is a natural extension of the technology. In a study of 50 patients undergoing laparoscopic evaluation of hepatic tumors, laparoscopic ultrasonography was performed in 43 patients.[28] Laparoscopy alone demonstrated that lesions shown to be resectable by preoperative imaging studies were unresectable in 23 (46%) patients. Hepatic lesions not visible by laparoscopic examination alone were identified by laparoscopic ultrasonography in 14 patients. Furthermore, the use of laparoscopic ultrasonography provided staging information in addition to that gained by laparoscopy in 18 (42%) patients.

A recent study of 420 patients with upper gastrointestinal malignancies evaluated the utility of combined laparoscopy and laparoscopic ultrasound in the staging of these tumors.[29] Patients underwent routine imaging studies and were felt to have resectable disease, and then underwent laparoscopy and laparoscopic ultrasound. The use of combined laparoscopic staging avoided laparotomy in 20% of patients, with a sensitivity of 70%. Whereas it was of little use in esophageal tumors, avoiding laparotomy in just 5% of patients and with 42% sensitivity, it appeared beneficial in patients with proximal bile duct tumors, liver tumors, and pancreatic tumors. This study supports the use of combined laparoscopy and laparoscopic ultrasound in the staging of patients with a variety of upper gastrointestinal malignancies.

Lymphoma

Indications and techniques for the performance of staging laparotomy in attempts to influence the associated morbidity and mortality have undergone considerable evolution over the last three decades. Although previously performed on 85% of all patients with Hodgkin's disease,[43] staging laparotomy is now performed in, at most, only 30% of patients.[44] With the refinement of non-invasive imaging techniques, as well as changes in the medical management of the disease, the value of surgical staging of lymphoma has been re-evaluated. Consequently, the subset of patients for whom surgical staging appears to be of value has become much smaller. This has resulted in significant decreases in the proportion of splenectomies performed for staging lymphoma. In a study of the frequency of splenectomy for Hodgkin's lymphoma, Marble et al. reported a rate of 44% during the period from 1979 to 1985, compared to only 26% during the period from 1986 to 1991.[45] The role of splenectomy, however, is still in evolution. There is some evidence that combined chemoradiation therapy for Hodgkin's lymphoma may be associated with a significantly increased risk of developing a second malignant disease.[46] If this risk proves to hold true, it follows that surgical staging may again provide significant benefits for patients with Hodgkin's lymphoma by reducing their need for combination therapy. Conversely, some centers are treating every patient with Hodgkin's disease using chemotherapy as a first-line modality, obviating the need for surgical staging.

Surgical staging of Hodgkin's lymphoma has been reported to change the pathological stage of the disease in 30–40% of patients. This resulted in significant alterations in both prognosis and treatment selection.[47,48] Invasive diagnostic and therapeutic maneuvers are attractive alternatives when the results of such interventions have a definable impact on the type of treatment given or on the course of the disease. All of these maneuvers, by their nature, are associated with a degree of morbidity and mortality. Staging laparotomy is associated with 18% morbidity and up to 0.7% mortality.[46,49] Late complications occur in 5–15% of patients.[49,50] These include partial small bowel obstruction in 9.8% of patients, which requires lysis of adhesions in 6.8%, and overwhelming post-splenectomy sepsis (OPSS) in 6.8% of patients.[50] Horowitz et al. reported a 52%

overall morbidity and a 9% mortality following splenectomy for hematological diseases. Splenic size was the only preoperative factor found to be predictive of postoperative complications.[51]

Minimal access surgery (laparoscopy) has become the procedure of choice for the surgical staging of abdominal lymphoma. The acknowledged benefits of laparoscopy for other major abdominal procedures should hold true for the staging of lymphoma and thus improve its risk–benefit profile. With the recent advances in video and instrument technology, especially the availability of clear, magnified, panoramic images and of laparoscopic staplers, a wider application of these techniques in the evaluation of abdominal lymphoma has developed. These new technologies have made the complete laparoscopic staging of lymphoma a reality.

The conventional technique for the surgical staging of lymphoma has been well described.[52,53] With the smaller incisions used in minimal access surgery, several potential advantages can be offered to patients undergoing laparoscopic staging of abdominal lymphoma. These include less postoperative pain, earlier ambulation, better breathing, and shorter recovery time. These can be translated into fewer postoperative complications and possibly the earlier administration of definitive therapy. However, the procedure remains a technically demanding operation with which no single surgeon will probably gain vast experience. With further advances in laparoscopic technology, and refinements in techniques, the laparoscopic staging of abdominal lymphoma will become an important tool in the surgical armamentarium.

The laparoscopic approach to this staging procedure follows the same principles as those delineated for the open procedure.[54] The indications, components, and sequence of components should remain the same. There are no true contraindications to laparoscopic staging. The relative contraindications include abdominal wall sepsis, gastrointestinal distention, intra-abdominal sepsis, and extensive adhesions.[55] Laparoscopic staging of abdominal lymphoma has been successfully performed by several groups.[54,56–59] A comparison of laparoscopic and open staging of Hodgkin's disease has demonstrated equivalent oncologic results, and functionally superior results with laparoscopic staging.[54] These investigators found a slightly longer operative time (202 versus 144 min), but significantly shortened postoperative ileus and postoperative hospitalization times. These data strongly support the use of laparoscopy for the accurate staging of Hodgkin's disease when indicated.

The morbidity and mortality associated with staging laparotomy are well established.[46,49–51,60] A review of staging laparotomy by Multani and Grossbard demonstrated a mortality of 0.3–1%, major morbidity of 3–18%, and minor morbidity of 6–19%. Delays to definitive treatment occurred in 5–10% of patients.[61] Jockovich et al. reported surgical complications in 26% of 133 consecutive patients; these included atelectasis in 13%, small bowel obstruction in 10% (requiring reoperation in 7%), sub-phrenic abscesses in 2%, and wound dehiscence in 1%.[50]

The use of laparoscopy in the management of a variety of abdominal lymphoproliferative diseases has recently been reported.[62] These investigators performed laparoscopic investigation in 64 patients with a number of diseases, including undiagnosed retroperitoneal adenopathy, staging for Hodgkin's disease and non-Hodgkin's disease. Laparoscopic ultrasound was used extensively. The authors concluded that the interval between diagnosis and treatment was significantly shortened by using a laparoscopic approach. Although this series does not necessarily provide the final word, it again demonstrates the utility of laparoscopy in the evaluation of these patients and suggests the need for further study.

Non-Hodgkin's lymphoma (NHL) is a diverse group of diseases with a wide range of biologic behaviors. The diseases may be very aggressive and rapidly fatal or behave as one of the most indolent and well-tolerated malignancies afflicting humans.[63] As the clinical course is variable, the pattern of spread is also unpredictable. Non-Hodgkin's lymphoma is classified into low-grade, intermediate, and high-grade pathologic groups according to the National Cancer Institutes (USA) working formulation. Each of these groups is further subdivided based on cell type (small cell, large cell, etc.). The therapy for these patients is still evolving, and surgical staging is generally reserved for the very small minority of patients who will receive radiation therapy alone if the disease is localized.

LAPAROSCOPY IN THE TREATMENT OF MALIGNANCY

Gastric cancer

The application of laparoscopic techniques to gastric resection has been made possible by the rapid advances in stapling technology over the last few years. The first laparoscopic gastric resection utilizing a Billroth II reconstruction performed intra-abdominally was reported in 1992.[64] Since that time, the same group has continued to apply laparoscopic surgical techniques to gastric surgery.[65] In this series of 16 patients, all were operated on for benign disease, although two patients had foci of cancer found at the time of histologic examination. These two patients later underwent open lymphadenectomy.

The use of laparoscopic techniques in the treatment of gastric cancer requires very careful selection of patients. Early gastric cancer involving the submucosa requires gastrectomy with removal of the greater omentum and level 1 lymph nodes. Techniques for this procedure have been fully described.[66] More advanced tumors that require further node dissections are not amenable to laparoscopic resection. Patients with stage IV disease but who require palliative gastric resections are good candidates for laparoscopic resection. Gastric lymphoma and gastric polyps requiring resection are also suitable for laparoscopic resection.[66] The inability to perform extensive lymphadenectomy may limit the applicability of laparoscopic gastric resection to malignancies, but it is clear that advances in technology may make this more feasible.

Colon cancer

Carcinoma of the colon is a very common disease in the USA, making it attractive to treat laparoscopically. Surgical resection of carcinoma of the colon is a well-established procedure. Thus, any surgical approach that can potentially treat this disease, with decreased postoperative pain and hospitalization, may result in considerable advantages, generating great interest in the laparoscopic resection of colon cancer. It is clear that laparoscopic colon resection is an 'advanced' procedure, requiring more training, experience, and time than for procedures such as appendectomy or cholecystectomy.[67] However, the principles of laparoscopic colon resection are similar to those used for open colon resection. In particular, the anastomosis is usually performed extracorporeally using conventional techniques, making the technique of laparoscopic colon resection less difficult to learn. Thus, the term 'laparoscopic-assisted colectomy' is often applied to this procedure. The use of animal models has facilitated the testing of some of these techniques and may be an important educational tool.[68] Intracorporeal anastomotic techniques may be used, but remain a greater technical challenge than extracorporeal anastomoses.

Indications for laparoscopic colon resection include segmental resections for diverticular disease, polyps, rectal prolapse, and intestinal volvulus.[69] The role of laparoscopic resections in the management of colonic malignancies remains undefined at this time, and these procedures should be carried out only in the setting of a prospective trial.[17,69–72] It is reasonable to resect colonic malignancies laparoscopically, with synchronous hepatic or pulmonary metastases as a palliative procedure. When performed appropriately, laparoscopic colon resection for cancer should include the following components, just as in open surgical resections:

1 resection of tumor in the bowel wall and adjacent soft tissues,
2 resection of an adequate margin of normal bowel,
3 an adequate lymph node resection with associated vascular pedicle.[73]

Some of the clinical trials performed to date are summarized in Table 5.3.

The preoperative factors affecting suitability for laparoscopic colonic surgery are similar to those that are important in other laparoscopic procedures. The lack of ability to use palpation in the abdominal cavity prompts

Table 5.3 *Clinical trials of laparoscopic colon resection*

Reference	Year	Number of patients	Indications	Outcomes
Hoffman et al.[86]	1996	238	39 with cancer	2-year follow-up with no adverse patterns of recurrence
Wexner et al.[85]	1996	140	IBD, cancer, diverticular disease, etc.	11% conversion rate, OR time 4 h, hospital stay 6.8 days
Phillips et al.[75]	1992	51	Cancer, diverticular disease, IBD, polyps	8% conversion to open, 2.3 h operative time, 4.6 days hospitalization, 2% mortality
Liberman et al.[82]	1996	14	Diverticular disease	Decrease in costs, postoperative stay
Gellman et al.[90]	1996	102	Cancer, diverticular disease	5.9 days for lap group, lymph node retrieval same as historical controls
Begos et al.[84]	1996	50	Cancer, diverticular disease	34% conversion rate, single surgeon, 8.3 days hospital stay
Huscher et al.[138]	1996	200	Cancer, diverticular disease, other	10.5% conversion, multicenter study, 208 min mean operation time, mean nodes = 12.1
Muckleroy et al.[80]	1999	38	Benign disease only	Compared to patients undergoing open colon surgery, decreased length of stay, slightly longer OR time
Lacy et al.[83]	1995	52	Colon cancer	Randomized to laparoscopic ($n = 25$) and open ($n = 26$); 16% conversion, longer OR time in lap cases
Ramos et al.[6]	1994	252	Cancer	All cases from a registry, 1% incidence of port-site recurrences (3/208)
Kwok et al.[87]	1996	83	Cancer	15.2 month follow-up
Poulin et al.[88]	1999	135	Cancer	Review of a prospective database, 24 month median follow-up, no trocar site recurrences, survival curves similar to historical controls
Dean et al.[67]	1994	122	Cancer, diverticular disease	48% conversion rate, longer OR time and shorter LOS in lap group compared to those opened
Franklin et al.[81]	1995	84	Cancer	Total of 194 patients, 84 had lap colon resection and 110 open in same group, non-randomized; node harvest similar, margins of resection similar, survival similar at 36 months
Milsom and Hammerhofer[92]	1995	42	Cancer	Follow-up of 18 months, 13% recurrences
Fielding et al.[139]	1997	149	Cancer	7% conversion, 33 month follow-up, 7% recurrence
Lacy et al.[140]	1998	31	Cancer	Range 11.5–21.4 months follow-up, 13% conversion, 16% recurrence

IBD, inflammatory bowel disease; OR, operating room; lap, laparoscopy; LOS, length of stay.

some to perform a more thorough preoperative evaluation with colonoscopy and CT scan.[73] Patients should undergo a routine mechanical and antibiotic bowel preparation. Intraoperative positioning of the patient and trocar placement is critical in laparoscopic colon resections. Poor trocar placement can prevent the successful completion of the operation. A Foley catheter and nasogastric tube are placed in every patient prior to the start of surgery. In general, the surgeon and assistant stand on the side opposite the bowel to be resected. Whereas some prefer the dorsolithotomy position,[73] others prefer the patient to be in the supine position.[67] The use of the dorsolithotomy position has two potential advantages:

1 intraoperative colonoscopy, facilitated by the use of low stirrups, may be necessary for localizing the lesion in the operating room;
2 a recently described technique demonstrates the utility of the colonoscope in dissecting the hepatic and splenic flexures.[74] The zero-degree laparoscope is used for these procedures.

In general, for a right hemicolectomy, two left-sided and one right-sided ports are used in addition to the umbilical camera port (Figure 5.4).[75] The abdomen is explored thoroughly, with special attention being paid to the liver just as with open surgical approaches. Ports are best placed as they are needed, allowing for flexibility, rather than using a static pattern placing all ports synchronously.[68,70] After mobilizing the right colon along the avascular plane, an incision is made in the periumbilical region and the bowel is brought extracorporeally. The bowel is resected, the anastomosis fashioned, and replaced in the abdominal cavity. A canine model was used to demonstrate the feasibility of an adequate right hemicolectomy for the treatment of cancer with an intracorporeal stapled anastomosis.[65]

For left colectomy, the patient is placed in the steep Trendelenburg position, with the right side of the operating table down. The zero-degree scope is passed through a supraumbilical port, and two 10–12-mm trocars are placed in the right upper and lower quadrants (see Figure 5.4). Commonly, a fourth trocar is placed in the left upper quadrant as well. The bowel is then mobilized, and the vascular pedicle to the sigmoid colon is divided using a stapler. The bowel is then exteriorized and an extracorporeal anastomosis fashioned.[76] A wide range of colonic resections have been performed laparoscopically,

including left colon resections, abdominoperineal resections, and sigmoid colectomies.

There are technical limitations to the performance of laparoscopic colon resections. In an attempt to define them, Pandya and colleagues examined indications for the intraoperative conversion of a laparoscopic colon resection to an open procedure.[77] Two hundred patients who underwent laparoscopic colon resection were reviewed, with 47/200 converted to an open operation. Indications for conversion included technical problems in 15 patients (hypercarbia, unclear anatomy, and stapler misfire), laparoscopic complications in 9 patients (bleeding, cystotomy, and enterotomy), and problems that 'exceeded the limits of laparoscopic dissection' in 23 patients (phlegmon, adhesions, obesity, and tumor invasion of adjacent organs). The investigators noted a decreasing conversion rate with experience. After the 'learning curve,' indications for conversion have included excessive tumor bulk, adhesions, and a massive diverticular phlegmon.

The safety and efficacy of laparoscopic colectomy have been studied retrospectively. In a series of 51 laparoscopic colon resections, 24 patients underwent surgery for cancer.[75] A majority of these operations were performed using intracorporeal anastomoses, but 14% were converted to laparoscopic-assisted cases, and 8% were converted to open procedures. This series included right, transverse, left, low anterior and abdominoperineal colon resections. Operative time averaged 2.6 h and hospitalization averaged 4.6 days. Complications were reported in 8% of patients.

In another series, 66 patients underwent attempted laparoscopic colon resections, with a conversion rate to open colectomy in 41%.[78] The length of hospitalization, hospital cost, and lymph node harvest were compared

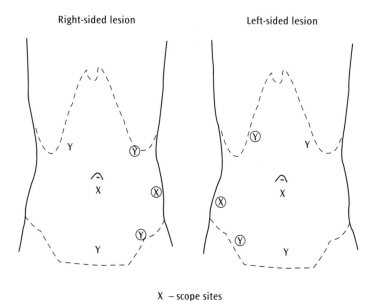

Right-sided lesion   Left-sided lesion

X – scope sites
Y – 10/11 mm
◯ – optional

Figure 5.4 *Port placement for laparoscopic colon resection is different for left and right colon procedures, as shown here. Reprinted with permission from reference 75.*

with those of patients who underwent open colon resection. The mean postoperative hospital stay was significantly shorter for patients with laparoscopic sigmoid and right colectomies than for those patients converted to open operation or those whose operations were performed using conventional open techniques. The total hospital cost for patients undergoing conventional open right hemicolectomy was less than that for the converted group, but not than that for those having a laparoscopic resection. Lymph node harvest was comparable in all three groups. These authors conclude that their results demonstrate that laparoscopic colectomy can be performed with acceptable morbidity and mortality, but that there is no definite cost saving.

Laparoscopic colon resection was performed in 80 patients and compared to a control group of 53 patients undergoing conventional open colectomy by the same group of surgeons.[79] Analysis included complications, rate of conversion, length of procedure, duration of postoperative ileus, hospital stay, hospital cost, and adequacy of the specimen obtained. Operations were converted to open procedures in 18 patients, which decreased to 12 patients in the second half of the series. The length of procedure was greater in those undergoing laparoscopic resection (mean 221 min) than in those undergoing open colectomy (mean 183 min). Operating room and total hospital charges were also greater for those patients undergoing laparoscopic resection compared to those having open colectomy. Patients having a laparoscopic colectomy had an average postoperative stay of 5.2 days, compared to 7.8 days for those having open colectomies. The pathology specimens were similar in all groups. This study further indicates that laparoscopic colectomy can be performed safely, with shorter hospitalization, but at higher overall cost. Perhaps, with greater experience, operating times will decrease, as was suggested by this study.

There have been a number of trials comparing laparoscopic colon resection to traditional open resection. Thirty-eight laparoscopic colon resections were compared to 39 open resections.[80] These authors found slightly longer operative time (161 min versus 131 min) in the laparoscopic group, with lower estimated blood loss (122 mL versus 192 mL), and significantly shorter length of stay (3.3 days versus 7.4 days), with similar complication rates. They conclude that laparoscopic colon resection for benign disease affords the patient the advantages of laparoscopic surgery, giving surgeons the opportunity to develop requisite skills while awaiting the results of trials of laparoscopic surgery for malignancy. In a prospective trial of 194 patients in San Antonio, Texas (USA), patients selected their own method of resection. Open colon resection was selected by 110 patients and laparoscopic by 84 patients.[81] The authors looked at a number of outcome variables, and observed that laparoscopic resection allows adequate margins and lymph node harvests that are no different

from those of open resection. In a brief follow-up, survival in the two groups was similar. In a study of 14 patients undergoing laparoscopic colon resection for diverticular disease, the patients were compared to a similar group who had undergone open resection.[82] Estimated blood loss, days to peroral liquids, and length of stay were significantly less in the laparoscopic group. The mean total hospital charges and costs were also less, suggesting the benefits of laparoscopic colon resection. In a randomized prospective trial, 51 patients underwent colon resection by laparoscopic means or by traditional open techniques.[83] Lymph node harvests were reported to be similar in the two groups, as were resection margins and adequacy of specimens. Also, patients were discharged earlier from hospital in the laparoscopic group. Although the follow-up was not long, this study suggests that the laparoscopic approach is preferable for patients requiring colon resection. Similar results have been observed by a number of authors.[84,85]

Some of the trials reported to date demonstrate excellent results, but lack lengthy follow-up. Hoffman et al. reported 238 patients who underwent laparoscopic colon resections, 39 of whom were available for just 24 months of follow-up.[86] They concluded that survival rates were similar to that observed for patients who underwent open colon resection. In a study of 100 patients, the median operative time for laparoscopic resection was 180 min, and the conversion rate was 31%,[87] although the conversion rate decreased relatively along the 'learning curve.' The median follow-up was just 15 months in this study, which demonstrated four distant recurrences and one pelvic recurrence. These authors assert the importance of longer follow-up and a randomized trial to establish the benefit of this procedure. In an excellent study of 172 patients who underwent laparoscopic resection for adenocarcinoma of the colon, 25 patients underwent conversion to open resection and 12 patients were lost to follow-up, leaving 135 patients in the study.[88] The median follow-up was 24 months, with observed 2-year survival rates of 100% stage I, 88% stage II, 81% stage III, and 29% stage IV. Survival rates at 4 years were 100% for stage I, 80% for stage II, 54% for stage III, and 0% for stage IV. No port-site recurrences were observed. While these authors correctly conclude that early survival curves for patients undergoing laparoscopic resection do not differ from those of historical controls, they also assert that '... further validation is needed.'

There is no question that laparoscopic colon resection is feasible. Some studies have pointed out that it remains a technically demanding procedure, considerably more difficult than laparoscopic cholecystectomy, with a 'learning curve.' However, the use of laparoscopic resection of the colon for the treatment of malignancies is currently under study. The American Society of Colon and Rectal Surgeons does not endorse the application of laparoscopic technology to cure carcinoma at this time.[69] The studies above have shown that laparoscopic colon resection is safe, feasible, and obtains pathologic specimens similar to those obtained from open surgery. While it is tempting to assume the same benefits of decreased hospitalization and recovery for patients undergoing colon resection as has been shown for patients undergoing cholecystectomy through the use of laparoscopy, there is no evidence at this time to conclude definitively that this is the case.

We must also consider the issue of the possibility of compromised cancer control and complications in this discussion.[72] Cancer control issues include the extent of lymph node resection, port-site recurrences, and the adequacy of intraperitoneal staging in the absence of tactile sensation. The series reviewed above suggest that a lymph node resection similar to that obtained by open surgery is possible. Others have made similar observations regarding lymph node harvests.[86–90] The issue of port-site metastases is discussed below, but rates from 0% to 3.2% have been reported, compared to less than 1% in open colon resection.[91] The problem with many of the anecdotal reports in the literature is that the overall denominator is not known, and only through a prospective trial can these issues be adequately studied. The 1-year port-site recurrence rate has been reported at less than 1% in the first 252 patients in the registry of the American Society of Colon and Rectal Surgeons.[6] In this series, all of the recurrences were in patients with node-positive disease. Sugarbaker has advocated the use of intraperitoneal chemotherapy based on his work with disseminated gastrointestinal malignancies.[16]

An attempt to evaluate some of the parameters of response to colon resection in an experimental model has been reported.[14] Two groups of ten pigs each underwent colon resection, one group with open techniques and one group undergoing laparoscopic colon resection. T-cell immune function as assayed by delayed-type hypersensitivity testing was better preserved after laparoscopic than after open colon resection.

While laparoscopic surgery has the potential to save hospitalization time and recovery time, such savings must not be made at the expense of overall survival. The prospective trial currently underway at many centers throughout the USA, funded by the National Institutes of Health, should address the issues of cancer control, costs, and quality of life.[72] The surgical community is awaiting the results of this carefully designed prospective trial, which will answer the significant questions regarding laparoscopic resection of colon cancer. The approach of waiting for the results of this study has been endorsed by a number of authors.[70,72,92]

Gallbladder

Although it is rare, the presence of a gallbladder malignancy is a possibility that must always be in the mind of the laparoscopic surgeon while performing a routine laparoscopic cholecystectomy. This disease, most common in older women, is the fifth most common malignancy of the gastrointestinal tract and is associated with a dismal prognosis.[93] It is estimated that carcinoma will be present in 1% of all cholecystectomy specimens.[93] Whereas laparoscopic cholecystectomy is the procedure of choice for patients with symptomatic cholelithiasis, the presence of gallbladder carcinoma remains a contraindication to the laparoscopic conduct of this procedure.[94,95] Preoperative diagnosis of this disease is difficult, because the sensitivity for ultrasonography in early cases is only about 20%. In view of the difficulty of preoperative diagnosis, it is not surprising that the diagnosis is often made only after histologic examination of the surgical specimen.

The optimal treatment for this rare disease remains elusive. In a large retrospective study of 724 patients from a number of European centers, although only 4% of patients presented with Tis lesions, these were the only patients with any hope of long-term survival.[96] Prognosis in stage T1 and T2 was markedly worse, although there are no data to support the use of extended surgical resections in these patients. Furthermore, others have shown that, at the present time, the use of adjuvant chemotherapy or radiation therapy does not significantly affect survival.[97]

The treatment of patients suspected of having carcinoma of the gallbladder preoperatively should include a definitive initial procedure performed by conventional open surgical techniques. Clinical data from ten patients with laparoscopically discovered gallbladder carcinoma have been reported.[98] All ten patients were felt to have resectable disease based on preoperative studies and intraoperative findings. The interval to exploration at the referral center was 14–74 days, with a median of 30 days. Gross intraperitoneal dissemination was found in four patients. These investigators conclude that patients in whom gallbladder carcinoma is suspected on visual examination of the gallbladder during attempted laparoscopic cholecystectomy should be converted immediately to an open procedure or the procedure terminated and the patient referred for definitive therapy. During the conduct of a laparoscopic cholecystectomy, any evidence of the presence of a carcinoma is cause for conversion to an open procedure. Routine examination of the specimen, with frozen section if suspicious areas are present, should also be carried out, with conversion to an open procedure if positive for malignancy.[95]

In summary, any patient with a lesion that is preoperatively suspect for malignancy should undergo conventional open cholecystectomy.[99] If the diagnosis is suspected during a laparoscopic cholecystectomy based on the appearance of the gallbladder, frozen section should be obtained and the procedure converted to an open cholecystectomy if the histology demonstrates malignancy. If the diagnosis is made only after laparoscopic cholecystectomy is completed, then port sites should be excised at a second procedure. Further surgical or adjuvant therapy may also be indicated.

Liver tumors

While the use of laparoscopy in the staging of hepatic lesions, either primary or metastatic, has become fairly widespread, laparoscopic treatment of hepatic malignancies is rarely performed. This is due to the technical difficulty of this procedure as well as to the scarcity of patients with lesions amenable to laparoscopic resection. The laparoscopic treatment of hepatic lesions has been reported. A benign liver cyst was fenestrated under laparoscopic guidance, providing effective therapy for a benign condition while avoiding the potential morbidity of a laparotomy.[100] A large series of 43 patients with benign solid and cystic lesions treated laparoscopically has been reported.[101] These authors concluded that laparoscopic surgery is indicated for patients with giant, solitary, hepatic cysts and for select patients with small, benign, solid tumors located in anterior liver segments.

There are a number of techniques which can be performed laparoscopically, including wedge excisions using a stapling device[22] or even laparoscopic hepatic segmentectomy. Figure 5.5 depicts the Couinaud classification of hepatic anatomy. In this figure, the areas of the segments in the anterolateral portions are shaded; these areas are amenable to laparoscopic resection because of their accessibility.[101]

Another application of laparoscopic technology to the treatment of liver lesions is cryotherapy. Cryosurgery has been shown to be effective in the treatment of some hepatic malignancies.[102] Ultrasound monitoring of this procedure is essential. With the advent of laparoscopic ultrasound probes and cryotherapy probes, it is possible to perform cryotherapy of hepatic lesions. However, anatomic limitations may prevent the use of this technology because of limited exposure of certain lesions. More recently, radiofrequency ablation (RFA) of tumors has been performed for metastatic and primary lesions of the liver.[103,104] This technique is often performed percutaneously, but there are situations in which a lesion is accessible only using laparoscopic techniques to ensure accurate positioning of the treatment probe. Of 30 patients who underwent RFA for primary and metastatic lesions of the liver in one series, 12 were treated laparoscopically, 12 at laparotomy, and six percutaneously.[104]

Spleen

Although the spleen rarely harbors primary or secondary tumors in humans, the surgical oncologist is often called upon to perform a splenectomy for hematologic diseases. The spleen is well within the reach of the laparoscopic surgeon and, by applying laparoscopic techniques, the patient is afforded the benefits of laparoscopic surgery, including shortened hospitalization and decreased postoperative pain. There are a number of series in the recent literature reporting laparoscopic removal of the spleen.[56,57,105–112] These operations have been performed for a number of indications, including staging of Hodgkin's lymphoma, idiopathic thrombocytopenia purpura (ITP), thrombotic thrombocytopenia purpura (TTP), acquired

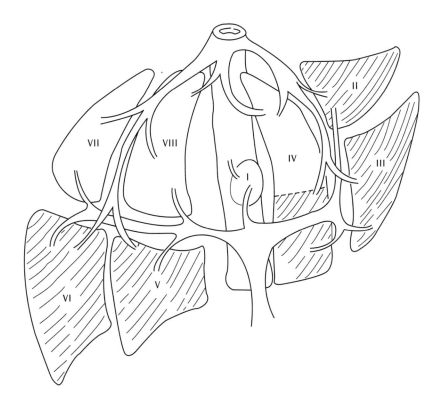

Figure 5.5 *The segmental anatomy of the liver suggests the scope of resections possible using laparoscopic means. The shaded parts of each segment, located anteriorly, are amenable to laparoscopic resection. Reprinted with permission from reference 101.*

immune deficiency syndrome (AIDS)-related thrombocytopenia, hereditary spherocytosis, autoimmune hemolytic anemia, leukemia, and splenic abscess. There may be particular subsets of patients for whom laparoscopic splenectomy is particularly beneficial. A case report of successful laparoscopic splenectomy on a patient who is human immunodeficiency virus (HIV) positive and a devout Jehovah's witness, refusing transfusion, with a preoperative hematocrit of 8.8%, highlights the attractiveness of this technique.[113] In general, laparoscopic splenectomy represents the 'gold standard' for removal of the spleen at this time.[114]

The laparoscopic conduct of this procedure should not alter the indications for operation. Once the decision to perform a splenectomy has been made, it is becoming clear that laparoscopic splenectomy may offer the patient advantages in terms of decreased postoperative hospitalization and recovery time. Splenectomy was commonly performed for the staging of lymphomas in the past, and in one series its use was demonstrated to have significantly increased in the time period 1963–82 compared to 1946–62.[45] However, recent trends show that splenectomies are now being performed more often for cytopenic/anemic diseases and less often for Hodgkin's disease.[115] The consequences of splenectomy are poorly understood at an immunologic level, but it is clear that the spleen plays a major role in a wide range of immune responses.[116] Patients should receive a pneumococcal vaccine preoperatively to help avoid the infectious complications of the asplenic state.[116]

The preoperative embolization of the splenic artery has been used in the management of patients with massive splenomegaly as an adjunct to surgery.[117] This measure has been adopted by some performing laparoscopic splenectomy.[107] However, it has not been adopted by all groups.[106] The patient can be positioned in several ways for this procedure, with some groups preferring a right decubitus position.[118]

In one large series, 43 patients were brought to the operating room for laparoscopic splenectomy, and 35 (81%) operations were successfully completed.[106] The remaining 19% underwent conversion to open splenectomy, usually for bleeding. Laparoscopic splenectomy has become the standard method for splenectomy in some centers. Conversion rates in other series have been reported as 2/22 (9%),[111] 2/17 (12%),[117] and 3/13 (23%).[109] The details of the technique have been adequately described elsewhere.[106] The patient is positioned on the operating table in the supine position, with a folded sheet under the left flank. While the lithotomy position is adequate for splenectomy, it is not useful for staging procedures because of limitations of access to the inguinal region.

It is important to make a thorough search for accessory splenic tissue, identified in 10% of the patients in one series.[106] Accessory spleens are identified in up to 18% of patients undergoing splenectomy.[119] The magnification afforded by the laparoscope may aid in this task. In a series of 100 patients undergoing open splenectomy for ITP, 13 had a poor response to splenectomy, of which five required accessory splenectomy.[120] In one large series of laparoscopic splenectomies for ITP, a positive response was observed in 18/22 (82%) patients with ITP.[106] It is difficult to predict who will respond to splenectomy, with no predictive factors being identified even in large series of patients with ITP.[120]

Mean blood loss in one series is 475 mL for laparoscopic splenectomy and 1250 mL for those converted to open splenectomy.[106] Transfusion was necessary in five of the 43 patients (12%). The mean operative time was 2.4 h (range 1.5–4.5 h) for laparoscopic splenectomy.[106] Postoperative nasogastric suction was not used in these patients, with no obvious deleterious effects. Most patients tolerated liquids the day following surgery and were discharged on the second postoperative day, with a mean hospital stay for the 43 patients of 2.7 days. Postoperative complications have included wound infections, a pleural effusion, and recurrent arrhythmias, but there have been no instances of postoperative hemorrhage or subphrenic abscess in the patients successfully undergoing laparoscopic splenectomy.

In a prospective study of operative outcomes, laparoscopic splenectomy using the lateral approach was performed on 147 patients and open splenectomy on 63 matched patients at three teaching centers.[109] Laparoscopic splenectomy resulted in longer operative times (145 min versus 77 min), reduced blood loss (162 mL versus 380 mL), shorter postoperative stay (2.4 days versus 9.2 days), and fewer complications compared to the open procedure. These authors also reported that the mean weighted cost of laparoscopic splenectomy was lower than that of the open procedure ($3311 versus $3861). The conversion rate in this series was 2.7%.

Although laparoscopic splenectomy is a technically demanding procedure, it offers the patient the potential for decreased postoperative pain and hospitalization, with more rapid return to the normal activities of living. Further prospective data will be needed to confirm these observations. Surgical alternatives to splenectomy have been offered as a way to reduce the incidence of postoperative infections, such as partial splenectomy.[121]

Adrenal tumors

Laparoscopic techniques have been used for the resection of adrenal lesions.[122–127] Whereas the anterior transabdominal approach is considered by some to be a source of postoperative morbidity, the laparoscopic approach may offer some advantages. Adrenal tumors are fairly common, having been found in 2% of patients in autopsy series.[128] Small, asymptomatic tumors are reported in as many as 0.6% of abdominal ultrasound and CT examinations. Those discovered that are less than 4 cm in diameter and in the absence of endocrine syndromes can be observed after a careful evaluation.[128] However, a fair proportion of these lesions may require extirpation, a procedure that has been performed laparoscopically, with the apparent advantages of decreased pain and a more rapid return to full activity.

Over a 14-month period, Takeda and coworkers removed seven left adrenal glands and three right adrenal glands from ten patients in operations ranging from 165 to 572 min (mean 295 min).[122] Conversion to open adrenalectomy was reported in one (10%) case. Takeda *et al.* concluded that laparoscopic adrenalectomy is applicable to cases of primary hyperaldosteronism, but application to other lesions requires further study.

Twenty-five consecutive laparoscopic adrenalectomies performed on 22 patients in a 1-year period were reported by Gagner *et al.*[124] These were performed through a lateral decubitus flank approach and four 11-mm trocars, and included 12 right and 13 left adrenal glands. The mean operative time for single adrenalectomy was 2.3 h and for bilateral adrenalectomy was 5.3 h. Diseases in this series included non-functional adenoma, pheochromocytoma, Cushing's disease, Cushing's adenoma, primary aldosteronism, angiomyolipoma, and medullary cyst. Lesions ranged in size from 1 to 15 cm, with a mean of 4.1 cm. Conversion to open laparotomy was required in one patient for lack of exposure, resulting in completion of the procedure in 96% of patients. The median postoperative stay was 4 days. These authors concluded that laparoscopic adrenalectomy results in less postoperative pain and a more rapid return to normal activity compared to open adrenalectomy.

A study compared laparoscopic adrenalectomy with a historical group of posterior adrenalectomies.[125] The two groups were comparable for patient demographics. The median time for posterior adrenalectomy was 120 min, versus a median of 160 min for laparoscopic adrenalectomy. Patients who underwent laparoscopic adrenalectomy had a mean hospital stay of 3 days, a shorter time to return to work, and a lower blood loss than those patients who underwent posterior adrenalectomy, with a mean hospital stay of 5 days. These authors conclude that laparoscopic adrenalectomy is the procedure of choice.

In recent report of the results of a case-controlled study of 40 laparoscopic and 40 open adrenalectomies,[126] statistically significant differences were found (laparoscopic versus open) in operative blood loss (40 mL versus 172 mL), operating time (147 min versus 79 min), hospital stay (12 days versus 18 days), and late morbidity (0% versus 48%). No statistically significant differences were found in time to oral intake, total cost, and early morbidity. The late morbidity in the 'open' group consisted of wound complications, which were absent in the 'laparoscopic' group. These authors conclude that the laparoscopic approach is the method of choice for adrenal masses less than 6 cm in diameter.

There have been no randomized prospective trials reported to date for this procedure. The studies noted above provide strong evidence that the procedure can be performed safely and effectively, affording patients with adrenal masses some of the benefits seen with laparoscopic cholecystectomy. Laparoscopic adrenalectomy is becoming the standard of care for patients with benign adrenal masses.[127] The use of minimally invasive surgery for adrenal malignancies remains controversial. The *SAGES manual* states that laparoscopy is not to be used in the treatment of patients with malignant lesions.[129] Other contraindications to laparoscopic adrenalectomy defined by these authors include masses larger than 10 cm, untreated coagulopathies, and surgeon inexperience. Further study of this technique is clearly needed.

LAPAROSCOPY IN THE PALLIATION OF MALIGNANCY

Laparoscopic stoma creation

Decompression of the intestinal tract may be an important procedure in the cancer patient, especially in those with carcinomatosis and resulting intestinal obstruction. The importance of colonic decompression in patients with obstructing carcinomas of the colon has been described.[130] The initial presentation of carcinoma of the colon is obstruction in 15–21% of patients, most commonly in the left colon. Five-year survival rates in these patients is significantly less than that in patients without obstruction. This common situation underscores the importance of palliative procedures which may decrease postoperative pain, incidence of ileus, and recovery time.

This procedure for loop colostomy creation was described recently with an associated decrease in postoperative pain and ileus and with a rapid recovery.[131] This technique utilizes creation of the stoma site in the desired area after mobilizing the intestine. The peritoneum at the stoma site is left intact, and a trocar is placed directly through this site (Figure 5.6). A grasper is then used to extract the intestine through the stoma site, which occludes the opening and allows recreation of the pneumoperitoneum (Figure 5.7). Alternatively, a stapling device can be introduced to divide the bowel and mesentery, allowing creation of an end stoma.

Whereas small laparotomy incisions may be used for the creation of intestinal stomas, the presence of metastatic disease or peritoneal implants may make such procedures difficult to perform. The use of a laparoscopic approach results in discharge from hospital within 24–48 h after surgery as well as the inspection of the abdominal cavity for other lesions. In one study, 17 of 19 (89%) patients were successfully diverted using laparoscopic techniques.[132] The remaining two patients had extensive adhesive disease that could not be managed

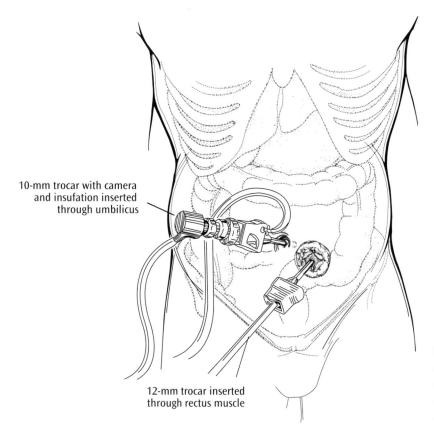

10-mm trocar with camera and insufation inserted through umbilicus

12-mm trocar inserted through rectus muscle

Figure 5.6 *Port placement and instrumentation for the laparoscopic creation of a loop colostomy. Reprinted with permission from reference 131.*

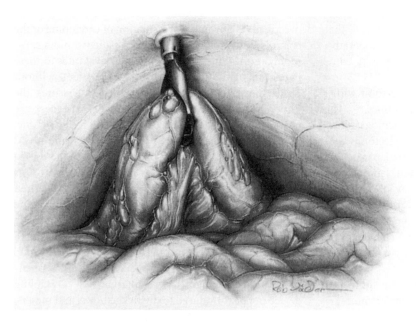

Figure 5.7 *Using a grasper to exteriorize a loop of colon for a palliative colostomy. Reprinted with permission from reference 131.*

laparoscopically and required conversion to open laparotomy. Other procedures, such as laparoscopic gastrostomy, may also be carried out as needed.

CONCLUSIONS

Exciting technology for laparoscopic surgery now under development will soon be in our operating rooms.

Cuschieri has pointed out that we need to 'see better, feel better, increase the precision of maneuverability and handling, reduce contamination, facilitate specimen extraction and bring order to the present ergonomic chaos in our operating rooms.'[133] New developments in the technology of imaging are being applied to laparoscopic surgery. Head-mounted displays have been tested, but they are probably less than optimal for the laparoscopic surgeon because of the isolation created by these devices.

Although three-dimensional imaging systems are not without their limitations at the present time, new systems may provide a true improvement in tissue visualization. Continued improvements in instrumentation will certainly be an important part of the evolution of laparoscopic surgery. New methods of tissue extraction include a sleeve system and an extracorporeal pneumoperitoneal access bubble.[133] Both of these systems have potential advantages, especially for the removal of large tumor specimens.

Training of surgeons in these newly emerging techniques remains a complicated process. Because hospitals decide what procedures may be performed by surgeons, criteria for training and furnishing credentials must be developed.[134] The Society of American Gastrointestinal Endoscopic Surgeons (SAGES) has suggested criteria for training and credentialling. It remains to be shown whether some advanced laparoscopic procedures result in true cost savings when the increased costs of instrumentation and operating room time are factored into the total expenses incurred.

The surgeon has traditionally been involved in the diagnosis, staging, treatment and palliation of patients with malignancies. Laparoscopy is rapidly becoming an important tool in each of these areas of the care of the cancer patient. The ultimate application of laparoscopic techniques depends on the imagination of surgical investigators as well as on careful analyses of risks and benefits. There may be uses of this technology which, over time, are not ultimately advantageous to the patient compared to traditional open surgical techniques. However, only by the conduct of carefully controlled studies will the facts be elucidated, allowing this methodology to be used where it will benefit the patient and avoided where it will not.

REFERENCES

1. Fusco MA, Paluzzi MW. Abdominal wall recurrence after laparoscopic-assisted colectomy for adenocarcinoma of the colon. Dis Colon Rectum 1993; 36:858–61.

2. Cava A, Roman J, Quintela AG, Martin F, Aramburo P. Subcutaneous metastasis following laparoscopy in gastric adenocarcinoma. Eur J Surg Oncol 1990; 16:63–7.

3. Nduka CC, Monson JRT, Menzies-Gow N, Darz A. Abdominal wall metastases following laparoscopy. Br J Surg 1994; 81:648–52.

4. Stockdale AD, Pocock TJ. Abdominal wall metastasis following laparoscopy. Eur J Surg Oncol 1985; 11:373–5.

5. Hughes ESR, McDermott FT, Polglase AL, Johnson WR. Tumor recurrence in the abdominal wall scar tissue after large-bowel cancer surgery. Dis Colon Rectum 1983; 26:571–2.

6. Ramos JM, Gupta S, Anthone GJ, Ortega AF, Simons AJ, Beart RW. Laparoscopy and colon cancer: is the port site at risk? Arch Surg 1994; 129:897–9.

7. Fleshman JW, Nelson H, Peters WR, et al. Early results of laparoscopic surgery for colorectal cancer. Dis Colon Rectum 1996; 39:S53–8.

8. Pearlstone DB, Mansfield PE, Curley SA, et al. Laparoscopy in 533 patients with abdominal malignancy. Surgery 1999; 125:67–72.

9. Ikramuddin S, Lucas J, Ellison EC, et al. Detection of aerosolized cells during carbon dioxide laparoscopy. J Gastrointest Surg 1998; 2:580–4.

10. Reymond MA, Wittekind C, Jung A, et al. The incidence of port site metastases might be reduced. Surg Endosc 1997; 11:902–6.

11. Tseng LN, Berends FJ, Wittich P, et al. Port site metastases: impact of local tissue trauma and gas leakage. Surg Endosc 1998; 12:1377–80.

12. Aoki Y, Shimura H, Li H, et al. A model of port site metastases of gallbladder cancer: the influence of peritoneal injury and its repair on abdominal wall metastases. Surgery 1999; 125:553–9.

13. Mutter D, Hajri A, Tassetti V, et al. Increased tumor growth and spread after laparoscopy vs laparotomy. Surg Endosc 1999; 13:365–70.

14. Bessler M, Whelan RL, Halverson A, Treat MR, Nowygrod R. Is immune function better preserved after laparoscopic versus open colon resection? Surg Endosc 1994; 8:881–3.

15. Allendorf JDF, Bessler M, Kayton ML, et al. Tumor growth after laparotomy or laparoscopy. Surg Endosc 1995; 9:49–52.

16. Sugarbaker PH. Wound recurrence after laparoscopic colectomy for cancer: new rationale for intraoperative intraperitoneal chemotherapy. Surg Endosc 1996; 10:295–6.

17. Johnstone PAS, Rohde DC, Swartz SE, et al. Port site recurrences after laparoscopic and thoracoscopic procedures in malignancy. J Clin Oncol 1996; 14:1950–6.

18. Foley EF, Kolecki RV, Schirmer BD. The accuracy of laparoscopic ultrasound in the detection of colorectal cancer liver metastases. Am J Surg 1998; 176:262.

19. Greene FL, Bianco JE. Laparoscopy's growing role in abdominal tumor diagnosis. Contemp Oncol January 1994; 14–20.

20. Lefor AT. Laparoscopic staging of abdominal lymphomas. In Greene F, ed. Minimal access surgical oncology. Oxford, Radcliffe, 1995, 31–44.

21. Cuschieri A. Diagnosis and staging of tumors by laparoscopy. Semin Laparosc Surg 1994; 1:3.

22. Lefor AT, Flowers JL. Laparoscopic wedge biopsy of the liver. J Am Coll Surg 1994; 178:307–8.

23. Lefor AT. Laparoscopic surgery for cancer. PPO Updates 1995; 9(7):1–19.

24. Jakimowicz J. Laparoscopic intraoperative ultrasonography, equipment, and technique. Semin Laparosc Surg 1994; 1:52–61.

25. Machi J, Sigel B. Intraoperative ultrasonography. Radiol Clin North Am 1992; 30:1085–103.

26. Stiegmann GV, McIntyre RC, Pearlman NW. Laparoscopic intracorporeal ultrasound. Surg Endosc 1994; 8:167–72.

27. Jakimowicz J. Review: intraoperative ultrasonography during minimal access surgery. J R Coll Surg Edinb 1993; 38:231–8.

28. John TG, Greig JD, Crosbie JL, Miles WF, Garden OJ. Superior staging of liver tumors with laparoscopy and laparoscopic ultrasound. Ann Surg 1994; 220:711–19.

29. Nieven van Dijkum EJ, de Wit LT, van Delden OM, et al. Staging laparoscopy and laparoscopic ultrasonography in more than 400 patients with upper gastrointestinal carcinoma. J Am Coll Surg 1999; 189:459–65.

30. Lightdale CJ. Laparoscopy for cancer staging. Endoscopy 1992; 24:682.

31. Hemming AW, Nagy AG, Scudamore CH, Edelman K. Laparoscopic staging of intraabdominal malignancy. Surg Endosc 1995; 9:325.

32. Salky BA. Laparoscopic staging of intra-abdominal malignancy. In Paterson-Brown S, Garden J, eds, *Principles and practice of surgical laparoscopy*. Philadelphia, WB Saunders, 1994.

33. Conlon KC, Dougherty E, Klimstra DG, et al. The value of minimal access surgery in the staging of patients with potentially resectable peripancreatic malignancy. Ann Surg 1996; 223:134.

34. Cuschieri A, Hall AW, Clark J. Value of laparoscopy in the diagnosis and management of pancreatic carcinoma. Gut 1978; 19:672–7.

35. Nishizaki T, Matsumata T, Adachi E, Sugimachi K. Laparoscopy is preferable to imaging procedures in detecting metastases of a pancreas carcinoma to the liver. Surg Endosc 1994; 8:1340–2.

36. John TG, Greig JD, Carter DC, Garden OJ. Carcinoma of the pancreatic head and periampullary region: tumor staging with laparoscopy and laparoscopic ultrasound. Ann Surg 1995; 221:156.

37. Luque de Leon E, Tsiotos GG, Balsiger B, et al. Staging laparoscopy for pancreatic cancer should be used to select the best means of palliation and not only to maximize the resectability rate. J Gastrointest Surg 1999; 3:111–18.

38. Rumstadt B, Schwab M, Schuster K, et al. The role of laparoscopy in the preoperative staging of pancreatic carcinoma. J Gastrointest Surg 1997; 1:245–50.

39. Steele GD, Bleday R, Mayer RJ, et al. A prospective evaluation of hepatic resection for colorectal carcinoma metastases to the liver: gastrointestinal Tumor Study Group Protocol 6584. J Clin Oncol 1991; 9:1105–12.

40. Lefor AT, Hughes K, Shiloni E, et al. Intra-abdominal extrahepatic disease in patients with colorectal hepatic metastases. Dis Colon Rectum 1988; 31:100–5.

41. Babineau TJ, Lewis WD, Jenkins RL, Bleday R, Steele GD. Role of staging laparoscopy in the treatment of hepatic malignancy. Am J Surg 1994; 167:151–5.

42. Solomon MJ, Stephen MS, Gallinger S, White GH. Does intraoperative hepatic ultrasonography change surgical decision making during liver resection? Am J Surg 1994; 168:307–10.

43. Bloomfield CD, DeCosse JJ. Staging laparotomy. Arch Surg 1978; 113:1135–42.

44. Urba WJ, Longo DL. Hodgkin's disease. N Engl J Med 1992; 326:678–87.

45. Marble KR, Deckers PJ, Kern KA. Changing role of splenectomy for hematologic disease. J Surg Oncol 1993; 52:169–71.

46. Williams SF, Golomb HM. Perspective on staging approaches in the malignant lymphomas. Surg Gynecol Obstet 1986; 163:193–201.

47. Martin JK, Clark SC, Beart RW, et al. Staging laparotomy in Hodgkin's disease, Mayo Clinic experience. Arch Surg 1982; 117:586–91.

48. Schneeberger AL, Girvan DP. Staging laparotomy for Hodgkin's disease in children. J Pediatr Surg 1988; 23:714–17.

49. Muskat PC, Johnson RA, Bowers GJ. Staging laparotomy in Hodgkin's lymphoma: 1979–1988. Am J Surg 1991; 162:603–7.

50. Jockovich M, Mendenhall NP, Sombeck MD, Talbert JL, Copeland EM, Bland KI. Long term complications of laparotomy in Hodgkin's disease. Ann Surg 1994; 219:615–24.

51. Horowitz J, Smith JL, Weber TK, et al. Postoperative complications after splenectomy for hematologic malignancies. Ann Surg 1996; 223:290–6.

52. Huang PP, Urist MM. Evaluation of abdominal Hodgkin's disease. Surg Oncol Clin North Am 1993; 2:207–11.

53. Grieco MB, Cady B. Staging laparotomy in Hodgkin's disease. Surg Clin North Am 1980; 60:369–79.

54. Baccarini U, Carroll BJ, Hiatt JR, et al. Comparison of laparoscopic and open staging in Hodgkin disease. Arch Surg 1998; 133:517–22.

55. Greene FL, Cooler AW. Laparoscopic evaluation of lymphomas. Semin Laparosc Surg 1994; 1:13–17.

56. Carroll BJ, Phillips EH, Semer CJ, et al. Laparoscopic splenectomy. Surg Endosc 1992; 6:183–5.

57. Tulman S, Holcomb GW, Karamanoukian HL, Reynhout J. Pediatric laparoscopic splenectomy. J Pediatr Surg 1993; 28:689–92.

58. Lefor AT, Flowers JL, Heyman M. Laparoscopic staging of Hodgkin's disease. Surg Oncol 1993; 2:217–20.

59. Cunneen SA, Lefor AT. Lymphoma surgery and nodal dissection. In Greene FL, Heniford BT, eds. *Minimally invasive cancer management*. New York: Springer-Verlag, 2001, 293–303.

60. Rosenberg SA. Annotation: splenectomy in the management of Hodgkin's disease. Br J Haematol 1971; 23:271–6.

61. Multani PS, Grossbard M. Staging laparotomy in the management of Hodgkin's disease: is it still necessary? Oncologist 1996; 1:41–55.

62. Silecchia G, Fantini A, Raparelli L, et al. Management of abdominal lymphoproliferative diseases in the era of laparoscopy. Am J Surg 1999; 177:325–30.

63. Rosenberg SA. Non-Hodgkin's lymphoma-selection of treatment on the basis of histologic type. N Engl J Med 1979; 301:924–8.

64. Goh PMY, Tekant Y, Kum CK. Totally intraabdominal laparoscopic Billroth II gastrectomy. Surg Endosc 1992; 6:160.

65. Goh P. Laparoscopic Billroth II gastrectomy. Semin Laparosc Surg 1994; 1:171–81.

66. Cuschieri A. Gastric resections. In Scott-Conner C, ed. *The SAGES manual.* New York: Springer-Verlag, 1999, 353–63.

67. Dean PA, Beart RW, Nelson H, Elftmann TD, Schlinkert RT. Laparoscopic assisted segmental colectomy: early Mayo Clinic experience. Mayo Clin Proc 1994; 69:834–40.

68. Böhm B, Milsom JW, Kitago K, Brand M, Stolfi VM, Fazio VW. Use of laparoscopic techniques in oncologic right colectomy in a canine model. Ann Surg Oncol 1995; 2:6–13.

69. Elftmann TD, Nelson H, Ota DM, Pemberton JH, Beart RW. Laparoscopic assisted segmental colectomy: surgical techniques. Mayo Clin Proc 1994; 69:825–33.

70. Cohen SM, Wexner SD. Laparoscopic right hemicolectomy. Surg Rounds November 1994; 627–34.

71. Milsom JW, Bohm B, Hammerhofer KA, et al. A prospective randomized trial comparing laparoscopic versus conventional techniques in colorectal cancer surgery: a preliminary report. J Am Coll Surg 1998; 187:46–54.

72. Ota DM. Laparoscopic colectomy for cancer: a favorable opinion. Ann Surg Oncol 1995; 2:3–5.

73. Jager RM, Ballantyne GH, Fleshman JW, Franklin ME. The technical nuances in laparoscopic colorectal surgery. Contemp Surg 1994; 45:355–9.

74. Reissman P, Teoh TA, Piccirillo M, Nogueras JJ, Wexner SD. Colonoscopic assisted laparoscopic colectomy. Surg Endosc 1994; 8: 1352–3.

75. Phillips EH, Franklin M, Carroll BJ, Fallas MJ, Ramos R, Rosenthal D. Laparoscopic colectomy. Ann Surg 1992; 216:703–7.

76. Weiss EG, Wexner SD. Laparoscopic segmental colectomies, anterior resection and abdominoperineal resection. In Scott-Conner C, ed. *The SAGES manual.* New York: Springer-Verlag 1999, 286–99.

77. Pandya S, Murray JJ, Coller JA, Rusin LC. Laparoscopic colectomy: indications for conversion to laparotomy. Arch Surg 1999; 134:471.

78. Falk PM, Beart RW, Wexner SD, et al. Laparoscopic colectomy: a critical appraisal. Dis Colon Rectum 1993; 36:28–34.

79. Hoffman GC, Baker JW, Fitchett CW, Vansant JH. Laparoscopic assisted colectomy: initial experience. Ann Surg 1994; 219:732–43.

80. Muckleroy SK, Ratzer ER, Fenoglio ME. Laparoscopic colon surgery for benign disease: a comparison to open surgery. J Soc Laparoendo Surg 1999; 3:33.

81. Franklin ME, Rosenthal D, Norem RF. Prospective evaluation of laparoscopic colon resection versus open colon resection for adenocarcinoma. Surg Endosc 1995; 9:811–16.

82. Liberman MA, Phillips EH, Carroll BJ, et al. Laparoscopic colectomy vs traditional colectomy for diverticulitis. Surg Endosc 1996; 10:15–18.

83. Lacy AM, Garcia-Valdecasa JC, Pique JM, et al. Short-term analysis of a randomized study comparing laparoscopic vs. open colectomy for colon cancer. Surg Endosc 1995; 9:1101–5.

84. Begos DG, Arsenault J, Ballantyne GH. Laparoscopic colon and rectal surgery at a VA hospital. Surg Endosc 1996; 10:1050–6.

85. Wexner SD, Reissman P, Pfeiffer J, et al. Laparoscopic colorectal surgery. Surg Endosc 1996; 10:133–6.

86. Hoffman GC, Baker JW, Doxey JB, et al. Minimally invasive surgery for colorectal cancer: initial follow-up. Ann Surg 1996; 223:790–8.

87. Kwok SP, Carey PD, Li AKC. Prospective evaluation of laparoscopic assisted large bowel excision for cancer. Ann Surg 1996; 223:170.

88. Poulin EC, Mamazza J, Schlachta CM, et al. Laparoscopic resection does not adversely affect early survival curves in patients undergoing surgery for colorectal adenocarcinoma. Ann Surg 1999; 229:487.

89. Greene FL. Laparoscopic management of colorectal cancer. CA 1999; 49:221.

90. Gellman L, Salky B, Edye M. Laparoscopic assisted colectomy. Surg Endosc 1996; 10:1041–4.

91. Berman IR. Laparoscopic colectomy for cancer: some cause for pause. Ann Surg Oncol 1995; 2:1–2.

92. Milsom JW, Hammerhofer KA. Role of laparoscopic techniques in colorectal cancer surgery. Oncology 1995; 9:393–405.

93. Abi-Rached B, Neugut AJ. Diagnostic and management issues in gallbladder carcinoma. Oncology 1995; 9:19–24.

94. Targarona EM, Pons MJ, Viella P, Trias M. Unsuspected carcinoma of the gallbladder: a laparoscopic dilemma. Surg Endosc 1994; 8:211–13.

95. Copher JC, Rogers JJ, Dalton ML. Trocar site metastasis following laparoscopic cholecystectomy for unsuspected carcinoma of the gallbladder. Surg Endosc 1995; 9:348–50.

96. Cubertafond P, Gainant A, Cucchiaro G. Surgical treatment of 724 carcinomas of the gallbladder. Ann Surg 1994; 219:275–80.

97. Sariego J, Aharonian A, Byrd M, Matsumoto T, Kerstein M. Adenocarcinoma of the gallbladder. Contemp Surg 1994; 44:91–6.

98. Fong Y, Brennan MF, Turnbull A, Coit DG, Blumgart LH. Gallbladder cancer discovered during laparoscopic surgery. Arch Surg 1993; 128:1054–6.

99. Lomis KD, Vitola JV, Delbeke D, et al. Recurrent gallbladder carcinoma at laparoscopy port sites diagnosed by positron emission tomography. Am Surg 1997; 63:341–5.

100. Tate JJ, Lau WY, Li AK. Transhepatic fenestration of liver cyst: a further application of laparoscopic surgery. Aust NZ J Surg 1994; 64:264–5.

101. Katkhouda N, Hurwitz M, Gugenheim J, et al. Laparoscopic management of benign solid and cystic lesions of the liver. Ann Surg 1999; 229:460–6.

102. Ravikumar TS, Kane R, Cady B, Jerkins R, Clouse M, Steele G Jr. A 5-year study of cryosurgery in the treatment of liver tumors. Arch Surg 1991; 126:1520–3.

103. Curley SA, Izzo F, Delrio P, et al. Radiofrequency ablation of unresectable primary and metastatic hepatic malignancies: results in 123 patients. Ann Surg 1999; 230:1–8.

104. Rose DM, Allegra DP, Bostick PJ, et al. Radiofrequency ablation: a novel primary and adjunctive ablative technique for hepatic malignancies. Am Surg 1999; 65:1009–14.

105. Lefor AT, Flowers JL, Bailey RW, Melvin WS. Laparoscopic splenectomy in the management of immune thrombocytopenia purpura. Surgery 1993; 114:613.

106. Flowers JL, Lefor AT, Steers JA, et al. Laparoscopic splenectomy in patients with hematologic diseases. Ann Surg 1996; 224:19–28.

107. Poulin E, Thibault G, Mamazza J, et al. Laparoscopic splenectomy: clinical experience and the role of preoperative splenic artery embolization. Surg Laparosc Endosc 1993; 3(6):445–50.

108. Schlinkert RT, Mann D, Weaver A. Laparoscopic splenectomy: reduction of hospital charges. J Gastrointest Surg 1998; 2:278–82.

109. Phillips EH, Carroll BJ, Fallas MJ. Laparoscopic splenectomy. Surg Endosc 1994; 8:931–3.

110. Poulin EC, Thibault C, Mamazza J. Laparoscopic splenectomy. Surg Endosc 1995; 9:172–7.

111. Cadiere GB, Verroken R, Himpens J, Bruyns J, Efira M, De Wit S. Operative strategy in laparoscopic splenectomy. J Am Coll Surg 1994; 179:668–72.

112. Park A, Marcaccio M, Sternbach M, et al. Laparoscopic vs. open splenectomy. Arch Surg 1999; 134:1263–9.

113. Ferzli GS, Hurwitz JB, Fiorillo MA, et al. Laparoscopic splenectomy in a Jehovah's witness with profound anemia. Surg Endosc 1997; 11:850–1.

114. Friedman RL, Fallas MJ, Carrol BJ, Phillips EH. Laparoscopic splenectomy for ITP: the gold standard. Surg Endosc 1996; 10:991.

115. Llende M, Santiago-Delpin EA, Lavergne J. Immunobiological consequences of splenectomy. J Surg Res 1986; 40:85–94.

116. Weintraub LR. Splenectomy: who, when and why. Hosp Pract 1994 June 15; 27–34.

117. Fujitani RM, Johs SM, Cobb SR, Mehringer CM, White RA, Klein SR. Preoperative splenic artery occlusion as an adjunct for high risk splenectomy. Am Surg 1988; 54:602–8.

118. Hashizume M, Sugimachi K, Kitano S, et al. Laparoscopic splenectomy. Am J Surg 1994; 167:611–14.

119. Akwari OE, Itani KMF, Coleman RE, Rosse WF. Splenectomy for primary and recurrent immune thrombocytopenia purpura. Ann Surg 1987; 206:529–41.

120. Coon WW. Splenectomy for idiopathic thrombocytopenic purpura. Surg Gynecol Obstet 1987; 164:225–9.

121. Hoekstra HJ, Tamminga RYJ, Timens W. Partial splenectomy in children: an alternative for splenectomy in the pathologic staging of Hodgkin's disease. Ann Surg Oncol 1994; 1:480–6.

122. Takeda M, Go H, Imai T, Nishiyama T, Morishita H. Laparoscopic adrenalectomy for primary aldosteronism: report of initial ten cases. Surgery 1994; 115:621–5.

123. Fernandez-Cruz L, Benarroch G, Torres E, Astudillo E, Saenz A, Taura P. Laparoscopic approach to adrenal tumors. J Laparoendosc Surg 1993; 3:541–6.

124. Gagner M, Lacroix A, Prinz RA, et al. Early experience with laparoscopic approach for adrenalectomy. Surgery 1993; 114:1120–4.

125. Ting ACW, Lo CY, Lo CM. Posterior or laparoscopic approach for adrenalectomy. Am J Surg 1998; 175:488.

126. Imai T, Kikumori T, Ohiwa M, et al. A case-controlled study of laparoscopic compared with open lateral adrenalectomy. Am J Surg 1999; 178:50–4.

127. Walther MM. Laparoscopic surgery for adrenal disease. PPO Updates 1997; 11(12):1–9.

128. Schmidt N. Strategic management of adrenal tumors. Oncology 1994; 8:73–81.

129. Arca MJ, Gagner M. Laparoscopic adrenalectomy. In Scott-Connor C, ed. The SAGES manual. New York: Springer-Verlag, 1999, 353–63.

130. Leitman IM, Sullivan JD, Brams D, DeCosse JJ. Multivariate analysis of morbidity and mortality from the initial surgical management of obstructing carcinoma of the colon. Surg Gynecol Obstet 1992; 174:513–18.

131. Lyerly HK, Mault JR. Laparoscopic ileostomy and colostomy. Ann Surg 1994; 219:317–22.

132. Ota DM. Laparoscopic management of colon cancer. Semin Laparosc Surg 1994; 1:18–25.

133. Cuschieri A. Whither minimal access surgery: tribulations and expectations. Am J Surg 1995; 169:9–19.

134. Soper NJ, Brunt LM, Kerbl K. Laparoscopic general surgery. N Engl J Med 1994; 330:409–19.

135. Jones DB, Guo LW, Reinhard MK, *et al*. Impact of pneumoperitoneum on trocar site implantation of colon cancer in hamster model. Dis Colon Rectum 1995; 38:1182–8.

136. Jacobi CA, Keller H, Monig S, Said S. Implantation metastasis of unsuspected gallbladder carcinoma after laparoscopy. Surg Endosc 1995; 9:351–2.

137. Bouvy ND, Marquet RL, Jeekel H, Bonjer HJ. Impact of gasless laparoscopy and laparotomy on peritoneal tumor growth and abdominal wall metastases. Ann Surg 1996; 224:694–701.

138. Huscher C, Silecchia G, Croce E, *et al*. Laparoscopic colorectal resection: a multicenter Italian study. Surg Endosc 1996; 10:875–9.

139. Fielding GA, Lumley J, Nathanson L, *et al*. Laparoscopic colectomy. Surg Endosc 1997; 11:745–9.

140. Lacy AM, Delgado S, Garcia-Valdecasas JC, *et al*. Port site metastases and recurrence after laparoscopic colectomy: a randomized trial. Surg Endosc 1998; 12:1039–42.

ANNOTATED BIBLIOGRAPHY

Baccarani U, Carroll BJ, Hiatt JR, *et al*. Comparison of laparoscopic and open staging in Hodgkin disease. Arch Surg 1998; 133:517–22.

This is a carefully performed analysis of outcomes in 15 patients who underwent laparoscopic staging for Hodgkin's disease. This study demonstrates oncologic equivalence and functional superiority over conventional open staging of Hodgkin's disease.

Greene FL. Laparoscopic management of colorectal cancer. CA. 1999; 49:221–8.

This review article addresses many of the significant issues in the application of laparoscopy to patients with colon cancer. Technical considerations are reviewed as well as cancer control issues such as lymph node harvest, margins of resection, etc. The author acknowledges early results in several trials, but emphasizes the importance of awaiting the results of ongoing clinical trials before considering the general use of laparoscopic colon resection for cancer.

Pearlstone DB, Mansfield PF, Curley SA, *et al*. Laparoscopy in 533 patients with abdominal malignancy. Surgery 1999; 125:67–72.

The issue of port-site recurrences has limited the wide application of laparoscopy to patients with malignancy. This large series from a major cancer referral center demonstrates that port-site recurrence is very rare (4/533) and, when it does occur, is much more common in patients with widespread tumor (3/71 patients) than in patients with localized disease (1/462, $p < 0.0003$).

Poulin EC, Mamazza J, Schlachta CM. Laparoscopic resection does not adversely affect early survival curves in patients undergoing surgery for colorectal adenocarcinoma. Ann Surg 1999; 229:487–92.

This is a carefully performed study of 177 consecutive laparoscopic resections of colorectal cancer performed by three surgeons in a university setting. There were 135 patients in the follow-up group, with a median 24 month follow-up. Observed 2-year survival rates were 100% stage I, 89% stage II, 81% stage III, and 29% stage IV. No port-site recurrences were identified. These authors conclude that their survival data are consistent with historical controls for open surgery, but that 'further validation is needed.'

Vittimberga FJ, Foley DP, Meyers WC, *et al*. Laparoscopic surgery and the systemic immune response. Ann Surg 1998; 227:326–34.

This excellent article reviews a large number of studies relating to the immune response to laparoscopic surgery as well as metabolic responses. Overall, it appears that there is less immune activation after laparoscopic surgery than after open surgery. Furthermore, the overall response is one of less activation rather than immunosuppression.

Commentary

NAMIR KATKHOUDA, ANDREAS M KAISER, STEVEN W GRANT, RAHILA ESSANI, KRANTHI ACHANTA, AND MELANIE H FRIEDLANDER

GENERAL CONSIDERATIONS

Even the role of open surgery for malignancy has not yet been completely defined, and such issues as the extent of lymph node dissection in gastric/pancreatic cancer surgery or total mesorectal resection for cancers of the rectum still require further clarification. Nevertheless, advances in laparoscopic surgery in the past few years have caused a major technical revolution in medicine and have resulted in a rapid expansion of its indications in many groups of patients, including those with cancer. Factors that have contributed to the success of laparoscopic surgery include rapid postoperative recovery with shorter lengths of hospitalization, reduced postoperative pain, faster return of bowel function, and fewer wound complications, such as infection, dehiscence, and incisional hernias. In accordance with these findings, acceptance of the laparoscopic approach has increased, and therefore the trend toward minimally invasive surgery has become inevitable in the management of benign disease. Defining the role of laparoscopy in the treatment of cancer is more complex, because concerns regarding cure, survival rates, and quality of life may overshadow the benefits of a minimally invasive approach. Nevertheless, in the era of laparoscopic surgery it is important to define the role of the minimally invasive approach for cancer, and to compare its feasibility, efficacy, and outcome relative to open surgery.

This commentary focuses on the acceptance of the laparoscopic approach in cancer patients, and is divided into the following three categories:

1 Patients with accepted or reasonable indications for laparoscopic surgery.
2 Patients in whom the role of laparoscopy needs further clarification or is still evolving.
3 Patients in whom laparoscopic surgery is contraindicated or inappropriate.

The acceptability of a given laparoscopic procedure may, of course, change with evolving technology, experience, and scientific evidence.

ACCEPTED/REASONABLE INDICATIONS FOR LAPAROSCOPIC SURGERY

Laparoscopic surgery is considered reasonable if its expected benefits outweigh the potential harm or risk. These interventions may either be purely diagnostic or therapeutic, or, more optimally, satisfy both goals simultaneously in order to limit the number of subsequent procedures.

Diagnostic procedures

Treatment strategies in cancer vary according to the histology and the extent of tumor spread, defined by the TNM staging classification. Such staging facilitates the standardization of treatment and outcome comparisons. Sophisticated imaging techniques now provide an increasing and often astonishing accuracy of information, which may be further enhanced by interventional tools, such as image-guided fine-needle aspiration. Despite these highly sensitive diagnostic modalities, lesions may be too small to detect (less than 0.5–1 cm), or there may remain a degree of uncertainty about the nature and extent of a neoplasm, warranting further evaluation. Under these circumstances, diagnostic laparoscopy (often combined with laparoscopic ultrasonography) may be indicated, provided that it will have an impact on the treatment.

The current concepts regarding the risk of port-site tumor implantation have been summarized by Dr. Lefor. Despite several early reports in the literature, the overall incidence of port-site metastasis does not appear to be significantly higher than that of wound recurrences in open procedures when matched for tumor stage. Regardless of the surgical approach, the incidence of implantation metastasis directly correlates with tumor stage, so that wound metastasis is an indicator of advanced disease. The overall risk of port-site metastasis appears to be acceptably low, given the valuable staging information obtained during exploratory laparoscopy. A breakdown in laparoscopic technique leading to tumor morcellation is another factor that unfavorably skewed early reported results.

Staging laparoscopy

For a number of gastrointestinal, hepatobiliary, and lymphatic malignancies, inspection of the peritoneal cavity allows determination of disease extent, distinguishing limited disease from locally advanced and metastatic disease. In addition, tumor resectability can often be assessed via laparoscopy. By identifying patients with advanced disease who are unresectable, the number of unnecessary open laparotomies is reduced. Besides guiding operative management, laparoscopy can also direct adjuvant treatment. For example, patients with supradiaphragmatic Hodgkin's lymphoma and absence of constitutional 'B' symptoms may benefit from staging laparoscopy to rule out concomitant infradiaphragmatic disease (stage III, IV), thereby allowing a radiation-only treatment protocol. In other cases, the purpose of the laparoscopic staging procedure is to detect evidence of intraperitoneal tumor seeding (peritoneal carcinomatosis), involvement of adjacent organs, or the presence of previously undetected liver or spleen involvement.

Staging laparoscopy has been shown to be beneficial in pancreatic cancer. Pancreatic resection with a curative intent is possible in less than one-third of patients, is associated with a considerable morbidity, and has a poor outcome if residual tumor is left behind. Attempts at curative resection are not indicated in patients considered to have an unresectable cancer due to extrapancreatic disease or significant vascular involvement. Very often, pancreatic cancer is associated with dispersed small liver metastases at the time of diagnosis, which may escape detection on computerized tomography (CT) or magnetic resonance imaging (MRI) scans. Even if the preoperative imaging studies suggest that the tumor is resectable, a diagnostic laparoscopy before the intended laparotomy appears to be justified, because it may accurately assess intraperitoneal evidence of incurability in 28–65% of patients in a quick and minimally invasive manner. The first step in laparoscopic staging consists of a general inspection of the peritoneal cavity via a single umbilical port in order to rule out obvious extrapancreatic disease such as peritoneal carcinomatosis or liver metastases. Additional trocars, which can be placed along the intended incision for the open operation, may become necessary, so that a sonographic probe and additional instruments can be utilized. Encasement of the portal or mesenteric vessels is assessed using the Doppler ultrasound probe. This approach reduces the number of unnecessary laparotomies and attempted resections, thus minimizing postoperative morbidity. For those patients who prove to have an unresectable tumor upon staging laparoscopy, there is reduced postoperative discomfort and a more rapid recovery due to the minimally invasive approach. Opponents of the laparoscopic pancreatic staging approach point out that some patients who initially avoided a laparotomy will eventually require a palliative operation for gastrointestinal or biliary obstruction, and therefore make an argument for an open operation at the outset. As previously noted, however, the laparoscopic strategy should include not only the diagnosis and staging, but also the ability to draw the right conclusions from the findings and to provide palliation (laparoscopic biliary and gastric bypass) to patients with intractable disease at the time of the diagnostic intervention (see below).

Establishing a histologic diagnosis

Patients found to have a mass, either solitary or associated with intra-abdominal (e.g., porta hepatis) or retroperitoneal lymph nodes, are candidates for laparoscopic exploration. While image-guided fine-needle aspiration cytology may discriminate between neoplasms of epithelial versus lymphatic origin, a definitive histologic assessment is commonly necessary to establish the final diagnosis and treatment plan. Laparoscopy permits large specimens and whole lymph nodes to be evaluated by the pathologist, enabling assessment of the intact architecture and providing ample tissue for immunohistochemical and tumor marker studies.

Discrimination of benign versus malignant liver tumors

The treatment of both primary liver neoplasms and hepatic metastases largely depends on the extent of liver involvement, the number of lesions, and the presence of an underlying liver condition, such as cirrhosis, hepatitis, or cholangitis. Benign and malignant lesions may be present in the same patient. An exact assessment of the nature of the lesion as well as of the liver morphology with regard to presence or absence of liver cirrhosis is therefore mandatory before a treatment plan is formulated. Diagnostic laparoscopy, particularly in combination with a Doppler-equipped ultrasound probe, has proved very useful in distinguishing benign tumors of the liver from metastases and in searching out small tumors of the liver that are not detectable by conventional imaging techniques. The use of laparoscopic ultrasound is of utmost importance, because it allows detection of deep parenchymal lesions and planning of the proper anatomic resection. Biopsies may be carried out by either laparoscopy-guided or laparoscopic ultrasound-guided percutaneous insertion of a Tru-cut® needle into a hepatic lesion or by performing a laparoscopic wedge resection.

Determination of the extent of peritoneal metastasis from ovarian cancer

Ovarian cancer is characterized by early metastases to the peritoneal surfaces (FIGO stages IC/IIC–IV). Considering that unselected women with cystic adnexal lesions have a very low incidence of malignancies, in the range of 2–4%, a laparoscopic exploration as a first-line approach is justified.[1] If a suspicious adnexal mass or peritoneal seeding is encountered, the tumor may be removed or sampled and sent for frozen sections. If malignancy is confirmed, a staging procedure is required that includes complete peritoneal visualization, multiple peritoneal washings and biopsies, omentectomy, lymph node sampling, as well as removal of the reproductive organs. There are advocates of a laparoscopic approach to the staging procedure, but conversion to an open operation should still be regarded as standard treatment.[2,3] Particularly in the presence of bulky disease, a meticulous cytoreduction is very important because there is a correlation between the residual tumor volume and response rates of postoperative chemotherapy.[4,5]

First-line treatment protocols for ovarian cancer include platinum-based chemotherapy following cytoreductive surgery. A surgical second-look procedure is considered to be the most sensitive way of detecting persistent disease after platinum chemotherapy. Almost 50% of patients with a complete clinical response do not have a pathological cure, and residual tumor may be detected during the surgical second-look operation.[6] Further studies will be necessary regarding the interpretation of the second look, as there is currently no standard second-line salvage regimen for a curative intent in patients with residual tumor. Furthermore, those patients who do have a complete pathological response as determined by second-look surgery still have a 50% chance of relapse.

Suspicion of malignant ascites

Malignant ascites is most frequently associated with gynecological or gastrointestinal malignancy.[7] Although ascites is associated with advanced cancer in 15–30% of patients, cytologic examination of the fluid as well as imaging studies may remain inconclusive. Diagnostic laparoscopy is indicated in those patients with suspected but undiagnosed malignant ascites, facilitating tissue diagnosis and ruling out other causes such as cirrhosis. In the presence of peritoneal carcinomatosis, an effort should be made to define the primary tumor and to take biopsies.

Palliative procedures

When a curative cancer operation is not possible, a palliative operation may be necessary to alleviate symptoms that compromise the patient's quality of life. Palliative surgery is usually undertaken to control metastatic disease, pain, obstruction, bleeding, or perforation. Laparoscopic procedures aim at providing a rapid approach to palliation while keeping postoperative recovery time at a minimum. As always, the goals in laparoscopic palliation should be safety, efficacy, and minimization of the postoperative recovery period. As the patient's remaining lifespan may be considerably shortened, every effort should be undertaken to assure a short hospital stay and to minimize complications.

Resection of liver metastases

Resection of a limited number of hepatic metastases, most frequently from a colorectal primary, has been shown to be a safe method that may prolong disease-free survival. Although a majority of patients will ultimately develop tumor recurrence, metastasectomy carries the potential for cure in up to 30% of selected individuals. The laparoscopic approach to resection of liver metastases has been shown to be safe and feasible as long as the operation is guided by the same standards followed in the open operation.[8,9] The patient should be free of cirrhosis, cholangitis, and extrahepatic disease. Ideally, there should be fewer than four metastases, and disease should be limited to one anatomic lobe. The masses should be less than 4 cm in maximal diameter, and allow for a resection margin of at least 1 cm. There are safe locations along the anterolateral segments of the liver that are favorable for a laparoscopic resection (segments II, III, IVa, V, and VIa), whereas the posterior areas of the liver (segments VII, VIII, I, IVb) are not amenable to the laparoscopic approach.[9]

In preparation for a laparoscopic liver resection, the patient is placed in the lithotomy position and four trocars are inserted. This modification to a 'four-hand' approach, by placement of two additional trocars, allows two surgeons to operate simultaneously. Following mobilization of the liver, Glisson's capsule is incised 2 cm from the lesion using electrocautery. The harmonic shears, based on high-frequency denaturation of proteins, is essential for laparoscopic liver surgery because it allows a parenchymal fracture technique while achieving hemostasis and biliostasis of small radicles. Larger vascular and biliary pedicles are divided between hemostatic clips. Hemostasis and control of bile leaks from the raw liver surface are achieved by wide application of fibrin sealant (Tisseel, Baxter, Deerfield, IL) or by means of the argon laser coagulator. The linear endovascular cutters are usually reserved for the hepatic veins. The specimen is placed in a puncture-resistant bag and brought out through the enlarged umbilical port. The conversion rate to laparotomy is about 7% and is due to inaccessibility of the lesion, insufficient distance to the main vascular structures, or to control bleeding. Following laparoscopic liver resection, the patient can expect a rapid recovery, with a regular diet being resumed on the first postoperative day, followed by a short length of stay in hospital.

Alleviation of gastrointestinal obstruction

In patients who present with a gastrointestinal or biliary obstruction from an advanced tumor that is not suitable for a curative resection, laparoscopic surgery may be used for palliation. A laparoscopic approach is reasonable for a relatively circumscribed obstruction that may be either resected with non-curative intent or bypassed. Patients with generalized peritoneal carcinomatosis and multiple sites of obstruction, however, are not candidates for a laparoscopic approach, if for surgery at all.

Pancreatic cancer often results in biliary and/or gastric outlet obstruction. Creation of a gastroenteric bypass may be performed by means of laparoscopy, optimally at the time of the staging procedure after determination of unresectability. An antecolic jejunal loop is approximated to the stomach in a side-to-side fashion, and the two limbs of a cutting endoscopic stapler are inserted through small enterotomies on each side. A 30-mm stapler is fired twice to produce a wide gastroenterostomy. The remaining opening is then closed with a running suture. Although biliary obstructions may often be addressed by means of endoscopic or percutaneous transhepatic stents, these may fail or suffer repeated complications. Patients with extrahepatic cholestasis due to pancreatic cancer should therefore be offered a laparoscopic bilio-enteric bypass at the time of staging laparoscopy and gastroenterostomy. Technically, this can be achieved by a cholecystojejunostomy, performed in an analogous manner to the gastroenterostomy. In some patients with a small or occluded cystic duct and a large common bile duct (>1 cm), a hand-sewn side-to-side choledochojejunostomy may be preferable.

Colon cancer may manifest as partial or complete large bowel obstruction, lower gastrointestinal bleeding, or tumor perforation, irrespective of distant metastases. Local tumor control is therefore of primary importance, whether for intent to cure (see section below) or for palliation. For curative intent, a standard resection of the involved colon including the respective lymph nodes is necessary. A limited segmental wedge resection of the colon is acceptable in patients with metastatic disease. Ease of bowel mobilization and subsequent tension-free anastomosis make tumors located in the sigmoid colon or cecum and ascending colon particularly suitable for a laparoscopic or laparoscopically assisted colectomy. Inoperable rectal or ovarian cancer can lead to colonic obstruction. Laparoscopic creation of a loop colostomy facilitates identification and mobilization of the appropriate colon segment through a minimal incision.[10]

Cancers of the oropharynx and upper gastrointestinal tract are often complicated by obstruction and insufficient oral intake. Although curative resection is possible in a minority of patients, most will still require surgery, endoscopic intervention, or chemoradiation in order to restore continuity. If those attempts fail, the next step is the creation of a feeding-tube gastrostomy or enterostomy. Whereas the former is preferably done as a percutaneous endoscopic gastrostomy, both may be performed laparoscopically, with the advantage that a catheter of larger diameter may be placed.[11]

Pain control

Pain is the most common complaint in patients with advanced cancer and is related to tumor infiltration or compression of sensitive structures. Malignancy causing intractable pain should be addressed, with the most common approaches being radiation therapy or surgery. Although pain management has generally become a complex issue that exceeds the scope of this review, it should be mentioned that surgery may offer pain relief in selected individuals with inoperable disease by blocking the neural pain transmission.

Patients with progressive pancreatic or gastric cancer may develop upper abdominal and back pain that may be alleviated by neurolysis at the level of the celiac plexus or splanchnic nerves.[12] This can be accomplished by image-guided percutaneous injection of alcohol or phenol into the plexus, or under direct vision at the time of staging laparoscopy. If a bulky tumor precludes the abdominal approach, thoracoscopic bilateral splanchnicectomy has the advantage of accessing the splanchnic nerves under direct view and away from the actual tumor site.[13]

THE EVOLVING ROLE OF LAPAROSCOPY

With improvements in technical ability and instrumentation, areas that once were thought to be inaccessible to the minimally invasive approach are now being tackled with success. While it is of primary importance in the advancement of medicine to explore the power of a new technology and therefore 'to push the envelope,' the process must adhere to sound scientific analysis. In contrast to the previous section, the operations described in this section are feasible, but there remains a lack of consensus regarding the indications or technique. Many of these issues are currently undergoing evaluation in study protocols. Both patients and the medical community may best be served by enrolling potential candidates in these important studies.

Laparoscopy in foregut cancer

The use of laparoscopy for the treatment of gastric cancer has evolved in the past decade along with other advanced laparoscopic procedures. The use of laparoscopic curative resection for gastric cancer is becoming more common, particularly in countries with a high incidence of the disease, such as Japan. Population screening programs in such high-risk countries result in earlier detection in 50–70% of gastric cancer patients. This is significantly higher than in Europe and in the USA, where patients more frequently present with advanced, symptomatic lesions at the time of diagnosis.[14,15] Prognosis in gastric cancer largely depends on the histological type, the stage, and the presence of lymph node involvement. The primary management of gastric cancer remains surgical resection, but the role of multimodal treatment needs to be better defined. The extent of the gastric resection depends on the location and the differentiation of the tumor and typically involves a subtotal or total gastrectomy. The extent of lymph node dissection is a matter of considerable controversy, where a more extensive resection must be weighed against its higher morbidity.[16,17] Early or superficial gastric carcinoma (T1) does not infiltrate beyond the muscularis mucosa of the gastric wall and presents with adjacent lymph node metastases in only 15.7% of patients.[18] Surgical resection of T1N0 lesions results in cure rates of more than 95%. These results and the detection of an increasing number of early lesions in Asian countries may lead to a trend toward minimizing the extent of the classical resection which originated on the basis of more advanced lesions.

Despite the lack of prospective randomized studies comparing open and laparoscopic gastric resections, laparoscopic resection of early gastric cancer has been shown to be safe and effective in a number of retrospective series.[19] Depending on the type, size, and location of the tumor, a local resection may be performed as a wall-lifting wedge resection using a laparoscopic EndoGIA stapler. However, this technique may cause a significant narrowing near the pylorus and cardia, with resultant outlet or inlet obstruction. Alternatively, the resection can be performed using an endogastric approach: three trocars are inserted through both the abdominal and the gastric wall, allowing more complete mobilization and resection of the gastric lesion by means of a stapler device.[20] There is concern that this localized type of T1 tumor resection does not adequately assess nodal involvement, so a subtotal gastrectomy may be preferable.

Despite much controversy, laparoscopic curative resection of advanced gastric cancer has been performed at several institutions with encouraging early results.[21,22] Five trocars are usually placed, resectability is determined, and the dissection begins outside of the gastroepiploic arcade, taking care to avoid injury to the transverse colon. The dissection proceeds along the greater curvature and ends with transsection of the right gastroepiploic artery between clips. The right gastric artery is divided at the superior aspect of the duodenum and the dissection behind the duodenum is completed to create a window for the introduction of a linear cutter to transsect the duodenum. The stomach may then be pulled up to expose and skeletonize the lesser curvature. For the resection and reconstruction, either an intra-abdominal gastrojejunostomy or a laparoscopically assisted exteriorized gastrojejunostomy may be performed.[22] Given the fact that gastric resection for benign diseases has become very rare, it will certainly require a steeper learning curve before laparoscopic gastric resections become routine. The appropriateness of the laparoscopic management of advanced gastric cancers remains to be elucidated.

Laparoscopy for colon cancer

Despite accumulating data on laparoscopic colon cancer resections,[23–26] it is still considered an evolving procedure, because there remains a lack of consensus regarding the indications and techniques. Although laparoscopic colon resections are increasingly performed for benign diseases such as diverticulitis or sessile colon polyps, there are concerns as to whether the laparoscopic technique compromises the quality of the cancer operation. Apart from the unquantified risk of developing port-site metastases, there has been concern about the adequacy of tumor margins, lymph node dissection, and the effect of the limited view on the length of dissection. Since 1990, a number of randomized studies have been initiated throughout the world. The largest among them is a USA multicenter study by the National Cancer Institute. This study will eventually enroll 1200 patients with colon tumors <T3 and no evidence of metastatic disease. To date, more than half of the required patients have already been accrued, although a few more years will be needed before conclusions can be made.

Laparoscopic colectomy is initiated by positioning three to four trocars according to the segment being removed. The colon should be mobilized to the same extent as in the open approach. The vascular pedicle is identified and transsected with an endovascular stapler. Although it is possible to perform a totally laparoscopic resection and anastomosis, it is questionable whether there is much of an advantage, because at some point an incision big enough to bring the specimen out must be made. The laparoscopically assisted technique therefore appears to be more rational, where the mobilized colon is exteriorized through a small abdominal incision, an extra-abdominal resection and anastomosis are performed, and the adjacent segment is returned to the abdomen. Upon fascial closure, pneumoperitoneum may be re-established to allow inspection of the anastomosis.

Laparoscopy for endocrine tumors

Neuroendocrine tumors of the pancreas are often small, with 80% being hormonally active. Insulin-producing tumors, which account for about 85% of all islet-cell tumors, are malignant in 10–30% of cases, whereas gastrin-producing or hormonally inactive tumors have a 60% incidence of malignancy. Control of the hormone imbalance, such as hypoglycemia due to an islet cell tumor, requires excision. If the preoperative localization studies reveal a tumor in the pancreatic tail, laparoscopic distal pancreatectomy can be performed. However, there are only a few small series to support this approach, probably due in part to the rarity of these endocrine tumors.[27–29]

CONTRAINDICATIONS TO LAPAROSCOPY FOR CANCER

The same general contraindications apply for both open and laparoscopic surgery, but a number of additional factors have to be considered specifically for laparoscopic procedures. Absolute contraindications to the minimally invasive approach include uncorrected coagulopathy or severe cardiopulmonary disease with inability to tolerate an abdominal surgical procedure under general anesthesia. Although laparoscopic procedures are considered to be better tolerated with respect to the postoperative period, this is not true during anesthesia. The maintenance of a pneumoperitoneum with increased intra-abdominal pressure causes a rise in blood CO_2 levels and a drop in cardiac index and pulmonary functional residual capacity. Relative contraindications to laparoscopic surgery are dependent on the surgeon's experience and commonly include pregnancy in the first and third trimester, bowel obstruction with significant intestinal distension leading to a lack of working space, and liver cirrhosis. Although liver cirrhosis is not an absolute contraindication to laparoscopy, the risk of bleeding complications from periportal collaterals due to portal hypertension is significant. Except for the assessment of liver pathology in patients with hepatic masses, the presence of liver cirrhosis should be regarded as a contraindication to the pursuit of a laparoscopic strategy in cancer patients.

CONCLUDING REMARKS

With increasing expertise and continued advancement in technology the diagnosis, treatment, and palliation of malignancy will more frequently be safely addressed by laparoscopic surgery. However, just because it *can* be done laparoscopically, does not necessarily mean it *should* be done. Despite abundant enthusiasm among surgeons and patients, we must proceed carefully. Many issues regarding the indications and extent of resection in oncologic surgery have yet to be resolved, and the central question remains: what should be done and when? The role of laparoscopic surgery in the *curative* treatment of cancer should be assessed in carefully designed, meticulous scientific studies that will include at least 5-year survival rates.

When Henri Bismuth, a well-known French liver surgeon and pioneer in liver transplantation, was asked to comment on the feasibility of laparoscopic liver resection for cancer, he simply answered: 'In my career as a liver surgeon, I never once had a patient ask me about the size of the incision, but rather, what are the chances of survival?'.

REFERENCES

1. Hidlebaough DA, Vulgaropulos S, Orr RK. Treating adnexal masses. Operative laparoscopy vs. laparotomy. J Repr Med 1997; 42:551–8.

2. Chi DS, Curtin JP. Gynecologic cancer and laparoscopy. Obstet Gynecol Clin North Am 1999; 26:201–15.

3. Cannistra SA. Medical progress: Cancer of the ovary. N Engl J Med 1993; 329:1550–9.

4. Hoskins WJ, McGuire WP, Brady MF, et al. The effect of diameter of largest residual disease on survival after primary cytoreductive surgery in patients with suboptimal residual epithelial ovarian carcinoma. Am J Obstet Gynecol 1994; 170:974–9.

5. McGuire WP, Hoskins WJ, Brady MF, et al. Assessment of dose-intensive therapy in suboptimally debulked ovarian cancer: a Gynecologic Oncology Group study. J Clin Oncol 1995; 13:1589–99.

6. Cacciari N, Zamagni C, Strocchi E, Pannuti F, Martoni A. Advanced ovarian cancer patients with no evidence of disease after platinum-based chemotherapy: retrospective analysis of the role of second-look. Eur J Gynaecol Oncol 1999; 20:56–60.

7. Parsons SL, Watson SA, Steele RH. Malignant ascites. Br J Surg 1996; 83:6–14.

8. Marks J, Mouiel J, Katkhouda N, Gugenheim J, Fabiani P. Laparoscopic liver surgery. A report on 28 patients. Surg Endosc 1998; 12:331–4.

9. Katkhouda N, Hurwitz M, Gugenheim J, et al. Laparoscopic management of benign solid and cystic lesions of the liver. Ann Surg 1999; 229:460–6.

10. Fuhrman GM, Ota DM. Laparoscopic intestinal stomas. Dis Colon Rectum 1994; 37:444–9.

11. Murayama KM, Johnson TJ, Thompson JS. Laparoscopic gastrostomy and jejunostomy are safe and effective for obtaining enteral access. Am J Surg 1996; 172:591–4.

12. Polati E, Finco G, Gottin L, Bassi C, Pederzoli P, Ischia S. Prospective randomized double-blind trial of neurolytic coeliac plexus block in patients with pancreatic cancer. Eur J Surg Oncol 1998; 85:199–201.

13. Ihse I, Zoucas E, Gyllstedt E, Lillo-Gil R, Andren-Sandberg A. Bilateral thoracoscopic splanchnicectomy: effects on pancreatic pain and function. Ann Surg 1999; 230:785–90.

14. Mok YJ, Koo BW, Whang CW, et al. Cancer of the stomach: a review of two hospitals in Korea and Japan. World J Surg 1993; 17:777–82.

15. Kitamura K, Yamaguchi T, Sawai K, et al. Chronologic changes in the clinicopathologic findings and survival of gastric cancer patients. J Clin Oncol 1997; 15:3471–80.

16. Cuschieri A, Fayers P, Fielding J, et al. Postoperative morbidity and mortality after D1 and D2 resections for gastric cancer: preliminary results of the MRC randomised controlled surgical trial. The Surgical Cooperative Group. Lancet 1996; 347:995–9.

17. Bonenkamp JJ, Hermans J, Sasako M, van de Velde CJ. Extended lymph-node dissection for gastric cancer. Dutch Gastric Cancer Group. N Engl J Med 1999; 340:908–14.

18. Kim JP, Hur YS, Yang HK. Lymph node metastasis as a significant prognostic factor in early gastric cancer: analysis of 1,136 early gastric cancers. Ann Surg Oncol 1995; 2(4):308–13.

19. Goh PM, So JB. Role of laparoscopy in the management of stomach cancer. Semin Surg Oncol 1999; 16:321–6.

20. Ohashi S. Laparoscopic intraluminal (intragastric) surgery for early gastric cancer. A new concept in laparoscopic surgery. Surg Endosc 1995; 9:169–71.

21. Goh PM, Alponat A, Mak K, Kum CK. Early international results of laparoscopic gastrectomies. Surg Endosc 1997; 11:650–2.

22. Katkhouda N. Advanced laparoscopic technique. In Techniques and tips. Philadelphia, Harcourt, Inc., 1997.

23. Bouvet M, Mansfield PF, Skibber J, et al. Clinical, pathological, and economic parameters of laparoscopic colon resection for cancer. Am J Surg 1998; 176:554–8.

24. Franklin ME Jr, Rosenthal D, Abrego-Medina D, et al. Prospective comparison of open vs. laparoscopic colon surgery for carcinoma. Five-year results. Dis Colon Rectum 1996; 39:S35–46.

25. Poulin E, Mamazza J, Schlachta CM, Grégoire R, Roy N. Laparoscopic resection does not adversely affect early survival curves in patients undergoing surgery for colorectal adenocarcinoma. Ann Surg 1999; 229:487–92.

26. Trebuchet G, Le Calve J, Launois B. Laparoscopic resection of the colon for adenocarcinoma. Report of a series of 218 cases. Chirurgie 1998; 123:343–50.

27. Vezakis A, Davides D, Larvin M, McMahon MJ. Laparoscopic surgery combined with preservation of the spleen for distal pancreatic tumors. Surg Endosc 1999; 13:26–9.

28. Collins R, Schlinkert RT, Roust L. Laparoscopic resection of an insulinoma. J Laparosc Adv Surg Tech 1999; 9:429–31.

29. Gagner M, Pomp A, Herrera MF. Early experience with laparoscopic resections of islet cell tumors. Surgery 1996; 120:1051–4.

Editors' selected abstracts (for Chapters 4 and 5)

Cancer and laparoscopy, experimental studies: a review.

Canis M, Botchorishvili R, Wattiez A, Pouly JL, Mage G, Manhes H, Bruhat MA.

Department of Obstetrics, Gynecology and Reproductive Medicine, Polyclinique, 13 Bd Charles de Gaulle, 63033, Clermont Ferrand, France.

European Journal of Obstetrics, Gynecology, & Reproductive Biology 91(1):1–9, 2000, July.

Objective: To review the experimental studies on laparoscopy and cancer and to propose guidelines for the clinical management of gynecologic cancer. *Methods:* The literature in MEDLINE was searched from January 1992 to December 1998 using the terms 'cancer', 'laparoscopy' and 'experimental or animal study'. Cross-referencing identified additional publications. Abstracts and letters to the editor were excluded. All the relevant papers were reviewed. *Results:* Depending on the model used, controversial results have been reported on the incidence of trocar site metastasis when comparing CO_2 laparoscopy and laparotomy. In contrast, the following conclusions can be proposed: (i) tumour growth after laparotomy is greater than after endoscopy; (ii) tumour dissemination is worse after CO_2 laparoscopy than after laparotomy; (iii) some of the disadvantages of CO_2 laparoscopy may be treated using local or intravenous treatments or avoided using other endoscopic exposure methods, such as gasless laparoscopy. *Conclusions:* The laparoscopic treatment of gynecologic cancer has potential advantages and disadvantages, and may only be performed in prospective clinical trials. The risk of dissemination appears high when a large number of malignant cells are present. Adnexal tumours with external vegetations, and bulky lymph nodes should be considered as contra-indications to CO_2 laparoscopy.

Laparoscopic versus open radical nephrectomy: a 9-year experience.

Dunn MD, Portis AJ, Shalhav AL, Elbahnasy AM, Heidorn C, McDougall EM, Clayman RV.

Departments of Surgery, Urology and Radiology, Mallinckrodt Institute of Radiology, Washington University School of Medicine, St Louis, MI, USA.

Journal of Urology 164(4):1153–9, 2000, October.

Purpose: The laparoscopic approach for renal cell carcinoma is slowly evolving. We report our experience with laparoscopic radical nephrectomy and compare it to a contemporary cohort of patients with renal cell carcinoma who underwent open radical nephrectomy. *Materials and methods:* From 1990 to 1999, 32 males and 28 females underwent 61 laparoscopic radical nephrectomies for suspicious renal cell carcinoma. Clinical data from a computerized database were reviewed and compared to a contemporary group of 33 patients who underwent open radical nephrectomy for renal cell carcinoma. *Results:* Patients in the laparoscopic radical nephrectomy group had significantly reduced, estimated blood loss (172 versus 451 mL, $p < 0.001$), hospital stay (3.4 versus 5.2 days, $p < 0.001$), pain medication requirement (28.0 versus 78.3 mg., $p < 0.001$) and quicker return to normal activity than patients in the open radical nephrectomy group (3.6 versus 8.1 weeks, $p < 0.001$). The majority of laparoscopic specimens (65%) were morcellated. Operating time and cost were higher in the laparoscopic than the open nephrectomy group. Average followup was 25 months (range 3 to 73) for the laparoscopic and 27.5 months (range 7 to 90) for the open group. Renal cell carcinoma in 3 patients (8%) recurred in the laparoscopic group versus renal cell carcinoma in 3 (9%) in the open group. When stratified patients with tumors larger than 4 to 10 cm experienced similar benefits and results as patients with tumors less than or equal to 4 cm. To date there have been no instances of trocar or intraperitoneal seeding in the laparoscopic radical nephrectomy group. *Conclusions:* Laparoscopic radical nephrectomy, although technically demanding, is a viable alternative for managing localized renal tumors up to 10 cm. It affords patients with renal tumors an improved postoperative course with less pain and a quicker recovery while providing similar efficacy at 2-year followup for patients with T1 and T2 tumors.

Hand-assisted laparoscopic liver resection: lessons from an initial experience.

Fong Y, Jarnagin W, Conlon KC, DeMatteo R, Dougherty E, Blumgart LH.

Department of Surgery, Memorial Sloan-Kettering Cancer Center, New York, NY, USA.

Archives of Surgery 135(7):854–9, 2000, July.

Background: Recent innovations in laparoscopic instrumentation make routine resection of solid organs a clinical possibility. *Hypothesis:* Hand-assisted laparoscopic liver resection is a safe and feasible procedure for solitary cancers requiring removal of 2 segments of liver or less. *Design and patients:* Eleven patients with liver tumors deemed technically resectable by laparoscopic techniques were subjected to laparoscopic evaluation and attempted hand-assisted laparoscopic resection between July 1998 and July 1999. During the same period, 230 patients underwent open liver resection. *Setting:* Tertiary care referral center for liver cancer. *Main outcome measures:* Success of laparoscopic resection, reasons for conversion to open liver resection, blood loss, tumor clearance margin, complications, and length of hospital stay. *Results:* Five patients underwent successful resection by the hand-assisted laparoscopic technique. Data from the 5 successful cases and the 6 aborted cases are presented to outline the issues and the lessons learned. *Conclusions:* In selected patients, hand-assisted laparoscopic liver resection can be safely performed and might have potential advantages over traditional liver resection if the tumor is limited to the left lateral segment or is at the margins of the liver.

Laparoscopic radical cystoprostatectomy with ileal conduit performed completely intracorporeally: the initial 2 cases.

Gill IS, Fergany A, Klein EA, Kaouk JH, Sung GT, Meraney AM, Savage SJ, Ulchaker JC, Novick AC.

Section of Laparoscopic and Minimally Invasive Surgery and Section of Urologic Oncology, Department of Urology, Cleveland Clinic Foundation, OH, USA.

Urology 56(1):26–9; discussion 29–30, 2000, July.

Objectives: To present the initial 2 patients who underwent laparoscopic radical cystoprostatectomy, bilateral pelvic lymphadenectomy, and ileal conduit urinary diversion, with the entire procedure performed exclusively by intracorporeal laparoscopic techniques. *Methods:* Two male patients, 78 and 70 years old, with muscle-invasive, organ-confined, transitional cell carcinoma of the urinary bladder underwent the procedure. The entire procedure, including radical cystoprostatectomy, pelvic node dissection, isolation of the ileal loop, restoration of bowel continuity with stapled side-to-side ileoileal anastomosis, retroperitoneal transfer of the left ureter to the right side, and bilateral stented ileoureteral anastomoses were all performed exclusively by intracorporeal laparoscopic techniques. Free-hand laparoscopic suturing and *in situ* knot-tying techniques were used exclusively. *Results:* The surgical time was 11.5 hours in the first patient and 10 hours in the second. The respective blood loss was 1200 mL and 1000 mL. In both patients, ambulation resumed on postoperative day 2, bowel sounds on day 3, and oral intake on day 4; the hospital stay was 6 days. Narcotic analgesia comprised 108.3 mg and 16.5 mg of morphine sulfate equivalent, respectively. Pathologic examination revealed pT4N0M0 (prostate) and pT2bN0M0 transitional cell carcinoma of the bladder with the surgical margins negative for cancer in both patients. No intraoperative or postoperative complications occurred in either patient. *Conclusions:* To our knowledge, this is the initial report of laparoscopic radical cystoprostatectomy with intracorporeal ileal conduit urinary diversion. We believe that with further experience and refinement in the operative technique, laparoscopic radical cystoprostatectomy with ileal conduit urinary diversion may become an attractive treatment option for selected candidates with localized muscle-invasive bladder cancer.

Retroperitoneal laparoscopic radical nephrectomy: the Cleveland Clinic experience.

Gill IS, Schweizer D, Hobart MG, Sung GT, Klein EA, Novick AC.

Section of Laparoscopic and Minimally Invasive Surgery, Department of Urology, The Cleveland Clinic Foundation, Cleveland, OH, USA.

Journal of Urology 163(6):1665–70, 2000, June.

Purpose: Laparoscopic radical nephrectomy is usually performed by the transperitoneal approach. At our institution the retroperitoneoscopic approach is preferred. We confirm the technical feasibility of retroperitoneoscopic radical nephrectomy, even for large specimens, and compare its results with open surgery in a contemporary cohort. *Materials and methods:* A total of 47 patients underwent 53 retroperitoneoscopic radical nephrectomies. Data from the most recent 34 laparoscopic cases were retrospectively compared with 34 contemporary cases treated with open radical nephrectomy. *Results:* For the 53 retroperitoneoscopic radical nephrectomies mean tumor size was 4.6 cm (range 2 to 12), surgical time was 2.9 hours (range 1.2 to 4.5) and blood loss was 128 cc. Mean specimen weight was 484 gm (range 52 to 1,328), and concomitant adrenalectomy was performed in 72% of patients. Mean analgesic requirement was 31 mg morphine sulfate equivalent. Average hospital stay was 1.6 days, with 68% of patients discharged from the hospital within 23 hours of the procedure. Minor complications occurred in 8 patients (17%) and major complications occurred in 2 (4%) who required conversion to open surgery. Various parameters, including patient age, body mass index, American Society of Anesthesiologists status, tumor size (5 versus 6.1 cm), specimen weight (605 versus 638 gm) and surgical time (3.1 versus 3.1 hours), were comparable between patients undergoing laparoscopic (34) and open (34) radical nephrectomy. However, laparoscopy resulted in decreased blood loss ($p < 0.001$), hospital stay ($p < 0.001$), analgesic requirements ($p < 0.001$) and convalescence ($p = 0.005$). Complications occurred in 13% of patients in the laparoscopic group and 24% in the open group. *Conclusions:* Retroperitoneoscopy is a reliable, effective and, in our hands, the preferred technique of laparoscopic radical nephrectomy. At our institution retroperitoneoscopy has emerged as an attractive alternative to open radical nephrectomy in patients with T1–T2N0M0 renal tumors.

Patterns of recurrence and survival after laparoscopic and conventional resections for colorectal carcinoma.

Hartley JE, Mehigan BJ, MacDonald AW, Lee PW, Monson JR.

University of Hull, Academic Surgical Unit, Castle Hill Hospital, Cottingham, East Yorkshire, UK.

Annals of Surgery 232(2):181–6, 2000, August.

Objective: To determine whether survival and recurrence after laparoscopic-assisted surgery for colorectal cancer is compromised by an initial laparoscopic approach. *Summary background data:* Laparoscopic colorectal resection for malignancy remains controversial 8 years after its first description. Fears regarding compromised oncologic principles and early recurrence (particularly the phenomenon of port-site metastases) have tempered enthusiasm for this approach. Long-term follow-up data are at present scarce. *Methods:* A prospective comparative trial was undertaken between December 1993 and May 1996, during which 114 patients had laparoscopic-assisted resection by a single laparoscopic colorectal surgeon or conventional open surgery by a second specialist colorectal surgeon. Intensive follow-up for at least 2 years is available on 109 patients. Analysis was performed on an intention-to-treat basis. *Results:* Recurrent disease has developed in 27 patients (25%), 16 of 57 in the laparoscopic group (28%) and 11 of 52 in the conventional group (21%). Crude death rates are 26/57 (46%) in the laparoscopic group and 24/52 (46%)

in the conventional group. No port-site metastases have occurred; however, wound metastases associated with disseminated disease have developed in three patients in the open group and one in the laparoscopic group. Stage-for-stage survival and recurrence figures are comparable. *Conclusion:* Oncologic outcome at a minimum of 2 years is not compromised by the laparoscopic approach. Wound recurrences are a feature of laparoscopic and conventional surgery for advanced disease.

The role of laparoscopy in preoperative staging of esophageal cancer.

Heath EI, Kaufman HS, Talamini MA, Wu TT, Wheeler J, Heitmiller RF, Kleinberg L, Yang SC, Olukayode K, Forastiere AA.

Department of Medical Oncology, Johns Hopkins Oncology Center, Baltimore, MD, USA.

Surgical Endoscopy 14(5):495–9, 2000, May.

Background: Diagnostic laparoscopy has been used to determine resectability and to prevent unnecessary laparotomy in patients with advanced esophageal cancer. The objective of this prospective study was to evaluate the role of laparoscopy in conjunction with computed tomography (CT) scan in staging patients with esophageal cancer. *Methods:* From March 1995 to October 1998, 59 patients with biopsy-proven esophageal cancer underwent diagnostic laparoscopy with concurrent vascular access device and feeding jejunostomy tube placement. *Results:* Laparoscopy changed the treatment plain in 10 of 59 patients (17%). Of the patients with normal-appearing regional or celiac nodes, 78% were confirmed by biopsy to be tumor free, whereas 76% of patients with abnormal-appearing nodes were confirmed by biopsy to have node-positive disease. *Conclusions:* Diagnostic laparoscopy is useful for detecting and confirming nodal involvement and distant metastatic disease that potentially would alter treatment and prognosis in patients with esophageal cancer.

Laparoscopy and peritoneal cytology in the staging of pancreatic cancer.

Jimenez RE, Warshaw AL, Fernandez-Del Castillo C.

Department of Surgery, Massachusetts General Hospital, Boston, MA, USA.

Journal of Hepatobiliary and Pancreatic Surgery 7(1):15–20, 2000.

Staging laparoscopy in patients with pancreatic cancer allows identification of metastatic disease which is beyond the resolution of computed tomography. Laparoscopic ultrasound, dissection, and/or peritoneal cytology may be used to enhance the sensitivity of the staging procedure. Our experience at Massachusetts General Hospital with staging laparoscopy and peritoneal cytology over the past 8 years ($n = 239$) reveals that approximately 30% of patients without metastases by computed tomography harbor occult metastatic disease at laparoscopy. Additionally, published series demonstrate accurate determination of resectability in greater than 75% of patients after staging laparoscopy. Staging laparoscopy in patients with pancreatic cancer allows optimization of resources and avoidance of unnecessary surgery.

Prospective, blinded comparison of laparoscopic ultrasonography vs. contrast-enhanced computerized tomography for liver assessment in patients undergoing colorectal carcinoma surgery.

Milsom JW, Jerby BL, Kessler H, Hale JC, Herts BR, O'Malley CM.

Department of Colorectal Surgery, The Cleveland Clinic Foundation, OH, USA.

Diseases of the Colon and Rectum 43(1):44–9, 2000, January.

Purpose: To prospectively and blindly compare intraoperative laparoscopic ultrasonography to preoperative contrast-enhanced computerized tomography in detecting liver lesions in colorectal cancer patients. Additionally, we compared conventional (open) intraoperative ultrasonography with bimanual liver palpation to contrast-enhanced computerized tomography in a subset of patients. *Methods:* From December 1995 to March 1998, 77 consecutive patients underwent curative ($n = 63$) or palliative ($n = 14$) resections for colorectal cancer. All patients undergoing curative resections were randomized to either laparoscopic ($n = 34$) or conventional ($n = 29$) surgery after informed consent. All patients underwent contrast-enhanced computerized tomography, diagnostic laparoscopy, and laparoscopic ultrasonography before resection. In those patients who had conventional procedures, intraoperative ultrasonography with bimanual liver palpation was also done. All laparoscopic ultrasonography and intraoperative ultrasonography evaluations were performed by one of two radiologists who were blinded to the CT results. All hepatic segments were scanned using a standardized method. The yield of each modality was calculated using the number of lesions identified by each imaging modality divided by the total number of lesions identified. *Results:* In 43 of the 77 patients, both the laparoscopic ultrasonography and CT scan were negative for any liver lesions. In 34 patients, a total of 130 lesions were detected by laparoscopic ultrasonography, CT, or both. When compared with laparoscopic ultrasonography, intraoperative ultrasonography with bimanual liver palpation identified one additional metastatic lesion and no additional benign lesions. Laparoscopic ultrasonography identified two patients with metastases who had negative preoperative contrast-enhanced computerized tomography. *Conclusions:* Laparoscopic ultrasonography of the liver at the time of primary resection of colorectal cancer yields more lesions than preoperative contrast-enhanced computerized tomography and should be considered for routine use during laparoscopic oncologic colorectal surgery.

Laparoscopy in patients following transverse rectus abdominus myocutaneous flap reconstruction.

Muller CY, Coleman RL, Adams WP Jr.

Department of Obstetrics and Gynecology, University of Texas Southwestern Medical Center, Dallas, TX, USA.

Obstetrics & Gynecology 96(1):132–5, 2000, July.

Background: We report our technique and experience performing laparoscopic pelvic surgery on four women after transverse rectus abdominus myocutaneous flap (TRAM). *Technique:* Examination under anesthesia is performed on all patients in the low lithotomy position parallel with the floor. The abdominal aorta is palpated and outlined. A pneumoperitoneum is created either by umbilical or left upper quadrant Veress placement. Patients with an acceptable umbilical location undergo port placement through the incision of the umbilical relocation. Other options include left upper quadrant or paramedian placement avoiding the ligamentum teres vessels. Lateral operative ports (5 mm) are placed with reference to the transverse incision present, the pelvic pathology, and the location of the umbilicus. Techniques of electrocautery, intra- and extracorporeal suturing and knot tying, and clips are preferred to minimize port size. *Experience:* Following unilateral or bilateral TRAM reconstruction, four consecutive breast cancer survivors underwent successful laparoscopic-assisted vaginal hysterectomy with oophorectomy using the periumbilical incision for trocar placement. The only complication was a superficial skin breakdown from an adhesive allergy that required 6 weeks for complete resolution. *Conclusion:* Laparoscopic pelvic surgery is feasible in women after TRAM reconstruction. Knowledge of anatomic and physiologic variations related to the TRAM procedure is necessary in planning a safe operation.

Laparoscopic cholecystectomy in the treatment of patients with gall bladder cancer.

Yoshida T, Matsumoto T, Sasaki A, Morii Y, Ishio T, Bandoh T, Kitano S.

Department of Surgery I, Oita Medical University, Japan.

Journal of the American College of Surgeons
191(2):158–63, 2000, August.

Background: Surgical procedures based on the depth of the primary tumor invasion (pT category) have been proposed in the treatment of gallbladder cancer (GBC). Trocar site metastases have been reported in patients who underwent laparoscopic cholecystectomy (LC) for preoperatively undiagnosed GBC. *Study design:* The aim of this study was to clarify the role of LC as a surgical strategy for GBC. From 1986 to 1998, 56 patients with GBC underwent surgical resection. Survival rates were compared retrospectively according to pT category and use of LC. *Results:* Five-year survival was 91% for pT1 ($n = 13$), 64% for pT2 ($n = 25$), 34% for pT3 ($n = 14$), and 0% for pT4 tumors ($n = 4$; $p < 0.0001$). LC was performed on 11 patients (4 with pT1, 5 with pT2, and 2 with pT3 tumors). Of the seven patients with pT2 or pT3 tumors, three underwent a second radical operation, three had an open radical operation to which the procedure was converted from LC, and one underwent no additional procedures. For pT1 tumors, one patient died of trocar site metastasis from bile spillage after LC. For pT2 or pT3 tumors, 5-year survival was 63% for radical surgery ($n = 35$) and 0% for cholecystectomy alone ($n = 4$; $p < 0.05$). For pT2 or pT3 tumors treated by radical surgery, 5-year survival was 75% for laparoscopic approach ($n = 6$) and 60% for open surgery ($n = 29$; not significant). *Conclusions:* LC may help to establish the diagnosis and to determine the surgical strategy for undiagnosed GBC. It is important to prevent spillage or implantation of malignant cells during LC. For pT2 or pT3 tumors diagnosed laparoscopically, a second or converted open radical surgery is necessary.

6

Organ transplantation and malignancy

STEVEN D COLQUHOUN, CRAIG A LIPKIN,* AND CAROLINE A CONNELLY

INTRODUCTION

Within the last 15 years, the field of solid organ transplantation has grown tremendously. Although kidney transplants have been performed for decades, within the last few years heart, liver, lung, and pancreas transplantations have all become the standard of care for end-stage organ disease. In addition, almost every conceivable combination of multi-organ transplants has been performed with success, and technical considerations no longer represent major obstacles to those in need. Currently, only small-bowel transplantation remains in the probationary realm. In the last decade, well over 220 000 organ transplants were performed in the USA. Most impressive is the magnitude of increase in the numbers of patients being added to organ transplant waiting lists. The United Network of Organ Sharing (UNOS) maintains the statistics regarding transplant volumes.[1] Considering all organs, the current UNOS waiting list now includes over 77 000 patients, with a new name added, on average, every 16 min.[1]

Perhaps the best representative example of the dramatic changes seen within the entire field of transplantation is the *exponential* growth in the number of patients awaiting liver transplants (Figure 6.1).[1] This increase can be attributed to both the expanded indications for liver transplantation and the heightened awareness of this therapeutic alternative on the part of both patients and physicians. However, the most important contribution to this dramatic expansion can be found in outcomes. Both patient and allograft survivals have continued to improve as individuals who previously faced death are returned to normal life.

Due to the current extent of transplantation in the USA, there is now an overwhelming likelihood that 'non-transplant' physicians will encounter either patients who have already received an organ transplant or those who may be future candidates. For this reason, there is a certain responsibility for all physicians to have

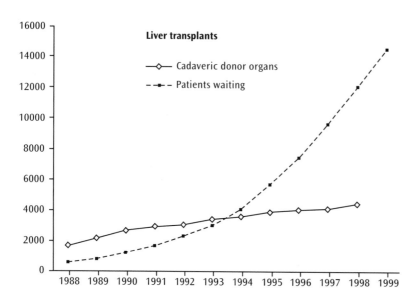

Figure 6.1 *Curves demonstrating growing disparity between number of patients needing a liver transplant and the availability of donor organs.*

---

*Deceased.

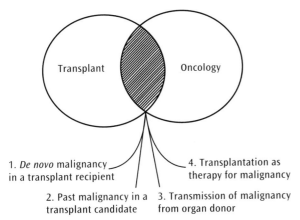

1. *De novo* malignancy in a transplant recipient

2. Past malignancy in a transplant candidate

3. Transmission of malignancy from organ donor

4. Transplantation as therapy for malignancy

Figure 6.2 *Areas of overlapping considerations in the fields of organ transplantation and oncology.*

some familiarity with the central issues, indications, and limitations of the field of organ transplantation. For the specialist in oncology, there are additional fascinating and instructive aspects in the simultaneous consideration of immunosuppression and malignancy. Indeed, surgical oncology and transplantation overlap in a number of areas, obligating physicians in each occupation to maintain an understanding of the issues common to both.

The fields of oncology and transplantation can be considered to overlap in four distinct areas (Figure 6.2). Three are clearly quite relevant to the practicing oncologist, whereas the last is mentioned for completeness and to illustrate further the profound interactions between malignancy and the immune response. Indeed, the function of the immune system is the issue central to both disciplines, promoting its function on the one hand and suppressing it on the other. The 'holy grail' of solid organ transplantation is the one-time permanent manipulation of the immune system to achieve the state of chimerism: the coexistence of host and allograft in the absence of ongoing immunosuppression. Research in this area is progressing with promise. We may therefore some day look forward to a greatly reduced concern with malignancy in the transplant population.

1 The first area of overlap is the setting in which a transplant recipient presents with a newly diagnosed malignancy. This circumstance could arise after any organ transplant in which the patient continues to receive immunosuppressive therapy. There may be *de novo* malignancies, probably related to the immunosuppression itself, as well as other more common malignancies that may arise in the general population, but which are exacerbated by immunosuppressive therapy.

2 Next is the consideration of transplant candidacy against the backdrop of a past malignancy. The questions faced center on the issue of potential residual

disease which may respond unfavorably in the environment of immunosuppression.

3 Another issue is the curious reality that a malignancy may be inadvertently acquired from the organ donor during transplantation. Transmission of malignancy has been described in most types of solid organ transplantation and illustrates the profound interaction between a malignancy and the immune system.

4 Last is the circumstance in which an existing malignancy may be the sole or partial indication for an organ transplant. This is an expectedly limited scenario; however, in certain settings, a transplant may provide results superior to those of other alternatives, even in the presence of immunosuppression.

This chapter discusses the principles guiding management decisions and the issues pertaining to specific tumors in each of these four areas.

IMMUNOSUPPRESSION AND MALIGNANCY

Introduction

Although the exact mechanisms are still incompletely understood, an appreciation of the profound interactions between the immune system and malignancy began in the earliest days of transplantation. Indeed, the clinical beginnings of transplantation predate much of what is now known about the immune system. Major contributions to our understanding of immunology have come from what has essentially been the human experiment of organ transplantation.[2] From this experience there have been three essential lessons learned regarding the impact of immunosuppressive drugs on malignancy:

1 The first and most dramatic is illustrated by a 1965 report describing the lethal outcome in a kidney transplant recipient when a pyriform sinus squamous-cell carcinoma was inadvertently transplanted along with the organ.[3] Through such impressive examples, it became clear that immunosuppression may allow more than just the organ of interest to be transplanted.

2 Next was a more gradual appreciation that certain malignancies appeared with greater than expected frequency in transplant recipients.[4]

3 Finally, the negative impact of immunosuppression on an existing malignancy in a transplant recipient was also fully recognized.[5]

Immunosuppression and *de novo* malignancy

It has been repeatedly observed that transplant recipients have a three–fourfold increased incidence of cancer compared with age-matched controls in the general population.[6] It has been estimated that 6% of all transplant recipients will develop a malignancy, but, for-tunately, overall only about 1% will die as a result.[4] Transplant recipients also develop tumors at younger ages than would be expected in the general population and often within a common time interval.[4,7] In one review, the average age at which transplant recipients were diagnosed with a cancer was 41 years. Although different malignancies are diagnosed within different time frames, there is a mean time to diagnosis of about 61 months from the time of transplant.[7] Interestingly, cancers that are common in the general population, such as carcinomas of the colon, breast, prostate, and lung, do not occur at any greater frequency in transplant recipients.[8–10] Rather, other, less common cancers, such as lymphomas, Kaposi's sarcoma, squamous-cell skin cancers, and anogenital tumors, are seen with greater frequency in transplant recipients.[4,5]

The first malignancies observed to appear with greater frequency in transplant recipients were those of the skin and lips. These are mostly squamous-cell cancers, which appear with up to a 20-fold greater incidence than expected.[6,11] Even more impressive increases have now been noted in the incidence of other tumors that are relatively uncommon in the general population. Non-Hodgkin's lymphoma has been reported to occur with an incidence 40-fold higher than expected. Kaposi's sarcoma is seen with a 400–500-fold increase, anogenital carcinoma (vulvar and anal) with a 20–100-fold increase, and uterine cervical carcinoma-in-situ with a 15-fold increase, while smaller increases have also been noted in non-Kaposi's sarcoma and renal cell carcinoma.[6,9] Finally, hepatocellu-lar carcinoma is seen with a 20–40-fold increased inci-dence compared to the general population.[11]

Although many of these increases are presumably due to the immunosuppressant drugs that are commonly used for all organ transplantations, the observed timing and incidence of tumors are not identical among recipi-ents of different organs. This certainly could be due to differences in the immunosuppression regimens used with different organs, or to a statistical effect resulting from the disproportionate numbers of the different transplanted organs. For example, the most accurate data may be available for renal transplants, which have been performed in greater numbers and for a greater number of years than transplants of any other organ. Whatever the reason, significant differences have been noted. For example, several recent reviews have concluded that, aside from skin cancers and post-transplant lymphopro-liferative disorders, the incidence of malignancy among liver transplant recipients is no higher than that of the general population.[12–14] On the other hand, heart trans-plant recipients often receive higher levels of immuno-suppression than some other organ recipients, and several reports continue to confirm higher rates of malignancy

among this population.[15–17] It has been suggested that lymphomas appear to be much more common among liver than renal transplant recipients (57% versus 12%), whereas the reverse is true for other de novo malignan-cies, including skin cancers.[18] Finally, some reports point to a disproportionately high incidence of lymphoma in cardiothoracic transplant recipients, representing 39% of all de novo malignancies, as compared to only 12% in renal recipients.[19]

Another difference among transplant recipients compared with the general population is the aggressive nature of the neoplasms that do occur. For example, skin cancers in immunosuppressed patients may not take the same indolent course typically seen. A basal-cell or squamous-cell cancer seen in a transplant recipient demands immediate definitive attention. This obviously extends to the more sinister forms of cancer as well. In one study of de novo malignancy in a group of over 2000 liver transplant recipients, the mortality was over 37%.[13]

The largest, worldwide repository for data on malignancies occurring in the transplant setting is the Cincinnati Transplant Tumor Registry (CTTR), which is under the direction of Dr Israel Penn. Although there is no mandatory reporting mechanism, the CTTR was the single most important instrument available to further our understanding of issues relating to malig-nancy and transplantation, and it remains the best source of data regarding the larger transplant population. Over the last 30 years, periodic reports from these data, and from the data of others, have consistently shown this increased incidence of specific cancers in transplant patients. Although discrepancies have been identified among data from smaller tumor registries, the voluntary nature of data reporting, in terms of age, gender, genetic, cultural, and environmental factors, may account for the observed differences.[20,21] In addition, there may be very significant differences amongst centers in the type and amount of immunosuppression administered as well as in the various organs transplanted. Reliable epi-demiological studies of malignancies in transplant recip-ients, including the ability to calculate risk ratios, are unavailable.

According to the most recent update from the CTTR, to date there have been 11 663 de novo malignancies recorded in 10 995 post-transplant patients. From those, 4406 were recorded to have various forms of skin cancer, meaning that about 38% of post-transplant malignan-cies arise from the skin.[22] Lip cancers have been found to occur at a rate of about 6%, compared to a 0.2% inci-dence in the general population.[9] In transplant patients, Kaposi's sarcoma also occurs in an estimated 6%, com-pared to a negligible incidence in the general popu-lation.[9] Carcinomas of the vulva and perineum also occur more frequently with an incidence of 3% com-pared to 0.7% (Table 6.1).[9]

Table 6.1 *Relative incidence of specific tumors*

Tumor	Incidence in general population (%)	Incidence in transplant recipients (%)
Lymphoma	5	24
Lip cancer	0.2	6
Kaposi's sarcoma	Negligible	6
Anogenital	0.4	3.5
Hepatobiliary	1.5	2.4
Vulva and perineum	0.7	3
Other sarcomas	0.5	1.8

Reference 135

Table 6.2 *Immunosuppressant-related malignancy*

Proposed mechanisms

Direct carcinogenic effects of immunosuppressant drugs
Facilitation of oncogenic viral mechanisms
Sensitization to other environmental carcinogens
Diminished immune surveillance
Chronic antigenic stimulation: hyperplasia to neoplasia
Impaired immunoregulation/unrestrained lymphoid
  proliferation
Decreased interferons/altered cytokine milieu

Immunosuppression: mechanisms of oncogenesis

As stated above, the exact mechanisms for the observed increased incidence of immunosuppressant-related malignancy are incompletely understood. However, a number of mechanisms have been proposed (Table 6.2). The most plausible include a possible direct carcinogenic effect of the immunosuppressant drugs, the facilitation of oncogenic viruses by the immunosuppressed state, sensitization to other carcinogenic conditions such as exposure to sunlight, viral infections, or hormonal factors, and a diminished immune surveillance facilitating malignant transformation.[23]

Drugs

Some of the primary agents used for immunosuppression in transplant recipients have been identified as probable carcinogens, including azathioprine, cyclophosphamide, and cyclosporin. It has also been proposed that cyclosporin and azathioprine may cause direct chromosomal injury.[9] Imidazole metabolites of azathioprine do sensitize skin to sunlight, and its 6-thioguanine metabolite may itself be a carcinogen.[24] At least one animal study has found that cyclosporin enhances the development and growth of hepatocellular carcinoma in particular.[25]

As more and better drugs have become available, the treatment of rejection has dramatically improved, but the incidence of post-transplant malignancies such as posttransplant lymphoproliferative disorders (PTLD) and Kaposi's sarcoma has increased disproportionately. For example, early drug regimens based on azathioprine or cyclophosphamide had an incidence of PTLD of about 11%, occurring on average within 48 months. After the introduction of cyclosporin, however, the incidence jumped to 26%, with an average occurrence in 15 months.[4] In a study of 1700 renal transplant recipients followed over a period of 25 years, the Kaplan–Meier estimates of cumulative cancer risk in those treated in the cyclosporin era were found to be nearly 6.6% at 5 years and nearly 14% by 10 years. Patients treated earlier without cyclosporin had a cumulative risk at 10 years of only 8.4%.[26] (It should be explained that comparisons of risks for malignancy between different eras can be interesting, but include a multitude of other factors and are not therefore completely valid.) The availability of cyclosporin brought a dramatic increase in the success of all organ transplants, essentially making non-renal transplantation feasible. The pre-cyclosporin data therefore reflect almost entirely renal transplant patients and a skewed population, considering the inferior rate of transplant success. Perhaps most telling on the issue of direct drug carcinogenesis is the incidence of tumors in patients receiving monoclonal antibody therapy, in which such a mechanism is difficult to imagine. Indeed, a direct effect of the drugs *per se* seems inadequate to account for the observed increases in malignancy, especially considering the array of different agents used and the evolution of new drugs with different mechanisms of action.

Oncogenic viruses

Viral infections have clearly been associated with the development of neoplasia in transplant recipients. In a study of skin lesions found in renal transplant patients, human papilloma virus DNA was found in 48% of premalignant skin lesions and in 54% of squamous-cell carcinomas.[27] In addition, the human papilloma virus probably plays a role in the increased incidence of uterine cervical and anogenital malignancies.[28,29] As discussed in greater detail below, the Epstein–Barr virus (EBV) is clearly related to the development of PTLDs. Hepatitis B and C are strongly related to the development of hepatocellular carcinoma. Finally, several viruses, including the herpes simplex 8 virus, are now strongly associated with Kaposi's sarcoma.[9]

Sensitization to other carcinogens

All organ transplant recipients are educated regarding the well-known sensitizing effects of their immunosuppressant drugs to sun exposure. As an addition to the genetic considerations, e.g., fair skin, there is some increased predisposition to ultraviolet-induced skin cancers.[11] Kaposi's sarcoma may also have a genetic component in that it appears with greater frequency in certain ethnic populations, which could be exacerbated by immunosuppression.[11]

Immunosurveillance

Some of the best suggestive evidence for diminished immunosurveillance leading to malignancy can be found in the non-transplant setting. Patients with acquired immunodeficiency syndrome (AIDS) suffer a 100-fold increase in both Kaposi's sarcoma and non-Hodgkin's lymphoma.[30] Other immunodeficiency disorders, such as Wiskott–Aldrich syndrome or ataxia-telangiectasia, are also associated with dramatically increased incidences of certain malignancies, especially non-Hodgkin's lymphoma.[9] The prevention of graft rejection with immunosuppression involves the inhibition of a response to non-self.[2] The immunogenicity of tumors and the presence of tumor-specific antigens (TSAs) and tumor-associated antigens (TAAs) are well established, and a great deal of work has been performed on the identification and characterization of the nature of such antigens.[31] Clearly, the immune system has some role to play in countering the development and/or spread of malignant cells. Indeed, at least four cellular elements of the immune system have been proven to interact with tumor cells, including natural killer (NK) cells, macrophages, and subpopulations of both B and T lymphocytes.[2] The evasion of immune surveillance remains a dominant theory of malignant transformation. If one subscribes to this paradigm, then it is simple to postulate that the increased incidence of malignancy associated with immunosuppression is due to the disruption of this mechanism.[2] Unfortunately, if this is indeed the case, one would expect an increased incidence of many other forms of cancer, rather than just the specific few that appear to be increased. Because many of the malignancies associated with immunosuppression appear to be virally associated or induced by environmental mutagens, perhaps the dysfunction specifically affects those mechanisms to a greater degree. Finally, if immunosurveillance plays a major role in suppressing the formation of tumors, one might expect a higher incidence of malignancy in immunologically privileged sites.

Other theories

A number of other theories regarding immunosuppressant-related oncogenesis have been proposed. Chronic antigenic stimulation leading to hyperplasia and ultimately to neoplasia, impaired immunoregulation leading to unrestrained lymphoid proliferation and lymphomas, and alterations in the milieu of cytokines have all been discussed.[32]

Finally, it should also be pointed out that several conditions that may lead to the need for transplantation may also be associated with the increased incidence of specific malignancies. For example, there is an association between primary sclerosing cholangitis and ulcerative colitis and both have associations with an increased incidence of malignancy. Therefore, a patient who undergoes liver transplantation for primary sclerosing cholangitis may also have related ulcerative colitis and be at risk for developing a subsequent colon cancer, and may further be at risk for cholangiocarcinoma. Analgesic nephropathy can lead to a need for a renal transplant, but is also associated with urinary tract malignancy. Similarly, acquired renal cystic disease has an associated increased incidence of renal cancer.[9]

Summary

The etiology of post-transplant malignancy is undoubtedly multifactorial. It is probably true that oncogenic viral activation within the environment of immunosuppression is a major etiologic factor; however, the other mechanisms discussed may also contribute.[7,10]

Increases in specific tumors *de novo*

Skin and lip tumors: basal-cell and squamous-cell carcinomas

Contrary to what is seen in the general population, in transplant patients there is a reverse trend in skin cancers toward more squamous-cell rather than basal-cell carcinomas.[28] One report noted the ratio of squamous-cell to basal-cell carcinoma to be as high as 5 : 1 in heart recipients.[16] Squamous-cell cancers, in fact, comprise 38% of those found in the CTTR, an incidence that increases with increasing length of follow-up.[28] Among a Norwegian cohort of over 2500 renal transplant recipients, the relative risk for developing squamous-cell cancer was increased 20-fold and 65-fold for the lip and skin, respectively.[15] Others have also noted that the frequency of skin cancer increases with time after transplant. In one study, 40–70% of patients had lesions after a follow-up of 20 years.[33] In an Australian study of almost 4000 renal transplant recipients, squamous-cell carcinomas were found in 11% at 5 years, 29% at 10 years, and 43% at 14 years post-transplant. Development of this tumor was calculated to occur in transplant patients at an average age that is 30 years younger than the age at which it occurs in the general population. In Spain, squamous-cell carcinomas developing in sun-exposed parts of the body tended to be multiple and more aggressive than those in the general population, even life threatening.[13] In the Australian study, although most lesions were found to be low grade, more than expected (7%) were aggressive, with lymph node metastases found at diagnosis. Overall, there was a tenfold increase in mortality from skin cancers over that seen in the general population.[28] Again, there have been noted to be differences among recipients of different organs. In a review of over 2000 liver transplant recipients, skin cancers comprised only 24% of de novo malignancies,[16] and skin cancers in heart recipients have been noted to be multiple and particularly aggressive in about half.

Melanoma

The most recent statistics from the American Cancer Society estimate the incidence of melanoma in the USA to be of the order of 4%.[34] The incidence of melanoma in transplant patients appears to be consistently higher than that seen in the general population, although one might intuitively expect a higher incidence of a disease so closely linked to the immune response. According to the CTTR, when the incidence nationwide was 2.7%, among transplant recipients it was 4.7%.[28] As the incidence of this disease in the general population continues to rise,[34,35] there will probably be at least a proportional increase among organ transplant recipients. Several retrospective reviews have suggested up to a fivefold increase in the incidence of malignant melanoma occurring among transplant recipients.[15,24,33,36] According to a report from the CTTR, of 8724 malignancies reported, 177 (or slightly over 2%) were malignant melanomas. At the time of analysis, 32% had died of this disease within an average follow-up of 42 months. It is interesting to note that, although the incidence of second malignancies among transplant recipients overall is about 6%, in those with melanoma, the figure for second malignancies was noted to be 35%. Not surprisingly, the majority of these second tumors were other non-melanoma skin cancers. As in the general population, transplant recipients with a history of non-melanoma skin lesions are also at risk for the development of melanoma.[24] In the same report it is also interesting to note that a relatively high proportion of melanomas occurred in pediatric-age recipients. In a study from Australia, with perhaps the highest overall incidence of skin cancer, only 8 out of 619 (1.3%) cardiothoracic transplant recipients developed melanoma within a 2-year minimum follow-up period.[37] Few comprehensive reports have noted the fate of transplant patients developing melanomas, although overall survival in the Australian group was quite poor.

Melanoma is especially intriguing to consider in the setting of immunosuppression, because of its long-appreciated interplay with the immune system. Unfortunately, to date, there have been few informative reports regarding the incidence and outcomes for patients with a history of melanoma who subsequently undergo organ transplantation. Penn reported 30 patients previously treated for melanoma who went on later to transplantation. In that series, 19% experienced recurrent disease after transplant; all died from the disease, on average 16 months after receiving their new organ.[24] Little information was available regarding the extent of these patient's primary tumors, but at least one was known to

have had a Clark's level IV lesion. Three had been treated less than 2 years before their transplant, but one had been clinically free of disease for 10 years. As the follow-up for the remaining patients was noted to be short, it seems likely that the true numerator is yet to be known.

Malignant melanoma has also been transmitted from the donor organ to the recipient.[38] This always inadvertent, and almost universally disastrous, circumstance has occurred on a number of occasions and has affected recipients of all types of organs. Although organ procurement professionals always obtain a meticulous and detailed medical history regarding any potential donor, errors can occur. Certainly, no individual with even a distant history of melanoma would ever be considered as a suitable candidate for organ or tissue donation. Therefore, in all cases, the donor's melanoma was previously unappreciated or misdiagnosed. Donor brain death has been attributed to either a primary brain tumor or a spontaneous cerebral hemorrhage, when the underlying pathology was actually a melanoma metastatic to the central nervous system (CNS).[24] Because this is a disease of neural crest origin, amelanotic melanomas have also been misinterpreted to be primary brain tumors. Penn reported the results of 20 organs transplanted from 11 different donors, all later appreciated to harbor occult malignant melanoma.[24] Errors were realized after donor autopsy, examination of organ explants, or when multiple recipients developed metastatic disease. Sixteen of the 20 recipients developed metastatic melanoma, on average 13 months after transplant. This indicates at least an 80% chance that an organ will contain occult malignant cells. As described above, the treatment alternatives for kidney and pancreas recipients include cessation of immunosuppression with donor organ explantation, an option that is essentially unavailable to heart, lung, or liver recipients. Indeed, in this series, 11 of the 16 died of the disease, including two liver and one heart recipient. Four renal allograft recipients had complete remissions after transplant nephrectomy and cessation of immunosuppression. Recently, an intriguing report described an advanced melanoma of donor origin in a renal transplant recipient. In this case, the disease was cured with cessation of immunosuppression, transplant nephrectomy, and immunotherapy. Surprisingly, the patient was subsequently retransplanted and has done well, with a 2-year disease-free follow-up.[39]

Merkel's cell carcinoma

It has recently been appreciated that the otherwise quite rare entity of Merkel's cell carcinoma (MCC) appears to be relatively more common among transplant recipients.[22,33] Penn and First found 41 cases of this type of tumor in the CTTR, with an additional 11 reported elsewhere in the literature. In this series, tumors were found at a mean of 91 months after transplant. The distribution was found to be the same as in the non-transplant setting, with the majority of lesions found in the head, neck, and upper extremities. However, significant differences do appear to exist. In the non-transplant setting, 95% of MCC occur in patients over the age of 50, whereas in this study almost 30% were found in younger patients. In addition, tumors were found to be more aggressive than in the general population. In this series, at the time of treatment, 68% of patients had lymph node metastasis and 56% had already died due to the tumor. With a short follow-up, another 33% still had active disease and therefore were seemingly at a very high risk of succumbing to the disease. Surprisingly, comparing these outcomes to the 29% mortality noted for transplant recipients developing malignant melanoma, it appears that patients with MCC fare even worse. The authors recommend a correspondingly aggressive approach to treatment, including wide local excision with a 2-cm margin when possible, radiation when feasible, and a strong consideration of systemic chemotherapy, especially in patients deemed to be at higher risk by virtue of location. A reduction of immunosuppression is almost always an additional consideration.

Kaposi's sarcoma

Although Kaposi's sarcoma was largely an obscure medical oddity prior to the onset of the AIDS epidemic, it was already appreciated to occur with increased frequency in transplant recipients.[40] An epidemiological study in 1979 found up to a 500-fold increase in Kaposi's sarcoma among renal transplant recipients.[41] The CTTR reported a 5.7% incidence of Kaposi's sarcoma in transplant recipients, which exceeded reports to that registry of tumors expected to be more common, such as colon and breast carcinomas.[9,42] Significant differences in genetic predisposition have also been suggested to play a part in the incidence of Kaposi's sarcoma after transplantation.[11] In Saudi Arabia, the Kaposi's sarcoma incidence is 5% rather than < 1%. In the USA, 6% of post-transplant malignancies are Kaposi's sarcoma, whereas in Saudi Arabia the figure is 76% of all *de novo* post-transplant malignancy.[43]

Sixty percent of Kaposi's sarcoma lesions have been found to involve only the skin, with rare conjunctival or mucosal involvement; visceral disease has been seen in the remaining 40%. In the latter group, two-thirds have also had skin involvement, but those without were found to be much more of a diagnostic challenge. The majority of cases of Kaposi's sarcoma reported in the literature appear to have occurred in renal allograft recipients, although this certainly may reflect the greater proportion of such transplants performed. The average age of afflicted patients has been reported to be 43 years, with tumors occurring on average 21 months after transplantation. As is true with the classic form of Kaposi's sarcoma, these lesions appear to be more common in patients with a Mediterranean or Middle Eastern background.[7,42] As a complication of immunosuppression, Kaposi's sarcoma has spared none of the widely used

agents, equally incriminating cyclosporin, tacrolimus, and mycophenolate mofetil.[42] The diagnosis of Kaposi's sarcoma in transplant recipients is usually based on the presence of characteristic reddish-blue lesions along with a high index of suspicion. Thorough imaging, including endoscopy, is required to pursue possible visceral involvement. The treatment of Kaposi's sarcoma in transplant recipients is tailored to the circumstances, but will almost always include a reduction of immunosuppression, and complete remissions have been reported in the absence of any other therapy.[9] In fact, nearly one-third of the complete remissions reported to the CTTR have occurred solely as the result of a reduction of immunosuppressive therapy.[9] This again suggests a central interaction between immunosurveillance and malignancy. As always, reduction or cessation of immunosuppression in transplant recipients is a double-edged sword. In the event of unsalvageable rejection, a renal or pancreas allograft can always be removed, with re-institution of dialysis or insulin therapy. However, the only option for heart, lung, and liver recipients is re-transplantation, with a very high risk of recurrence or death. Out of 11 liver transplant patients with Kaposi's sarcoma treated with a reduction of immunosuppression, only two displayed complete remission, while four were unchanged, five progressed, and two died as a result of chronic rejection.[44] Transplant patients with Kaposi's sarcoma tend to fare better than those with AIDS, probably due in part to the fact that modulation of immunosuppression is possible. Failure to make a timely diagnosis may lead to poor outcomes; in the CTTR records, nearly 60% of patients with visceral disease died.[42] Overall, complete remission has been reported to occur in about 40% of patients. Both local and systemic treatments, including immunotherapy, chemotherapy, and antiviral therapy, as well as surgery have all been utilized.[42] The etiology of Kaposi's sarcoma has long been suspected to be at least in part due to viral infection. Once linked by epidemiology to cytomegalovirus,[10] most recently the herpes virus HSV-8 has become strongly associated with Kaposi's sarcoma and has now been sequenced.[45] A better understanding of the pathogenesis of Kaposi's sarcoma and of its interactions with the immune system and improved strategies for treatment should follow soon.

Other sarcomas

There is some evidence to suggest an increased incidence of sarcomas other than Kaposi's sarcoma in transplant recipients.[46] Although some are probably related to a pre-transplant disease, exposure, or treatment, there still appears to be some increased association. Similar observations have been made in patients with AIDS. Among the most prevalent histologic types of sarcoma reported in transplant patients has been leiomyosarcoma.[46] A possible etiology may be emerging with findings of latent EBV infection in such tumors.[47,48]

Hepatobiliary/pancreatic malignancies

Malignancies of the hepatobiliary and pancreatico-duodenal (HBPD) tract have been noted with some increased frequency in transplant recipients. However, given what we know of immunosuppressed patients, the histologic types are not unexpected. In a review of the CTTR, Penn has described the overall incidence of lesions in this vicinity to be of the order of 7%.[49] Of that total, over half (63%) were PTLDs. Interestingly, the vast majority (82%) of such lesions were not actually confined to the HBPD tract, but also included other sites. In the preponderance of such instances, it was, not surprisingly, the allograft that was involved: 84% liver and 59% pancreas. The remaining 37% non-PTLD malignancies were comprised mostly of hepatocellular carcinoma (15%), pancreatic carcinoma (11%), Kaposi's sarcoma (3%), and cholangiocarcinoma (3%). In the cases of Kaposi's sarcoma, only one was confined to the HBPD tract. Interestingly, among the 25 total instances of cholangiocarcinoma, apparently only one occurred in a patient who underwent liver transplantation for primary sclerosing cholangitis and who was therefore at risk for developing this tumor. Perhaps the most striking finding in this study was the proportion of non-lymphomatous pancreaticoduodenal tumors identified. While lymphomas are now appreciated to be related to EBV, hepatocellular carcinomas to recurrent hepatitis, and Kaposi's sarcoma to immunosuppression, adenocarcinomas of the distal bile duct and pancreas have no such associations aside from primary sclerosing cholangitis and were apparently not associated with any such predisposing circumstance. Further observations will be required before ascribing a specific increased risk of such tumors in transplant recipients.

Post-transplant lymphoproliferative disorders

General

Both inherited and acquired forms of immunodeficiency are associated with an increased incidence of lymphoma. It is therefore not surprising that pharmacological immunosuppression has the same association, and a PTLD is well described in this setting.[4] PTLD is a non-Hodgkin's B-cell lymphoma which has an EBV association similar to that of Burkett's lymphoma and probably the same pathophysiology as AIDS-associated B-cell lymphoma.[50] However, PTLD differs from non-Hodgkin's lymphoma in the general population in several ways. PTLD has a higher incidence of extra-nodal distribution (nearly 70% versus 24+%) and CNS involvement (28% versus 1%), where it may be confined. Finally, the transplanted organ is involved in about 20% of cases.[4] PTLD strikes rather unpredictably, although it is generally associated with more potent immunosuppressive regimens and a higher cumulative dose.[51] It is therefore more likely to arise in patients who have undergone intensive therapy for episodes of rejection or who have received aggressive antibody induction therapy. The outcome of PTLD in transplant patients is frequently fatal, although it is certainly dependent upon specific circumstances, some of which determine therapeutic options. Increased sophistication in managing immunosuppressants, newer, more effective means of diagnosis, pre-emptive interventions, and better treatment strategies are evolving that may soon significantly alter the nature of this problem.

Incidence

PTLD is the second most common malignancy arising in transplant recipients as recorded in the CTTR.[7] An impression of an increasing incidence of this disease may be difficult to discern from improvements in recognition and diagnosis. In a recent study of *de novo* malignancy among more than 2000 liver transplant recipients, lymphomas accounted for 21% (0.82% incidence).[13] Overall, PTLD appears to develop in 2–5% of all organ transplant recipients.[52] Perhaps due to the different immunosuppressant strategies required for different organs, the reported incidences differ amongst organs. According to one report, renal transplant recipients had an estimated incidence of about 1%, liver recipients 2.7%, heart recipients 3.3%, and heart/lung recipients 3.8%.[53] Another report found the lowest incidence among patients with liver transplants, followed by heart, kidney/pancreas, and finally lung.[51] As noted above, regimens utilizing higher cumulative doses of immunosuppression are associated with a higher incidence, explaining the higher observed rates seen with lung and small-bowel transplantation.[54] This may be particularly devastating in pediatric programs, which have reported incidences in the 8%–10% range.[55,56]

Head and neck occurrences of PTLD have been described mostly in the pediatric population.[54] In one study, five of eight pediatric liver recipients with PTLD developed head and neck disease, primarily in Waldeyer's ring.[57,58]

As noted, CNS involvement is more common than with non-Hodgkin's lymphoma in the general population. In one large report, the CNS was involved in 22% of cases and PTLD was confined to the CNS in 12%.[54] Regardless of the location at diagnosis, PTLD is generally regarded to be a systemic disease.

Most PTLD manifests within the first year and is rare after 2 years from the time of transplant.[51] One review found 47% occurred within the first year, and in a separate report from a pediatric liver program, the mean time to occurrence was 1.2 years.[13,56]

Risks

As noted above, the risk of developing PTLD appears to be in part related to the cumulative dose and potency of the immunosuppression regimen administered.[51] The propensity of organs to undergo rejection differs and accounts for some variation in immunosuppressive regimens and, therefore, in the rates of occurrence of PTLD in different organs. Antibody therapy is generally considered more potent and has an increased association with PTLD. The exact immunosuppressive agent may also play a role, and drugs such as OKT3 and ATG may increase risk by up to sixfold.[51,54] Tacrolimus is a more potent calcineurin inhibitor than cyclosporin and has been noted to have a higher associated incidence of PTLD.[56,59,60] However, this may also be due to differences in the early dosing regimens utilized with this drug. Different age groups may also require more or less immunosuppression. Children usually receive higher doses of drugs because they metabolize and absorb differently from adults, and display more frequent and severe rejection episodes.

Age is perhaps even more important as it relates to prior exposure to EBV. Clearly, the individuals at highest risk for PTLD are those naïve to EBV receiving an organ from a seropositive donor.[54,57] A study from the Mayo Clinic found a very strong correlation between seronegativity and the incidence of PTLD, with an increasing significance in those with fatal PTLD and those in whom it occurred primarily in the CNS.[51] This study also noted that about 95% of the adult population should be expected to be EBV seropositive (this obviously includes donors). In one pediatric liver transplant program, 87% of PTLD occurred in those with primary EBV infection occurring after transplant, with a mortality rate in this study of 60%.[56] All PTLD, however, does not occur in those experiencing a primary infection, as reactivation of EBV clearly plays a major role.

Recent studies have also suggested a possible role for hepatitis C (HCV) infection in the development of PTLD.[61] This is made more significant by the fact that HCV is the most common indication for liver transplantation in the USA.

Pathophysiology

EBV infects only B lymphocytes in the peripheral blood.[62,63] It is specific to epithelial cells and B lymphocytes via the CD21 receptor. After initial infection, EBV becomes latent and can lead to B-cell transformation. In the immunocompetent individual, CTL effectively clear EBV-infected cells. In the immunosuppressed individual, clearance is ineffective and can favor EBV-infected B-cell transformation.[63] Of course, this process would be exacerbated if the initial infection occurred in the absence of a competent immune response.

Solid organs have the potential to carry lymphocytes from the organ donor.[64–66] Indeed, numerous studies have documented the presence of donor lymphocytes distant from the allograft. Donor-origin PTLD is rare, but has been described.[64–66]

Diagnosis

The diagnosis of PTLD requires an appreciation of the disease correlations and a high index of suspicion. PTLD can be quite protean in its presentation, ranging from that found in asymptomatic individuals discovered on routine imaging or biopsy to that of generalized symptoms of malaise, fever, diarrhea, lymphadenopathy, or rash. More specific localized findings such as pain, mass, or obstruction can also occur. Allograft dysfunction may also be the presenting finding.[54,59,63] Examples of more unusual presentations can include biliary obstruction in post-liver transplant patients,[67] or urinary obstruction in renal transplant recipients.[54]

Diagnosis is confirmed by biopsy. Most recently, peripheral blood EBV DNA has been correlated with PTLD. Kenagy et al. have shown a correlation between EBV DNA levels in peripheral blood leukocytes as determined by polymerase chain reaction (PCR). They found that patients with PTLD had very high levels of EBV, and that levels fell dramatically with response to therapy.[62] It is generally believed that rising EBV DNA levels precede the development of PTLD. Others have found a predictive correlation between the development of monoclonal proteins (M proteins: monoclonal antibodies) in the serum or urine and the subsequent development of PTLD.[63]

Treatment

The treatment options available for PTLD include:

1 reduction of immunosuppression,
2 antiviral therapy using ganciclovir,
3 local therapy, if feasible, utilizing either resection or radiation therapy,[68]
4 other systemic therapy, including anti-B-cell treatment, interferon, chemotherapy, e.g., cyclophosphamide, doxorubicin, vincristine, and prednisone (CHOP),[68]
5 organ removal and/or re-transplantation.

To date, in the CTTR, there have been 399 cases of complete remission in patients with PTLD.[9] In that group, 65% had a reduction of immunosuppression as a part of therapy, including 17% for whom reduced immunosuppression was the sole therapy.[9]

When PTLD is diagnosed, a number of options are usually exercised. The first step is a reduction of immunosuppression. If the transplanted organs can be removed (e.g., kidney and/or pancreas), then strong consideration is given to complete cessation of immunosuppression. Obviously, for life-saving organs (e.g., heart, lung, and liver), this is not an option. Although generally considered to be systemic, if the disease appears to be localized, it may be amenable to either resection or radiation therapy. If the disease is confined to the transplanted organ but resolution is incomplete and/or rejection follows reduction of immunosuppression, then re-transplantation may be a consideration. Antiviral therapy with ganciclovir is usually instituted empirically, although EBV testing is now generally available to guide this treatment. Davis et al. have proposed a stepwise approach including:

1 reduced immunosuppression and local therapy, if feasible,

2 interferon therapy, and finally,

3 systemic chemotherapy.[69]

However, treatment is most often tailored to the specific circumstances. Studies monitoring viral EBV load during therapy for PTLD have shown a correlation between clearance of EBV and regression of disease.[70]

In high-risk recipients (EBV-seronegative recipient receiving an EBV-seropositive donor organ), intravenous ganciclovir combined with serial monitoring of peripheral blood for EBV by PCR can be used. Pre-emptive therapy consisted of lowering immunosuppression in light of a rising EBV titer, and cessation of immunosuppression and re-administration of ganciclovir in the presence of PTLD.[55] Alternatives include administration of intravenous immunoglobulin and 'adoptive' immunotherapy using activated autologous EBV-specific cytotoxic T-cells (CTL).[71]

Some success with autologous lymphokine-activated killer (LAK) cell therapy in transplant recipients with both EBV-positive and EBV-negative LPD has been reported. Using leukapheresis, Nalesnik et al. treated autologous peripheral blood leukocytes with interleukin 2 (IL2), providing a single-dose treatment administered without systemic IL2 after about 10 days.[52]

Summary of treatments

In general, any malignancy arising in a transplant recipient can be responded to with a reduction in immunosuppression. Depending upon the nature of the neoplasm, such a manipulation can occasionally lead to remission. More often than not, additional therapy is required. In the circumstance of a life-threatening malignancy and a lifestyle-influencing transplant, i.e., kidney or pancreas, complete cessation of immunosuppressants can be considered. In the event of severe organ rejection, the organs can be removed. As pointed out above, such a 'luxury' is unavailable to the recipient of a life-saving transplant, i.e., lung, heart, or liver. Chemotherapy, radiation therapy, and local therapy including excision or resection should be contemplated as in any non-transplant patient.

Issues regarding patient selection and past malignancy

Because of the severe organ shortage, there is an additional burden for transplant centers to ensure that patients with a pre-existing malignancy who are listed for transplant are not at an inappropriately high risk for recurrence of their disease. Therefore, a past history of malignancy is always of great concern when assessing the candidacy of a potential transplant recipient. Even in the absence of detectable disease, there must be concern regarding the effects of immunosuppression on the growth of any persistent tumor cells.[72] Many tumors common in the general population, such as breast and colon cancer, may clearly recur years after definitive treatment, even in the absence of immunosuppression. The concept of tumor dormancy[73] and the complexity of the microenvironments that influence metastases[74] are both active areas of research, which may eventually provide a better understanding of these issues.

Generally, the two most significant factors considered in the selection process for transplant candidacy are tumor histology and the interval between treatment and transplantation. Unfortunately, very few data exist to help guide this process. Empirically, most centers attempt to avoid treating histologically more aggressive tumors in close temporal proximity to the time of transplant/immunosuppression. On the other hand, the waiting interval required of a patient with a history of a prior malignancy who is in need of a transplant must be balanced against the consequences of waiting. In one recent circumstance experienced by one of the authors, a young woman presented with fulminant liver failure and a recently treated stage II breast cancer. Under optimal circumstances, a waiting period of at least 2 years without recurrence would be expected before committing to a transplant. Unfortunately, in this circumstance, the patient's mortality risk without an immediate transplant was 100%. Clearly, each patient's circumstances need to be considered individually.

On occasion, there have been patients transplanted with unappreciated and therefore untreated malignancies. Penn has reported on 92 such individuals with pre-existing tumors, treated, on average, 3 months post-transplantation. Histologic types included skin cancers (non-melanoma), prostate cancer, renal-cell cancer, and other miscellaneous cell types.[72] Only about one-third of these patients developed recurrent disease within the average follow-up period of 43 months.[72]

According to one report from the CTTR data, there had been 855 individuals transplanted with a history of a previously treated malignancy, and overall 22% developed recurrent disease.[75] Of all recurrences, 53% were in patients treated less than 2 years prior to transplant. Another 34% of recurrences were in those treated for their malignancy from 2 to 5 years prior to transplant. Finally, 13% of those with recurrences were treated more than 5 years prior to transplant. The time interval from transplant to recurrence was less than 2 years in 60%, between 2 and 5 years in 26%, and more than 5 years in 14%. Various tumor cell types can be classified as low (0–10%), intermediate (11–22%), or high (≥23%), based on the propensity to recur after transplantation (Table 6.3).[75–77] Considering these data, decisions are made based on the stage and grade of a tumor. For example, with tumors such as malignant melanoma, colon and breast cancer, a 5-year waiting period would be ideal, but in most cases is unrealistic. In most circumstances encountered in the CTTR database, a 2-year wait would have eliminated 54% of recurrences. However, there are significant differences based on tumor histology.

Table 6.3 *Tumor recurrence following transplant*

Low (0–10%)	Intermediate (11–22%)	High (≥ 23%)
Incidental renal cell (1%)	Any lymphoma (11%)	Breast (23%)
Uterine (4%)	Wilm's tumor (13%)	Bladder (29%)
Testicular tumors (5%)	Prostate (18%)	Symptomatic renal cell (27%)
Uterine cervix (6%)	Colon (21%)	Sarcoma (29%)
Papillary thyroid (7%)	Melanoma (21%)	Non-melanoma skin cancer (53%)
		Myeloma (67%)

In summary, when accepting transplant candidacy for patients with a prior malignancy, one must consider:

1 the histology, stage, and natural history of the specific tumor,
2 other non-transplant-related comorbid conditions,
3 the indications and relative urgency for transplant.

Excluding the influence of an end-stage organ failure, if a patient has an excellent chance of a 5-year tumor-free survival, then transplant candidacy should be viewed favorably. On the other hand, if a patient has only a small chance of a 5-year tumor-free survival, then transplant candidacy should be reconsidered. Other practical issues, such as the average waiting time for the particular organ required, should also be considered; the average waiting time for a cadaveric renal allograft in some areas, for example, may be as long as 4 years.

Issues regarding transmission

Tumor transmission with donor organs has been mentioned as a part of earlier discussions in some detail. Most reports of tumor transmission are, by definition, small and anecdotal. An early tumor registry study of 240 donors with malignancies showed an overall 40% rate of tumor transmission to renal transplant recipients.[6] In 67% of cases, there was either local invasion or distant metastases, and in only 33% was the tumor confined to the allograft at diagnosis. Although some patients recovered after transplant nephrectomy and cessation of immunosuppression, the majority did not.[6] Extreme care must always be taken when assessing the suitability of a potential donor. All measures to avoid such a disastrous occurrence must be taken.

Summary

A high index of suspicion should be maintained for the development of malignancy in post-transplant recipients. Regular visits to a dermatologist, with a complete examination, are prudent. Any premalignant or questionable skin lesions must be removed. Specific groups should undergo more frequent and involved examinations. Renal transplant patients for analgesic nephropathy should have regular urinary tract imaging as well

as urine cytology.[29] Liver transplant recipients with a history of hepatocellular carcinoma should be imaged frequently as well. Similarly, those with primary sclerosing cholangitis and associated ulcerative cholitis should undergo regular colonoscopy with biopsies. The presentation of patients with PTLD can be protean. Given the proper time frame, a diagnosis of lymphoma should be entertained and sought for any patient presenting with unusual or persistent symptoms, including CNS complaints.

TRANSPLANTATION IN THE TREATMENT OF MALIGNANCY

Introduction

In general, the utilization of solid organ transplantation for the treatment of an existing malignancy is severely limited by the need for subsequent immunosuppressive therapy. As discussed in detail above, immunosuppression *per se* will favor the growth of any occult malignant cells and can often lead to an accelerated recurrence of disease.[25,78] In this setting, treatment must be based on the assumption that the patient will be rendered completely free of disease by the removal and replacement of an organ. In practice, the only area in which this applies is that of liver transplantation. With exceptions, the vast majority of such patients will have a diagnosis of hepatocellular carcinoma. Although liver transplantation has been performed for hepatocellular carcinoma from the earliest days of its use, it is still an area in evolution, and continues to be the focus of much interest and debate. For these reasons, this topic is addressed first and in the greatest detail. With the availability of dialysis, renal transplantation is essentially never performed in the direct treatment of malignancy. Although special circumstances may exist in both heart and lung transplantation, transplantation of these organs in the treatment of malignancy remains exceptionally rare. Small-bowel transplants have been utilized as a part of 'cluster' transplants in the treatment of foregut tumors, but only on a limited investigational basis, and with less than encouraging results.[79] To be complete in mentioning all organs, there are essentially no plausible circumstances in which a patient might receive a pancreas transplant in the treatment of malignancy.

Liver transplantation and the treatment of hepatic malignancy

Liver transplant indications and organ allocation

Outcomes in liver transplantation have continually improved over the last decade as a result of advances in organ preservation, surgical technique, perioperative management, control of infection, and immunosuppressive therapy. Orthotopic liver transplantation (OLT) is now a well-established standard of care for the treatment of end-stage liver disease and, when considering involvement with tumor, makes possible the most radical form of liver resection. Indeed, in the earliest days of liver transplantation, patients with advanced hepatic malignancy not amenable to conventional resection were considered ideal candidates for OLT due to their overall better health than those with end-stage cirrhosis and portal hypertension.[80] Currently, in a variety of circumstances, including the management of malignancy, the appropriate role for OLT is still in evolution. To understand fully the role of transplantation in the treatment of primary hepatic malignancy, it is appropriate to review the criteria utilized for determining liver transplant candidacy in general. Even when the presence of a tumor may be the primary indication for liver transplantation, there is usually also an underlying associated liver disease.[81]

Under the guidelines of the Organ Procurement and Transplantation Network (OPTN), UNOS is the government contracted agency that governs the procurement and distribution of all organs for transplantation in the USA. In the USA, literally no one can obtain a cadaveric organ for transplantation without notification of UNOS and, therefore, without adhering to the UNOS guidelines.

The accepted UNOS-sanctioned listing criteria and requirements are well documented.[1,82] The standard indications for determining 'end-stage' liver disease are also well described and time honored.[83] Progressive hyperbilirubinemia, hepatic encephalopathy, portal hypertension, and diminished synthetic function are the primary determinants. Portal hypertension is most often apparent as any combination of variceal bleeding, ascites, and hypersplenism, as evidenced by splenomegaly and thrombocytopenia. Because of the extreme shortage of organs, the high costs of transplantation, the magnitude of the liver transplant procedure, the need for vigilant, continued medical care and life-long immunosuppression, it is necessary for both medical and psychosocial contraindications to transplantation to be weighted equally. Additional well-recognized criteria include specific circumstances in which a malignancy is confined to the liver, even in the absence of end-stage parenchymal disease.

Although in place for many years, the guidelines outlined above unfortunately suffered from relative subjectivity. As liver transplantation grew, indications greatly expanded, while many contraindications, such as extremes of age or certain technical considerations, became irrelevant. Finally, the number of physicians trained in the 'era' of liver transplantation affected the acceptance of this alternative and greatly increased patient referrals to transplant centers. These factors all had the effect of dramatically increasing the number of patients qualifying for liver transplantation. As a result, waiting lists grew ever longer. As advocates for their individual patients, most transplant centers felt obliged to compensate for longer waiting times by placing patients on waiting lists earlier in the course of their disease. Those listed earlier would stand a better chance of receiving an organ before succumbing to their disease. The obvious effect of this practice was to increase the overall size of the waiting list, thus further increasing the average waiting time. This vicious circle largely ended in January of 1998, when UNOS instituted new, more objective, liver-allocation criteria.[82]

The current UNOS criteria are based on modifications of the original Child's classification. The Child–Turcotte–Pugh (CTP) scoring system includes five specific parameters: encephalopathy, ascites, albumin, International normalized ratio/prothrombin time (INR/PT), and bilirubin. UNOS requires that a potential recipient must have a score of at least seven points to be listed for a transplant. In general, these listing criteria are based on the assumption that, overall, the chance of 1-year survival after OLT is about 90%. If an individual's disease may lead to the chance of a survival of less than 90% at 1 year, then transplant becomes reasonable. As alluded to above, the purposes of instituting these new criteria were several:

1 to increase objectivity and therefore consistency to listing for OLT,
2 to stop the trend toward early listing which had the effect of further increasing overall list size and waiting times,
3 to avoid unnecessary transplants.

In the absence of seven CTP points, patients can still be listed, with certain well-defined exceptions, such as a prior variceal hemorrhage, the onset of hepatorenal dysfunction, or advanced hepatic encephalopathy. Specifically, patients with hepatocellular carcinoma can be listed for transplantation regardless of their CTP score. Whether due to the nature of referrals to transplant centers or to the nature of this disease, it is the minority of patients with hepatocellular carcinoma who do not otherwise meet minimal listing criteria based on their underlying liver disease.

In the USA, organs for transplantation are allocated to those who have waited the longest, but more importantly to those who are the 'sickest.' For the allocation of livers, patients are stratified according to their CTP score and clinical symptoms into one of four categories, from the most acute to those who are chronic and relatively well compensated.

Status 1 patients are those with acute liver failure, which, by definition, excludes any patient with chronic liver disease.

Status 2 was found to be too inclusive and was divided into 2A and 2B. Status 2A patients are those with chronic liver disease who are hospitalized in an intensive care unit and have a predicted survival of less than 7 days.

Status 2B patients are those with chronic liver disease who have at least ten CTP points or an acute medical problem relating to their liver disease.

Status 3 patients are those who simply meet minimal listing criteria and are generally the most well-compensated patients. Again due to the extreme shortage of organs, currently only those patients who are at a 'higher' status are likely to receive a new organ. As their liver disease advances, most patients tend to progress to a higher status before receiving an organ offer.

Despite the more objective listing criteria, currently in the USA the number of patients waiting for transplants is growing exponentially, while waiting times grow correspondingly ever longer. With some regional variation, the average waiting time for a liver transplant in the USA is now well over 1 year.[82] The implications for a patient with a tumor are obvious. Until relatively recently, patients who did not qualify for a higher waiting status based on their underlying liver disease were not allowed any special consideration or status elevation based on the presence of tumor. However, since November 1998, UNOS has allowed those individuals with stage I or II hepatocellular carcinoma an increase to status 2B, based solely on the presence of tumor. Despite the greater sense of urgency associated with more advanced disease, patients with stage III or IV tumor are not allowed this luxury. Although this may appear somewhat counterintuitive, as a group, those patients with more extensive disease are expected to have poorer outcomes. As the ultimate goal of UNOS and the transplant community is to optimize the utilization of a scarce resource, facilitating organ transplants in patients with advanced disease cannot be justified.[84] A visit to the UNOS web site can be used to update the latest statistics or answer other questions regarding organ allocation and transplantation.[1] As long as the shortage exists, the allocation of all organs, especially livers, will be an emotionally charged area, subject to public and government interpretation and change. From the earliest days, transplant physicians have recognized the ongoing moral and ethical issues related to this field and have facilitated open dialog for their resolution.

In the ensuing discussion regarding liver transplantation in the treatment of malignancy, it should be emphasized that the time spent waiting for a cadaveric organ may be the most important determinant of outcome. Outside the transplant field, the surgeon, the oncologist, and the patient are all compelled to act with haste when the diagnosis of a neoplasm has been made. Imagine the frustration when the evaluation is complete, the plan of action is set, and the reality of waiting for an unknown, often prolonged period of months is considered. The shortage of organs is the greatest limitation to the use of liver transplantation in the treatment of malignancy.

Liver transplants for the treatment of hepatocellular carcinoma

Perspective on hepatocellular carcinoma and liver disease

Hepatocellular carcinoma is by far the most common primary hepatic malignancy, accounting for approximately 90% of such tumors.[85,86] At the same time, it is also one of the most common malignancies worldwide, ranking eighth in incidence among all cancers.[87] In high-risk regions of the world, such as parts of Asia and the African continent, hepatocellular carcinoma has an incidence as great as 150 cases per 100 000.[85] The frequency in Western Europe and the USA is much lower; in the range of 1–5 cases per 100 000.[86] The annual occurrence in the USA is estimated to be in the order of about 7000 new cases per year,[87] but this too has been shown to be on the rise.[88]

A number of risk factors have been associated with the development of hepatocellular carcinoma. In some endemic regions, an environmental contribution is associated with exposure to the mycotoxin aflatoxin B. This agent can be present in poorly stored grains and is one of the most potent carcinogens known. Worldwide, however, the incidence of hepatocellular carcinoma is primarily related to the prevalence of cirrhosis due to chronic viral hepatitis, the highest incidence being found in those areas endemic for hepatitis B (HBV) and C (HCV). Although the mechanisms are incompletely understood, both HBV and HCV are associated with a relative risk several hundred-fold greater than the risk for those unaffected.[85] The common contributing feature appears to be the presence of chronic inflammation and actively dividing hepatocytes. In addition, HBV can lead directly to the development of hepatocellular carcinoma, even in the absence of cirrhosis. In this case, hepatocarcinogenesis is thought to be due to DNA intermediates in the replicative cycle of the hepatitis B virus. These intermediates can integrate into the host genome and cause mutations that lead to the development of tumor.[85,89] This mechanism may alter the relationship between suppressor genes and oncogenes. Roles for both the suppressor gene $p53$ and host proto-oncogenes such as C-fos and C-jun have been suggested.[90]

In the USA, HCV is unequivocally the most common indication for orthotopic liver transplantation, accounting for about 40% of transplants at most centers[1] and up to half of all cases of hepatocellular carcinoma.[87] It has also now been appreciated that HCV appears to have the highest associated incidence of hepatocellular carcinoma.[91] HCV may be primarily responsible for the increasing incidence of hepatocellular carcinoma in the USA and other Western countries.[88] Although viral hepatitis heads the list, essentially any cause of chronic inflammation and cirrhosis can also lead to the development of hepatocellular carcinoma.[87] An obvious and prevalent association is chronic alcohol consumption, accounting for an estimated 15% of hepatocellular carcinoma in the USA. Interestingly, alcohol and HCV appear to act synergistically in the development of both cirrhosis and tumor.[87] In one Japanese study, over 80% of patients with a history of both alcoholism and HCV exposure developed hepatocellular carcinoma within a 10-year period.[92] Other less common conditions are also associated with hepatocellular carcinoma. Patients with genetic hemochromatosis and hereditary tyrosinemia can be particularly prone to the development of hepatocellular carcinoma, with an incidence as high as 40% or more.[85,87] Entities such as cryptogenic cirrhosis, autoimmune hepatitis, alpha-1-antitrypsin deficiency, and even primary biliary cirrhosis can also be associated with tumor development.[85,87] Cirrhosis in general is associated with a 1–4% per year incidence in the development of hepatocellular carcinoma and clearly should be considered a premalignant state.[87]

Although there are rare exceptions, such as tumors associated with oral contraceptive use,[87,93] the overwhelming majority (80–90%) of hepatocellular carcinoma in developed parts of the world arises in the context of chronic liver disease and cirrhosis.[81,85,87] It is this point that presents the greatest dilemma in the treatment of hepatocellular carcinoma: with underlying disease and impaired hepatic reserve, those who present with hepatocellular carcinoma are often the least well suited for definitive treatment with partial resection. Even in the presence of small lesions, bilobar or critically located disease will preclude even partial wedge resection. Indeed, when considering all patients, it has been estimated that only 5–15% of those presenting with hepatocellular carcinoma are candidates for definitive resection.[94]

Yet another problem is that partial hepatic resection for hepatocellular carcinoma is predicated on the assumed focality of this disease, when clearly it is a multifocal process. Studies of hepatectomy specimens from patients undergoing OLT for presumed solitary lesions frequently show the presence of multifocal, often bilobar, disease.[95–97] Indeed, many studies assessing the role of OLT for hepatocellular carcinoma describe 'incidental' tumors found in the hepatectomy specimen that escaped vigorous preoperative assessments.[95,97,98] In the context of cirrhosis, gross clearance of tumor still permits the possibility of small, yet unidentified lesions to remain, and allows the persistence of 'fertile soil' for the development of future lesions.[89,99] In fact, the nature of recurrent hepatocellular carcinoma after partial resection is poorly understood, as it could represent previously undetected disease, intrahepatic metastases, or new tumor development.[100,101] Even in the absence of cirrhosis, one major study found no difference in the recurrence rates from those of patients who were cirrhotic, implying either tumor dissemination during resection or inadequate clearance of unappreciated multifocal disease.[102] Indeed, recurrences after resections for hepatocellular carcinoma have been found to be as high as 20–25% per year,[103] with an additional long-term mortality associated with the underlying cirrhosis. The 5-year disease-free survival for those few patients successfully resected is quite low, at about 27%.[104] Depending on patient selection, those undergoing a definitive resection could conceivably fare worse as a group than their untreated cohort.[105,106] With these considerations, liver transplantation for the treatment of hepatocellular carcinoma has great intuitive appeal: it simultaneously addresses both the tumor and the underlying associated liver disease.

The final, and perhaps the most confounding, issue regarding the treatment of hepatocellular carcinoma is the biologic inhomogeneity of the disease. With a spectrum of presentations, the variability in size, number, and location of tumors can be remarkable. Tumor doubling times can vary tremendously, with more than one study documenting extremes in the range of 30 to over 600 days.[106–108] An overall average of 3–6 months now seems well accepted.[87,106,107] Not surprisingly, tumor doubling time has also been found to correlate with both disease-free interval and survival, regardless of treatment modality.[78,106,108] Histologic subtypes are also well described and clearly influence treatment options and the potential for cure.[85] Therefore, the presentation of any one patient with hepatocellular carcinoma can fall anywhere on a rather large continuum, such that no one therapy is always correct. In this regard, orthotopic liver transplantation is only one of several options available in the armamentarium against a disease for which treatment must always be individualized.

Fortunately, with improvements in screening and diagnosis, a greater number of patients with hepatocellular carcinoma are presenting with treatable and, therefore, potentially curable disease.[105,109]

Overview of treatment options

The optimal treatment for hepatocellular carcinoma clearly entails the complete removal of all tumor; with either partial hepatic resection or total hepatic resection and subsequent transplantation. In addition, there are a number of alternative therapeutic options available for the treatment of hepatocellular carcinoma, including percutaneous alcohol injection, chemoembolization, cryoablation, and radiofrequency ablation. Notwithstanding the ever-present promise of new experimental drugs, systemic chemotherapy is also available, but notoriously ineffective. In certain settings, the outcomes utilizing alternative treatments may be comparable to those for surgery.[110] However, regardless of how encouraging, any treatment short of complete resection cannot offer cure. Nevertheless, several of these therapies may serve as adjuncts to resection in the treatment of this disease.

As is true for other malignancies, such as breast cancer, one must be aware of the potential influence of early diagnosis on outcome interpretation. Screening of at-risk populations and the availability of improved, high-resolution imaging modalities may allow tumors to be diagnosed at an earlier stage and may manifest as lead-time bias suggesting improved survival due to treatment interventions.

Screening, diagnosis, and staging in transplant candidates

As noted earlier, hepatocellular carcinoma represents over 80% of primary hepatic malignancies. In the patient with known cirrhosis and no prior history of other malignancy, an hepatic mass is overwhelmingly likely to be hepatocellular carcinoma. Hepatocellular carcinoma often shows a characteristic hypervascularity, which may be correlated with more aggressive growth.[111] In the proper clinical setting, CT, MRI and, on occasion, Doppler ultrasound may all strongly suggest the diagnosis of hepatocellular carcinoma based on this vascularity. With properly timed dye administration during CT, early-phase images will distinguish an hepatocellular carcinoma lesion. On the other hand, poorly timed dye administration may miss a large lesion entirely. CT portography or spiral CT scanning usually provides superior images compared to conventional modalities. Although the mechanism is not well understood, Lipiodol and related agents concentrate and persist in tumors. The role of 'lipiodol CT' in the diagnosis of hepatocellular carcinoma is not well defined. MRI is also very sensitive and is often used to confirm the diagnosis, especially in the absence of normal renal function, which may preclude nephrotoxic dye administration. With the quality and accuracy of modern imaging techniques, biopsies are avoided in patients under consideration for OLT. Again, depending upon the clinical setting, imaging almost invariably furnishes adequate information without the need for histologic confirmation. In addition, most transplant centers have anecdotal experience with needle-track seeding and local recurrence seen after transplantation and the administration of immunosuppression.[112] A recent study has validated the diagnosis of hepatocellular carcinoma without biopsy, showing an accuracy of 99.6%, a sensitivity of 100%, and a specificity of 98.9%.[113] Although it is usually too late for intervention when a patient presents with clinical signs and symptoms, classically, hepatocellular carcinoma presents in one of two ways:

1 right upper quadrant pain and mass,
2 deterioration in a known cirrhotic.

Given that hepatocellular carcinoma occurs in cirrhotic patients at a rate of about 3% per year,[87] it would seem reasonable to regularly screen those at risk. Clearly, there is little to offer patients presenting with symptoms and advanced disease; therefore, the only real hope is in finding disease at an earlier stage. However, given the large numbers of patients with cirrhosis, the cost effectiveness of screening programs is a matter of some debate. Defining not only which populations are at risk but also those in whom definitive intervention will be feasible are both persistent issues. Candidates for regular screening include patients with HBV and HCV and those with hemochromatosis. The exact modality or combination of tests that are most reasonable has yet to be precisely defined. For example, the addition of color Doppler to the ultrasound assessment of liver lesions can certainly increase sensitivity, but also adds complexity and cost. Alfa-fetoprotein (AFP) determinations clearly have a role, but only about 70% of hepatocellular carcinoma are associated with this marker, while a flare of hepatitis without tumor can also be associated with a markedly increased AFP.[90] Furthermore, the fibrolamellar variant is never associated with AFP, whereas hepatoblastomas have a correlation of virtually 100%. Finally, it has been appreciated that screening itself may carry some social stigma and long-term negative psychosocial impact for those requiring such testing.

The historical role of transplantation for hepatocellular carcinoma

One of the first liver transplants ever performed was for the treatment of a primary hepatocellular carcinoma. The tumor recurred after 3 months and the patient died of disseminated metastatic disease.[114] In 1983, the National Institutes of Health Consensus Conference on Liver Transplantation took place, which essentially authorized this new therapeutic modality. With the exception of Starzl's pioneering program, all other liver transplant programs in the USA were initiated subsequent to this meeting. During that conference, based on the results to date, the official stance regarding primary hepatic malignancy as an indication for transplantation was already equivocal.[115] As liver transplantation has evolved, the indications and contraindications have continued to be refined; some have broadened, while others have narrowed. The latter is true for transplantation in patients with malignancies. Indeed, the initial enthusiasm for such indications waned rather quickly as up to

80% of patients had early recurrences,[116] with 5-year survivals not better than 20%.[87]

The immunosuppressant drug cyclosporin was in large part responsible for the improved results that led to the broader application of liver transplantation in general. The 'early days' of liver transplantation may be defined to include the first decade after the availability of this drug (*circa* 1980). In the earliest part of that period, the procedure itself often proved still to be a major obstacle. The technical aspects of the procedure were gradually refined and the collective learning curve reached a plateau. Patient selection practices changed as it was increasingly appreciated that patients with hepatocellular carcinoma and other hepatic malignancy fared much worse than others. The European Liver Transplant Registry (ELTR) showed a dramatic decrease in transplants for tumor: from 46% before 1982 down to only 15% between 1988 and 1992,[117] with similar trends noted elsewhere.[87] In 1990, about 10 years into the 'modern' or 'cyclosporin era' of liver transplantation, a study by Olthoff *et al.* documented the results and attitudes from that period.[118] In this early experience, the primary indication for transplantation in patients with hepatocellular carcinoma was extensive 'otherwise unresectable' (stage III or IV) disease. In that report, the longest survivor died at 31 months and the 2-year actuarial survival was 22.5%. At that time, although essentially anecdotal, the common finding in a review of the world's literature was long-term survival not greater than about 20% for patients with hepatocellular carcinoma. However, the far superior outcomes among patients with very small or 'incidental' tumors discovered only after the hepatectomy were becoming appreciated.[118,119] It was further recognized that the occasional patient fared extremely well, with survivals measured in decades.[120] In a 1994 review from the ELTR, the 10-year period from 1972 to 1982 was compared to the later period from 1982 to 1992. There was a noticeable shift toward treating patients with lower stage tumors as the disappointing results with those at higher stages were realized.[117] A careful look at subsequent reports reveals a progressive shift from treating patients with larger tumors toward treating those with smaller tumors, with an increasing appreciation for optimal patient selection resulting in steadily improving results.[121] Further refinements gradually began to define the parameters in which patients fared best, e.g., tumor size less than 3 or 4 cm, with greater appreciation of the effects of tumor multiplicity, histology, and vascular invasion.[112,122] Small studies using strict selection criteria suggested more acceptable results could be achieved, with survivals near 70% at 3 years.[123]

Despite the overall initial poor results with liver transplantation for hepatocellular carcinoma, interest in this area has persisted due to the lack of alternatives. Although the use of scarce cadaveric donor organs in patients with tumors may appear without justification, like all other aspects of medicine and surgery, the essence of good results is in the proper selection of patients. Indeed, defining optimal parameters for the treatment of hepatocellular carcinoma with OLT remains the central question.

Current role: resection versus transplantation

The debate over partial resection versus total resection and subsequent transplantation in the treatment of hepatocellular carcinoma is ongoing, but mostly of little merit. There have been no prospective randomized trials to compare the two approaches, nor will there probably ever be such a trial. It is clearly the minority of patients in whom a partial resection is possible. In most circumstances, partial resection is precluded by underlying liver disease, bilobar extension, critically placed lesions, extrahepatic spread, or other comorbid conditions. On the other hand, transplantation may also be contraindicated based on the size and location of the tumor, the possibility of micrometastases, comorbid conditions that might limit the extent of the procedure, or psychosocial considerations that are an integral part of the transplant evaluation for the proper utilization of this limited resource. Transplantation also has an even larger disadvantage in that the wait for a cadaver organ may be considerably longer than a particular patient can afford. With the popularization of living-donor adult-to-adult liver transplants, this latter issue may be of less consequence. Obviously, all of these factors need consideration in each patient's individual circumstance. However, with all other factors equal, in that small minority of patients for whom either approach seems possible, which form of therapy is superior?

Patients with hepatocellular carcinoma can present with disease and circumstances that may fall anywhere on a rather broad spectrum. The size, number, and location of tumors can certainly vary considerably. In addition, the doubling times of hepatocellular carcinomas can also be quite inconsistent, from those that grow quite slowly to those clearly expanding rapidly. The degree of underlying liver disease can vary from none to that of severe cirrhosis. Age, gender, and comorbid conditions can also weigh heavily in the process of choosing the best therapy for a given individual. The mainstay of surgical intervention for hepatocellular carcinoma remains resection when feasible. Unfortunately, in developed countries, hepatocellular carcinoma arises almost exclusively in the setting of chronic liver disease, often with significant cirrhosis, which may preclude a major hepatic resection. These issues all contribute to the notoriously low rates of resectability in hepatocellular carcinoma.

In the treatment of hepatocellular carcinoma, liver transplantation holds great intuitive appeal. Total hepatectomy with OLT not only allows for the complete removal of malignant disease, but also avoids the limitations posed by major resections in the presence of underlying liver disease and the attendant potential for postoperative dysfunction or failure. As noted above, it is the clear minority of patients who present with resectable disease by virtue of either limited tumor or minimal parenchymal disease. At the same time, those with more extensive tumor and/or parenchymal disease may not be candidates for resection short of total hepatectomy with transplantation. This reality frequently makes it exceedingly difficult to directly compare outcomes between those patients undergoing resection and those who are transplanted.

There are decidedly few reports in the literature that appropriately compare the relative merits of resection versus transplantation in patients with hepatocellular carcinoma; however, at least one reasonable comparison of these two groups has been made.

In summary:

1 OLT has evolved considerably and many of the general impressions regarding this as a therapy for hepatocellular carcinoma may be outdated; overall results in OLT are excellent, the procedure itself, the postoperative care, and the prophylactic and immunosuppressive regimens have been greatly refined and continue to be refined.

2 In the past, 'otherwise unresectable' hepatocellular carcinomas have usually been considered appropriate for OLT; outcomes have been suboptimal.

3 It now seems appropriate that OLT may be the superior treatment for smaller hepatocellular carcinomas which otherwise recur with a remarkably high incidence.

4 The cadaver organ shortage and the long waiting times – especially for candidates with tumor – may largely be relieved by the perfection of living-donor liver transplantation, which provides for scheduled elective OLT and superior outcomes.

5 The role of adjuvant therapies in the treatment of hepatocellular carcinoma has yet to be defined; only multicenter studies will provide volumes large enough and only prospective randomized trials will be able truly to provide answers.

The role of adjuvant therapies with transplantation

As stated above, the nationwide average waiting time for suitable cadaveric allografts is now well over 1 year.[1] In patients with hepatocellular carcinoma, strategies for utilizing 'marginal' allografts to shorten this period have been adopted, but only after appropriate informed consent. Surgeons can afford to be selective in accepting a donor organ for many potential recipients, whereas they may accept higher risk donors for those with tumor. Such donors include those who are older, are at higher risk for non-function, those with hepatitis, which the recipient may or may not already have, or those at risk for transmitting hepatitis. Aside from these tactics, some other temporizing adjuvant therapy must be invoked. Depending upon

circumstances, a number of different adjuvant therapies have been employed in this manner, including chemoembolization, cryoablative therapy, ethanol injection, radiofrequency ablation, and systemic chemotherapy.

Chemoembolization with orthotopic liver transplantation

In general, hepatocellular carcinoma is a hypervascular tumor primarily fed by branches of the hepatic artery.[86] During angiography, selective access to the feeding vessels of a tumor can be utilized to administer chemotherapeutic agents in high concentration. Thrombotic agents delivered in the same way can be used to induce ischemic necrosis. The combination is often performed for hepatocellular carcinoma and is termed 'chemoembolization.' Usually, an emulsion of iodized oil is also administered, which, for reasons unknown, persists in hepatocellular carcinoma lesions and aids in diagnosis and may add a therapeutic advantage. A variety of single and combination chemotherapeutic regimens have been utilized, with none showing a clear advantage. Not without risk, a number of complications may result from this procedure. Abscess formation, jaundice, increased encephalopathy, fever, and pain have all been reported.[87] In one study of transplant candidates,[124] 15% of patients suffered major complications related to chemoembolization, including gastric perforation and gangrenous cholecystitis; the latter has also been reported by others.[125] Finally, most series have reported deaths due to hepatic failure precipitated by chemoembolization. Indeed, due to the risk of hepatic failure, Child's C cirrhosis and portal vein thrombosis are two commonly accepted contraindications to this procedure. Despite literally hundreds of articles in the literature, the true role of chemoembolization in the treatment of hepatocellular carcinoma remains to be defined. Indeed, some have suggested an overall negative impact on survival.

In the non-transplant setting, a prospective, randomized, multicenter European trial with strict entry criteria was terminated early due to a lack of benefit, increased liver failure, and longer hospitalizations with higher resource utilization in chemoembolization-treated patients compared to those receiving supportive therapy alone.[126] Other randomized trials have had similar discouraging results.[87] In partial resection candidates, at least one study has failed to discern any survival advantage to preoperative chemoembolization while showing a significantly shorter time to recurrence.[127]

Despite the results of chemoembolization in the non-transplant setting, many believe this procedure may have an appropriate neoadjuvant role in candidates for either partial or total resection. This attitude is based on the obviously different end-point with eventual tumor removal. Indeed, chemoembolization is commonly utilized in the transplant setting due to the compelling need to temporize patients while on long cadaveric organ waiting lists, which now average well over 1 year.[1,82] Depending upon the circumstances, chemoembolization may be performed on multiple occasions in the same patient.[128] In addition, it has been speculated that manipulation during transplant hepatectomy may disseminate tumor cells,[129] suggesting that preoperative chemoembolization may help to alleviate this potential problem.[125,128] Unfortunately, some studies have conversely suggested that chemoembolization itself may serve to facilitate tumor metastases. Nevertheless, dramatic results can be achieved with chemoembolization in the transplant setting, with many reports indicating extensive or total tumor necrosis at the time of subsequent hepatectomy. A study from Milan found that 36% of lesions treated with chemoembolization responded, with more than 90% necrosis found at the time of hepatectomy.[128] Another more recent series found no viable tumor in the majority of resection specimens, with up to 93% of tumors showing extensive or total necrosis.[130] Another small, prospective study in the transplant setting has suggested a survival advantage may be attributable to chemoembolization.[125] Chemoembolization has also been utilized in an effort to 'downstage' larger tumors, facilitating transplant candidacy patients who might otherwise not qualify. Thus far, this practice remains unproven.[87] Many variables will continue to add confusion to the potential role of chemoembolization in the transplant setting, e.g., the nature and extent of underlying liver disease and the size, number, and location of tumors. In addition, the biology of lesions, including the doubling time, vascular invasion, and degree of differentiation, is obviously relevant to outcome. Finally, perhaps the most significant variable and the most difficult to control is the interval between listing for transplant and receiving an organ. Until these problems are solved, the appropriateness of chemoembolization in the transplant setting will remain speculative. However, at least one prospective, randomized trial is underway. It will be only through such coordinated studies that there will be any hope of defining the role for this (or other) adjuvant therapy.

Ethanol injection (with OLT)

Ethanol injection has most often been described as a primary therapy for hepatocellular carcinoma and less often as an adjuvant to OLT. This technique is best suited to lesions of less than 4.5 cm.[131]

Cryosurgical ablation (with OLT)

This standard surgical technique has often been utilized for patients with hepatocellular carcinoma on transplant waiting lists. It is most successful when tumors are less than 5 cm, which corresponds to that group of patients who are best suited for transplantation.[131]

Systemic therapy (with OLT)

Systemic chemotherapy is notoriously ineffective in the treatment of hepatocellular carcinoma. A variety of single and combination regimens have been attempted, but with an almost universal lack of success. The presence of hormone receptors in hepatocytes has inspired some efforts to influence tumor growth by utilizing hormonal therapy.[87] Tamoxifen has been found to be ineffective, whereas results with octreotide and agents such as thalidomide may be more promising. The most recent efforts center on the mechanisms of hepatocarcinogenesis and the possibility of intervention utilizing approaches involving gene therapy.[87]

Variants of hepatocellular carcinoma

Hepatoblastoma

Hepatoblastoma is the third most common intra-abdominal malignant tumor of childhood, typically occurring in children under 3 years of age, with an early peak incidence and 50% of diagnoses made by the age of 1 year.[132] Achilleos et al. reported two cases of hepatoblastoma. One patient had multifocal, bilobar disease while the other had unifocal disease. Both were well at the time of their report at 37 and 25 months post OLT, respectively.[132] A report of CTTR data included a total of 18 patients.[133] Patients ranged in age from 1.5 to 24 years, with an average of 7 years. At the time of the report, there was a recurrence rate of 33%, all within 18 months of transplant. The actuarial survival at 2 years was only 50%.[133] Much more data will be required to determine the true role of OLT in the treatment of this disease.

Fibrolamellar

The fibrolamellar subtype (FLC) of hepatocellular carcinoma has been recognized as a distinct clinical and pathologic variant of this disease. FLC is thought to account for between 5% and 24% of the total incidence of hepatocellular carcinoma.[134] As noted earlier, the more common form of hepatocellular carcinoma occurs in older patients and almost exclusively in the setting of underlying cirrhosis or other chronic liver disease. In rather striking contrast, however, FLC occurs in younger patients and in the absence of underlying liver disease. It follows that, compared to resection rates well below 20% for common hepatocellular carcinoma, the resectability of FLC is as high as 75%. Although close to 80% of the common forms of hepatocellular carcinoma are associated with an elevation of the AFP tumor marker, there is no such associated elevation in FLC. Characteristic findings on imaging can also help distinguish this tumor. Due both to the lack of underlying parenchymal disease and to the younger age group of those involved, a greater proportion of patients with FLC are candidates for resection, which remains the mainstay of therapy. However, as one might expect in a disease presenting in young, otherwise healthy individuals, patients with FLC tend initially to present with rather large, higher stage tumors, and local recurrences are common. In this setting, total hepatectomy with OLT has great appeal in the sense that patients are definitively rendered free of the primary tumor. Unfortunately, due to the relative rarity of this variant, no single center has extensive experience with resection versus transplant, and for the same reasons no prospective randomized trials are likely to emerge.

The early experience with resection versus transplantation for fibrolamellar hepatocellular carcinoma was reported from Pittsburgh.[135] A more recent single-center review has also looked at resection versus transplantation as part of a retrospective analysis of FLC in general.[134] In this study of 20 patients with FLC, tumors ranged in size from 4 cm to 20 cm, with an average size of nearly 8 cm. Ages ranged from 13 to 38 years, with a mean of about 22 years. Neither the transplant group nor those undergoing resection were found to have a clear survival advantage. As is often true with such studies, the two groups were not truly comparable and the earliest patients were treated in the pretransplant era, strongly suggesting that treatment options were not equally available. Not surprisingly, the transplant group had higher stage disease and were considered for transplantation only because they were otherwise unresectable. This study went on to compare the survivals seen in FLC versus those seen in the more common form of hepatocellular carcinoma. Given that the majority of FLCs are resectable, as opposed to the extreme minority of other hepatocellular carcinoma, one might intuitively expect a better long-term survival. In this study, the overall long-term survivals for patients undergoing resection for FLC or for common hepatocellular carcinoma appeared to be surprisingly similar. This is probably true, despite the generally regarded 'favorable' status of FLC, and can be attributed to the fact that FLC often presents as higher stage disease.[134] Indeed, it appears that the overall prognosis for patients with either form of hepatocellular carcinoma is related to stage at presentation rather than to the particular cell type. What is not known with any certainty is the stage-for-stage survival in patients with FLC versus common hepatocellular carcinoma. Due to the higher rate of 'resectability,' many patients with this disease who have come to OLT have done so only after a local recurrence. It is conceivable that early consideration of total hepatectomy with OLT may influence long-term outcome in FLC. Currently, FLC remains an indication for OLT in selected circumstances. Due to the rarity of this disease, it seems unlikely that a definitive algorithm for its treatment and the role of OLT will surface in the near future.

A report from the CTTR showed the results of 33 patients.[133] Overall, 39% developed recurrent disease but 10 survived disease free for more than 2 years. Life-table analysis indicated a 2-year survival of 60%, with a survival at 5 years of 55%.[133]

Summary: treatment of hepatocellular carcinoma with liver transplantation

In summary, then, one might consider that the treatment of hepatocellular carcinoma is a study of contradictions. Almost by definition, those who acquire the disease are the least amenable to definitive treatment. Among surgical candidates, it appears that those who may appear best suited for resection are the same group as those who might benefit most from transplantation in the long term. In the current era, it seems that transplant centers are best equipped to treat patients with hepatocellular carcinoma, offering a full spectrum of treatments available in the setting of a multidisciplinary team consisting of hepatobiliary/transplant surgeons, hepatologists, medical oncologists, and interventional radiologists. Specifically regarding the indications for and utilization of OLT, no individual or group of physicians outside of a transplant center is qualified to determine the appropriateness and candidacy for OLT in a particular setting, exposing a significant medical–legal risk when patients are not referred.

Liver transplantation for the treatment of other tumors

Cholangiocarcinoma

In general, cholangiocarcinoma is considered to be an absolute contraindication to liver transplantation. The early results utilizing OLT for the treatment of this disease were almost universally dismal.[78]

All forms of cholangiocarcinoma have been treated with total hepatectomy and transplantation, with some differences in the apparent biology of the disease in different locations favoring survival in those with extrahepatic disease.[131,136] One report noted a 25% 5-year survival in the absence of both vascular invasion and nodal metastases.[137] However, in the presence of either factor, there were no survivors beyond 2 years after transplantation. Despite very careful selection, aggressive surgery with transplantation and both chemotherapy and radiotherapy postoperatively, the Dallas group achieved only 33% disease-free survival at 2 years.[131,138]

Special consideration must be given to cholangiocarcinoma arising in the presence of primary sclerosing cholangitis. Although an association had been recognized some years earlier, a 10% incidence of cholangiocarcinoma among patients with primary sclerosing cholangitis was noted in the context of the early transplant experience at Pittsburgh.[136] In that report, ten patients were transplanted with cholangiocarcinoma, three with known disease, and the remainder were incidental. Presumably due to the effects of immunosuppression, several patients transplanted with cholangiocarcinoma succumbed to 'florid carcinomatosis' rather than the slowly progressive process typically associated with this tumor. As a group, even those with incidental disease did not fare well. Unfortunately, cholangiocarcinoma complicating primary sclerosing cholangitis can be exceedingly difficult to diagnose pre-transplant.[139,140] In fact, cholangiocarcinomas arising in patients with primary sclerosing cholangitis are often small and multifocal, although the signs and symptoms of the two conditions mimic one another. The incidence of occult cholangiocarcinoma in patients undergoing OLT for primary sclerosing cholangitis has been found to be as high as 40%.[141,142] Various prognostic indices have been developed to predict survival in patients with primary sclerosing cholangitis, but none accounts for, or predicts, the development of cholangiocarcinoma.[143] The tumor marker CA19-9 has been associated with the development of cholangiocarcinoma, but is also elevated in primary sclerosing cholangitis, and this has been shown to have a poor predictive value.[144] Brush cytology at ERCP has been shown to have yields as low as 30%.[142] Because of frequent perineural and submucosal tumor spread, those transplanted with cholangiocarcinoma have a high incidence of recurrence. Long-term survival, even among patients transplanted with incidental disease, is not good: 28% 2-year survival,[136] 30% 1-year survival, and 0% 6-year survival.[142] One more recent single-center retrospective study included ten patients with incidental (<1 cm) tumors found only at the time of pathologic sectioning. This group appeared to fare as well as those without tumor, with survivals of 100%, 83%, and 83% at 1, 2, and 5 years.[145] Some long-term survivors have been reported.[146] A recent update of the Pittsburgh experience notes a 50% 5-year survival when margins and lymph nodes are negative and tumor depth is ≤ T2, conditions that, unfortunately, are largely determined postoperatively.[147] A prospective multicenter trial could help to determine if there is any role for OLT in the treatment of cholangiocarcinoma. However, considering the increasingly severe shortage of cadaveric donors, the justification of such a study seems difficult.

Even when an experienced group instituted an aggressive stance using multimodality postoperative therapy, 1-year and 2-year disease-free survivals after OLT were only 40% and 33%, respectively.[138]

The biology of tumors arising in peripheral versus hilar locations have been suggested.[131] In the absence of nodal disease and vascular invasion, one group showed a 25% 5-year survival after transplantation, as compared to 0% 2-year survival when these factors were present.[137]

Upper-abdominal exenteration procedures have been performed with liver transplantation for the treatment of cholangiocarcinomas.[79] Unfortunately, even with such a radical procedure, 3-year survivals are not better than 20%. The CTTR data showed 109 patients undergoing OLT for this tumor.[133] Patients ranged in age from 21 to 72 years. Seven patients survived disease free for more than 2 years, while three survived longer than 5 years.[133] Life-table analysis showed a 2-year survival of 30%,

with a 17% survival at 5 years. Considering both the overall discouraging results and the extreme shortage of cadaveric organs, cholangiocarcinoma is now generally accepted to be an absolute contraindication to liver transplantation.[131]

Neuroendocrine tumors

As with all other aspects of transplantation for malignant disease, there is significant controversy regarding the appropriate role for OLT, if any, in the treatment of metastatic neuroendocrine tumors. Due to the more indolent nature of such tumors and their propensity to cause significant hormone-related symptoms, early attempts were made to treat such patients with total hepatectomy and OLT, with encouraging results.[148,149] In fact, considering the dismal outcomes with other tumors metastatic to the liver, the results with transplantation for neuroendocrine tumors looked particularly promising. This led many to conclude that such tumors represented an exception. Most of the early reports were anecdotal case reports of only a handful of patients.[148–153] However, the encouraging aspects of this early experience were primarily based on the technical achievement itself and on the early symptomatic relief experienced by such patients. Unfortunately, most patients were found to have relatively early recurrence of their disease, sometimes with an aggression that suggested a negative impact of immunosuppression.[152] Because most such tumors are slowly progressive and survival can be long without resection, the wisdom of transplantation, with its requisite immunosuppression, can be questioned, especially in light of the extreme shortage of donor organs.

A review of the world's literature up to 1994 revealed 30 patients transplanted for neuroendocrine tumors, with a 1-year survival of 52%, and a death rate of 17% in the first year related to tumor recurrence. Caution and great attention to individual patient selection were emphasized.[80] In a more recent single-center experience, 11 patients with no evidence of extrahepatic spread underwent OLT for the treatment of various metastatic hepatic neuroendocrine tumors.[154] All patients were relieved of their symptoms, but six experienced early recurrence, five died of their recurrence, and an additional patient experienced a late recurrence. In this report, the overall 1-year and 5-year actuarial survivals were 82% and 57%, respectively. From this small experience, the authors also concluded that patients with non-carcinoid tumors fare better. In another similar single-center report, 15 patients were considered for OLT; only eight were found to be acceptable, and only three survived without recurrence at 6, 15, and 52 months.[120] Two more recent retrospective studies, one French and one German, attempted to assess the role of OLT for neuroendocrine tumors. Le Treut et al. found 15 cases of metastatic carcinoid and 16 cases of islet-cell carcinoma that had been treated with OLT.[155]

Many patients underwent aggressive surgical therapy, e.g., Whipple procedures, to control the primary at the time of transplantation. Overall actuarial survivals were 59%, 47%, and 36% at 1, 3, and 5 years, respectively, with a 17% disease-free survival at 5 years. This group observed that, while patients with carcinoid tended to have recurrence in the same time frame as the non-carcinoid, they tended to fare better. In the German experience, 3 of 12 patients (25%) had long-term disease-free follow-up. An update of these data has recently been published, with no improvement in overall outcomes.[156] The largest compilation to date includes data from the literature on 103 patients.[157] Overall survivals at 2 and 5 years were found to be 60% and 47%, but disease-free survival was 24%. A poorer prognoses was found to be associated with patients requiring foregut resection or Whipple's procedure combined with the transplant.

In summary, liver transplantation may continue to play some role in the treatment of neuroendocrine tumors metastatic to the liver. Currently, it is probably most appropriate for young, otherwise healthy patients in whom the primary has been controlled, in whom other alternatives are unavailable or have failed, and who suffer from significant symptomatic hormone-related syndromes, mass effect, or other sequelae such as portal hypertension. Under certain favorable circumstances, excellent palliation and even cure have been achieved with OLT in patients with metastatic neuroendocrine tumors. However, utilization of the scarce resource of cadaveric organs must be considered. Each liver transplanted into one individual is an organ denied to another. The acceptance of living-donor liver transplantation by such patients and its impact on them will be interesting to follow and raise many additional ethical questions.

Upper-abdominal exenteration has been done in conjunction with liver transplantation for the treatment of metastatic neuroendocrine tumors.[79,158] The most recent results reported for this operation are better with neuroendocrine tumors (64% at 3 years) than for other cell types, but the overall results of such operations at 5 years have only a 21% disease-free, 30% overall survival.[79]

Hepatic epithelioid hemangioendothelioma

Epithelioid hemangioendothelioma is a rare vascular neoplasm of intermediate malignancy which, among other locations, can occur as a primary hepatic disease. While it usually affects younger adults, it is to be distinguished from the also rare, but almost exclusively benign, infantile hemangioendothelioma.[86,159] It has no obvious associations or etiologic factors, except for the frequently invoked potential relation to oral contraceptives, and at least one report incriminating vinyl chloride.[86,160]

The first difficulty presented by hepatic epithelioid hemangioendothelioma (HEHE) is its diagnosis. Its vascular nature is often concealed from both radiologic and pathologic examination,[161] and misdiagnosis is common.[162] Histologic diagnosis is confirmed by immunohistochemical staining for factor VIII,[161] but a recent report suggests CD34 may be even more sensitive.[162] Clinically, the course of HEHE is highly unpredictable, but almost always progressive. Patients may present with widely variable circumstances in terms of size, number, location of tumors, and overall progression of their disease. Survival can be long term, even in the presence of metastases. The largest reported series of 32 patients included nine untreated patients surviving from 5 to 28 years, and many survive 5–10 years after diagnosis.[163] On the other hand, more rapidly progressive or even fulminant courses are known to occur.

Due to its rarity and unpredictable nature, the optimal treatment of HEHE remains unclear. Systemic chemotherapy is generally ineffective. Surgical resection is often precluded by the location or multiplicity of lesions. This has led to the utilization of total hepatectomy with OLT for many patients.[161,164–166] However, the appropriate roles of both primary resection and liver transplantation in the treatment of this tumor remain elusive. Unfortunately, the literature is comprised almost exclusively of small, single-center, retrospective reviews.

When determining the best treatment option, all aspects of the patient's circumstance must be considered, as a significant number may be asymptomatic. Conversely, associated manifestations such as portal hypertension, obstructive jaundice, ascites, and pain,[160,163,166] often occurring in a young individual, may compel some intervention. Gelin et al. reported the case of a 34-year-old man presenting with the recent onset of non-specific symptoms followed by massive upper gastrointestinal bleeding from portal hypertensive varices.[160] Imaging revealed clearly unresectable bilobar disease, but no extrahepatic spread. The patient underwent transplantation, but died of locally recurrent disease 2 years later. An autopsy showed that the tumor remained confined to the allograft. In an another report from Pittsburgh, a total of ten patients underwent transplantation for HEHE.[164] Five patients had evidence of extrahepatic spread at the time of surgery. Interestingly, of those with metastases at transplant, all were alive at the time of the report, while two of those with no apparent spread had died of metastases. In this report, there was an apparently optimistic projected actuarial survival of 76%. Long-term results from the same institution for a total of 16 patients appeared in a subsequent report.[167] In that study, with follow-up ranging from 1 to 15 years, actual patient survivals at 1, 3, and 5 years were 100%, 87.5%, and 71.3%. Disease-free survivals at the same time points were 81.3%, 68.8%, and 60.2%. A report based on the CTTR data of 21 OLT patients indicated an 82% 2-year survival and a 43% survival at 5 years.[133] Such results do suggest a role for OLT in the treatment of this disease. Most recently, the group at Mount Sinai has attempted to address the question of resection versus transplantation in a retrospective review of their experience with 11 patients.[166] In that series, patients were divided into three groups: resection (two with one crossover to OLT), OLT (five), and observation only (five). The two patients with localized disease who underwent resection both experienced early aggressive local recurrence in the residual liver. Interestingly, of the five patients who underwent OLT, two had extrahepatic disease at the time of transplant. However, one of those two remained alive at 8 years, even after an additional resection for recurrent disease. Overall, three of five OLT patients were alive, but only one was free of recurrence. Finally, four of the five treated with observation were alive with stable disease. In this study the authors found resection to be most disappointing and speculated that the hepatic regenerative process may stimulate tumor growth. Surprisingly, this group suggests that extrahepatic disease should not contraindicate OLT.

In summary, the optimal treatment of this rare and biologically unpredictable tumor remains uncertain. With the data available to date, it would seem impossible meaningfully to compare the various therapeutic alternatives. On the one hand, in light of the increasing shortage of cadaveric donor organs, the increasing waiting times, and the undesirable influence of immunosuppression, it is easy to be critical of OLT as an option. On the other hand, patients may be young and resection may not be feasible. Indeed, resection could ultimately be found to stimulate tumor growth. Finally, it is also true that many patients may have extended survival even without treatment. It seems logical, therefore, to advocate individualization of treatment options, with each considered a potential tool for use when clinically appropriate. In well-selected patients, however, it appears likely that liver transplantation may remain the best option.

Primary hepatic sarcoma

A CTTR report of patients transplanted for either hemangiosarcoma or epithelioid endotheliosarcoma indicates an expectedly poor overall survival.[133] The longest surviving patient lived just over 27 months. Except under a new experimental protocol, these diseases should represent contraindications to OLT.

Generally, it is now accepted that primary hepatic sarcoma is no longer an acceptable indication for a liver transplant.[131]

Metastatic disease

When a tumor has spread from its primary location to another organ, the disease is considered systemic by definition. Nevertheless, resection of metastatic disease can be warranted, for example, in the circumstance of hepatic colorectal metastases, with which one-third of patients undergoing resection survive for more than 5 years.[168] However, removal and replacement of the entire involved organ, although technically feasible, are confounded by the need for subsequent immunosuppressive therapy and its profound affect on tumor recurrence. The early liver transplant experience with secondary malignancy was poor enough for this to be excluded as an indication during the 1983 National Institutes of Health Consensus Development Conference, which allowed broader application of this procedure in the USA.

The CTTR reports data on 41 patients undergoing OLT for tumors metastatic to the liver.[133] These were comprised of several different histologic types, including colon carcinoma (ten), carcinoid (nine), small-bowel leiomyosarcoma (five), breast cancer (three), gastrinoma (two), glucagonoma (two), meningioma (one), neuroblastoma (one), renal-cell carcinoma (one), pancreatic cystosarcoma (one), hemangiopericytoma (one), seminoma (one), vipoma (one), malignant melanoma (one), and an unknown primary carcinoma. One patient with metastatic colon cancer survived for just over 5 years after undergoing OLT followed by high-dose chemotherapy, total-body irradiation, and autologous bone marrow transplantation. A similar strategy was used on two patients with breast cancer, but they survived only 9 and 10 months.[133] Altogether, there was a 70% recurrence rate amongst those transplanted for metastatic colon carcinoma, and 100% for those with breast cancer. Life-table analysis showed a 2-year survival of 38% and a 5-year survival of 21%.

To summarize, that early experience showed outcomes that, although reasonable from an oncology perspective, were dismal compared to the outcomes for other transplant indications. Considering the utilization of resources, unfortunately, such poor results were not justified from any perspective. As stated above, it was the National Institutes of Health Consensus Development Conference in 1983 that allowed for the wider utilization of OLT as a therapeutic option in the USA.[115] Due to the collectively poor outcomes with transplantation for metastatic tumors to the liver, secondary malignancies were excluded as indications for OLT at that conference. Consequently, few such transplants have subsequently taken place.

Again, from certain perspectives, the outcomes for patients transplanted with metastatic tumors may not appear unreasonable, especially when considering the certainty of the alternatives. However, in light of the extreme shortage of cadaveric donor organs, as well as the utilization of other resources in general, metastatic tumors spread to the liver continue to be absolute contraindications to OLT.

Except for isolated, specific circumstances involving some neuroendocrine tumors and possibly leiomyosarcoma, any malignancy metastatic to the liver is considered to be an unequivocal contraindication to liver transplantation.[131]

Isolated reports from single centers in the past have appeared to advocate the use of OLT for metastatic colon carcinoma.[169] However, 1-year survival of 45% is clearly unacceptable in an era of 90% 1-year survival and a critical organ shortage.

From the oncologic perspective, the outcomes after liver transplantation may appear quite acceptable, with survivals clearly superior to those of alternative therapies.[170] However, when considering the distribution of the scarce resource of donor organs and the dramatically superior survival of recipients without secondary malignancy, this indication for transplant becomes unacceptable.

To summarize: long-term palliation and even potential cures have been reported using liver transplantation in the treatment of tumor metastatic to the liver. Furthermore, the overall results for liver transplantation in the treatment of hepatic metastases may be superior to those of other treatment options available and therefore appear quite acceptable. However, the vastly superior survival of recipients without metastatic tumor and the extreme shortage of donor organs prohibit the widespread utilization of the scarce resource of donor organs for this purpose. The only role for such treatment is in the context of a prospective randomized trial of other new therapies.

Premalignant and benign lesions

There are a number of histologically benign conditions that have been appropriate indications for liver transplantation. These include lesions which may be premalignant or effectively malignant in their impact on the patient. The dramatically increased incidence of hepatic adenomas is widely acknowledged to have been linked with the use of oral contraceptives,[171] although less common associations exist, such as type Ia glycogen storage disease.[172] Although adenomas can cause pain, the primary indication for removal is the potential for spontaneous life-threatening hemorrhage and malignant degeneration.[171,173,174] In the rare event that an adenoma is not otherwise resectable due to its size, location, or multiplicity, liver transplantation may be the best alternative. A number of transplant centers have reported this uncommon indication for OLT.[175–178] For those with otherwise unresectable disease, the alternative of observation with serial scans and AFP determinations would now appear indefensible.[174] As one might expect, in the absence of end-stage parenchymal liver disease and portal hypertension, these patients fare well with the transplant procedure.[176–178]

Other benign conditions have also been reported as indications for liver transplantation. Tepetes *et al.* have reported not only a series of six adenomas, but a case of diffuse focal nodular hyperplasia, two patients with mesenchymal hamartoma, one cavernous hemangioma with Kasselbach–Merritt syndrome, one inflammatory pseudotumor, and a case of massive hepatic lymphangiomatosis.[176] A number of other liver transplant programs in the USA have also transplanted patients with adenomas and other benign conditions, such as biliary papillomatosis, another premalignant condition (personal experience).

Probably the most common histologically benign condition leading to liver transplantation has been symptomatic, massive hepatomegaly due to adult polycystic liver disease. Aspiration is essentially unhelpful, and fenestration or resection is appropriate when cysts are confined and significant uninvolved parenchyma exists.[179,180] Even when amenable to interventions short of transplantation, significant morbidity may be associated and relief from symptoms is always temporary.[180] Liver transplantation in appropriately selected patients can provide excellent outcomes, with a dramatic resolution to an often dramatic problem.[181]

Summary: transplantation in the treatment of malignancy

Currently, then, OLT is contraindicated in the presence of cholangiocarcinoma, sarcoma, and any non-neuroendocrine tumor metastatic to the liver. In certain ideal circumstances, OLT may be indicated for the treatment of hepatocellular carcinoma, epithelioid hemangioendothelioma, hepatoblastoma, metastatic neuroendocrine, leiomyosarcoma, 'incidental' cholangiocarcinoma, and benign but otherwise unresectable lesions.[131] In the field of transplantation, there are essentially no organs, other than the liver, for which a transplant may be performed as part of the treatment for a malignancy.

CONCLUSION

The role of organ transplantation continues to expand rapidly, saving the lives and lifestyles of thousands each year in the USA alone. Many of the technical problems of the past have now been mastered. Improvements in organ preservation, patient management, and infection control and a broader, more effective array of immunosuppressive agents have all contributed to the dramatic successes of organ transplantation. Nevertheless, immunosuppression changes the balance of forces in favor of malignancy: it increases the incidence of new tumors, it favors the recurrence of prior malignancy, and it can allow the transmission of cancer from an organ donor. Only under limited and very specific circumstances can transplantation be utilized to treat a malignancy. However, in the future, the ability to induce specific tolerance may be achieved, eliminating the need for current strategies. When this occurs, the indications for transplantation may expand again, further increasing the overlap in the fields of oncology and transplantation.

ACKNOWLEDGMENT

The authors wish to acknowledge their appreciation to Livio Romani, MD, for invaluable assistance in reviewing this manuscript.

REFERENCES

1. www.unos.org 1999 (unpublished).
2. Elgert KD. *Immunology: understanding the immune system*. New York, Wiley-Liss, 1996.
3. McPhaul JJ, McIntosh DA. Tissue transplantation still vexes. N Engl J Med 1965; 272:105.
4. Penn I. Cancers complicating organ transplantation. N Engl J Med 1990; 323:1767.
5. Penn I. Cancer is a complication of severe immunosuppression. Surg Gynecol Obstet 1986; 162:603.
6. Penn I. Neoplasia: an example of plasticity of the immune response. Transplant Proc 1996; 28:2089.
7. First MR, Peddi VR. Malignancies complicating organ transplantation. Transplant Proc 1998; 30:2768.
8. Penn I. Malignancy. Horizons in organ transplantation. Surg Clin North Am 1994; 74:1247–57.
9. Penn I. Posttransplant malignancies. Transplant Proc 1999; 31:1260.
10. El-Sabrout R, Gruber SA. Etiology and pathogenesis of posttransplant tumors: new insights into viral oncogenesis. Ann Transplant 1997; 2:67.
11. Sillman FH, Sentovich S, Shaffer D. Ano-genital neoplasia in renal transplant patients. Ann Transplant 1999; 2:59 (Abstract).
12. Kelly DM, Emre S, Guy SR, Miller CM, Schwartz ME, Sheiner PA. Liver transplant recipients are not at increased risk for nonlymphoid solid organ tumors. Cancer 1998; 83:1237.
13. Galve V, Cuervas-Mons V, Figueras J, *et al*. Incidence and outcome of de novo malignancies after liver transplantation. Transplant Proc 1999; 31:1275.
14. Peyregne V, Ducerf C, Adham M, *et al*. De novo cancer after orthotopic liver transplantation. Transplant Proc 1998; 30:1484.
15. Jensen P, Hansen S, Moller B, *et al*. Skin cancer in kidney and heart transplant recipients and different long-term immunosuppressive therapy regimens. J Acad Dermatol 1999; 40:177.
16. Adamson R, Obispo E, Dychter S, *et al*. High incidence and clinical course of aggressive skin cancer in heart transplant patients: a single-center study. Transplant Proc 1998; 30:1124.
17. Lanza RP, Cooper DKC, Cassidy MJD, Barnard CN. Malignant neoplasms occurring after cardiac transplanation. JAMA 1983; 249:1746.
18. Penn I. Post-transplantation de novo tumors in liver allograft recipients. Liver Transpl Surg 1996; 2:52.
19. Penn I. Solid tumors in cardiac allograft recipients. Ann Thorac Surg 1995; 60:1559.
20. Birkeland SA, Storm HH, Lamm LU, *et al*. Cancer risk after renal transplantation in the Nordic countries, 1964–1986. Int J Cancer 1995; 60:183.
21. Hoshida Y, Tsukuma H, Yasunaga Y, *et al*. Cancer risk after renal transplantation in Japan. Int J Cancer 1997; 16:517.
22. Penn I, First MR. Merkel's cell carcinoma in organ recipients. Transplantation 1999; 68:1717.
23. Penn I. Overview of the problem of cancer in organ transplant recipients. Ann Transplant 1999; 2:5.
24. Penn I. Malignant melanoma in organ allograft recipients. Transplantation 1996; 61:274.
25. Masuhara M, Ogasawara H, Katyal SL, Nakamura T, Shinozuka H. Cyclosporin stimulates hepatocyte proliferation and accelerates development of hepatocellular carcinoma in rats. Carcinogenesis 1993; 14:1579.
26. Hiesse C, Rieu P, Kriaa F, *et al*. Malignancy after renal transplantation: analysis of incidence and risk factors in 1700 patients followed during a 25 year period. Transplant Proc 1997; 29:831.
27. Euvrard S, Chardonnet Y, Pouteil-Noble CP, Kanitakis J, Thivolet J, Touraine JL. Skin malignancies and human papillomaviruses in renal transplant recipients. Transplant Proc 1993; 25:1392.
28. Penn I. Why do immunosuppressed patients develop cancer? Clin Rev Oncogen 1999; 1:27.
29. Penn I. Transplantation oncology: the next frontier. In Sher L, Makowka L, eds. *Intra-abdominal organ transplantation 2000*. R.G. Landes Company, 1994, 189.
30. Shipp MA, Mauch PM, Harris NL. Lymphomas. In DeVita VT, Hellman S, Rosenberg SA, eds. *Cancer principles and practice of oncology*. Philadelphia, Lippincott-Raven, 1997, 2165.
31. Rosenberg SA. Principles of cancer management: biologic therapy. In DeVita VT, Hellman S, Rosenberg SA, eds. *Cancer principles and practice of oncology*. Philadelphia, Lippincott-Raven, 1997, 349.
32. Penn I. Cancers in cyclosporine-treated vs azathioprine-treated patients. Transplant Proc 1996; 28:876.
33. Euvrard S, Kanitakis J, Pouteil-Noble C, Claudy A, Touraine JL. Skin cancers in organ transplant recipients. Ann Transplant 1997; 2:28.
34. Greenlee RT, Murray T, Bolden S, Wingo PA. Cancer statistics, 2000. CA Cancer J Clinic 2000; 50:7.
35. www.seer Cancer Statistics. 2000 (unpublished).
36. Sheil AG. Cancer after transplantation. World J Surg 1986; 10:389.
37. Veness MJ, Quinn DI, Ong CS, *et al*. Aggressive cutaneous malignancies following cardiothoracic transplantation: the Australian experience. Cancer 1999; 85:1758.
38. Jeremy D, Farnsworth RH, Robertson MR, Annetts DL, Murnaghan GF. Transplantation of malignant melanoma with a cadaver kidney. Transplantation 1972; 13:619.
39. Suranyi MG, Hogan PG, Falk MC, *et al*. Advanced donor-origin melanoma in a renal transplant recipient: immunotherapy, cure, and retransplantation. Transplantation 1998; 66:655.

40. Siegel JH, Janis R, Alper JC, Schutte H, Robbins L, Blaufox MD. Disseminated visceral Kaposi's sarcoma. Appearance after human renal homograft operation. JAMA 1969; 207:1493.

41. Harwood AR, Osoba D, Hofstader SL, et al. Kaposi's sarcoma in recipients of renal transplants. Am J Med 1979; 67:759.

42. Penn I. Kaposi's sarcoma in transplant recipients. Transplantation 1997; 64:669.

43. Shaheen F, Al-Sulaiman MH, Ramprasad KS, Al-Khader AA. Kaposi's sarcoma in renal transplant recipients. Ann Transplant 1999; 2:49 (Abstract).

44. Bismuth H, Samuel D, Venancie PY, Menouar G, Szekely AM. Development of Kaposi's sarcoma in liver transplant recipients: characteristics, management, and outcome. Transplant Proc 1991; 23:1438.

45. Russo JJ, Bohenzky RA, Chien M-C, et al. Nucleotide sequence of the Kaposi sarcoma-associated herpesvirus (HHV8). Proc Natl Acad Sci USA 1996; 93:14862.

46. Penn I. Sarcomas in organ allograft recipients. Transplantation 1995; 60:1485.

47. Timmons CF, Dawson DB, Richards CS, Andrews WS, Katz JA. Epstein–Barr virus-associated leiomyosarcomas in liver transplantation recipients. Origin from either donor or recipient tissue. Cancer 1995; 76:1481.

48. McClain KL, Leach CT, Jenson HB, et al. Association of Epstein–Barr virus with leiomyosarcoma in children with AIDS. N Engl J Med 1995; 332:12.

49. Penn I. Primary malignancies of the hepato-biliary-pancreatic system in organ allograft recipients. J Hepatobiliary pancreat Surg 1998; 5:157–64.

50. Babcock GL, Decker LL, Freeman RB, Thorley-Lawson DA. Epstein–Barr virus-infected resting memory B cells, not proliferating lymphocytes, accumulate in the peripheral blood of immunosuppressed patients. J Exp Med 1999; 190:567.

51. Walker RC, Paya CV, Marshall WF, et al. Pretransplantation seronegative Epstein–Barr virus status is the primary risk factor for posttransplantation lymphoproliferative disorder in adult heart, lung, and other solid organ transplantations. J Heart Lung Transplant 1995; 14:214.

52. Nalesnik MA, Rao AS, Furukawa H, et al. Autologous lymphokine-activated killer cell therapy of Epstein–Barr virus-positive and -negative lymphoproliferative disorders arising in organ transplant recipients. Transplantation 1997; 63:1200.

53. Nalesnik M, Locker J, Jaffe R. Experience with posttransplant lymphoproliferative disorders in solid organ transplant patients. Clin Transplant 1992; 6:249.

54. Harmon W. Posttransplant lymphoproliferative disorder: literature scan. Transplantation 1996; 12:1.

55. McDiarmid SV, Jordan S, Lee GS, et al. Prevention and preemptive therapy of posttransplant lymphoproliferative disease in pediatric liver recipients. Transplantation 1998; 66:1604.

56. Newell KA, Alonso EM, Whitington PF, et al. Posttransplant lymphoproliferative disease in pediatric liver transplantation. Transplantation 1996; 62:370.

57. Lattyak BV, Rosenthal P, Mudge C, et al. Posttransplant lymphoproliferative disorder presenting in the head and neck. Laryngoscope 1998; 108:1195.

58. Oda D, Persson GR, Haigh WG, Sabath DE, Penn I, Aziz S. Oral presentation of posttransplantation lymphoproliferative disorders. An unusual manifestation. Transplantation 1996; 61:435.

59. Cox K, Lawrence-Miyasaki LS, Garcia-Kennedy R, et al. An increased incidence of Epstein–Barr virus infection and lymphoproliferative disorder in young children on FK506 after liver transplantation. Transplantation 1995; 59:524.

60. Sokal EM, Antunes H, Beguin C, et al. Early signs and risk factors for the increased incidence of Epstein–Barr virus-related posttransplant lymphoproliferative diseases in pediatric liver transplant recipients treated with tacrolimus. Transplantation 1997; 64:1438.

61. Hezode C, Duvoux C, Germanidis G, et al. Role of hepatitis C virus in lymphoproliferative disorders after liver transplantation. Hepatology 1999; 30:775.

62. Kenagy DN, Schlesinger Y, Weck K, Ritter JH, Gaudrealt-Keener MM, Storch GA. Epstein–Barr virus DNA in peripheral blood leukocytes of patients with posttransplant lymphoproliferative disease. Transplantation 1995; 60:547.

63. Badley AD, Portela DF, Patel R, et al. Development of monoclonal gammopathy precedes the development of Epstein–Barr virus-induced posttransplant lymphoproliferative disorder. Liver Transplant Surg 1996; 5:375.

64. Personal communication.

65. Ribas Y, Rafecas A, Figeras J, et al. Post-transplant lymphoma in a liver allograft. Transplant Int 1995; 8:488.

66. Cherqui D, Duvoux C, Plassa F, et al. Lymphoproliferative disorder of donor origin in a liver transplant recipient: complete remission after drastic reduction of immunosuppression without graft loss. Transplantation 1993; 56:1023.

67. Navarro F, Pyda P, Pageaux GP, et al. Lymphoproliferative disease after liver transplantation: primary biliary location. Transplant Proc 1998; 30:1486.

68. Tsai DE, Stadtmauer EA, Canaday DJ, Vaughn DJ. Combined radiation and chemotherapy in posttransplant lymphoproliferative disorder. Med Oncol 1998; 15:279.

69. Davis CL, Wood BL, Sabath DE, Joseph JS, Stehman-Breen C, Broudy VC. Interferon-alpha treatment of posttransplant lymphoproliferative disorder in recipients of solid organ transplants. Transplantation 1998; 66:1770.

70. Green M, Cacciarelli TV, Mazariegos GV, et al. Serial measurement of Epstein–Barr viral load in peripheral blood in pediatric liver transplant recipients during treatment for posttransplant lymphoproliferative disease. Transplantation 1998; 66:1641.

71. Khanna R, Bell S, Sherritt M, et al. Activation and adoptive transfer of Epstein–Barr virus-specific cytotoxic T cells in solid organ transplant patients with posttransplant lymphoproliferative disease. Proc Natl Acad Sci 1999; 96:10391.

72. Penn I. Evaluation of the candidate with a previous malignancy. Liver Transplant Surg 1996; 2:109.

73. Stewart TH, Hollinshead AC, Raman S. Tumour dormancy: initiation, maintenance and termination in animals and humans. Can J Surg 1991; 34:321.

74. Fidler IJ. Critical determinants of cancer metastasis: rationale for therapy. Cancer Chemother Pharmacol 1999; 43:S3.

75. Penn I. Effect of immunosuppression on perplexing cancers. Transplant Proc 1993; 25:1380.

76. Penn I. The effect of immunosuppression on pre-existing cancers. Transplantation 1993; 55:742.

77. Penn I. Evaluation of transplant candidates with pre-existing malignancies. Ann Transplant 1997; 2:14 (Abstract).

78. Yokoyama I, Carr B, Saitsu H, et al. Accelerated growth rates of recurrent hepatocellular carcinoma after liver transplantation. Cancer 1991; 68:2095.

79. Alessiani M, Tzakis A, Todo S, Demetris AJ, Fung JJ, Starzl TE. Assessment of five-year experience with abdominal organ cluster transplantation. J Am Coll Surg 1995; 180:1.

80. Bechstein WO, Neuhaus P. Liver transplantation for hepatic metastases of neuroendocrine tumors. Ann N Y Acad Sci 1994; 733:507.

81. Kew MC, Popper H. Relationship between hepatocellular carcinoma and cirrhosis. Semin Liver Dis 1984; 4:136.

82. United Network of Organ Sharing. 1997 annual report. Washington, D.C., US Scientific Registry of Transplant Recipients and the Organ Procurement and Transplant Network, 1998.

83. Weisner RH. Current indications, contraindications, and timing for liver transplantation. In Busuttil RW, Klintmalm GB, eds. Transplantation of the liver. Philadelphia, W.B. Saunders Company, 1996, 71.

84. Clavien P-A. Orthotopic liver transplantation for stage II and stage IV hepatocellular carcinoma. Liver Transplant Surg 1997; 3:S52.

85. Crawford JM. The liver and the biliary tract. In Cotran RS, Kumar V, Collins T, eds. Robbins pathologic basis of disease. Philadelphia, W.B. Saunders Company, 1999, 845.

86. Kew MC. Tumors of the liver. In Zakim D, Boyer TD, eds. Hepatology: a textbook of liver disease. Philadelphia, W.B. Saunders, 1996, 1513.

87. Schafer DF, Sorrell MF. Hepatocellular carcinoma. Lancet 1999; 353:1253.

88. El-Serag HB, Mason AC. The increasing incidence of hepatocellular carcinoma in the United States. N Engl J Med 1999; 340:745.

89. Moradpour D, Wands JR. Hepatic oncogenesis. In Zakim D, Boyer TD, eds. Hepatology: a textbook of liver disease. Philadelphia, W.B. Saunders, 1996, 1490.

90. Martin P. Hepatocellular carcinoma: risk factors and natural history. Liver Transplant Surg 1998; 5:S87.

91. Di Bisceglie AM. Hepatitis C and hepatocellular carcinoma. Hepatology 1997; 26:34s.

92. Yamauchi M, Nakahara M, Maezawa Y, Satoh S, Nishikawa F, Ohata M. Prevalence of hepatocellular carcinoma in patients with alcoholic cirrhosis and prior exposure to hepatitis C. Am J Gastroenterol 1993; 88:39.

93. Schafer DF, Sorrell MF. Hepatocellular carcinoma (Letter). Lancet 1999; 354:253.

94. Bismuth H, Majno PE, Adam R. Liver transplantation for hepatocellular carcinoma. Semin Liver Dis 1999; 19:311.

95. Schwartz ME, Sung M, Mor E, et al. A multidisciplinary approach to hepatocellular carcinoma in patients with cirrhosis. J Am Coll Surg 1995; 180:596.

96. Tan KC, Rela M, Ryder SD, et al. Experience of orthotopic liver transplantation and hepatic resection for hepatocellular carcinoma of less than 8 cm in patients with cirrhosis. Br J Surg 1995; 82:253.

97. Mion F, Grozel L, Boillot O, Paliard P, Berger F. Adult cirrhotic liver explants: precancerous lesions and undetected small hepatocellular carcinomas. Gastroenterology 1996; 111:1587.

98. Achkar J-P, Araya V, Baron RL, Marsh JW, Dvorchik I, Rakela J. Undetected hepatocellular carcinoma: clinical features and outcome after liver transplantation. Liver Transplant Surg 1998; 4:477.

99. Borzio M, Bruno S, Roncalli M, et al. Liver cell dysplasia is a major risk factor for hepatocellular carcinoma in cirrhosis: a prospective study. Gastroenterology 1995; 108:812.

100. Barbu V, Bonnand AM, Hillaire S, et al. Circulating albumin messenger RNA in hepatocellular

carcinoma: results of a multicenter prospective study. Hepatology 1997; 26:1171.

101. Gion T, Taketomi A, Shimada M, *et al.* Perioperative change in albumin messenger RNA levels in patients with hepatocellular carcinoma. Hepatology 1998; 28:1663.

102. Otto G, Heuschen U, Hofmann WJ, Krumm G, Hinz U, Herfarth C. Survival and recurrence after liver transplantation versus liver resection for hepatocellular carcinoma: a retrospective analysis. Ann Surg 1998; 227:424.

103. Nagasue N, Uchida M, Makino Y, *et al.* Incidence and factors associated with intrahepatic recurrence following resection of hepatocellular carcinoma. Gastroenterology 1993; 105:488.

104. Fan ST, Ng IO, Poon RT, Lo CM, Liu CL, Wong J. Hepatectomy for hepatocellular carcinoma: the surgeon's role in long-term survival. Arch Surg 1999; 134:1124.

105. Llovet JM, Bustamante J, Castells A, *et al.* Natural history of untreated nonsurgical hepatocellular carcinoma: rationale for the design and evaluation of therapeutic trials. Hepatology 1999; 29:62.

106. Barbara L, Benzi G, Gaiani S, *et al.* Natural history of small untreated hepatocellular carcinoma in cirrhosis: a multivariant analysis of prognostic factors of tumor growth rate and patient survival. Hepatology 1992; 16:132.

107. Ebara M, Hatano R, Fukuda H, Yoshikawa M, Sugiura N, Saisho H. Natural history of small hepatocellular carcinoma with underlying cirrhosis. A study of 30 patients. Hepatogastroenterology 1998; 45:1214.

108. Okazaki N, Yoshino M, Yoshida T, *et al.* Evaluation of the prognosis for small hepatocellular carcinoma based on tumor volume doubling time. A preliminary report. Cancer 1989; 63:2207.

109. Lai EC, Fan ST, Lo CM, Chu KM, Liu CL, Wong J. Hepatic resection for hepatocellular carcinoma. An audit of 343 patients. Ann Surg 1995; 221:291.

110. Castells A, Bruix J, Bru C, *et al.* Treatment of small hepatocellular carcinoma in cirrhotic patients: a cohort study comparing surgical resection and percutaneous ethanol injection. Hepatology 1993; 18:1121.

111. Okazaki N, Kosuge T, Takayama T, *et al.* Accelerated tumor growth and changes in images concomitant with vascularization in a patient with hepatocellular carcinoma. Hepatogastroenterology 1991; 38:160.

112. McPeake JR, O'Grady JG, Zaman S, *et al.* Liver transplantation for primary hepatocellular carcinoma: tumor size and number determine outcome. J Hepatol 1993; 18:226.

113. Torzilli G, Minagawa M, Takayama T, *et al.* Accurate preoperative evaluation of liver mass lesions without fine-needle biopsy. Hepatology 1999; 30:889.

114. Starzl TE. *The puzzle people*. Pittsburg, University of Pittsburg, 1992.

115. NIH Consensus Development Conference Statement on Liver Transplantation: June 20–23, 1983. Hepatology 1983; 4S:107S.

116. Stone MJ. Transplantation for primary hepatic malignancy. In Busuttil RW, Klintmalm G, eds. *Liver transplantation*. 1995, 120.

117. Pichlmayr R, Weimann A, Ringe B. Indications for liver transplantation in hepatobiliary malignancy. Hepatology 1994; 20:33s.

118. Olthoff KM, Millis JM, Rosove MH, Goldstein LI, Ramming KP, Busuttil RW. Is liver transplantation justified for the treatment of hepatic malignancies? Arch Surg 1990; 125:1261.

119. Iwatsuki S, Gordon RD, Shaw BW, Starzl TE. Role of liver transplantation in cancer therapy. Ann Surg 1985; 202:401.

120. Dousset B, Houssin D, Soubrane O, Boillot O, Baudin F, Chapuis Y. Metastatic endocrine tumors: is there a place for liver transplantation? Liver Transplant Surg 1995; 1:111.

121. Gonzalez EM, Gomez R, Garcia I, *et al.* Liver transplantation in malignant primary hepatic neoplasms. Am J Surg 1992; 163:395.

122. Haug CE, Jenkins RL, Rohrer RJ, *et al.* Liver transplantation for primary hepatic cancer. Transplantation 1992; 53:376.

123. Chung SW, Toth JL, Rezieg M, *et al.* Liver transplantation for hepatocellular carcinoma. Am J Surg 1994; 167:317.

124. Colquhoun SD, Ghobrial RM, Farmer DG, *et al.* Effectiveness of preoperative chemo-embolization for hepatocellular carcinoma in liver transplant candidates. Transplantation 1998; (Abstract).

125. Venook AP, Ferrell LD, Roberts JP, *et al.* Liver transplantation for hepatocellular carcinoma: results with preoperative chemoembolization. Liver Transplant Surg 1995; 1:242.

126. Groupe d'Etude et de Traitement du Carcinome Hepatocellulaire. A comparison of lipiodol chemoembolization and conservative treatment for unresectable hepatocellular carcinoma. N Engl J Med 1995; 332:1256.

127. Negasue N, Galizia G, Kohno H, *et al.* Adverse effects of preoperative hepatic artery chemoembolization for resectable hepatocellular carcinoma: a retrospective comparison of 138 liver resections. Surgery 1989; 106:81.

128. Spreafico C, Marchiano A, Regalia E, *et al.* Chemoembolization of hepatocellular carcinoma in patients who undergo liver transplantation. Radiology 1994; 192:687.

129. Yamanaka N, Okamoto E, Fujihara S, *et al.* Do the tumor cells of hepatocellular carcinomas dislodge into the portal venous stream during hepatic resection? Cancer 1992; 70:2263.

130. Colquhoun SD, Ghobrial RM, Seu P, *et al.* Chemo-embolization preceding orthotopic liver

transplantation in patients with hepatocellular carcinoma. Transplantation 1997; (Abstract).

131. Testa G, Klintmalm GB. Liver transplantation for primary and metastatic liver cancers. Ann Transplant 1997; 2:19.

132. Achilleos OA, Buist LJ, Kelly DA, et al. Unresectable hepatic tumors in childhood and the role of liver transplantation. J Pediatr Surg 1996; 31:1563.

133. Penn I. Hepatic transplantation for primary and metastatic cancers of the liver. Surgery 1991; 110:726.

134. Ringe B, Wittekind C, Weimann A, Tusch G, Pichlmayr R. Results of hepatic resection and transplantation for fibrolamellar carcinoma. Surg Gynecol Obstet 1992; 175:299.

135. Starzl TE, Iwatsuki S, Shaw BW. Treatment of fibrolamellar hepatocellular carcinoma. Am J Surg 1986; 162:145.

136. Stieber AC, Marino IR, Iwatsuki S, Starzl TE. Cholangiocarcinomas in sclerosing cholangitis. The role of liver transplantation. Int Surg 1989; 74:1.

137. Pichlmayr R, Weimann A, Oldhafer KJ, et al. Role of liver transplantation in the treatment of unresectable liver cancer. World J Surg 1995; 19:807.

138. Goldstein RM, Stone M, Tillery GW, et al. Is liver transplantation indicated for cholangiocarcinoma? Am J Surg 1993; 166:768.

139. Miros M, Kerlin P, Walker N, Harper J, Lynch S, Strong R. Predicting cholangiocarcinoma in patients with primary sclerosing cholangitis before transplantation. Gut 1991; 32:1369–73.

140. Abu-Elmagd KM, Selby R, Iwatsuki S, et al. Cholangiocarcinoma and sclerosing cholangitis: clinical characteristics and effect on survival after liver transplantation. Transplant Proc 1993; 25:1124.

141. Delcore R, Eisenach JB, Payne KM, Bhatia P, Forster J. Risk of occult carcinomas in patients undergoing orthotopic liver transplantation for end-stage liver disease secondary to primary sclerosing cholangitis. Transplant Proc 1993; 25:1883.

142. Nashan B, Schlitt HJ, Tusch G, et al. Biliary malignancies in primary sclerosing cholangitis: timing for liver transplantation. Hepatology 1996; 23:1105.

143. Broome U, Eriksson LS. Assessment for liver transplantation in patients with primary sclerosing cholangitis. J Hepatol 1994; 20:654.

144. Fisher A, Theise ND, Min A, et al. CA19-9 does not predict cholangiocarcinoma in patients with primary sclerosing cholangitis undergoing liver transplantation. Liver Transplant Surg 1995; 1:94.

145. Goss JA, Shackleton RR, Farmer DG, et al. Orthotopic liver transplantation for primary sclerosing cholangitis. Ann Surg 1997; 225:472.

146. Casavilla FA, Marsh JW, Iwatsuki S, et al. Hepatic resection and transplantation for peripheral cholangiocarcinoma. J Am Coll Surg 1997; 185:429.

147. Iwatsuki S, Todo S, Marsh JW, et al. Treatment of hilar cholangiocarcinoma (Klatskin tumors) with hepatic resection or transplantation. J Am Coll Surg 1998; 187:358.

148. Arnold JC, O'Grady JG, Bird GL, Calne RY, Williams R. Liver transplantation for primary and secondary hepatic apudomas. Br J Surg 1989; 76:248.

149. Makowka L, Tzakis AG, Mazzaferro V, et al. Transplantation of the liver for metastatic endocrine tumors of the intestine and pancreas. Surg Gynecol Obstet 1989; 168:107.

150. Schweizer RT, Alsina AE, Rosson R, Bartus SA. Liver transplantation for metastatic neuroendocrine tumors. Transplant Proc 1993; 25:1973.

151. Alsina AE, Bartus S, Hull D, Rosson R, Schweizer RT. Liver transplant for metastatic neuroendocrine tumor. J Clin Gastroenterol 1990; 12:533.

152. Gulanikar AC, Kotylak G, Bitter-Suerman H. Does immunosuppression alter the growth of metastatic liver carcinoid after orthotopic liver transplantation? Transplant Proc 1991; 23:2197.

153. Frilling A, Rogiers X, Knofel WT, Broelsch EE. Liver transplantation for metastatic carcinoid tumors. Digestion 1994; 55:104.

154. Routley D, Ramage JK, McPeake J, Tan KC, Williams R. Orthotopic liver transplantation in the treatment of metastatic neuroendocrine tumors of the liver. Liver Transplant Surg 1995; 1:118.

155. Le Treut YP, Delpero JP, Cherqui D, et al. Results of liver transplantation in the treatment of metastatic neuroendocrine tumors. A 31-case French multicentric report. Ann Surg 1997; 225:355.

156. Lang H, Schlitt HJ, Schmidt H, et al. Total hepatectomy and liver transplantation for metastatic neuroendocrine tumors of the pancreas – a single center experience with ten patients. Langenbeck's Arch Surg 1999; 384:370.

157. Lehnert T. Liver transplantation for metastatic neuroendocrine carcinoma: an analysis of 103 patients. Transplantation 1998; 66:1307.

158. Tzakis AG, Todo S, Madariaga J, Tzoracoeleftherakis E, Fung JJ, Starzl TE. Upper-abdominal exenteration in transplantation for extensive malignancies of the upper abdomen – an update. Transplantation 1991; 51:727.

159. Calder CJ, Buckels JAC, Kelly DA. Orthotopic liver transplantation for type 2 hepatic infantile haemangioendothelioma. Histopathology 1996; 28:271.

160. Gelin M, Van de Stadt J, Rickaert F, et al. Epithelioid hemangioendothelioma of the liver following contact with vinyl chloride. Recurrence after orthotopic liver transplantation. J Hepatol 1989; 8:99.

161. Scozec J-Y, Lamy P, Degott C, et al. Epithelioid hemangioendothelioma of the liver. Gastroenterology 1988; 94:1447.

162. Demetris AJ, Minervini M, Raikow RB, Lee RG. Hepatic epithelioid hemangioendothelioma. Am J Surg Pathol 1997; 21:263.

163. Ishak KG, Sesterhenn IA, Goodman ZD, Rabin L, Stromeyer FW. Epithelioid hemangioendothelioma of the liver: a clinicopathologic and follow-up study of 32 cases. Hum Pathol 1984; 15:839.

164. Marino IR, Todo S, Tzakis AG, et al. Treatment of hepatic epithelioid hemangioendothelioma with liver transplantation. Cancer 1988; 15:2079.

165. Kelleher MB, Iwatsuki S, Sheahan DG. Epithelioid hemangioendothelioma of liver. Am J Surg Pathol 1989; 13:999.

166. Ben-Haim M, Roayaie S, Ye MQ, et al. Hepatic epithelioid hemangioendothelioma: resection or transplantation, which and when? Liver Transplant Surg 1999; 5:526.

167. Madariaga JR, Marino IR, Karavias DD, et al. Long-term results after liver transplantation for primary hepatic epithelioid hemangioendothelioma. Ann Surg Oncol 1995; 2:483.

168. Iwatsuki S. Liver transplantation for metastatic hepatic malignancy. In Busuttil RW, Klintmalm G, eds. Liver transplantation. 1998, 130.

169. Muhlbacher F, Piza F. Orthotopic liver transplantation for secondary malignancies of the liver. Transplant Proc 1987; 19:2396–8.

170. Muhlbacher F, Huk I, Steininger R, et al. Is orthotopic liver transplantation a feasible treatment for secondary cancer of the liver? Transplant Proc 1991; 23:1567.

171. Tesluk H, Lawrie J. Hepatocellular adenoma. Arch Pathol Lab Med 1981; 105:296.

172. Coire CI, Qizilbash AH, Castelli MF. Hepatic adenomata in type Ia glycogen storage disease. Arch Pathol Lab Med 1987; 111:166.

173. Gyorffy EJ, Bredfeldt JE, Black WC. Transformation of hepatic cell adenoma to hepatocellular carcinoma due to oral contraceptive use. Ann Int Med 1989; 110:489.

174. Foster JH, Berman MM. The malignant transformation of liver cell adenomas. Arch Surg 1994; 129:712.

175. Leese T, Farges O, Bismuth H. Liver cell adenomas. Ann Surg 1988; 208:558.

176. Tepetes K, Selby R, Webb M, Madariaga JR, Iwatsuki S, Starzl TE. Orthotopic liver transplantation for benign hepatic neoplasms. Arch Surg 1995; 130:153.

177. Mueller J, Keefe EB, Esquivel CO. Liver transplantation for the treatment of giant hepatocellular adenomas. Liver Transplant Surg 1995; 1:99.

178. Faivre L, Houssin D, Valayer J, Brouard J, Hadchouel M, Bernard O. Long-term outcome of liver transplantation in patients with glycogen storage disease type Ia. J Inherit Metab Dis 1999; 22:723.

179. Que F, Nagorney DM, Gross JB, Torres VE. Liver resection and cyst fenestration in the treatment of severe polycystic liver disease. Gastroenterology 1995; 108:487.

180. Gigot JF, Jadoul P, Que F, et al. Adult polycystic liver disease: is fenestration the most adequate operation for long-term management? Ann Surg 1997; 225:286.

181. Swenson K, Seu P, Kinkhabwala M, et al. Liver transplantation for adult polycystic liver disease. Hepatology 1998; 28:412.

Commentary

ACHILLES A DEMETRIOU

With the advent of organ transplantation, it has become apparent that there is an increased incidence of tumor formation in organ recipients. The true incidence of malignant tumors in transplanted patients is not known, but it appears to be greater than 6%.[1]

The above observation has profound implications regarding patient care in two respects:

1 The true incidence and type of malignancies need to be defined so that future organ recipients have a better understanding of the risks they face and how they need to be monitored for early tumor detection.

2 The mechanism and etiology of this phenomenon need to be clarified to determine whether the risk can be either lowered or eliminated and to guide the development of rational therapeutic regimens.

Regarding the incidence of cancer and the clinical implications of carcinogenesis for transplant recipients, it is clear that many new cancers in the post-transplant setting are easily treatable if detected early through aggressive monitoring. These include low-grade skin tumors, in situ carcinoma of the cervix, and in situ carcinoma of the vulva and perineum.[2] The average age of patients developing malignant tumors in this setting is relatively young (42 years), and the ratio of males to females is 2 : 1, reflecting the demographic characteristics of organ recipients in general.[1] The incidence of malignancy increases with the length of the post-transplant period.[3]

In general, in this group of patients there is no increased incidence of the types of carcinomas commonly seen in the general population (i.e., carcinomas of the breast, prostate, colon, and lung).[4] However, cancers that are relatively uncommon in the general population appear with increased frequency in the transplanted patient population. These include lymphomas, lip carcinoma, Kaposi's sarcoma, renal carcinoma, carcinoma of the vulva and perineum, hepatobiliary tumors, and sarcomas.[1,4] Significant differences in the incidence of malignancy have been observed among recipients of different types of organs. Liver transplant recipients have a higher incidence of lymphomas than renal allograft recipients.[2,5]

The intriguing primary questions are:

Why is there an increase in the incidence of cancer in allograft recipients?

Why is there an increased incidence of relatively less common types of cancer and cutaneous types of tumors in these patients?

Why are there differences in terms of incidence and types of tumors between kidney and liver allograft recipients?

The most important contribution to our understanding of some of the issues and to attempts to obtain answers to the above questions came out of epidemiological data analyses made possible by the establishment of the Cincinnati Transplant Tumor Registry, initiated and maintained by Dr Israel Penn.

Immunosuppression has been offered as one possible explanation for the increased incidence of malignancies in the transplant recipient population.[6,7] Intuitively, this would seem logical, considering that in other immunosuppression settings a similar pattern has been observed (i.e. Kaposi's sarcoma in acquired immunodeficiency syndrome). It is felt that the immune surveillance system is impaired secondary to the immunosuppressive therapeutic agents and, as a result, there is an increased incidence of tumor development. It is also believed that there is a loss of normal regulatory mechanisms controlling the immune response secondary to chronic graft antigen stimulation.

It has been proposed, based on the types of malignancies transplant recipients develop as well as on the relatively short induction time, that many of the observed tumors may be of viral etiology. If this were true, strategies to develop antiviral vaccines could be used to prevent and treat these patients. It is also possible that some

of the immunosuppressive agents used to treat transplant recipients may directly cause cancer or indirectly potentiate the effects of other carcinogens and result in cancer development. These issues are discussed in the comprehensive monograph by Colquhoun and colleagues.

It is clear, from a review of the literature in the field, that there is limited understanding of the etiology of enhanced susceptibility to cancer in the post-transplant setting. As a result, there is little hope for developing rational therapeutic strategies to prevent cancer development. Most efforts at reducing the risk of cancer have focused on attempts to minimize the use of immunosuppressive agents, to eliminate exposure to cofactors (i.e. sunlight), and on aggressive tumor-detection surveillance.

Most of what is known in this area to date is a result of the analysis of historic data and clinical correlations. There have been very few attempts to carry out randomized clinical trials examining the role of the type of immunosuppressive regimen on incidence and type of tumor development in a prospective setting. Moreover, there has been very little work, either experimental animal or basic *in vitro*, focusing on specific questions in controlled settings to generate meaningful data to guide future therapeutic strategies. This is an important and exciting area, offering opportunities for future research contributions.

REFERENCES

1. Penn I. Why do immunosuppressed patients develop cancer? Crit Rev Oncogen 1986; 1:27–52.
2. Penn I. Cancers complicating organ transplantation. N Engl J Med 1990; 323:1767–72.
3. Sheil AGR, Disney APS, Mathew TH, *et al.* Cancer development in cadaveric donor renal allograft recipients treated with azathioprine or cyclosporine or both. Transplant Proc 1986; 23:1111–12.
4. Penn I. Post-transplantation de novo tumors in liver allograft recipients. Liver Transpl Surg 1996; 2:52–60.
5. Nalesnik MA, Makowka L, Starzl TE. The diagnosis and treatment of posttransplant lymphoproliferative disorders. Curr Probl Surg 1988; 25:371–472.
6. Harwood AR, Osoba D, Hofstader SL, *et al.* Kaposi's sarcoma in recipients of renal transplants. Am J Med 1979; 67:759–65.
7. Hanto DW, Birkenbach M, Frizzera G, *et al.* Confirmation of the heterogeneity of post-transplant Epstein–Barr virus-associated B cell proliferations by immunoglobulin gene rearrangement analyses. Transplantation 1989; 47:458–64.

Editors' selected abstracts

Solid cancers after bone marrow transplantation.

Bhatia S, Louie AD, Bhatia R, O'Donnell MR, Fung H, Kashyap A, Krishnan A, Molina A, Nademanee A, Niland JC, Parker PA, Snyder DS, Spielberger R, Stein A, Forman SJ.

Divisions of Hematology and Bone Marrow Transplantation, Pediatric Oncology, Biostatistics, and Pathology, City of Hope National Medical Center, Duarte, CA, USA.

Journal of Clinical Oncology 19:464–71, 2001.

Purpose: To evaluate the incidence and associated risk factors of solid cancers after bone marrow transplantation (BMT). *Patients and methods:* We analyzed 2,129 patients who had undergone BMT for hematologic malignancies at the City of Hope National Medical Center between 1976 and 1998. A retrospective cohort and nested case-control study design were used to evaluate the role of pretransplantation therapeutic exposures and transplant conditioning regimens. *Results:* Twenty-nine patients developed solid cancers after BMT, which represents a two-fold increase in risk compared with a comparable normal population. The estimated cumulative probability ($\pm$ SE) for development of a solid cancer was 6.1% $\pm$ 1.6% at 10 years. The risk was significantly elevated for liver cancer (standardized incidence ratio [SIR], 27.7; 95% confidence interval [CI], 1.9 to 57.3), cancer of the oral cavity (SIR, 17.4; 95% CI, 6.3 to 34.1), and cervical cancer (SIR, 13.3; 95% CI, 3.5 to 29.6). Each of the two patients with liver cancer had a history of chronic hepatitis C infection. All six patients with squamous cell carcinoma of the skin had chronic graft-versus-host disease. The risk was significantly higher for survivors who were younger than 34 years of age at time of BMT (SIR, 5.3; 95% CI, 2.7 to 8.6). Cancers of the thyroid gland, liver, and oral cavity occurred primarily among patients who received total-body irradiation. *Conclusion:* The risk of radiation-associated solid tumor development after BMT is likely to increase with longer follow-up. This underscores the importance of close monitoring of patients who undergo BMT.

Management of recipients of hepatic allografts harvested from donors with malignancy diagnosed shortly after transplantation.

Detry O, Honore P, Jacquet N, Meurisse M.

Department of Surgery and Transplantation, CHU Sart Tilman, Liege, Belgium.

Clinical Transplantation 12(6):579–81, 1998, December.

Transmission of undiagnosed malignancy with the graft is a dramatic complication of liver transplantation. Alternatives in the management of the recipients of livers, harvested from donors with malignancy diagnosed shortly after transplantation, are either early re-transplantation or close follow-up without re-operation. We reported 4 cases of liver recipients whose allografts were harvested from donors who were diagnosed with malignancy shortly after the liver transplantation. One recipient underwent re-transplantation, and the three other allografts were not removed. No recipient developed recurrence in the follow-up. While graft removal may be the only way to avoid tumor recurrence in recipients of liver graft harvested from donor with malignancy, close follow-up without re-operation may also be considered. The risk of tumor transferral may depend on the histopathological aggressiveness and metastatic potential of the donor tumor, and may be low for low-grade, local tumors. This risk should be evaluated by analyzing large series, using databases of Eurotransplant or United Network for Organ Sharing.

Colon carcinoma in patients undergoing liver transplantation.

Fabia R, Levy MF, Testa G, Obiekwe S, Goldstein RM, Husberg BS, Gonwa TA, Klintmalm GB.

Baylor University Medical Center, Transplantation Services, Dallas, TX, USA.

American Journal of Surgery 176(3):265–9, 1998, September.

Background: Organ recipients are at risk for certain neoplasms. Ulcerative colitis (UC) is itself a strong risk factor for the development of colon carcinoma (CCa). Transplant patients with UC might be at higher risk for CCa. We analyzed these patients to compare the incidence and pattern of CCa development in these and non-UC patients following liver transplantation (OLTX). *Patients and methods:* Retrospective study of 1,085 OLTX patients. *Results:* In 1,022 patients without UC, 1 patient ($<0.1\%$) developed adenocarcinoma in a colonic polyp 46 months after OLTX. Sixty-three of 108 (60%) patients undergoing OLTX simultaneously had UC. Five OLTX patients (8%) with UC developed colon adenocarcinoma 22 to 66 (mean 48) months after OLTX. Two have died. *Conclusions:* Coexistent UC in patients requiring OLTX constitutes a potentially high risk for the development of colonic cancer, a late-appearing event. These patients require close observation and frequent colonoscopic/histologic screening of the colon.

Liver transplant recipients are not at increased risk for nonlymphoid solid organ tumors.

Kelly DM, Emre S, Guy SR, Miller CM, Schwartz ME, Sheiner PA.

Department of Surgery, King's College Hospital, London, UK.

Cancer 83(6):1237–43, 1998, September 15.

Background: Organ transplant recipients are at higher risk for developing lymphoid tumors, skin carcinomas, and sarcomas. Whether liver transplant recipients are at higher risk for developing more common cancers is unclear. *Methods:* All patients with a history of malignancy prior to liver transplantation and those who developed malignancy, either de novo or recurrent, after transplantation were identified retrospectively. The following parameters were examined: age at diagnosis; indication for transplant;

interval from transplant to tumor diagnosis; tumor treatment received; predisposing factors for the development of cancer; immunosuppression regimen, including the use of OKT3; number and treatment of rejection episodes; and survival. *Results:* Of 888 patients, 29 (3.2%) had 31 previous malignancies; of these 29 patients, 4 developed a recurrence in the posttransplant period. Thirty-nine patients (4.3%) developed 43 de novo nonlymphoid malignancies. Alcoholic cirrhotic patients had a significantly higher incidence of de novo carcinomas. Except for skin carcinomas, tumors did not occur with greater frequency than in the general population, and recurrent tumors were not more aggressive than reported for that disease. One patient had an unrecognized renal cell carcinoma at the time of transplant that progressed rapidly; this patient died 64 days after transplantation. *Conclusions:* With current immunosuppressive regimens, liver transplant patients do not appear to be at an increased risk for developing nonlymphoid solid organ tumors. However, longer follow-up will be necessary to confirm these results.

Liver transplantation for cholangiocarcinoma: results in 207 patients.

Meyer CG, Penn I, James L.

Department of Surgery, University of Cincinnati Medical Center, OH, USA.

Transplantation 69(8):1633–7, 2000, April 27.

Background: Because of the high incidence of recurrent tumor, many surgeons have become disenchanted with transplantation as a treatment for cholangiocarcinoma. *Methods:* The Cincinnati Transplant Tumor Registry database was used to examine 207 patients who underwent liver transplantation for otherwise unresectable cholangiocarcinoma or cholangiohepatoma. Specific factors evaluated included tumor size, presence of multiple nodules, evidence of tumor spread at surgery, and treatment with adjuvant chemotherapy and/or radiation therapy. Incidentally found tumors were compared to tumors that were known or suspected to be present before transplantation. *Results:* The 1, 2, and 5-year survival estimates using life table analysis were 72, 48, and 23%. Fifty-one percent of patients had recurrence of their tumors after transplantation and 84% of recurrences occurred within 2 years of transplantation. Survival after recurrence was rarely more than 1 year. Forty-seven percent of recurrences occurred in the allograft and 30% in the lungs. Tumor recurrence, and evidence of tumor spread at the time of surgery, were negative prognostic variables. There were no positive prognostic variables. Patients with incidentally found cholangiocarcinomas did not have improved survival over patients with known or suspected tumors. A small number of patients survived for more than 5 years without recurrence. However, this group had no variable in common that would aid in the selection of similar patients in the future. *Conclusions:* Because of the high rate of recurrent tumor and lack of positive prognostic variables, transplantation should seldom be used as a treatment for cholangiocarcinoma. For transplantation to be a viable treatment in the future, more effective adjuvant therapies are necessary.

Ulcerative colitis has an aggressive course after orthotopic liver transplantation for primary sclerosing cholangitis.

Papatheodoridis GV, Hamilton M, Mistry PK, Davidson B, Rolles K, Burroughs AK.

Liver Transplantation and Hepatobiliary Medicine, Royal Free Hospital, London, UK.

Gut 43(5):639–44, 1998, November.

Background: The course of inflammatory bowel disease after liver transplantation has been reported as variable with usually no change or improvement, but there may be an increased risk of early colorectal neoplasms. In many centres steroids are often withdrawn early after transplantation and this may affect inflammatory bowel disease activity. *Aims:* To evaluate the course of inflammatory bowel disease in primary sclerosing cholangitis transplant patients who were treated without long term steroids. *Methods:* Between 1989 and 1996, there were 30 patients transplanted for primary sclerosing cholangitis who survived more than 12 months. Ulcerative colitis was diagnosed in 18 (60%) patients before transplantation; two had previous colectomy. All patients underwent colonoscopy before and after transplantation and were followed for 38 (12–92) months. All received cyclosporin or tacrolimus with or without azathioprine as maintenance immunosuppression. *Results:* Ulcerative colitis course after transplantation compared with that up to five years before transplantation was the same in eight (50%) and worse in eight (50%) patients. It remained quiescent in eight and worsened in four of the 12 patients with pretransplant quiescent course, whereas it worsened in all four patients with pretransplant active course ($p = 0.08$). New onset ulcerative colitis developed in three (25%) of the 12 patients without inflammatory bowel disease before transplantation. No colorectal cancer has been diagnosed to date. *Conclusions:* Preexisting ulcerative colitis often has an aggressive course, while de novo ulcerative colitis may develop in patients transplanted for primary sclerosing cholangitis and treated without long term steroids.

Hepatic arterial complications in liver transplant recipients treated with pretransplantation chemoembolization for hepatocellular carcinoma.

Richard HM 3rd, Silberzweig JE, Mitty HA, Lou WY, Ahn J, Cooper JM.

Department of Radiology, Mount Sinai Hospital, New York, NY, USA.

Radiology 214(3):775–9, 2000, March.

Purpose: To compare the prevalence of hepatic arterial complications in patients who underwent hepatic arterial chemoembolization for hepatocellular carcinomas before orthotopic liver transplantation with the prevalence of hepatic arterial complications in the total population of liver transplant recipients. *Materials and methods:* Forty-seven patients underwent selective hepatic arterial chemoinfusion with mitomycin C, doxorubicin hydrochloride, and cisplatin combined with embolization. The prevalence rates for hepatic arterial complications, including pseudoaneurysm, stenosis, anastomotic disruption, and thrombosis, were tabulated and compared with results in

1,154 patients who underwent orthotopic liver transplantation but not chemoembolization. *Results:* Of the 47 patients who had undergone preoperative hepatic arterial chemotherapy, 13% developed hepatic arterial complications within a mean of 7 days after transplantation; an 8% prevalence of hepatic arterial thrombosis was observed. Of the 1,154 patients who underwent orthotopic liver transplantation but not chemotherapy, 6% developed hepatic arterial complications; a 5% prevalence of hepatic arterial thrombosis was observed. There was no statistically significant difference in the prevalence rates for thrombosis and complications between the patients who underwent chemoembolization before orthotopic liver transplantation and those who did not. The mean interval between chemotherapy and orthotopic liver transplantation was 111 days (range, 3–428 days). *Conclusion:* Patients who undergo hepatic arterial chemotherapy are not at an increased risk of developing hepatic arterial thrombosis or other hepatic arterial complications after orthotopic liver transplantation.

7

Peritoneal carcinomatosis, sarcomatosis, and mesothelioma: surgical responsibilities

PAUL H SUGARBAKER

INTRODUCTION

As surgical oncology expanded in the midst of a technological revolution in patient care, this discipline accepted responsibilities not only for the resection of primary tumor, but also for the surgical management of metastatic disease. For gastrointestinal cancer, early success with this new concept was with complete resection of locally recurrent colon and rectal cancer.[1,2] Then the resection of isolated liver metastases from the same diseases was shown to be of benefit to a selected group of patients.[3] Aggressive management strategies to bring about long-term survival for patients with peritoneal surface malignancy have been pioneered by our group.[4] The treatment of abdominal and pelvic malignancies that disseminate to peritoneal surfaces has grown out of extensive experience with appendiceal cancer. Appendiceal cancer became the paradigm for the successful treatment of peritoneal carcinomatosis.[5] This chapter reviews the background, the technique for cytoreduction, the standardized regional chemotherapy currently in use, and the results of the treatment of peritoneal surface malignancy. The selection factors leading to long-term benefit with acceptable morbidity and mortality are a central focus. The peritoneal surface malignancies discussed include appendiceal cancer and pseudomyxoma peritonei, colon cancer with carcinomatosis, gastric cancer with carcinomatosis, abdominopelvic sarcoma with sarcomatosis, and primary peritoneal surface malignancy including peritoneal mesothelioma, papillary serous cancer, and primary peritoneal adenocarcinoma. A discussion of the palliative treatments for debilitating ascites is included.

PRINCIPLES OF MANAGEMENT

The successful treatment of peritoneal surface malignancy requires a combined approach that utilizes cytoreductive surgery and perioperative intraperitoneal chemotherapy. In addition, proper patient selection is mandatory. The complete resection of all visible malignancy is essential for the treatment of peritoneal surface malignancy to result in long-term survival. Up to six peritonectomy procedures may be required.[6] The visceral and parietal peritonectomy procedures that one must utilize to adequately resect all visible evidence of disease are illustrated below. Their utilization depends on the distribution and extent of invasion of the malignancy disseminated within the peritoneal space. Normal peritoneum is not excised, only that which is implanted by cancer.

PERITONECTOMY PROCEDURES

If a surgeon elects to manage patients with peritoneal surface malignancy, a requirement is that he or she should be knowledgeable regarding the dissemination of cancer on peritoneal surfaces. It is imperative that the surgeon develops the technical skills and is proficient in dissection using electrosurgery.

The rationale for peritonectomy procedures

Peritonectomy procedures are necessary if one is successfully to treat peritoneal surface malignancies with curative intent. Peritonectomy procedures are used in the areas of visible cancer progression in an attempt to leave the patient with only microscopic residual disease. Isolated tumor nodules are removed using electroevaporation; involvement of the visceral peritoneum frequently requires resection of a portion of the stomach, small intestine, or colorectum. Layering of cancer on a peritoneal surface or a portion of the bowel requires peritonectomy or bowel resection for complete removal.

Locations of peritoneal surface malignancy

Peritoneal surface malignancy tends to involve the visceral peritoneum in greatest volume at three definite sites. These are sites where the bowel is anchored to the retroperitoneum and peristalsis causes less motion of the visceral peritoneal surface.

1 The rectosigmoid colon, as it emerges from the pelvis, is a non-mobile portion of the bowel. Also, it is located in a dependent site and is therefore frequently layered by carcinomatosis. Usually, a complete pelvic peritonectomy requires stripping of the abdominal sidewalls, the peritoneum overlying the bladder, the cul-de-sac, and resection of the rectosigmoid colon.
2 The ileocecal valve is another area where there is limited mobility. Resection of the terminal ileum and a small portion of the right colon is often necessary.
3 A final site often requiring resection is the antrum of the stomach, which is fixed to the rectoperitoneum at the pylorus. Tumor coming into the foramen of Winslow accumulates in the subpyloric space and may cause intestinal obstruction as a result of gastric outlet obstruction. Large volumes of tumor in the lesser omentum combined with disease in the subpyloric space will cause a confluence of disease that requires a total gastrectomy for complete cytoreduction.

Electroevaporative surgery

In order adequately to perform cytoreductive surgery, the surgeon must use electrosurgery. Peritonectomies and visceral resections using the traditional scissor and knife dissection will unnecessarily disseminate a large number of tumor cells within the abdomen. High-voltage electrosurgery leaves a margin of heat necrosis that is devoid of viable malignant cells. Not only does electroevaporation of tumor and normal tissue at the margins of resection minimize the likelihood of persistent disease, but it also minimizes blood loss. In the absence of electrosurgery, profuse bleeding from stripped peritoneal surfaces may occur; this may be specially prominent during the intraperitoneal wash with chemotherapy.

Conversion of peritoneal surface to invasive malignancy by surgery

Cancer surgery in the absence of perioperative intraperitoneal chemotherapy may actually harm patients in the long run rather than help them. If peritoneal surface malignancy is present, cancer resection without intraperitoneal chemotherapy will cause tumor cells to become implanted within a deeper layer of the abdomen and pelvis. This may contribute to obstruction of vital structures such as the ureter or common bile duct. Also, deep involvement of the pelvic sidewall and tissues along vascular structures will occur. If surgeons attempt to treat peritoneal surface malignancy, they must become thoroughly familiar with the techniques of intraperitoneal chemotherapy. Complete cytoreduction combined with aggressive perioperative intraperitoneal chemotherapy and proper patient selection are the three essential requirements of treatment for peritoneal surface malignancy.

Position and incision (Figure 7.1)

The patient is placed in the supine position with the gluteal fold advanced to the end of the operating table to allow full access to the perineum during the surgical procedure. In the lithotomy position, the weight of the legs must be directed to the soles of the feet. Myonecrosis within the gastrocnemius muscle may occur unless the legs are protected properly.

Abdominal skin preparation is from mid-chest to mid-thigh. The external genitalia are prepared in male patients and a vaginal preparation is used in female patients. A Foley catheter is placed and a silastic 18-gauge nasogastric sump tube is placed within the stomach.

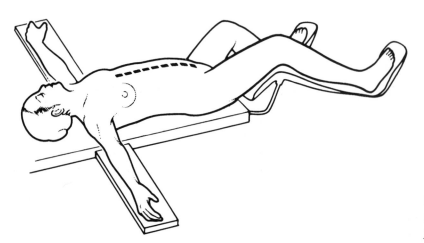

Figure 7.1 *Modified lithotomy position and maximal midline incision for cytoreductive surgery.*

Abdominal exposure, greater omentectomy, and splenectomy (Figure 7.2)

The abdomen is opened through a midline incision from xiphoid to pubis. Generous abdominal exposure is achieved through the use of a Thompson Self-Retaining Retractor (Thompson Surgical Instruments, Inc., Traverse City, MI). The standard tool used to dissect tumor on peritoneal surfaces from the normal tissues is a 3-mm ball-tipped electrosurgical handpiece (Valleylab, Boulder, CO). The ball-tipped instrument is placed at the interface of tumor and normal tissues. The focal point for further dissection is placed on strong traction. The electrosurgical generator is used on pure cut at high voltage. Electroevaporative surgery is used cautiously for tumor removal on tubular structures, especially the ureters, small bowel, and colon. Dissection of parietal peritoneal surfaces causes less risk for heat necrosis and fistula formation.

Using ball-tipped electrosurgery on pure cut creates a large volume of plume because of the electroevaporation (carbonization) of tissue. To maintain visualization of the operative field and to preserve a smoke-free atmosphere, a smoke filtration unit is used. The vacuum tip is maintained 5–8 cm from the field of dissection whenever electrosurgery is performed.

To free the mid-abdomen of a large volume of tumor, the greater omentectomy–splenectomy is performed. The greater omentum is elevated and then separated from the transverse colon using electrosurgery. This dissection continues beneath the peritoneum that covers the transverse mesocolon in order to expose the lower border of the pancreas. The branches of the gastro-epiploic arcade to the greater curvature of the stomach are clamped, ligated, and divided. Also, the short gastric vessels are transected. With traction on the spleen, the peritoneum superior to the pancreas is stripped from the gland using electrosurgery. This freely exposes the splenic artery and vein at the tail of the pancreas. These vessels are ligated in continuity and proximally suture ligated.

Left subphrenic peritonectomy (Figure 7.3)

To begin the peritonectomy procedure in the left upper quadrant, the epigastric fat and peritoneum at the edge of the abdominal incision are stripped off the posterior rectus sheath. Strong traction is exerted on the tumor specimen throughout the left upper quadrant in order to separate tumor from the diaphragmatic muscle, the left adrenal gland, and the superior half of perirenal fat. The splenic flexure of the colon is severed from the left abdominal gutter and moved medially by dividing the peritoneum along Toldt's line. Dissection beneath the peritonium covering the hemidiaphragm muscle must be performed with ball-tipped electrosurgery, not blunt dissection. Numerous blood vessels between the diaphragm muscle and its peritoneal surface must be electrocoagulated before their transection or unnecessary bleeding will occur as the divided blood vessels retract into the muscle of the diaphragm. The plane of dissection is defined using ball-tipped electrosurgery on pure cut, but all blood vessels are electrocoagulated before their division.

Left subphrenic peritonectomy completed (Figure 7.4)

When the left upper quadrant peritonectomy is completed, the stomach may be reflected medially. Numerous branches of the gastroepiploic arteries that have been ligated are evident. The left adrenal gland, pancreas, and left perinephric fat are visualized completely, as is the anterior surface of the transverse mesocolon. The surgeon must avoid the left gastric artery and vein to preserve the sole remaining vascular supply to the stomach.

Right subphrenic peritonectomy (Figure 7.5)

Peritoneum is stripped from the right posterior rectus sheath to begin the peritonectomy in the right upper quadrant of the abdomen. Strong traction on the specimen is used to elevate the hemidiaphragm into the operative field. Again, ball-tipped electrosurgery on pure cut is used to dissect at the interface of tumor and normal tissue. Coagulation current is used to divide the blood vessels as they are encountered and before they bleed.

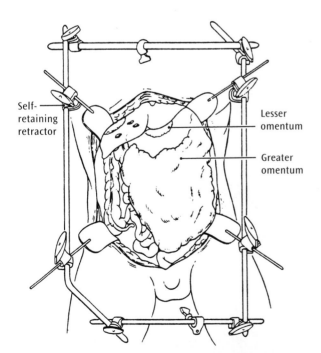

Self-retaining retractor

Lesser omentum

Greater omentum

Figure 7.2 *Abdominal exposure using a self-retaining retractor, complete greater omentectomy, and splenectomy.*

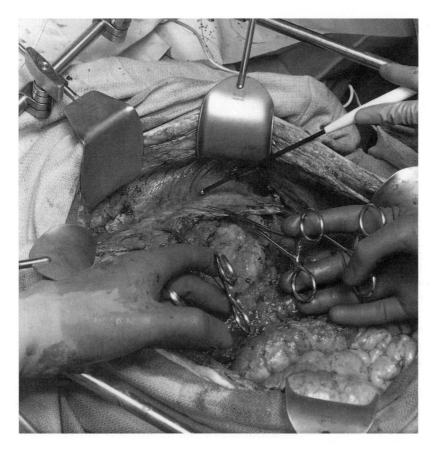

Figure 7.3 *Peritoneal stripping from the left diaphragm.*

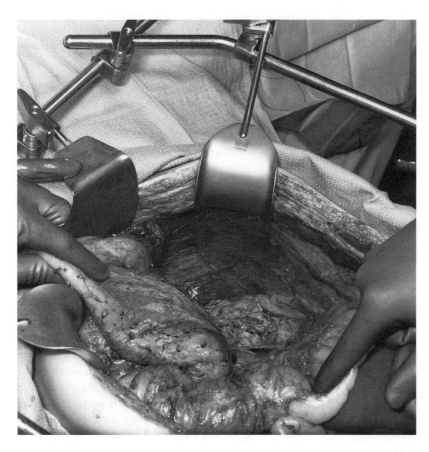

Figure 7.4 *Left subphrenic peritonectomy completed.*

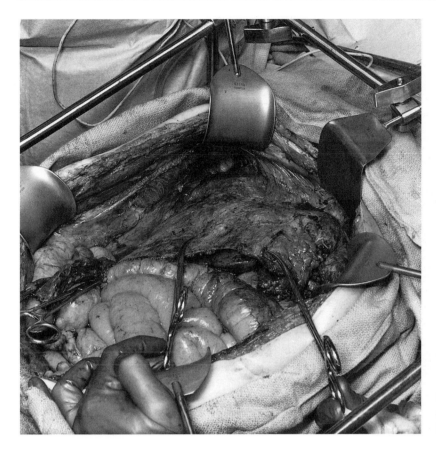

Figure 7.5 *Peritoneal stripping of the undersurface of the right hemidiaphragm.*

Stripping of tumor from Glisson's capsule (Figure 7.6)

The stripping of tumor from the undersurface of the right hemidiaphragm continues until the bare area of the liver is encountered. At that point, tumor on the superior surface of the liver is electroevaporated until the liver surface is cleared. With ball-tipped electroevaporative dissection, a thick layer of tumor may be lifted off the liver surface by moving beneath Glisson's capsule. Isolated patches of tumor on the liver surface are electroevaporated with the distal 2 cm of the ball tip bent and stripped of insulation ('hockey-stick' configuration). Ball-tipped electrosurgery is also used to extirpate tumor from the attachments of the falciform ligament and round ligament.

Tumor from beneath the right hemidiaphragm, from the right subhepatic space, and from the surface of the liver forms an envelope as it is removed *en bloc*. The dissection is greatly facilitated if the tumor specimen can be maintained intact. The dissection continues laterally on the right to encounter the perirenal fat covering the right kidney. Also, the right adrenal gland is visualized and carefully avoided as tumor is stripped from the right subhepatic space. Care is taken not to traumatize the vena cava or to disrupt the caudate lobe veins that pass between the vena cava and segment 1 of the liver.

Completed right subphrenic peritonectomy (Figure 7.7)

With strong upward traction on the right costal margin by the self-retaining retractor and medial displacement of the right liver, one can visualize the completed right subphrenic peritonectomy. The anterior branches of the phrenic artery and vein on the hemidiaphragm are seen and have been preserved. The right hepatic vein and the vena cava below have been exposed. The right subhepatic space, including the right adrenal gland and perirenal fat covering the right kidney, constitutes the base of the dissection.

If the malignancy is invasive, tumor is densely adherent to the tendinous central portion of the left or right hemidiaphragm. If this occurs, the normal tissue infiltrated by tumor must be resected. This usually requires an elliptical excision of a portion of the hemidiaphragm on either the right or the left side. The defect in the diaphragm is closed with interrupted sutures after the intraoperative chemotherapy of both chest and abdomen is completed.

Lesser omentectomy and cholecystectomy with stripping of the hepatoduodenal ligament (Figure 7.8)

The gallbladder is removed in a routine fashion from its fundus toward the cystic artery and cystic duct. These

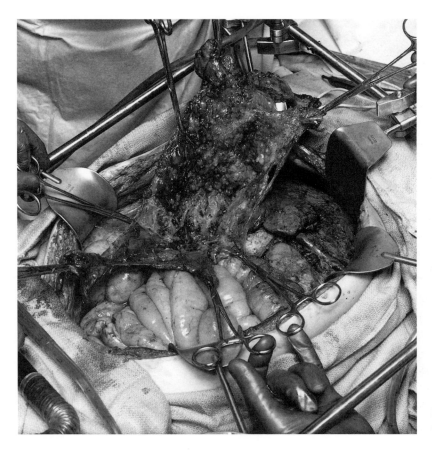

Figure 7.6 *Stripping of tumor from Glisson's capsule.*

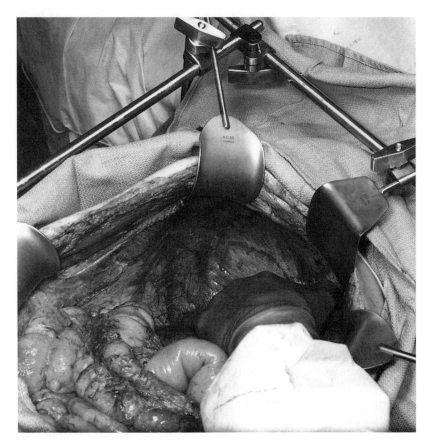

Figure 7.7 *Completed right subphrenic peritonectomy.*

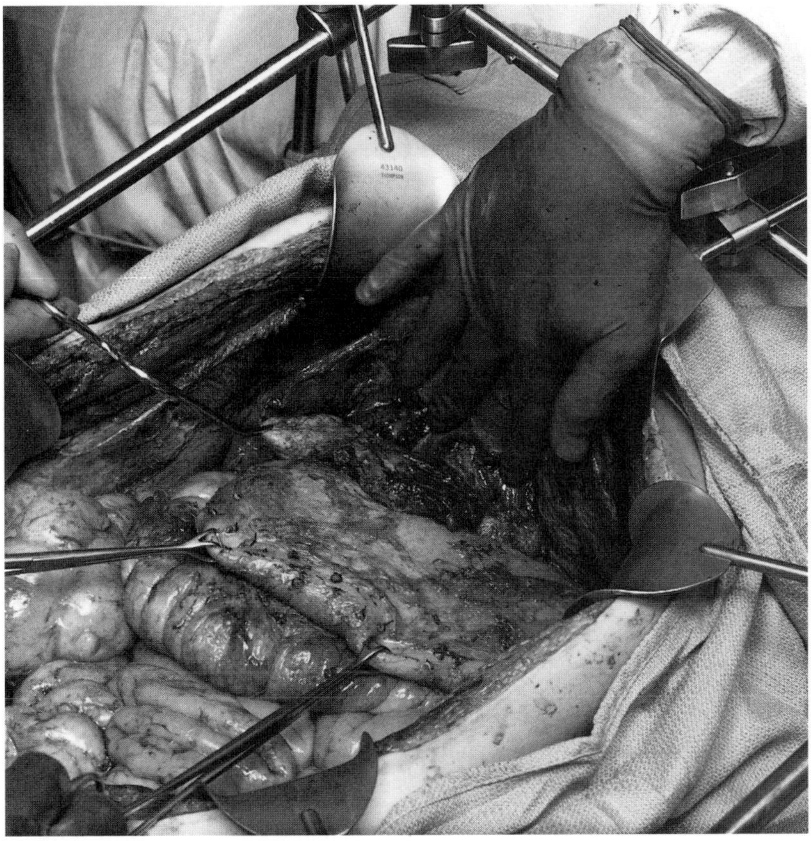

Figure 7.8 *Lesser omentectomy and cholecystectomy with stripping of the porta hepatis.*

structures are ligated and divided. The hepatoduodenal ligament is characteristically heavily layered with tumor. Using strong traction, the cancerous tissue that coats the porta hepatis is bluntly stripped from the base of the gallbladder bed toward the duodenum. The right gastric artery going to the lesser omental arcade is preserved. To continue resection of the lesser omentum, the surgeon separates the gastrohepatic ligament from the fissure that divides liver segments 2, 3, and 4 from segment 1. Ball-tipped electrosurgery is used to electroevaporate tumor from the surface of the caudate process. Care is taken not to traumatize the anterior surface of the caudate process, for this can result in excessive and needless blood loss. The segmental blood supply to the caudate lobe is located on the anterior surface of this segment of the liver, and hemorrhage may occur with only superficial trauma. Also, care must be taken to avoid an accesory left hepatic artery, which may arise from the left gastric artery and cross through the hepatogastric fissure.

Stripping of the omental bursa (Figure 7.9)

As one clears the left side of liver segment 1 of tumor, the vena cava is visualized beneath. To begin to strip the omental bursa, strong traction is maintained on the tumor, and ball-tipped electrosurgery is used to divide the fibrous tissue between liver segment 1 and the vena cava. The phrenoesophageal ligament is incised in order for the peritoneum to be elevated away from the crus of the right hemidiaphragm. The common hepatic artery and the left gastric artery are skeletonized and lymph nodes in this region are avoided. The branches of the left gastric artery and vein are identified and avoided. Separation of tumor from lesser omental fat by compressing tissue between the thumb and index finger helps identify the major branches of the left gastric artery. Omental fat not involved by tumor is preserved to ensure adequate blood supply to the stomach. At least two major branches of the left gastric artery to the lesser curvature of the stomach are required to provide blood supply to the stomach.

The surgeon dissects in a clockwise direction along the lesser curvature of the stomach, attempting to preserve the arcade between the right and left gastric arteries. Care is taken to preserve as much omental fat as possible and to attempt to remove tumor tissue only. Efforts are made to spare the anterior vagus nerve going toward the antrum of the stomach.

A pyloroplasty or gastrojejunostomy must be performed if a truncal vagotomy was necessary. As a result of the anterior vagotomy and in the absence of a gastric drainage procedure, gastric stasis may occur.

Complete pelvic peritonectomy (Figure 7.10)

The tumor-bearing peritoneum is stripped from the posterior surface of the lower abdominal incision, exposing

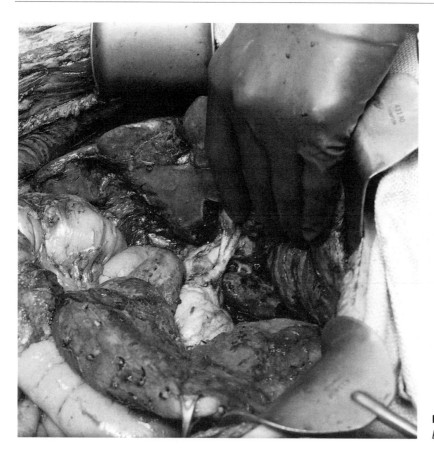

Figure 7.9 *Stripping of the omental bursa.*

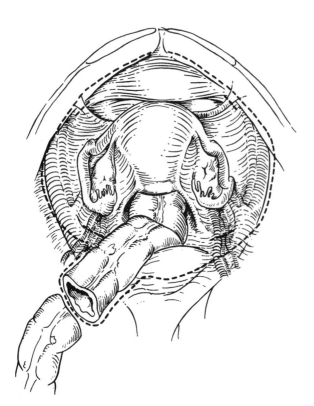

Figure 7.10 *Complete pelvic peritonectomy.*

the rectus muscle. The muscular surface of the bladder is revealed as ball-tipped electrosurgery strips peritoneum and preperitoneal fat from this structure. The urachus must be divided and is then elevated on a clamp as the leading point for this dissection. In women, the round ligaments are divided as they enter the internal inguinal ring.

The peritoneal incision around the pelvis is connected to the peritoneal incisions of the right and left paracolic sulci. The right and left ureters are identified and preserved. In women, the right and left ovarian veins are ligated at the level of the lower pole of the kidney and divided. A linear stapler is used to divide the sigmoid colon just above the limits of the pelvic tumor. The vascular supply of the distal portion of the bowel is traced back to its origin on the aorta. The inferior mesenteric artery is suture ligated and divided. This allows one to pack all the viscera, including the proximal sigmoid colon, in the upper abdomen.

Resection of rectosigmoid colon and cul-de-sac of Douglas (Figure 7.11)

Electrosurgery is used to dissect at the limits of the mesorectum. The surgeon works in a centripetal fashion. Extraperitoneal ligation of the uterine arteries is performed just above the ureter and close to the base of the

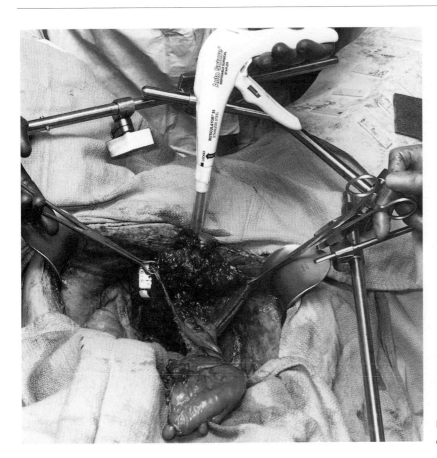

Figure 7.11 *Resection of rectosigmoid colon and cul-de-sac of Douglas.*

bladder. The bladder is moved gently off the cervix and the vagina is entered. The vaginal cuff anterior and posterior to the cervix is transected using electrosurgery, and the rectovaginal septum is entered. The perirectal fat is divided beneath the peritoneal reflection so that all tumor that occupies the cul-de-sac is removed intact with the specimen. The rectal musculature is skeletonized using electrosurgery so that a stapler can be used to close off the rectal stump. The rectum is sharply divided above the stapler.

Vaginal closure and low colorectal anastomosis (Figure 7.12)

One of the few suture repairs performed prior to the intraoperative chemotherapy is the closure of the vaginal cuff. If one fails to close the vaginal cuff, chemotherapy solution will leak from the vagina. The circular stapled colorectal anastomosis occurs after the intraoperative chemotherapy has been completed. A circular stapling device is passed into the rectum, and the trochar penetrates the staple line. A purse-string applier is used to secure the staple anvil in the proximal sigmoid colon. The body of the circular stapler and anvil are mated and the stapler is activated to complete the low colorectal anastomosis.

Descending colon mobilization for a tension-free low colorectal anastomosis (Figure 7.13)

An absolute requirement for a complication-free low colorectal anastomosis is the absence of tension on the staple line. Adequate mobilization of the entire left colon is needed, and several steps may be required to accomplish this. The inferior mesenteric artery is ligated on the aorta, and then its individual branches are resected as they arise from this vascular trunk. The Y-configuration of the sigmoidal vessels is converted to a V-configuration to keep the intermediate arcade intact. The inferior mesenteric vein is divided as it courses around the duodenum. The mesentery of the transverse colon and splenic flexure are completely elevated from the perirenal fat surrounding the left kidney. Taking care to avoid the left ureter, the surgeon divides the left colon mesentery from all its retroperitoneal attachments. These maneuvers allow the junction of the sigmoid and descending colon to reach to the low rectum or anus for a tension-free anastomosis. Redundant descending colon should fall into the hollow of the sacrum.

To assess the stapled colorectal anastomosis, the proximal and distal tissue rings are examined for completeness. Air is insufflated into the rectum with a water-filled pelvis to check for an airtight circle of staples. Two hands

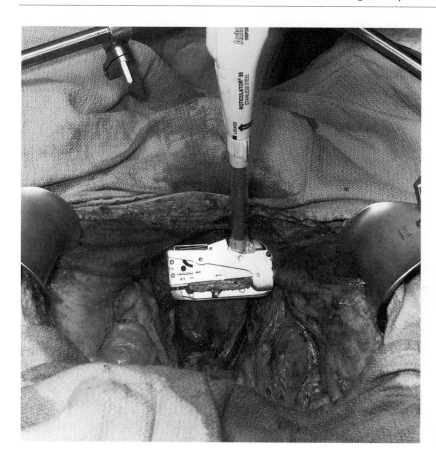

Figure 7.12 *Vaginal closure and low colorectal anastomosis.*

should easily pass beneath the sigmoid colon to ensure there is no tension on the stapled anastomosis. A rectal examination is done to check for staple-line bleeding at the anastomosis.

Total gastrectomy with staged reconstruction (Figure 7.14)

In approximately 10% of patients with appendiceal mucinous tumors, a total gastrectomy will be needed to clear the left upper quadrant of mucinous tumor. In most instances, this indicates that the tumor has an aggressive character. Alternatively, the patient may have had many prior surgical procedures with prior extensive dissection in the left upper quadrant.

To perform the gastrectomy, the esophagus is closed off with a linear stapler and is then transected. The left gastric artery is ligated and suture ligated. Final attachments of the stomach to the superior portion of the head of the pancreas are divided using electrosurgery. Great care is taken not to damage the anterior surface of the pancreas.

In order to reconstruct the gastrointestinal tract after gastrectomy as part of a complete cytoreduction, a duodenal exclusion operation is performed which protects the esophagojejunal anastomosis. Approximately 20 cm below the ligament of Treitz, a portion of jejunum is transected with a linear stapler and brought in a retrocolic

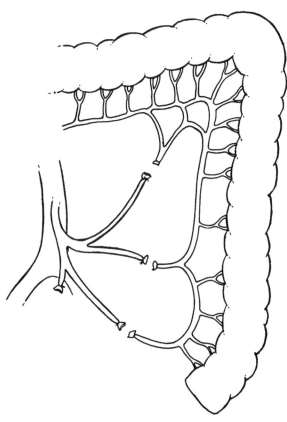

Figure 7.13 *Left colon mobilization for a low colorectal anastomosis.*

fashion up to the esophagus. The esophageal staple line is removed and a purse-string applier is used to secure the anvil of a circular stapler in the distal esophagus. The staple line closing the proximal jejunum is removed and the stapler is passed approximately 5 cm into the jejunum and then out through the jejunal wall. It is mated with the anvil within the esophagus, and the staple line is completed. The proximal jejunum is stapled off, and then the staple line is inverted with interrupted sutures. This reconstruction is performed after the intraoperative chemotherapy is complete.

The portion of jejunum proximal to the linear staple line is now brought out in the left upper quadrant as an endostomy in order to divert all bile and digestive

enzymes from the gastrointestinal tract. This diverting jejunostomy is closed between 6 and 9 months postoperatively as part of a second-look procedure.

Tubes and drains required for intraoperative and early postoperative intraperitoneal chemotherapy (Figure 7.15)

Four closed-suction drains are placed in the dependent portions of the abdomen: one in the right subhepatic space, one in the left subdiaphragmatic space, and two in the pelvis. A Tenckhoff catheter is placed through the abdominal wall and positioned within the abdomen at the site that is thought to be the area of greatest risk for recurrence. All transabdominal drains and tubes are secured to the skin in a watertight fashion with purse-string suture. Temperature probes are placed at the inflow site (Tenckhoff catheter) and at a remote site. The temperature probes are removed after the intraoperative chemotherapy has been completed, but all closed suction drains are retained. Right-angle thoracostomy tubes (Deknatel, Floral Park, NY) are inserted on both the right and left sides to prevent abdominal fluid from accumulating in the chest as a result of the subphrenic peritonectomy.

INTRAPERITONEAL CHEMOTHERAPY

Conceptual changes with intraperitoneal chemotherapy

Modifications in the use of chemotherapy in patients with peritoneal carcinomatosis, peritoneal sarcomatosis,

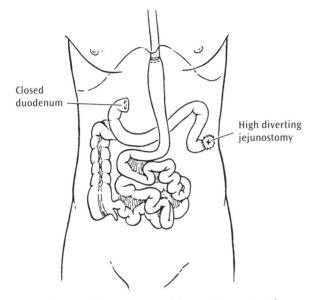

Figure 7.14 *Total gastrectomy with staged reconstruction.*

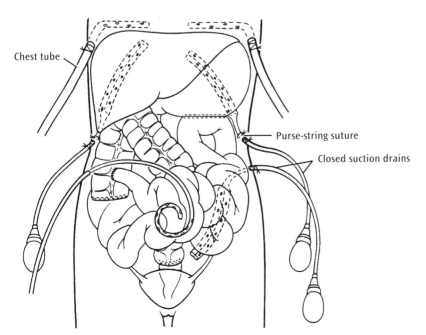

Figure 7.15 *The tubes and drains required for intraoperative and early postoperative intraperitoneal chemotherapy.*

and peritoneal mesothelioma have occurred and have shown favorable results of treatment.

1 A change in the *route* of drug administration has occurred. Chemotherapy is given intraperitoneally, or by combined intraperitoneal and intravenous routes. Intravenous chemotherapy alone is rarely indicated and has shown minimal benefits.

2 A change in *timing* has occurred in that chemotherapy begins in the operating room and may be continued for the first 5 postoperative days.

3 A change in the *selection* criteria for treatment of cancer has occurred. The non-aggressive peritoneal surface malignancies are selected for complete cytoreduction because they are minimally invasive of the peritoneal surfaces. For other malignancies, the lesion size and the distribution of peritoneal implants are of crucial importance. Patients with small intraperitoneal tumor nodules that have a limited distribution within the abdomen and pelvis and can be completely cytoreduced are likely to show prolonged benefit.

Aggressive treatment strategies for an advanced and invasive intraperitoneal malignancy will not produce long-term benefits, and are often the cause of excessive morbidity or mortality. The initiation of treatments for peritoneal surface malignancy must occur as early as possible in the natural history of these diseases in order to achieve the greatest benefits. A significant proportion of these patients are cured with the early application of combined treatments.

Background

Cancers that occur within the abdomen or pelvis will disseminate by three different routes: by hematogenous metastases, lymphatic metastases, and spread through the peritoneal space to surfaces within the abdomen and pelvis. In a substantial number of patients with abdominal or pelvic malignancy, surgical treatment failure is isolated to the resection site or to peritoneal surfaces. This suggests that the effective treatment of peritoneal surface malignancy may have an impact on the survival of these cancer patients. Also, it would eliminate a leading cause of suffering in patients with these malignancies. Prior to the use of cytoreductive surgery and intraperitoneal chemotherapy, these conditions were uniformly fatal, eventually resulting in intestinal obstruction. Occasionally, patients with low-grade malignancies such as pseudomyxoma peritonei and cystic mesothelioma have survived for several years, but all reports of end results show a fatal outcome.

Current technology for the administration of intraperitoneal chemotherapy demands that it be used as an integral part of the surgical procedure. Several crucial technological modifications of chemotherapy administration are required:

1 An intraperitoneal rather than an intravenous route for chemotherapy is used. The intraperitoneal route, when properly utilized, will allow uniform distribution of a high concentration of anticancer therapy at the site of the malignancy. This is achieved by the surgeon intraoperatively manipulating the intestinal contents to distribute the chemotherapy uniformly. In the early postoperative period, the patient's position is repeatedly changed to assist gravity in maintaining an optimal chemotherapy distribution.

2 The chemotherapy administration is timed so that all of the malignancy, except for microscopic residual disease, will have been removed prior to the chemotherapy treatments. This means that the limited penetration of chemotherapy into tissues, which is approximately 1 mm, will be adequate to eradicate all tumor cells. Also, the chemotherapy will be used prior to the construction of any anastomosis. This means that suture-line recurrences should also be eliminated. Finally, because all adhesions were resected during cytoreduction, there will be no surfaces in the abdomen or pelvis excluded by scar tissue from contact with chemotherapy solutions.

The combined treatments of cytoreductive surgery and intraperitoneal chemotherapy must be used as early in the natural history of the cancer as is possible. No longer can the clinician wait for the patient with peritoneal carcinomatosis to become symptomatic to begin treatments. The treatment of patients with an invasive malignancy that has a wide distribution of a large mass of cancer will not produce long-term benefits. Peritoneal surface malignancy can be cured, but an optimal result requires these aggressive treatments to be initiated in a timely fashion.

Peritoneal–plasma barrier

Intraperitoneal chemotherapy gives high response rates within the abdomen because the 'peritoneal–plasma barrier' provides dose-intensive therapy.[7] Many chemotherapy agents are large molecular weight substances, so they are confined to the abdominal cavity for long time periods.[8] This means that the exposure of peritoneal surfaces to pharmacologically active molecules can be greatly increased by giving the drugs via the intraperitoneal route rather than the intravenous route.

For the chemotherapy agents used to treat peritoneal carcinomatosis or peritoneal sarcomatosis, the area under the curve ratios of intraperitoneal to intravenous exposure are favorable. Table 7.1 presents the area under the curve (intraperitoneal/intravenous) for the drugs in routine clinical use for patients with peritoneal seeding. In our studies, these include 5-fluorouracil, mitomycin C, doxorubicin, cisplatin, paclitaxel, and gemcitabine.

One should not assume that the intraperitoneal administration of chemotherapy eliminates the systemic

Table 7.1 *Area under the curve (concentration of drug times the duration of exposure) ratios of peritoneal surface exposure to systemic exposure for drugs used to treat intra-abdominal cancer*

Drug	Molecular weight (Da)	Area under the curve ratio
5-Fluorouracil	130	250
Mitomycin C	334	75
Doxorubicin	544	500
Cisplatin	300	20
Paclitaxel	808	1000
Gemcitabine	263	50

toxicities of the drugs used. Although the drugs are sequestered within the peritoneal space, they are eventually cleared into the systemic circulation. For this reason, the safe doses of most drugs instilled into the peritoneal cavity are identical to the intravenous dose. The exceptions are drugs with hepatic metabolism such as 5-fluorouracil and gemcitabine. An increased dose of approximately 50% is usually possible with 5-fluorouracil. The dose for a 5-day course of intravenous 5-fluorouracil is approximately 500 mg/m^2; for intraperitoneal 5-fluorouracil, the dose is 750 mg/m^2 per day. This increase (approximately 50%) in the dose of 5-fluorouracil is of great advantage in treating peritoneal carcinomatosis.

Tumor-cell entrapment

Tumor-cell entrapment may explain the rapid progression of peritoneal surface malignancy in patients who undergo treatment using surgery alone. This theory relates the high incidence and rapid progression of peritoneal surface implantation to the fibrin entrapment of intra-abdominal tumor emboli on traumatized peritoneal surfaces and to the progression of these entrapped tumor cells through growth factors involved in the wound-healing process. Tumor-cell entrapment may cause a high incidence of surgical treatment failure in patients treated for primary gastrointestinal cancer. Also, the reimplantation of malignant cells into peritonectomized surfaces in a reoperative setting must be expected unless intraperitoneal chemotherapy is used.

Chemotherapy employed in the perioperative period not only directly destroys tumor cells, but also eliminates viable platelets, white blood cells, and monocytes from the peritoneal cavity. This diminishes the promotion of tumor growth associated with the wound-healing process. Removal of the leukocytes and monocytes also decreases the ability of the abdomen to resist an infectious process. For this reason, strict aseptic technique is imperative when administering the chemotherapy or handling abdominal tubes and drains.

In order to eradicate the implantation of tumor cells on abdominal and pelvic surfaces, the abdominal cavity is flooded with chemotherapy in a large volume of fluid during the operation as heated intraoperative intraperitoneal chemotherapy, and in the postoperative period as early postoperative intraperitoneal chemotherapy.

Prior limited benefits with intraperitoneal chemotherapy

The use of intraperitoneal chemotherapy in the past has met with limited success and acceptance by oncologists. There have been three major impediments to greater benefits:

1 Intracavitary instillation allows very *limited penetration* of drug into tumor nodules. Only the outermost layer (approximately 1 mm) of a cancer nodule is penetrated by the chemotherapy. This means that only minute tumor nodules can be definitely treated. In most trials, oncologists have attempted to treat established disease, and this improper selection of patients has resulted in disappointment with intraperitoneal drug use. Microscopic residual disease is the ideal target for intraperitoneal chemotherapy protocols.

2 A second cause for disappointment with intraperitoneal chemotherapy is a *non-uniform drug distribution*. A majority of patients treated by drug instillation into the abdomen or pelvis have had prior surgery, which invariably causes scarring between peritoneal surfaces. The adhesions create multiple barriers to the free access of fluid. Although the instillation of a large volume of fluid will partially overcome the problems created by adhesions, large surface areas will often have no access to chemotherapy. Limited access from adhesions is impossible to predict and may increase with repeated instillations of chemotherapy.

Not only do adhesions interfere with chemotherapy distribution, they also sequester cancer cells away from chemotherapy. Surgery causes fibrin deposits on surfaces that have been traumatized by the cancer resection. Free intraperitoneal cancer cells become trapped within the fibrin. The fibrin is infiltrated by platelets, neutrophils, and monocytes as part of the wound-healing process. As collagen is laid down, the tumor cells are entrapped within scar tissue. The scar tissue is dense and is not penetrated by intraperitoneal chemotherapy.

Non-uniform drug distribution may be caused by gravity. Intraperitoneal fluid does not uniformly distribute itself to anterior peritoneal surfaces. Gravity pulls the fluid to dependent areas, especially the pelvis, paracolic gutters, and right retrohepatic space. Unless the patient actively pursues frequent changes in position, the surfaces between the bowel loops and the anterior abdominal wall will remain relatively untreated.

3 A final obstacle to success in the past is the *difficulty* and *dangers* of *long-term peritoneal access*. There has

been no technical solution to the requirement for reliable access to the peritoneal space. Repeated instillations of large volumes of chemotherapy solution cause great inconvenience and can result in a large number of serious complications. Whether the oncologist chooses repeated paracentesis or an indwelling catheter, complications such as pain upon instillation, bowel perforation, instillation into soft tissues, or inability to infuse or drain occur repeatedly. At this time, prolonged peritoneal access is a technical challenge without a known solution.

The limitations of penetration, distribution, and repeated access have led to the development of surgically directed chemotherapy. All visible abdominal or pelvic cancer should be completely extirpated by surgery. Then, in the operating room, a high dose of heated chemotherapy is delivered with manual distribution to eradicate tiny tumor nodules and microscopic cancer cells. This means that all abdominal and pelvic components of the cancer, including persistent peritoneal surface malignancy, are eliminated. Systemic components of the disease now become the responsibility of the medical oncologist.

Clinical evidence that cytoreductive surgery and intraperitoneal chemotherapy are of benefit to patients with peritoneal surface malignancy

Treatments for peritoneal carcinomatosis and sarcomatosis have been shown to provide prolonged survival, with some patients alive at 5 years and considered cured. As discussed above, the strategy for treating these patients has always involved three essential components:

1 The first component is a *complete cytoreduction*, utilizing peritonectomy procedures with an attempt to remove all visible tumor.
2 Assuming that microscopic residual disease will eventuate in recurrence in all these patients, the second component involves *perioperative intraperitoneal chemotherapy*.
3 It is becoming increasingly clear that *proper patient selection* is the third essential component of these treatment strategies.

Although no one questions the essential need for complete cytoreduction and for accurate patient selection, many oncologists are not convinced that the intraperitoneal chemotherapy is of benefit to prevent the recurrence of peritoneal surface disease. There are data from prospective trials and from clinical observations that show that intraperitoneal chemotherapy is effective in reducing or eliminating the recurrence of peritoneal carcinomatosis after surgery.

The first data come from prospective clinical trials. Sugarbaker and coworkers conducted a trial in patients with poor prognosis colon cancer.[9] Intravenous 5-fluorouracil was randomized against intraperitoneal 5-fluorouracil. Each cycle of treatment was given for 5 days, and the treatments were repeated on a monthly basis for 1 year. Patients who recurred were explored, and the status of their disease was assessed during the surgery. A statistically significant decrease in the incidence of peritoneal carcinomatosis occurred in patients who had received intraperitoneal 5-fluorouracil ($p = 0.003$). In this small group of poor prognosis patients, there was no improvement in survival, but there was a great reduction in the incidence of recurrence of peritoneal carcinomatosis in the patients receiving intraperitoneal 5-fluorouracil.

Several prospective, randomized studies of peritoneal carcinomatosis from gastric cancer have been reported. In all but one of these trials, the intraperitoneal chemotherapy was given in the perioperative period. There was an improved survival in all seven trials utilizing perioperative intraperitoneal chemotherapy.[10]

In the study by Yu *et al.*, perioperative intraperitoneal mitomycin C and 5-fluorouracil were used for the first 5 days following gastrectomy. This combined treatment was compared to gastrectomy alone, with a statistically significant survival advantage ($p = 0.02$). In patients with stage III disease, the survival advantage was even more impressive ($p = 0.001$). These data strongly suggest that microscopic residual disease can be eliminated by adjuvant perioperative intraperitoneal chemotherapy.[11]

Data provided by Gough and coworkers at the Mayo Clinic of patients with pseudomyxoma peritonei suggested that intraperitoneal chemotherapy was effective in this patient population. In their report on 56 patients, the only long-term survivors were those who had both surgery and intraperitoneal chemotherapy. Patients who had only repeated surgeries had a median survival of 3 years, and only 5% of these patients were alive at the end of 5 years.[12]

The patterns of recurrence in patients treated with intraperitoneal chemotherapy have shown marked differences in the incidence of recurrence in the abdomen as compared to other anatomic sites. Zoetmulder and colleagues demonstrated that diaphragm perforation in patients with pseudomyxoma peritonei that occurred at the time of cytoreduction was associated with disease progression within the pleural space in 10 of 11 patients.[13] In contrast, there was disease control within the abdomen where intraperitoneal chemotherapy was used in these patients. Small-volume disease that entered the chest through a diaphragm perforation without intrapleural chemotherapy resulted in progression. Much larger residual disease found in the abdomen was controlled with perioperative intraperitoneal chemotherapy. Likewise, if drain tracts are used in patients with known peritoneal carcinomatosis, they will become involved by disease. Drain tracts in patients undergoing cytoreductive surgery with intraperitoneal chemotherapy seldom, if ever, develop abdominal wall recurrence. Similarly, the abdominal incision is frequently involved if surgery only is used to treat peritoneal carcinomatosis or sarcomatosis. If the surgery is combined with intraperitoneal chemotherapy, disease within the abdominal incision is not seen. This is also true in ovarian cancer patients with vaginal cuff recurrence. If the vaginal cuff is closed without intraperitoneal chemotherapy, ovarian cancer is inoculated into this anatomic site. If intraperitoneal chemotherapy is used after an ovarian cancer cytoreduction, no recurrence within the vaginal cuff has been observed.[14]

There is a very definite correlation of the pattern of failure in patients receiving early postoperative intraperitoneal chemotherapy with dye studies that show non-uniform distribution of intraperitoneal chemotherapy in a closed abdomen. Zoetmulder found that recurrence in patients with appendiceal mucinous tumors was most likely to occur within the abdominal incision, within colorectal or gastrojejunal suture lines, and at the base of the small bowel mesentery.[13] In patients given early postoperative intraperitoneal chemotherapy, the closure of the abdominal incision and suture lines prevents adequate chemotherapy access at these sites. Another common area for recurrence was the anterior surface of the stomach. Dye studies have shown that the left lobe of the liver almost invariably becomes adherent to the anterior surface of the stomach in patients treated with a closed intraperitoneal chemotherapy technique. Also, dye studies have demonstrated poor chemotherapy access to the base of the small bowel mesentery. These data strongly suggest that peritoneal surface malignancy recurs where there is imperfect exposure to the intraperitoneal chemotherapy. Other sites that have been noted to have a high incidence of recurrence after the use of intraperitoneal chemotherapy are the inverted appendiceal stump and umbilical fissure.

Elias and coworkers reported an interesting pattern of recurrence in those patients who were treated using a peritoneal expander to deliver intraperitoneal chemotherapy. They observed a high incidence of recurrent disease where the peritoneal expander contacted the peritoneal surface at the edges of the abdominal incision. Cancer cells were pressed into the peritoneal surface at this site and were prevented from coming into contact with the heated chemotherapy solution (personal communication).

Finally, surgery has been used for many decades in an attempt to treat patients with recurrent intra-abdominal cancer; but surgery alone has always been unsuccessful. Not a single report in the surgical literature suggests long-term survival by surgery alone. Data presented in this review clearly show that there is a high salvage rate in properly selected patients who are treated with cytoreductive surgery combined with adequate intraperitoneal chemotherapy. These data taken together strongly suggest that intraperitoneal chemotherapy is an essential component of treatment protocols for peritoneal surface malignancies.

PATIENT SELECTION FOR TREATMENT

The greatest impediment to lasting benefits from intraperitoneal chemotherapy should be attributed to improper patient selection. A great number of patients with advanced intra-abdominal disease have been treated, with minimal benefit. Excluding pseudomyxoma peritonei patients, extensive cytoreductive surgery and aggressive intraperitoneal chemotherapy are not likely to produce a lasting benefit. Rapid recurrence of peritoneal surface cancer combined with progression of lymph nodal or systemic disease are likely to interrupt long-term survival in these patients. Patients who benefit must have minimal peritoneal surface disease isolated to peritoneal surfaces so that complete cytoreduction can occur. Uniform access to chemotherapy is required so that complete eradication of disease can occur. In the natural history of this disease, the early initiation of treatment has a great bearing on the benefits achieved. Asymptomatic patients with small-volume peritoneal surface malignancy must be selected for the combined treatment.

Clinical assessments of peritoneal surface malignancy

In the past, peritoneal carcinomatosis was considered to be a fatal disease process. The only assessment used was either carcinomatosis *present*, with a presumed fatal outcome, *or* carcinomatosis *absent*, with curative treatment options available. Currently, there are four important clinical assessments of peritoneal surface malignancy that need to be used to select patients who will benefit from treatment protocols:

1 the histopathology to assess the invasive character of the malignancy;
2 the preoperative computerized tomography (CT) scan of abdomen and pelvis;
3 the Peritoneal Cancer Index;
4 the completeness of cytoreduction (CC) score.

Histopathology to assess invasive character

The biological aggressiveness of a peritoneal surface malignancy will have a profound influence on its treatment options. Non-invasive tumors such as pseudomyxoma peritonei or cystic mesothelioma may have extensive spread on peritoneal surfaces and yet be completely resectable by peritonectomy procedures. Also, these non-invasive malignancies are extremely unlikely to metastasize by the lymphatics to lymph nodes and by the blood to the liver and other systemic sites. Therefore, protocols for cytoreductive surgery and intraperitoneal chemotherapy may have a curative intent in patients with a large mass of widely disseminated pseudomyxoma peritonei and well-differentiated peritoneal mesothelioma.[15,16] Also, some

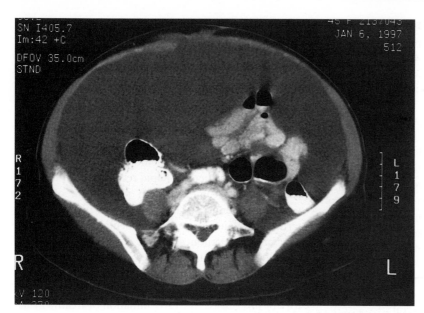

Figure 7.16 *A patient with adenomucinosis of appendiceal origin (pseudomyxoma peritonei syndrome) who had a complete cytoreduction and remains disease free at 2 years postoperatively. The mucinous tumor is very extensive, but the small bowel loops are of normal caliber and are not distended by air. Also, the small bowel has become 'compartmentalized' by the mucinous tumor. The small bowel surfaces and small bowel mesentery remain tumor free.*

low-grade sarcomas, despite extensive disease progression, may be aggressively treated with cure as a goal using cytoreductive surgery and intraperitoneal chemotherapy. Pathology review and an assessment of the invasive or non-aggressive nature of a malignancy are essential to treatment planning.

Preoperative CT scan

The preoperative CT scan of the chest, abdomen, and pelvis may be of great value in planning treatments for peritoneal surface malignancy. Systemic metastases can be clinically excluded and pleural surface spread ruled out. Unfortunately, the CT scan should be regarded as an inaccurate test by which to quantitate the intestinal type of peritoneal carcinomatosis from adenocarcinoma. The malignant tissue progresses on the peritoneal surfaces and its shape conforms to the normal contours of the abdominopelvic structures. This is quite different from the metastatic process in the liver or lung, which progresses as three-dimensional tumor nodules and can be accurately assessed by CT.[17]

However, the CT scan has been of great help in locating and quantitating *mucinous* adenocarcinoma within the peritoneal cavity.[18] These tumors produce large volumes of mucoid material that is readily distinguished by shape and density from normal structures. Using two distinctive radiologic criteria, those patients with a high likelihood of complete cytoreduction can be selected from those with non-resectable malignancy. This prevents patients who are unlikely to benefit from undergoing expensive cytoreductive surgical procedures. The two radiologic criteria found to be most useful are:

1 segmental obstruction of small bowel,
2 the presence of tumor nodules greater than 5 cm in diameter on small bowel surfaces or directly

adjacent to small bowel mesentery of jejunum and upper ileum.

These criteria reflect radiologically the biology of the mucinous adenocarcinoma. Obstructed segments of bowel signal an invasive character of malignancy on small bowel surfaces that would be unlikely to be completely cytoreduced. Mucinous cancer on small bowel or small bowel mesentery indicates that the mucinous cancer is no longer redistributed. This means that small bowel surfaces or small bowel mesentery will have residual disease after cytoreduction, because these surfaces are impossible to peritonectomize (Figures 7.16 and 7.17).

The CT scan is also of great help in the identification of nodules of recurrent sarcoma and sarcomatosis. The recurrences on peritoneal surfaces are nodular and the result of fibrin entrapment of traumatically disseminated sarcoma cells. In a CT scan with maximal filling of bowel with oral contrast, even small, 1 cm, nodular sarcoma recurrences are imaged.

Peritoneal cancer index

The third assessment of peritoneal surface malignancy is the Peritoneal Cancer Index. This is a clinical integration of both peritoneal implant size and distribution of nodules on the peritoneal surface (Figure 7.18). It should be used in the decision-making process as the abdomen is completely explored. To arrive at a score, the size of intraperitoneal nodules must be assessed. The lesion size (LS) score should be used. An LS-0 score means that no malignant deposits are visualized. An LS-1 score signifies that tumor nodules less than 0.5 cm are present. The number of nodules is not scored, only the size of the largest nodule. An LS-2 score signifies that tumor nodules between 0.5 and

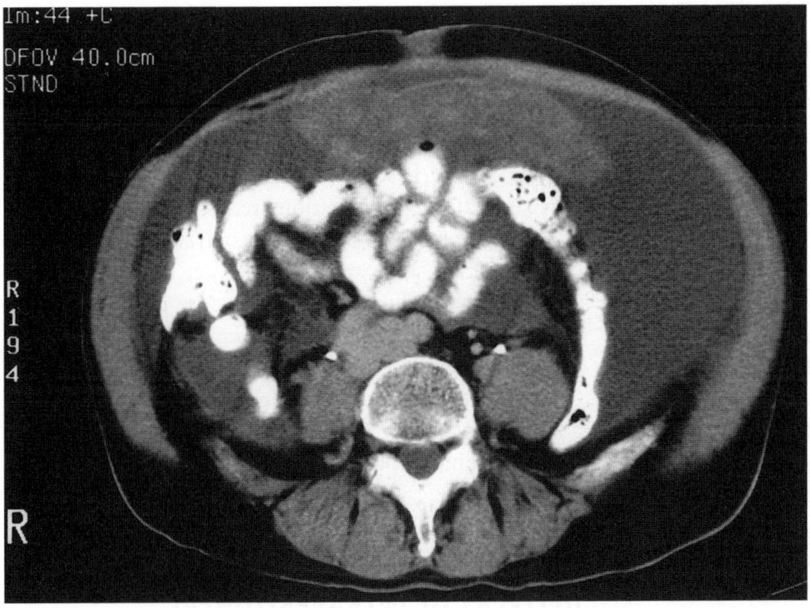

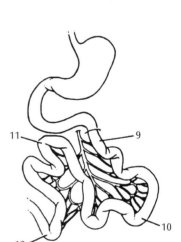

Figure 7.17 *A patient with intermediate-grade mucinous adenocarcinoma which has recurred after extensive prior cytoreductive surgery. Small bowel loops are slightly distorted and contain small volumes of air; the mesenteric surface is coated by mucinous tumor nodules. This patient has less than a 5% likelihood of a complete cytoreduction.*

Peritoneal Cancer Index

Regions	Lesion size	Lesion size score
0 Central	_____	LS 0 No tumor seen
1 Right upper	_____	LS 1 Tumor up to 0.5 cm
2 Epigastrium	_____	LS 2 Tumor up to 5.0 cm
3 Left upper	_____	LS 3 Tumor > 5.0 cm
4 Left flank	_____	or confluence
5 Left lower	_____	
6 Pelvis	_____	
7 Right lower	_____	
8 Right flank	_____	
9 Upper jejunum	_____	
10 Lower jejunum	_____	
11 Upper ileum	_____	
12 Lower ileum	_____	

Horizontal abdomino-pelvic sectors

1 2 3 Upper
8 0 4 Middle
7 6 5 Lower

Vertical abdomino-pelvic sectors

Right   Axial   Left

PCI

Figure 7.18 *The Peritoneal Cancer Index is a composite score of lesion size 0–3 in abdominopelvic regions 0–12.*

5.0 cm are present. LS-3 signifies the presence of tumor nodules greater than 5.0 cm in any dimension. If there is a confluence of tumor, the lesion size is scored as 3.

In order to assess the distribution of peritoneal surface disease, the abdominopelvic regions are utilized. For each of these 13 regions, an LS score is determined. The summation of the LS scores for each of the 13 abdominopelvic regions is the Peritoneal Cancer Index for that patient. A maximal score is 39 (13 × 3).

To date, the Peritoneal Cancer Index has been validated in three separate situations:

1 Steller used it successfully to quantitate intraperitoneal tumor in a murine peritoneal carcinomatosis model.[19]
2 Gomez Portilla and coworkers showed that it could be used to predict long-term survival in patients with peritoneal carcinomatosis from colon cancer undergoing a second cytoreduction.[20]

3 Berthet and coworkers showed that it predicted benefits for the treatment of peritoneal sarcomatosis from recurrent visceral or parietal sarcoma.[21]

In these clinical studies, patients with a favorable prognosis had a score of less than 13.

There are some exceptions to the rules established for the use of the Peritoneal Cancer Index:

1 Non-invasive malignancy on peritoneal surfaces may be completely cytoreduced even though the index is up to 39. Diseases such as pseudomyxoma peritonei, cystic peritoneal mesothelioma, and grade 1 sarcoma are in this category. With these minimally invasive tumors, the status of the abdomen and pelvis after cytoreduction may have no relationship to the status at the time of abdominal exploration. In other words, even though the surgeons may find an abdomen with a Peritoneal Cancer Index of 39, it can be converted to an index of 0 by cytoreduction. In these diseases, the prognosis will only be related to the condition of the abdomen after the cytoreduction (completeness of cytoreduction score).

2 A second caveat for the Peritoneal Cancer Index regards cancer at crucial anatomic sites. For example, invasive cancer not cleanly resected on the common bile duct will result in a poor prognosis despite a low Peritoneal Cancer Index. Invasion of the base of the bladder or unresectable disease on a pelvic sidewall may, by itself, result in residual invasive cancer after cytoreduction and eventuate in a poor prognosis. Also, unresectable cancer at numerous sites on the small bowel may, by itself, confer a poor prognosis. In other words, invasive cancer at crucial anatomic sites may function as systemic disease in the assessment of the prognosis with invasive cancer. Because long-term survival can only occur in patients with a complete cytoreduction, residual disease at anatomically crucial sites may override a favorable score with the Peritoneal Cancer Index.

Completeness of cytoreduction score

The most definitive assessment of prognosis to be used with peritoneal surface malignancy is the CC score. This information is of less value to the surgeon in planning treatments than the Peritoneal Cancer Index. The CC score is not available until after the cytoreduction is complete, whereas the Peritoneal Cancer Index is available at the time of abdominal exploration. If, during exploration, it becomes obvious that cytoreduction will not be complete, the surgeon may decide that a palliative debulking, which will provide symptomatic relief, is appropriate and may discontinue plans for an aggressive cytoreduction with intraperitoneal chemotherapy. In both non-invasive and invasive peritoneal surface malignancy, the CC score is the major prognostic indicator. It has been shown to function with accuracy in pseudomyxoma

peritonei, peritoneal carcinomatosis from colon cancer, sarcomatosis, and peritoneal mesothelioma.[15,16,20,21]

For gastrointestinal cancer, the CC score has been defined as follows. A CC-0 score indicates that no peritoneal seeding was exposed during the complete exploration. A CC-1 score indicates that tumor nodules persisting after cytoreduction are less than 2.5 mm. This is a nodule size thought to be penetrable by intracavity chemotherapy and would, therefore, be designated a complete cytoreduction. A CC-2 score indicates tumor nodules between 2.5 mm and 2.5 cm. A CC-3 score indicates tumor nodules greater than 2.5 cm or a confluence of unresectable tumor nodules at any site within the abdomen or pelvis. CC-2 and CC-3 cytoreductions are considered incomplete.

CURRENT METHODOLOGY FOR THE DELIVERY OF INTRAPERITONEAL CHEMOTHERAPY

Heated intraoperative intraperitoneal chemotherapy administration

In the operating room, heated intraoperative intraperitoneal chemotherapy is used. Thermal targeting is part of the optimizing process and is used to bring dose intensity to the abdominal and pelvic surfaces. Hyperthermia with intraperitoneal chemotherapy has several advantages:

1 Heat by itself has more toxicity for cancerous tissue than for normal tissue. This predominant effect on cancer increases as the vascularity of the malignancy decreases.

2 Hyperthermia increases the penetration of chemotherapy into tissues. As tissues soften in response to heat, the elevated interstitial pressure of a tumor mass may decrease and allow improved drug penetration.

3 Probably most important, heat increases the cytotoxicity of selected chemotherapy agents. This synergism occurs only at the interface of heat and body tissue at the peritoneal surface.

The rationale for using heated chemotherapy as a surgically directed modality in the operating room is presented in Table 7.2.

After the cancer resection is complete and prior to performing any anastomoses, the Tenckhoff catheter and closed suction drains are placed through the abdominal wall and made watertight with a purse-string suture at the skin. Temperature probes are secured to the skin edge. Using a long, running No. 2 monofilament suture, the skin edges are secured to the self-retaining retractor. A plastic sheet is incorporated into these sutures to create a covering for the abdominal cavity. A slit in the plastic cover is made to allow the surgeon's double-gloved hand

Table 7.2 *Rationale for the use of heated intraoperative intraperitoneal chemotherapy*

Heat increases drug penetration into tissue

Heat increases the cytotoxicity of selected chemotherapy agents

Heat has an antitumor effect by itself

Intraoperative chemotherapy allows manual distribution of drug and heat uniformly to all surfaces of the abdomen and pelvis

Renal toxicities of chemotherapy given in the operation room can be avoided by careful monitoring of urine output during chemotherapy perfusion

The time that elapses during the heated perfusion allows a normalization of many physiologic parameters (temperature, blood clotting, hemodynamic, etc.)

Access to the peritoneal cavity over 90 min allows time for debridement of tumor nodules from small bowel surfaces and mechanical disruption of cancer from within blood clots and fibrin accumulations

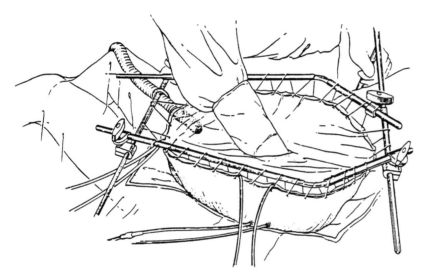

Figure 7.19 *The Coliseum technique for heated intraoperative intraperitoneal chemotherapy. Surgical manipulation of the abdominal contents after complete resection of cancer assures uniform distribution of heat and chemotherapy.*

access to the abdomen and pelvis (Figure 7.19). During the 90 min of perfusion, all the anatomic structures within the peritoneal cavity are uniformly exposed to heat and to chemotherapy. The surgeon continuously manipulates all viscera to eliminate adherence of peritoneal surfaces. Roller pumps force the chemotherapy solution into the abdomen through the Tenckhoff catheter and pull it out through the drains. A heat exchanger keeps the fluid being infused at 42–46 °C to maintain the intraperitoneal fluid at 41–42 °C. A diagram of the apparatus used for the administration of heated intraoperative intraperitoneal chemotherapy is shown in Figure 7.20. The smoke evacuator is used to pull air from beneath the plastic cover through activated charcoal, preventing contamination of air in the operating room by chemotherapy aerosols.

After the intraoperative perfusion is complete, the abdomen is suctioned dry of fluid. The abdomen is then reopened, the retractors are repositioned, and reconstructive surgery is performed. It should be re-emphasized that no suture lines are constructed until after the chemotherapy perfusion is complete. One exception to this rule is

the closure of the vaginal cuff to prevent intraperitoneal chemotherapy leakage. The standardized orders for heated intraoperative intraperitoneal chemotherapy are given in Table 7.3.

Mitomycin C

Mitomycin C is used intraoperatively to treat appendiceal, colonic, and gastric cancer. Occasionally, this drug may be appropriate for patients with pancreas cancer or small bowel adenocarcinoma. It is appropriate for ovarian cancer patients who have cisplatin neuropathy.

Cisplatin and doxorubicin

A combination of doxorubicin and cisplatin is used to treat sarcomatosis, peritoneal mesothelioma, and ovarian cancer. Also, papillary serous cancer and primary peritoneal adenocarcinoma are treated with the doxorubicin and cisplatin regimen.

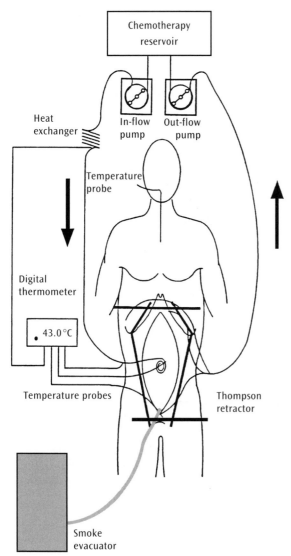

Figure 7.20 *The circuit for heated intraoperative intraperitoneal chemotherapy perfusion. All plastic tubes are positioned in a standardized fashion except the Tenckhoff catheter for the heated intraoperative perfusion. It is placed at the anatomic site at which the surgeon thinks there is the greatest likelihood of recurrence. This allows for regional dose intensity of the heated chemotherapy.*

Immediate postoperative abdominal lavage

Most patients with adenocarcinoma who receive intraperitoneal chemotherapy are also given early postoperative intraperitoneal 5-fluorouracil. Therefore, the catheters for drug instillation and abdominal drainage must be kept clear of blood clots and tissue debris. To accomplish this, an abdominal lavage, which utilizes the same tubes used for heated intraoperative intraperitoneal chemotherapy, is begun in the operating room. Large volumes of fluid are rapidly infused and then drained from the abdomen after a short dwell time. The standardized orders for immediate postoperative

abdominal lavage are given in Table 7.4. All intra-abdominal catheters are withdrawn after fluid drainage is substantially reduced but before the patient is discharged from the hospital.

Early postoperative intraperitoneal 5-fluorouracil

The standardized orders for early postoperative intraperitoneal 5-fluorouracil are presented in Table 7.5. After the patient stabilizes postoperatively, and after the drainage from the immediate postoperative abdominal lavage is no longer blood stained, the 5-fluorouracil instillation occurs. The patients treated are those with carcinomatosis from adenocarcinoma. In some patients who have extensive small bowel trauma from the lysis of adhesions, the early postoperative 5-fluorouracil is withheld because of the risk of fistula formation.[22,23] These patients are usually recommended for second-look surgery.

Adjuvant treatment with intravenous mitomycin C and intraperitoneal 5-fluorouracil

Patients should be carefully selected to receive additional cycles of intraperitoneal chemotherapy. Intestinal adhesions are the most frequent contraindication to its use. Usually, adjuvant intraperitoneal chemotherapy is not recommended in patients with extensive prior peritonectomy. The treatment is directed at the small bowel surfaces and is designed to eradicate large numbers of minute peritoneal implants. Parietal peritoneal surfaces, stomach surfaces, and the large bowel can usually be completely cytoreduced. Small bowel surfaces are the most common site for residual disease that prevents the CC-0 or CC-1 cytoreduction. Table 7.6 presents the standardized orders for adjuvant cycles of chemotherapy for adenocarcinoma.

Reoperative surgery plus additional intraperitoneal chemotherapy

As the clinical data regarding the treatment of peritoneal surface malignancy become available, the need for a more aggressive approach in selected patients has become clear. This seems most evident for tumors that do not have a tumor marker by which to monitor for recurrent disease. Peritoneal carcinomatosis from colon cancer is now routinely managed with a second-look surgery at 6–9 months. Also, primary peritoneal surface malignancy, especially mesothelioma, has a scheduled second-look surgery at 6–9 months.

At the second-look surgery, the abdomen is widely opened and all of the peritoneal surfaces are visualized,

Table 7.3 *Standardized orders for heated intraoperative intraperitoneal chemotherapy*

Mitomycin orders
1. For adenocarcinoma from appendiceal, colonic, rectal, gastric, and pancreatic cancer: add mitomycin ___ mg to 2 L of 1.5% peritoneal dialysis solution
2. Dose of mitomycin: for males, 12.5 mg/m^2; for females, 10 mg/m^2
3. Use a 33% dose reduction for heavy prior chemotherapy, marginal renal function, age greater than 60, extensive intraoperative trauma to small bowel surfaces, or prior radiotherapy
4. Send 1 L of 1.5% peritoneal dialysis solution to test the perfusion circuit
5. Send 1 L of 1.5% peritoneal dialysis solution for immediate postoperative lavage
6. Send the above to operating room ___ at ___ o'clock

Cisplatin and doxorubicin orders
1. For sarcoma, ovarian cancer, and mesothelioma: add cisplatin ___ mg to 2 L of 1.5% peritoneal dialysis solution; the dose of cisplatin is 50 mg/m^2
2. Add doxorubicin ___ mg to the same 2 L of 1.5% peritoneal dialysis solution; the dose of doxorubicin is 15 mg/m^2.
3. Use a 33% dose reduction for heavy prior chemotherapy, marginal renal function, age greater than 60, extensive intraoperative trauma to small bowel surfaces, or prior radiotherapy
4. Send 1 L of 1.5% peritoneal dialysis solution to test the perfusion circuit
5. Send 1 L of 1.5% peritoneal dialysis solution for immediate postoperative lavage
6. Send the above to operating room ___ at ___ o'clock

Table 7.4 *Immediate postoperative abdominal lavage*

Day of operation
1. Run in 1000 mL 1.5% dextrose peritoneal dialysis solution as rapidly as possible; warm to body temperature prior to instillation; clamp all abdominal drains during infusion
2. No dwell time
3. Drain as rapidly as possible through the Tenckhoff catheter and abdominal drains
4. Repeat irrigations every 1 h for 4 h, then every 4 h until returns are clear; then every 8 h until chemotherapy begins
5. Change dressing at Tenckhoff catheter and abdominal drain skin sites using sterile technique once daily and as required
6. Standardized precautions must be used for all body fluids from this patient

Table 7.5 *Early postoperative intraperitoneal chemotherapy with 5-fluorouracil*

Postoperative days 1–5
1. Add to ___ mL 1.5% dextrose peritoneal dialysis solution:
   (a) ___ mg 5-fluorouracil (650 mg/m^2, maximal dose 1300 mg)
   (b) 50 mEq sodium bicarbonate
2. Intraperitoneal fluid volume: 1 L for patients <2.0 m^2, 1.5 L for >2.0 m^2
3. Drain all fluid from the abdominal cavity prior to instillation, then clamp abdominal drains
4. Run the chemotherapy solution into the abdominal cavity through the Tenckhoff catheter as rapidly as possible; dwell for 23 h and drain for 1 h prior to next instillation
5. Use gravity to maximize intraperitoneal distribution of the 5-fluorouracil; instill the chemotherapy with the patient in a full right lateral position; after $\frac{1}{2}$ hour, direct the patient to turn to the full left lateral position; change position right to left every $\frac{1}{2}$ hour; if tolerated, use 10 degrees of Trendelenburg position; continue turning for the first 6 h after instillation of chemotherapy solution
6. Continue to drain abdominal cavity after final dwell until Tenckhoff catheter is removed
7. Use 33% dose reduction for heavy prior chemotherapy, age greater than 60, or prior radiotherapy

with a complete take-down of all adhesions. Additional cytoreduction is performed, and additional visceral resections may be required. If a CC-1 cytoreduction can again be achieved, then the treatment with heated intraoperative intraperitoneal chemotherapy is repeated. Also, if the patient has adenocarcinoma, early postoperative intraperitoneal 5-fluorouracil is again recommended.

If it appears from the re-operation that the initial heated chemotherapy and early postoperative chemotherapy

Table 7.6 *Intraperitoneal 5-fluorouracil and intravenous mitomycin chemotherapy for adjuvant treatment or for debilitating ascites from adenocarcinoma*

Cycle # ___

1. Platelets, complete blood chemistries (CBC), and appropriate tumor marker prior to treatment; CBC and platelets 10 days after initiation of treatments
2. 5-Fluorouracil ___ mg (750 mg/m^2, maximum dose 1600 mg) and 50 mEq sodium bicarbonate in 1000 mL 1.5% dextrose peritoneal dialysis solution via intraperitoneal catheter every day × 5 days; last dose ___; dwell for 23 h, drain for 1 h; continue with next administration even if no drainage obtained
3. On day 3 (Date _____): 500 mL lactated Ringer's solution intravenously over 2 h prior to mitomycin infusion; mitomycin ___ mg (10 mg/m^2 in women; 12.5 mg/m^2 in men) in 200 mL 5% dextrose and water intravenously over 2 h
4. Follow routine procedure for peripheral extravasation of a vesicant if extravasation should occur
5. Compazine 25 mg per rectum every 4 h as required for nausea; **outpatient only:** May dose × 4 for use at home
6. Percocet 1 tablet peroral every 3 h as required for pain; **outpatient only:** May dose × 4 for use at home
7. Routine vital signs
8. Out of bed at lib
9. Diet: regular as tolerated
10. Daily dressing change to intraperitoneal catheter skin exit site
11. Use 33% dose reduction for age greater than 60 or prior radiotherapy
12. Total lifetime dose of mitomycin is 100 mg.

treatments were successful at most anatomic sites, then the same regimen will be employed again. If there is a 'chemotherapy failure' and recurrent disease is seen in areas that have been previously peritonectomized, then a chemotherapy change would be initiated.

Indications for heated intraoperative intraperitoneal chemotherapy as an oncologic emergency

As a primary gastrointestinal cancer is resected, unexpected dissemination of cancer cells on peritoneal surfaces may be documented. Resections of gastrointestinal cancers may occur in which there is disruption of the cancer specimen resulting in 'intraoperative tumor spill.' In women, ovarian involvement of a gastrointestinal cancer indicates peritoneal contamination. A small volume of localized cancer seeding on the specimen or in the omentum that would be resected as part of the removal of the primary tumor signals generalized peritoneal contamination. Another indication would be a perforated intra-abdominal malignancy when that perforation is through the cancer itself. Positive peritoneal cytology and malignant ascites would also be considered an indication for the oncologic emergency. A majority of these patients will be recommended for second-look surgery at 6–9 months after the appropriate adjuvant chemotherapy is completed.

CLINICAL RESULTS OF TREATMENT

Reliable relief of debilitating ascites

Patients with a large volume of malignant ascites are frequently encountered as a cancerous process moves toward its terminal phase. This may be caused by breast cancer, gastric cancer, mucinous malignancies of the colon or appendix, and primary peritoneal surface cancers. Intraperitoneal chemotherapy is uniformly successful in eliminating the debilitating ascites.[24,25] Success usually requires three or four cycles of a systemic dose of appropriate chemotherapy into the abdomen. Combinations of both systemic and intraperitoneal chemotherapy are selected (see Table 7.6). Also, Link and colleagues used mitoxantrone in this clinical situation.[26]

It is important to inform patients that intraperitoneal chemotherapy as treatment for malignant ascites is for symptomatic relief and should not be considered curative. The mass of solid tumor will remain unchanged or will progress during treatment. Only the ascites will disappear. The mechanism of action of intraperitoneal chemotherapy on large-volume malignant ascites is the destruction of surface cancer. It is thought that intraperitoneal chemotherapy results in a layer of fibrosis over all malignant deposits and also on normal parietal and visceral peritoneal surfaces. This fibrotic layer of tissue prevents the formation of both normal peritoneal fluid and malignant fluids.

Technique for chemotherapy instillation for the treatment of malignant ascites

The technique used for repeated instillations of intraperitoneal chemotherapy to palliate malignant ascites is crucial for success. First, paracentesis using a temporary, all-purpose drain should provide access to the peritoneal space. A long-term indwelling (Tenckhoff) catheter should not be used to provide access because of the high incidence of infection with a foreign body located within a large-volume intra-abdominal fluid over a long time period. Also, an intraperitoneal subcutaneous port should not be used because of the difficulties it creates with the drainage of intraperitoneal fluid. Repeated paracentesis is safe if CT or ultrasound is used to select the site on the abdominal wall for puncture. When the ascites is gone or greatly diminished, the paracentesis becomes more dangerous. Of course, because these treatments are palliative, if the malignant ascites is greatly reduced, then the treatments are discontinued.

Schedule and dose of intraperitoneal chemotherapy for the treatment of ascites

The all-purpose drain is kept in place for 5 days. Each day, the ascites fluid is drained as completely as possible. Multiple changes in the patient's position may facilitate drainage. Then the intraperitoneal chemotherapy solution is instilled for a 23-h dwell. For adenocarcinoma, intravenous mitomycin C and intraperitoneal 5-fluorouracil may be appropriate. In some patients, a combination of cisplatin ($15 \, mg/m^2/day$) and doxorubicin ($3 \, mg/m^2/day$) is instilled. As soon as the chemotherapy solution has entered the abdomen, the patient is instructed to turn from front to back and from side to side every half an hour. Alternatively, mitoxantrone can be used at $3 \, mg/m^2/day$ for 5 days in a row. The cycle of treatments is repeated at 3-week intervals. In a few patients, persistent ascites may require a surgical procedure (debulking) in order to separate adherent bowel loops, remove bulk disease, and allow the use of a single cycle of heated intraoperative intraperitoneal chemotherapy. During the debulking, the large masses of tumor are removed and any obstructing portions of bowel are resected. This generally includes the greater and lesser omentum and pedunculated tumor masses. No attempt at a complete cytoreduction is made. The responses achieved in patients who are debulked and then given intraoperative chemotherapy may be more lasting than those in patients given chemotherapy only.

The treatment of mucinous ascites

If the intraperitoneal fluid is mucinous, it cannot be drained through a tube. Relief of mucinous ascites can only be achieved by laparotomy and manual removal of mucinous tumor. Usually, a greater omentectomy is performed as part of the debulking. Liposuction apparatus may greatly facilitate the complete evacuation of the viscous material. If the tumor mass can be reduced to a low level, intraoperative and early postoperative intraperitoneal chemotherapy may slow the re-accumulation of mucinous tumor.

Appendix cancer and pseudomyxoma peritonei

The paradigm for the treatment of peritoneal carcinomatosis is appendiceal malignancy. The experience with

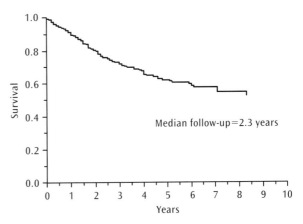

Figure 7.21 *The survival of 450 patients with established peritoneal surface malignancy from a perforated appendiceal malignancy. Patients were treated by cytoreductive surgery and intraperitoneal chemotherapy.*

approximately 450 patients treated over a 15-year time span is presented in this chapter. The survival of all patients is approximately 50% (Figure 7.21).

Appendiceal malignancy as a paradigm

The concepts gained from treating peritoneal surface malignancy from an appendiceal primary tumor can be applied to the management of other gastrointestinal cancers. There are unique clinical features of the appendiceal malignancies that have facilitated the extraordinary favorable results of treatment documented with this tumor:

1 Spread from appendiceal tumors usually occurs in the absence of lymph node and liver metastases. The primary tumor occurs within a tiny lumen. Even small tumors early in the natural history of the disease will cause appendiceal obstruction and perforation. This results in a release of tumor cells into the free peritoneal cavity. The seeding of the abdomen occurs in almost every patient before lymph node metastases or liver metastases have occurred.

2 There is a wide spectrum of invasion exhibited by these tumors. Mucinous tumors that are minimally invasive can be totally resected using peritonectomy procedures to achieve a CC-1 cytoreduction.

3 The majority of these tumors are mucinous. The texture of the implants allows greater penetration by chemotherapy than with solid tumors.

4 The malignancy disseminates so that all of the disease is within the regional chemotherapy field. If the intraperitoneal chemotherapy is successful in eradicating microscopic residual disease on peritoneal surfaces, the patient will be a long-term survivor.

In these patients, the response achieved by the intraperitoneal chemotherapy determines the outcome, assuming, of course, that a CC-1 cytoreduction was possible.

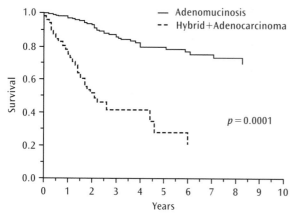

Figure 7.22 *The survival of appendiceal malignancy with peritoneal surface disease established by histologic appearance.*

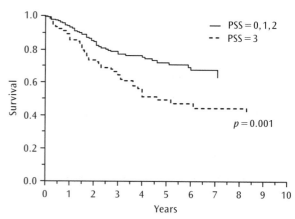

Figure 7.24 *The survival of appendiceal malignancy with peritoneal surface disease established by the extent of prior surgical interventions. Both patients with and without complete cytoreduction are included. If the prior surgical score is 3 (PSS-3) at least five of the nine abdominopelvic regions had been previously dissected without the use of intraoperative or early postoperative intraperitoneal chemotherapy. For PSS-2, two to five abdominopelvic regions had been dissected. For PSS-1, only one region had been dissected. These patients had exploratory surgery but no major organ or tissue dissection. For PSS-0, patients had biopsy only. Patients with a prior surgical score showing little or moderate dissection are compared to patients who had a prior attempt at a complete cytoreduction without perioperative intraperitoneal chemotherapy.*

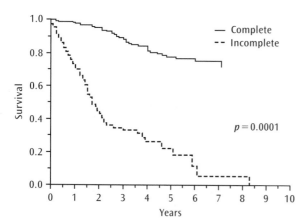

Figure 7.23 *The survival of appendiceal malignancy with peritoneal surface disease established by completeness of cytoreduction.*

The treatment strategies used included peritonectomy procedures combined with perioperative intraperitoneal chemotherapy with mitomycin C and 5-fluorouracil. Survival was significantly correlated with the invasive character of the mucinous tumor (Figure 7.22), the completeness of cytoreduction (Figure 7.23), and the prior surgical score (Figure 7.24). In contrast to most studies with gastrointestinal cancer patients, lymph node involvement was not a determinate prognostic factor in patients with peritoneal dissemination of malignancy if intraperitoneal chemotherapy was used.

Peritoneal carcinomatosis from colon cancer

Approximately 150 patients have been treated who presented with peritoneal carcinomatosis from colon cancer. In this disease, the Peritoneal Cancer Index provided a score that was valuable in the selection of patients for treatment (Figure 7.25). In patients who had a complete cytoreduction, there was marked improvement in survival; patients with residual disease showed the short survival expected with peritoneal carcinomatosis from colon cancer (Figure 7.26). These data suggest that an early aggressive approach to the peritoneal surface spread of adenocarcinoma of the colon is indicated in selected patients. Patients with positive lymph nodes at the time of resection of the primary cancer have a reduced prognosis ($p = 0.0251$). With positive lymph nodes and peritoneal carcinomatosis, only approximately 15% of patients showed prolonged survival.

Sarcomatosis

Berthet and colleagues have reviewed their experience with cytoreductive surgery and intraperitoneal chemotherapy for the treatment of selected patients with sarcomatosis.[21] If the Peritoneal Cancer Index at the time of abdominal exploration was less than 13, there was a 75% 5-year survival. In those who had a Peritoneal Cancer Index of 13 or more, the 5-year survival was only 13% (Figure 7.27). The completeness of cytoreduction was also statistically significant for an improved prognosis. The 5-year survival rate for 27 patients with a complete cytoreduction was 39%, and 14% for 16 patients with a CC-2 or CC-3 resection (Figure 7.28).

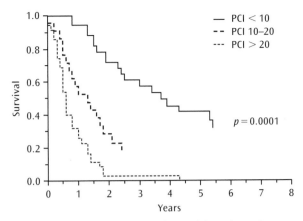

Figure 7.25 *The survival of patients with peritoneal carcinomatosis from colon cancer by Peritoneal Cancer Index (PCI).*

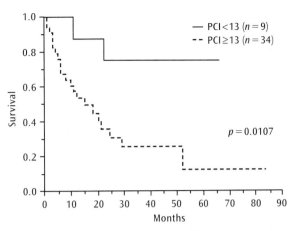

Figure 7.27 *The survival of patients with recurrent abdominopelvic sarcoma by Peritoneal Cancer Index.*

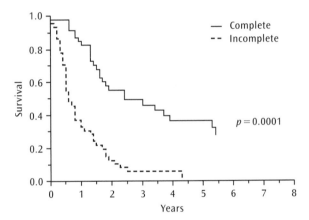

Figure 7.26 *The survival of patients with peritoneal carcinomatosis from colon cancer established by completeness of cytoreduction.*

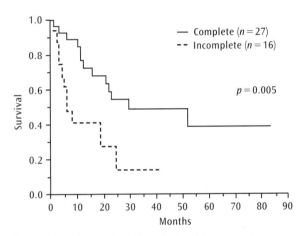

Figure 7.28 *The survival of patients with recurrent abdominopelvic sarcoma established by completeness of cytoreduction.*

Peritoneal seeding from gastric cancer

Extensive studies with peritoneal seeding from gastric cancer have been conducted in Japan. The survival rates for patients in Japan who underwent heated intraoperative intraperitoneal chemotherapy at the time of gastrectomy vary from 10% to 43%.[27,28] The results of treatment of a group of Western patients have not yet been reported; however, a theoretical and clinical basis for treatment has been established.[29]

Primary peritoneal surface malignancy

A confusing and poorly understood group of tumors that have been successfully treated with peritonectomy and perioperative intraperitoneal chemotherapy is the primary peritoneal surface malignancies. These diseases include peritoneal mesothelioma, papillary serous adenocarcinoma, primary peritoneal adenocarcinoma, and desmoplastic small round cell tumor. Currently, all patients are being treated with heated intraoperative cisplatin and doxorubicin and adjuvant intraperitoneal paclitaxel. A second-look procedure with initiation of these same treatments is performed after 6–9 months. The survival was heavily dependent upon the invasive character of the tumor and on the completeness of cytoreduction. The median survival in a group of 41 patients with primary peritoneal tumors was 18 months (Figure 7.29). Further experience with this group of patients is necessary.

Recurrent and obstructing gastrointestinal cancer

Averbach and Sugarbaker examined their experience with a poor prognosis group of patients. These were patients with intestinal obstruction from recurrent gastrointestinal malignancy. With aggressive treatments using a

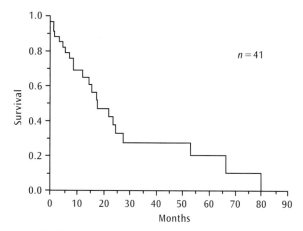

Figure 7.29 *The survival of 41 patients with primary peritoneal surface malignancy.*

second-look surgery, peritonectomy procedures, and intraperitoneal chemotherapy, a complete cytoreduction resulted in a 5-year survival in 60% of the patients, and an incomplete resection resulted in no patient surviving 5 years. The patients with appendiceal malignancy had a greatly improved survival as compared to those with colon cancer or other diagnoses. A recurrence-free interval of greater than 2 years between primary malignancy and the onset of obstruction also correlated favorably with prolonged survival.[30]

MORBIDITY AND MORTALITY OF PHASE 2 STUDIES

The morbidity and mortality of 200 consecutive patients who had cytoreductive surgery and heated intraoperative intraperitoneal chemotherapy for peritoneal carcinomatosis have been reported.[31] In these patients, there were three treatment-related deaths (1.5%). Peripancreatitis (7.1%) and fistula (4.7%) were the most common major complications. Grade III or IV complications occurred in 25.3% of patients.

ALTERNATIVE APPROACHES

Peritoneal carcinomatosis has been treated in the past with systemic chemotherapy. No long-term survivors have been described in the literature. Palliative surgery can give temporary relief of intestinal obstruction. These efforts have always been categorized as low-value surgery because long-term survival was rarely achieved. Other therapies that included intraperitoneal immunotherapy, intraperitoneal isotopes, and intraperitoneal labeled monoclonal antibody have not shown reproducible beneficial results. In summary, alternative approaches to cytoreductive surgery and intraperitoneal chemotherapy for peritoneal carcinomatosis have not been reported.

POSTOPERATIVE MANAGEMENT

The major management issue postoperatively with combined cytoreductive surgery and intraperitoneal chemotherapy is prolonged ileus. Patients may have a nasogastric tube in place, with large volumes of secretions being aspirated for 2–4 weeks postoperatively. The length of time required for nasogastric suctioning is dependent upon the extent of the peritonectomy procedures and of the prior abdominal adhesions requiring lysis.

A life-threatening postoperative complication is the fistula. Fistulas are almost always sidewall perforations of the small bowel, but colon and stomach perforations have occurred. Patients need to be made aware of the possibility of a fistula before cytoreductive surgery and intraperitoneal chemotherapy are contemplated. As mentioned above, the anastomotic leak rate is low.

Pancreatitis occurs in approximately 30% of patients who have an extensive upper abdominal cytoreduction. Prolonged nutritional support, antibiotics, and serial CT to drain peripancreatic fluid collections may be necessary. The process is self-limited, but may cause fever and persistent nausea for up to a month.

Following these treatments, the patient is usually maintained on parenteral feeding for 2–4 weeks. Approximately 20% of patients, especially those who have had extensive prior surgery or who have a short bowel, will need parenteral feeding for several months after they leave the hospital.

ETHICAL CONSIDERATIONS IN CLINICAL STUDIES WITH PERITONEAL SURFACE MALIGNANCY

The sequence of events that should accompany a new program for peritoneal surface malignancy have not yet been defined. The requirements for formal institutional review board approval will vary from one institution to another. Guidelines for an evolution of treatment strategies that allows for reliable clinical research may occur as follows.

Without exception, adjuvant intraperitoneal chemotherapy studies in patients with primary gastrointestinal cancer must be randomized and require review by a research board. An exception to the need for randomization is resected pancreas cancer. Also, when a group first attempts to initiate treatment plans with intraperitoneal chemotherapy, the learning curve associated with a new technology is best approached by a start-up protocol approved by an institutional review board. This forces members of the group to standardize the methods and familiarize themselves with the experience of others. Selection criteria to treat patients with a reasonable likelihood of benefit must be determined. An omnibus protocol is suggested, which allows aggressive cytoreduction and perioperative intraperitoneal chemotherapy in patients without systemic dissemination and with small-volume peritoneal seeding from peritoneal carcinomatosis, peritoneal sarcomatosis, and mesothelioma. This omnibus protocol should be utilized for a limited time period to treat 10–20 patients.

Formal protocols should not be required for the treatment of debilitating ascites because of the marked quality-of-life benefits demonstrated.[32] Also, the long-term survival of patients with peritoneal surface malignancy that has a small volume and limited distribution has been established. After completing the start-up protocols, the treatment of this group of patients by an oncologic team that has demonstrated experience should proceed without the need for further institutional review board approval. The peritoneal surface spread of most gastrointestinal cancers that have a low Peritoneal Cancer Index and that have a CC score of 0 or 1 after surgery should be routinely treated according to standardized intraperitoneal chemotherapy protocols. The treatment of peritoneal carcinomatosis, sarcomatosis, and mesothelioma definitively at the time of initial diagnosis will always be preferred over the treatment of recurrence.[33]

REFERENCES

1. Gunderson LL, Sosin H. Areas of failure found at reoperation (second or symptomatic look) following 'curative surgery' for adenocarcinoma of the rectum: clinicopathologic correlation and implications for adjuvant therapy. Cancer 1974; 34:1278–92.

2. Sugarbaker PH. Surgical management of locally recurrent and metastatic colorectal cancer. In Karakousis CP, Copeland EM, Bland QUI, eds. *Atlas of surgical oncology*. Philadelphia, Saunders, 1995, 671–92.

3. Sugarbaker PH, Hughes KA. Surgery for colorectal metastasis to liver. In Wanebo H, ed. *Colorectal cancer*. St Louis, Mosby-Year Book, 1993, 405–13.

4. Sugarbaker PH. *Peritoneal carcinomatosis: principles of management*. Boston, Kluwer, 1996.

5. Sugarbaker PH. Peritoneal carcinomatosis from appendiceal cancer: a paradigm for treatment of abdominopelvic dissemination of gastrointestinal malignancy. Acta Chir Austriaca 1996; 28:4–8.

6. Sugarbaker PH. Peritonectomy procedures. In Sugarbaker PH, ed. *Peritoneal carcinomatosis: principles of management*. Boston, Kluwer, 1996, 235–62.

7. Jacquet P, Vidal-Jove J, Zhu BW, Sugarbaker PH. Peritoneal carcinomatosis from intraabdominal malignancy: natural history and new prospects for management. Acta Belgica Chirurgica 1994; 94:191–7.

8. Sugarbaker PH, Graves T, DeBruijn EA, *et al.* Rationale for early postoperative intraperitoneal chemotherapy (EPIC) in patients with advanced gastrointestinal cancer. Cancer Res 1990; 50:5790–4.

9. Sugarbaker PH, Gianola FJ, Speyer JL, Wesley R, Barofsky I, Meyers CE. Prospective randomized trial of intravenous versus intraperitoneal 5-fluorouracil in patients with advanced primary colon or rectal cancer. Surgery 1985; 98:414–21.

10. Begossi G, Caprino P, Tentes AA, Chang D, Sugarbaker PH. Management of peritoneal seeding from gastric cancer: palliative gastrectomy, peritonectomy and perioperative intraperitoneal chemotherapy. Acta Chir Austriaca 1999; 31(155):35–8.

11. Yu W, Whang I, Shu I, Averbach A, Chang D, Sugarbaker PH. Prospective randomized trial of early postoperative intraperitoneal chemotherapy as an adjuvant for resectable gastric cancer. Ann Surg 1998; 228(3):347–54.

12. Gough DB, Donahue JH, Schutt AJ, *et al.* Pseudomyxoma peritonei: long-term survival with an aggressive regional approach. Ann Surg 1994; 219:112–19.

13. Zoetmulder FAN, Sugarbaker PH. Patterns of failure after complete cytoreduction and early postoperative intraperitoneal chemotherapy. Eur J Cancer 1996; 32A(10):1727–33.

14. Sugarbaker TA, Chang D, Koslowe P, Sugarbaker PH. Pathobiology of peritoneal carcinomatosis from ovarian malignancy. In Sugarbaker PH, ed. *Peritoneal carcinomatosis: drugs and diseases*. Boston, Kluwer, 1996, 63–74.

15. Sugarbaker PH, Ronnett B, Archer A, *et al.* Management of pseudomyxoma peritonei of appendiceal origin. Adv Surg 1997; 30:233–80.

16. Sebbag G, Yan H, Shmookler BM, Chang D, Sugarbaker PH. Results of treatment of 33 patients with peritoneal mesothelioma. Br J Surg 2000; 87:1587–93.

17. Archer A, Sugarbaker PH, Jelinek J. Radiology of peritoneal carcinomatosis. In Sugarbaker PH, ed. *Peritoneal carcinomatosis: principles of management*. Boston, Kluwer, 1996, 263–88.

18. Jacquet P, Jelinek J, Sugarbaker PH. Abdominal computed tomographic scan in the selection of patients with mucinous peritoneal carcinomatosis for cytoreductive surgery. J Am Coll Surg 1995; 181(6):530–8.

19. Steller EP. Comparison of four scoring methods for an intraperitoneal immunotherapy model. Enhancement and Abrogation: Modifications of Host Immune Influence IL-2 and LAK Cell Immunotherapy, PhD Thesis, Erasmus University, Rotterdam, 1988.

20. Gomez Portilla A, Sugarbaker PH, Chang D. Second-look surgery after cytoreductive and intraperitoneal chemotherapy for peritoneal carcinomatosis from

colorectal cancer: analysis of prognostic features. World J Surg 1999; 23(1):23–9.

21. Berthet B, Sugarbaker TA, Chang D, Sugarbaker PH. Quantitative methodologies for selection of patients with recurrent abdominopelvic sarcoma for treatment. Eur J Cancer 1999; 35:413–19.

22. Murio EJ, Sugarbaker PH. Gastrointestinal fistula following cytoreductive procedures for peritoneal carcinomatosis: incidence and outcome. J Exp Clin Cancer Res 1993; 12:153–8.

23. Fernandez-Trio V, Sugarbaker PH. Diagnosis and management of postoperative gastrointestinal fistulas: a kinetic analysis. J Exp Clin Cancer Res 1994; 13:233–41.

24. Gilly FN, Sayag AC, Carry PY, et al. Intraperitoneal chemohyperthermia (CHIP): a new therapy in the treatment of the peritoneal seedings. Int Surg 1991; 76:164–7.

25. Fujimoto S, Shrestha RD, Kokubun M, et al. Intraperitoneal hyperthermic perfusion combined with surgery effective for gastric cancer patients with peritoneal seeding. Ann Surg 1988; 208(1):36–41.

26. Link K, Hepp G, Staib L, Butzer U, Bohm W, Beger HG. Intraperitoneal regional chemotherapy (IPRC) with mitoxantrone. In Sugarbaker PH, ed. *Peritoneal carcinomatosis: drugs and diseases*. Boston, Kluwer, 1996, 31–40.

27. Yonemura Y, Fujimura T, Nishmura G, et al. Effects of intraoperative chemohyperthermia in patients with

gastric cancer with peritoneal dissemination. Surgery 1996; 119(4):437–44.

28. Fujimoto S, Shrestha RD, Kokubin M, et al. Positive results of combined therapy of surgery and intraperitoneal hyperthermia perfusion for far-advanced gastric cancer. Ann Surg 1990; 212(5):592–6.

29. Sugarbaker PH, Yonemura Y. Clinical pathway for the management of resectable gastric cancer with peritoneal seeding: best palliation with a ray of hope for cure. Oncology 2000; 58:96–107.

30. Averbach AM, Sugarbaker PH. Recurrent intraabdominal cancer with intestinal obstruction. Int Surg 1995; 80(2):141–6.

31. Stephens AD, Alderman R, Chang D, et al. Morbidity and mortality of 200 treatments with cytoreductive surgery and heated intraoperative intraperitoneal chemotherapy using the Coliseum technique. Ann Surg Oncol 1999; 6(8):790–6.

32. McQuellon RP, Loggie BW, Fleming RA, et al. Quality of life after intraperitoneal hyperthermic chemotherapy (IPHC) for peritoneal carcinomatosis. Am Soc Clin Oncol 1997; 16:76.

33. Pestieau SR, Sugarbaker PH. Treatment of primary colon cancer with peritoneal carcinomatosis: a comparison of concomitant versus delayed management. Dis Colon Rectum 2000; 43:1341–8.

Commentary

ALLAN W SILBERMAN

As to diseases, make a habit of two things – to help, or at least, to do no harm.

Extreme remedies are very appropriate for extreme diseases.

Hippocrates, 460–370 BC

Operating upon patients with metastatic disease carries added responsibility for the surgeon. Complications in this setting, which might be considered minor in an otherwise healthy patient, can be devastating to the cancer patient because recovering from the operation and caring for the complication can intrude upon any remaining quality time. The indication for surgery in the patient with metastatic disease must be clear to both the doctor and the patient.

Is the operation potentially curative?

Is the operation palliative (keeping in mind that you cannot palliate an asymptomatic patient)?

Does the operation offer staging information that may alter subsequent non-surgical therapy?

Is the proposed procedure experimental or part of an experimental protocol?

Does the patient understand the experimental nature of the procedure?

These questions must be asked and answered prior to any planned surgical procedure.

The concept of surgical tumor debulking, or cytoreductive surgery, has been a controversial topic for over 25 years. One reason for the controversy is that resection of tumors without the preoperative expectation of complete removal violates traditional surgical principles and obscures the concept of operability. Another reason is that the definition of surgical cytoreduction has often been misunderstood. Cytoreductive surgery is not curative; it is not palliative; it is not a staging operation. Surgical cytoreduction is a procedure whereby a surgically incurable malignant neoplasm is partially or grossly removed *without curative intent* in order to make subsequent therapy with drugs, radiation, or other adjunctive measures more effective and thereby improve the length of patient survival.[1] The adjunctive therapy, usually chemotherapy, is the primary therapeutic method and is used with curative intent against the residual gross or microscopic tumor. The debulking or cytoreductive operation is, in effect, a preliminary adjuvant to the chemotherapy. The reductive operation should not be confused or compared with palliative surgical procedures, the purpose of which is to improve the patient's quality of life, or with staging procedures, the goal of which is to assess accurately the extent of disease and thereby effect subsequent non-surgical therapy. These latter procedures may involve a considerable reduction in tumor burden; however, they do not constitute a debulking procedure. To add to the confusion, what is considered a palliative operation today may be considered a debulking procedure in the future as adjunctive therapy improves.

Is the removal of a malignant melanoma in conjunction with a positive lymphadenectomy a debulking procedure? Is the resection of a Dukes' C colon cancer or a right hepatic lobectomy for an isolated metastasis to the liver a debulking procedure? In none of these situations is there anywhere near a 100% 5-year survival; thus, all these procedures could be considered debulking because regional or systemic micrometastases, or both, are present in many, if not all, of these patients. As Morton pointed out years ago, in many patients, the major role of the surgeon is to remove the bulk of tumor to lower the level of immunosuppression induced by the neoplasm. The immune defenses of the host can then eradicate any microscopic foci of tumor cells scattered throughout the body. Surgery, then, can be viewed as immunotherapy.[2] However, most operations for solid tumors do not constitute a debulking procedure because some patients are cured by the procedure alone and the surgical *intent* is curative. Although post-surgical adjuvant therapy has improved the length of survival for patients with some types of solid cancers, for example breast and colon cancer, therapeutic chemotherapy or other adjunctive therapy is *required* to achieve improved survival time or cure with neoplasms that are surgically debulked. Thus, the definition of a surgical debulking procedure is an operation which, by itself, has no chance for cure, often leaves gross tumor behind, and depends upon other non-surgical therapy to effect a cure or improve survival time.

This combination of reductive surgery and chemotherapy is a rational, although unproved, method for the treatment of advanced solid cancers. The approach is based upon the general biologic characteristics of solid tumors. Large tumors have a high percentage of cells in the rest period of their cell cycle; moreover, they have a relatively poor central blood supply. These factors make the tumor relatively insensitive to cytotoxic drugs, because most chemotherapeutic agents are cycle specific or phase specific. In better perfused, smaller tumors that have a larger percentage of cells that are actively dividing, chemotherapy becomes more effective. Theoretically, then, tumor debulking, by removing a large proportion of the resting cells, could promote a more effective response to chemotherapy.

Ovarian cancer has been the disease for which surgical cytoreduction has been used most extensively. Most authorities believe that primary cytoreductive surgery is the standard of care in patients with epithelial ovarian carcinoma.[3] However, the value of cytoreductive surgery in the management of ovarian cancer has been debated for years. Several non-randomized studies have shown improved survival of patients with ovarian cancer whose residual tumors after debulking surgery were < 1.0 cm in diameter.[4–6] However, other studies[7,8] have noted that, despite optimal cytoreduction, the survival of patients with large intra-abdominal metastases before resection was significantly worse than that of patients with small initial intra-abdominal lesions. Thus, in addition to the size of residual disease after cytoreduction, intrinsic tumor factors also appear to be of prognostic significance. In fact, it may well be that the biologically less aggressive tumors are the ones that lend themselves to optimal cytoreduction and therefore the reason those patients do better is more related to their intrinsic tumor biology than to surgical cytoreduction. These non-randomized studies are also difficult to evaluate because most of the patients also received chemotherapy in the postoperative period. In 1987, the European Organization for Research and Treatment of Cancer (EORTC) initiated a randomized phase III study to establish the effect on survival of debulking surgery *after* induction chemotherapy with three cycles of cyclophosphamide and cisplatin. Following the induction chemotherapy, the patients were randomized to either debulking surgery or no surgery. All patients then received an additional three cycles of chemotherapy. Progression-free and overall survival were both significantly longer in the group undergoing debulking surgery.[3] Most of the patients in this study had undergone hysterectomy and bilateral oophorectomy prior to entering the study. Thus, the debulking surgery, although occurring after induction chemotherapy, was part of a second-look operation. It may be that it is now time to study the effect of chemotherapy given before any surgical manipulation.

Ovarian cancer lends itself to debulking surgery because it tends to spread along peritoneal surfaces without metastasizing to the liver and other intra-abdominal viscera and outside the abdominal cavity. Other tumors, often of gastrointestinal origin, can also spread in a similar fashion. Symptomatic peritoneal carcinomatosis causes marked deterioration in quality of life and is associated with short survival. Bowel obstruction is common, caused by malignant adhesions or the presence of mass lesions. Malignant ascites often reflects widespread peritoneal surface dissemination and often results in dyspnea, discomfort lying or standing, and pseudo-obstruction.

Dr Sugarbaker and his group from Washington Hospital Center in Washington, DC, have pioneered an aggressive management strategy designed to bring about long-term survival to patients with peritoneal surface malignancies. Their approach is outlined in the preceding chapter. It is stressed that the successful treatment of peritoneal surface malignancy requires three components: cytoreductive surgery that *completely* removes all visible malignancy; perioperative intraperitoneal chemotherapy including hyperthermic intraoperative intraperitoneal chemotherapy; and, equally importantly, proper patient selection. The rationale and technical details of peritonectomy procedures are discussed. The importance of intraperitoneal chemotherapy is emphasized because of the belief that this type of surgery, without perioperative intraperitoneal chemotherapy, may actually harm patients rather than help them because tumor cells can become implanted within a deeper layer of the abdomen and pelvis, contributing to obstruction of vital structures. Of interest is the fact that the heated, intraoperative intraperitoneal chemotherapy is used *prior* to the construction of any gastrointestinal anastomosis in an effort to eliminate suture-line recurrences. However, the vaginal cuff is closed prior to the chemotherapy to prevent the drugs leaking from the vagina.

Peritoneal carcinomatosis secondary to appendiceal carcinoma has been the malignancy most often treated with this technique. Sugarbaker's group has treated more than 450 patients over a 15-year period, with a survival of approximately 50%. There are unique features of appendiceal malignancies that lend themselves to Sugarbaker's technique:

1 the seeding of the abdomen often occurs before the development of either lymph node or liver metastases;
2 tumors that are minimally invasive can be totally resected using the peritonectomy procedures;
3 all of the remaining residual disease is within the regional chemotherapy field.

The concepts gained from this huge experience have been applied to the management of other malignancies, including colon cancer, gastric cancer, sarcomatosis, mesothelioma, and other primary peritoneal surface malignancies.

Morbidity and mortality are a major concern when a procedure of this magnitude is undertaken, particularly in a population of patients with metastatic disease. In 10% of the patients with appendiceal mucinous tumors, a total gastrectomy was necessary to accomplish an adequate cytoreduction. Patients undergoing total gastrectomy are diverted with a jejunostomy, which is closed about 6–9 months postoperatively as part of a second-look procedure. In 385 patients studied by Sugarbaker,

the morbidity was 27%, with a mortality of 2.7%.[9,10] Pancreatitis and fistula were the most common major complications. In addition, prolonged ileus with large nasogastric tube outputs can last as long as a month postoperatively. Prolonged nutritional support with total parenteral nutrition (TPN), antibiotics, and serial CT scans with percutaneous drainage of fluid collections are commonly used in the postoperative setting. Approximately 20% of patients will require TPN support for several months following discharge from the hospital. Despite the morbidity involved in offering these patients this aggressive treatment approach, the results obtained by Dr Sugarbaker in a group of patients with an otherwise uniformly fatal prognosis are quite impressive. Other groups have also published preliminary promising results using the Sugarbaker approach.[11–14] It seems clear that patients with mucinous tumors of uncertain malignant potential and those with low-grade appendiceal adenocarcinomas have the best response to this aggressive approach. However, in those patients with a high-grade malignant form of the disease, aggressive attempts at surgical debulking do not seem to translate into a survival benefit. In addition, survival data for patients with peritoneal carcinomatosis from non-appendiceal gastrointestinal malignancies (colon and gastric cancer) have not been nearly as impressive as those from appendiceal carcinoma.[11] Defining the subset of patients that will have a survival advantage using this aggressive technique of surgical cytoreduction and hyperthermic intraperitoneal chemotherapy needs to be a priority. Beaujard and associates from Lyon, France, pointed out five problem areas with this technique that need to be improved upon:[14]

1 obtaining homogeneous diffusion of heat and drugs inside the abdominal cavity;
2 defining the indications for repeat intraperitoneal chemotherapy;
3 using multidrug therapy intraperitoneally as is done in systemic chemotherapy;
4 improving upon the morbidity associated with extensive debulking, particularly in the face of intraperitoneal chemotherapy;
5 using intraperitoneal chemotherapy in the *adjuvant* setting for patients with gastrointestinal carcinomas with serosal involvement.

The approach offered by Dr Sugarbaker for the treatment of patients with peritoneal carcinomatosis requires a committed team, dedicated to both the patient and the technique. Physicians who only rarely see these types of problems should refer their patients to centers where the required interest and expertise are available. I believe that a national trial at a limited number of centers under the direction of Dr Sugarbaker would be the best way to study this technique and better define its indications and contraindications.

REFERENCES

1. Silberman AW. Surgical debulking of tumors. Surg Gynecol Obstet 1982; 155:577–85.

2. Morton DL. Changing concepts of cancer surgery; surgery as immunotherapy. Am J Surg 1978; 135:367–71.

3. van der Burg MEL, van Lent M, Buyse M, et al. The effect of debulking surgery after induction chemotherapy on the prognosis in advanced epithelial ovarian cancer. N Engl J Med 1995; 332:629–34.

4. Vogl SE, Pagano M, Kaplan BH, et al. Cis-platin based combination chemotherapy for advanced ovarian cancer: high overall response rate with curative potential only in women with small tumor burdens. Cancer 1983; 51:2024–30.

5. Neijt JP, ten Bokkel Huinink WW, van der Burg MEL, et al. Long-term survival in ovarian cancer: mature data from the Netherlands Joint Study Group for Ovarian Cancer. Eur J Cancer 1991; 27:1367–72.

6. Omura GA, Bundy BN, Berek JS, et al. Randomized trial of cyclophosphamide plus cisplatin with or without doxorubicin in ovarian carcinoma: a Gynecologic Oncology Group study. J Clin Oncol 1989; 7:457–65.

7. Hacker NF, Berek JS, Lagasse LD, et al. Primary cytoreductive surgery for epithelial ovarian carcinoma. Obstet Gynecol 1983; 61:413–20.

8. Hoskins WJ, Bundy BN, Thigpen JT, et al. The influence of cytoreductive surgery on recurrence-free interval and survival in small-volume stage III epithelial ovarian cancer: a Gynecologic Oncology Group study. Gynecol Oncol 1992; 47:159–66.

9. Sugarbaker PH, Chang D. Results of treatment of 385 patients with peritoneal surface spread of appendiceal malignancy. Ann Surg Oncol 1999; 6:727–31.

10. Stephens AD, Alderman R, Chang D, et al. Morbidity and mortality analysis of 200 treatments with cytoreductive surgery and hyperthermic intraoperative intraperitoneal chemotherapy using the Coliseum technique. Ann Surg Oncol 1999; 6:790–6.

11. Loggie BW, Fleming RA, McQuellon RP, et al. Cytoreductive surgery with intraperitoneal hyperthermic chemotherapy for disseminated peritoneal cancer of gastrointestinal origin. Am Surg 2000; 66:561–8.

12. Mansfield PF. Appendiceal malignancy: where do we stand? Ann Surg Oncol 1999; 6:715–16.

13. Wirtzfeld DA, Rodriguez-Bigas M, Weber T, Petrelli NJ. Disseminated peritoneal adenomucinosis: a critical review. Ann Surg Oncol 1999; 6:797–801.

14. Beaujard AC, Glehen O, Caillot JL, et al. Intraperitoneal chemohyperthermia with mitomycin C for digestive tract cancer patients with peritoneal carcinomatosis. Cancer 2000; 88:2512–19.

Editors' selected abstracts

Adult respiratory distress syndrome occurring in two patients undergoing cytoreductive surgery plus perioperative intraperitoneal chemotherapy: case reports and a review of the literature.

Alonso O, Sugarbaker PH.

Surgery Oncology Service, The Washington Cancer Institute, Washington Hospital Center, Washington, DC, USA.

American Surgeon 66:1032–6, 2000.

Cytoreductive surgery and perioperative intraperitoneal chemotherapy with mitomycin C and 5-fluorouracil may be considered as an accepted treatment for appendiceal malignancy with mucinous peritoneal carcinomatosis or for pseudomyxoma peritonei. This aggressive approach has been successfully utilized in approximately 500 patients with an acceptable mortality (1.5%) and morbidity (27%). Although pulmonary complications are frequently recorded, life-endangering acute respiratory failure in the absence of pulmonary infection or an obvious source of systemic sepsis has not been previously described. An extensive clinical review of two patients who had a clinical course compatible with acute respiratory distress syndrome without obvious cause except for the cytoreductive surgery and perioperative intraperitoneal chemotherapy itself was undertaken. These two patients developed gradually increasing respiratory distress in the postoperative period. No bacterial or fungal infections of lungs or intra-abdominal sites or sepsis were discovered. These two patients were unusual in that they had extensive cytoreduction, maximal heat with the mitomycin C chemotherapy, and perfusion of both the abdominal cavity and the right pleural space. Reoperation in both patients failed to show a septic source within the abdomen for progressive adult respiratory distress syndrome. We conclude that aggressive cytoreductive surgery plus perioperative intraperitoneal and intrapleural chemotherapy was associated with life-endangering respiratory failure in two patients. No other cause for this condition was evident from an exhaustive review of the clinical course of these two patients. It is possible that this aggressive approach to appendix malignancy with carcinomatosis is sufficiently traumatic to be considered a cause of adult respiratory distress syndrome.

Treatment of peritoneal carcinomatosis with intent to cure.

Cavaliere F, Perri P, Di Filippo F, Giannarelli D, Botti C, Cosimelli M, Tedesco M, Principi F, Laurenzi L, Cavaliere R.

First Department of Surgical Oncology, Regina Elena National Cancer Institute, Rome, Italy.

Journal of Surgical Oncology 74(1):41–4, 2000, May.

Background and objectives: Low-grade malignant tumors arise in the abdomen, do not infiltrate, and 'redistribute' on the peritoneum with no extraregional spreading. In these cases, aggressive surgery combined with localized chemotherapy may provide cure. *Methods:* After removing the tumor with the regional peritoneum en bloc, intra-abdominal hyperthermic chemoperfusion was performed throughout the abdominopelvic cavity. Alternatively, early intraabdominal chemotherapy, starting on the first post-operative day, was administered for 5 days. *Results:* Forty patients affected with extensive peritoneal carcinomatosis underwent peritonectomy, with no residual macroscopic disease except in four cases. Seventy-five percent of the patients underwent locoregional chemotherapy. Major complications were observed in 40% of the patients and led to death in five; there was a direct correlation to the duration of surgery ($p = 0.03$). At a mean follow-up of 20 months, the overall 2-year survival was 61.4%, with a median survival of 30 months. *Conclusions:* After a learning curve of 18 months, the feasibility of the integrated treatment increased to greater than 90%, and mortality dramatically decreased. The combined treatment resulted in a high survival rate in patients with extensive carcinomatosis who were no longer responsive to traditional therapies.

Hyperthermic intraperitoneal chemoperfusion in the treatment of locally advanced intra-abdominal cancer.

Ceelen WP, Hesse U, de Hemptinne B, Pattyn P.

Department of Abdominal Surgery 2P4, Ghent University Hospital, Ghent, Belgium.

British Journal of Surgery 87(8):1006–15, 2000, August.

Background: Surgical treatment of intra-abdominal cancer is often followed by local recurrence. In a subgroup of patients, local recurrence is the sole site of disease, reflecting biologically low-grade malignancy. These patients might, therefore, benefit from local treatment. Recently, debulking surgery followed by hyperthermic chemoperfusion has been proposed in the treatment of locally advanced or recurrent intra-abdominal cancer. This paper reviews the rationale and assesses the currently accepted indications for and results of this novel treatment. *Methods:* A systematic web-based literature review was performed. Information was also retrieved from handbooks, congress abstracts and ongoing clinical trials. *Results:* A growing body of experimental evidence supports the use of hyperthermia combined with chemotherapy as an adjunct to cytoreductive surgery. Randomized clinical trials are available to support its use in the treatment and prevention of peritoneal carcinomatosis following resection of pathological tumour stage pT3 or pT4 gastric cancer; several other phase III trials are ongoing. Numerous phase I and II trials have reported good results for various other indications, with acceptable morbidity and mortality rates. Case mix, limited patient numbers and absence of a standardized technique are, however, a drawback in many of these series. *Conclusion:* For a subgroup of patients with peritoneal cancer without distant disease, debulking surgery followed by hyperthermic chemoperfusion may offer a chance of cure or palliation in this otherwise untreatable condition. This novel therapy should, however, be considered experimental until further results from ongoing phase III trials become available.

A critique of surgical cytoreduction in advanced ovarian cancer.

Covens AL.

Department of Obstetrics and Gynecology, Sunnybrook and Women's College Health Sciences Center, Toronto, Ontario, Canada.

Gynecologic Oncology 78(3 Pt 1):269–74, 2000, September.

Due in most part to the abundant retrospective evidence suggesting that surgical cytoreduction is essential to the management of advanced ovarian cancer, most clinicians do not question its application. Irrespective, there are many who still doubt its value, given its unique role in ovarian cancer, in comparison to other solid tumors. While many papers have extolled the virtues of debulking surgery, few have taken the opposing view. This paper attempts to expose the weaknesses in the current available data regarding surgical cytoreduction in advanced ovarian cancer. By reviewing the retrospective data, the theoretical benefits of surgery, cellular kinetics, the fallacies of residual disease, interval debulking surgery, and neoadjuvant chemotherapy, a critique of debulking surgery is made. Issues surrounding perioperative morbidity and its impact on quality of life have not been adequately addressed. Despite the need for randomized trials of surgery in advanced ovarian cancer, they are unlikely to occur. The window of opportunity with respect to studying the questions on the optimal timing, degree of aggressiveness, and patient selection for surgery has likely passed. Biases and ethical issues based upon the data cited in this paper have and will continue to hamper our ability to fully elaborate the benefits of surgery with respect to survival and quality of life.

Surgical cytoreduction during second-look laparotomy in patients with advanced ovarian cancer.

Gadducci A, Iacconi P, Fanucchi A, Cosio S, Teti G, Genazzani AR.

Department of Procreative Medicine, University of Pisa, Italy.

Anticancer Research 20(3B):1959–64, 2000, May–June.

Background: The impact of surgical cytoreduction performed during second-look on the survival of patients with advanced ovarian cancer is still under debate. *Materials and methods:* The present retrospective investigation assessed 81 patients with advanced ovarian cancer who underwent second-look laparotomy after initial cytoreductive surgery and six cycles of platinum-based chemotherapy. *Results:* At the beginning of the second-look, 31 patients were in pathological complete response, 7 had microscopic residual disease, 22 had macroscopic residual disease <2 cm and 21 had a larger residuum. Twenty-two

(51.2%) of the 43 patients with macroscopic disease underwent surgical cytoreduction during the second-look: 11 patients were completely cytoreduced, whereas 11 were debulked from residuum >2 cm to macroscopic residuum <2 cm. Patients with microscopic residual disease after the second-look had improved survival when compared to those with macroscopic residuum after re-exploration (median survival, 43 months versus 19.5 months, $p = 0.002$). Among the former, no difference in survival was detected between the patients who had microscopic disease at the beginning of the second-look and those who were surgically cytoreduced to microscopic disease. Moreover, the patients with macroscopic residuum <2 cm after the second-look had a better survival than those with a larger residuum after re-exploration (median survival, 24 months versus 10 months, $p = 0.0001$). Among the former, no difference in survival was seen between the patients who had residual disease <2 cm at the beginning of the second-look and those who were surgically cytoreduced to <2 cm. However, ovarian cancer recurred in all the patients with small or large macroscopic residuum after the second-look. *Conclusion:* The complete resection of macroscopic persistent tumor seems to give ovarian cancer patients the highest likelihood of long-term survival and should represent the goal of surgical cytoreduction during second-look laparotomy.

Use of ultrasonic surgical aspirator in operative cytoreduction of pseudomyxoma peritonei.

Keating JP, Frizelle FA.

Department of Surgery, Wellington School of Medicine, New Zealand.

Diseases of the Colon & Rectum 43(4):559–60, 2000, April.

Pseudomyxoma peritonei presents a unique challenge to the surgical oncologist. Residual gelatinous tumor with varying degrees of adherence always remains on the abdominal viscera after standard excisional therapy. Traditionally, this has been removed by 'electroevaporation' with ball-tip diathermy, but this is associated with an extensive peritoneal burn and associated ileus. We describe the use of an ultrasonic surgical aspirator as a safe and efficient method of tumor removal in this condition.

Laparoscopic management of pseudomyxoma peritonei secondary to adenocarcinoma of the appendix.

Raj J, Urban LM, ReMine SG, Raj PK.

Department of Surgery, Fairview Hospital, Cleveland Clinic Health System, OH, USA.

Journal of Laparoendoscopic & Advanced Surgical Techniques Part A, 9(3):299–303, 1999, June.

Pseudomyxoma peritonei is a rare disease in which the abdominal cavity fills with thick mucoid material secondary to either benign or malignant conditions. We discuss a case where pseudomyxoma peritonei secondary to adenocarcinoma of the appendix was diagnosed and managed laparoscopically. The laparoscopic approach allows thorough exploration of the abdomen, as well as irrigation and aspiration of the thick mucinous material using a 10-mm suction cannula and the instillation of mucolytic agents

such as 5% dextrose solution. Appendectomy or right hemicolectomy can be performed with minimal disturbance of the anterior abdominal wall, thus minimizing future adhesions as well as possible tumor-cell implantation. Intraperitoneal catheters for chemotherapy can be placed easily through the port sites. These measures offer an alternative to radical peritoneal dissection and can be accomplished during the initial laparoscopic exploration.

Peritoneal carcinomatosis from non-gynecologic malignancies: results of the Evocape 1 Multicentric Prospective Study.

Sadeghi B, Arvieux C, Glehen O, Beaujard AC, Rivoire M, Baulieux J, Fontaumard E, Brachet A, Caillot JL, Faure JL, Porcheron J, Peix JL, Francois Y, Vignal J, Gilly FN.

Surgical Department, Centre Hospitalo Universitaire (CHU) Lyon Sud, Lyon Pierre Benite, France.

Cancer 88(2):358–63, 2000, January 15.

Background: Peritoneal carcinomatosis (PC) is a common evolution of digestive cancer, associated with a poor prognosis. Yet it is poorly documented in the literature. *Methods:* Three hundred seventy patients with PC from non-gynecologic malignancies were followed prospectively: the PC was of gastric origin in 125 cases, of colorectal origin in 118 cases, of pancreatic origin in 58 cases, of unknown origin in 43 cases, and of miscellaneous origins in 26 cases. A previously reported PC staging system was used to classify these 370 patients. *Results:* Mean and median overall survival periods were 6.0 and 3.1 months, respectively. Survival rates were mainly affected by the initial PC stage (9.8 months for Stage I with malignant peritoneal granulations less than 5 mm in greatest dimension, versus 3.7 months for Stage IV with large, malignant peritoneal masses more than 2 cm in greatest dimension). The presence of ascites was associated with poor survival of patients with gastric or pancreatic carcinoma. Differentiation of the primary tumor did not influence the prognoses of patients with PC. *Conclusions:* A better knowledge of the natural history of PC is needed, in view of the many Phase I, II, and III trials currently being conducted to evaluate aggressive multimodal therapeutic approaches to treating patients with PC from non-gynecologic malignancies.

Neoadjuvant chemotherapy versus primary debulking surgery in advanced ovarian cancer.

Vergote IB, De Wever I, Decloedt J, Tjalma W, Van Gramberen M, van Dam P.

Department of Gynecologic Oncology, University Hospitals Leuven, Belgium.

Seminars in Oncology 27(3 Suppl. 7):31–6, 2000, June.

Primary surgical cytoreduction followed by chemotherapy usually is the preferred management of advanced (stage III or IV) ovarian cancer. The presence of residual disease after surgery is one of the most important adverse prognostic factors for survival. Neoadjuvant chemotherapy has been proposed as an alternative approach to conventional surgery as initial management of bulky ovarian cancer, with the goal of improving surgical quality. Since 1989, we have been treating advanced epithelial ovarian cancer with neoadjuvant chemotherapy instead of primary cytoreductive surgery in approximately half of the patients with stage III–IV disease. Selection of neoadjuvant chemotherapy was based on disease-related characteristics (e.g., metastatic tumor load, stage of disease, performance status). Since 1993, open laparoscopy also has been used to aid in evaluating operability. A retrospective analysis of 338 patients was conducted to compare outcomes during 1989 to 1998, when neoadjuvant chemotherapy was used, with those observed during 1980 to 1988, when all patients underwent primary cytoreductive surgery. Crude 3-year survival rates were higher and postoperative mortality rates were lower during the second time period compared with the first. Overall, the results suggest that neoadjuvant chemotherapy results in survival rates in selected patients with advanced ovarian cancer that are comparable with those associated with primary cytoreductive surgery. Patients with stage IV disease, total metastatic tumor load greater than 1,000 g, uncountable plaque-shaped peritoneal metastases, and/or a poor performance status are probably the best candidates for this alternative approach. A prospective randomized study of neoadjuvant chemotherapy and primary cytoreductive surgery is ongoing.

Whole-body PET with (fluorine-18)-2-deoxyglucose for detecting recurrent primary serous peritoneal carcinoma: an initial report.

Wang PH, Liu RS, Li YF, Ng HT, Yuan CC.

Department of Obstetrics and Gynecology, National Yang-Ming University School of Medicine, Taipei, 112, Taiwan. phwang@vghtpe.gov.tw

Gynecologic Oncology 77(1):44–7, 2000, April.

Objective: Because of the limited sensitivity and specificity of conventional tools such as computerized tomography (CT) or magnetic resonance imaging (MRI) for detecting persistent or recurrent primary serous peritoneal carcinoma (PSPC), a reliable means of diagnosis remains elusive. Positron emission tomography (PET) scanning may offer another approach to this problem. *Methods:* A prospective study of three patients requiring surgical exploration for suspected recurrence of PSPC received a whole-body PET (fluorine-18)-2-deoxyglucose (FDG) scanning in a teaching hospital from July 1995 to December 1998. The suspected recurrence was based upon clinical findings including a detailed physical examination, serum CA-125 marker ultrasound, CT, and MRI. Three patients were enrolled in this study. *Results:* In all three patients, PET images demonstrated increased FDG uptake in a distribution that correlated with surgical-pathologic findings (100%); on the contrary, CT can detect 33.3% of these patients with malignant diseases and MRI can detect two-thirds of cases. Serum CA-125 was also elevated in all three patients, although one patient showed an equivocal elevation of 25.7 IU/mL. *Conclusions:* Conventional imaging studies are neither sensitive nor specific for detecting recurrent PSPC. In contrast, besides CA-125, PET might offer a relatively effective tool for detecting recurrent primary serous peritoneal carcinoma. Due to the very small number of patients available in this study, considerable research must be performed to clarify the impact of PET on detecting recurrence of PSPC.

Disseminated peritoneal adenomucinosis: a critical review.

Wirtzfeld DA, Rodriguez-Bigas M, Weber T, Petrelli NJ.

Division of Surgical Oncology, Roswell Park Cancer Institute, State University of New York at Buffalo, NY, USA.

Annals of Surgical Oncology 6(8):797–801, 1999, December.

Background: The term pseudomyxoma peritonei has been used in reference to any condition, benign or malignant, in which the peritoneal cavity becomes filled with a gelatinous substance. The term is nonspecific and does not denote therapeutic or prognostic significance. Controversy centers around which patients benefit from and should be treated by aggressive surgical debulking. *Methods:* A review of the current literature pertaining to the classification, treatment, and prognosis of patients with pseudomyxoma peritonei was undertaken. *Results:* Disseminated peritoneal adenomucinosis refers to a subset of patients with pseudomyxoma peritonei who derive the greatest long-term benefit from multimodality therapy including aggressive surgical debulking. These patients have a benign form of the disease in which the peritoneal implants are derived from the extrusion of epithelial cells from an adenoma of the appendix. The pathophysiology of mucin deposition is defined by the redistribution phenomenon. The adenomatous cells are distributed according to the fluid flow and gravitational forces within the peritoneal cavity. The small bowel is relatively spared until late in the disease (visceral sparing), and therefore aggressive surgical debulking should be attempted at the first laparotomy by an experienced surgeon. Preoperative computed tomographic imaging can establish the diagnosis and aid in defining which groups of patients are resectable for cure. *Conclusions:* Attempts at curative treatment should include aggressive debulking and intraperitoneal chemotherapy. Those patients with a high-grade malignant process should be treated symptomatically, because aggressive therapy is associated with high morbidity rates and no long-term improvement in survival.

8

Intraperitoneal drug therapy for intra-abdominal spread of cancer

FRANCO M MUGGIA, GILA HORNREICH, AND YURI PARISKY

INTRODUCTION

Tumors arising in the ovaries and in the gastrointestinal tract – particularly appendiceal and gastric tumors – have a high incidence of intraperitoneal (IP) spread as the most prominent manifestation of disease. Following resection of the primary site, many of the gastrointestinal (GI) tumors may, in fact, initially show little tendency to invade adjacent organs or spread beyond the abdomen. In some instances, such as low-grade adenocarcinomas that produce vast amounts of mucin, the clinical picture consists solely of serosal spread, giving rise to the entity known as pseudomyxoma peritonei.

Gynecologic oncologists have emphasized the pattern of spread shared by most epithelial ovarian cancers, and have incorporated cytologic washings, multiple peritoneal biopsies, and omentectomy as part of routine initial surgical staging. After a decade of small phase I and pilot studies, phase II and III studies have been carried out to address the role of IP cisplatin in upfront treatment and as part of consolidation treatment for advanced epithelial ovarian carcinoma.[1–3] On the other hand, surgical oncologists have seldom ventured beyond descriptive analyses of colorectal malignancies spreading to the ovaries in women as an indication of peritoneal spread of cancer. Routine oophorectomy at the time of colectomy for bowel cancers beyond T1 stage occurring in women is still controversial; however, this issue has only recently been addressed in a systematic manner and preliminary data suggest a possible recurrence-free survival advantage.[4] The role of IP-directed therapy in other GI malignancies (gastric, appendiceal) has also been addressed over the past few years.[5–7] This chapter provides information on the type of IP-directed therapies that should be considered for such circumstances, and emphasizes

how clinical trials beyond pilot studies are required to establish a role for IP therapy. Such data should be applicable not only to gynecologic cancers, but also to primary peritoneal malignancies, to GI tract malignancies, including pancreatic and biliary tract cancers, and to the occasional metastatic malignancy, such as some breast cancers that at times share a predominant peritoneal spread. Although the focus to date has been IP drug therapy, the IP route is also being explored as a mode for the delivery of different genetic materials (i.e., gene therapy)[8,9] as well as biologic materials.[10,11]

Drugs administered intraperitoneally have been studied primarily to determine their 'pharmacologic advantage' at peritoneal surfaces versus what could be achieved by their systemic administration at maximally tolerated doses. This pharmacologic advantage is usually expressed as a ratio of drug exposure (concentration × time) in the peritoneal fluid (IP) over the plasma (PL) drug exposure. Occasionally, the ratio of peak levels in peritoneal fluid and in plasma has also been compared, because such levels may be predictive of certain toxicities. The concentration × time plot yields an area-under-the-curve (AUC) with the resulting pharmacologic advantage for a given drug at the recommended IP doses expressed by:

$$\text{IP drug advantage} = AUC_{IP}/AUC_{PL}.$$

Maximal exposure of all peritoneal surfaces is ensured by delivering the drug in large volumes, usually 2 L, but best standardized as 1 L/m^2.

Despite many pharmacologic studies, however, IP drug delivery has not been widely adopted into surgical practice. This chapter begins with a historical perspective and a discussion of issues regarding the IP delivery of drugs. Review of phase II and III studies and our own therapeutic experience follows, ending with an overview of the ideal clinical setting for IP therapy.

HISTORICAL PERSPECTIVE

Intraperitoneal chemotherapy has had a firm pharmacologic basis since studies in the late 1970s, initially carried out at the National Cancer Institute and subsequently at the University of California at San Diego, Memorial Sloan-Kettering Cancer Center, New York University, University of Arizona, Netherlands Cancer Institute, and other institutions. Due to the fact that these studies have been primarily of a pharmacological nature and the assessment of peritoneal disease is difficult, the therapeutic accomplishments of IP chemotherapy obtained with various drugs and combinations have been uncertain. The reasons for therapeutic failure other than extraperitoneal disease progression probably include extreme drug resistance, initial or subsequent failure of drug distribution, selection of a suboptimal drug schedule, and improper patient entry. However, much of this is inferential and, even after nearly two decades of study, the basic principles leading to more widespread clinical application remain controversial.

Studies in the late 1970s by Dedrick, Myers, Collins, DeVita, and other colleagues at the National Cancer Institute (USA) first worked out the pharmacologic principles of IP chemotherapy.[12,13] The studies from the outset had in mind the possible therapeutic application of IP chemotherapy in the management of minimal residual ovarian cancer, but had not formulated constraints in relation to the extent or type of spread of disease. Its original modeling utilized timed 'dwells' of large (2 L) volumes of fluid containing the selected drug. Subsequent principles were elaborated on by Howell at the University of California, San Diego, who, with his coworkers in gynecologic oncology, introduced implantable IP devices, concepts of systemic neutralization, combination chemotherapy, and the first claim for a role of IP cisplatin in the treatment of ovarian cancer.[14,15] Cisplatin's lack of schedule dependency eliminated the need for the cumbersome 'dwell' (often not feasible because of outflow obstruction) and it became utilized alone or in combination with other cytotoxic drugs given in one volume (usually 2 L) of dialysate every 3 weeks. King's studies also first suggested therapeutic benefit from IP cytosine arabinoside – a drug not otherwise active by the systemic route.[16] Speyer and colleagues first studied 5-fluorouracil (5-FU) and described the non-linear pharmacokinetics of systemic exposure (e.g., plasma AUCs) resulting from IP administration.[17–20] With Sugarbaker, they demonstrated an effect of 5-FU against IP recurrences of colon cancer, and against the recurrence of pseudomyxoma peritonei after aggressive debulking.[18,20] In 1985, at a meeting of the Gastrointestinal Tumor Study Group, Myers hypothesized that IP floxuridine (FUDR) would have very favorable pharmacologic characteristics for IP administration.[21] This hypothesis generated the studies conducted at the New York University and at the University of Southern California by us,[22–24] and subsequently taken up by the Southwest Oncology Group, in a randomized phase II study[25] testing IP consolidation with FUDR or mitoxantrone following positive second-look laparotomies for ovarian cancer.

Phase III studies of IP cisplatin by cooperative groups were designed after 1986, but did not yield definitive analyses until a decade later.[2] A consistent advantage for IP over intravenous (IV) cisplatin for the progression-free survival of epithelial ovarian cancer (EOC) was documented in this study, and in a subsequent study by the Gynecologic Oncology Group.[3] For other drugs or regimens, the rationale for the use of IP-administered drugs in minimal residual disease has not evolved much beyond phase I and pharmacologic studies.[25] The clinical information is mostly confined to issues of tolerance and short-term outcome as determined by a subsequent reassessment laparotomy. The paucity of comparative clinical information has led to negative editorials in the medical literature applicable to gynecologic cancer.[26–28] These negative attitudes have arisen in large part from initially unrealistic expectations of such therapy in a somewhat clinically resistant population, frequent technical problems encountered, and – in retrospect – an unsatisfactory choice of drugs and doses in some trials. The recent and ongoing randomized studies may lead to a more critical consideration of the potential for IP therapy in gynecologic and surgical oncology.[2,3] It is hoped that this will facilitate renewed interest in optimal IP devices and techniques, and foster studies in gene therapy as well as other therapeutic innovations.

ISSUES IN INTRAPERITONEAL DRUG DELIVERY

Drug-related variables

In addition to important pharmacologic properties which determine the pharmacologic advantage of IP over systemic drug administration, there are other important and poorly understood variables in the selection of a drug for IP therapy. Slow clearance from the peritoneal cavity leading to prolonged IP exposure has been advocated as an attractive feature favoring IP paclitaxel.[29–31] On the other hand, diffusivity (penetrance) into tumors and into juxtaperitoneal lymphatics is likely to be relevant to the common spread of malignant disease, and therefore to affect the therapeutic results that may be achieved. Such issues have been studied in some animal models, and cisplatin has been identified as having better penetrance than carboplatin into tumor nodules,[32] and doxorubicin as having minimal penetrance.[33] Cannulation of the thoracic duct in rabbits has indicated high concentrations are achieved following IP administration of cisplatin and 5-FU, but not etoposide.[34]

Scheduling

Scheduling has been almost universally single dose and intermittent because it was most practical for cisplatin, but it may not be optimal for antimetabolites, podophyllotoxins (etoposide or teniposide), or topoisomerase I inhibitors. Paclitaxel was initially introduced in the usual once every 3 weeks schedule,[31] but more recently has been given on a weekly schedule to improve peritoneal tolerance.[35] Obvious chemical peritonitis may affect the ability to administer a drug repeatedly and this has been seen with doxorubicin, mitoxantrone, as well as paclitaxel. However, subclinical changes in peritoneal permeability may occur as a result of treatment and affect drug pharmacokinetics and the 'pharmacologic advantages' in subsequent cycles. Such changes have been documented with the otherwise well-tolerated fluoropyrimidines.[23,36]

Catheter complications

Catheter complications may be indicative of chemical peritonitis because they occurred at a much greater rate with mitoxantrone than with FUDR in a randomized study.[25]

Tumor sensitivity

Tumor sensitivity has been the overriding rationale in IP drug selection. For example, IP cisplatin is the major drug used for ovarian cancer despite a pharmacologic advantage between 10- and 20-fold, which is not as remarkable as for many other drugs.[15,37] However, the pharmacologic advantage does lend support to the use of some drugs that play little or no role by the systemic route. Cytarabine has yielded well-documented remissions in platinum-resistant ovarian cancer, presumably because of its 3-log pharmacologic advantage despite playing no role by the systemic route.[16,38,39]

Intraperitoneal dose-limiting factors

IP dose-limiting factors vary with drugs and may differ from toxicities resulting from their systemic administration. Again, cisplatin is not representative of many other drugs: the same dosing by the IP or IV route yields virtually identical toxicities (the exception being lesser ototoxicity for IP cisplatin). For fluoropyrimidines, systemic toxicity from IP drug administration becomes evident only when the capacity of the liver to thoroughly metabolize the drugs is exceeded – a feature subject to marked interindividual variation. Therefore, consistent systemic effects from IP fluoropyrimidines may require the concomitant administration of systemic therapy. A similar situation is applicable to drugs regularly leading to clinical chemical peritonitis, with which systemic dose-limiting toxicities may not be reached.[40]

Disease-related variables

As already noted, the intrinsic susceptibility of ovarian cancer to platinum compounds renders IP cisplatin one of the preferred drugs for treatment selection. Interest in IP paclitaxel has been generated for the same reason (in addition to its prolonged half-life in the peritoneal cavity). For colon or appendiceal cancer metastases, the fluoropyrimidines are the drugs of major interest. In gastric cancer, both fluoropyrimidines and cisplatin are believed to play a role.[41] The type of disease in the peritoneum is also likely to be a key factor in both drug-regimen selection and treatment outcome: microscopic disease or nodules with tumor volumes not exceeding 5 mm are the best targets for IP drug therapy.[42] Such features may be even more important for trials including biological agents. The Gynecologic Oncology Group identified a category of patients with poor outcome following IP therapy: both platinum resistance (i.e., evidence of unresponsiveness to this initial therapy or regrowth of disease within 6 months) and/or diffuse rather than patchy peritoneal seeding.[43] Disease exceeding 1 cm in cross-sectional area would not be expected to preferentially yield to IP therapy vis-à-vis systemic drug administration. Moreover, in such patients, the interval between treatments may be crucial, because the circumstances for optimal therapy become progressively more unfavorable if the tumor is allowed to grow before treatment cycles are repeated.

Technique/catheter-related factors

Catheters for IP drug administration evolved from experience with peritoneal dialysis, but their use for cancer treatment soon faced other issues related to prior surgeries, recent surgical exploration and resections, and dynamic changes in the peritoneum as a result of drug effects.

Outflow obstruction

Outflow obstruction is a common problem that probably results from peritoneal tissue growing into and partially blocking the catheter opening, and, paradoxically, may be more common with multiple openings.

Blockage and maldistribution

More serious are total blockage and/or maldistribution of the infused fluid into a small loculated pocket rather than throughout the peritoneal cavity. Unfortunately, factors predisposing to such occurrences or methods to avoid them have been inadequately studied. Multiple surgeries and resections certainly increase the incidence of complications. Erosions of the catheter opening into the site of bowel anastomoses or into a partially blocked ureter have been recorded by the authors. As noted earlier, some drugs – such as mitoxantrone in one randomized trial – may be associated with a greater frequency of problems.

Placement of the catheter

Placement of the catheter in some areas, such as infradiaphragmatic surfaces, is done only rarely, but in our experience may have a greater propensity to malfunction. We recently noted a tendency toward bleeding upon lavaging a catheter that had been placed on the pancreatic head upon gastrectomy and lymph node dissection for gastric cancer. Also, the placement of multiple catheters may be counterproductive, because factors leading one catheter to malfunction frequently lead to obstruction in the other.

Catheter maintenance

Catheter maintenance, especially during early postoperative periods, may be important. Initially, frequent irrigations were carried out. Whereas this may not be necessary, early use of the catheter is recommended. Outflow obstruction was less frequent with the Tenckhoff catheter than with implantable ones,[44] and this may just be a function of the frequent flushing that is routinely carried out with the Tenckhoff catheter. Following uneventful use for several cycles of IP therapy, flushing the catheter every 6 weeks has been sufficient to maintain its function if it is deemed desirable not to remove it immediately after the completion of contemplated therapy.

Type of catheter

The type of catheter, i.e., one with multiple openings rather than only a distal opening, and/or valve-like openings, may also have an impact on complication rates, but data are not available. A Groshong-type collapsable tip may be advantageous in preventing growth into the catheter. On the other hand, multiple openings have been noted to become occluded by peritoneal connective tissue growing into the catheter, which, upon its removal, resembles a centipede. IP therapy may also be delivered via percutaneously introduced catheters. Repeat administration, however, is labor intensive for the operator and often difficult for the patient.

Finally, the use of IP drugs immediately following resection for colon cancer or pseudomyxoma peritonei has been advocated by Sugarbaker[20] and has been utilized following gastrectomy by Japanese and Korean surgeons.[45–48] A one-time exposure to chemotherapy, even at the 'optimal' time, is unlikely to prove curative under most circumstances, and therefore such practices must be evaluated in randomized clinical trials.

Distribution studies

Distribution studies using IP contrast (and IV plus oral) with computerized tomography (Figure 8.1) have been routinely used at our institution for the purposes of obtaining baseline pretreatment staging/disease-assessment information and of confirming adequate distribution for IP drug delivery.[49] Such a step is a wise investment in guiding treatment for other circumstances, such as for

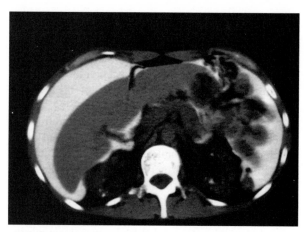

Figure 8.1 *Intraperitoneal contrast with normal distribution seen on a mid-abdomen CT scan. Contrast is distributed over the surface of the right lobe of the liver and between loops of small bowel and mesentery.*

patients who have had prior surgeries and may have other metastatic sites not detected by the surgeon. Other techniques for assessing distribution have included the introduction of radionuclides[50] and magnetic resonance imaging with saline administration.[51]

SPECIFIC MODALITIES OF INTRAPERITONEAL THERAPY

Table 8.1 lists chemotherapeutic drugs that have had some evaluation for their potential when given via the IP route. Most of these remain in the experimental realm, and only those drugs that have current therapeutic relevance are described in detail.

Fluoropyrimidines

In various publications, we have outlined why the deoxyribose of 5-FU, FUDR, is the preferred fluoropyrimidine for IP administration.[21–24] Although the two drugs share many pharmacologic properties and FUDR actually yields substantial IP and plasma levels of 5-FU, they differ in their potency for surface cytotoxicity, their solubility in slightly acidic pH, and the extent of their hepatic (first-pass) metabolism. In all these characteristics, FUDR is more advantageous for IP administration, and a tolerable dose schedule has been devised and tested in both multi-institutional[25] and other single-institution studies.[52] However, 5-FU has been the subject of more clinical studies (see below, 'Clinical settings for intraperitoneal therapy'), probably due to cost and drug availability issues. The systemic toxicities from both drugs are identical, and relate to plasma levels resulting in mucosal and marrow toxicities. Sclerosing peritonitis, however, has been reported for 5-FU.[53] Efforts to enhance their therapeutic effects have included modulating their

Table 8.1 *The pharmacological advantage* and tolerance of intraperitoneal drugs*

Agent (reference)	Peak concentrations	AUC	Major toxicities
Cisplatin (15)	20	12	Emesis, renal
Carboplatin (87)		6–10	Bone marrow
Melphalan (88)	93	65	Bone marrow
Thiotepa (89)		4	Bone marrow
Mitomycin (90)		32	IP (pain), bone marrow
Doxorubicin (91)	474	400	IP, peritonitis
Mitoxantrone (40)		1400	Peritonitis
Methotrexate (92)		92	Bone marrow
Fluorouracil (17)	298	376	Peritonitis, bone marrow
Floxuridine (21)	>1000	>1000	Stomatitis
Cytarabine (39)	664	300–1000	Bone marrow
Etoposide (59)		65	Alopecia, bone marrow
Paclitaxel (34)	780–1255	–	Peritonitis
Bleomycin (71)		4	Peritonitis, fever
Interleukin-2 (73)		200–1000	Sclerosis, edema
Interferon-alpha (60)	?	?	Flu symptoms
Interferon-gamma (74)	?	?	Flu symptoms
Gemcitabine (70)			Bone marrow[a]
Topotecan (71)			Bone marrow

*See definition in Introduction. Numbers refer to this ratio and therefore do not have the customary units for concentrations or AUC.
[a]In combination with cisplatin.
AUC, area under the curve.

action with IP leucovorin (folinic acid)[23,24] or by concurrent IV hydroxyurea,[54] supplementing systemic exposure by concurrent IV 5-FU,[55] or by combining them with IP cisplatin.[41,56] The millimolar concentrations in the peritoneal cavity for either fluoropyrimidine should be cytotoxic to most tumor cells and unlikely to be enhanced further through modulation.

Platinum compounds

Cisplatin is the drug that has received the widest trial via the IP route. IP cisplatin has been advocated in ovarian cancer following the initial induction with systemic carboplatin and paclitaxel. At the University of Southern California, it has also been used postoperatively (together with FUDR) following a neoadjuvant systemic regimen of 5-FU plus cisplatin and curative gastrectomy for gastric cancer.[7,41] The toxicities of IP cisplatin are dose related and analogous dose per dose with systemic administration. Peak plasma levels of the drug are lower after IP administration and a slightly improved tolerance for IP cisplatin over IV cisplatin has been noted in a randomized study.[57] In patients with pre-existing neuropathy, partial substitution of cisplatin by carboplatin may allow the maintenance of dose intensity of a platinum regimen at a cost of slightly greater myelosuppression from carboplatin.[58] Local signs and symptoms are generally mild with either platinum; however, subcutaneous extravasation from a malfunctioning delivery system may result in sloughing of the abdominal wall (Figure 8.2). Sodium thiosulfate IV

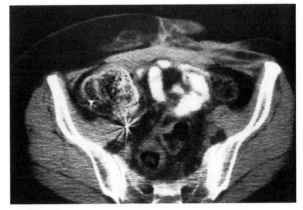

Figure 8.2 *Left lower abdominal wall defect seen on a mid-pelvis CT scan. The defect was caused by cisplatin administered into a blocked IP catheter, resulting in extravasation into the soft tissues of the left abdomen wall, with subsequent necrosis.*

has been given to protect against the nephrotoxicity of IP cisplatin in doses of up to 200 mg/m²;[15] this maneuver renders the treatment more complex and its usefulness remains to be established. Cisplatin has often been given in combination with other drugs such as cytarabine[38] or etoposide,[1,59] or as part of chemoimmunotherapy with interferon,[43,60–62] but the contribution of the other drugs has been uncertain and the popularity of many of these regimens has waned. Trials of IP cisplatin with local hyperthermia have been difficult, in part because of erratic renal toxicity.[63] Carboplatin IP has also been combined with hyperthermia in order to avoid such potential aggravation of nephrotoxicity.[64]

Other chemotherapeutic drugs

The taxane paclitaxel is currently attracting interest for possible IP use in gynecologic cancer.[29,65,66] Mitomycin C IP is subjectively not well tolerated, but has been extensively used during operations for gastric cancer in Japan, alone[46] or with hyperthermia.[67] Cytarabine is an antimetabolite with little activity against solid tumors, but concentrations achievable in the peritoneal cavity have shown activity in clinical studies including patients with ovarian cancer.[14,16] An analogue of doxorubicin, AD-32, that had a brief trial systemically[68] and has now been approved for intravesical use, has shown activity against ovarian cancer in an IP phase I trial.[69] Both topotecan and gemcitabine are currently being investigated in phase I trials for their possible role in IP therapy.[70,71] A number of drugs such as bleomycin[72,73] and mitoxantrone[40] have been given for the palliation of ascites, but this does not necessarily recommend their use as an adjuvant to surgery and for the containment and/or eradication of peritoneal metastases.

Other modalities

Biological compounds

Biological compounds such as interferon-alpha and interferon-gamma have been given intraperitoneally in several clinical studies, and positive results in ovarian cancer have stimulated subsequent trials alone and in combination with cisplatin.[60,62,74] Direct cytotoxicity or indirect antiangiogenic actions have been postulated to explain these therapeutic effects. Interleukin-2 was initially given with lymphokine-activated killer cells and subsequently by itself in several trials.[10,11,75] Peritoneal fibrosis was a major problem, but interest has rekindled in view of some long-term survivals in the largest trial with this agent. Monoclonal antibodies tagged with radionuclides have had extensive trial in ovarian cancer,[76] but their role remains uncertain, even though delivery of radioactivity and the physics of the radionuclide used (yttrium, rhenium) have considerable theoretical advantages over colloidal solutions of ^{32}P. T-cells coated with bispecific antibodies represent yet another IP-administered modality.[77]

Hyperthermia

Hyperthermia may be provided by radiofrequency to the abdomen containing fluid plus drugs, or may be achieved, usually intraoperatively, by administering warm dialysate.[63,64,67]

Gene therapy

Gene therapy by the IP route has been tested in animal models, and clinical trials are ongoing using the herpes simplex thymidine kinase gene transduction, and relying on the 'bystander effect' also killing non-transduced cells following the administration of ganciclovir.[9] Another approach already in phase II and III trials combined with chemotherapy in ovarian cancer is the use of p53 transduction following the rationale that chemoresistance is mediated in part by p53 mutations.

CLINICAL SETTINGS FOR INTRAPERITONEAL THERAPY

Ovarian cancer

The intergroup (INT 0051, SWOG 8501) phase III study of IP versus IV cisplatin (100 mg/m^2) plus IV cyclophosphamide has provided the best data to date in terms of efficacy and treatment tolerance.[2] INT 0051 demonstrated that optimally debulked (defined in this study, initiated in 1985, as $\leqslant 2$ cm greatest diameter of residual lesions) stage III ovarian cancer patients treated with IP cisplatin (100 mg/m^2) at 3-week intervals, had a better outcome than those treated with IV cisplatin at the same dose and schedule (both groups also received IV cyclophosphamide). The median survival on the IP arm was 49 months, as compared to 41 months on the IV arm. Other observations in this trial also support greater efficacy for IP cisplatin in patients with all gross disease resected initially. For the 83 patients in this category who underwent second-look laparotomy, 80% on the IP arm versus 56% on the IV arm were documented to have pathological complete responses ($p = 0.02$ by the two-sided Fisher's Exact Test). The pathological complete responses, including only patients who agreed to undergo second-look laparotomies, were 47% on the IP arm versus 36% on the IV arm ($p = 0.06$). Most patients entered (72% and 73% respectively) had disease at entry classified as either microscopic or $\leqslant 0.5$ cm; however, differences are not significant in subset analysis. In this respect, the results suggest a contribution of IP therapy with cisplatin even in tumor residua $\geqslant 0.5$ cm, which was not expected from a number of pilot phase II studies. On the other hand, these other studies dealt with patients previously exposed to platinum compounds. In considering a role for IP consolidation, it would seem appropriate to confine patient eligibility to residua not exceeding 1 cm.[14]

Unexpected findings in INT 0051 were toxicologic differences favoring lesser ototoxicity and neutropenia in the IP arm. In both arms, tolerance was excellent, and allowed the maintenance of equivalent cisplatin dose intensity for the six cycles of treatment. In this respect, the study differs from the attenuation in dose of IV cisplatin observed in the Southwest Oncology Group study comparing cisplatin to carboplatin in suboptimally debulked disease (SWOG No. 8412), both given with cyclophosphamide.[78] Although there are differences in schedule and in dose-adjustment measures between the two studies, it is likely that the better tolerance in the IP/IV study relates to lack of disease progression during therapy and a lesser impact of adverse organ dysfunction that presumably occurs in the presence of the more advanced ovarian cancer in patients on study No. 8412.

Attention is drawn to several ongoing phase III trials:

1 The recently completed GOG No. 114, which utilized IP cisplatin and IV paclitaxel following IV carboplatin induction in its 'dose-intense' arm to be compared with the 'standard' arm of IV cisplatin and paclitaxel.[3]
2 The EORTC IP cisplatin consolidation versus observation.
3 GOG No. 93 of IP chromic phosphate-32 suspension versus observation.
4 SWOG No. 8790 of IP recombinant interferon alpha-2 versus observation, all of them following negative second-look reassessment surgery.
5 A study by the Gruppo Oncologico Nord-Ovest (GONO) comparing IV cyclophosphamide, epirubicin, and cisplatin versus the same with the cisplatin IP. This study was interrupted early because of poor compliance with the IP regimen, but showed an advantage of progression-free survival for the IP arm even if the median number of IP courses was two.

In addition to these data that are and will be available on IP cisplatin, our own institutional experience utilizing IP FUDR[22,56] positioned this drug within the SWOG study No. 8835, which utilized a randomized phase II selection design comparing it to IP mitoxantrone, for patients with ≤1 cm residual disease at second-look laparotomy.[25] In this study, catheter complications or abdominal pain leading to treatment discontinuation occurred in 12 of 39 patients on mitoxantrone, versus 3 of 28 patients on FUDR. The high incidence of complications associated with IP mitoxantrone had not been attributable to the drug in preceding studies. The randomized phase II design not only selected FUDR for further study based on a superior time-to-failure (median of 24 months versus 11 months for mitoxantrone), but also improved the interpretation of toxicologic findings.

Newer drugs that have been emerging over the past few years for the IV treatment of epithelial ovarian cancer are being explored for their potential role in the IP setting as well. These include paclitaxel,[35,79] topoisomerase I inhibitors,[71] and gemcitabine,[70] among others.

Taken together, randomized phase II and III data serve as a key background for future uses of IP consolidation in epithelial ovarian cancer. Out of 11 ovarian cancer

patients with minimal residual disease treated from July 1993 to September 1994 in the pilot study of IP FUDR/ leucovorin,[24] three remain free of disease at 20+ to 26+ months. We subsequently combined FUDR with cisplatin or carboplatin in a pilot study and the preliminary results are favorable.[56] It is worth emphasizing that there is a 'window of opportunity' for IP therapy at the time of first assessment, and that a normal plasma CA-125 may identify a favorable population for considering IP treatment.[80]

Gastric cancer

The selection of IP FUDR for further study as a consolidation treatment in gastric cancer was in part based on vast experience at the University of Southern California in phase I and pharmacologic studies, and subsequently in a pilot program of neoadjuvant therapy, gastrectomy, and intraperitoneal consolidation.[41] We initially established tolerance to repeated daily × three courses of FUDR by itself or with leucovorin and then used IP FUDR with cisplatin without leucovorin for postoperative consolidation in resected gastric cancer. This last trial yielded a very favorable median survival exceeding 4 years, compared to less than 1 year for historical controls of resected gastric cancer patients over a 2-year period at the Los Angeles County Hospital.[7]

Studies from Japan and Europe have utilized IP and intra-arterial mitomycin C at the time of surgery[45] and, more recently, IP carbon-absorbed mitomycin C.[6,46] Of the two latter studies, one indicated a survival advantage for patients randomized to receive such IP therapy, whereas the other did not find any advantage to the IP therapy. In another Japanese institution, patients with peritoneal seeding and no liver metastases were treated with IP cisplatin 50 mg during surgery. Their survival was better than that of a similar group of patients who received only systemic adjuvant therapy consisting of mitomycin C and tegafur.[47] Another phase II study from England, however, led to the opposite interpretation of no benefit.[81] A more complex IP regimen containing cisplatin, etoposide, and interferon-alpha was interpreted as superior to historical controls in a study from Italy: 20 deaths in 44 IP-treated patients compared to 36 deaths of 47 historical controls at median follow-up of 44 and 97 months, respectively.[61] At Memorial Sloan-Kettering Cancer Center, IP cisplatin plus 5-FU with systemic 5-FU has been given as a postoperative adjuvant 14–28 days after potentially curative resections to 35 patients with gastric cancer. At a median follow-up of 2 years, 51% of the patients remained alive and disease free; a major complication in five patients was sclerosing encapsulating peritonitis.[53] A later study from Memorial Sloan-Kettering Cancer Center, looking at the neoadjuvant therapy of high-risk gastric cancer utilizing fluorouracil, doxorubicin, and metrotrexate (FAMTX) as a preoperative regimen and intraperitoneal 5-FU–cisplatin plus intravenous 5-FU postoperatively, concluded that IP therapy can be successfully delivered to most resected patients and that the intra-abdominal failure pattern appears to be decreased compared with that expected.[82] With a median follow-up time of 29 months, the median survival duration was 15.3 months. For patients who underwent potentially curative resections, the median survival duration was 31 months. Peritoneal failure was seen in 16% of patients. Because peritoneal recurrences are a major route for the dissemination of gastric cancer, studies of IP drug administration should be considered high priority.

Colorectal and appendiceal cancers, and pseudomyxoma peritonei

Occasional colorectal and many appendiceal cancers have as a prominent clinical manifestation intraperitoneal spread of cancer, at times also accumulating vast amounts of mucin. If this peritoneal spread is detected at the initial surgical resection, postoperative IP therapy is an attractive therapeutic modality because systemic therapy is often ineffective.[83] On the other hand, if peritoneal recurrences become the dominant clinical picture in the absence of invasiveness to other intra-abdominal viscera, symptomatic relief may be obtained through surgical debulking. IP therapy has been advocated under these circumstances in order to delay or even eliminate potential regrowth.[84,85] The prognosis in this last instance appears to be dependent on the intrinsic invasiveness of the cancer. Although several drugs (5-FU, mitomycin C, doxorubicin) have been used as adjuncts to surgical debulking, their relative contributions to a favorable outcome are unclear. In our experience with FUDR, some prolonged control of the disease has been observed in patients with colorectal cancer or pseudomyxoma peritonei of appendiceal origin.[22,23] IP 5-FU and IP FUDR have also been used in resected colorectal cancer as adjuvant therapy in patients at high risk for recurrence. This approach was initially conceived during the pharmacologic studies by Speyer and Sugarbaker at the National Cancer Institute.[17–20] In a randomized study, no improvement in survival was noted with IP 5-FU, but the tolerance was excellent, and the peritoneal recurrences were less than with 5-FU IV. In view of these results, in 1985 this approach was considered a promising area for study. A subsequent pilot study in very high-risk resected patients at Memorial Sloan-Kettering Cancer Center utilizing FUDR was deemed promising.[86] Finally, a randomized study from Vienna indicates superior survival in 58 patients receiving IP 5-FU plus leucovorin (days 1 and 3), as well as the same drugs IV on days 1–4 for six cycles as compared to 60 patients randomized to observation. This study was stopped early because of ethical concerns regarding the control arm, and a new study was initiated with 5-FU plus levamisole as the control.[55]

CONCLUSIONS

Review of the status of IP drug therapy may be timely, because the treatment of intra-abdominal malignancies over the last decade has increasingly been refined through improvements in diagnosis and surgery. Such improvements have identified the questions to be asked in clinical trials. In addition, pharmacologic principles are helping us to optimize the use of the available anticancer drugs. IP therapy, particularly with fluoropyrimidines and cisplatin, is emerging as a most rational approach to deal with small or microscopic peritoneal metastases. The peritoneal route may also be useful in the future detection of peritoneal recurrences and in the delivery of new therapeutic approaches such as gene therapy.

In ovarian cancer treatment, the newly recognized contribution of IP cisplatin has been followed by a trial (GOG 114) utilizing IP cisplatin and IV paclitaxel following the induction with two cycles of high-dose carboplatin.[3] While this study evaluates a high-dose strategy versus the now standard IV paclitaxel and cisplatin, the inclusion of IP cisplatin in this trial will be a confirmation of an advantage for this drug provided by the IP route of administration in optimally debulked ovarian cancer. Interest has also been generated by the pharmacologic properties of paclitaxel when given by the IP route.[29,66] However, the experience with FUDR, and previously with cytosine arabinoside, suggests that repeated administration may lead to remarkable therapeutic effects with drugs that are not usually part of ovarian cancer therapies. The near absence of chemical peritonitis may be another prerequisite. In addition, not only the pharmacologic advantage provided by concentrations at the peritoneal surfaces but also a sustained, high concentration in juxtaperitoneal lymphatics may be responsible for lasting antitumor effects. Strategies should test IP consolidation with cisplatin or with cisplatin and FUDR in the presence of persistent disease at the time of initial reassessment. With 50% recurrences at 5 years, patients presenting with stage III disease who obtain pathological complete responses should also be targets for IP consolidation.

Similarly, in cancers of gastric origin, the neoadjuvant approach followed by surgery and IP consolidation must be tested in clinical trials versus surgery alone. Such studies should have greater priority than postoperative adjuvant studies because, potentially, they will apply to a greater patient population than those selected by having had curative resections. In colorectal cancer, awareness of peritoneal disease and the potential for IP drug administration must be enhanced in order to stimulate adjuvant trials in patients at high risk for recurrence.

The evolution of IP drug administration (see Table 8.1) into a useful treatment modality has been long and arduous. The pharmacologic basis underlying such treatment is still evolving,[93] and the optimal circumstances for therapeutic effects in ovarian cancer and in other cancers with prominent peritoneal spread remain far from clear. Nevertheless, recent randomized phase II and III trials provide new, important reference points: cisplatin is better tolerated and has greater efficacy by the IP than the IV route in small-volume residual disease; FUDR is well tolerated on a daily × three schedule and has shown promising antitumor activity by itself and in combination with cisplatin for gastric and ovarian cancers. Gene therapies and biological approaches are extending beyond phase I. It is imperative that surgical oncologists be aware of the results achievable with IP therapy, and consider IP port placement during both curative and palliative surgical interventions.

REFERENCES

1. Barakat RR, Almadrones L, Venkatraman ES, *et al.* A phase II trial of intraperitoneal cisplatin and etoposide as consolidation therapy in patients with stage II–IV epithelial ovarian cancer following negative surgical assessment. Gynecol Oncol 1998; 69:17–22.

2. Alberts DS, Liu PY, Hannigan EV, *et al.* Intraperitoneal cisplatin plus intravenous cyclophosphamide versus intravenous cisplatin plus intravenous cyclophosphamide for stage III ovarian cancer [see comments]. N Engl J Med 1996; 335:1950–5.

3. Markman M, Bundy BN, Alberts DS, *et al.* Phase III trial of standard dose intravenous paclitaxel and intraperitoneal cisplatin in small-volume stage III ovarian carcinoma: an intergroup study of the Gynecologic Oncology Group, Southwestern Oncology Group, and Eastern Cooperative Oncology Group. J Clin Oncol 2001; 19:1001–7.

4. Young-Fadok TM, Wolff BG, Nivatvongs S, Metzger PP, Ilstrup DM. Prophylactic oophorectomy in colorectal carcinoma: preliminary results of a randomized, prospective trial. Dis Colon Rectum 1998; 41:277–83; discussion 283–5.

5. Sugarbaker PH. Patient selection and treatment of peritoneal carcinomatosis from colorectal and appendiceal cancer. World J Surg 1995; 19:235–40.

6. Rosen HR, Jatzko G, Repse S, *et al.* Adjuvant intraperitoneal chemotherapy with carbon-adsorbed mitomycin in patients with gastric cancer: results of a randomized multicenter trial of the Austrian Working Group for Surgical Oncology. J Clin Oncol 1998; 16:2733–8.

7. Crookes P, Leichman CG, Leichman L, *et al.* Systemic chemotherapy for gastric carcinoma followed by postoperative intraperitoneal therapy: a final report. Cancer 1997; 79:1767–75.

8. Cao G, Kuriyama S, Gao J, *et al.* Effective and safe gene therapy for colorectal carcinoma using the cytosine deaminase gene directed by the carcinoembryonic antigen promoter. Gene Ther 1999; 6:83–90.

9. Misawa T, Chiang MH, Pandit L, Gordon EM, Anderson WF, Parekh D. Development of systemic immunologic responses against hepatic metastases during gene therapy for peritoneal carcinomatosis with retroviral HS-tk and ganciclovir. J Gastrointest Surg 1997; 1:527–33.

10. Freedman RS, Ioannides CG, Mathioudakis G, Platsoucas CD. Novel immunologic strategies in ovarian carcinoma. Am J Obstet Gynecol 1992; 167:1470–8.

11. Edwards RP, Gooding W, Lembersky BC, *et al.* Comparison of toxicity and survival following intraperitoneal recombinant interleukin-2 for persistent ovarian cancer after platinum: twenty-four-hour versus 7-day infusion. J Clin Oncol 1997; 15:3399–407.

12. Dedrick RL, Myers CE, Bungay PM, DeVita VT Jr. Pharmacokinetic rationale for peritoneal drug administration in the treatment of ovarian cancer. Cancer Treat Rep 1978; 62:1–11.

13. Myers CE, Collins JM. Pharmacology of intraperitoneal chemotherapy. Cancer Invest 1983; 1:395–407.

14. Howell SB, Zimm S, Markman M, *et al.* Long-term survival of advanced refractory ovarian carcinoma patients with small-volume disease treated with intraperitoneal chemotherapy. J Clin Oncol 1987; 5:1607–12.

15. Howell SB, Pfeifle CL, Wung WE, *et al.* Intraperitoneal cisplatin with systemic thiosulfate protection. Ann Intern Med 1982; 97:845–51.

16. King ME, Pfeifle CE, Howell SB. Intraperitoneal cytosine arabinoside therapy in ovarian carcinoma. J Clin Oncol 1984; 2:662–9.

17. Speyer JL, Sugarbaker PH, Collins JM, Dedrick RL, Klecker RW Jr, Myers CE. Portal levels and hepatic clearance of 5-fluorouracil after intraperitoneal administration in humans. Cancer Res 1981; 41:1916–22.

18. Sugarbaker PH, Gianola FJ, Speyer JC, Wesley R, Barofsky I, Meyers CE. Prospective, randomized trial of intravenous versus intraperitoneal 5-fluorouracil in patients with advanced primary colon or rectal cancer. Surgery 1985; 98:414–22.

19. Speyer JL, Collins JM, Dedrick RL, *et al.* Phase I and pharmacological studies of 5-fluorouracil administered intraperitoneally. Cancer Res 1980; 40:567–72.

20. Sugarbaker PH, Graves T, DeBruijn EA, *et al.* Early postoperative intraperitoneal chemotherapy as an adjuvant therapy to surgery for peritoneal

carcinomatosis from gastrointestinal cancer: pharmacological studies. Cancer Res 1990; 50:5790–4.

21. Group GTS. Gastrointestinal Tumor Study Group, Workshop on Intraperitoneal Chemotherapy, Orlando, Florida. Semin Oncol 1985; 12(Suppl. 4).

22. Muggia FM, Chan KK, Russell C, *et al.* Phase I and pharmacologic evaluation of intraperitoneal 5-fluoro-2′-deoxyuridine. Cancer Chemother Pharmacol 1991; 28:241–50.

23. Muggia FM, Tulpule A, Retzios A, *et al.* Intraperitoneal 5-fluoro-2′-deoxyuridine with escalating doses of leucovorin: pharmacology and clinical tolerance. Invest New Drugs 1994; 12:197–206.

24. Israel VK, Jiang C, Muggia FM, *et al.* Intraperitoneal 5-fluro-2′-deoxyuridine (FUDR) and (S)-leucovorin for disease predominantly confined to the peritoneal cavity: a pharmacokinetic and toxicity study. Cancer Chemother Pharmacol 1995; 37:32–8.

25. Muggia FM, Liu PY, Alberts DS, *et al.* Intraperitoneal mitoxantrone or floxuridine: effects on time-to-failure and survival in patients with minimal residual ovarian cancer after second-look laparotomy – a randomized phase II study by the Southwest Oncology Group. Gynecol Oncol 1996; 61:395–402.

26. Ozols RF. Intraperitoneal therapy in ovarian cancer: time's up [editorial; comment] [see comments]. J Clin Oncol 1991; 9:197–9.

27. Vogl SE. Ovarian cancer: diagnostic second laparotomy and salvage intra-peritoneal chemotherapy fail again. Eur J Cancer 1995; 5:651–3.

28. Ozols RF. Intraperitoneal salvage chemotherapy in ovarian cancer: who is left to treat? [editorial; comment]. Gynecol Oncol 1992; 45:1–2.

29. Markman M. Intraperitoneal paclitaxel in the management of ovarian cancer. Semin Oncol 1995; 22:86–7.

30. Markman M, Brady MF, Spirtos NM, Hanjani P, Rubin SC. Phase II trial of intraperitoneal paclitaxel in carcinoma of the ovary, tube, and peritoneum: a Gynecologic Oncology Group study. J Clin Oncol 1998; 16:2620–4.

31. Markman M, Rowinsky E, Hakes T, *et al.* Phase I trial of intraperitoneal taxol: a Gynecologic Oncology Group study. J Clin Oncol 1992; 10:1485–91.

32. Los G, Mutsaers PH, Lenglet WJ, Baldew GS, McVie JG. Platinum distribution in intraperitoneal tumors after intraperitoneal cisplatin treatment. Cancer Chemother Pharmacol 1990; 25:389–94.

33. Ozols RF, Locker GY, Doroshow JH, Grotzinger KR, Myers CE, Young RC. Pharmacokinetics of adriamycin and tissue penetration in murine ovarian cancer. Cancer Res 1979; 39:3209–14.

34. Lindner P, Heath DD, Shalinsky DR, Howell SB, Naredi P, Hafstrom L. Regional lymphatic drug exposure following intraperitoneal administration of 5-fluorouracil, carboplatin, and etoposide. Surg Oncol 1993; 2:105–12.

35. Francis P, Rowinsky E, Schneider J, Hakes T, Hoskins W, Markman M. Phase I feasibility and pharmacologic study of weekly intraperitoneal paclitaxel: a Gynecologic Oncology Group pilot study. J Clin Oncol 1995; 13:2961–7.

36. Sugarbaker PH, Klecker RW, Gianola FJ, Speyer JL. Prolonged treatment schedules with intraperitoneal 5-fluorouracil diminish the local–regional nature of drug distribution. Am J Clin Oncol 1986; 9:1–7.

37. Howell SB, Pfeifle CE, Wung WE, Olshen RA. Intraperitoneal cis-diamminedichloroplatinum with systemic thiosulfate protection. Cancer Res 1983; 43:1426–31.

38. Markman M, Hakes T, Reichman B, *et al.* Intraperitoneal cisplatin and cytarabine in the treatment of refractory or recurrent ovarian carcinoma [see comments]. J Clin Oncol 1991; 9:204–10.

39. Kirmani S, Zimm S, Cleary SM, Mowry J, Howell SB. Extremely prolonged continuous intraperitoneal infusion of cytosine arabinoside. Cancer Chemother Pharmacol 1990; 25:454–8.

40. Alberts DS, Surwit EA, Peng YM, *et al.* Phase I clinical and pharmacokinetic study of mitoxantrone given to patients by intraperitoneal administration. Cancer Res 1988; 48:5874–7.

41. Leichman L, Silberman H, Leichman CG, *et al.* Preoperative systemic chemotherapy followed by adjuvant postoperative intraperitoneal therapy for gastric cancer: a University of Southern California pilot program. J Clin Oncol 1992; 10:1933–42.

42. Markman M. Intraperitoneal therapy of ovarian cancer. Semin Oncol 1998; 25:356–60.

43. Markman M, Berek JS, Blessing JA, McGuire WP, Bell J, Homesley HD. Characteristics of patients with small-volume residual ovarian cancer unresponsive to cisplatin-based IP chemotherapy: lessons learned from a Gynecologic Oncology Group phase II trial of IP cisplatin and recombinant alpha-interferon [see comments]. Gynecol Oncol 1992; 45:3–8.

44. Piccart MJ, Speyer JL, Markman M, *et al.* Intraperitoneal chemotherapy: technical experience at five institutions. Semin Oncol 1985; 12:90–6.

45. Jinnai D, Higashi H. Extended radical operation with preoperative chemotherapy for gastric cancer. In Hirayama T, ed. *Cancer in Asia.* Baltimore, University Park Press, 1976, 111–19.

46. Hagiwara A, Takahashi T, Kojima O, *et al.* Prophylaxis with carbon-adsorbed mitomycin against peritoneal recurrence of gastric cancer [see comments]. Lancet 1992; 339:629–31.

47. Tsujitani S, Okuyama T, Watanabe A, Abe Y, Maehara Y, Sugimachi K. Intraperitoneal cisplatin during surgery for gastric cancer and peritoneal seeding. Anticancer Res 1993; 13:1831–4.

48. Yu W, Whang I, Suh I, Averbach A, Chang D, Sugarbaker PH. Prospective randomized trial of early

postoperative intraperitoneal chemotherapy as an adjuvant to resectable gastric cancer. Ann Surg 1998; 228:347–54.

49. Muggia FM, LePoidevin E, Jeffers S, *et al.* Intraperitoneal therapy for ovarian cancer: analysis of fluid distribution by computerized tomography. Ann Oncol 1992; 3:149–54.

50. Wahl RL, Gyves J, Gross BH, *et al.* SPECT of the peritoneal cavity: method for delineating intraperitoneal fluid distribution. Am J Roentgenol 1989; 152:1205–10.

51. Magre GR, Terk M, Colletti P, Muggia F, Boswell W. Saline MR peritoneography. Am J Roentgenol 1996; 167:749–51.

52. Reichman B, Markman M, Tong W, *et al.* Phase I trial of intraperitoneal (IP) FUDR and leucovorin (LV) given every other week. Proc Am Soc Clin Oncol 1991; 10:100.

53. Atiq OT, Kelsen DP, Shiu MH, *et al.* Phase II trial of postoperative adjuvant intraperitoneal cisplatin and fluorouracil and systemic fluorouracil chemotherapy in patients with resected gastric cancer. J Clin Oncol 1993; 11:425–33.

54. Koda R, Parimoo D, Spears C, *et al.* Hydroxyurea (HU) IV 72-hour infusion during intraperitoneal (IP) floxuridine (FUDR) and leucovorin (LV): pharmacologic/clinical correlates. Proc Am Assoc Clin Res 1996; 37.

55. Scheithauer W, Kornek G, Rosen H, *et al.* Combined intraperitoneal plus intravenous chemotherapy after curative resection for colonic adenocarcinoma. Eur J Cancer 1995; 31A:1981–6.

56. Muggia F, Muderspach L, Roman L, *et al.* Phase I/II study of intraperitoneal (IP) floxuridine (FUDR) with either cisplatin or carboplatin or both. Proc Am Soc Clin Oncol 1995; 14:270.

57. Markman M. Intraperitoneal cisplatin chemotherapy in the management of ovarian carcinoma. Semin Oncol 1989; 16:79–82.

58. Alberts DS. Carboplatin versus cisplatin in ovarian cancer. Semin Oncol 1995; 22:88–90.

59. Howell SB, Kirmani S, Lucas WE, *et al.* A phase II trial of intraperitoneal cisplatin and etoposide for primary treatment of ovarian epithelial cancer. J Clin Oncol 1990; 8:137–45.

60. Repetto L, Chiara S, Guido T, *et al.* Intraperitoneal chemotherapy with carboplatin and interferon alpha in the treatment of relapsed ovarian cancer: a pilot study. Anticancer Res 1991; 11:1641–3.

61. Frasci G, Iaffaioli RV, Comella G, *et al.* Intraperitoneal adjuvant immunochemotherapy in operable gastric cancer with serosal involvement. Clin Oncol 1994; 6:364–70.

62. Berek JS, Markman M, Blessing JA, *et al.* Intraperitoneal alpha-interferon alternating with cisplatin in residual ovarian carcinoma: a phase II Gynecologic Oncology Group study. Gynecol Oncol 1999; 74:48–52.

63. Leopold KA, Oleson JR, Clarke-Pearson D, *et al.* Intraperitoneal cisplatin and regional hyperthermia for ovarian carcinoma. Int J Radiat Oncol Biol Phys 1993; 27:1245–51.

64. Formenti SC, Shrivastava PN, Sapozink M, *et al.* Abdomino-pelvic hyperthermia and intraperitoneal carboplatin in epithelial ovarian cancer: feasibility, tolerance and pharmacology. Int J Radiat Oncol Biol Phys 1996; 35:993–1001.

65. Alberts DS. Treatment of refractory and recurrent ovarian cancer. Semin Oncol 1999; 26:8–14.

66. Muggia F. Role of intraperitoneal consolidation in ovarian cancer. Israel J Obstet Gynecol 1996; 7(2):17–22.

67. Fujimoto S, Takahashi M, Kobayashi K, *et al.* Cytohistologic assessment of antitumor effects of intraperitoneal hyperthermic perfusion with mitomycin C for patients with gastric cancer with peritoneal metastasis. Cancer 1992; 70:2754–60.

68. Blum RH, Garnick MB, Israel M, Canellos GP, Henderson IC, Frei E III. Initial clinical evaluation of N-trifluoroacetyladriamycin-14-valerate (AD-32), an adriamycin analog. Cancer Treat Rep 1979; 63:919–23.

69. Markman M, Homesley H, Norberts DA, *et al.* Phase I trial of intraperitoneal AD-32 in gynecologic malignancies. Gynecol Oncol 1996; 61:90–3.

70. Aghajanian C, Sabbatini P, Hensley M, *et al.* A phase I trial of intraperitoneal (IP) cisplatin with IP gemcitabine in patients with epithelial ovarian cancer. Proc Am Soc Clin Oncol 1999; 18:Abstract 1428.

71. Plaxe SC, Christen RD, O'Quigley J, *et al.* Phase I and pharmacokinetic study of intraperitoneal topotecan. Invest New Drugs 1998; 16:147–53.

72. Ostrowski MJ. An assessment of the long-term results of controlling the reaccumulation of malignant effusions using intracavity bleomycin. Cancer 1986; 57:721–7.

73. Alberts DS, Chen HS, Mayersohn M, Perrier D, Moon TE, Gross JF. Bleomycin pharmacokinetics in man. II. Intracavitary administration. Cancer Chemother Pharmacol 1979; 2:127–32.

74. Allavena P, Peccatori F, Maggioni D, *et al.* Intraperitoneal recombinant gamma-interferon in patients with recurrent ascitic ovarian carcinoma: modulation of cytotoxicity and cytokine production in tumor-associated effectors and of major histocompatibility antigen expression on tumor cells. Cancer Res 1990; 50:7318–23.

75. Lotze MT, Custer MC, Rosenberg SA. Intraperitoneal administration of interleukin-2 in patients with cancer. Arch Surg 1986; 121:1373–9.

76. Epenetos AA, Hooker G, Krausz T, Snook D, Bodmer WF, Taylor-Papadimitriou J. Antibody-guided irradiation of malignant ascites in ovarian cancer: a new

therapeutic method possessing specificity against cancer cells. Obstet Gynecol 1986; 68:71–4S.

77. Stoter G, Bolhuiis R, Arienti F, Nooy M, Bolis G, Canevari S. Intraperitoneal (IP) therapy of ovarian cancer with infusion of T-lymphocytes coated with the bispecific monoclonal antibody (bs-mAB) OCTR. Proc Am Soc Clin Oncol 1994; 13:230.

78. Alberts DS, Green S, Hannigan EV, et al. Improved therapeutic index of carboplatin plus cyclophosphamide versus cisplatin plus cyclophosphamide: final report by the Southwest Oncology Group of a phase III randomized trial in stages III and IV ovarian cancer [published erratum appears in J Clin Oncol 1992; 10(9):1505] [see comments]. J Clin Oncol 1992; 10:706–17.

79. Markman M, Francis P, Rowinsky E, Hoskins W. Intraperitoneal paclitaxel: a possible role in the management of ovarian cancer? Semin Oncol 1995; 22:84–7.

80. Muggia F, Liu P, Alberts D, et al. Elevated CA-125: an adverse prognostic factor for survival in epithelial ovarian cancer with minimal residual disease after second-look laparotomy. Proc Am Soc Clin Oncol 1995; 14:270.

81. Jones AL, Trott P, Cunningham D, et al. A pilot study of intraperitoneal cisplatin in the management of gastric cancer. Ann Oncol 1994; 5:123–6.

82. Kelsen D, Karpeh M, Schwartz G, et al. Neoadjuvant therapy of high-risk gastric cancer: a phase II trial of preoperative FAMTX and postoperative intraperitoneal fluorouracil–cisplatin plus intravenous fluorouracil. J Clin Oncol 1996; 14:1818–28.

83. Cintron JR, Pearl RK. Colorectal cancer and peritoneal carcinomatosis. Semin Surg Oncol 1996; 12:267–78.

84. Sugarbaker P, Chang D. Treatment of peritoneal surface malignancy from appendiceal primary tumors using cytoreductive surgery and perioperative intraperitoneal mitomycin C and 5-fluorouracil: report of all patients treated over 15 years. Proc Am Soc Clin Oncol 1998; 17:Abstract 1077.

85. Sugarbaker PH, Schellinx ME, Chang D, Koslowe P, von Meyerfeldt M. Peritoneal carcinomatosis from adenocarcinoma of the colon. World J Surg 1996; 20:585–91; discussion 592.

86. Kelsen DP, Saltz L, Cohen AM, et al. A phase I trial of immediate postoperative intraperitoneal floxuridine and leucovorin plus systemic 5-fluorouracil and levamisole after resection of high risk colon cancer [see comments]. Cancer 1994; 74:2224–33.

87. McVie JG, ten Bokkel Huinink W, Dubbelman R, Franklin H, van der Vijgh W, Klein I. Phase I study and pharmacokinetics of intraperitoneal carboplatin. Cancer Treat Rev 1985; 12(Suppl. A):35–41.

88. Howell SB, Pfeifle CE, Olshen RA. Intraperitoneal chemotherapy with melphalan. Ann Intern Med 1984; 101:14–18.

89. Garcia Moore ML, Savaraj N, Feun LG, Donnelly E. Successful therapy of peritoneal mesothelioma with intraperitoneal chemotherapy alone. A case report. Am J Clin Oncol 1992; 15:528–30.

90. Monk BJ, Surwit EA, Alberts DS, Graham V. Intraperitoneal mitomycin C in the treatment of peritoneal carcinomatosis following second-look surgery. Semin Oncol 1988; 15:27–31.

91. Ozols RF, Young RC, Speyer JL, et al. Phase I and pharmacological studies of adriamycin administered intraperitoneally to patients with ovarian cancer. Cancer Res 1982; 42:4265–9.

92. Howell SB, Chu BB, Wung WE, Metha BM, Mendelsohn J. Long-duration intracavitary infusion of methotrexate with systemic leucovorin protection in patients with malignant effusions. J Clin Invest 1981; 67:1161–70.

93. Dedrick RL, Flessner MF. Pharmacokinetic problems in peritoneal drug administration: tissue penetration and surface exposure. J Natl Cancer Inst 1997; 89:480–7.

Commentary

JOHN J KAVANAGH

Intraperitoneal antineoplastics have been used for approximately 25 years. The principles of such use have been elucidated by Dedrick et al. in a classic paper describing the pharmacokinetic theoretical rationale.[1] These principles led to mathematical calculations of favorable differential exposure of neoplastic cells in the peritoneum compared to concentrations obtained in the systemic circulation. However, it is implicit in this construct that the optimal compound would have a linear dose–response curve; evidence of synergy if used in combination; immediate cytotoxic activity without intermediary metabolism; and exit from the peritoneal cavity that is slow but, upon occurring, results in rapid clearance, thereby minimizing systemic toxicity. There is the obvious pragmatic counterpart that the compound should not have characteristics that result in poor patient compliance, and it should be able to be given in a repeated fashion, with minimal pain and inflammatory peritonitis. Unfortunately, no such 'ideal' compound currently exists.

The term 'intraperitoneal' therapy may be inappropriate. The consensus is that the peritoneal cavity is a dynamic environment where compounds diffuse directly across the peritoneal surface, are preferentially absorbed into the lymphatic system, and also enter the portal venous circulation.[2,3] These issues make the contribution of the intraperitoneal modality a conundrum. This is particularly true in the adjunctive therapies of gastric cancer, for which lymphatic metastases are considered of paramount importance. Unfortunately, there is very limited information on the newer compounds in terms of their disposition by the three major routes. Therefore, it becomes very difficult to attribute a positive outcome to a concentration-related phenomenon or a simple modification of the area under the curve in the systemic sense. As we use non-classical chemotherapy agents, pharmacy-modified drugs, or biologics, understanding the pharmacodynamics will become essential in developing rational clinical strategies.

A second aspect of intraperitoneal chemotherapy as discussed by Dr Muggia and his colleagues is the mechanics. Over the years, a multitude of infusates, volumes, and catheter devices have been utilized with this modality. Previous trials were handicapped by catheter-related problems and an inability to evaluate the suitability of the peritoneal cavity for therapy. However, technical advances in catheter technology, increased surgical experience in the placement of such devices, and the utilization of computerized tomography or radionuclide scanning for the evaluation of the peritoneal cavity have allowed the proper treatment and selection of patients. Many early trials must be considered compromised because of the lack of the evolution of these factors.[4–6] Although not mentioned in the chapter, the careful education of the patient and all medical personnel is crucial to the success of the trials. In addition, established standardized protocols of catheter care and the administration of compounds are a *sine qua non* of minimizing complications.

As the years have progressed, certain tumor types commonly associated with residual disease after surgery seem to warrant further study. The depth of penetration of the classical chemotherapy agents in the tumor tissue is 3 mm or less. As pointed out in the chapter, there is little evidence to substantiate the treatment of so-called bulky disease with an intraperitoneal modality. From the information available, one would have to assume that an advantage gained in the latter situation is due to an incidental phenomenon other than direct tumor–drug interaction, i.e., systemic absorption. Several tumor types continue to be attractive for intraperitoneal therapy. Patients with epithelial ovarian cancer who have minimal or no residual disease after primary surgery and/or chemotherapy seem an ideal group. This can be intellectually justified as a result of the cooperative group trial that randomized approximately 600 patients to either

intravenous or intraperitoneal cisplatinum, with both arms receiving intravenous cyclophosphamide. Survival increased by 8 months for the intraperitoneally treated patients.[7] However, paclitaxel became a standard therapy after this trial was finished and, therefore, it is unknown whether simple systemic paclitaxel and a platin compound would accomplish the same outcome. There is now another cooperative trial that randomizes optimally cytoreduced patients to intravenous cisplatin and paclitaxel versus intraperitoneal and intravenous paclitaxel and intraperitoneal cisplatin. If this trial shows no significant benefit, intraperitoneal modalities utilizing chemotherapy agents in epithelial ovarian cancer will enter a quiescence. The converse is, of course, true.

A tumor that warrants a creative intraperitoneal approach is pseudomyxoma peritonei. There is no established systemic therapy for this tumor. In the initial stages of this disease, surgical cytoreduction is often optimal. Patients usually die of disease that is confined strictly to the peritoneum and require multiple surgeries to remove the mucinous deposits. Yet, there is very little information in the literature, and there has been no focused effort to conduct pilot trials with this disease when a new intraperitoneal modality is reported. A therapeutic advance in this disease could result in a significant clinical benefit to patients who have the misfortune to have indolent progressive recurrences after their primary diagnosis.

The utilization of intraperitoneal therapy in gastric cancer is somewhat perplexing. The chapter nicely summarizes the conflicting therapy data about the subject. It should be noted that the vast majority of studies use some other form of adjunctive therapy in addition to the intra-abdominal treatment. However, if the trend toward lower intraperitoneal recurrence is seen in such patients, there is the possibility of a palliative advance. However, one must consider that, pending the discovery of a more active agent in the disease, the utilization of an intraperitoneal approach will be limited.[8]

Another tumor that has not been well studied and yet may be a logical area of endeavor is mesothelioma. Although an uncommon disease, surgical resection is a possibility in the primary setting. In addition, if there were a means of inducing a significant cytotoxic tumor reduction, a secondary or delayed surgical approach could be helpful. The tumor often remains confined to the intra-abdominal cavity, with a slowly advancing course. Pilot trials in this area could be of great potential benefit to this subset of patients.

A crucial issue that is indirectly approached in the chapter is that of trial design. Critics of intra-abdominal chemotherapy correctly point out that the vast majority of trials have been either single arm or randomized, with insufficient power to detect meaningful differences. Often, systemic therapy is also administered. However, in fairness, this criticism of the historical experience does not prove negativity; there are simply inadequate definitive trial data. The somewhat unexpected results of the intraperitoneal platinum trial in ovarian cancer by the cooperative groups demonstrated the importance of careful prospective planning of these clinical studies.[7] It is difficult to argue that, after initial dose-finding studies, the next step should be randomized trials that set a high benchmark with very detailed knowledge of the participants. This would allow prognostic criteria to be carefully analysed. Unfortunately, the cost and duration of such randomized trials are often perceived as excessive. Advances in the statistical methodology of trial design are required when dealing with a relatively costly and inconvenient therapy. There is a need to move quickly in view of the newer classes of compounds being discovered that are applicable for an intraperitoneal evaluation.

The final critical issue in considering an intraperitoneal approach is that of agent selection. Clearly, because of scientific limitations, the work has largely involved classical chemotherapy agents. However, it is difficult to imagine that this is the future of developmental therapies. Indeed, compounds that have pharmacy modifications, such as liposomal doxorubicin or polyglutamated paclitaxel, may increase activity and/or modify toxicity. Such aspects are intuitively obvious choices for intraperitoneal experimentation. In addition, these are part of the selective uptake retention compounds which should be pursued for intraperitoneal study.

Monoclonal antibodies are another area of obvious interest. The reference provided within the chapter is that of an earlier radioisotope of murine origin.[9] Clearly, we have advanced in terms of the technology of humanized antibodies and multiple active components on the antibody. The difficulty will be in determining the appropriate volumes of disease to be treated and the trial designs necessary to prove efficacy. The general consensus in ovarian cancer is that such therapy would be best suited to those patients with minimal or no detectable residual tumor.

Also to be considered are the biological therapies, which include intraperitoneal cytokines and cellular therapies. As published by Freedman and associates, the intraperitoneal cavity represents a rich environment of cytokines and cellular expression. Indeed, it may be that an autologous tumor vaccine coupled with a cytokine would be the optimal intra-abdominal approach, both solving the local therapeutic issue and inducing a systemic response.[10]

Another rapidly advancing area of experimental antineoplastic therapy concerns compounds that target molecular endpoints. These would include such drugs as tyrosine kinase inhibitors. A difficult issue in the evaluation of such drugs is how to determine their surrogate endpoint efficacy, i.e., the positive molecular change that parallels the clinical response. Perhaps such an approach would have an advantage in intraperitoneal therapy in view of the available technology for repeated access for the analysis of the constituents of the abdominal microenvironment. Indeed, the so-called molecular compounds may provide an ideal opportunity for a better understanding in terms of cellular and molecular kinetics of the intra-abdominal environment of neoplasms.

In summary, Dr Muggia and his colleagues have provided a very reasonable and well-balanced overview of intraperitoneally administered therapies. One must recognize that, despite the sound theoretical foundation, there has been no compound found that equals the ideal model. Many investigators have contributed to the evolution of what is now a functional, though relatively cumbersome, form of therapy. The results of various trials now justify a continuation of the modality in an investigational setting. A consensus has been reached that gross abdominal cancer does not benefit from this approach. Tumor types that appear to be most promising are epithelial ovarian cancer, gastric cancer, pseudomyxoma peritonei, and possibly intra-abdominal mesotheliomas. Pending the outcome of randomized cooperative group trials in ovarian cancer, perhaps the wisest direction of research would be innovative pilot studies involving non-classical chemotherapy and biologic agents with a translational emphasis.

REFERENCES

1. Dedrick RL, Myers CE, Bungay PM, DeVita VT Jr. Pharmacokinetic rationale for peritoneal drug administration in the treatment of ovarian cancer. Cancer Treat Rep 1978; 62:1–11.

2. Wolf BE, Sugarbaker PH. Intraperitoneal chemotherapy and immunotherapy. Recent Results Cancer Res 1988; 110:254–73.

3. Sugarbaker PH, Cunliffe WJ, Belliveau J, et al. Rationale for integrating early postoperative intraperitoneal chemotherapy into the surgical treatment of gastrointestinal cancer. Semin Oncol 1989; 16(Suppl. 6):83–97.

4. Piccart MJ, Speyer JL, Markman M, et al. Intraperitoneal chemotherapy: technical experience at five institutions. Semin Oncol 1985; 12(3) (Suppl. 4):90–6.

5. Muggia FM, LePoidevin E, Jeffers S, et al. Intraperitoneal therapy for ovarian cancer: analysis of fluid distribution by computerized tomography. Ann Oncol 1992; 3:149–54.

6. Wahl RL, Gyves J, Gross BH, et al. SPECT of the peritoneal cavity: method for delineating intraperitoneal fluid distribution. Am J Roentgenol 1989; 152:1205–10.

7. Alberts DS, Liu PY, Hannigan EV, et al. Intraperitoneal cisplatin plus intravenous cyclophosphamide versus intravenous cisplatin plus intravenous cyclophosphamide for stage III ovarian cancer. N Engl J Med 1996; 335:1950.

8. Kelsen D, Karpeh M, Schwartz G, *et al*. Neoadjuvant therapy of high-risk gastric cancer: a phase II trial of preoperative FAMTX and postoperative intraperitoneal fluorouracil–cisplatin plus intravenous fluorouracil. J Clin Oncol 1996; 14:1818–28.

9. Epenetos AA, Hooker G, Krausz T, Snook D, Bodmer WF, Taylor-Papadimitriou J. Antibody-guided irradiation of malignant ascites in ovarian cancer: a new therapeutic method possessing specificity against cancer cells. Obstet Gynecol 1986; 68:71–4S.

10. Freedman RS, Kudelka AJ, Kavanagh JJ, *et al*. Clinical and biological effects of intraperitoneal injections of recombinant interferon-γ and recombinant interleukin 2 with or without tumor-infiltrating lymphocytes in patients with ovarian or peritoneal carcinoma. Clin Cancer Res 2000; 6:2268–78.

Editors' selected abstracts

Hemodynamic and cardiac function parameters during heated intraoperative intraperitoneal chemotherapy using the open 'coliseum technique'.

Esquivel J, Angulo F, Bland RK, Stephens AD, Sugarbaker PH.

The Washington Cancer Institute, Washington, DC, USA.

Annals Surgical Oncology 7(4):296–300, 2000, May.

Background: Heated intraoperative intraperitoneal chemotherapy achieves high peritoneal concentrations with limited systemic absorption and has become an important tool in the management of patients with peritoneal carcinomatosis from low-grade malignancies such as pseudomyxoma peritonei and in selected cases of high-grade tumors such as colon adenocarcinoma. When the closed abdomen technique is used, its perioperative toxicity seems to be related to the hemodynamic and cardiac function changes associated with increased body temperature and increased intra-abdominal pressure. *Methods:* Hemodynamic and cardiac function variables during heated intraoperative intraperitoneal chemotherapy, using an open abdomen 'coliseum technique,' were measured in 15 patients with the use of a noninvasive esophageal Doppler monitor. *Results:* The hemodynamic and cardiac function changes were characterized by an increased heart rate, increased cardiac output and decreased systemic vascular resistance associated with an increased body temperature, and decreased effective circulating volume with the urinary output tending to decrease as the therapy progressed. *Conclusion:* Heated intraoperative intraperitoneal chemotherapy with the open abdomen coliseum technique induces a hyperdynamic circulatory state with an increased intravenous fluid requirement and avoids changes because of increased intra-abdominal pressure. Hemodynamic and cardiac stability, as documented by normal blood pressure and adequate urinary output, can be achieved by liberal intravenous fluids, titrated to frequent urinary output determination.

Intra-abdominal fibrosis after systemic and intraperitoneal therapy containing fluoropyrimidines.

Fata F, Ron IG, Maluf F, Klimstra D, Kemeny N.

Gastrointestinal Oncology Service, Departments of Medicine and Pathology, Memorial Sloan-Kettering Cancer Center and the Cornell University Medical College, New York, NY, USA.

Cancer 88(11):2447–51, 2000, June 1.

Background: Intra-abdominal and retroperitoneal fibrosis has been described as secondary to intraperitoneal (IP) administration of several chemotherapeutic agents, including carboplatin, mitoxantrone, and the combination of 5-fluorouracil and cisplatin. The IP administration of floxuridine (FUDR) is an effective and minimally toxic treatment for patients with metastases to the peritoneum. An increasing number of patients with colorectal, gastric, or ovarian carcinoma are treated with IP chemotherapy. *Methods:* The authors report two patients with metastatic colon carcinoma who experienced severe intra-abdominal fibrosis presenting as an intra-abdominal mass mimicking recurrence in one patient and diffuse encasement of the bowel in the other, after the administration of IP FUDR and leucovorin. *Results:* Two patients with Stage III colon adenocarcinoma received postoperative adjuvant 5-fluorouracil and levamisole. They subsequently presented with a rise in carcinoembryonic antigen level and isolated liver metastasis. They underwent hepatic lobectomy with postoperative intra-arterial hepatic FUDR and systemic 5-fluorouracil and leucovorin. They each had an intra-abdominal recurrence, which was resected and treated with postoperative IP FUDR and leucovorin. They then presented with a diffuse pattern of IP fibrosis with no tumor identified. *Conclusions:* IP FUDR and leucovorin therapy can be associated with diffuse IP fibrosis, which in this study caused an intra-abdominal mass that was indistinguishable from recurrent malignancy in one patient and encasement of the bowel in the other.

Phase II trial of combination intraperitoneal cisplatin and 5-fluorouracil in previously treated patients with advanced ovarian cancer: long-term follow-up.

Morgan RJ Jr, Braly P, Leong L, Shibata S, Margolin K, Somlo G, McNamara M, Longmate J, Schinke S, Raschko J, Nagasawa S, Kogut N, Najera L, Johnson D, Doroshow JH.

Department of Medical Oncology and Therapeutics Research, City of Hope National Medical Center, Duarte, CA, USA.

Gynecology and Oncology 77(3):433–8, 2000, June.

Objectives: This trial was performed to determine the response rate and progression-free and overall survivals of patients with advanced recurrent ovarian cancer who were treated with intraperitoneal cisplatin and 5-fluorouracil.

Methods: Twenty-four patients with ovarian cancer were entered on this trial and treated with intraperitoneal (ip) cisplatin (DDP) and ip 5-fluorouracil, every 3 weeks for eight cycles. Following iv hydration, the cisplatin and 5-fluorouracil were administered through an ip catheter in 2 liters of 0.9% normal saline with a 4-h dwell. *Results:* All patients were evaluable for progression-free and overall survival and toxicity analysis, and 22 patients for response. The median age was 59 (range, 35–71); initial disease status included 9 patients with residual disease following chemotherapy prior to entry on this study; 5 patients had progressed, and 10 patients had recurrent disease more than 6 months following initial chemotherapy. Of the 9 patients with residual disease, 1 complete response and 3 partial responses were observed; of 10 patients with recurrent disease, 1 complete and 1 partial response were observed for an overall response rate of 27%. No objective responses were seen in the 7 patients who were platinum-refractory on protocol entry. The median progression-free and overall survivals are 7.0 (range, 0.5–137) and 15.5 (range, 3–147) months, respectively. Toxicity included hypomagnesemia, vomiting, abdominal pain, and mild anemia. Only one patient required a dosage adjustment of cisplatin for a serum creatinine elevation >2.0 mg/dL. *Conclusions:* We conclude that the combination of ip cisplatin and 5-FU is an effective regimen for patients with residual or relapsed epithelial ovarian cancer with survival durations, response rates, and toxicity profiles that compare favorably with those of other second-line ovarian cancer regimens. Patients who are primarily platinum-refractory are unlikely to benefit from these agents administered into the peritoneal cavity.

Phase II trial of adjuvant radiation and intraperitoneal 5-fluorouracil for locally advanced colon cancer: results with 10-year follow-up.

Palermo JA, Richards F, Lohman KK, Lovelace JV, Atkinson J, Case LD, White DR, Blackstock AW.

Department of Radiation Oncology, Wake Forest University Baptist Medical Center, Winston-Salem, NC, USA.

International Journal of Radiation Oncology, Biology, Physics 47(3):725–33, 2000, June 1.

Purpose: To determine the toxicity, disease-free survival, and overall survival for patients with Modified Astler-Coller (MAC) B2-3 or C1-3 colon cancer receiving adjuvant radiation and sequential intraperitoneal 5-fluorouracil (5-FU). *Methods and materials:* From August 1984 to June 1989, 45 patients were accrued to this Phase II trial and received a 21-week course of intraperitoneal 5-FU (20 mg/kg/d × 5) and external beam radiation. The radiation was delivered to the tumor bed and para-aortic lymph nodes in two split-courses of 22.5 Gy, alternating with the first two cycles of chemotherapy. All patients then received 4 additional cycles of intraperitoneal 5-FU. *Results:* The therapy was well tolerated with 4 patients experiencing Grade 3 peritonitis.

Four patients developed small bowel obstruction requiring surgery; in each instance, recurrent tumor was found at the time of laparotomy. The median and overall survivals at 10 years were 9.3 months and 53% respectively. Local failures were infrequent, occurring in only 11% of patients treated. *Conclusions:* Sequential intraperitoneal 5-FU and tumor-bed/para-aortic irradiation is tolerable in patients with resected colon cancer. Although the incidence of local and regional relapse appeared to be lower than anticipated, this did not appear to translate into improved survival.

Adjuvant intraperitoneal 5-fluorouracil in high-risk colon cancer: a multicenter phase III trial.

Vaillant JC, Nordlinger B, Deuffic S, Arnaud JP, Pelissier E, Favre JP, Jaeck D, Fourtanier G, Grandjean JP, Marre P, Letoublon C.

Centre de Chirurgie Digestive, Hopital Saint Antoine et Service de Chirurgie Digestive et Hepato-Biliaire, Groupe Hospitalier Pitie-Salpetriere, Paris, France.

Annals of Surgery 231(4):449–56, 2000, April.

Objective: To evaluate the results of a prospective multicenter randomized study of adjuvant intraperitoneal 5-fluorouracil (5-FU) administered during 6 days shortly after resection of stages II and III colon cancers. *Summary background data:* Systemic adjuvant chemotherapy improves the survival of patients with stage III colon cancer receiving treatment for 6 months. Intraperitoneal chemotherapy theoretically combines peritoneal and hepatic effects. *Methods:* After resection, 267 patients were randomized into two groups. Patients in group 1 (*n* = 133) underwent resection followed by intraperitoneal administration of 5-FU (0.6 g/m^2/day) for 6 days (day 4 to day 10). These patients also received intravenous 5-FU (1 g) during surgery. Patients in group 2 underwent resection alone (*n* = 134). *Results:* In group 1, 103 patients received the total dose, 18 received a partial dose as a result of technical or tolerance problems, and 12 did not receive the chemotherapy. Rates of surgical death and complications were similar in both groups. Tolerance to treatment was excellent or fair in 97% of the patients and poor in 3%. After a median follow-up of 58 months, 5-year overall survival rates were 74% in group 1 and 69% in group 2; disease-free survival rates were 68% and 62%, respectively. Survival curves were superimposed until 3 years after treatment and began diverging thereafter. Among patients receiving the full treatment, the 5-year disease-free survival rate was improved in the treatment group in patients with stage II cancers but was unchanged in patients with stage III cancers. *Conclusions:* Chemotherapy with intraperitoneal 5-FU administered during a short period after surgery was well tolerated but was not sufficient to reduce the risk of death significantly. However, it reduced the risk of recurrence in stage II cancers. These results suggest that it should be associated with systemic chemotherapy to reduce both local and distant recurrences.

9

Surgical consequences of abdominal irradiation

LEON MORGENSTERN

INTRODUCTION

Radiation to the abdomen or pelvis, administered in therapeutic doses for neoplastic disease, can adversely affect the structure and function of any organ system or viscus in the path of the radiation beam.[1–5] The severity of the damage incurred is determined by the radiation dose, the radiosensitivity of the tissue, the volume exposed, and a number of other factors that influence tissue vulnerability. This chapter reviews the broad spectrum of radiation injury to the intra-abdominal viscera, the factors influencing its occurrence and severity, the underlying pathologic processes, the clinical manifestations of radiation damage and their surgical management. Preventive measures that can limit or obviate injury to vulnerable structures are also discussed.

Abdominal irradiation as a primary therapeutic modality for neoplastic disease is less frequently employed today than previously. Nevertheless, injuries secondary to prior irradiation continue to be seen, albeit more rarely. Radiation changes in tissues are lifelong, and clinical manifestations of injury may occur many years after the completion of therapy.

There is a large group of neoplastic diseases for which abdominal or abdominopelvic radiation may be given. These are listed in Table 9.1.

Although radiation injuries may be seen in any of the conditions listed, the most frequent sequelae are seen with gynecological neoplasms, and include carcinoma of the ovary, carcinoma of the uterus, and carcinoma of the uterine cervix. Also not uncommon are radiation injuries after treatment of carcinoma of the prostate, anus, and rectum.

Radiation injuries in the remaining conditions listed are seen sporadically, but with considerably less frequency than those mentioned above.

PREVALENCE OF RADIATION INJURY

The most widely accepted figure for expected radiation injury after treatment in the usual dosage range

Table 9.1 *Neoplasms treated by abdominal or abdominopelvic irradiation*

Condition	Dosage range (cGy)
Bile duct carcinoma	3000–5000
Pancreatic carcinoma	4500–6000
Hodgkin's disease	4000–4500
Seminoma	3000
Lymphoma	4500
Wilms' tumor	4500–6000
Neuroblastoma	4500
Rhabdomyosarcoma	4500
Liposarcoma	4500–5000
Carcinoma of the ovary	4500–8000
Carcinoma of the uterus	4500–8000
Carcinoma of the uterine cervix	4500–8000
Carcinoma of the prostate	5000
Carcinoma of the anus	5000–8000
Carcinoma of the rectum	4500–6000
Carcinoma of the bladder	4000–6000

(4500 cGy, or 150–200 cGy five times weekly for 5–6 weeks) is 5%. This is often expressed as the minimum tolerance dose (TD 5/5), the dosage at which 5% of patients will manifest symptoms of radiation injury within 5 years.[6] As dosage is increased for specific indications, such as salvage therapy in ovarian or uterine carcinoma, the prevalence of injury may be expected to rise to 20% or higher.[7,8] The expression denoting the maximal tolerance dose (TD 50/5) is that dosage at which 50% of the patients treated will exhibit manifestations of injury within 5 years. Although this figure is approached in certain salvage regimens,[9] no current therapeutic regimen results in such a high rate of injury.

ORGANS OR ORGAN SYSTEMS INVOLVED IN RADIATION INJURY AFTER ABDOMINAL IRRADIATION

The gastrointestinal tract is the organ system by far the most vulnerable to abdominal irradiation. This is a function of its high rate of cell replication. It is this system that is chiefly discussed in this chapter.

Other structures which may incur injury are the liver, pancreas, kidneys, ureter, and bladder. The surgical consequences of injuries to these structures are much less prevalent and are discussed briefly after injuries to various portions of the gastrointestinal tract.

GASTROINTESTINAL TRACT: RELATIVE VULNERABILITY

The duodenum, jejunum, and ileum are the most radiosensitive segments of the gastrointestinal tract. Although the colon is moderately sensitive, significant injury to the ascending, transverse, and descending colon is relatively rare. The sigmoid, more likely to be included in the radiation field for pelvic malignancies, may incur significant damage. The rectum is the least radiosensitive of the gastrointestinal segments, but because it is frequently in the direct path of the radiation beam for gynecologic, prostatic, and rectal malignancies, it is often the site of significant injury.

The comparative radiation tolerances of the various components of the gastrointestinal tract are listed in Table 9.2.

PATHOLOGY OF RADIATION INJURY TO THE INTESTINE

All elements of the intestinal wall suffer damage with ionizing radiation.[10-14] The earliest injury is to the mucosa, where the cellular replication rate is the highest. The early changes are diffuse or multifocal ulceration, with varying degrees of damage to the surface and crypt epithelium. These early changes seldom, if ever, require surgical intervention. The regenerated mucosa, in all

parts of the irradiated gastrointestinal tract, exhibits cells with bizarre nuclear changes and varying degrees of structural aberration. The permanently altered mucosa results in decreased absorptive capacity and increased susceptibility to mechanical injury, especially in the stomach and colon, which are subject to friction by the solid contents within them. Trauma to the vulnerable mucosa may be the initiating event in the development of ulceration leading to surgical complications. In the small intestine, the villi are blunted and irregular, with altered absorptive capacity.

Radiation-induced changes in the submucosa are of greater surgical consequence than the mucosal changes (Figure 9.1). The submucosa undergoes diffuse hyalinization, and telangiectasia of lymphatic, venous, and arterial channels. Bizarre fibroblasts known as 'radiation fibroblasts' are scattered in the collagenous matrix. It is the dense collagenization of the submucosa that gives the 'stiffened' character to the radiation-damaged intestine.

All vascular elements, including capillaries, arteries, and veins of all sizes, suffer the effects of irradiation. The principal damage is to the endothelium, which responds by intimal proliferation and progressive hyalinization,

Table 9.2 *Radiation tolerances of parts of the gastrointestinal tract*

Organ	Injury	Min./max. tolerance dose (cGy) (TD 5/5) (TD 50/5)
Esophagus	Ulcer, stricture, perforation	6000–7500
Stomach	Ulcer, perforation	4500–5500
Small intestine	Ulcer, stricture, fistula, infarction, perforation	4500–6500
Colon	Ulcer, stricture, fistula	4500–6500
Rectum	Ulcer, stricture, fistula	5500–8000

Adapted from Rubin and Casarett.[6]

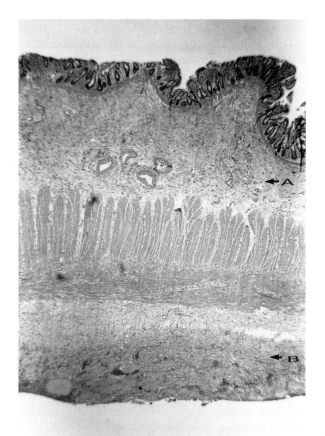

Figure 9.1 *Histologic section of irradiated ileum. In addition to altered villous architecture, note the thickening and hyalinization of the submucosa (A), with ectatic vasculature. The thickened serosa or 'peel', (B) is also well illustrated in this section.*

often to the point of luminal obliteration. Recent work[15] has postulated a decrease in endothelial anticoagulant substances, normally present in endothelium, as a factor leading to the vascular damage. Progressive endarteritic changes are responsible for the late occurrence of ischemic necrosis and segmental infarction of the bowel wall, a catastrophic complication.

The muscularis propria does not exhibit the severe changes seen in the mucosa and submucosa. There are scattered foci of collagen deposition, radiation fibroblasts, and some disruption of the normal architecture. The basic structural integrity of the muscularis, however, is not significantly altered.

Alterations of the serosal surface also have major surgical consequences. These are probably the most frequent pathologic change encountered by the surgeon upon opening the abdomen for a complication of radiotherapy. The serosa, which has a normal thickness of 1–2 µ, may, in its altered state, measure 10 µ or more. The thickened serosa, or 'peel,' is dense collagenous tissue, infiltrated with radiation fibroblasts (Figure 9.1). In the presence of surgically induced adhesions, the serosal reaction promotes an agglutination of adjacent loops, rendering them difficult or impossible to separate without serious risk of inadvertent enterotomy. The serosal thickening also gives the radiation-injured bowel its 'parboiled' appearance (Figure 9.2), with occasional mottling due to the irregular deposition of collagen and areas of telangiectasia. The tightly coiled, agglutinated loops are most frequently encountered within or just above the pelvis (Figure 9.3). Dense fibrotic adherence to all structures within the pelvis can render the dissection extraordinarily difficult. At risk are the bladder, rectum, iliac vessels, and ureters, which may be involved in the fibrotic process or 'fused' to the fibrotic 'peel' of the affected intestinal loops. Fistulization may occur as enterocutaneous entero-enteral, enterovesical, enterovaginal, or enterorectal fistulas.

STOMACH

The stomach, though not as radiosensitive as the small intestine, can be the site of sequelae which require surgical intervention. The two most frequent complications are bleeding and ulceration.

Bleeding may occur from diffuse focal erosions or small ulcerations, chiefly in the distal stomach (Figure 9.4). Beneath the atrophic mucosa, embedded in the hyalinized submucosa, lies a complex of telangiectatic vessels that are subject to exposure and erosion. Bleeding from this source is not massive, but constant, requiring increasingly frequent blood replacement by transfusion. This type of intractable bleeding from diffuse injury requires surgical intervention if it does not respond to medical measures, discussed below.

Chronic gastric ulcer, manifested clinically by intractable pain and occasionally by massive bleeding episodes, may also require surgical intervention. The chronic radiation ulcer can resemble the chronic peptic ulcer, but is characterized by the typical radiation-induced changes seen on histologic examination. Bleeding, at times of massive proportions, results if a major arterial or venous vessel is exposed deep within the ulcer. The radiation-induced ulcer is most commonly seen in the distal stomach, the usual site of maximal exposure to radiation. It does not ordinarily respond to medical measures. Perforation due to radiation injury is not a frequent occurrence, although it has been reported. In contrast to the small intestine, the vascular supply of the stomach is more extensive, generally precluding infarction, necrosis,

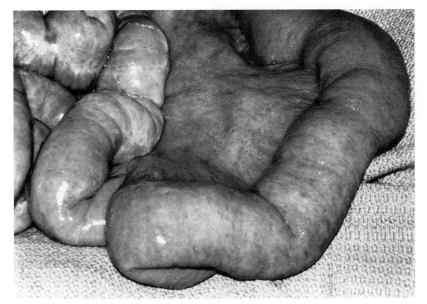

Figure 9.2 *Irradiated loops of jejuno-ileum showing late changes of serosal thickening and parboiled, grayish appearance. Dilatation is a result of chronic obstruction.*

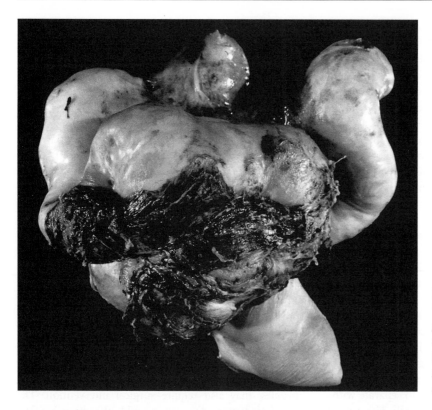

Figure 9.3 *Resected complex of 'agglutinated' ileal loops, freed from pelvis, which had been the source of chronic obstruction. Radiation had been administered after abdominal surgery. Note the dense, fibrotic fusion of adjacent loops.*

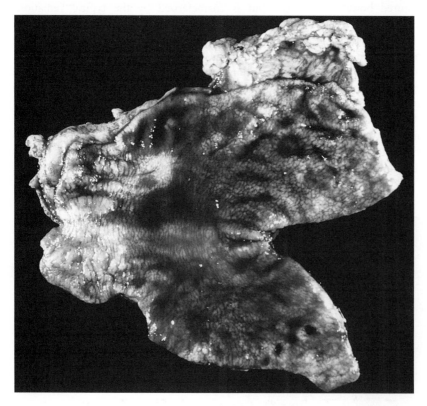

Figure 9.4 *Stomach resected for intractable bleeding due to diffuse erosive gastritis, with extensive telangiectasia of submucosal vessels. The patient received 5000 cGy to the upper abdomen for pancreatic carcinoma.*

and perforation due to endovascular occlusion. The thickness of the gastric wall and decreased acid-pepsin levels are also factors in the less than expected incidence of free perforation from radiation-induced ulcer. Worthy of mention, however, is the perforation of the stomach that occurs following irradiation of some gastric lymphomas in which the radiosensitive neoplasm, involving the full thickness of stomach wall, is totally destroyed. The surgical consequence, free perforation of the involved stomach, is an acute abdominal catastrophe.

Gastric erosions and ulcers in the irradiated stomach are not exactly analogous to their acid-peptic counterparts in the non-irradiated stomach. A treatment for peptic ulcer earlier in the twentieth century was gastric irradiation in a dosage range of 25 cGy. This effectively decreased gastric acidity by causing sufficient damage to the parietal cells to heal some peptic ulcers. At higher dosage levels in the irradiated stomach, the acid-peptic factors are still operative, but to a lesser extent. Equally important factors favoring ulceration in the irradiated stomach are the atrophic, easily injured mucosa with its impaired reparative ability, the pre-existent hyalinization of the submucosa, and the vascular changes within the gastric wall, all accentuating the tendency to extend the destructive process.

For bleeding or ulceration, intense medical measures should be employed before surgical treatment is undertaken. These include all current therapies such as H2 blockers, omeprazole, sucralfate, and endoscopic coagulation of focal bleeding sites, where accessible. For chronic blood loss unresponsive to iron therapy, occasional transfusions are of lesser risk than major extirpative surgery, especially in elderly or debilitated patients.

When intractable pain, progressive blood loss, or episodes of massive bleeding are unmanageable with medical measures, resection of the affected gastric segment is the surgical treatment of choice. Distal gastrectomy should include as much of the damaged stomach as possible or feasible, from the pylorus to grossly proximal normal stomach. The choice between a Billroth I or Billroth II type of reconstruction will depend on the conditions at operation. Anastomoses constructed with irradiated tissues are always precarious and should be done meticulously, whether hand-sewn or stapled. Carefully done, there is no advantage of one type of anastomosis over the other. Anastomoses, whether of the Billroth I or Billroth II type, should be under no tension whatsoever. Ease of approximation without tension may influence the decision between a Billroth I and Billroth II reconstruction. Hand-sewn anastomoses should be marked at their extremities with hemoclips for ease of radiologic identification later. Postoperative nasogastric suction is advisable for 48–72 h to ensure decompression of the stomach and to detect postoperative bleeding. Resumption of oral intake is not recommended before 5 days. Thereafter, progression to the usual post-gastrectomy dietary regimen should be allowed as tolerated.

SMALL INTESTINE

The small intestine is the most common site of radiation-induced injuries which require surgical intervention within the abdomen.[16,17] The indications for surgical intervention include intractable bleeding, obstruction, ulceration, fistulization, and infarction–necrosis with perforation. Any or all of these may exist alone or in combination.

Bleeding as a primary reason for operation in the irradiated small intestine is rare, though possible, from either a focal or a diffuse source. Bleeding from a unifocal site is generally due to deep ulceration into a major vessel. Recently, a primary aortoduodenal fistula was reported between the fourth portion of the duodenum and the abdominal aorta 20 years following radiotherapy and para-aortic lymph node dissection for seminoma.[18]

The most common indication for surgical intervention in the irradiated small intestine is obstruction, usually occurring within 6 months to 2 years after radiotherapy, but possible even decades later. The obstructive episode may be acute, complete, and strangulating or, as more commonly encountered, multiple recurrent episodes, finally unmanageable by non-operative therapy.

The etiologic mechanism is described above under 'Pathology of radiation injury to the intestine.' The hyalinized, stiffened submucosa and serosa impair motility; the presence of adhesions secondary to prior operations sets the stage for an adhesive enteropathy in which loops of bowel become entrapped in a complex of narrowed, convoluted loops (Figure 9.5), with progressive endoluminal compromise as the fibrosis advances. The initiating mechanism of individual obstructive episodes is often difficult to identify, as is also the case with non-irradiated bowel. But, once initiated, the obstructive process feeds on itself and worsens, with progressive dilatation of proximal fluid-filled loops. Impaired peristaltic ability fails to propel their contents beyond the constricted lumina. If the obstruction is acute, complete, or strangulating, early or immediate surgical intervention is indicated. More often, the obstructive episodes are chronic, recurrent, and increasingly difficult to resolve by medical measures.

The most common site for the obstruction just described is in the pelvis, because this is the site where the small bowel is subjected to most irradiation in the more commonly used regimens. It is also the site where postoperative adhesions and confinement of the small bowel within a small space predispose to radiation injury. Similar phenomena of 'agglutinated,' obstructive loops may be found adherent to the anterior abdominal wall along the site of surgical incision, or to the retroperitoneum, where the bowel has become adherent to deperitonealized areas. Such adhesions occur with paraortic lymph node dissection or resection of retroperitoneal tumors.

If strangulation is not suspected on the basis of physical findings, the first therapeutic measures should be conservative. Cessation of oral intake and intubation–suction may be all that is necessary to circumvent operation when the obstruction is early or incomplete. The long intestinal tube (Cantor or Miller–Abbot) was an effective means of intestinal decompression before the use of metallic mercury was prohibited. Barium has proved a poor substitute for mercury in the weighted bag, but it works occasionally. Nasogastric intubation is second best in this situation (not a universally accepted

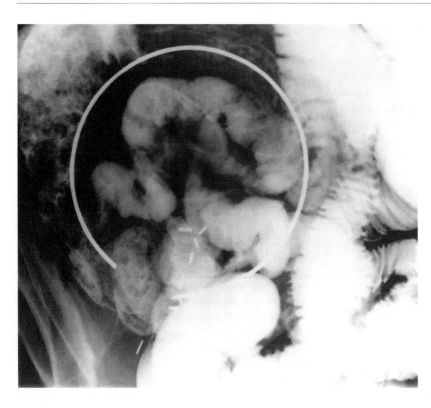

Figure 9.5 *Radiograph of narrowed, convoluted loops of terminal ileum, 12 years after abdominal irradiation for fallopian tube carcinoma (4800 cGy to pelvis; 3000 cGy to midplane of abdomen). Surgery was performed for chronic recurrent obstruction.*

evaluation), but may suffice to override the acute situation and avoid operation.

If operation cannot be avoided, the administration of broad-spectrum antibiotics preoperatively is recommended. Informed consent should always include possible intestinal resection and the possibility of an enteric stoma, if there is any likelihood of such a necessity in the surgeon's judgment. If the obstructive mechanism is in the pelvis or near the pelvic brim, the ureters should be catheterized.

It is best to avoid incision into heavily irradiated skin to prevent postoperative wound-healing problems. Entry into the peritoneal cavity should be exceedingly cautious to avoid inadvertent enterostomy. The laparoscopic approach to radiation-induced intestinal obstruction is not recommended.

The course of action after the offending pathology is identified depends on the individual situation. In the rare event that the obstructive mechanism is simple and involves lysis of some adhesions easily amenable to lysis, resection of bowel should be avoided. In such situations, particular attention should be paid to the possibility of small enterotomies or fistulas which may be difficult to discern on casual inspection, but which, if overlooked, can be catastrophic postoperatively. The long tube also served a useful purpose following lysis of adhesions, inasmuch as methylene blue could be instilled into the intestinal lumen and extravasation could easily be identified.

More commonly, the finding is one of an aggregation of tightly coiled loops, densely adherent to one another in a conglomerate mass, through which no plane can be identified. It is a mistake in this setting to proceed with lengthy, extensive, difficult lysis of adhesions, often with multiple accidental superimposed enterotomies. Even if successful, this mode of dealing with radiation-induced obstruction only sets the stage for a later intervention, which is rendered even more difficult and of greater risk to the patient. If a discrete group of involved loops can be seen and dissected from contiguous tissues as a unit, it is preferable to resect this obstructive complex and anastomose unobstructed, relatively uninvolved bowel to its distal counterpart. If the obstructive mass is in the vicinity of the ileocecal valve, it is wiser to resect the terminal ileum and perform an ileocolic anastomosis rather than to preserve a small segment of ileum proximal to the ileocecal valve. The latter type of anastomosis does not function well. Anastomoses may be hand-sewn in the usual fashion or constructed with intestinal staplers. They may be end-to-end, if the lumina are adequate, or side-to-side (functional end-to-end), depending on the operator's preference. Both reconstructions function well. The extremities of the anastomosis should be marked with hemoclips.

Bypass of the affected, obstructive loops should be performed only in the rare circumstance in which resection poses unacceptable risks of morbidity and mortality. Leaving the bypassed, radiation-damaged intestine poses a life-long risk for later complications.

There should be no undue hurry in discontinuing nasogastric suction in the postoperative period. Only when there is indication of effective peristalsis through the newly constructed anastomosis should oral feeding be begun, usually not before a minimum of 5 days. If delay for longer than 7 days is necessary for any reason before oral feeding is resumed, supplemental parenteral nutrition should be considered. In nutritionally depleted patients, parenteral nutrition should be initiated preoperatively and continued until caloric intake is adequate.

FISTULIZATION

The radiation-damaged small intestine is prone to fistulization in a manner akin to that seen with granulomatous enteritis. Although not as common as obstruction, fistulization may occur between loops, into the colon, rectum, vagina, bladder, or through the skin. Entero-entero fistulas in themselves need not be an indication for surgery if they are asymptomatic. Fistulas at the other sites mentioned require surgical intervention. Enterocutaneous fistulas may occur in the immediate or late postoperative period from anastomotic leaks or minute enterotomies. If the source is from a radiation-damaged loop, they rarely close spontaneously.

A principle to remember in radiation-induced enteric fistulas is that they cannot be managed by simple closure. Such closures inevitably fail after a short, delusive, apparently successful interlude, and a larger fistula usually results. The loop involved in the fistula must be resected and the bowel segments carefully approximated in the manner mentioned above. Enterocutaneous fistulas secondary to radiation injury and associated operative procedures rarely close with non-operative therapy, unless they are minute. When enterocutaneous fistulas occur in the context of advanced malignancy, management by enterostomal therapy and nutritional support is kinder than an aggressive resective approach to therapy.

ULCER

Small-intestinal ulcers as a consequence of irradiation are rare. They are probably due to focal vascular compromise, generally extending deep into the muscularis propria. In this setting, they may be the source of an intractable bleed, or, by associated cicatrization and luminal constriction, the cause of obstruction (Figure 9.6). In either event, the indication is for segmental resection. Conservative measures are of little avail.

INFARCTION, NECROSIS, AND PERFORATION

This trio of complications represents the ultimate catastrophe in radiation injury to the small intestine. It is the end-stage of progressive endoluminal vascular occlusion of larger feeding vessels to an intestinal segment or segments. Infarction may be in a single segment or in multiple segments (Figure 9.7).

The natural history of infarcted intestine is well known. The sequelae are full-thickness necrosis and ultimate perforation. There is no room for expectant treatment, because the clinical picture is one of an acute abdomen with progressive sepsis. Infarction, necrosis, and perforation are usually a late complication with severe radiation damage. They are more frequent in the pelvis than in the upper abdomen. The only definitive treatment is resection of the affected segment or segments.

PREDISPOSING FACTORS

Among the factors that are considered conducive to radiation injury are body habitus, malnutrition, generalized

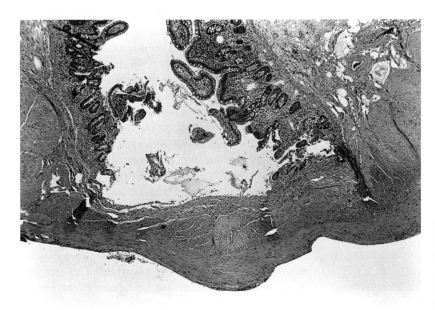

Figure 9.6 *Histologic section of irradiated ulcer of mid-ileum occurring many years after abdominopelvic irradiation for uterine carcinoma. The ulcer caused recurrent obstruction and bleeding.*

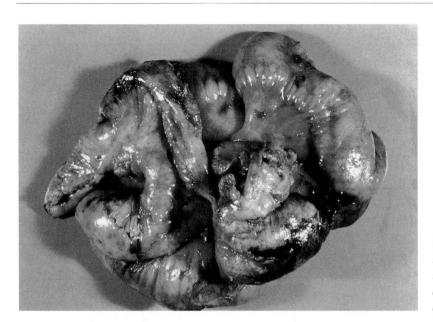

Figure 9.7 *Loops of irradiated pelvic ileum resected for multiple, segmental infarctions and perforations years after radiation therapy for cervical carcinoma.*

vascular disease (e.g., diabetes, arteriosclerosis), concomitant chemotherapy, and rare genetic syndromes (e.g., ataxia-telangiectasia, Fanconi's anemia). The most important factor by far, however, is postoperative fixation and decrease in the mobility of loops by postoperative adhesions. This is most pronounced in the pelvis, in the region of the incision, and in the retroperitoneum. The pelvis is by far the most common site.

Obesity may be a contributing factor if it interferes with accurate delineation of the ports and direction of the beam. Ultimately, the most potent factor influencing radiation damage is the radiation dosage. As the dose approaches levels above 4500–5000 cGy, increasing degrees of radiation damage can be predicted with certainty.

Although some relationship of late radiation injuries to severe symptoms encountered during the original therapy has been suspected, evidence for this is anecdotal and difficult to document. There are no convincing long-term studies to substantiate such a conclusion. On the basis of anecdotal evidence, however, it is advisable to interrupt therapy in the face of severe adverse symptoms which occur early in the treatment regimen.

PREVENTIVE MEASURES

Preventive measures should begin before the institution of radiotherapy, principally in the operating room. Areas of peritoneal denudation should be reperitonealized as completely as possible in the pelvis and retroperitoneum. Although this does not obviate postoperative adhesions, it lessens their number and density.

Various measures have been tried to exclude the small bowel from the pelvis, all with questionable success and some with serious shortcomings. Among the simplest, if omentum is available, is the positioning of as much omentum into the pelvis as possible, with fixation to pelvic sidewalls or pelvic brim.[19] This maneuver, however, is helpful only if the omentum is plentiful and mobile. In some operations for pelvic malignancy, it is not available, because of either prior removal or indicated removal concurrent with the operation.

The placing of packing or prosthetic devices in the pelvis to exclude the small intestine during the course of radiotherapy has not been widely accepted. Among the devices used have been plain packing, silicone prostheses,[20] and foam-rubber prostheses shaped to conform to and fill the pelvis. These are removed in a second stage after the completion of radiotherapy. They are not recommended.

In vogue in recent years has been the construction of an absorbable mesh barrier at the pelvic brim to exclude the intestine from the pelvis.[21–23] The sheet of mesh, either polyglycolic acid or polyglactin, is tacked to the edges of the pelvic inlet as tautly as possible. It has been shown to retain its tautness for sufficient time to complete the radiotherapy, after which the absorption of the material allows the small bowel to descend again into the pelvis. No convincing evidence of the effectiveness of this maneuver based on a large series of cases has been published, and the method has some disadvantages. The mesh itself is desmoplastic, inducing a dense fibrous reaction to structures with which it is in contact. This can render future operation extraordinarily difficult. Also, defects in the mesh barrier can and do occur, either at the sutured edges or in the substance of the mesh itself, allowing herniation of loops through dangerously small openings. Nevertheless, it is an operative maneuver still in the process of evaluation, and deserves continuing consideration.

During radiotherapy, several steps have been suggested or adopted to lessen the likelihood of injury. It is now routine in a number of treatment centers to perform a small-bowel series with a mixture of barium and gastrografin during the planning simulation of therapy. With predetermined knowledge of areas of small-bowel fixation, it is possible to alter the position, ports, and radiation fields, or to interpose blocks or other barriers to avoid (if possible) direct irradiation of fixed, immobile loops.

Fractionation of radiation treatments (e.g., divided doses twice daily rather than a single dose daily) has had limited acceptance in a few centers only. The difficult logistics of multiple daily treatments for a questionable benefit ratio have not yet justified a more generalized use of fractionation.

There has been a plethora of radioprotective substances suggested, many of which have not had demonstrated practical benefit or are still being tested.[24] These substances include the thiophosphates (WR2721), glutamine, prostaglandin antagonists, anti-proteases, interleukin-1α, and others. These have not yet been generally accepted as practical or useful. Directed against the known factor of free oxygen radicals, an important element in the deleterious effect of ionizing radiation has been the oral administration of an antioxidant regimen including vitamin E, betacarotene, and vitamin C. Evidence for the usefulness of any of these regimens is still anecdotal.

Similarly, elemental diets,[25] total parenteral nutrition, cholestyramine, and other nutrition modifiers have not been shown to be unequivocally useful.

COLON AND RECTUM

The ascending, transverse, and descending segments of the colon are seldom the site of radiation damage, except in instances of extreme radiosensitivity or unusually high dosage. The sigmoid and rectosigmoid colons, however, may suffer the same sequelae and surgical consequences as indicated for the small intestine, but with much less frequency. Conditions in which the rectosigmoid or sigmoid colon may be damaged during radiotherapy are in the management of gynecological malignancies and carcinoma of the rectum, anal canal, and prostate.

The rectum is the most frequently injured segment of the lower gastrointestinal tract, despite its lesser sensitivity to radiation damage as compared with the small intestine.[26] The vulnerability of the rectum is a consequence of its fixation, its high exposure to the radiation beam, and the frequent use of booster dosages in the treatment of pelvic malignancies.[27]

The most frequently encountered consequence of radiation injury to the rectum is bleeding. Radiation proctitis is best diagnosed by proctoscopy and is recognized by the granular, hyperemic, and friable rectal mucosa. Such proctitis occurring soon after the initiation of therapy is usually well managed by topical therapy or endoscopic treatment of focal bleeding points with laser or electrocoagulative therapy. Late, persistent, or chronic proctitis is more difficult to manage. Pain, tenesmus, and steady blood loss may require surgical intervention in addition to all medical measures.

There are many topical agents useful in radiation proctitis which may be effective in controlling mild or moderate cases. These include sucralfate,[28] hydrocortisone enemas, sodium pentosanpolysulfate (PPS), and even formalin.[29] Severe proctitis may not be relieved and may require fecal diversion, although colostomy alone may still not fully alleviate symptoms or control blood loss. Focal ulceration with bleeding has been managed successfully with laser or electrocoagulation. Medical measures as mentioned above should also be employed concurrently.

In order of severity, the next major complication in the rectum is the chronic rectal ulcer. This ulcer is located characteristically on the anterior rectal wall, is shallow in depth, circumscribed by a zone of induration, and exhibits a necrotic greyish-yellow base. The ulcer may bleed or give rise to severe pain. Conversely, it may be entirely asymptomatic. Most ulcers respond to topical therapy in time, but others may require fecal diversion.

Radiation-induced strictures may be found in the rectum or rectosigmoid colon as a consequence of ulceration with healing or more diffuse circumferential injury. Neoplastic involvement should always be suspected and sought endoscopically during study of the stricture. Strictures of early onset usually have an acute inflammatory component, which will respond to non-surgical measures. Higher grade strictures of later onset require fecal diversion or an extirpative procedure.

Rectovaginal fistula is the most common fistula complicating radiation injury to the rectum. More severe grades of fistulization involve the bladder, buttocks, and even the retroperitoneum (Figure 9.8). Radiation-induced fistulas do not respond to non-operative measures. The least extensive surgical procedure is a diverting colostomy, which may result in the healing of the less severe cases. The more severe cases require complex reconstructive tissue transfer procedures for permanent cure, in addition to fecal diversion, if permanent closure of the fistula is to be obtained. Details of these procedures are beyond the scope of this chapter and can be found in surgical texts on these subjects.

PROCTECTOMY AND COLOSTOMY

The radiation-damaged rectum, whether involved with intractable bleeding, ulceration, stricture, or fistula, may

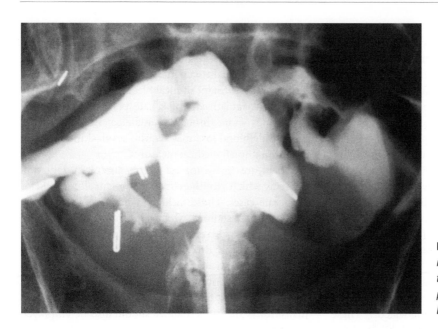

Figure 9.8 *Extensive fistulization of mid-rectum following radiation therapy for carcinoma of the prostate. Fistulas extended into the buttocks and true pelvis.*

require proctectomy as the definitive procedure. Low rectal anastomoses in the presence of radiation injury are always precarious and in the majority of instances should be protected with a proximal colostomy.

If the colostomy is performed in the sigmoid colon, which is generally the most easily accessible and the best functional site for such a stoma, there is a likelihood that the sigmoid colon may also have been in the path of the radiation beam. Special attention must therefore be given to the creation of the stoma to avoid serious complications.

If at all possible, the stoma should not be placed in an area of skin which has been irradiated. The colonic mucosa should not be sutured flush with the abdominal wall, but at least 2 or 3 cm should be allowed to protrude as a rosette. Stomata within irradiated bowel have a great tendency to retract and segmental or circumferential necrosis may occur if there has been vascular compromise or there is tension on the exteriorized bowel.

The rules of postoperative colostomy care then pertain as usual. The stoma should be observed daily for circulatory sufficiency and viability. Excessive digital examination and dilatation should be avoided.

DAMAGE TO OTHER INTRA-ABDOMINAL OR RETROPERITONEAL STRUCTURES

Collateral damage secondary to radiation to organs or structures outside the gastrointestinal tract during abdominal irradiation is rarely of surgical consequence.

The liver, pancreas, kidneys, and bone marrow may be affected to a greater or lesser degree, depending on the radiation dosage absorbed by them. For a detailed discussion of the effects on these organs, the reader is referred to other sources.[1,2,4,5]

MAXIMS IN THE MANAGEMENT OF RADIATION ENTEROPATHY

1 Operation should always be a measure of last resort.
2 Optimal nutritional status should be achieved preoperatively.
3 Incision into heavily irradiated areas of skin should be avoided.
4 Dilated bowel should be decompressed preoperatively, by long tube if possible.
5 Antibiotic bowel preparation should be done preoperatively and broad-spectrum, parenteral antibiotics should be given postoperatively.
6 Resection of severely damaged bowel is more definitive than bypass, but judgment at the time of operation should determine this decision.
7 Excessive adhesiolysis should be avoided. It is rarely definitive treatment for obstructive enteropathy; it may aggravate it and risks fistula formation.
8 Hand-sewn, stapled, end-to-end, or side-to-side anastomoses are equally effective, but each requires meticulous fashioning. Anastomoses in radiation-damaged bowel are precarious.
9 Anastomoses should be identifiable, either by staple lines in stapled anastomoses or by hemoclips in hand-sewn anastomoses.
10 Oral feeding should be delayed until effective peristalsis returns and the anastomosis is functional. A minimum 5-day delay is recommended.
11 Low rectal anastomosis in irradiated bowel should be protected against leaks with a proximal colostomy for maximum safety.
12 Intestinal stomata made with irradiated bowel or in irradiated skin are prone to complications. An ample segment should be exteriorized.

13 Radiation-induced fistulas rarely respond to non-operative therapy or simple closure. Resection or tissue transfer is usually necessary. Bypass exclusion is an option, though less desirable.

REFERENCES

1. Trott K-R, Herrmann T. Radiation effects on abdominal organs. In Scherer E, Streffer C, Trott K-R, eds. *Medical radiology*. New York, Springer-Verlag, 1991, 313–46.

2. Fajardo L-GLF. Sequelae. Morphology of radiation effects on normal tissues. In Perez CA, Brady LW, eds. *Principles and practice of radiation oncology*, 2nd edn. Philadelphia, JB Lippincott Co., 1992, 50–63, 114–23.

3. Morgenstern L. Radiation enteropathy. In Bouchier IAD, Allan RN, Hodgson HJF, Keighley MRB, eds. *Gastroenterology: clinical science and practice,* 2nd edn. London, WB Saunders Co., 1993, 688–97.

4. Basic radiation physics, chemistry, and biology. Direct effects of radiation. Perception and acceptance of risk. In Mettler FA Jr, Upton AC, eds. *Medical effects of ionizing radiation*, 2nd edn. Philadelphia, WB Saunders Co., 1995, 1–23, 214–95, 375–83.

5. Coia LR, Myerson RJ, Tepper JE. Late effects of radiation therapy on the gastrointestinal tract. Int J Radiat Oncol Biol Phys 1995; 31(5):1213–36.

6. Rubin P, Casarett G. A direction for clinical radiation pathology: the tolerance dose. In Vaeth JM, ed. *Frontiers of radiation therapy and oncology*, Vol. 6. Baltimore, University Park Press, 1972, 1–16.

7. Hacker NF, Berek JS, Burnison CM, Heintz PM, Juillard GJF, Lagasse LD. Whole abdominal radiation as salvage therapy for epithelial ovarian cancer. Obstet Gynecol 1985; 65(1):60–6.

8. Reddy S, Lee M-S, Yordan E, Graham J, Sarin P, Hendrickson FR. Salvage whole abdomen radiation therapy: its role in ovarian cancer. Int J Radiat Oncol Biol Phys 1993; 27(4):879–84.

9. Fine BA, Hempling RE, Piver MS, Baker TR, McAuley M, Driscoll D. Severe radiation morbidity in carcinoma of the cervix: impact of pretherapy surgical staging and previous surgery. Int J Radiat Oncol Biol Phys 1995; 31(4):717–23.

10. Warren S, Friedman NB. Pathology and pathologic diagnosis of radiation lesions in the gastrointestinal tract. Am J Pathol 1942; 18:499–513.

11. White DC. Intestines. In White DC, ed. *An atlas of radiation histopathology*. Oakridge, TN, Technical Information Center, Office of Public Affairs, US Energy Research and Development Administration, Washington, DC, 1975, 141–60.

12. Berthrong M, Fajardo LF. Radiation injury in surgical pathology. Part II. Alimentary tract. Am J Surg Pathol 1981; 5:153–78.

13. Fajardo LF. General morphology of radiation injury. In *Pathology of radiation injury*. New York, Masson, 1982, 6–14.

14. Berthrong M. Pathologic changes secondary to radiation. World J Surg 1986; 10(2):155–70.

15. Richter KK, Fink LM, Hughes BM, *et al.* Differential effect of radiation on endothelial cell function in rectal cancer and normal rectum. Am J Surg 1998; 176(6):642–7.

16. Morgenstern L, Thompson R, Friedman NB. The modern enigma of radiation enteropathy: sequelae and solutions. Am J Surg 1977; 134:166–72.

17. Morgenstern L, Hart M, Lugo D, Friedman NB. Changing aspects of radiation enteropathy. Arch Surg 1985; 120:1225–8.

18. Kalman DR, Barnard GF, Massimi GJ, Swanson RS. Primary aortoduodenal fistula after radiotherapy. Am J Gastroenterol 1995; 90(7):1148–50.

19. O'Leary DP. Use of the greater omentum in colorectal surgery. Dis Colon Rectum 1999; 42(4):533–9.

20. Sezur A, Martella L, Abbou C, *et al.* Small intestine protection from radiation by means of a removable adapted prosthesis. Am J Surg 1999; 178(1):22–5.

21. Devereaux DF, Chandler JJ, Eisenstat T, Zinkin L. Efficacy of an absorbable mesh in keeping the small bowel out of the human pelvis following surgery. Surg Gynecol Obstet 1984; 159:162–3.

22. Dasmahapatra KS, Anangur PS. The use of biodegradable mesh to prevent radiation-associated small-bowel injury. Arch Surg 1991; 126:366–9.

23. Bazán A, Hontanilla B. The use of the rectus abdominis muscle and a vicryl mesh to protect the small intestine and the rectus in radiation treatments to the lower pelvis. Plast Reconstr Surg 1999; 103(2):746–7.

24. Spitzer TR. Clinical aspects of irradiation-induced alimentary tract injury. In Dubois A, King GL, Livengood DR, eds. *Radiation and the gastrointestinal tract*. Boca Raton, Florida, CRC Press, 1995.

25. Craighead PS, Young S. Phase II study assessing the feasibility of using elemental supplements to reduce acute enteritis in patients receiving radical pelvic radiotherapy. Am J Clin Oncol 1998; 21(6):573–8.

26. Otchy DP, Nelson H. Radiation injuries of the colon and rectum. In Wolff BG, ed. Inflammatory disorders of the colon. Surg Clin North Am 1993; 73(5):1017–35.

27. Ogino I, Kitamura T, Okamoto N, *et al.* Late rectal complication following high dose rate intracavitary brachytherapy in cancer of the cervix. Int J Radiat Oncol Biol Phys 1995; 31(4):725–34.

28. Kochhar R, Sriram PVJ, Sharma SC, Goel RC, Patel F. Natural history of late radiation proctosigmoiditis treated with topical sucralfate suspension. Dig Dis Sci 1999; 44(5):973–8.

29. Rubinstein E, Ibsen T, Rasmussen RB. Formalin treatment of radiation-induced hemorrhagic proctitis. Am J Gastroenterol 1986; 81:44–5.

ANNOTATED BIBLIOGRAPHY

Coia LR, Myerson RJ, Tepper JE. **Late effects of radiation therapy on the gastrointestinal tract. Int J Radiat Oncol Biol Phys 1995; 31(5):1213–36.**
Summary of Consensus Conference on Late Radiation Injuries to the Gastrointestinal Tract, held in 1992. Includes severity grading scales of radiation oncology societies and suggested treatment of clinical syndromes.

Fajardo L-GLF. **Morphology of radiation effects on normal tissues. In** *Principles and practice of radiation oncology.* **Philadelphia, JB Lippincott Co., 1992, 50–63, 114–23, 996–7.**
An authoritative text on early and late sequelae of radiation. Tabulated morbidity scoring criteria; extensive bibliography.

Mettler FA, Upton AC. **Direct effects of radiation. In** *Medical effects of ionizing radiation,* **2nd edn. Philadelphia, WB Saunders Co., 1995, 215–95.**
Excellent descriptions of low-dose and high-dose response of various organs to radiation. Extensive, scholarly bibliography of older and current literature.

Morgenstern L. **Radiation enteropathy. In Bouchier IAD, Allan RN, Hodgson JF, Keighley MRB, eds.** *Gastroenterology: clinical science and practice,* **2nd edn. Philadelphia, WB Saunders Co., 1993, 668–97.**
Clinically oriented summary of radiation injuries of the gastrointestinal tract. Based on author's observations on more than 100 cases.

Trott K-R, Herrmann T. **Radiation effects on abdominal organs. In** *Radiopathology of tissues and organs.* **New York, Springer-Verlag, 1991, 313–46.**
A comprehensive survey of individual abdominal organ responses to radiation, including clinical effects and histopathology.

Commentary

BERNARD S LEWINSKY

INTRODUCTION

In this chapter, Dr Morgenstern has eloquently summarized the known pathways that can lead to radiation damage of organs in the abdomen. The pitfalls of performing surgery on irradiated tissues have also been outlined. The pathophysiology of radiation damage has been studied, not only in the laboratory, but also in clinical scenarios that are encountered in the management of common malignancies. After all, therapeutic ionizing radiation has been utilized in one form or other since the discovery of the X-ray by Roentgen in 1895 and its first use on a patient in 1896.[1]

The important issue, however, is what we are currently learning and applying in radiation oncology to reduce the incidence and severity of complications when ionizing radiation is applied in the modern era. More sophisticated equipment with higher and higher energy levels is not likely to produce a significant improvement, but the application of computer technology into the design and capabilities of new accelerators and in the planning phase of therapy may well be the hallmark of a new era in radiation oncology.

A brief review of 'the state of the art' is appropriate so that the surgical oncologist can interact with the radiation oncologist in a meaningful way in the vastly expanded computerized age.

THE TEAM

It may be a naïve, but intuitively obvious, concept that all the members of the oncology team must be working together in the management of the patient. With the integration of chemotherapy into the management of most malignancies, both surgeons and radiation oncologists must understand the added morbidity in the application of their craft. Radiation doses must be adjusted in accordance with the chemical agent used, and surgical techniques as well as the timing of surgery must be augmented.

The dialogue between radiation oncologist and surgeon is crucial in all phases of care.

In the preoperative stage, when the diagnosis may not even have been made but there is suspicion of malignancy, the patient will benefit most from this type of discussion. Should a specific patient with rectal cancer receive preoperative or postoperative radiation therapy? Should the radiation oncologist examine the patient prior to surgery to assist in this decision as he or she will probably be called upon to treat the patient later? The answer to this question is a definite yes.

A second simple example is the suggested possibility of a sarcoma by virtue of location, size, or organ site. If the radiation oncologist is made aware of this possibility, he or she may be available to place catheters in the tumor bed for brachytherapy, whereas if the tumor is resected and a decision is subsequently made that a brachytherapy approach is indicated, a second surgical procedure will be necessary. This is not only costly, but also adds to the morbidity by virtue of the increased adhesions due to repeated surgeries.

Another obvious advantage to the patient in this type of interchange is the discussion of surgical and radiotherapeutic techniques that may eventually lead to decreased morbidity and complications. Reminding the surgeon to place copious clips at the tumor bed or residual tumor, or to perform an omental sling, if needed, is a simple example that makes treatment planning and the delivery of specific concentrated therapy more accurate, precise, and effective. Placement of two clips at the apex of the vaginal stump after the uterus has been resected provides a landmark to shield the rectum when the vaginal canal is treated with high-dose brachytherapy to boost the vaginal dose. Details of these techniques are given below.

In the post-irradiation setting, the discussion between the surgeon and radiation oncologist is perhaps even more important. Not only are there management issues, but medicolegal implications become important, especially if complications ensue.

Before the surgeon embarks on a surgical procedure, he or she should be well versed as to the exact treatment the patient received. Knowing that the patient 'received radiation' is not sufficient. The surgeon should know when, where, the dose, total dose, technique of delivery, site, approach to therapy, fractionation, time from last dose, and nutritional status of the patient. How often is a surgical procedure done without the benefit of these crucial data?

If this information is not sought, how can the surgeon know the segment of bowel that perhaps received a very high dose by virtue of an intracavitary treatment for gynecologic malignancy? Should one be surprised if a colostomy done at that site falls apart in the postoperative period? Who is at fault – the radiation oncologist who placed the sources to treat the cancer appropriately, or the surgeon who did not know where the radiation oncologist placed the sources, and who could easily have done a colostomy at a different site?

These are all the issues that are basic in the management of patients in a multidisciplinary approach. A single oncologist cannot possibly know the details of all therapies to direct all cancer care for patients. In most communities, it is virtually impossible to have all modalities present for each patient in a tumor board setting at all times. However, it is certain that verbal communication by telephone or e-mail can be achieved in modern practices and it is the most efficient way of decreasing potential disasters.

MODERN ONCOLOGIC PROTOCOLS

In reviewing Table 9.1 in the chapter, one can select diseases and sites that are now treated with either a combined-modality approach or with modified doses. These changes have occurred as a result of aggressive new studies and data or the development of new drugs that have significantly changed the treatment parameters.

Hodgkin's disease became a curable disease when the extended radiotherapeutic approach yielded high cure rates.[2,3] As cures became the norm in this disease, and long-term side-effects became evident, the availability of new drugs and treatment regimens spawned new studies that have led to the inclusion of combination chemotherapy in even the earliest and most radiocurable stages.[4] The role of radiation therapy in many cases has been relegated to consolidation therapy after primary chemotherapy. The advantage in this setting is the reduced volume treated and total doses required. Doses of 2400, 3000, or 3600 cGy are more frequently delivered than the previous doses of 4000–4500 cGy. Naturally, all cases must be individualized, but the reduction in total dose results in decreased radiation morbidity.[5]

In seminoma of the testis, treatment of the para-aortic nodes and ipsilateral pelvic nodes that included the surgical scar was common in the not too distant past. The radiosensitivity of this malignancy is such that dose de-escalation has been possible, along with a reduction in the primary target size. The risk of recurrence and the chance of subsequent control in this disease are such that fields are now limited to the para-aortic nodes and the upper ipsilateral iliac nodes. Not only does this approach reduce bowel irradiation, but it also decreases gonadal exposure to preserve fertility. The doses to treat this disease have been reduced from 3500–4000 cGy to 2400 cGy.[6] The role of radiation for non-seminoma testicular tumors is extremely limited due to the enormously successful chemotherapy for this entity.

In carcinoma of the esophagus and anus, as well as some cases of bladder carcinoma, the chemoradiation approach has not only reduced the doses of radiation, but has also allowed the preservation of organs by eliminating the need for surgery.[7]

These are areas of progress in the oncology arena that have markedly impacted the quality of life of the cancer patient. Communication between treating members of the team is the hallmark that results in appropriate and modern care.

STATE-OF-THE-ART EQUIPMENT: THE PRESENT AND THE FUTURE

In the early 1960s, the era of megavoltage therapy began, first with the introduction of cobalt-60 units and then with the introduction of linear accelerators. The introduction of higher and higher energies allowed the treatment of deep-seated tumors to be undertaken, with decreased morbidity to the skin and subcutaneous tissues. This was a great advantage to obese and large patients, but had virtually no effect on tumor-cell kill or cure rates. In fact, glottis cancer treatment results diminish with increasing energy.[8] Many departments still treat head and neck diseases with cobalt-60 or with 4 or 6 meV units.

If higher energies have not improved results with regard to cell kill, what can we anticipate to achieve with ionizing radiation? The key is still the radiosensitivity of the tissues surrounding the tumor. One could easily predict that all cancer could be cured if we could deliver the doses that are needed to kill the cancer cells. Unfortunately, normal tissues would be damaged with these doses. Particulate beams (protons and neutrons) have different physical and radiobiological properties that theoretically would increase cell kill, but in clinical studies they have fallen short of expectations. However, individual cases may warrant the use of these beams.

If higher energies do not provide the answer, decreasing the morbidity of therapy will not only improve quality of life, but may also allow the delivery of higher doses to the tumor while protecting surrounding organs.

Multi-leaf collimation

Multi-leaf collimation (MLC) is a mechanical, electronic device that is attached beneath the collimator of the unit. It consists of 80–120 slim metal collimators attached to individual motors (Figure 1). The motors can be programmed to move the collimators a specific distance, thus creating different shapes. It allows the isolation of the tumor for treatment as seen on computerized tomography (CT) or magnetic resonance imaging (MRI) scans taken in the treatment position. The tumor can be isolated from its surrounding organs and the radiation field is custom shaped. By virtue of computer treatment planning programs, the MLC can change into infinite shapes to conform to the various tumor sizes and shapes.

If one imagines a tumor on a CT scan and a shaped field (by virtue of MLC) around the tumor, and if one scans through the subsequent CT scans and electronically changes the MLC to conform to that subsequent shape, one can envision the MLC jaws opening and closing to conform to the shape of the tumor in three dimensions. This is similar to a cartoon animation that shows motion with rapid sequencing. Taking into consideration the changing outer contour of the patient, i.e., the tumor extends from within a thin portion of the patient to a thicker one, physics would dictate that a different energy intensity could deliver the dose to tissues at different depths, thus effectively pinpointing and killing cancer cells while sparing normal tissues and organs (Plate 1). The dynamic change of intensities to compensate for body size together with three-dimensional treatment planning and verification comprise the next generation of technology, known as intensity modulated radiation therapy (IMRT). Long-term data on this modality are still scarce, but certainly dose escalation with decreasing morbidity is the expected end-result of this innovation.

High dose rate

High dose rate (HDR) is a method of delivering interstitial or intracavitary treatment remotely in rapid, sustained pulses or fractionated therapy. Not only does this approach decrease radiation exposure to personnel, but it also allows interstitial or intracavitary treatments to be given in the outpatient setting. Doses to tumor beds, organs, or other sites can be given intraoperatively if appropriate shielding is available in the operating suites. This method is the ultimate in delivering the dose to the tumor with the least normal-tissue interference.

Intraoperative radiation therapy and intraoperative electron radiation therapy

Intraoperative radiation therapy (IORT) and intraoperative electron radiation therapy (IOERT)[9] are modalities that allow the use of ionizing or electron-beam treatments directly in the tumor while the tumor or tumor bed is exposed in the operating room. New techniques with radio-immunoguidance help localize the area for treatment.[10] Both of these modalities are costly, requiring the treatment vault to be in the operating room or converted into an operating room, or that the operating room is shielded to allow portable HDR technology. Whereas this modality is quite novel, the practicality of this approach for the average radiation oncology department is quite limited, and thus not very popular. Intraoperative, mobile electron units are available, but the cost of the equipment is difficult to justify for the majority of institutions.

Radiosurgery

Radiosurgery is the technique of combining CT scan data, computerization, immobilization of the patient, and treatment planning for the delivery of, usually high, concentrated external-beam doses to the tumor. Because the planning and delivery are so prolonged and time consuming, the treatment is usually delivered in one or more high-dose fractions. This modality is particularly effective in treating intracranial or other central nervous system lesions, where normal tissue preservation is critical. Cost containment issues limit its use to highly curable cases or for maximal palliative potential.[11]

There are obviously a great number of steps being taken in several fields that are collaborating to develop a new generation of units whose aim is to treat more precisely in order to decrease morbidity.

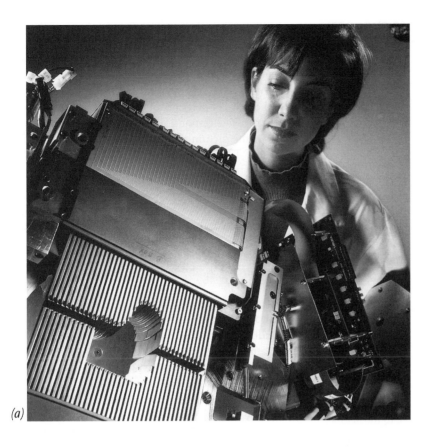

(a)

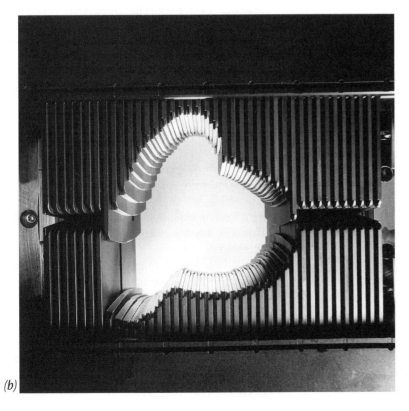

(b)

Figure 1 *(a) Collimator head with multi-leaf collimator. (b) Close-up of multi-leaf collimator with configuration of an object. Photographs courtesy of Varian Medical Systems, Palo Alto, CA.*

ADVANCES IN RADIATION PHYSICS SUPPORT

The radiation oncologist's partner in planning therapy is the simulator. Treatment simulators are usually converted X-ray tubes on a gantry that simulate the beam from the treatment unit. The simulator allows for the rudimentary treatment parameters to be established and then transferred to the treating accelerator for the actual therapy. Computerization of the simulator by incorporation of software to regular CT scans allows for a CT scan to be done with the patient in the treatment position. The patient can then go home and the tumor can be outlined at a later time by the radiation oncologist. By using treatment-planning programs, the fields and other treatment parameters can be set up without the presence of the patient – thus the term virtual simulation. This methodology therefore combines the data from the CT scan with the treatment-planning program to produce the best treatment plan for that specific site.

In similar fashion, programs have been developed that provide non-coplanar fields (i.e., fields that do not oppose each other) around a tumor that will limit the doses to the surround tissues while delivering the designated dose to the tumor. An example would be treating the prostate to 7800 cGy or more while limiting the dose to the bladder to 6000 cGy, the rectum to 4500 cGy, and the femoral heads to 3000 cGy. Standard fields could not achieve this dose distribution, but with multiple (six or more) fields and at various angles and entry points, this conformal, computer-devised, precise treatment can be delivered. Naturally, daily duplication of treatments, organ mobility, breathing, and heart movement must all be taken into account in the final treatment plan. This process is known as three-dimensional conformal therapy.

Lastly, computerization and imaging modalities have allowed the development of programs that look at volumes of normal or abnormal tissues that receive a particular dose. With these data, dose–volume histograms can be generated, which in turn correlate to the volume of normal to abnormal tissue being treated in a particular treatment plan. This aid provides information that will predict normal-tissue complications, and thus the treatment plan can be altered to deliver a more favorable course of therapy.[12]

CONCLUSION

The chapter on the surgical management of irradiated abdominal structures provides the reader with a concise review of the problems and pitfalls that may be encountered by the oncologic surgeon. As a radiation oncologist, I have tried to expound on the areas in radiation oncology that will complement the surgeon's knowledge of this field. Whereas what goes on behind the concrete vaults (mostly in basements) may seem obscure and frightening, I have tried to outline the strides taken to increase tumor control and cure rates without sacrificing normal tissue and, at the same time, decreasing the morbidity of therapy. This ultimate goal can only be achieved with the full cooperation of all involved on the team, whose true, sole responsibility is to the patient. It is wise to follow the dictum that 'the best treatment is the first treatment.' Thus, we owe it to the patient to make his or her cancer treatment the **best** treatment.

REFERENCES

1. del Regato J. *Radiological oncologists: the unfolding of a medical specialty.* Reston, VA, Radiology Centennial, Inc., 1993.
2. Kaplan HS. Prognosis. In *Hodgkin's disease.* Cambridge, MA, Harvard University Press, 1972, 360–88.
3. Smithers D, Peckham MJ. Assessment of the results of treatment. In *Hodgkin's disease.* Edinburgh, London, Churchill Livingstone,1973, 236–48.
4. Specht L. Limited radiation therapy for selected patients with pathological stage 1A and 2A Hodgkin's disease. In *Seminars in radiation oncology*, Vol. VI, No. 3. Philadelphia, WB Saunders Co., 1996, 162–71.
5. Hoppe RT. Hodgkin's disease. In Liebel S, Phillips T, eds. *Textbook of radiation oncology.* Philadelphia, WB Saunders Co., 1998, 1079–94.
6. Small EJ, Torti FM. Testes. In Abeloff MD, Armitage JO, Lichter AS, Niederhuber JE, eds. *Clinical oncology.* Edinburgh, London, Churchill Livingstone, 1995, 1504–26.
7. Meyer JL, Vaeth JM. Organ conservation in curative cancer treatment – indications, contraindications, methods. In *Frontiers of radiation therapy and oncology*, Vol. 27. Basel, Karger Press, 1993, 103–17, 118–29, 143–65.
8. Wang CC. *Radiation therapy for head and neck neoplasms*, 3rd edn. New York, Wiley & Sons, 1997, 231–2.
9. Wolkov HB. Intraoperative radiation therapy. In Leibel S, Phillips T, eds. *Textbook of radiation oncology.* Philadelphia, WB Saunders Co., 1998, 276–90.
10. Nag S. Radioimmunoguided IORT for colorectal carcinoma. Adv Admin Radiol Radiat Oncol 1999; 9(9):39–40.
11. Kondziolka D, Patel A, Lunsford LD, *et al.* Stereotactic radiosurgery plus whole brain radiotherapy vs radiotherapy alone for patients with multiple brain metastases. Int J Radiat Oncol Biol Phys 1999; 45(2):427–34.
12. Kutcher GJ, Mageras GS, Burman CM. Three dimensional radiation therapy. In Leibel S, Phillips T, eds. *Textbook of radiation oncology.* Philadelphia, WB Saunders Co., 1998, 141–9.

Editors' selected abstracts

CT of radiation-induced injury of the gastrointestinal tract: spectrum of findings with barium studies correlation.

Boudiaf M, Soyer P, Pelage JP, Kardache M, Nemeth J, Dufresne AC, Rymer R.

Department of Radiology, Hopital Lariboisiere-AP-HP, Paris, France.

European Radiology 10(6):920–5, 2000.

Because of improvement in survival rate of patients with abdominal cancer, gastrointestinal complications following external radiation therapy are becoming more frequent. Thus, an increased number of patients are commonly investigated with imaging because of suspected radiation-induced injury of the gastrointestinal tract. This pictorial review highlights the spectrum of CT and barium study manifestations of radiation-induced injury of the gastrointestinal tract. The major role of CT in the evaluation and management of patients with radiation injury of the gastrointestinal tract is highlighted. Emphasis is placed on CT imaging signs that may help in distinguishing between radiation-induced injury and recurrent disease.

Intestinal failure after surgery for complicated radiation enteritis.

Girvent M, Carlson GL, Anderson I, Shaffer J, Irving M, Scott NA.

Intestinal Failure Unit, Hope Hospital, Manchester, UK.

Annals of the Royal College of Surgeons of England 82(3):198–201, 2000, May.

Between 1983 and 1997, a total of 16 patients were referred to a tertiary Intestinal Failure Unit (IFU) following surgery elsewhere for complications of radiation enteritis. Eleven were female with a mean age of 43 years (range 21–71 years) and the most common primary site of malignancy was genitourinary ($n = 13$). Patients had undergone an average of two laparotomies (range 1–7 laparotomies) for complications of radiation enteritis prior to transfer to the IFU. On admission, the principal problem in eight patients was persisting intestinal fistulation, four patients had continuing intestinal obstruction and four had the short bowel syndrome after extensive intestinal resection. Only one patient had evidence of residual malignancy; this patient with short bowel syndrome was allowed home without invasive therapy. Of the remaining 15 patients, 12 required an abdominal surgical procedure, while three were discharged without further surgery after training for home parenteral nutrition (HPN). Following abdominal surgery, five patients died in hospital, but the remaining seven patients went home alive – including two further patients on HPN. Overall, of the 15 patients referred with intestinal failure after surgery for complications of radiation enteritis and actively treated, one-third died in hospital and a further third required institution of HPN before being able to be discharged home.

Natural history of late radiation proctosigmoiditis treated with topical sucralfate suspension.

Kochhar R, Sriram PV, Sharma SC, Goel RC, Patel F.

Department of Gastroenterology, Postgraduate Institute of Medical Education and Research, Chandigarh, India.

Digestive Diseases & Sciences 44(5):973–8, 1999, May.

Rectal bleeding due to radiation proctosigmoiditis is often difficult to manage. We had earlier shown the efficacy of short-term therapy with topical sucralfate in controlling bleeding in the radiation proctosigmoiditis. We now report our long-term results with this form of therapy. The study comprised 26 patients with radiation proctosigmoiditis. Sigmoidoscopically, 9 (34.6%) patients had severe changes, 15 (57.69%) had moderate, and 2 (7.69%) had mild changes. Severity of bleeding was graded as severe (>15 episodes per week), moderate (8–14 episodes per week), mild (2–7 episodes per week), negligible (≤ 1 episode per week), or nil (no bleeding). Ten patients had moderate rectal bleeding, while 16 had severe bleeding. All patients were treated with 20 mL of 10% rectal sucralfate suspension enemas twice a day until bleeding per rectum ceased or failure of therapy was acknowledged. Response to therapy was considered good whenever the severity of bleeding showed improvement by a change of two grades. Rectally administered sucralfate achieved good response in 20 (76.9%) patients at 4 weeks, 22 (84.6%) patients at 8 weeks, and 24 (92.3%) patients at 16 weeks. This change was significant by Wilcoxon matched-pairs signed-ranks test. Two patients required surgery due to poor response. Over a median follow-up of 45.5 months (range 5–73 months) after cessation of bleeding, 17 (70.8%) patients had no further bleeding while 7 (22.2%) had recurrence of bleeding. All recurrences responded to short-term reinstitution of therapy. No treatment-related complications were observed. Ten patients had other associated late toxicity due to pelvic irradiation in the form of asymptomatic rectal stricture ($n = 3$), rectovaginal fistula ($n = 1$), intestinal stricture ($n = 1$), vaginal stenosis ($n = 1$), and hematuria ($n = 6$). Three patients had progression of the primary disease in the form of pelvic recurrence ($n = 2$) and hepatic metastases ($n = 1$). We conclude that topical sucralfate induces a lasting remission in a majority of patients with moderate to severe rectal bleeding due to radiation proctosigmoiditis.

Review article: new insights into the pathogenesis of radiation-induced intestinal dysfunction.

MacNaughton WK.

Gastrointestinal Research Group and Department of Physiology and Biophysics, University of Calgary, Canada.

Alimentary Pharmacology & Therapeutics 14(5):523–8, 2000, May.

Exposure of the abdomino-pelvic region to ionizing radiation, such as that received during radiotherapy, is associated with the development of a number of untoward symptoms which may limit the course of therapy or which may involve serious chronic intestinal disease. While the mucosal dysfunction surrounding acute radiation enteritis is generally ascribed to the effects of ionizing radiation on the cell cycle of epithelial stem cells of the intestinal crypts and subsequent epithelial loss, recent evidence suggests that other, earlier events also play a role. The severity of these early events may determine the incidence and severity of chronic enteritis. The mechanism for this is unclear, but may relate to radiation-induced compromise of host defence responses to luminal pathogens or antigens. This review will address the current state of knowledge of the pathogenesis of radiation-induced intestinal dysfunction, focusing on events which occur in the mucosa, and will discuss what the future may hold with respect to the treatment of radiation-associated diseases of the intestinal tract.

Late radiogenic small bowel damage: guidelines for the general surgeon.

Meissner K.

Department of General Surgery, District Hospital, Tamsweg, Austria.

Digestive Surgery 16(3):169–74, 1999.

Background/aims: The majority of late radiogenic small bowel injuries present with obstruction or peritonitis. Owing to an average latency period of years, many of these patients are admitted to community hospitals and treated by general surgeons, who in turn see only a few pertinent patients in their professional lifetime. This study intends to provide the general surgeon with comprehensive guidelines for safer surgical management. *Material and methods:* Forty-one publications were analyzed in a search for clinical, procedural and outcome data. *Results:* After a mean interval of 3.4 years following radiotherapy, patients with a mean age of 57 years present with obstruction (71%), fistula (17%), perforation (10%) or hemorrhage (2%) due to small bowel radiation injury. 22% have associated colorectal injury. The intestinal compartments most frequently affected are lower ileum, cecum, and rectosigmoid, whereas the midgut and transverse colon are usually free. Consequently, the dehiscence rate of resection and ileoileostomy is 26%, jejunoileostomy 12%, ileoascendostomy 9% and ileotransversostomy 4%, and the pertinent rate of progressive radiation injury is 9.1%. Bypass procedures yield an overall dehiscence rate of 9%, ileotransverse bypass 1.6%, and the rate of progressive radiation injury is 37%. The lethality of suture line insufficiency is 85%. Lysis carries a lethal perforation rate of 6%. Only 58% of patients survive over 2 years, and of those not succumbing to unrelated disease, 37% die from progressive radiation injury and 63% from tumor progression. *Conclusion:* If resection is warranted, a reasonably extended ileal resection, right hemicolectomy and ileotransversostomy, is safe. Likewise, ileotransverse anastomosis is the best choice for bypass. Lysis should not be enforced in radiation-injured bowel compartments. Terminal enterostomy with distal mucous fistula alleviates otherwise untreatable fistulae.

The incidence and clinical consequences of treatment-related bowel injury.

Miller AR, Martenson JA, Nelson H, Schleck CD, Ilstrup DM, Gunderson LL, Donohue JH.

Division of Gastroenterologic and General Surgery, Mayo Clinic and Mayo Foundation, Rochester, MN, USA.

International Journal of Radiation Oncology, Biology, Physics 43(4):817–25, 1999.

Objective: To assess the frequency and clinical features of treatment-induced bowel injury in rectal carcinoma patients receiving perioperative external beam radiotherapy (EBRT). The frequency of and factors associated with treatment-induced intestinal injury have previously not been well quantified for rectal cancer patients. Postoperative adjuvant chemoirradiation is recommended for Stage II and III rectal cancers, making such data of significant interest. *Methods and materials:* The records of 386 consecutive patients undergoing radiotherapy with or without chemotherapy (CT) for rectal carcinoma between 1981–90 were reviewed. Eighty-two patients were excluded for receiving nontherapeutic EBRT or modalities other than EBRT. *Results:* Symptomatic acute treatment-related enteritis (within 30 days of EBRT +/− CT) was diagnosed in 13 patients, 3 of whom developed chronic bowel injury. Chronic treatment-related enteritis was identified in 18 patients and reoperation was required in 17 (5% of the 304 patients with complete follow-up). Chronic proctitis was documented in 38 patients, including 3 patients with small bowel injury. The probability of developing treatment-induced bowel injury at 5 years following treatment was 19%. Variables associated with an increased risk of bowel injury using multivariate analysis were transanal excision ($p = 0.002$), escalating radiation dose ($p = 0.005$), and increasing age ($p = 0.01$). Twenty of the affected patients required operative treatment, and 2 deaths resulted from treatment-induced enteritis. *Conclusion:* Patients with rectal carcinoma treated with EBRT +/− CT have the risk of developing treatment-induced bowel injury. The pelvic radiation dose should be limited to ≤ 5040 cGy unless small bowel can be displaced. Reperitonealization of the pelvis, or other surgical methods of excluding the small intestine should be used whenever possible.

Acute and late toxicity of patients with inflammatory bowel disease undergoing irradiation for abdominal and pelvic neoplasms.

Willett CG, Ooi CJ, Zietman AL, Menon V, Goldberg S, Sands BE, Podolsky DK.

Department of Radiation Oncology, Massachusetts General Hospital, Boston, MA, USA.

International Journal of Radiation Oncology, Biology, Physics 46(4):995–8, 2000, March 1.

Purpose: Little data exists in the medical literature describing the response of patients with inflammatory bowel disease (IBD) to abdominal and pelvic irradiation. To clarify the use of this modality in this setting, this study assesses the short- and long-term tolerance of 28 patients with IBD to abdominal and pelvic irradiation. *Methods and materials:* From 1970 to 1999, 28 patients with IBD (10 patients – Crohn's disease, 18 patients – ulcerative colitis) were identified and underwent external beam abdominal or pelvic irradiation. Mean follow-up time after radiation therapy was 32 months. Patients were treated either by specialized techniques (16 patients) to minimize small and large bowel irradiation or by more conventional approaches

(12 patients). Acute and late toxicity was scored. *Results:* The overall incidence of severe toxicity was 46% (13/28 patients). Six of 28 patients (21%) experienced severe acute toxicity necessitating cessation of radiation therapy. Late toxicity requiring hospitalization or surgical intervention was observed in 8 of 28 patients (29%). One patient experienced both an acute as well as late toxicity. For patients undergoing radiation therapy by conventional approaches, the 5-year actuarial rate of late toxicity was 73%. This figure was 23% for patients treated by specialized techniques ($p = 0.02$). *Conclusions:* Because of the potentially severe toxicity experienced by patients with IBD undergoing abdominal and pelvic irradiation, judicious use of this modality must be employed. Definition of IBD location and activity as well as careful attention to irradiation technique may allow treatment of these patients with acceptable rates of morbidity.

10

Management of women at high risk for the development of breast cancer

DARCY V SPICER, VALERIE ISRAEL, ROBIN D CLARK AND MALCOLM C PIKE

In this chapter, the known risk factors are reviewed as they relate to our understanding of breast cancer etiology. The current options for prevention, including surveillance, prophylactic surgery, chemoprevention, and participation in prevention studies, are discussed.

NON-HEREDITARY RISK FACTORS FOR BREAST CANCER

Age

Most common non-hormone-dependent adult cancers (such as colon cancer) arise from a multistage process for which the rate of change from stage to stage is relatively independent of age;[1] thus, incidence increases with advancing age, and the incidence of the cancers rises continuously and increasingly rapidly with age. This is consistent with modern molecular biology concepts that view cancer as a multi-step process. While the risk of breast cancer also increases with advancing age, the relationship between age and breast cancer risk is more complex. Breast cancer risk rises throughout life, but the rate at which risk rises abruptly declines at approximately the age of 50. Thus, elements important in the genesis of breast cancer decline at approximately the age of 50, and the menopause is the proximate cause of the complex relationship between age and breast cancer risk. In all likelihood, if the menopause did not occur, the incidence curve for breast cancer would be similar to that for other adult malignancies.

Age at menopause

An early natural menopause is associated with a reduced breast cancer risk,[2,3] as is bilateral oophorectomy at a young age.[4] As early surgical oophorectomy reduces breast cancer risk, a cause-and-effect relationship between ovarian function and breast cancer risk is established. The

hormonal pattern of premenopausal women with the cyclic production of relatively large amounts of estradiol and progesterone causes a greater rate of increase in breast cancer risk than the constant low estradiol and very low progesterone of postmenopausal women. The age at menopause provides no information concerning the relative importance of either ovarian hormone in determining breast cancer risk.

Age at menarche

The age at menarche determines the time of exposure to the mitogenic effect of ovarian hormones and, as expected, later menarche decreases breast cancer risk: there is an approximately 15% decrease in breast cancer risk with each year that menarche is delayed.[5]

Breast epithelial cell proliferation

To interpret these observations of breast cancer risk, an understanding of the specific effects of sex steroids on the rates of normal breast cell proliferation is necessary. Sex steroids influence cell division rates, and their effects on the genesis of breast cancer are likely to be through their effects on normal breast epithelial cell proliferation. Repetitive cell proliferation is central to the risk of many common human cancers, and factors that increase cell proliferation in a tissue can result in malignant transformation by increasing the probability of converting DNA damage, however caused, into stable mutations.[6–10] The kinetics of normal breast epithelial proliferation have been studied using both mitotic counts and ^{3}H-thymidine labeling index and correlate breast cell proliferation rates with the menstrual cycle. In premenopausal women, breast epithelial cell proliferation is low during the follicular phase of the menstrual cycle, increasing twofold to threefold in the luteal phase.[11–15] These results suggest that the estrogen levels of the follicular phase (estradiol level approximating 50 pg/mL) induce some breast cell proliferation, and the combined effect of estrogen and progesterone together produces greater breast cell proliferation, i.e., both estrogen and progesterone are mitogens in the normal human breast epithelial cell. In the postmenopausal breast, the rate of cell proliferation is substantially less than in the premenopausal breast.[16] The very low proliferative rate of postmenopausal women undoubtedly accounts for the small relative increase in breast cancer risk seen during the postmenopausal years.

Use of combination oral contraceptives and depot medroxyprogesterone acetate

The available data show that the amount of sex steroid necessary to provide acceptable contraception appears to produce breast cell proliferation equivalent to a normal ovulatory cycle.[14,15] This is consistent with the epidemiologic studies demonstrating a small or no effect of combination oral contraceptive use on breast cancer risk.[17,18] Studies of breast cancer risk and combination oral contraceptive use before first full-term pregnancy have shown a small increase in breast cancer risk.[17,19–22] Whether the increased risk seen in young women will continue as these women age is unknown.[17,23]

The long-lasting (90-day) injectable progestogen contraceptive depot medroxyprogesterone acetate (DMPA) provides a method of contraception that is increasingly utilized throughout the world. Despite the reduction in estradiol levels that occurs in women using DMPA, epidemiological studies of the effect of DMPA on breast cancer risk have found no evidence for a reduction in breast cancer risk.[24,25] This is consistent with the proliferative effect of progestogens (MPA in this case) on breast cells and in the genesis of breast cancer.

Postmenopausal hormone replacement

Current trends in the use of replacement therapy are for its long-term use for the prevention of osteoporosis, the control of menopausal symptoms, and possibly to decrease the risk of cardiovascular disease. Based on the effects of ovarian hormones on breast cancer risk, the effect of postmenopausal replacement therapy on breast cancer risk can be predicted. The relative risks of remaining premenopausal for 5 or 10 years (versus being postmenopausal) during the perimenopausal age range are approximately 1.3 and 1.6, respectively. Given the low-dose replacement therapy currently utilized, it is unlikely that such therapy would have effects on breast cancer risk greater than that of endogenous hormones, and the effects of estrogen replacement alone would be predicted to be even less. In a previous meta-analysis of population-based studies by Pike *et al.*,[17] the use 0.625 mg of conjugated estrogens as estrogen replacement therapy was found to increase the risk of breast cancer by 2.1% per year above the baseline increase of 2.0% per year of

a normal postmenopausal woman. This increase in breast cancer risk is in agreement with the relative effective estradiol levels: the non-sex hormone-binding, globulin-bound estradiol levels of conjugated estrogen users is approximately twice that of a normal postmenopausal woman. A similar increase in breast cancer risk was found by some meta-analyses.[26]

The addition of a progestin to estrogen replacement therapy has only been practiced with any frequency in the past decade. The addition of the progestin further increases breast cancer risk.[27]

Obesity

Postmenopausal obesity increases breast cancer risk, but obesity during the premenopausal years actually reduces risk.[28] This inverse relationship can be explained in terms of the differential effects of premenopausal and postmenopausal obesity on endogenous hormone levels. Although premenopausal obesity decreases sex hormone-binding globulin and minimally increases exposure to estrogen,[29] it actually decreases breast exposure to progesterone.[30] Postmenopausally, the decrease in risk associated with premenopausal obesity is gradually eliminated and, eventually, the increased bioavailable estrogen levels associated with postmenopausal obesity produce an increased risk for breast cancer.

Exercise

Endogenous sex-steroid levels are associated with differences in physical activity (exercise). Strenuous exercise by premenarcheal girls delays the onset of the menarche. The frequency of anovulatory cycles increases with moderate exercise.[31] In premenopausal women, breast cancer risk has been shown to be inversely related to exercise.[32] In this study, an odds ratio of 0.42 was found for women who spent 3.8 h or more per week doing physical exercise activities compared to inactive women.

Age at first term pregnancy

Most epidemiological studies have identified a clear association between age at first full-term pregnancy and risk of breast cancer. Women who have a late (after the age of 30) first full-term pregnancy have a greater breast cancer risk than nulliparous women, and nulliparous women have a greater breast cancer risk than parous women.[33] How full-term pregnancy alters subsequent breast cancer risk is unknown, but it has been suggested that pregnancy alters the susceptibility of breast tissue to carcinogenic exposure,[34] or that hormone levels are decreased permanently following first pregnancy.[35] The sparse available information shows that breast cell proliferation increases during the first half of pregnancy and then decreases during the second half of pregnancy, when cell differentiation occurs.[36] This may explain why breast cancer risk is not reduced by non-term pregnancy.

Breast-feeding

Patterns of breast-feeding have undergone substantial change over time and differ considerably by region. Epidemiological studies relating breast cancer risk to breast-feeding patterns have not drawn clear conclusions. No association was found between history of breast-feeding and subsequent risk of breast cancer in a recent USA prospective study, except for woman who had given birth only once and breast-fed.[37] In studies from Asian countries, where the duration of breast-feeding is substantially greater than in the USA, protective associations between breast-feeding and breast cancer risk have been found.[38]

Race

The incidence of breast cancer in Japan is substantially lower than in the USA. In Japan, the average age at menarche is approximately 2 years greater, and postmenopausal Japanese women weigh substantially less than postmenopausal women in the USA. These two characteristics partially explain the lowered incidence in Japanese women living in Japan.[5] The low postmenopausal weight of Japanese woman will lead to low estrogen levels, and therefore to no increase in breast cancer risk postmenopausally. In premenopausal Asian women who maintain a traditional lifestyle, urinary conjugated estrogens[39] and serum estradiol levels[40–42] are substantially lower, which in all probability accounts for the remaining lowered risk of Asian women. Asian immigrants to the USA show a doubling of incidence rates within 10 years of arrival.[43]

Benign breast disease

Women with a history of prior breast biopsy for benign breast disease have an increased risk of breast cancer. This increase in risk is associated with specific epithelial abnormalities, and those without proliferative breast disease do not have an increase in risk. Atypical hyperplasia is associated with an approximately fivefold increase in breast cancer risk, and proliferative lesions without atypica are associated with a twofold increase in risk.[44,45]

Mammographic parenchymal pattern

Breast cancer risk has been shown to be associated with the parenchymal pattern seen on mammography. The majority of the breast consists of adipose and fibrous tissue. In the premenopausal breast, less than 15% of the volume of the breast consists of epithelial cells, and this decreases to less than 5% by the age of 60.[46] The relative amounts of fibrous and adipose tissue are what determine the appearance of the mammographic image, because fibrous tissue is radio-opaque and adipose tissue is radiolucent. Increased fibrous tissue equates to increased mammographic densities. Classification of mammograms into different breast cancer risk patterns, essentially based on radiographic densities, has been done by a number of investigators. Although mammographic appearance is a poor predictor of individual breast cancer risk, epidemiologic studies have consistently found that these classification schemes are associated with breast cancer risk, independent of other breast cancer risk factors, with increased densities being associated with greater risk.[47–49] An important point to note is that mammographic densities decrease, while breast cancer risk increases, with age: the association of increased densities with greater breast cancer risk is for women of the same age.

HEREDITARY BREAST CANCER

Breast cancer is a common disease that ultimately will affect 11% of American women. However, hereditary breast/ovarian cancer is relatively rare, causing only 5–10% of all breast cancers. Although sporadic breast cancer is most common in postmenopausal women, younger premenopausal women face the greatest risk of hereditary breast cancer and affected family members tend to have earlier onset of disease. Families that carry a hereditary or 'germline' mutation often present with a cluster of cases of early-onset breast cancer or breast and ovarian cancer. Fewer families with late-onset disease have been linked to germline mutations.

BRCA1 and BRCA2

Approximately 1 in 400 women in the general population carry an inherited mutation in one of the two recognized breast cancer predisposition genes: BRCA1 and BRCA2 (BRCA1/2).[50] Possibly a quarter of the cases of breast cancer in women under the age of 30 are due to inherited genetic alterations. Germline mutations in BRCA1 and BRCA2 account for about 70% of hereditary breast cancer cases. Additional genes that contribute to hereditary breast cancer are likely to be discovered in the future.[51,52] While germline mutations are implicated in familial cases, somatic mutations in BRCA1 and BRCA2 appear to be rare events in both sporadic breast and ovarian cancers.[53–57]

BRCA1

The first of these breast cancer susceptibility genes, BRCA1, was linked to chromosome 17 in early-onset breast cancer families. The gene, located at 17q21, has now been fully characterized.[58–60] Up to 45% of breast cancer and 70–90% of breast/ovarian cancer families exhibit linkage to BRCA1.[59–61] The probability that families with three or more breast or ovarian cancers are linked to BRCA1 increases with the number of ovarian cancers within the family.[62–64] Women with a germline mutation in BRCA1 face increased risks of 50–85% for breast cancer, 40–60% for a second breast cancer, and 15–45% risk for ovarian cancer by the age of 70.[65,66]

BRCA2

Further genetic analysis in breast cancer families that were not linked to the BRCA1 locus on 17q21 revealed a second breast cancer susceptibility locus, BRCA2, located on chromosome 13q12-13.[51,67] BRCA2 mutations account for up to 35–40% of familial breast cancer. Women who are BRCA2 mutation carriers face a lifetime risk of breast cancer similar to that seen in female BRCA1 mutation carriers: 50–85%. The risk for ovarian cancer is somewhat less, at 10–27%. There is also a significant risk of 6% for breast cancer in males who carry mutations in BRCA2.[65,66,68]

Molecular biology of BRCA1/2

BRCA1 is made up of 22 exons that encompass more than 100 kb.[67,69,70] The data support a tumor-suppressor mechanism for BRCA1 and the gene fits the Knudson 'two-hit hypothesis' for hereditary cancer.[71–74]

The BRCA2 coding sequence is even larger than that of BRCA1. The cloning and characterization of BRCA2 revealed 27 exons.[57,68] Like BRCA1, BRCA2 is a tumor-suppressor gene rather than a dominant oncogene.[75,76]

Other genetic predisposition syndromes

There are other familial cancer syndromes associated with an increased risk of breast cancer, but these are rare. The Li–Fraumeni syndrome is caused by germline mutations in the p53 tumor-suppressor gene TP53 on chromosome 17p13. This rare disorder is associated with a wide range of neoplasms in young adults and children, including early-onset breast cancer, lung cancer, soft-tissue sarcomas, brain tumors, rhabdomyosarcomas, leukemias, and adrenocortical cancer.[77] Although breast cancer is seen in about half of Li–Fraumeni families, it is not a necessary element in the family history. The diagnostic criteria for classical Li–Fraumeni syndrome require a bone or soft-tissue sarcoma in a proband prior to the age of 45, and two other close relatives (two first-degree relatives or a first-degree and a second-degree relative) with a related cancer also under the age of 45. When these strict criteria are met, there is a 75% chance of a mutation in TP53. However, it is significant that only 50% of families with germline mutations in TP53 will meet the strict criteria. Many families with clusters of these types of cancers do not meet these criteria. For instance, a threefold excess of breast cancer has been noted in mothers of children with bone or soft-tissue sarcomas. Such so-called Li–Fraumeni-like families demonstrate defects in TP53 in only about 10% of cases. The overall contribution of TP53 mutations to breast cancer is unknown, but probably accounts for no more than 1% of all breast cancers, although it may be higher when breast cancer occurs prior to the age of 30.

Heterozygotes for a mutation on the ataxia telangiectasia gene on chromosome 11q have an increased risk of breast cancer.[78–81] Some rare abnormalities of androgen receptors can be associated with breast cancer in men.[82] Cowden disease (multiple hamartoma syndrome) is a rare autosomal, dominant, familial cancer syndrome which is associated with an increased risk for breast cancer. The gene responsible for Cowden disease, PTEN, is on chromosome 10q22-23.[83] Other hereditary syndromes with a breast cancer predisposition include Muir–Torre syndrome (mutations in MSH2 or MLH1) and Peutz–Jeghers syndrome (STK11).[84]

Estimating the gene penetrance of BRCA1/2 mutations

The likelihood that a mutation carrier will develop the disease for which he or she is at risk is the gene penetrance. The BRCA1/2 genes have incomplete penetrance, meaning that not all individuals with a BRCA1/2 mutation will develop cancer. Gene penetrance is influenced by other genes and environmental factors. In fact, different combinations of gene–gene (G×G) and gene–environment (G×E) interactions modify the phenotypic expression of BRCA1/2 mutations differently in different individuals. Thus, there are high-penetrance families and low-penetrance families. Estimating gene penetrance in a particular family is important when counseling mutation carriers.

The original families collected by the Breast Cancer Linkage Consortium were chosen for gene mapping because of large kinships with many affected individuals, factors that favored high penetrance of a gene predisposing for breast cancer. Thus, original risk estimates generated from this biased sample gave penetrance estimates at the high end of the range. The original studies estimated the lifetime risk for breast cancer in women who carry a BRCA1 mutation at 70–80% and 40–60% for ovarian cancer.[50,62,85] Although these values overestimate breast cancer risks for the entire population of BRCA1/2 mutation carriers, they may still be useful when counseling a large breast/ovarian cancer family with many affected relatives.

Other data from subsequent population-based studies give lower risk estimates. In 121 Ashkenazi Jewish BRCA1/2 mutation carriers, the penetrance was 56% for breast cancer by the age of 70 and 16% for ovarian cancer.[86] In an Australian study, BRCA1/2 mutations were sought in a population of relatives of 388 women with breast cancer under the age of 40. The risk to mutation carriers for breast cancer was estimated to be about 40% to the age of 70, or about half the original estimates of 70–80%.[87] As gene penetrance estimates are revised downward, patients without a strong family history become candidates for gene testing. In the Australian study, family history was not a strong predictor of mutation status: only 5 of 18 mutation carriers had at least one affected relative. This illustrates the need to consider *BRCA1/2* mutations in the absence of a striking family history.

Factors that influence gene penetrance

Pregnancy and hormone use may affect breast cancer risk in *BRCA1/2* mutation carriers. Although pregnancy, especially pregnancy at an early age, is associated with a decreased risk of breast cancer in the general population, an early first pregnancy does not confer protection for carriers of *BRCA1/2* mutations.[88] This matched, case-control study of 236 pairs (189 *BRCA1* case-control pairs and 47 *BRCA2* case-control pairs) demonstrated that women with *BRCA1/2* mutations who had full-term pregnancies were significantly more likely than nulliparous carriers to develop breast cancer by the age of 40. Each birth, up to three, further increased the risk. This suggests that *BRCA1/2* mutations interfere with the normal maturation and differentiation of pluripotent, undifferentiated breast epithelial cells in late pregnancy. Poor milk production has also been reported in carriers of *BRCA1* mutations, possibly reflecting abnormal breast epithelial differentiation.[89]

Oral contraceptive use and its relationship to breast and ovarian cancer has been studied in carriers of *BRCA1/2* mutations. In a group of 207 women with hereditary ovarian cancer and 161 of their sisters as controls, any past oral contraceptive use was associated with a decreased risk (adjusted odds ratio 0.5) of ovarian cancer.[90] This trend became stronger with increasing duration of use, with a 60% reduction in risk when oral contraceptives were used for 6 or more years.

The limited data available on breast cancer and oral contraceptive use from one small study noted an increased risk in *BRCA1/2* mutation carriers. In this small, population-based sample of 50 young Ashkenazi women with breast cancer, 14 had *BRCA1/2* mutations. The long-term use of oral contraceptives before first full-term pregnancy correlated with an increased risk of being a *BRCA1/2* mutation carrier in this group.[91] This association needs further study before any conclusions can be drawn.

Clinical characteristics of the hereditary breast cancers

Clinically, inherited forms of breast cancer differ little from sporadic breast cancer, except for earlier age at diagnosis, bilaterality, and occurrence in males.[58,60,92]

Table 10.1 *Frequency of* BRCA1 *mutations by average age at diagnosis of familial breast cancer*

Average age at diagnosis (years)	Number of families	Number of mutations	Percentage of total families
<35	5	1	3.7
35–39	27	7	25.9
40–44	32	5	18.5
45–49	24	5	18.5
50–54	34	4	14.8
55–59	24	1	3.7
>59	23	4	14.8
Total	169	27	99.9

Adapted from Couch *et al.* (1997).[95]
These data illustrate the trend for a decreased likelihood of *BRCA1* mutation with increasing average age at diagnosis. However, it is noteworthy that, in this sample, 9 of 27 mutations were found in families with an average age of onset of 50 years or above.

The proportion of breast cancer cases that are attributable to mutations in *BRCA1/2* decreases markedly with age. For women whose breast cancer is diagnosed at the age of 20–29, up to 33% of cases may be due to a genetic predisposition, compared with 2% in women diagnosed at the age of 70–79. The age of onset of ovarian cancer associated with *BRCA1* is about 10 years younger than that of sporadic cases.[93] The median ages of onset of breast cancer and ovarian cancer in one large familial cluster kindred studied were 48 and 53 years, respectively.[94] The relationship between average age at diagnosis in breast cancer families and *BRCA1/2* mutation status[95] is summarized in Table 10.1.

Although male breast cancer is rare, it is significantly increased in families linked to *BRCA2* mutations.[51,76,96,97] *BRCA2* may account for 14% of all male breast cancer cases.[96]

The pathology of breast cancer cases related to *BRCA1* appears to have increased S-phase and mitotic rates (growth rates), but tends to be associated with better survival and recurrence rates.[98,99] Tubular-lobular histology may be more common in *BRCA2*-linked individuals than in sporadic tumors.[99]

Specific histologic types of ovarian cancer may also correlate with hereditary predisposition. Mucinous carcinomas of the ovary appear to be less common and serous tumors more common in familial ovarian cancer than in sporadic cases.[93,100,101] Patients with ovarian cancer and *BRCA1* mutations appear to have significantly longer overall survival compared with matched controls.[93]

Other tumors associated with *BRCA1* and *BRCA2*

Prostate cancer has been linked to *BRCA1/2* mutations.[102] Men with a *BRCA1* mutation have three times the risk of prostate cancer of non-carriers.[102,103] Men and women with a *BRCA1* mutation have four times the risk of developing colon cancer. *BRCA2* also appears to be associated with an increased risk of ocular melanoma, pancreatic, and other malignancies. Based on data from the Breast Cancer Linkage Consortium, a cohort of 3728 individuals with *BRCA2* mutations and their close relatives revealed significant increases in risk for prostate cancer (relative risk [RR] = 4.65), pancreatic cancer (RR = 3.51), gallbladder and bile duct cancer (RR = 4.97), stomach cancer (RR = 2.59), and malignant melanoma (RR = 2.58). The RR for prostate cancer in men under the age of 65 is 7.33. For women who had already developed breast cancer, the cumulative risk of a second contralateral breast cancer by the age of 70 was 52.3% and for ovarian cancer was 15.9%.[104]

Risk assessment for hereditary breast/ovarian cancer

As outlined in this chapter, two major genes responsible for hereditary breast/ovarian cancer are *BRCA1* and *BRCA2*. When mutated, these genes confer an increased risk of breast and ovarian cancer in women, and with *BRCA2* gene mutations there is also an increased risk for male breast cancer. Although a family history of breast/ovarian cancer is often seen, there is no specific guideline that can reliably predict which family may harbor a germline mutation. Pedigrees with multiple early-onset breast cancers, bilateral breast cancer, ovarian cancers, breast and ovarian cancer in the same individual, or male breast cancers suggest an increased likelihood that the family carries a genetic mutation. However, some women with *BRCA1/2*-related cancers do not have a striking family history of early-onset breast cancer. Because particular *BRCA1/2* mutations are more common in Ashkenazi Jews, patients should be asked about the ethnic and religious background in their families (see below).

Taking a family history for breast/ovarian cancer

Autosomal dominant genes are responsible for the majority of familial malignancy syndromes. Importantly, the term autosomal indicates that these genes, which are *not* located on the sex chromosomes, are just as likely to be inherited from the maternal as from the paternal side of the family. A complete family history for cancer includes information (age of onset, laterality, pathology) on both sides of the family for at least three generations. This can be accomplished quickly with a cancer family history questionnaire completed by the patient (Figure 10.1). This is less time consuming than constructing a pedigree (Figure 10.2) and yet provides a written record of the family members with cancer and their ages of onset. However, a pedigree can convey complex relationships clearly and provides a concise graphic representation of a cancer family history.

Interpreting the family history

The possibility of hereditary breast/ovarian cancer deserves serious consideration when:

- Two or more relatives on the same side of the family have early-onset (premenopausal) breast cancer.
- Ovarian cancer occurs in a family with two or more breast cancers at any age.
- One family member has both breast and ovarian cancer.
- Breast cancer occurs in a male.

The familial nature of hereditary breast/ovarian cancer is more likely to be appreciated when a first-degree relative[1] is affected, especially when the patient's mother has breast cancer. A paternal family history of hereditary breast/ovarian cancer may become cryptic when there are no affected first-degree or second-degree relatives. For instance, in Figure 10.2, the proband's daughter has no sisters and her closest affected female relatives are her first cousins. A family history of two or more paternal first cousins with early-onset breast cancer should not be dismissed because the relationships are too distant to be significant. When the pattern of autosomal dominant inheritance is obvious, the degree of relationship between the proband and her affected relatives is less important (Figure 10.2).

Ashkenazi Jewish heritage

When a breast/ovarian cancer family is of Ashkenazi Jewish descent, there is an even greater concern as Jewish women face a higher risk of hereditary breast and ovarian cancers.[105,106] Approximately 1 in 40 Ashkenazi individuals carry one of three founder mutations in the *BRCA1/2* genes. This compares with a general population frequency of *BRCA1/2* mutations of fewer than 1/400.

The three founder mutations, 185delAG and 5382insC in *BRCA1*[85] and 6174delT in *BRCA2*,[107] are found in up to 30% of Ashkenazi Jewish women with breast cancer under the age of 40.[108,109] Because these three mutations are so common in Jews, they should always be measured together. A negative test for any one of these mutations could be falsely reassuring, because the patient could have inherited one of the other common founder mutations.

[1]First-degree relatives: parents, siblings, and offspring, share 50% of the proband's genes. Second-degree relatives: half-siblings, aunts, uncles, nieces, nephews, grandparents, and grandchildren, share 25% of the proband's genes. Third-degree relatives: cousins, great aunts/uncles, greatgrandparents, share about 12% of the proband's genes.

FAMILY CANCER HISTORY

Some cancers can run in families. Information about all the cancer cases in your family can help us explore your potential risk to develop certain types of cancer. Please answer the following questions.

Please check boxes that best describe YOU: ☐ Male ☐ Female
☐ African-American ☐ Asian/Pacific Islander ☐ Ashkenazi (Eastern European) Jewish
☐ Latino/Hispanic ☐ European descent ☐ Native American ☐ Other:_____

Are you interested in discussing your family history of cancer with a genetic counselor? ☐ **YES** ☐ **NO**

For **EACH PERSON** who had cancer in your family (**YOU** and your **BLOOD relatives ONLY**) please write the **AGE** when the cancer was found under the appropriate **CANCER TYPE** column (the place where the cancer started).

CANCER TYPE → AGE OF ONSET →	BREAST Age?	OVARIAN Age?	PROSTATE Age?	COLON Age?	OTHER CANCER TYPE and Age
YOU					
Your SPOUSE					
Your MOTHER			N/A		
Your FATHER		N/A			
Your SISTERS			N/A		
			N/A		
			N/A		
Your BROTHERS		N/A			
		N/A			
		N/A			
Your DAUGHTERS			N/A		
			N/A		
			N/A		
Your SONS		N/A			
		N/A			
		N/A			
Your MOTHER'S SIDE OF THE FAMILY					
GRANDMOTHER			N/A		
GRANDFATHER		N/A			
Your AUNTS			N/A		
			N/A		
			N/A		
Your UNCLES		N/A			
		N/A			
		N/A			
Your COUSINS					
Your FATHER'S SIDE OF THE FAMILY					
GRANDMOTHER			N/A		
GRANDFATHER		N/A			
Your AUNTS			N/A		
			N/A		
			N/A		
Your UNCLES		N/A			
		N/A			
		N/A			
Your COUSINS					

Figure 10.1 *A cancer family history questionnaire. This is an example of a patient questionnaire that provides key information about the cancer history in the patient's first-degree, second-degree, and third-degree relatives.*

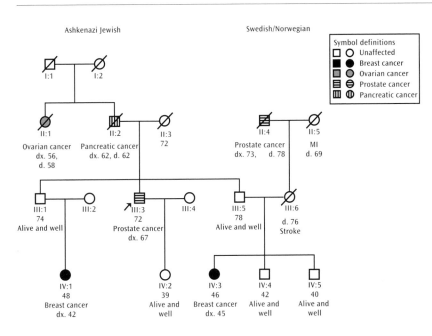

Figure 10.2 *A pedigree showing hereditary breast ovarian cancer. This pedigree illustrates a positive family history of breast/ovarian cancer in two first cousins and their paternal great aunt. Although the relationships are more distant, the pattern is consistent with autosomal dominant transmission in the paternal lineage. Using the BRCAPro risk model, the proband (arrow) has an estimated risk of 44% for a mutation in BRCA1/2, and his unaffected daughter has a risk estimate of 22%. If this family were not Ashkenazi Jewish, the risk estimate for the proband would be substantially less, at about 10%.*

The significant contribution of Ashkenazi Jewish heritage to the risk is illustrated in Figure 10.3, where a variety of family history scenarios are compared between a proband who is Ashkenazi Jewish and one who is not.[110] For this reason, information should be sought from every breast and/or ovarian cancer patient or at-risk relative about Jewish background in any of her four grandparents.

MODELS THAT ESTIMATE BREAST CANCER RISK

Various models attempt to estimate an individual's risk for invasive breast cancer by integrating relevant risk factors (Table 10.2). The two most widely known breast cancer risk-assessment methods are the Gail model and the Claus model.[84,111] They are widely used for women at low risk for hereditary breast cancer. The Couch model and the Parmigiani–Berry model estimate the likelihood of carrying a deleterious mutation of *BRCA1* and *BRCA1/2*, respectively. These two models incorporate more specific family history and ethnic information relevant to risk assessment in hereditary breast/ovarian cancer. Information about predisposing conditions such as lobular carcinoma *in situ* (LCIS), ductal carcinoma *in situ* (DCIS), or atypical hyperplasia is not included in these four models.

Gail model

The Gail model uses data from the Breast Cancer Detection Demonstration Project (BCDDP) to calculate the risk for breast cancer.[112] This model considers age, age at menarche, age at first live birth, number of previous breast biopsies, and number of first-degree relatives with breast cancer in risk analysis. It does not address early-onset breast cancer in relatives or other familial cancer characteristics. The Gail model is useful in the assessment of breast cancer risk in those at low risk for hereditary breast/ovarian cancer.[84]

Claus model

Claus attempts to quantify risk in individuals with a family history of breast cancer.[113] Using data from the Cancer and Steroid Hormone (CASH) data set, this model is based on the premise that an autosomal dominant gene produces a lifetime risk of 80% and that the lifetime risk of sporadic breast cancer alone is 6%.[113,114] This model incorporates the age of affected family members at diagnosis, the number of affected relatives, and the degree of relationship (first or second). However, the Claus model does not incorporate ovarian cancer, bilateral breast cancer, or male breast cancer cases within the family into the calculated risk. Breast/ovarian cancer in third-degree relatives also appears to increase the relative risk (1.35), as do cases of colon cancer; however, they are not included in the Gail model.[115]

Couch model

Based on empiric data collected from 263 women with breast cancer who attended clinics that evaluate the risk of breast cancer, Couch *et al.*[95] developed a model for estimating *BRCA1* mutation risk. The median age at diagnosis was 41 years in families with *BRCA1* mutations

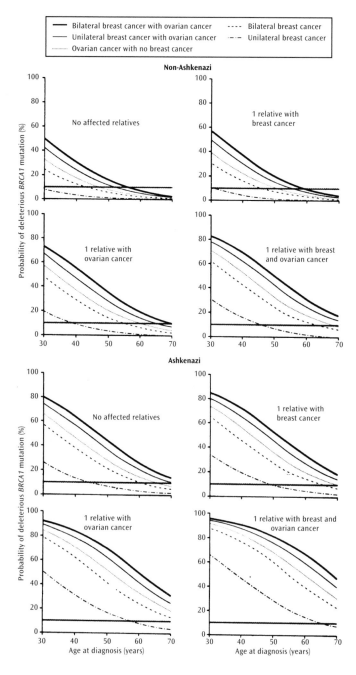

Figure 10.3 *Ashkenazi Jewish heritage and BRCA1 mutation estimates. These graphs, adapted from Shattuck-Eidens et al.,[110] illustrate the impact that an Ashkenazi Jewish background has on the probability of encountering a deleterious mutation in BRCA1 given a particular personal and family history of breast/ovarian cancer. Even without any family history of breast or ovarian cancer, a 40-year-old Jewish woman with breast cancer has a greater than 10% probability of a BRCA1 mutation.*

and 50.7 years in families without *BRCA1* mutations. *BRCA1* mutations were found in 7% of breast cancer families without ovarian cancer, in 18% of families with bilateral breast cancer, in 40% of families with both breast and ovarian cancer, and in 67% of families with breast and ovarian cancer in the same individual. This model incorporates the average age of onset of breast cancer in a family, the presence of ovarian cancer, of breast and ovarian cancer in the same individual, and Ashkenazi Jewish ancestry. The authors concluded that the number of breast cancers in a family, the average age of onset of ovarian cancer, and the presence of bilateral disease were not independent predictors of *BRCA1* mutation status.

Parmigiani–Berry model

The Parmigiani–Berry model[116] incorporates pertinent cancer family history for all first-degree and second-degree relatives in a family, including the ages of affected and unaffected relatives. Bilateral breast cancer, males with breast cancer, women with both breast and ovarian cancer, other cancers, Ashkenazi Jewish background, and results of *BRCA* mutation testing are considered in the model. This model does not take into account the cancer history in more distant third-degree or fourth-degree relatives, which will underestimate the number of families with significant histories in the paternal lineage. The chance of mutations in other breast cancer susceptibility genes

Table 10.2 *Breast cancer risk-assessment models*

Model	Estimates risk of	Includes family history of breast cancer	Includes family history of bilateral breast cancer	Includes family history of ovarian cancer	Includes Ashkenazi Jewish heritage
Gail	Breast cancer	Number of affected first-degree relatives	No	No	No
Claus	Breast cancer	Number and age of affected first-degree and second-degree relatives	No	Yes	No
Couch	BRCA1 carrier status	Average age at diagnosis in affected relatives	No	Yes	Yes
Parmigiani–Berry (BRCAPro)	BRCA1/2 carrier status	Affected and unaffected first-degree and second-degree relatives	Yes	Yes	Yes

The Gail and Claus models are used to estimate breast cancer risk in women at low risk for hereditary breast/ovarian cancer. The Couch model estimates the probability of a *BRCA1* mutation in an at-risk family. The Parmigiani–Berry model is the most comprehensive risk model for estimating the probability of a *BRCA1/2* mutation in breast/ovarian cancer families.

(Li–Fraumeni, Cowden syndromes) and spontaneous mutations in *BRCA1/2* are not incorporated into the model. Finally, it does not account for other environmental or genetic factors that could influence the penetrance of *BRCA1/2*, such as pregnancy or oral contraceptive use. Even with these limitations, this model provides a clinically useful estimate of the likelihood of a *BRCA1/2* mutation in a given family. It is available as BRCAPro in a CD-ROM format from the authors.

GENETIC COUNSELING AND TESTING FOR BREAST/OVARIAN CANCER PREDISPOSITION

Predictive genetic testing with DNA sequencing analysis is available for *BRCA1* and *BRCA2*. When there is a significant pattern of breast/ovarian cancer in a family or when there is a risk estimate of 10% or more for a *BRCA1/2* mutation, genetic counseling should be offered to the patient. The patient must be thoroughly informed about the issues in order to give an informed consent prior to DNA testing. The issues surrounding genetic testing are complex and are best communicated in a formal genetic counseling session with an experienced cancer genetic counselor.[117] Cancer genetic counseling includes many components, which are summarized in Table 10.3. A cancer genetic services directory is available online at the National Cancer Institute's web site: http://cnetdb.nci.nih.gov/genesrch.shtml

An accurate, complete, and up-to-date pedigree is essential for appropriate cancer genetic counseling. The medical history of family members, especially from generations past, may not always be reliably recollected.[111]

It is often advisable to confirm the reported cases of malignancy within a family by obtaining pathology reports. A benign breast biopsy in a relative can be mistakenly recalled as a malignancy; what was explained to relatives as 'stomach cancer' in a grandmother may in fact have been ovarian cancer. Such misinformation can cause erroneous diagnosis, inaccurate risk assessment, and inappropriate testing and medical/surgical intervention.

Psychosocial aspects

Genetic testing can produce unexpected psychological consequences, even when results are normal. Ongoing support may be needed after receiving both abnormal and normal genetic test results. An organization of individuals at risk for hereditary breast/ovarian cancer, Facing Our Risk of Cancer Empowered (FORCE), maintains an on-line support group at www.facingourrisk.org

An abnormal genetic test result can bring with it a profound sense of loss, hopelessness, and anxiety. Depression, fear, guilt, and anger may develop.[118,119] This response can be anticipated by using psychological screening measures during the genetic counseling process to identify patients at risk for depression, anxiety, and lack of support. In these individuals, genetic testing can either be postponed or coordinated with mental health professionals who can provide psychological support. Even well-adjusted individuals may experience so-called *survivor guilt* when they have a normal test result and other family members have an abnormal test result or develop cancer. When parents feels guilty about the possibility of transmitting a mutation to their children, they can pressure the clinician to test or treat a minor child (see below).

Table 10.3 *Components of cancer genetic counseling*

1. A cancer risk assessment based on the personal and family history of cancer
2. Recommendation of appropriate genetic tests based on the likelihood of cancer susceptibility syndromes
3. Discussion of limits of DNA testing, including abnormal and uninterpretable results, false-positive and false-negative rates
4. Discussion of the possibility that family relationships may be altered by genetic testing (e.g., the discovery of non-paternity)
5. Review of the likelihood of developing cancer based on an abnormal result (gene penetrance)
6. Review of options for and effectiveness of cancer surveillance protocols and how genetic test results would affect those options
7. Review of efficacy of chemoprevention, prophylactic surgery, and other risk-reduction strategies and how genetic test results would affect those options
8. Discussion of the psychosocial impact of normal and abnormal results on the patient and family members
9. Review of confidentiality of the test results and implications for insurance and employment

Because of the complexity of the cancer genetic counseling process, patients should be referred to a certified genetic counselor with specific expertise in oncology.

Genetic testing for *BRCA1/2*

Hundreds of deleterious mutations have been identified in *BRCA1/2*, making gene sequencing the preferred method of testing. However, this technique may miss mutations outside the coding sequence as well as inversions and very large deletions that require other techniques (Southern blots, RT-PCR) for detection.[120] The interpretation of results can be complicated by the identification of genetic variants of unknown significance, some of which may represent benign polymorphisms. In these situations, further testing of other family members is indicated to determine that the mutation tracks with the cancer in affected individuals. For these reasons, clinicians who thoroughly understand the limits and best uses of available technology and are able to interpret the sometimes complex results of gene sequencing are best equipped to order *BRCA1/2* mutation analysis.

Genetic testing should begin with a family member who has had cancer. This establishes that a specific genetic mutation is associated with cancer in a given family. After the association between the gene mutation and cancer has been established, the results of genetic testing can be used to assess cancer risks in unaffected family members. When a mutation associated with cancer runs in the family, either a positive test or a negative test result provides clinically useful information for at-risk relatives. However, when DNA testing is initiated in a family member who has never had cancer, the association between a gene mutation and cancer cannot be established. In this situation, a negative test result cannot be used to reduce risk.

Legal, ethical, and social issues

Genetic predisposition testing for malignant conditions raises a number of complex ethical, psychological, social,

legal, financial, and health insurance issues. These issues deserve due consideration and are reviewed as part of the genetic counseling process. Several important points need to be stressed.

1 Predisposition testing for adult-onset disease is not recommended in childhood. At this time, there is no effective preventative strategy that warrants genetic diagnostic testing for hereditary breast/ovarian cancer prior to the age of majority. Children and even some young adults may not be able to withstand the psychological impact of a positive test. There is a real risk of harm from inappropriate or premature medical or surgical intervention.

2 Prenatal diagnosis for hereditary breast/ovarian cancer is discouraged, for several reasons. First, all fetuses have some inherited risk factors that will contribute to their risk of adult-onset diseases such as cancer, stroke, and heart disease. It is virtually impossible to conceive a risk-free fetus. Second, we cannot properly assess the real risks faced by the adult this fetus will become, given that their adulthood will be spent in a more sophisticated medical future.

3 The genetic discrimination remains a concern, but it may be diminishing as there are few, if any, reports of documented cases of insurance or employment discrimination based on genetic predisposition testing in general or specifically for cancer susceptibility syndromes.[119,121,122] It is still important that patients are fully informed of the potential for discriminatory policies.

INTERVENTION

Women at increased risk for breast cancer or ovarian cancer look to physicians for recommendations. The options available for these patients are intensified surveillance, prophylactic surgeries, chemoprevention, and participation in clinical trials. Standards of care for these recommendations do not exist, and the efficacy currently has limited data. Whenever possible, patients should be placed on research protocols so that the statistical representation of the characteristics of these conditions will be more meaningful.

Surveillance

Recommendations for the surveillance of high-risk women with genetic predisposition vary among institutions. It is unknown whether increased surveillance will detect premalignant lesions and reduce mortality in high-risk women.[123] Recommended surveillance schedules generally include monthly breast self-exams. Mammograms are recommended at 6-month intervals by some and at yearly intervals by others in high-risk women, and physician breast examinations are often recommended biannually.[84,124] The increased exposure to radiation is an unknown variable, particularly with genetic factors involved; however, this has not been a strong argument against screening mammography.[119] The age at which to begin mammographic testing is also a debated issue in this population, in part due to the increased breast density in younger women, which makes radiologic interpretation more difficult. Generally, beginning mammograms at least 5–10 years before the youngest breast cancer in the family is reasonable, because there is some indication that breast cancer may occur at earlier ages in successive generations.[111,124]

Screening for ovarian cancer is not done routinely in populations without a family history. Although no standards exist for high-risk women, guidelines have been set by institutions in an effort to detect disease earlier.[111,124] Transvaginal ultrasounds and bimanual examination every 6 months are a common recommendation. The tumor marker CA125 may or may not be recommended with the ultrasound, or it may be recommended in postmenopausal women only.

Chemoprevention

Although there has been substantial interest in chemoprevention strategies for more than a decade, data concerning preventive approaches have only recently begun to mature. The most significant single study in this regard is the National Surgical Adjuvant Breast and Bowel Project (NSABP) P1 trial of tamoxifen as a chemopreventive agent for women at increased risk for breast cancer.[125] This study was designed to determine if the use of tamoxifen by these women would be beneficial, based on the substantial evidence that adjuvant tamoxifen reduced the incidence of contralateral primary malignancy. The P1 trial included more than 13 000 women

who were at increased breast cancer risk because they were: aged 60 years or more; had a history of lobular carcinoma *in situ*; or had a 5-year risk predicted by the Gail model to be at least 1.66% and were aged 35–59. Participants were randomized to receive either tamoxifen 20 mg per day or a placebo for 5 years. Tamoxifen reduced the risk of invasive breast cancer by 49% and of non-invasive breast cancer by 50%.[125] In women at increased risk based on a prior history of lobular carcinoma *in situ*, tamoxifen reduced the risk by 56%. In women with atypical hyperplasia on a prior biopsy, tamoxifen reduced the risk by 86%. The reduction in risk occurred in all age groups, including those in the premenopausal ranges, and in those with first-degree relatives with breast cancer. Tamoxifen reduced the risk for estrogen-receptor-positive tumors, but had no effect on the risk of estrogen-receptor-negative tumors; whether a decrease in the risk of such tumors will be seen with long-term follow-up is unknown. Since the presentation and publication of the P1 study, two additional trials testing the role of tamoxifen in breast cancer have been published, both showing no reduction in risk with tamoxifen.[126,127] The reasons for the differences are unknown, but may relate to differences in the populations included in the studies, such as relatively low-risk women in the Italian trial and a more extensive family history in the UK study. These differences do not substantially detract from the important results of the P1 study. In addition, the P1 study provides important information concerning the side-effects and safety of tamoxifen use by women at increased risk for breast cancer. The side-effect profile of tamoxifen has been well established. As expected, tamoxifen was found to reduce the risk of hip, radius, and spine fractures. An increase in the risk of endometrial cancer (risk ratio 2.53) was seen, predominantly in women over 50 years of age. The risk of thromboembolic phenomena, including stroke, pulmonary embolism, and deep-vein thrombosis, was greater in women receiving tamoxifen.[125] Given the effects of tamoxifen, both positive and negative, weighing the risks and benefits of tamoxifen use by an individual woman is complex. To assist in this regard, tables and aids have been developed to identify classes of women for whom the benefits of tamoxifen outweigh the risks.[128]

In addition to tamoxifen, interest in other selective estrogen receptor modulators (SERMs) as potential breast cancer preventive agents has arisen. The most fully developed of the new SERMs is raloxifene. The recent Multiple Outcomes of Raloxifene Evaluation (MORE) trial demonstrated a substantial reduction in breast cancer in women randomized to receive raloxifene primarily for osteoporosis.[129] These provocative results and the potential for raloxifene to have less effect on the uterus (and less risk of endometrial cancer) have led to the Study of Tamoxifen and Raloxifene (STAR) trial to determine the relative benefits of tamoxifen and raloxifene in women at increased risk for breast cancer.

Prophylactic surgery

Although prophylactic mastectomy has been considered an appropriate option for some women at increased risk for breast cancer, data concerning the efficacy of such surgery in the prevention of breast cancer have been lacking. Recently, however, Hartmann et al.[130] have provided important data from a retrospective study of women with a family history of breast cancer who underwent bilateral prophylactic mastectomy at the Mayo Clinic, Rochester, Minnesota. With a median follow-up of 14 years following prophylactic mastectomy at a mean age of 42 years, a 89.5% reduction in risk was seen (using the Gail model to estimate risk). The acceptance of prophylatic mastectomy by both patients and physicians is highly variable.

Prophylactic oophorectomy has been recommended in women at increased risk for ovarian cancer on the basis of family history and, more recently, on the basis of genetic testing. Among cancer-free women with *BRCA1* mutations, prophylactic oophorectomy carried out for the prevention of ovarian cancer may decrease the incidence of breast cancer.[131] The risk reduction was greatest in women who were followed for more than 5 years after the procedure. The observation of this risk reduction is of enormous importance, in terms of both the potential for benefit to individual patients and of our understanding of the hormonal dependence of the disease process of breast cancer in *BRCA1* carriers. Thus, although breast cancers arising in *BRCA1* carriers have a lower frequency of estrogen-receptor positivity, the genesis of breast cancer in such individuals would appear to be a hormone-dependent event.

Clinical trials

In addition to the STAR trial of tamoxifen and raloxifene discussed above, there are other SERMs under development for breast cancer prevention. Retinoids are another class of compounds in clinical trials for cancer prevention. The retinamide fenretinide has undergone testing in a phase III trial to prevent contralateral breast cancer.[132] Although there was no overall benefit found in this study, subset analysis suggested reduced breast cancer rates in premenopausal women and an opposite effect in postmenopausal women. Previously, we evaluated the potential for an approach utilizing a potent agonist of gonadotropin-releasing hormone (GnRHA) plus low-dose add-back hormone replacement in women at increased breast cancer risk (primarily on the basis of family history). In that study, the regimen was found to be well tolerated,[133] and a substantial reduction in mammographic density was identified.[134] Currently, a similar regimen is undergoing further evaluation in high-risk women. GnRHA has also been demonstrated to reduce contralateral breast cancer risk in the adjuvant setting,[135] and additional studies of the potential role of GnRHA are underway or under discussion.

REFERENCES

1. Peto R. Epidemiology, multistage models, and short-term mutagenicity tests. In Hiatt HH, Watson JD, Winsten JE, eds. *Origins of human cancer: Book C, human risk assessment.* Cold Spring Harbor, NY, Cold Spring Harbor Laboratory; 1977, 1403–28.
2. Lilienfeld A. The relationship of cancer of the female breast to artificial menopause and marital status. Cancer 1956; 9:927–34.
3. Kelsey J. A review of the epidemiology of human breast cancer. Epidemiol Rev 1979; 1:74–109.
4. Trichopoulos D, MacMahon B, Cole P. Menopause and breast cancer risk. J Natl Cancer Inst 1972; 48:605–13.
5. Pike M, Krailo M, Henderson B, Casagrande J, Hoel D. 'Hormonal' risk factors, 'breast tissue age' and the age-incidence of breast cancer. Nature 1983; 303:767–70.
6. Henderson B, Ross RK, Pike M, Casagrande J. Endogenous hormones as a major factor in human cancer. Cancer Res 1982; 42:3232–9.
7. Ames BN, Gold LS. Too many rodent carcinogens: mitogenesis increases mutagenesis. Science 1990; 249:970–1.
8. Cohen SM, Ellwein L. Cell proliferation in carcinogenesis. Science 1990; 249:1007–11.
9. Preston-Martin S, Pike MC, Ross RK, Jones PA, Henderson BE. Increased cell division as a cause of human cancer. Cancer Res 1990; 50:7415–21.
10. Butterworth B, Slaga T. Chemically induced cell proliferation: implications for risk assessment. New York, Wiley-Liss, 1991.
11. Meyer JS. Cell proliferation in normal human breast ducts, fibroadenomas, and other duct hyperplasias, measured by nuclear labeling with tritiated thymidine. Hum Pathol 1977; 8:67–81.
12. Anderson TJ, Ferguson DJP, Raab GM. Cell turnover in the 'resting' human breast: influence of parity, contraceptive pill, age and laterality. Br J Cancer 1982; 46:376–82.
13. Longacre TA, Bartow SA. A correlative morphologic study of human breast and endometrium in the menstrual cycle. Am J Surg Pathol 1986; 10:382–93.
14. Anderson TJ, Battersby S, King RJB, McPherson K, Going JJ. Oral contraceptive use influences resting breast proliferation. Hum Pathol 1989; 20: 1139–44.
15. Williams G, Anderson E, Howell A. Oral contraceptive (OCP) use increases proliferation and decreases oestrogen receptor content of epithelial cells in the

normal human breast. Int J Cancer 1991; 48:206–10.

16. Meyer JS, Connor RE. Cell proliferation in fibro-cystic disease and postmenopausal breast ducts measured by thymidine labeling. Cancer 1982; 50:746–51.

17. Pike MC, Bernstein L, Spicer DV. Exogenous hormones and breast cancer risk. In Niederhuber JE, ed. *Current therapy in oncology*. BD Decker. St Louis, MI, Mosby Year Book, 1993, 292–303.

18. Pike MC, Spicer DV. Oral contraceptives and cancer. In Shoupe D, Haseltine F, eds. *Contraception*. New York, Springer-Verlag, 1993, 67–84.

19. Meirik O, Lund E, Adami H. Oral contraceptive use and breast cancer in young women. Lancet 1986; 2:650–3.

20. Stadel B, Schlesselman J, Murray P. Oral contraceptives and breast cancer. Lancet 1989; 1:1257–8.

21. UK National Case-Control Study Group. Oral contraceptive use and breast cancer risk in young women. Lancet 1989; 1:973–82.

22. Bernstein L, Pike M, Krailo M, Henderson B. Update of the Los Angeles Study of Oral Contraceptives and Breast Cancer: 1981 and 1983. In Mann R, ed. *Oral contraceptives and breast cancer*. Park Ridge, NJ, Parthenon Publishing Group, 1990, 169.

23. Vessey MP. The Jephcott Lecture, 1989. An overview of the benefits and risks of combined oral contraceptives. In Mann RD, ed. *Oral contraceptives and breast cancer*. Park Ridge, NJ, Parthenon Publishing Group, 1990, 121–32.

24. Lee NC, Rosero-Bixby L, Oberle MW, Grimaldo C, Whately AS, Rovira EZ. A case-control study of breast cancer and hormonal contraception in Costa Rica. J Natl Cancer Inst 1987; 79:1247–54.

25. Paul C, Skegg DCG, Spears GFS. Depot medroxyprogesterone (Depo-Provera) and risk of breast cancer. Br Med J 1989; 299:759–62.

26. Steinberg K, Thacker S, Smith S, Stroup D, Zack M, Flanders W. A meta-analysis of the effect of estrogen replacement therapy on the risk of breast cancer. JAMA 1991; 265:1985–90.

27. Ross RK, Paganini-Hill A, Wan PC, Pike MC. Effect of hormone replacement therapy on breast cancer risk: estrogen versus estrogen plus progestin. J Natl Cancer Inst 2000; 92(4):328–32.

28. Hunter DJ, Willett WC. Diet, body size, and breast cancer. Epidemiol Rev 1993; 15:110–32.

29. Zumoff B. Relationship of obesity to blood estrogens. Cancer Res 1982; 42:3289–94s.

30. Shoupe D. Effect of body weight on reproductive function. In Mishell DR Jr, Davajan V, Lobo RA, eds. *Infertility, contraception and reproductive endocrinology*. Boston, Blackwell Scientific Publications, 1991, 288–316.

31. Bernstein L, Ross RK, Lobo R, Hanisch R, Krailo M, Henderson BE. The effects of moderate physical activity on menstrual cycle patterns in adolescence: implications for breast cancer prevention. Br J Cancer 1987; 55:681–5.

32. Berstein L, Henderson BE, Hanisch R, Sullivan-Halley J, Ross RK. Physical exercise and reduced risk of breast cancer in young women. J Natl Cancer Inst 1994; 86:1403–8.

33. Kelsey JL, Gammon MD, John EM. Reproductive factors and breast cancer. Epidemiol Rev 1993; 15:36–47.

34. Russo J, Tay L, Russo I. Differentiation of the mammary gland and susceptibility to carcinogenesis. Breast Cancer Res Treat 1982; 2:5–73.

35. Bernstein L, Pike MC, Ross R, *et al*. Estrogen and sex hormone-binding globulin levels in nulliparous and parous women. J Natl Cancer Inst 1985; 74:741–5.

36. Battersby A, Anderson TJ. Proliferative and secretory activity in the pregnant and lactating human breast. Virchows Archiv A Pathol Anat 1988; 413:189–96.

37. Michels KB, Willett WC, Rosner A, *et al*. Prospective and secretory activity in the pregnant and lactating human breast. Virchows Archiv A Pathol Anat 1996; 413:189–96.

38. Tao S, Yu M, Ross M, Ziu K. Risk factors for breast cancer in Chinese women in Beijing. Int J Cancer 1988; 42:459–598.

39. MacMahon B, Cole P, Brown JB, *et al*. Urine estrogen profiles of Asian and North American women. Int J Cancer 1974; 14:161–7.

40. Goldin BR, Adlercreutz H, Gorbach SL, *et al*. The relationship between estrogen levels and diets of Caucasian American and Oriental immigrant women. Am J Clin Nutr 1986; 44:945–53.

41. Bernstein L, Yuan J-M, Ross RK, *et al*. Serum hormone levels in premenopausal Chinese women in Shanghai and white women in Los Angeles: results from two breast cancer case-control studies. Cancer Causes Control 1990; 1:51–8.

42. Key TJA, Chen J, Wang DY, Pike MC, Boreham J. Sex hormones in women in rural China and in Britain. Br J Cancer 1990; 62:631–6.

43. Zeigler R, Hoover R, Pike M, *et al*. Migration patterns and breast cancer risk in Asian-American women. J Natl Cancer Inst 1993; 85:1819–27.

44. Dupont W, Page D. Risk factors for breast cancer in women with proliferative breast disease. N Engl J Med 1985; 312(3):146–51.

45. Page D, Dupont W, Rogers L, Rados M. Atypical hyperplastic lesions of the female breast. Cancer 1985; 55:2698–708.

46. Hutson SW, Cowen PN, Bird CC. Morphometric studies of age related changes in normal human breast and their significance for evolution of

mammary cancer. J Clin Pathol 1985; 38:281–7.

47. Saftlas AF, Szklo M. Mammographic parenchymal patterns and breast cancer risk. Epidemiol Rev 1987; 9:146–74.

48. Boyd NF, Byng JW, Jong RA, et al. Quantitative classification of mammographic densities and breast cancer risk: results from the Canadian National Breast Screening Study. J Natl Cancer Inst 1995; 87:670–5.

49. Oza AM, Boyd NF. Mammographic parenchymal patterns: a marker of breast cancer risk. Epidemiol Rev 1993; 15:196–208.

50. Claus E, Risch N, Thompson W. Genetic analysis of breast cancer in the Cancer and Steroid Hormone Study. Am J Hum Genet 1991; 48:232–42.

51. Wooster R, Neuhausen S, Mangion J, et al. Localization of a breast cancer susceptibility gene, BRCA2, to chromosome 13q12-13. Science 1994; 265:2088–90.

52. Rebbeck T, Couch F, Kant J, et al. Genetic heterogeneity in hereditary breast cancer: role of BRCA1 and BRCA2. Am J Hum Genet 1996; 59:547–53.

53. Futreal P, Liu Q, Shattuck-Eidens D, et al. BRCA1 mutation in primary and ovarian carcinomas. Science 1994; 226:120–2.

54. Lancaster J, Wooster R, Mangion J, et al. BRCA2 mutations in primary breast and ovarian cancers. Nat Genet 1996; 13:238–40.

55. Miki Y, Katagiri T, Kasumi F, Yoshimoto T, Nakamura Y. Mutation analysis in the BRCA2 gene in primary breast cancers. Nat Genet 1996; 13:245–7.

56. Takahashi H, Behbakht K, McGovern P, et al. Mutation analysis of the BRCA1 gene in ovarian cancers. Cancer Res 1995; 55:2998–3002.

57. Teng D, Bogden R, Mitchell J, et al. Low incidence of BRCA2 mutations in breast carcinoma and other cancers. Nat Genet 1996; 13:241–4.

58. Hall J, Lee M, Newman B, et al. Linkage of early-onset familial breast cancer to chromosome 17q21. Science 1990; 250:1684–9.

59. Narod S, Feunteun J, Lynch H, et al. Familial breast–ovarian cancer locus on chromosome 17q12-q23. Lancet 1991; 338:82–3.

60. Easton D, Bishop D, Ford D, Crockford C. The Breast Cancer Linkage Consortium: genetic linkage analysis in familial breast and ovarian cancer: results from 214 families. Am J Hum Genet 1993; 52:678–701.

61. Lynch H, Watson P. Genetic counseling and hereditary breast/ovarian cancer (Letter). Lancet 1992; 339:1181.

62. Easton D, Ford D, Bishop D, and the Breast Cancer Linkage Consortium. Breast and ovarian cancer incidence in BRCA1-mutation carriers. Am J Hum Genet 1995; 56:265–71.

63. Narod S, Ford D, Devilee P, et al. An evaluation of genetic heterogeneity in 145 breast–ovarian cancer families. Am J Hum Genet 1995; 56:254–64.

64. Phelan C, Rebbeck T, Weber B, et al. Ovarian cancer risk in BRCA1 carriers is modified by the HRAS1 variable number of tandem repeat (VNTR) locus. Nat Genet 1996; 12:309–11.

65. Burke W, Daly M, Garber J, et al. Recommendations for follow-up care of individuals with an inherited predisposition to cancer: II. BRCA1 and BRCA2. JAMA 1997; 277:997–1003.

66. Ford D, Easton D, Stratton M, et al. Genetic heterogeneity and penetrance analysis of the BRCA1 and BRCA2 genes in breast cancer families. Am J Hum Genet 1998; 62:676–89.

67. Miki Y, Swensen J, Shattuck-Eidens D, et al. A strong candidate for the breast and ovarian cancer susceptibility gene BRCA1. Science 1994; 266:66–71.

68. Tavtigian S, Simard J, Rommens J, et al. The complete BRCA2 gene and mutations in chromosome 13q-linked kindreds. Nat Genet 1996; 12:333–7.

69. Cannon-Albright L, Skolnick M. The genetics of familial breast cancer. Semin Oncol 1996; 23 (Suppl.):1–5.

70. Shattuck-Eidens D, McClure M, Simard J, et al. A collaborative survey of 80 mutations in the BRCA1 breast and ovarian cancer susceptibility gene. JAMA 1995; 273:535–41.

71. Castilla D, Couch F, Erdos M, et al. Mutations in the BRCA1 gene in families with early-onset breast and ovarian cancer. Nat Genet 1994; 8:387–91.

72. Kelsell D, Black D, Bishop D, Spurr N. Genetic analysis of the BRCA1 region in a large breast/ovarian family: refinement of the minimal region containing BRCA1. Hum Mol Genet 1993; 2:1823–8.

73. Merajver S, Pham T, Caduff R, et al. Somatic mutations in the BRCA1 gene in sporadic ovarian tumours. Nat Genet 1995; 9:439–43.

74. Smith S, Easton D, Evans D, Ponder B. Allele losses in the region 17q12-21 in familial breast and ovarian cancer involve the wild-type chromosome. Nat Genet 1992; 2:128–31.

75. Schutte M, da Costa L, Hahn S, et al. Identification by representational difference analysis of a homozygous deletion in pancreatic carcinoma that lies with the BRCA2 region. Proc Natl Acad Sci USA 1995; 92:5950–4.

76. Wooster R, Bignell G, Lancaster J, et al. Identification of the breast cancer susceptibility gene BRCA2. Nature 1995; 378:789–92.

77. Malkin D. The Li–Fraumeni syndrome. Principle Practice Oncology 1993; 7:1–14.

78. Swift M, Sholman L, Perry M, *et al*. Malignant neoplasms in the families of patients with ataxia-telangiectasia. Cancer Res 1976; 36:209–15.

79. Swift M, Morrell D, Massey R, *et al*. Incidence of cancer in 161 families affected by ataxia-telangiectasia. N Engl J Med 1991; 326:1831–6.

80. Easton D. Cancer risks in A-T heterozygotes. Int J Radiat Biol 1994; 66:S177–82.

81. Savitsky K, Bar-Shira A, Gilad S, *et al*. A single ataxia telangiectasia gene with a product similar to PI-3 kinase. Science 1995; 268:1749–53.

82. Wooster R, Mangion J, Eeles R, *et al*. A germline mutation in the androgen receptor gene in two brothers with breast cancer and Reifenstein syndrome. Nat Genet 1992; 2:132–4.

83. Nelen M, Padberg G, Peeters E, *et al*. Localization of the gene for Cowden disease to chromosome 10q22-23. Nat Genet 1996; 13:114–16.

84. Hoskins K, Stopfer J, Calzone K, *et al*. Assessment and counseling for women with a family history of breast cancer: a guide for clinicians. JAMA 1995; 273:577–85.

85. Struewing J, Abeliovich D, Peretz T, *et al*. The carrier frequency of the *BRCA1* 185delAG mutation is approximately 1 percent in Ashkenazi Jewish individuals. Nat Genet 1995; 11:198–200.

86. Struewing JP, Hartge P, Wacholder S, *et al*. The risk of cancer associated with specific mutations of *BRCA1* and *BRCA2* among Ashkenazi Jews. N Engl J Med 1997; 336:1401–8.

87. Hopper J, Southey M, Dite G, *et al*. Population-based estimate of the average age-specific cumulative risk of breast cancer for a defined set of protein-truncating mutations in *BRCA1* and *BRCA2*: Australian Breast Cancer Family Study. Cancer Epidemiol Biomarkers Prev 1999; 8:741–7.

88. Jernstrom H, Lerman C, Ghadirian P, *et al*. Pregnancy and risk of early breast cancer in carriers of *BRCA1* and *BRCA2*. Lancet 1999; 354:1846–50.

89. Jernstrom H, Johannsson O, Borg A, Olsson H. Do *BRCA1* mutations affect the ability to breast-feed? Breast 1998; 7:320–4.

90. Narod S, Risch R, Moslehi R, *et al*. Oral contraceptives and the risk of hereditary ovarian cancer. N Engl J Med 1998; 339:424–8.

91. Ursin G, Henderson B, Haile R, *et al*. Does oral contraceptive use increase the risk of breast cancer in women with *BRCA1/BRCA2* mutations more than in other women? Cancer Res 1997; 57:3678–81.

92. Anderson D, Badziocil M. Risks of familial breast cancer. Cancer 1985; 56:383.

93. Rubin S, Benjamin I, Behbakht K, *et al*. Clinical and pathological features of ovarian cancer in women with germ-line mutations of *BRCA1*. N Engl J Med 1996; 335:1413–16.

94. Goldgar D, Fields P, Lewis C, *et al*. A large kindred with 17q-linked susceptibility to breast and ovarian cancer: relationship between genotype and phenotype (Abstract). Am J Hum Genet 1992; 51 (Suppl.):A27.

95. Couch F, DeShano M, Blackwood M, *et al*. *BRCA1* mutations in women attending clinics that evaluate the risk of breast cancer. N Engl J Med 1997; 336:1409–15.

96. Couch F, Farid L, DeShano M, *et al*. *BRCA2* germline mutations in male breast cancer cases and breast cancer families. Nat Genet 1996; 13:123–4.

97. Thorlacius S, Tryggvadottir L, Olatsdottir G, *et al*. Linkage to *BRCA2* region in hereditary male breast cancer. Lancet 1995; 346:544–5.

98. Lynch H, Marcus J, Watson P, Page D. Distinctive clinicopathologic features of *BRCA1*-linked hereditary breast cancer. Proc ASCO 1994; 7:103–7.

99. Marcus J, Watson P, Page D, *et al*. Hereditary breast cancer: pathobiology, prognosis, and *BRCA1* and *BRCA2* gene linkage [see comments]. Cancer 1996; 77:697–709.

100. Piver M, Baker T, Jishi M, *et al*. Familial ovarian cancer: a report of 658 families from the Gilda Radner Familial Ovarian Cancer Registry 1981–1991. Cancer 1993; 71:582–8.

101. Narod S, Madletisby L, Bradley L, *et al*. Hereditary and familial ovarian cancer in Southern Ontario. Cancer 1994; 74:2341–6.

102. Ford D, Easton D, Bishop D, Narod S, Goldgar D, B.C.L. Consortium, Risks of cancer in *BRCA-1* mutation carriers. Lancet 1994; 343:692–5.

103. Arason A, Barkardottir R, Egilsson V. Linkage analysis of chromosome 17q markers and breast–ovarian cancer in Icelandic families, and possible relationship to prostatic cancer. Am J Hum Genet 1993; 52:711–17.

104. Consortium B.C.L., Cancer risks in *BRCA2* mutation carriers. J Natl Cancer Inst 1999; 91:1310–16.

105. Egan K, Newcomb P, Longnecker M, *et al*. Jewish religion and risk of breast cancer. Lancet 1996; 347:1645–6.

106. Steinberg K, Pernarelli J, Marcus M, Khoury M, Schildkraut J, Marchbanks P. Increased risk for familial ovarian cancer among Jewish women: a population-based case-control study. Genet Epidemiol 1998; 15:51–9.

107. Neuhausen S, Gilewski T, Norton L, *et al*. Recurrent *BRCA2* 6174delT mutations in Ashkenazi Jewish women affected by breast cancer. Nat Genet 1996; 13:126–8.

108. Fitzgerald M, MacDonald D, Krainer M, *et al*. Germ-line *BRCA1* mutations in Jewish and non-Jewish women with early-onset breast cancer. N Engl J Med 1996; 334:143–9.

109. Offit K. Breast cancer and *BRCA1* mutations [Letter]. N Engl J Med 1996; 334:1197–8; 1199–200.

110. Shattuck-Eidens D, Oliphant A, McClure M, *et al.* *BRCA1* sequence analysis in women at high risk for susceptibility mutations. Risk factor analysis and implications for genetic testing [see comments]. JAMA 1997; 278:1242–50.

111. Offit K, Brown K. Quantitating familial cancer risk: a resource for clinical oncologists. J Clin Oncol 1994; 12:1724–36.

112. Gail M, Brinton L, Byar D, *et al.* Projecting individualized probabilities of developing breast cancer for white females who are being examined annually. J Natl Cancer Inst 1989; 81:1879–86.

113. Claus E, Risch N, Thompson W. Autosomal dominant inheritance of early-onset breast cancer. Cancer 1994; 73:643–51.

114. Claus E, Risch N, Thompson W. The calculation of breast cancer risk for women with a first degree family history of ovarian cancer. Breast Cancer Res Treat 1993; 28:115–20.

115. Slattery M, Kerber R. A comprehensive evaluation of family history and breast cancer risk. JAMA 1993; 270:1563–8.

116. Parmigiani G, Berry DA, Aguilar O. Determining carrier probabilities for breast cancer-susceptibility genes *BRCA1* and *BRC2*. Am J Hum Genet 1998; 62:145–58.

117. Struewing J, Lerman C, Kase R, Giambarresi T, Tucker M. Anticipated uptake and impact of genetic testing in hereditary breast and ovarian cancer families. Cancer Epidemiol Biomarkers Prev 1995; 4:169–73.

118. Lynch H, Lynch J, Conway T, Severin M. Psychological aspects of monitoring high risk women for breast cancer. Cancer 1994; 74:1184–92.

119. Weber B, Giusti R, Liu E. Developing strategies for intervention and prevention in hereditary breast cancer. J Natl Cancer Inst Monogr 1995; 17:99–102.

120. Petrij-Bosch A, Peelen T, van Vliet M, *et al.* *BRCA1* genomic deletions are major founder mutations in Dutch breast cancer patients (Letter). Nat Genet 1997; 17:341–5.

121. Natowicz MR, Alper JK, Alper JS. Genetic discrimination and the law. Am J Hum Genet 1992; 50:465–75.

122. Billings P, Kohn M, de Cuevas M, *et al.* Discrimination as a consequence of genetic testing. Am J Hum Genet 1992; 50:476–82.

123. Weber B. Genetic testing for breast cancer. Sci Am 1996; 17:12–21.

124. Olopade O, Cummings S. Genetic counseling for cancer: part 1. Principle Practice Oncology 1996; 10:1–13.

125. Fisher B, Costantino JP, Wickerham DL, Redmond CK. Tamoxifen for prevention of breast cancer: report of the National Surgical Adjuvant Breast and Bowel Project P-1 Study. J Natl Cancer Inst 1998; 90(18):1371–88.

126. Veronesi U, Maisonneuve P, Costa A, *et al.* Prevention of breast cancer with tamoxifen: preliminary findings from the Italian randomised trial among hysterectomised women. Italian Tamoxifen Prevention Study. Lancet 1998; 352:93–7.

127. Powles T, Eeles R, Ashley S, *et al.* Interim analysis of the incidence of breast cancer in the Royal Marsden Hospital Tamoxifen Randomised Chemoprevention Trial. Lancet 1998; 352:98–101.

128. Gail MH, Costantino JP, Bryant J, Croyle R, Freedman L. Weighing the risks and benefits of tamoxifen treatment for preventing breast cancer. J Natl Cancer Inst 1999; 91(21): 1829–46.

129. Cummings S, Eckert S, Krueger K, *et al.* The effect of raloxifene on risk of breast cancer in postmenopausal women: results from the MORE randomized trial. Multiple Outcomes of Raloxifene Evaluation. JAMA 1999; 281:2189–97.

130. Hartmann LC, Schaid DJ, Woods JE, Crotty TP, Myers JL. Efficacy of bilateral prophylactic mastectomy in women with a family history. N Engl J Med 1999; 340(2):77–84.

131. Rebbeck R, Levin A, Eisen A, *et al.* Breast cancer risk after bilateral prophylactic oophorectomy in *BRCA1* mutation carriers. J Natl Cancer Inst 1999; 91:1475–9.

132. Veronesi U, De Palo G, Marubini E, Costa A, Formelli F. Randomized trial of fenretinide to prevent second breast malignancy in women. J Natl Cancer Inst 1999; 91(21):1847–56.

133. Spicer DV, Pike MC, Pike A, Rude R, Shoupe D, Richardson J. Pilot trial of a gonadotropin hormone agonist with replacement hormones as a prototype contraceptive to prevent breast cancer. Contraception 1993; 47:427–44.

134. Spicer D, Ursin G, Parisky Y, *et al.* Changes in mammographic densities induced by a hormonal contraceptive designed to reduce breast cancer risk. J Natl Cancer Inst 1994; 86:431–6.

135. Baum M. Adjuvant treatment of premenopausal breast cancer with zoladex and tamoxifen: results from the ZIPP trial organized by the Cancer Research Campaign Breast Cancer Trials Group, the Stockholm Breast Cancer Study Group, the South East Sweden Breast Cancer Group and Gruppo Interdisciplinare Valutazione Intervention Oncologia (GIVIO). Breast Cancer Res Treat 1999; 57:30.

Commentary

M WILLIAM AUDEH

INTRODUCTION: THE NEW ERA OF CANCER RISK ASSESSMENT

Why do some women develop breast cancer, while others do not? Is it possible to predict who is at greatest risk for developing breast cancer, and intervene in the process of carcinogenesis? These are questions of primary importance to clinicians as we enter the twenty-first century, and there is great hope that the era of 'genomic medicine'[1] will provide answers to them.

Traditional epidemiology has been the mainstay of cancer risk assessment, with observed associations leading to numerical estimates of risk, as in the Gail model.[2] This approach is insufficient to allow a full understanding of the true causes of breast cancer, as this can only be gained from the study of breast carcinogenesis at the molecular, cellular, and organismal level.

The very concept of 'risk factors' for cancer will be changed dramatically by the complete sequencing of the human genome, as we approach the identification of all genes which may play a role in cancer development. It is already apparent, from the nearly 200 genes now known to play a role in cancer development,[3] that 'risk factors' for cancer will not be understood as single genes or environmental factors, but rather as the end-result of complex interactions between multiple genes and numerous environmental factors. The terms 'hereditary' and 'sporadic,' now used to mark a seemingly clear distinction between cancers due to genetic versus environmental causes, will be supplanted by the understanding that cancer develops on a continuum of gene–environment effects. It will soon no longer be adequate, therefore, to rely upon traditional epidemiology to identify risk factors for breast cancer, particularly because the key to effective prevention will require a functional understanding of gene–environment interactions that only genomic medicine, through molecular epidemiology, can provide.[4] The accurate identification and appropriate management of women at high risk for breast cancer will depend on the application of this emerging knowledge to the clinic as rapidly as possible.

In this chapter, Drs Spicer, Israel, and Clark provide an excellent summary of the 'known risk factors,' as culled from traditional epidemiology, followed by an in-depth discussion of the most highly penetrant known genes associated with breast cancer, and the current status of genetic counseling for high-risk women. The chapter closes with a brief description of 'options for prevention.' While the authors' focus is understandably limited to a broad overview of this rapidly developing field, it is the purpose of this commentary to provide a somewhat different perspective on the understanding of risk factors for breast cancer, and on the promise this approach holds for the management of women at high risk.

RISK FACTORS FOR BREAST CANCER: THE BIOLOGICAL PERSPECTIVE

In order to move beyond traditional epidemiology, the clinician must approach the identified risk factors for breast cancer from a biological perspective. Which factors are specific to breast cancer, and which are universal factors relevant to carcinogenesis in general?

It is now understood that all cancer (including breast cancer) develops as the result of the acquisition, within a cell, of multiple genetic lesions which confer a survival advantage to that cell.[3] It is also recognized that these genetic lesions, i.e., somatic mutations, must occur in key cellular pathways which regulate critical functions such as the control of proliferation, programmed cell death, response to intercellular communication, etc. A key cellular step driving the overall process of carcinogenesis is the loss of genetic stability, thereby accelerating the mutation rate, an event that leads to the markedly aberrant genome of the cancer cell – the 'mutator phenotype.'[5] Loss of genetic stability results from mutations in genes responsible for the detection and repair of DNA damage, and may be in the form of acquired somatic mutations, or inherited genetic polymorphisms in DNA repair pathways.

It is readily apparent, therefore, that any factors that increase the likelihood of the acquisition of somatic mutations will be important risk factors for the development of cancer. It is now known, for example, that inherited mutations in BRCA1 and BRCA2 increase the risk of breast cancer, in part by reducing the repair of DNA damage. It is also apparent that they are not the only genes with relevance to breast cancer. Genetic variation in other DNA-repair enzymes, in carcinogen-metabolizing enzymes, and in hormone-metabolizing enzymes, for example, may be added to the growing list of genes with importance in determining an individual's risk of breast cancer.

Hormonal carcinogenesis

Breast cancer falls within the category of 'hormone-related cancers,' for which the process of 'hormonal carcinogenesis' is a major causative factor.[6] Hormonal carcinogenesis is the process by which hormones provide a significant mitogenic stimulus to a tissue at risk, causing multiple rounds of cell proliferation and the associated risk of acquired somatic mutation. The breast tissue is present from the time of birth as a dormant rest of stem cells, stimulated by hormones to develop rapidly in a burst of proliferation at menarche, and then undergoing cyclic proliferation due to hormones until menopause. In a general sense, cell proliferation in the breast is driven by endogenous and exogenous hormones, estrogen and progesterone, and, with each round of proliferation, there is the attendant risk of DNA mutation. This mutation risk may be the result of random errors in replication (as is inherent in our error-prone system[7]) or of inadequate repair of DNA damage acquired from other sources, such as oxidative damage, or exogenous genotoxic agents such as environmental and dietary carcinogens.[8]

Reassessing breast cancer risk factors

It is useful to reassess certain of the traditional epidemiological risk factors cited by Spicer *et al.* from a biological perspective, as they may be seen to represent surrogate markers for biological processes relevant to cancer development.

Age

Age may be thought of as a surrogate marker for the total burden of somatic mutations acquired by an individual, as the result of proliferative cycles and unrepaired DNA damage. Greater age implies a greater burden of somatic mutations, with an estimated increase of mutations of approximately 1% per year as individuals age.[7]

Age at menopause/menarche

Age at menopause and age at menarche may be thought of as surrogate markers for the total length of estrogen exposure or, more accurately, for the total number of proliferative cycles in the breast epithelium deriving from ovarian estrogen exposure. While both of these hormonal 'landmarks' may well have a hereditary component, it is clear that dietary and societal factors significantly alter their impact. Women in 'modern' societies, where breast cancer is epidemic, consume Westernized diets, experience earlier menarche, later menopause, and fewer pregnancies than the average woman in traditional hunter–gatherer societies, where breast cancer is rare.[9] The result is that the actual number of ovulatory cycles in women in modern societies is estimated to be approximately 450, compared to approximately 145 in hunter–gatherer societies.

Exogenous hormones/obesity/exercise

These may be thought of as factors that modulate absolute hormone levels and/or, in the case of obesity and exercise, total numbers of ovulatory cycles.

Hormonal risk factors may best be understood in terms of factors that *increase* hormone exposure, thereby increasing risk (e.g., early menarche, late menopause, postmenopausal obesity, hormone replacement therapy), and those that *decrease* hormone exposure, thereby reducing risk (e.g., young age at first pregnancy, prolonged breast-feeding, exercise).[6]

Benign breast disease

Benign breast disease is identified as a risk factor by traditional epidemiology (and by Spicer *et al.*), due to the fact that women who have undergone breast biopsy for any reason have an increased likelihood of developing breast cancer.[2] However, it is clear that not all 'benign' breast disease is truly benign, and that the more accurate risk marker is 'proliferative' breast disease such as atypical ductal hyperplasia, which carries a twofold to fivefold increase in risk of breast cancer,[10] and appears to be clonally related to invasive breast cancer.

Proliferative breast disease may actually be a marker for a genetic predisposition to breast cancer, as suggested by studies of the first-degree relatives of women with breast cancer from breast cancer kindreds.[11] This study analysed breast aspirate specimens and found proliferative breast disease in 35% of first-degree relatives, compared to only 13% in unrelated controls. It is significant as well that women with proliferative breast disease may reduce their risk of developing breast cancer by over 50% with the use of tamoxifen, as evidenced by the NSABP Breast Cancer Prevention Trial.[12]

Race

Race is a complex epidemiological factor, which is, in reality, an imperfect surrogate for a variety of genetic and environmental factors:

1 Genetic cofactors, in the form of low-penetrance genes that are highly represented in a particular ethnic group and that may affect cancer risk, such as polymorphisms in estrogen-metabolizing enzymes[6] or carcinogen-metabolizing enzymes.[4]
2 Environmental factors specific to a geographical region (such as diet) when 'race' is equated with a common geographic location such as Japanese living in Japan.
3 Cultural factors that accompany members of an ethnic group despite geographical separation, such as exported dietary or cultural practices which impact upon cancer risk. In the most accurate sense, 'race' is perhaps best replaced by 'genetic background' to remove the confounding factors of culture, diet, and geography.

The ability to analyse an individual's genetic background as part of a cancer risk assessment is a major benefit to be derived from the completion of the Human Genome Project.[1]

Hereditary versus non-hereditary factors

Spicer, Israel, and Clark classify a variety of epidemiological risk factors as 'non-hereditary,' in distinction to clearly hereditary factors such as the inheritance of highly penetrant genes such as *BRCA1* and *BRCA2*. These factors classified as 'non-hereditary' include age, age at menopause, age at menarche, obesity, race, and benign breast disease, as well as the use of exogenous hormones for contraception or postmenopausal hormone replacement, exercise, age of first pregnancy, and breast-feeding. It can be argued that many of these risk factors are indeed the result of an interplay between genes (i.e., 'hereditary' factors) and environmental factors. Unfortunately, the term 'hereditary' risk factors for cancer has been applied only to highly penetrant mutated genes which clearly display Mendelian inheritance patterns, whereas the majority of cancers can be attributed to the interaction of multiple low-penetrance genes with environmental factors. These low-penetrance genes are exceedingly common in the population, and represent genetic polymorphisms which form the basis for the observed variation in drug metabolism, and may well explain the variation in the risk of cancer development.[13] Therefore, it is no longer useful to draw sharp distinctions between hereditary and non-hereditary risk factors for breast cancer, for the action of nearly all known environmental, or non-hereditary, factors will be affected by genetic variation.

THE TRUE GENETICS OF BREAST CANCER

All breast cancer may be understood as the result of gene–environment interactions. By examining the known epidemiological risk factors for their biologic basis, our understanding of breast cancer development is improved. For example, it is now clear that hormonal exposure, as indicated by a variety of traditional epidemiological observations, is important in the process of hormonal carcinogenesis. However, hormone exposure is not uniform throughout the human species, but is highly variable due to genetic variation in hormone production and metabolism. These genes may be thought of as low-penetrance, high-frequency genes, which may affect the risk of breast cancer in the absence of strongly positive family histories. Conversely, studies of families with breast cancer have allowed the identification of highly penetrant genes, such as *BRCA1*, which confer a lifetime risk of breast cancer of 55% or greater.[14] Our growing understanding of the universal features of cancer development leads to the realm of molecular epidemiology, where genetic variability in both low-penetrance and high-penetrance genes contributes to the overall cancer risk.

The types of genes affecting breast cancer risk

While hormonal carcinogenesis offers the mitogenic stimulus of hormone exposure as the driving force for cancer development,[6] cancer will not develop unless DNA damage is acquired in the process. Which germline, inherited, genetic factors affect whether or not DNA damage develops in the breast epithelium? Are there other genes that affect the ability of endogenous or exogenous genotoxic agents to damage DNA?

Genes involved in DNA repair

BRCA1 and *BRCA2* are involved in DNA repair, and participate in the formation of a large protein complex that is important for the maintenance of genomic integrity.[15] Mutations that inactivate these functions will accelerate the acquisition and fixation of DNA mutations in the breast epithelium. Other genes involved in the detection or correction of DNA damage that have been implicated in familial breast cancer, as outlined by Spicer *et al.*, include *ATM* and *p53*. These are rare, high-penetrance genes, and may significantly underestimate the importance of inherited variation in DNA repair in the general population at risk for breast cancer.

Many other genes are involved in the maintenance of genomic integrity, and they may be a factor in the inherited predisposition to breast cancer.[8] Mammalian cells possess at least four mechanisms for DNA repair, which are distinguished by the type of lesion they repair:

base excision repair (BER) repairs single base lesions produced by oxygen radicals, X-rays and alkylating agents;

mismatch repair (MMR) repairs replication errors leading to A-G and T-C mismatch;

nucleotide excision repair (NER) repairs lesions produced by ultraviolet light and polycyclic aromatic hydrocarbons such as bulky DNA adducts;

recombinational repair repairs double-strand breaks and interstrand crosslinks due to a variety of factors.[16] Nearly all genes identified within this repair system are polymorphic within the population, and underlie interindividual variation in DNA repair capacity.

It may be hypothesized that certain individuals who develop breast cancer may do so as the result of inadequate DNA-repair mechanisms. Recent evidence supports this hypothesis. A review of 64 epidemiological studies of DNA-repair capacity in cancer patients revealed the consistent finding of an inherited deficiency of DNA repair in cancer patients (including breast cancer) versus controls, with the odds ratio being on average a twofold to tenfold increased risk of cancer.[8] This low but common level of risk is consistent with the action of low-penetrance, high-frequency genes. At present, there is inconsistency in the manner in which DNA-repair capacity is measured, and only a small number of specific genes identified which may be analysed for mutation or polymorphisms. Modern cancer risk assessment will eventually include the rapid assessment of DNA-repair capacity, by either functional assays or genetic analysis.[17]

Genes involved in carcinogen metabolism

Are chemical carcinogens involved in the development of breast cancer? To date, no consistent factor, other than estrogen, has been implicated as a causative agent, although carcinogen-induced DNA damage has been detected in human breast epithelium.[18] The implication is that chemical carcinogens may well play a role in breast cancer development, depending on individual variation in the metabolism of DNA-damaging agents.

Polycyclic aromatic hydrocarbons (PAHs) and heterocyclic amines (HCAs) are organic compounds derived from a variety of sources, including cigarette smoke, products of combustion, and dietary sources. They are potent mammary carcinogens in animal models and, in humans, their metabolism is determined by enzymes such as the cytochrome p450 system (CYP), glutathione-S-transferase (GST), and N-acetyltransferase (NAT2), which are polymorphic in the general population.[19] Polymorphisms in genes encoding metabolizing enzymes have functional consequences, with a wide range of enzyme activity between individuals. Such interindividual variation may play a role in the development of breast cancer.

Carcinogens which bind directly to DNA deform its structure, producing a DNA–carcinogen adduct. DNA adducts due to PAH have been detected in normal breast tissue from breast cancer patients at significantly higher levels than in the breast tissue from controls.[18] In subsequent studies controlling for exposure, breast cancer patients were again found to have significantly higher levels of DNA adducts than controls, suggesting that, with equal exposure, these patients may be metabolizing carcinogens differently than controls.

Specific genetic polymorphisms have been associated with increased breast cancer risk when appropriate exposure to chemical carcinogens is encountered. For example, a specific polymorphism in CYP1A1 may predispose women who smoke at an early age to the development of breast cancer, accounting for as much as 5% of all breast cancer cases.[20] The GST M1 null polymorphism, present in 50% of the Caucasian population, has been significantly associated with higher levels of PAH–DNA adducts in breast tissue.[4] NAT2, which detoxifies carcinogenic HCAs by N-acetylation, is present as slow and rapid acetylator genotypes, with slow acetylators being less effective at clearing the carcinogen; 50–60% of Caucasians and 30–40% of African-Americans carry the slow acetylator genotype. Smoking appears to increase the risk of breast cancer in postmenopausal women who possess the slow acetylator genotype of NAT2.[21]

Genes involved in hormone metabolism

Steroid hormones implicated in the development of breast cancer are produced, metabolized, bound, and transported by a number of cellular proteins, most of which are encoded by genes which are polymorphic. Genetic variants with minor differences in the activity of their protein product may, over a period of decades, and in association with other hormonally related genes, significantly alter the hormonal milieu to which the breast epithelium is exposed.[6] Critical genes in these pathways are the 17-beta-hydroxysteroid dehydrogenase 1 gene (HSD17β1), the cytochrome 17 gene (CYP17), the aromatase gene (CYP19), the estrogen receptor alpha gene (ER), and the progesterone receptor gene (PR). To date, results have shown a genetic basis for wide variation in endogenous hormone levels, but association with breast cancer has been inconsistent.

ASSESSING BREAST CANCER RISK IN THE AGE OF GENOMIC MEDICINE

Inherited genetic variation is an essential component of breast cancer risk. A growing number of genes have been identified with relevance to the development of breast cancer, ranging from common, low-penetrance genes to rare, high-penetrance genes, all of which lead to the development of cancer through their interaction with other genes and with environmental factors. The optimal approach to breast cancer risk assessment would therefore be the analysis of all relevant genes and environmental exposures for a given individual. At the present time, only rare, high-penetrance genes such as BRCA1 and BRCA2 are routinely analysed in the clinic, leaving the bulk of meaningful genetic variation in an individual (such as genes for DNA repair, carcinogen and hormone metabolism) unknown and unexamined. While Spicer et al. provide a complete summary of our current knowledge of BRCA1 and BRCA2, it is clear that the vast majority of genetic information with relevance to cancer risk has yet to be added to the general approach to risk assessment for breast cancer.

At the present time, genotyping is technically simpler and more accurately reflective of cancer risk than the assessment of environmental exposure, although this may soon change.[22] The objective assessment of exposure currently includes techniques such as DNA adduct detection in breast tissue, but primarily still relies upon historical recall of exposure such as smoking frequency and diet.[23] As the Human Genome Project expands the list of genes relevant to cancer development, expanded genotyping of individuals will become technically feasible and clinically useful. Although microarray technology[1] is removing the technical impediments to the rapid analysis of large numbers of genes, significant social impediments to genotyping remain.[24] Efforts to control access to genetic testing for clinical use have been the subject of intense debate, centered around the issue of whether patients and clinicians are sufficiently informed to avoid the misuse and misinterpretation of genetic information.[25–27]

The implications of genetic information about cancer risk

Concerns regarding the emotional, social and economic impact of genetic information abound, and the problem is exemplified by the discussion of genetic counseling offered by Spicer *et al*. These authors suggest that 'the issues surrounding genetic testing are complex and are best communicated in a formal genetic counseling session with an experienced cancer genetic counselor.' This statement appears to be in conflict with the recommendation of the American Society of Clinical Oncology, which, as the leading organization of physicians who treat people with cancer, 'affirms the role of clinical oncologists in … providing counseling regarding familial cancer risk, and options for prevention and early detection, and recognizing those families for which genetic testing is appropriate.'[28] Is the assessment of cancer risk, which includes the analysis of genetic information, the province of genetic counselors or clinical oncologists?

The model of genetic counseling offered by genetic counselors was initially developed in prenatal and pediatric settings, and has traditionally offered psychological support for families dealing with rare, high-penetrance genetic syndromes, whereas the realm of cancer genetics, with its growing emphasis on high-frequency, low-penetrance predisposition genes acting in concert with environmental factors, is entirely different.[29] The clinical utility of cancer risk assessment is not simply the identification of individuals at increased risk of breast cancer, but also the application of this information to a rational strategy for prevention. As the mechanisms of carcinogenesis become more clearly understood, the approach to prevention will need to be tailored to an individual's genotype and environment, a complex clinical intervention based on knowledge of molecular biology, epidemiology, and medicine that is most appropriately the responsibility of the clinical oncologist.

MANAGING THE WOMAN AT RISK FOR BREAST CANCER

Cancer prevention may only be achieved by intervening in the process of carcinogenesis. The identification of individuals possessing a genetic predisposition to cancer is essential to defining and applying appropriate intervention, although general approaches based on estimates of epidemiological risk, as with the Tamoxifen Breast Cancer Prevention Trial, have yielded positive results.[12] Currently, the approach to women at increased risk is screening, surgical removal of the tissue at risk (mastectomy), and/or medical therapy (chemoprevention). The management of women with *BRCA1* and *BRCA2* mutations is well described by Spicer *et al*. and is not addressed further here. The general approach to women at risk for breast cancer merits discussion, however, as it too will change with the application of new information from genomics and molecular epidemiology.

Screening and the surgical removal of the tissue at risk (mastectomy) have been well summarized by Spicer *et al*. These methods are appropriate and, in the case of prophylactic mastectomy, proven to be effective.[30] However, these are the only options for prevention when no ability to intervene in the process of carcinogenesis exists. One may argue that this is no longer the case, as our understanding of the mechanism of carcinogenesis points the way to targeted intervention for the purpose of cancer prevention.[31]

Chemoprevention is the only method of targeted intervention based on an understanding of the process of carcinogenesis. Tamoxifen, the first known chemoprevention agent for breast cancer, is a selective estrogen receptor modulator (SERM), intervening in the process of hormonal carcinogenesis, which is essential to the development of breast cancer. A number of new SERMs are in development, offering the possibility of more selective intervention with fewer side-effects. The effect of genotype on the action of SERMs is not currently known, although it is likely that genetic variation in hormone-related genes, as well as *BRCA1* and *BRCA2*, may modify the effect of SERMs.

Other mechanism-based chemoprevention agents include inhibitors of cyclo-oxygenase 2 (COX 2), an enzyme that is clearly implicated in the development of colorectal cancer, but may be involved in a variety of cancers, suggesting the application of COX 2 inhibitors in other epithelial tumors, such as breast cancer.[31] Retinoids, which bind nuclear hormone receptors, may alter gene expression and interfere with the development of breast cancer, as has been suggested in animal studies with the synthetic retinoid Targretin.[32] Clinical trials in Europe with another retinoid, fenretinide, as a breast cancer prevention agent have been equivocal, although there is a suggestion of a beneficial effect for premenopausal women at risk.[33]

With the identification of low-penetrance genes predisposing to breast cancer, additional methods of prevention will be required. Individuals with deficient DNA repair or unfavorable metabolism of carcinogens may need to practice the diligent avoidance of ubiquitous but obvious carcinogenic or genotoxic factors such as cigarette smoke and X-irradiation. Appropriate dietary manipulation may lead to a significant reduction in the intake of dietary carcinogens and increase the intake of genoprotective factors such as antioxidants. There is also evidence that diet may affect the biology of the breast, as the reduction of saturated fat and cholesterol has been shown to reduce mammographic breast density in postmenopausal women,[34] a factor associated with increased estrogen effect and the risk of breast cancer. While these interventions may be of minor or inconsequential benefit as preventive measures for the general population, they may be highly protective for individuals with a genetic susceptibility to cancer.

SUMMARY

Understanding the causes of breast cancer at the biological level is essential to cancer prevention. Identifying women at increased risk of breast cancer, and intervening in the process of cancer development, will soon be possible with greater certainty. The application of sophisticated genetic information in every-day clinical practice will allow targeted intervention for women at increased risk of cancer. Chemoprevention holds the promise of expanding efforts at cancer prevention beyond the current choices of screening or mastectomy, into the realm of low-toxicity, mechanism-based intervention. Participating in this 'revolution' in medicine will require that clinical oncologists possess an understanding of cancer genetics and molecular epidemiology, in addition to traditional aspects of medicine.

REFERENCES

1. Collins F. Medical and societal consequences of the Human Genome Project. N Engl J Med 1999; 341:28–37.
2. Gail M, Brinton LA, Byer DP, et al. Projecting individualized probabilities of developing breast cancer for white females who are being examined annually. J Natl Cancer Inst 1989; 81:1879–86.
3. Hanahan D, Weinberg R. The hallmarks of cancer. Cell 2000; 100:57–70.
4. Perera F. Molecular epidemiology: on the path to prevention? J Natl Cancer Inst 2000; 92:602–12.
5. Loeb K, Loeb L. Significance of multiple mutations in cancer. Carcinogenesis 2000; 21:379–85.
6. Henderson B, Feigelson H. Hormonal carcinogenesis. Carcinogenesis 2000; 21:427–33.
7. Simpson A. The natural somatic mutation frequency and human carcinogenesis. Adv Cancer Res 1997; 71:209–40.
8. Berwick M, Vineis P. Markers of DNA repair and susceptibility to cancer in humans: an epidemiologic review. J Natl Cancer Inst 2000; 92:874–97.
9. Greaves M. Cancer: the evolutionary legacy. Oxford, Oxford University Press, 2000.
10. Dupont W, Page D. Risk factors for breast cancer in women with proliferative breast disease. N Engl J Med 1985; 312:146–51.
11. Skolnick M, Cannon-Albright LA, Goldgar DE, et al. Inheritance of proliferative breast disease in breast cancer kindreds. Science 1990; 250:1715–20.
12. Fisher B, Constantino JP, Wickersham D, et al. Tamoxifen for prevention of breast cancer: report of the NSABP Project P-1 study. J Natl Cancer Inst 1998; 90:1371–88.
13. Evans W, Relling M. Pharmacogenomics: translating functional genomics into rational therapeutics. Science 1999; 286:487–91.
14. Ford D, Easton D, Stratton M, et al. Genetic heterogeneity and penetrance analysis of the BRCA1 and BRCA2 genes in breast cancer families. Am J Hum Genet 1998; 62:676–89.
15. Kato M, Yano K, Matsuoi F, et al. Identification of Rad51 alterations in patients with bilateral breast cancer. J Hum Genet 2000; 45:133–7.
16. De Boer J, Hoeijmakers J. Nucleotide excision repair and human syndromes. Carcinogenesis 2000; 21:453–60.
17. Sarasin A, Stary A. Human cancer and DNA repair-deficient diseases. Cancer Detect Prev 1997; 1:406–11.
18. Perera F, Estabrook A, Hewer A, et al. Carcinogen–DNA adducts in human breast tissue. Cancer Epidemiol Biomarkers Prev 1995; 4:233–8.
19. Guengerich F. Metabolism of chemical carcinogens. Carcinogenesis 2000; 21:345–51.
20. Ishibe N, Harkinson S, Colditz G, et al. Cigarette smoking, cytochrome p450 1A1 polymorphisms, and breast cancer risk in the Nurses' Health Study. Cancer Res 1998; 58:667–71.
21. Ambrosone C, Freudenheim J, Graham S, et al. Cigarette smoking, N-acetyltransferase 2 polymorphisms and breast cancer risk. JAMA 1996; 276:1494–501.
22. Poirier M, Santella R, Weston A. Carcinogen macromolecular adducts and their measurement. Carcinogenesis 2000; 21: 353–9.
23. Lai C, Shields P. The role of interindividual variation in human carcinogenesis. J Nutr 1999; 129(2S Suppl.): 552S–5S.
24. Secretary's Advisory Committee on Genetic Testing. Adequacy of oversight of genetic tests: preliminary conclusions of the SACGT. Bethesda, MA, National Institutes of Health, 2000.
25. Schulman J, Stern H. Genetic predisposition testing for breast cancer. Cancer J Sci Am 1996; 2:244–9.
26. Burke W, Kahn M, Garber J, Collins F. et al. 'First do no harm' also applies to cancer susceptibility testing. Cancer J Sci Am 1996; 2:250–2.
27. Audeh MW. Genetic predisposition testing for breast cancer. Cancer J Sci Am 1997; 3:254–5.
28. Statement of the American Society of Clinical Oncology: genetic testing for cancer susceptibility. J Clin Oncol 1996; 14:1730–40.

29. Offit K. *Clinical cancer genetics.* New York, Wiley-Liss, 1998, 9–19.

30. Eisen A, Rebbeck T, Wood W, Weber B. Prophylactic surgery in women with a hereditary predisposition to breast and ovarian cancer. J Clin Oncol 2000; 18:1980–95.

31. Sporn M, Suh N. Chemoprevention of cancer. Carcinogenesis 2000; 21:525–30.

32. Gottardis M, Martin L, Greenberg W, *et al.* Chemoprevention of mammary carcinoma by LGD1069

(Targretin): an RXR-selective ligand. Cancer Res 1996; 56:5566–70.

33. Veronesi U, De Palo G, Marubini E, *et al.* Randomized trial of fenretinide to prevent second breast malignancy in women with early breast cancer. J Natl Cancer Inst 1999; 91:1847–56.

34. Knight J, Martin L, Greenberg W, *et al.* Macronutrient intake and change in mammographic density at menopause: results from a randomized trial. Cancer Epidemiol Biomarkers Prev 1999; 8:123–8.

Editors' selected abstracts

Primary care: reducing the risk of breast cancer.

Chlebowski RT.

Harbor-UCLA Research and Education Institute, Torrance, CA, USA.

New England Journal of Medicine 343(3):191–8, 2000, July 20.

A technology assessment by the American Society of Clinical Oncology recently reviewed the use of tamoxifen and raloxifene to reduce the risk of breast cancer. The report recommended that women at increased risk for breast cancer (defined as a risk of at least 1.7% over five years) 'may be offered tamoxifen (20 mg/d) to reduce their risk' after an informed decision-making process, with careful consideration of risks and benefits. Because the overall benefits to health and survival have not been established, the decision to use tamoxifen for risk reduction depends on an individual woman's perception of her breast-cancer risk and her reaction to this risk. On the basis of current information, the routine use of raloxifene should be reserved for its approved indication, the prevention or treatment of bone loss in postmenopausal women.

The identification of appropriate candidates for tamoxifen therapy requires assessment of breast-cancer risk, estimation of the risks and benefits of tamoxifen, and informed decision making, with full participation by the patient. A recent comprehensive review outlines methods for the assessment of breast-cancer risk. Risk–benefit indexes for general tamoxifen use for breast-cancer risk reduction can be estimated from published tables that incorporate breast-cancer risk, age, race, and the presence or absence of a uterus. This projection is then adjusted by considering individual risk factors for endometrial cancer, stroke, vascular events, and fractures such as obesity, smoking, and hypertension. Although there is hope for future improvement, the inexact nature of the current process should be recognized, and the information should be discussed in the context of a patient's individual concerns and circumstances. Efforts are under way to develop methods of conveying this complex medical and numerical information.

The use of tamoxifen in combination with raloxifene or other hormonal agents (such as estrogen), or the sequential use of such agents, has not been well studied and should be avoided in clinical practice.

Observational results suggest that prophylactic surgery, including bilateral mastectomy or bilateral oophorectomy, reduces breast-cancer risk, although there have been no prospective clinical trials of these procedures. Prophylactic surgery is a reasonable approach only in women at substantial risk for breast cancer who are willing to accept its irreversible consequences. Lifestyle change is a prudent approach to reducing the risk of breast cancer but is currently supported only by observational studies and preclinical evidence.

Risk reduction in women at greatly increased risk for breast cancer because of germ-line mutations remains a dilemma. The use of tamoxifen in women with *BRCA1* or *BRCA2* mutations is currently based on inference, since current studies have yet to identify a sufficient number of women with mutations to evaluate efficacy. Observational studies suggest that prophylactic mastectomy and oophorectomy are beneficial in women with *BRCA1* and *BRCA2* mutations. Although published decision analyses compare predicted outcomes of various interventions, their value is limited by the uncertainty surrounding the estimates of the magnitude of the reduction in risk associated with the interventions. Further studies in this important population are critically needed.

The era of risk reduction with respect to breast cancer has arrived. Although many questions remain, current evidence is sufficient to support the informed application of selected interventions in women at risk for this disease.

Prophylactic surgery in women with a hereditary predisposition to breast and ovarian cancer.

Eisen A, Rebbeck TR, Wood WC, Weber BL.

Department of Medicine, Biostatistics and Epidemiology, and Genetics, University of Pennsylvania School of Medicine, Philadelphia, PA, USA.

Journal of Clinical Oncology 18(9):1980–95, 2000, May.

Purpose: To review the published literature on the efficacy and adverse effects of prophylactic mastectomy (PM) and prophylactic oophorectomy (PO) in women with a hereditary predisposition to breast and ovarian cancer and to provide management recommendations for these women. *Methods:* Using the terms 'prophylactic,' 'preventive,' 'bilateral,' 'mastectomy,' 'oophorectomy,' and 'ovariectomy,' a MEDLINE search of the English-language literature for articles related to PM and PO was performed. The bibliographies of these articles were reviewed to identify additional relevant references. *Results:* There have been no prospective trials of PM or PO for the reduction of breast cancer or ovarian cancer incidence or mortality. Most of the available retrospective studies are composed of women who had surgery for a variety of indications and in whom genetic risk was not well characterized. However, some reports in women at increased risk of breast or ovarian cancer have shown that PM and PO can reduce cancer incidence. *Conclusion:* Interest in and use of PM and PO are high among physicians and high-risk women. PM and PO seem to be associated with considerable reduction in the risk of breast and ovarian cancer, albeit incomplete. The surgical morbidity of PM and PO is low, but the complications of premature menopause may be significant, and few studies address quality-of-life issues in women who have opted for PM and PO. Management recommendations for high-risk individuals are presented on the basis of the available evidence.

Short-term breast cancer prediction by random periareolar fine-needle aspiration cytology and the Gail risk model.

Fabian CJ, Kimler BF, Zalles CM, Klemp JR, Kamel S, Zeiger S, Mayo MS.

Division of Clinical Oncology, Department of Internal Medicine, University of Kansas Medical Center, Kansas City, KS, USA.

Journal of the National Cancer Institute 92(15):1217–27, 2000, August 2.

Background: Biomarkers are needed to refine short-term breast cancer risk estimates from epidemiologic models and to measure response to prevention interventions. The purpose of our study was to determine whether the cytologic appearance of epithelial cells obtained from breast random periareolar fine-needle aspirates or molecular marker expression in these cells was associated with later breast cancer development. *Methods:* Four hundred eighty women who were eligible on the basis of a family history of breast cancer, prior precancerous biopsy, and/or prior invasive cancer were enrolled in a single-institution, prospective trial. Their risk of breast cancer according to the Gail model was calculated, and random periareolar fine-needle aspiration was performed at study entry. Cells were characterized morphologically and analyzed for DNA aneuploidy by image analysis and for the expression of epidermal growth factor receptor, estrogen receptor, p53 protein, and HER2/NEU protein by immunocytochemistry. All statistical tests are two-sided. *Results:* At a median follow-up time of 45 months after initial aspiration, 20 women have developed breast cancer (invasive disease in 13 and ductal carcinoma in situ in seven). With the use of multiple logistic regression and Cox proportional hazards analysis, subsequent cancer was predicted by evidence of hyperplasia with atypia in the initial fine-needle aspirate and a 10-year

Gail projected probability of developing breast cancer. Although expression of epidermal growth factor receptor, estrogen receptor, p53, and HER2/NEU was statistically significantly associated with hyperplasia with atypia, it did not predict the development of breast cancer in multivariable analysis. *Conclusion:* Cytomorphology from breast random periareolar fine-needle aspirates can be used with the Gail risk model to identify a cohort of women at very high short-term risk for developing breast cancer. We recommend that cytomorphology be studied for use as a potential surrogate end point in prevention trials.

Risk of breast cancer with oral contraceptive use in women with a family history of breast cancer.

Grabrick DM, Hartmann LC, Cerhan JR, Vierkant RA, Therneau TM, Vachon CM, Olson JE, Couch FJ, Anderson KE, Pankratz VS, Sellers TA.

Department of Health Sciences Research, Mayo Clinic, Rochester, MN, USA.

Journal of the American Medical Association 284(14): 1791–8, 2000, October 11.

Context: Oral contraceptive (OC) use is weakly associated with breast cancer risk in the general population, but the association among women with a familial predisposition to breast cancer is less clear. *Objective:* To determine whether the association between OC use and risk of breast cancer is influenced by family history of the disease. *Design and setting:* Historical cohort study of 426 families of breast cancer probands diagnosed between 1944 and 1952 at the Tumor Clinic of the University of Minnesota Hospital. Follow-up data on families were collected by telephone interview between 1991 and 1996. *Participants:* A total of 394 sisters and daughters of the probands, 3002 granddaughters and nieces, and 2754 women who married into the families. *Main outcome measure:* Relative risk (RR) of breast cancer associated with history of OC use by relationship to proband. *Results:* After accounting for age and birth cohort, ever having used OCs was associated with significantly increased risk of breast cancer among sisters and daughters of the probands (RR, 3.3; 95% confidence interval [CI], 1.6–6.7), but not among granddaughters and nieces of the probands (RR, 1.2; 95% CI, 0.8–2.0) or among marry-ins (RR, 1.2; 95% CI, 0.8–1.9). Results were essentially unchanged after adjustment for parity, age at first birth, age at menarche, age at menopause, oophorectomy, smoking, and education. The elevated risk among women with a first-degree family history of breast cancer was most evident for OC use during or prior to 1975, when formulations were likely to contain higher dosages of estrogen and progestins (RR, 3.3; 95% CI, 1.5–7.2). A small number of breast cancer cases ($n = 2$) limited the statistical power to detect risk among women with a first-degree relative with breast cancer and OC use after 1975. *Conclusions:* These results suggest that women who have ever used earlier formulations of OCs and who also have a first-degree relative with breast cancer may be at particularly high risk for breast cancer. Further studies of women with a strong family history who have used more recent lower-dosage formulations of OCs are needed to determine how women with a familial predisposition to breast cancer should be advised regarding OC use today.

Gene-expression profiles in hereditary breast cancer.

Hedenfalk I, Duggan D, Chen Y, Radmacher M, Bittner M, Simon R, Meltzer P, Gusterson B, Esteller M, Raffeld M, Yakhini Z, Ben-Dor A, Dougherty E, Kononen J, Bubendorf L, Fehrle W, Pittaluga S, Gruvberger S, Loman N, Johannsson O, Olsson H, Wilfond B, Sauter G, Kallioniemi OP, Borg A, Trent J.

Cancer Genetics Branch (IH, DD, YC, MB, PM, O-PK, JT) and the Medical Genetics Branch (BW), National Human Genome Research Institute, and the Division of Cancer Treatment and Diagnosis, National Cancer Institute (MR, RS), National Institutes of Health, Bethesda, MD, USA; the Department of Oncology, University of Lund, Lund, Sweden (IH, AB); the Department of Pathology, Western Infirmary, University of Glasgow, Glasgow, Scotland, UK (BG); and the Division of Tumor Biology, Johns Hopkins Oncology Center, Baltimore, MD, USA (ME).

New England Journal of Medicine 344:539–48, 2001 February.

Background: Many cases of hereditary breast cancer are due to mutations in either the *BRCA1* or the *BRCA2* gene. The histopathological changes in these cancers are often characteristic of the mutant gene. We hypothesized that the genes expressed by these two types of tumors are also distinctive, perhaps allowing us to identify cases of hereditary breast cancer on the basis of gene-expression profiles. *Methods:* RNA from samples of primary tumors from seven carriers of the *BRCA1* mutation, seven carriers of the *BRCA2* mutation, and seven patients with sporadic cases of breast cancer was compared with a microarray of 6512 complementary DNA clones of 5361 genes. Statistical analyses were used to identify a set of genes that could distinguish the *BRCA1* genotype from the *BRCA2* genotype. *Results:* Permutation analysis of multivariate classification functions established that the gene-expression profiles of tumors with *BRCA1* mutations, tumors with *BRCA2* mutations, and sporadic tumors differed significantly from each other. An analysis of variance between the levels of gene expression and the genotype of the samples identified 176 genes that were differentially expressed in tumors with *BRCA1* mutations and tumors with *BRCA2* mutations. Given the known properties of some of the genes in this panel, our findings indicate that there are functional differences between breast tumors with *BRCA1* mutations and those with *BRCA2* mutations. *Conclusions:* Significantly different groups of genes are expressed by breast cancers with *BRCA1* mutations and breast cancers with *BRCA2* mutations. Our results suggest that a heritable mutation influences the gene-expression profile of the cancer.

Intention to undergo prophylactic bilateral mastectomy in women at increased risk of developing hereditary breast cancer.

Meiser B, Butow P, Friedlander M, Schnieden V, Gattas M, Kirk J, Suthers G, Haan E, Tucker K.

Hereditary Cancer Clinic and Department of Liaison Psychiatry, Prince of Wales Hospital, New South Wales, Australia.

Journal of Clinical Oncology 18(11):2250–7, 2000, June.

Purpose: To assess intention to undergo prophylactic bilateral mastectomy and psychologic determinants in unaffected women at increased risk of developing hereditary breast cancer. *Patients and methods:* Three hundred and thirty-three women who were awaiting their initial appointments for risk assessment, advice about surveillance, and prophylactic options at one of 14 familial cancer clinics participated in a cross-sectional, questionnaire-based survey. *Results:* Nineteen percent of women would consider and 47% would not consider a prophylactic mastectomy, should genetic testing identify a mutation in a breast cancer-predisposing gene, whereas 34% were unsure and 1% had already undergone a prophylactic mastectomy. In a bivariate analysis, women at a moderately increased risk of developing breast cancer had the highest proportion of subjects reporting that they would consider a prophylactic mastectomy (25%), compared with women at high risk (16%) (χ^2 = 7.79; p = 0.051). In multivariate analyses, consideration of prophylactic mastectomy strongly correlated with high levels of breast cancer anxiety (odds ratio [OR] = 17.4; 95% confidence interval [CI], 4.35 to 69.71; p = 0.0001) and overestimation of one's breast cancer risk (OR = 3.01; 95% CI, 1.43 to 6.32; p = 0.0036), whereas there was no association with objective breast cancer risk (p = 0.60). *Conclusion:* A significant proportion of women at increased risk of developing hereditary breast cancer would consider prophylactic mastectomy. Although prophylactic mastectomy may be appropriate in women at high risk of developing breast cancer, it is perhaps less so in those who have a moderately increased risk. Such moderate-risk women are likely to benefit from interventions aimed at reducing breast cancer anxiety and correcting exaggerated breast cancer risk perceptions.

Prophylactic mastectomy.

Newman LA, Kuerer HM, Hung KK, Vlastos G, Ames FC, Ross MI, Singletary SE.

Department of Surgical Oncology, The University of Texas MD Anderson Cancer Center, Houston, TX, USA.

Journal of the American College of Surgeons 191(3): 322–30, 2000, September.

The Society of Surgical Oncology has developed a position statement that lists conditions warranting consideration of prophylactic mastectomy. It must be stressed that there are no absolute indications for prophylactic mastectomy. The data are limited about the efficacy of prophylactic mastectomy in humans, but recent studies suggest that it results in up to 90% reduction in the risk for breast cancer. Total mastectomy is technically a more definitive procedure, although reported series have had a predominance of patients undergoing subcutaneous, nipple-sparing procedures. Prophylactic mastectomy may improve longevity in BRCA mutation carriers, but this must be balanced against the impact on quality of life. The benefits of prophylactic mastectomy relative to chemoprevention are unclear because there are no prospective randomized studies comparing these two strategies. Contralateral prophylactic mastectomy in patients with a unilateral cancer is unlikely to improve survival, but this approach may be considered for high-risk or difficult-to-observe patients, to facilitate breast reconstruction, and for the psychologic benefits. Patients considering prophylactic mastectomy should be well informed of risk-reduction alternatives and the limitations in the efficacy and cosmetic results of the procedure.

Women's regrets after bilateral prophylactic mastectomy.

Payne DK, Biggs C, Tran KN, Borgen PI, Massie MJ.

Barbara White Fishman Center for Psychological Counseling of the Department of Psychiatry and Behavioral Sciences, Memorial Sloan-Kettering Cancer Center, New York, NY, USA.

Annals of Surgical Oncology 7(2):150–4, 2000, March.

Background: Primary prevention strategies such as chemopreventive agents (e.g., tamoxifen) and bilateral prophylactic mastectomy (PM) have received increasingly more attention as management options for women at high risk of developing breast cancer. *Methods:* A total of 370 women, who had registered in the Memorial Sloan-Kettering Cancer Center National Prophylactic Mastectomy Registry, reported having undergone a bilateral PM. Twenty-one of these women expressed regrets about their decision to have a PM. A psychiatrist and psychologist interviewed 19 of the women about their experiences with the PM. *Results:* A physician-initiated rather than patient-initiated discussion about the PM represented the most common factor in these women. Psychological distress and the unavailability of psychological and rehabilitative support throughout the process were the most commonly reported regrets. Additional regrets about the PM related to cosmesis, perceived difficulty of detecting breast cancer in the remaining breast tissue, surgical complications, residual pain, lack of education about the procedure, concerns about consequent body image, and sexual dysfunction. *Conclusions:* Although a PM statistically reduces the chances of a woman developing breast cancer, the possibility of significant physical and psychological sequelae remains. Careful evaluation, education, and support both before and after the procedure will potentially reduce the level of distress and dissatisfaction in these women. We discuss recommendations for the appropriate surgical and psychiatric evaluation of women who are considering a PM as risk-reducing surgery.

Uncommon high-risk lesions of the breast diagnosed at stereotactic core-needle biopsy: clinical importance.

Philpotts LE, Shaheen NA, Jain KS, Carter D, Lee CH.

Department of Diagnostic Radiology, Yale University School of Medicine, New Haven, CT, USA.

Radiology 216(3):831–7, 2000, September.

Purpose: To assess the outcome of papillary lesions, radial scars, or lobular carcinoma in situ (LCIS) diagnosed at stereotactic core-needle biopsy (SCNB). *Materials and methods:* Retrospective review of 1,236 lesions sampled with SCNB yielded 22 papillary lesions, nine radial scars, and five LCIS lesions. Diffuse lesions such as papillomatosis, papillary ductal hyperplasia, papillary ductal carcinoma in situ (DCIS), and atypical lobular hyperplasia were not included. The mammographic findings, associated histologic features, and outcome were assessed for each case. *Results:* Sixteen papillary lesions were diagnosed as benign at SCNB. Of these, five were benign at excision, and 10 were unremarkable at mammographic follow-up. At excision of an unusual lesion containing a microscopic papillary lesion, DCIS was found. Three of four papillary lesions suspicious at SCNB proved to be papillary carcinomas; the fourth had no residual carcinoma at excision. Eight of nine radial scars were excised, which revealed atypical hyperplasia in four scars but no malignancies. One LCIS lesion was found at excision to contain DCIS. *Conclusion:* Benign or malignant papillary lesions were accurately diagnosed with SCNB in the majority of cases. Cases diagnosed as suspicious for malignancy or with atypia or unusual associated histologic findings should be excised. No malignancies were found at excision of radial scars diagnosed at SCNB. Surgical removal of these lesions following SCNB may not be routinely necessary. DCIS was found in one lesions diagnosed as LCIS at SCNB, which suggests that removal of these lesions may be prudent.

Estimation of tamoxifen's efficacy for preventing the formation and growth of breast tumors.

Radmacher MD, Simon R.

Biometric Research Branch, Division of Cancer Treatment and Diagnosis, National Cancer Institute, Bethesda, MD, USA.

Journal of the National Cancer Institute 92(1):48–53, 2000, January 5.

Background: Several randomized clinical trials have tested the hypothesis that tamoxifen is effective in preventing breast cancer. The largest such trial, the National Surgical Adjuvant Breast and Bowel Project's Breast Cancer Prevention Trial (BCPT), reported a 49% reduction in risk of invasive breast cancer for the tamoxifen group. However, it is unclear whether the effect of tamoxifen in this trial was mainly due to prevention of newly forming tumors or to treatment of occult disease. *Methods:* We used various tumor growth models (i.e., exponential and Gompertzian [growth limited by tumor size]) and a computer simulation to approximate the percentage of detected tumors that were initiated after study entry. Maximum likelihood techniques were then used to estimate separately the efficacy of tamoxifen in treating occult disease and in preventing the formation and growth of new tumors. *Results:* Under the assumptions of most of the growth models, the trial was sufficiently long for substantial numbers of new tumors to form, grow, and be detected during the trial. With the Gompertzian model and all available incidence data from the BCPT, it was estimated that 60% (95% confidence interval [CI] = 40%–80%) fewer new tumors were detected in the tamoxifen group than in the placebo group. Likewise, 35% (95% CI = 6%–63%) fewer occult tumors were detected in the tamoxifen group. With this model, the estimated incidence rate of invasive breast cancer among women in the placebo group of the BCPT was 7.7 (95% CI = 6.6–8.9) per 1000 women per year. Similar results were obtained with three exponential tumor growth models. *Conclusions:* These results support the concept that tamoxifen reduced cancer incidence in the BCPT through both treatment of occult disease and prevention of new tumor formation and growth. However, data from prevention trials may never be sufficient to completely distinguish prevention of new tumor formation from treatment of occult disease.

Comment in: *J Natl Cancer Inst* 92(11):943–4, 2000, June 7.

Familial invasive breast cancers: worse outcome related to *BRCA1* mutations.

Stoppa-Lyonnet D, Ansquer Y, Dreyfus H, Gautier C, Gauthier-Villars M, Bourstyn E, Clough KB, Magdelenat H, Pouillart P, Vincent-Salomon A, Fourquet A, Asselain B.

Departments of Oncology Genetics, Biostatistics, Radiotherapy, Surgery, Pharmacology, Medical Oncology, and Pathology, Institut Curie, Paris, France.

Journal of Clinical Oncology 18(24):4053–9, 2000, December 15.

Purpose: Although all studies confirm that *BRCA1* tumors are highly proliferative and poorly differentiated, their outcomes remain controversial. We propose to examine, through a cohort study, the pathologic characteristics, overall survival, local recurrence, and metastasis-free intervals of 40 patients with *BRCA1* breast cancer. *Patients and methods:* A cohort of 183 patients with invasive breast cancer, treated at the Institut Curie and presenting with a familial history of breast and/or ovarian cancer, were tested for *BRCA1* germline mutation. Tumor characteristics and clinical events were extracted from our prospectively registered database. *Results:* Forty *BRCA1* mutations were found among the 183 patients (22%). Median follow-up was 58 months. *BRCA1* tumors were larger in size ($p = 0.03$), had a higher rate of grade 3 histoprognostic factors ($p = 0.002$), and had a higher frequency of negative estrogen ($p = 0.003$) and progesterone receptors ($p = 0.002$) compared with non-*BRCA1* tumors. Overall survival was poorer for carriers than for noncarriers (5-year rate, 80% v 91%, $p = 0.002$). Because a long time interval between cancer diagnosis and genetic counseling artificially increases survival time due to unrecorded deaths, the analysis was limited to the 110 patients whose diagnosis-to-counseling interval was less than 36 months (19 *BRCA1* patients and 91 non-*BRCA1* patients). The differences between the *BRCA1* and non-*BRCA1* groups regarding overall survival and metastasis-free interval were dramatically increased (49% v 85% and 18% v 84%, respectively). Multivariate analysis showed that *BRCA1* mutation was an independent prognostic factor. *Conclusion:* Our results strongly support that among patients with familial breast cancer, those who have a *BRCA1* mutation have a worse outcome than those who do not.

Breast cancer prevention: a review of current evidence.

Vogel VG.

Comprehensive Breast Program, Magee-Womens Hospital, University of Pittsburgh Cancer Institute, PA, USA.

CA: A Cancer Journal for Clinicians 50(3):156–70, 2000, May–June.

The National Cancer Institute has created a breast cancer risk assessment tool that quickly estimates a woman's individualized absolute risk of developing breast cancer. Understanding the magnitude of risk is important because recent data show that breast cancer incidence may be reduced. All women may improve their overall health and thus perhaps minimize breast cancer risk by maintaining a healthy weight, avoiding cigarettes, limiting alcohol consumption, getting regular exercise, and avoiding nondiagnostic ionizing radiation. Nevertheless, no lifestyle modifications have yet been proven to prevent or definitively lower the risk of breast cancer. In addition, women whose personal breast cancer risk is high may consider reducing risk by pharmacologic or surgical means. In such women, a five-year course of tamoxifen reduced the risk of invasive breast cancer by 49%; women with lobular carcinoma in situ or atypical hyperplasia experienced even greater risk reductions. Because of the potential for vascular and endometrial side effects, women who are candidates for a preventive course of tamoxifen must be counseled regarding its relative risks and benefits. Prophylactic mastectomy offers at least a 90% reduction in the risk of breast cancer, but the physical and psychological changes involved in such a procedure make it a difficult choice for many women. Breast cancer risk assessment and appropriate counseling are becoming standard components of breast cancer screening and overall health maintenance.

11

Ductal carcinoma *in situ* of the breast

MELVIN J SILVERSTEIN, KRISTIN A SKINNER, AND JAMES R WAISMAN

INTRODUCTION

As two of the authors are surgeons, the majority of this chapter is surgical in its orientation. It does, however, briefly review the incidence, biology, natural history, and pathology of ductal carcinoma *in situ* (DCIS) before discussing diagnostic and treatment considerations. It also deals briefly with lobular carcinoma *in situ* (LCIS). Although we review the work of others, our opinions are biased by our own experiences.

Our personal data and experience come from The Van Nuys Breast Center in Van Nuys California,[1,2] and the Harold E. and Henrietta C. Lee Breast Center at Kenneth Norris Comprehensive Cancer Center on the campus of the University of Southern California School of Medicine. Our personal DCIS series includes 821 patients treated from 1979 through mid-1999 and we refer to that series frequently.

Until 1980, the treatment for most patients with DCIS was mastectomy. Currently, the data suggest that most patients with DCIS can be successfully treated with breast preservation, with or without radiation therapy. In this chapter, we attempt to show you how we use easily available data to help in the complex treatment-selection process.

Terms, definitions, and incidence

Ductal carcinoma *in situ* is most commonly referred to as DCIS. It is also often called intraductal carcinoma, non-invasive ductal carcinoma, or *in situ* duct carcinoma. We believe that ductal carcinoma *in situ* or *in situ* duct carcinoma are the preferred terms. The words *in situ* connote a less aggressive concept. Conversely, the words intraductal carcinoma, to a patient not schooled in the subtleties of breast cancer, evoke the same fear as colon carcinoma or lung carcinoma.

DCIS is a heterogeneous group of lesions,[3,4] in which, presumably, malignant epithelial cells proliferate within the ductal system but no evidence of invasion through the basement membrane is demonstrable by light microscopy. The lesion generally begins in the small to moderate-sized ducts. It is highly variable in its appearance, biology, and behavior. It is a disease so confusing that it is not uncommon for patients to seek second, third, and fourth opinions, and to receive a diverse spectrum of advice ranging from biopsy only, to wide excision, segmental resection, quadrant resection, mastectomy, or even bilateral mastectomy. With all treatments other than mastectomy, radiation therapy may or may not be advised. In other words, the advice ranges from nothing to everything, and there are physicians willing to support most of these options.[5]

Prior to 1980, DCIS was a rare disease, representing about 1% of all breast cancer and generally presenting as a palpable mass, nipple discharge, or Paget's disease.[6] Since 1980, with the acceptance and increased use of mammography, the clinical presentation of DCIS has changed dramatically. Today, most DCIS is non-palpable and discovered mammographically.

From 1979 to 1981, the Van Nuys group treated a total of only 15 patients with DCIS, five per year. Only two lesions (13%) were detected by mammography. Van Nuys added two state-of-the-art mammography units and a full-time experienced mammographer in 1982 and suddenly we were diagnosing more than 30 new DCIS cases per year, most of them non-palpable. When third and fourth machines were added, the group began diagnosing 40–50 cases per year. Analysis of the entire series of 821 patients reveals that 701 (85%) lesions were detected by mammography alone. If we look at only those diagnosed since 1992, 91% were non-palpable.

Today, DCIS represents at least 15–20% of all newly diagnosed cases of breast cancer,[7,8] and as much as 20–40% of cases diagnosed by mammography.[9,10] In 1999, there were more than 40 000 new cases of DCIS.[11]

It is not clear whether the entire increase in breast cancer incidence can be explained by increased and improved mammography, or whether there is also a true increase in the incidence of breast cancer.

NATURAL HISTORY

Because most patients with DCIS have been treated with mastectomy, our knowledge of the natural history of this disease is relatively scant. The main questions revolve around which lesions will become invasive and when that will happen. In a study of 110 consecutive, medicolegal autopsies of young and middle-aged women between the ages of 20 and 54 years, 14% were found to have DCIS,[12] suggesting that the subclinical prevalence of DCIS is significantly higher than the clinical expression of the disease.

The studies of Page et al.[13] and Rosen et al.[14] enlighten us regarding the non-treatment of lower grade DCIS. In these studies, patients with non-comedo DCIS were initially misdiagnosed with benign lesions and therefore went untreated. Subsequent analysis of these patients revealed that approximately 25% developed invasive breast cancer, generally during the first 10 years. Had the lesions been high-grade comedo DCIS, we would expect that the invasive breast cancer rate would have been significantly higher than 25%. With few exceptions, in both of these studies, the invasive breast carcinoma was of the ductal type and located at the site of the original DCIS. These findings and the fact that autopsy series have revealed up to a 14% incidence of DCIS show that not all DCIS lesions progress to invasive breast cancer or become clinically significant.[12,15]

Page and associates recently updated their series.[16] Of 28 women with low-grade DCIS misdiagnosed as benign lesions and treated with biopsy only between 1950 and 1968, ten have recurred locally, nine with invasive breast cancer. This is a 42% actuarial local recurrence rate projected to 30 years of follow-up. Five of these patients have died of metastatic breast cancer, a 22% actuarial breast cancer-specific mortality rate at 30 years. At first, these recurrence and mortality rates are alarming. However, they are only slightly worse than what can be expected with long-term follow-up of patients with lobular carcinoma in situ, a disease that most clinicians are willing to treat with careful clinical follow-up. In addition, these patients were treated with biopsy only. No attempt was made to excise these lesions with a clear surgical margin.

PATHOLOGY

The concept of pre-invasive carcinoma of the breast was recognized by Cheatle as early as 1906.[17] In 1932, Broders used the term in situ to describe the non-invasive stage of breast cancer.[18] The difficulty in diagnosing intraductal lesions was discussed by Foote and Stewart in 1946.[19] The challenge of differentiating between highly atypical proliferative lesions and in situ carcinoma remains today.[20,21] Page and associates reviewed the pathology of over 10 000 breast biopsies and were able to establish qualitative and quantitative criteria differentiating proliferative lesions with and without atypia and DCIS.[22,23]

Although there is no universally accepted histopathologic classification, most pathologists divide DCIS into five architectural subtypes (papillary, micropapillary, cribriform, solid, and comedo), and often compare the first four (non-comedo) with comedo.[9,24,25] Comedo DCIS is frequently associated with high nuclear grade,[9,24,25] aneuploidy[26] a higher proliferation rate,[27] HER2/neu gene amplification or protein overexpression,[28-33] and clinically more aggressive behavior.[34-37] Non-comedo lesions tend to be just the opposite. The division by architecture between comedo are non-comedo lesions, however, is an oversimplification, because high nuclear grade non-comedo lesions may express similar markers to high-grade comedo lesions and, as discussed later in this chapter, such lesions may require more aggressive treatment. Adding to the confusion is the fact that frequent admixtures of the various architectural subtypes within a single biopsy specimen are common. In our series, 72% of all lesions had significant amounts of two or more architectural subtypes. It is clear, however, that lesions exhibiting a predominant comedo DCIS pattern are generally more aggressive and more likely to recur if treated conservatively than non-comedo lesions.

Recently, the concept of high nuclear grade has assumed greater importance. Nuclear grade, which is more of a biologic mirror than architecture, is emerging as a key histopathologic factor for identifying aggressive behavior.[24,25,34,36,38-41] With this in mind, in 1995 we introduced a new histopathologic DCIS classification.[38] Three groups of DCIS patients were defined (Plates 2–4) by the presence of high nuclear grade (nuclear grade 3) to select the most aggressive group, group 3. The remaining non-high-grade lesions (nuclear grades 1 or 2) were then divided by the presence (group 2) or absence (group 1) of comedo-type necrosis (Figure 11.1), which has also been shown to be a marker of more aggressive behavior.[9,41]

Nuclear grade was scored in the following manner. Essentially, low-grade nuclei (grade 1) were defined as nuclei 1–1.5 red blood cells in diameter, with diffuse chromatin and unapparent nucleoli. Intermediate nuclei (grade 2) were defined as nuclei 1–2 red blood cells in diameter, with coarse chromatin and infrequent nucleoli. High-grade nuclei (grade 3) were defined as nuclei with a diameter > 2 red blood cells, with vesicular chromatin and one or more nucleoli.[9]

Traditional comedo-type DCIS with central lumina containing necrotic debris surrounded by large pleomorphic viable cells in solid masses was classified as showing comedo-type necrosis.[41] Other architectural patterns of DCIS, such as cribriform or micropapillary, with substantial amounts of necrotic neoplastic cells of duct origin within duct lumina were also classified as showing comedo-type necrosis.

No requirement was made for a specific amount of high nuclear grade DCIS. In other words, the presence of any amount of high-grade DCIS, no matter how little, warrants classification as a group 3 lesion. Similarly, there was no requirement for a minimum amount of comedo-type necrosis. Occasional desquamated or individually necrotic cells were ignored and were not scored as comedo-type necrosis.

We chose high nuclear grade as the most important factor in our classification because there is general agreement that patients with high nuclear grade lesions are likely to do worse than patients with low nuclear grade lesions.[24,25,34,38–41] Comedo-type necrosis was chosen because it is easy to recognize[42] and its presence suggests a poor prognosis.[35–37,43] In addition, it has been suggested

that there is an association between the differentiation of DCIS and the histological grade of coexistent invasive cancer;[44] this proposal could imply that nuclear grade is a factor in the progression of *in situ* breast cancers to invasive disease, although proof is lacking.

The most difficult part of most classifications is nuclear grading, particularly the intermediate grade lesions. The subtleties of the intermediate grade lesion are not important to our classification; only nuclear grade 3 need be recognized. The cells must be large and pleomorphic, lack architectural differentiation and polarity, have prominent nucleoli and coarse clumped chromatin, and generally show mitoses.[9,24,25,41]

The classification is useful because it divides DCIS into three groups with different risks of local recurrence after breast conservation therapy (Figure 11.2). This histopathologic classification, when combined with tumor size and margin status, is an integral part of the Van Nuys Prognostic Index, a system that is explained in more detail below.

MICROINVASION AND OCCULT INVASION

The incidence of microinvasion is difficult to quantitate because, until recently, there was no formal and universally accepted definition of exactly what constitutes microinvasion. The most recent edition of the *Breast tumors in TNM atlas* now defines microinvasion as one or more foci of invasion, none of which is more than 1 mm in diameter.[45]

Using this strict definition, relatively few lesions are considered DCIS with microinvasion (DCIS-Mi). If a lesion measures 1.1–5 mm, it is classified as a T1a invasive breast carcinoma with an extensive intraductal component (EIC). If it measures 1 mm or less, the area of invasion must be unequivocal. If the focus of invasion is

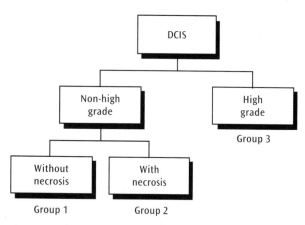

Figure 11.1 *Pathologic classification. DCIS patients are sorted into high nuclear grade and non-high nuclear grade. Non-high nuclear grade cases are then sorted by the presence or absence of comedo-type necrosis. Lesions in group 3 (high nuclear grade) may or may not show comedo-type necrosis.*

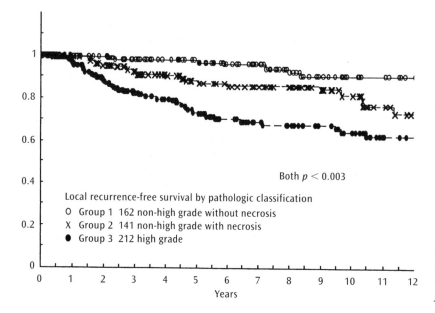

Figure 11.2 *The probability of local recurrence-free survival using the Van Nuys DCIS pathologic classification for 515 breast conservation patients.*

not unequivocal, the lesion is classified as DCIS without microinvasion.

The reported incidence of occult invasion (invasive disease at mastectomy in patients with a biopsy diagnosis of DCIS) varies highly, ranging from as little as 2% to as much as 21%.[39,46] This problem was elegantly addressed in the investigations of Lagios et al.,[34,39] who performed a meticulous serial subgross dissection correlated with specimen radiography. Occult invasion was found in 13 of 111 mastectomy specimens from patients who had initially undergone excisional biopsy of DCIS. All occult invasive cancers were associated with DCIS greater than 45 mm in diameter; the incidence of occult invasion approached 50% for DCIS greater than 55 mm. In the study of Gump et al.,[47] foci of occult invasion were found in 11% of patients with palpable DCIS but in no patients with clinically occult DCIS. These results suggest a correlation between the size of the DCIS lesion and the incidence of occult invasion.

MULTICENTRICITY AND MULTIFOCALITY

Multicentricity is defined as DCIS in a quadrant other than the quadrant in which the original DCIS was diagnosed (index quadrant). There must be normal breast tissue separating the two foci. However, definitions of multicentricity vary from author to author. Hence, the reported incidence of multicentricity also varies. Rates from zero to 78%,[39,48–51] averaging about 30%, have been reported.

Holland evaluated 119 mastectomy specimens by taking a whole organ section every 5 mm.[52,53] Each section was radiographed. Paraffin blocks were made from every radiographically suspicious spot. In addition, an average of 25 blocks was taken from the quadrant containing the index cancer; random samples were taken from all other quadrants, the central subareolar area, and the nipple. The microscopic extension of each lesion was verified on the radiographs. This technique permitted a three-dimensional reconstruction of each lesion. This elegant study demonstrated that most DCIS lesions were larger than expected (50% greater than 50 mm), involved more than one quadrant by continuous extension (23%), but, most importantly, were unifocal (99%). Only 1 of 119 mastectomy specimens (0.8%) had 'true' multicentric distribution with a separate lesion in a different quadrant. From this, it is clear that complete excision of a DCIS lesion is possible due to unifocality, but may be extremely difficult due to larger than expected size. This information, when combined with the fact that most local recurrences are at or near the original DCIS (91% in our series), suggests that the concept of multicentricity per se is not important in the treatment decision-making process.

Multifocality is defined as separate foci of DCIS within the same quadrant. The studies of Holland et al.[52,53] and Noguchi et al.[54] suggest that multifocality

may be artifactual, resulting from looking at a three-dimensional arborizing entity in two dimensions on a glass slide. It would be analogous to saying that the branches of a tree were not connected if the branches were cut through one plane, placed separately on a slide, and viewed in cross-section.

DETECTION AND DIAGNOSIS

Mammography

During the last 5 years, 91% of our DCIS patients presented with non-palpable lesions. A few percent were detected as random findings during a biopsy for a breast thickening or some other benign fibrocystic change; most lesions, however, were detected by mammography. The most common mammographic findings were microcalcifications, frequently clustered and generally without an associated soft-tissue abnormality. Eighty percent of our DCIS patients exhibited microcalcifications on preoperative mammography. The patterns of these microcalcifications may be focal, diffuse, or ductal, with variable size and shape. Patients with comedo DCIS tend to have 'casting calcifications.' These are linear, branching, or bizarre and are almost pathognomonic for comedo DCIS (Figure 11.3a).[55] Almost all comedo lesions, 90% in our series, have calcifications, that can be visualized on mammography.

Fifty percent of non-comedo lesions in our series did not have mammographic calcifications, making them more difficult to find and the patients more difficult to follow, if treated conservatively. When non-comedo lesions are calcified, they tend to have fine, granular, punctate calcifications (Figure 11.3b).

A major problem confronting surgeons relates to the fact that calcifications do not always map out the entire DCIS lesion, particularly those of the non-comedo subtype. Even though all the calcifications are removed, the surgeon may be leaving some DCIS behind. Sometimes, the majority of the calcifications are benign. In other words, the DCIS lesion may be smaller, larger, or the same size as the calcifications that lead to its identification. Calcifications more accurately approximate the size of comedo lesions than that of non-comedo lesions.[52] Despite these difficulties, the mammographic detection of suspicious microcalcifications in an asymptomatic patient has become extremely important in our understanding of the natural history of DCIS.

Before mammography was common or of good quality, most DCIS was clinically apparent, diagnosed by palpation or inspection; it was gross disease. Gump et al.[47] divided DCIS by method of diagnosis into gross and microscopic disease. Similarly, Schwartz et al.[37] divided DCIS into two groups: clinical and subclinical. Both groups felt patients presenting with a palpable mass, a nipple discharge, or Paget's disease of the nipple required

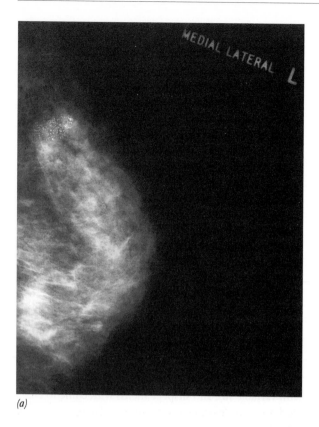

(a)

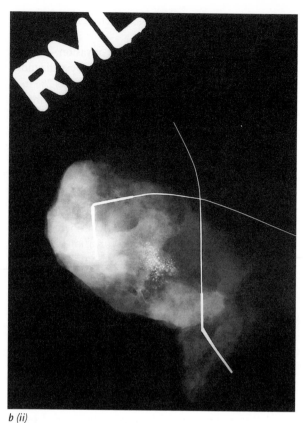

b (ii)

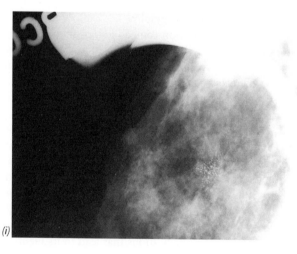

b (i)

Figure 11.3 *(a) Mediolateral mammography in a 43-year-old woman revealed irregular branching calcifications. Histopathology revealed high-grade comedo DCIS, Van Nuys' Group 3. (b) (i) Magnification mammography revealed finely stippled, punctate microcalcifications in a 41-year-old woman. Histopathology revealed a low-grade micropapillary DCIS with necrosis, Van Nuys' Group 2. (ii) Specimen radiography after bracketed wire-directed excision of the lesion. The margin appears widely clear.*

more aggressive treatment. Schwartz believes that palpable DCIS should be treated as though it were an invasive lesion. He suggests that the pathologist simply has not found the area of invasion. Whereas it makes perfect sense to believe that the change from non-palpable to palpable disease is a poor prognostic sign, our group has not been able to demonstrate this for DCIS. In our series, when equivalent patients with palpable and non-palpable DCIS are compared, they do not differ in the rate of local recurrence or mortality. In other words, palpability is not a significant predictor of local recurrence in patients with DCIS. We have, however, demonstrated a poorer prognosis for palpable invasive breast cancer when compared with similarly sized non-palpable invasive breast cancer.[56]

Further mammographic work-up

Most patients with DCIS are identified when their screening mammogram reveals an abnormality. This will probably be microcalcifications, but it could be a non-palpable mass or a subtle architectural distortion. At this point, additional radiologic work-up needs to be done. This may include cone-down compression mammography, magnification views, or ultrasonography. Based on the results of these diagnostic studies, the radiologist will recommend biopsy or short-interval follow-up studies in 3–6 months, depending on how suspicious the abnormality appears. Personally, we do not like putting a patient on hold for 3–6 months if there is significant suspicion about the mammographic abnormality; we think it is anxiety provoking. If it is at all possible, we prefer that a diagnosis, benign or malignant, be made reasonably soon, particularly given the low morbidity of minimally invasive breast biopsy.

Biopsy

If the radiologist suggests biopsy, there are four types:

1 fine-needle aspiration (FNA),
2 stereotactic biopsy,
3 ultrasound-guided biopsy (a more comfortable alternative to stereotactic biopsy if the lesion is discernible on ultrasound),
4 wire-directed open (surgical) biopsy.

FNA is generally of little help for non-palpable DCIS. With FNA, it is possible to obtain cancer cells, but as there is no tissue, there is no architecture. So, whereas the cytopathologist can say that malignant cells are present, the cytopathologist, generally, cannot say whether or not the lesion is invasive.

Stereotactic core biopsy is relatively new and its importance has increased dramatically over the last few years. Dedicated tables with digital attachments (Lorad and Fischer Imaging) make this a precise tool in experienced hands. For DCIS, stereotactic 14-gauge core biopsy presents some problems. Because the biopsy sample is small, one cannot always rule out invasion. Decisions that require a knowledge of whether or not invasion is present, such as axillary node dissection, may need to be based on excision of the entire lesion rather than core biopsy. If multiple core biopsies have been performed and the lesion is subsequently surgically removed, the area of the core biopsies (which were done with a large 14-gauge needle) might be disrupted, making it difficult to tell whether there is true invasion.

This problem was remedied, to a major extent, in the mid-1990s, with the development of a number of new, larger core tissue-acquisition systems for percutaneous minimally invasive breast biopsy. We have experience with one of these, the 11-gauge vacuum-assisted Mammotome probe (Ethicon Endo-Surgery, Cincinnati, OH). This tool takes significantly larger cores of tissue when compared with the 14-gauge needle and affords the ability to sample tissue contiguously. Consequently, upgrading or changing the diagnosis at the time of definitive surgery is far less frequent, only about 5% in large series (personal communication, S Parker, 1999).

If the diagnosis cannot be made with a minimally invasive technique, wire-directed breast biopsy is the next step. We believe that the first attempt to remove this lesion is the most important: the first excision is the best chance to remove the entire lesion and to achieve the best possible cosmetic result. Currently we prefer two to four wires to bracket the lesion (Plates 5 and 6).[57–59] This technique makes complete removal during the initial biopsy more likely. We seldom remove a possible DCIS using a single wire, because it may lead to incomplete removal of the abnormality, calcifications at the edge of the specimen, positive histologic margins, and the need to re-excise the lesion (Plate 7). If a single wire is used, the surgeon should make certain that the excision is adequate by personally reviewing the intraoperative specimen radiography with the radiologist and inspecting the gross margins with the pathologist. The bigger problem, however, is that the distribution of microcalcifications does not always accurately map out the extent of disease. Multiple wires does not help with this problem.

Needle localization, intraoperative specimen radiography, and correlation with the preoperative mammogram should be performed in every non-palpable case. Margins should be inked or dyed and specimens should be serially sectioned at 2–3-mm intervals. The tissue sections should be arranged and processed in sequence. Pathologic evaluation should include a description off all architectural subtypes, nuclear grade, polarization, an assessment of necrosis, the measured or estimated size or extent of the lesion, and the margin status with measurement of the closest margin.

Tumor size should be determined by direct measurement or ocular micrometry from stained slides for smaller lesions. For larger lesions, a combination of direct measurement and estimation, based on the distribution of the lesion in a sequential series of slides, should be used. The proximity of DCIS to an inked margin should be determined by direct measurement or ocular micrometry. The closest single distance between any involved duct containing DCIS and an inked margin should be reported.

If the lesion is large and the diagnosis unproven, we would suggest stereotactic Mammotome biopsy as a first step, to prove that malignant cells are present and to obtain enough tissue to make a definitive diagnosis. If the patient is motivated for breast conservation, a multiple wire-directed excision can be planned. This will give the patient her best chance at two opposing goals: clear margins and good cosmesis. Our best chance at completely removing a large lesion is with a large initial excision. Our best chance at good cosmesis is with a small biopsy. It is the surgeon's job to optimize these opposing goals. A large-quadrant resection should not be performed unless there is cytologic or histologic proof of malignancy or an extremely suspicious (unequivocal) mammogram. This type of resection may lead to breast deformity and, should the diagnosis prove to be benign, the patient will be quite unhappy.

The removal of non-palpable lesions is best performed with an integrated team of surgeon, radiologist, and pathologist. The radiologist who places the wires must be experienced, as must the surgeon who removes the lesion, and the pathologist who processes the tissue.

At Van Nuys Breast Center, we developed an optimal set-up for wire-directed breast biopsy. A pathologist was always with us in the operating room to receive the specimen and to be oriented as to its exact position in the patient. Our pathologist then took the specimen to our radiology department, only 30 m away and on the same floor, where specimen radiology was carried out under the direction of the radiologist who placed the wires. We believe it is a mistake for the pathologist to perform the specimen radiology in the pathology department, particularly if the mammographic abnormality is a subtle mass or an architectural distortion. The pathologist should not be responsible for determining whether or not the surgeon has properly removed an area that was initially identified by another physician, the radiologist.

Ideally, the radiologist who identified the lesion initially should place the wires, read the specimen radiogram, and inform the surgeon and the pathologist that the proper area has been removed and that the margins appear adequate by specimen radiography. When several physicians are involved, passing the case from one to another, there is a greater risk of error.

Once our radiologist confirms that the proper area has been removed, our pathologist returns to the pathology laboratory and dyes the specimen, using a different color for each surface (Plate 8). Should the red surface show involved margins on final histopathologic evaluation, we know it is the superior surface of the biopsy specimen and it will be relatively easy to re-excise. The entire specimen should be serially sectioned and submitted for histologic evaluation (Plate 9). No tissue should be discarded. No frozen sections should be performed on non-palpable lesions. Hormone receptors, DNA analysis, *HER2/neu*, etc. can be determined on the paraffin-fixed blocks.

Once the surgeon has been told that the proper area has been removed, the biopsy cavity should be marked with metallic clips (Plate 10). This will identify the area of the biopsy if radiation therapy is elected or if there is a local recurrence.

Counseling the patient with biopsy-proven DCIS

It is never easy to tell a patient that she has breast cancer; but is DCIS really cancer? When we think of cancer, we generally think of a disease that, if untreated, runs an inexorable course toward death. That is certainly not the case with DCIS. We must emphasize to the patient that she has a borderline cancerous lesion, a 'preinvasive' lesion, which, at this time, is not a threat to her life. In our series of 821 patients with DCIS, the mortality rate is less than 0.8%. Numerous other DCIS series confirm an extremely low mortality rate.[6,9,60,61]

One of the most frequent concerns expressed by patients once a diagnosis of cancer has been made is the fear that the cancer has spread throughout her body. We are able to assure patients with DCIS that no invasion was seen microscopically and the likelihood of systemic spread is minimal.

The patient needs to be educated that the term breast cancer encompasses a multitude of lesions of varying degrees of aggressiveness and lethal potential. The patient with DCIS needs to be reassured that she has a minimal lesion and that she is probably going to need some additional treatment, which may include surgery or radiation therapy, or both. She needs reassurance that she will not need chemotherapy, that her hair will not fall out, and that, in all likelihood, she is not going to die from this lesion. She will, of course, need careful clinical follow-up for the rest of her life.

TREATMENT

Let us start by saying that for most patients there will be no single correct answer. Right or wrong, there will generally be a choice. As the choices increase and become more complicated, frustration will increase for both the patient and her physician.[5]

Mastectomy

Until the 1980s, most breast cancer, including DCIS, was treated with mastectomy. As clinicians began using breast conservation (excision of the tumor, axillary dissection, and whole-breast irradiation) for small invasive lesions, the treatment of DCIS lagged behind. Surgeons continued to perform mastectomies for DCIS while recommending breast conservation for more aggressive invasive lesions. Because of this, there is a large amount of data available regarding outcome after mastectomy for DCIS, although most mastectomy studies reflect lesions that were palpable and generally larger than those routinely discovered today.

Swain, in a review of DCIS, constructed a table consisting of 12 series of DCIS patients with a total of 723 patients treated with mastectomy.[62] The local recurrence rate was 5% (range 0–10%), and the mortality rate was 1.3% (range 0–8%). As you would expect, most of these patients had palpable DCIS. Fowble, in her review, constructed a table of 14 studies containing 1061 patients treated with mastectomy.[63] The local recurrence rate was 1%, and the mortality rate was 1.7%. Barth *et al.*, in their review, constructed a table consisting of 15 studies with 1342 patients. The local recurrence rate was 1.1%, and the mortality rate was 1.3%.[64] There is, of course, significant patient overlap in these three reviews.

In our series, there are 306 patients treated with mastectomy, two of whom (0.7%) have recurred locally (both with invasive lesions), neither of whom (0%) has died from breast cancer. Mastectomy clearly works for DCIS. However, for many patients it represents too much treatment. Mastectomy is deforming and may be psychologically mutilating, even with breast reconstruction. Our challenge is to select for mastectomy only those patients who require it because a lesser procedure will lead to an unacceptably high local recurrence rate.

Mastectomy is indicated for large diffuse lesions, for patients:

with documented multicentric disease (biopsy proof of DCIS in multiple quadrants),

unwilling to take even the slightest increased risk of death due to an invasive recurrence,

who have no interest in breast conservation or who are medically unsuited for breast conservation,

who are unwilling and/or unable to undergo careful clinical follow-up.

In a subsequent section, entitled 'The Van Nuys Prognostic Index,' our guidelines and patient selection process will become clearer.

When mastectomy is required and reconstruction desired, we generally perform a procedure that we call glandular replacement therapy (GRT).[65] This is a combination of skin-sparing mastectomy and autologous tissue reconstruction. Because DCIS does not invade the skin, there is no reason to discard large amounts of skin, as when a mastectomy is performed for a large invasive breast cancer close to or involving overlying skin (Figure 11.4). By saving most of the skin, the original skin envelope is preserved. When this is filled with autologous tissue, it generally yields a breast of similar size, shape, and consistency when compared with the remaining contralateral breast (Figure 11.5). We do not save the nipple. Our usual choice for autologous tissue is a transrectus abdominus myocutaneous (TRAM) flap, either free with microvascular anastomoses or pedical. Reconstruction with latissimus dorsi flaps or implants should be considered for appropriate patients.

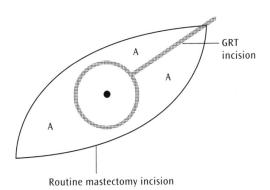

Figure 11.4 *Skin incision for glandular replacement therapy (GRT): skin-sparing mastectomy and immediate reconstruction.*

The danger of local recurrence

Before we go any further, a few words are required about the dangers of local recurrence. If all local recurrences were non-invasive, there would be little indication for mastectomy as the initial procedure. In our own series and in most other reported series, approximately half of all local recurrences are invasive.[9,36,66] Local recurrences are, therefore, extremely important. When they occur in patients who have struggled to save their breasts, they are both demoralizing and, theoretically, a threat to life. By avoiding mastectomy, we gain both psychological and physical advantages, but when there is an invasive recurrence, we have allowed a totally curable, non-invasive lesion to advance to a potentially less curable form. At some point in time, this may translate to a higher mortality rate for patients treated conservatively.

Breast conservation for DCIS

Today, we live in an era in which breast conservation therapy for small invasive tumors is being used more and more frequently. With this in mind, it becomes extremely difficult to justify the continued use of mastectomy for less aggressive, non-invasive disease.

Breast conservation for DCIS is performed differently from breast conservation for invasive lesions. An invasive breast cancer requires excision of the primary lesion with clear margins, axillary node dissection, or at least sentinel node biopsy, whole-breast irradiation, a possible radiation boost to the area of the tumor, and chemotherapy, if nodes are positive or if the primary tumor has poor prognostic features. Breast conservation for DCIS is different. It requires, at a minimum, excision of the primary tumor, generally with clear histologic margins. Radiation therapy may or may not be added. There is no need for chemotherapy or formal axillary dissection.

Because of the serial subgross work of Holland et al.,[52,53] described in the section on multicentricity and multifocality, we now know that, theoretically, many DCIS lesions can be completely excised. Unfortunately, in 23% of Holland et al.'s cases, the lesion occupied more than a full quadrant of the breast. Nevertheless, in a large percentage of cases, it is potentially possible to remove the entire lesion while achieving acceptable cosmetic results. High-quality mammography and an aggressive biopsy policy utilizing stereotactic cores and multiple hooked wires will yield a higher percentage of smaller lesions that can be completely excised with excellent cosmetic results.

What constitutes a clear margin?

We have already talked about how tissues should be processed and how important it is to mark (ink or dye) all margins. When this has been done and the pathologist

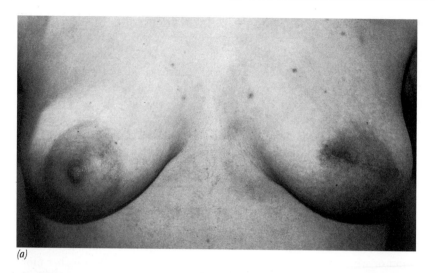

(a)

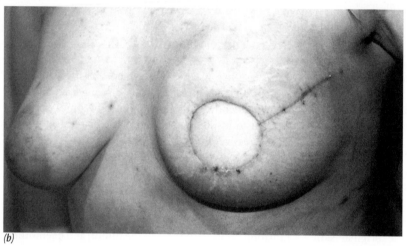

(b)

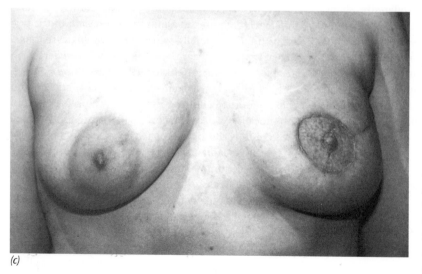

(c)

Figure 11.5 *Cosmetic results of glandular replacement therapy (GRT). (a) A preoperative photograph of a 34-year-old woman. The left nipple had been removed 2 years earlier for Paget's disease. She presented with a 8 cm recurrence of high-grade comedo DCIS. (b) A reconstructed breast after skin-sparing mastectomy and TRAM flap reconstruction (GRT). The island of skin that has been replaced is circular and exactly the same size as the nipple/areolar complex that has been removed. (c) The nipple/areolar complex has been reconstructed.*

tells us that the margins are free of disease, what does that mean? Does it really mean that we have excised the entire lesion? First, we must define clear margins. Our initial problem is that there is no consensus on what constitutes a clear margin; different researchers use different criteria. In the past, our group has used 1 mm. Shortly,

we will show that 1 mm is inadequate. Solin *et al.* have used 2 mm.[36] The National Surgical Adjuvant Breast and Bowel Project (NSABP)[48] requires that the tumor has not been transected; only a few adipose cells between the tumor and the inked margin are needed to call the margin clear. Holland and associates require normal breast structures between the tumor and the margin.[67] The Nottingham group has required 10 mm in all directions.[68] The work of Faverly et al. suggests that 10 mm would be an excellent choice for clear margins.[69] Using the serial subgross technique, they showed that only 8% of DCIS lesions have gaps (skip lesions) greater than 10 mm.

We have looked at the importance of margins in our series. Figure 11.6 compares the local recurrence rates when 1 mm or more is used as the definition of a clear margin. Figure 11.7 compares the local recurrence rates when 10 mm or more is used as the definition of a clear margin. The local recurrence rate drops dramatically when 10 mm is required in every direction. As mentioned above, the three-dimensional work of Faverly and associates[69] suggests that skip areas are generally less than 10 mm and that 10-mm margins may be the gold standard.

However, we must acknowledge that 10 mm in every direction is difficult to achieve while obtaining good cosmesis. In the operating room, the surgeon is faced with a difficult problem: DCIS is a lesion that generally

can neither be seen nor felt. The surgeon's best chance for a complete excision with widely clear margins comes only with the placement of multiple hooked wires in a lesion whose extent is well marked by calcifications. If the lesion extends significantly beyond the calcifications, complete excision is far less likely and will only occur if the surgeon is not only highly competent but lucky.

Can DCIS be completely removed using a cosmetic wide excision?[70]

Do clear margins mean that no residual DCIS has been left behind? Do involved margins mean that we are certain to find residual DCIS if we perform a mastectomy? No matter how exhaustive the evaluation of the margins, it is not perfect. Thousand of slides could be made from a 50-mm biopsy specimen. Generally, our group will submit about 20–30 cassettes from a 50-mm excision; this is a mere sampling. The evaluation of margins is, at best, a scientific approximation.

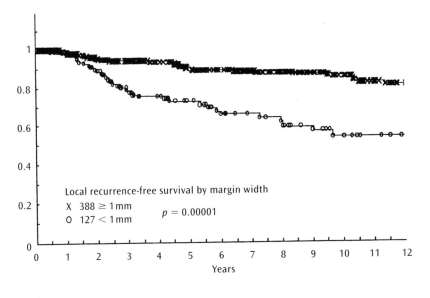

Figure 11.6 *The probability of local recurrence-free survival comparing margins ⩾1 mm with margins <1 mm for 515 breast conservation patients.*

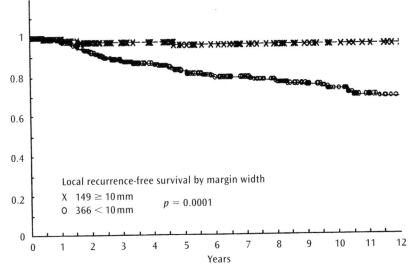

Figure 11.7 *The probability of local recurrence-free survival comparing margins ⩾10 mm with margins <10 mm for 515 breast conservation patients.*

We have unpublished data on 498 patients with DCIS in whom an initial excision was performed and who subsequently underwent mastectomy or re-excision of the initial biopsy site. This allowed us to evaluate histologically how much DCIS was left behind, and to correlate whether or not the initial margin status was a good predictor of residual DCIS. As expected, 71% (278/390) of patients with involved margins had residual DCIS; surprisingly, 37% (40/108) of patients with clear margins of 1 mm or more also had residual DCIS. Similar data are available from the NSABP Protocol B-06. In this study, 22 patients with negative margins underwent mastectomy; residual DCIS was found in 41%.[48]

From this, we can conclude that DCIS is difficult to excise completely using a cosmetic, wide, local excision. If the object is completely to excise DCIS while preserving the breast, a true quadrantectomy may be required in many cases. We can also conclude that our evaluation of the initial biopsy margins leaves something to be desired. Despite a thorough evaluation, with color coding of all margins, 37% of patients with what we thought were clear margins (using 1 mm or more as the definition of clear margins) had residual disease. Although we believe factors like nuclear grade and comedo-type necrosis are important, inadequate excision of the primary lesion is probably the most important cause of local failure after conservative treatment for intraductal breast carcinoma.

When re-excision of the entire biopsy cavity is required because of positive histologic margins, one of us (MJS) generally waits 2–4 months for the induration and inflammatory response to subside, because there is no biologic urgency with DCIS. In his experience, immediate re-excision often yields an inferior cosmetic result when compared with delayed re-excision.

On the other hand, one of us (KAS) generally re-excises immediately. Using this technique, it is easier to define the biopsy cavity and it is often possible to re-excise only the involved or close margins.

Wide excision only

Lagios and associates[9,34,39] have been leaders in breast conservation without radiation therapy for more than a decade. In the 1970s, they began treating selected patients with DCIS by excision only. Their strict criteria for eligibility required that all lesions be non-palpable, discovered mammographically, 25 mm or less in maximum size, and free of microcalcifications on postoperative mammography. Lagios reported a 12% actuarial local recurrence rate at 5 years and 16% at 10 years.[66] There were no breast cancer-related deaths and no patients have developed distant metastases. These are among the lowest local recurrence rates reported to date for DCIS treated by excision only.

A number of other investigators have reported similar but slightly higher rates of local recurrence for DCIS treated by excision only.[37,61,71] The NSABP (whose study is discussed below) has reported an actuarial local recurrence rate of 20.9% at 5 years.[61] Schwartz *et al.* have reported a 15.3% (absolute rate) at 4 years.[37] On an actuarial basis, this is likely to be about 20% at 5 years, similar to the NSABP.

The average size of Lagios' tumors was only 7 mm. In addition, Lagios used the strictest criteria for inclusion in his protocol, explaining why his local recurrence rate is lower, despite longer follow-up.

We believe that excision only is an acceptable form of treatment for carefully selected patients with DCIS. We elaborate on our selection process in the section entitled 'The Van Nuys Prognostic Index.'

Wide excision plus radiation therapy

Numerous retrospective analyses of patients with DCIS treated with breast-conserving surgery and radiation therapy have been published.[36,40,72–80] Follow-up is relatively short. Local recurrence rates average about 8–10% at 5 years. The largest of these retrospective radiation analyses is that of Solin *et al.*[36,72,80] This study combined the data of nine institutions in the USA and Europe: 261 DCIS lesions were treated with excision plus breast irradiation. The 15-year actuarial local recurrence rate was 19%. Half of the recurrences were DCIS and half were invasive. The 15-year breast cancer-specific survival rate was 96%.[80]

In 1985, the NSABP began a prospective randomized study to evaluate the value of postoperative breast irradiation after excision of the DCIS lesion. After excision of the lesion with clear margins (NSABP non-transection definition), patients were randomized to receive ipsilateral breast irradiation or no further therapy. Axillary node dissection was required until June 1987. Thereafter, it was optional, at the surgeons' discretion. If an axillary dissection was performed, the nodes had to be negative.

In 1993, the first NSABP report was published.[61] A total of 790 patients was evaluable, 391 treated by excision only and 399 treated by excision plus breast irradiation. The 5-year actuarial local recurrence rates were 10.4% for excision plus irradiation and 20.9% for excision only. The difference was highly significant. There was a total of 64 recurrences in the excision-only group, exactly half of which were invasive. There were 28 recurrences in the excision plus irradiation group, only eight of which were invasive (29%). The NSABP concluded that excision plus breast irradiation was more appropriate than excision only for patients with localized DCIS and, if there was a local recurrence, irradiation statistically decreased the likelihood that it would be invasive. After years of retrospective analyses, this was the first prospective, randomized, clinical trial for patients with DCIS and it is of profound importance.

The NSABP recommended excision of the lesion and irradiation for all conservatively treated patients with localized DCIS and clear margins (by their definition), regardless of histologic subtype, nuclear grade, or size of the DCIS lesion. In other words, they concluded that excision alone for DCIS was inappropriate. While we give great credit to the NSABP for organizing and conducting an outstanding study, it is difficult for clinicians to use global recommendations in an age of sophisticated consumer medicine.

The NSABP gave no recurrence analysis by subset. Readers were told that almost 50% of the patients had comedo necrosis, that more than 85% of the patients had lesions 20 mm or smaller, and that 81% of the lesions were non-palpable. However, physicians were not told how any of these parameters affected outcome. We were told that radiation-treated patients had a 5-year actuarial local recurrence rate of 10.4% and non-irradiated patients had a 20.9% actuarial local recurrence rate. We were told how many recurrences were invasive and how many were non-invasive in each group. However, because there was no subset analysis, there was no way for us to see whether the outcome was different for a 3-mm low-grade micropapillary lesion with widely clear margins compared with a 20-mm high-grade comedo DCIS with minimally clear margins. The NSABP did not tell us whether patients with palpable DCIS recurred at a higher rate than patients with non-palpable lesions. Because of these shortcomings, the paper was criticized.[81,82]

In 1995, the NSABP published a second report, from a pathologic perspective.[83] This was updated in 1999.[84] Approximately three-quarters of the patients had microscopic slides available for central pathology review. In the 1995 analysis, both comedo-type necrosis and margin status (close/involved) were found to be significant predictors of an increased likelihood of local recurrence. In the 1999 update, only comedo-type necrosis was significant as an independent predictor of local recurrence. The NSABP continued to recommend that all patients with DCIS electing breast conservation receive radiation therapy, in addition to excision with clear margins. At the 6th St Gallen Adjuvant Therapy of Primary Breast Cancer Conference (St Gallen, Switzerland, March 1998), both Dr Fisher and Dr Margolese independently reiterated the NSABP position that all conservatively treated patients with DCIS should receive postoperative radiation therapy.

The outcome results of B-17 were updated in 1998.[85] At 8 years, 27% of patients treated with excision only had recurred locally, whereas, only 12% of those treated with excision plus irradiation had recurred. There was a significant decrease in local recurrence of both DCIS and invasive breast cancer among the irradiated patients. The 8-year data led the NSABP to reconfirm their 1993 position and to continue to recommend postoperative radiation therapy for all patients with DCIS who choose to save their breasts.

The favorable results of B-17, in support of radiation therapy for patients with DCIS, led the NSABP to perform protocol B-24.[86] In this trial, 1804 patients with DCIS were treated with excision and radiation therapy, and then randomized to receive either tamoxifen or placebo. At 5 years of actuarial follow-up, 9% of patients treated with placebo had recurred locally, compared with 6% of those treated with tamoxifen. When all breast cancer events were analysed (this included new contralateral breast cancers as well as regional and distant recurrences), the cumulative rate was 8.2% for those who received tamoxifen and 13.4% for those who received placebo ($p = 0.0009$). The results of B-17, B-24, and P-1 (the NSABP Chemoprevention Study)[87] led the NSABP to recommend both radiation therapy and tamoxifen for all patients with DCIS treated with breast preservation.[88]

Recently, the EORTC announced the results of its prospective, randomized DCIS study,[89] a trial with a similar randomization to B-17. This trial included more than 1000 patients: at 4 years, 9% of patients treated with excision plus radiation therapy had recurred locally compared with 16% of patients treated with excision alone.

Despite these prospectively collected data which show that radiation therapy reduces local recurrence in patients with DCIS, many physicians do not want to use radiation therapy in all patients with DCIS who elect breast preservation. Radiation therapy is expensive, time consuming, and accompanied by side-effects in a small percentage of patients.[90] Radiation fibrosis of the breast is a somewhat more common side-effect, particularly with the type of radiation therapy given during the 1980s. Radiation fibrosis changes the texture of the breast and skin, may make mammographic follow-up more difficult, and could result in delayed diagnosis if there is a local recurrence. Should there be an invasive recurrence at a later date, radiation therapy cannot be used again (although some have tried this). Should there be significant skin and vascular changes following radiation therapy, skin-sparing mastectomy, if needed in the future, is clearly more difficult to perform, with flap necrosis more likely. Physicians must be sure that the benefits of radiation therapy significantly outweigh the side-effects, complications, inconvenience, and costs for a given subgroup of patients.

Should all conservatively treated patients with DCIS receive postoperative radiation therapy? We believe that the answer is no. We think it is clear that breast irradiation reduces the local recurrence rate by about 50% at 5 years (from around 20% to around 10%). Series with longer follow-up, however, suggest that, as time passes, recurrences will continue to accrue in the patients treated with radiation.[72,80] This raises speculation that, at least in some patients, radiation merely delays rather than prevents an inevitable recurrence. We believe that there is now sufficient, easily available information that can aid clinicians in differentiating patients who require radiation therapy after excision versus those who do not.

These same data can point out patients who are better served by mastectomy because recurrence rates with breast conservation are unacceptably high with or without radiation therapy.

The Van Nuys Prognostic Index

There are numerous clinical, pathologic, and laboratory factors that might aid clinicians and patients wrestling with the difficult treatment decision-making process. Our research[38,40] and the research of others has shown that various combinations of nuclear grade, the presence of comedo-type necrosis, tumor size, and margin status are all important factors in predicting local recurrence in patients with DCIS who elect breast conservation.[9,34,36,37,39,41,43,66,71,83,91] By using a combination of these factors, it may be possible to select subgroups of patients who do not require irradiation or to select patients whose recurrence rate is potentially so high, even with breast irradiation, that mastectomy is preferable.

We used the first two of these prognostic factors (nuclear grade and necrosis) to develop the histopathologic classification described earlier in this chapter.[38] However, nuclear grade and comedo-type necrosis are inadequate as the sole guidelines in the treatment-selection process; tumor size and margin status are also important.

The Van Nuys Prognostic Index (VNPI)[92–96] was devised by combining three statistically significant predictors (by multivariate analysis) of local tumor recurrence in patients with DCIS: tumor size, margin status, and pathologic classification.[38] A score of 1 (best prognosis) to 3 (worst prognosis) was given for each of the three predictors. The objective with all three predictors was to create three statistically different subgroups for each predictor, using local recurrence as a marker of treatment failure. Cut-off points were determined by statistical analyses, using the log rank test with an optimum *p*-value approach.

- *Size score.* A score of 1 was given for small tumors of 15 mm or less, 2 was given for intermediate-size tumors of 16–40 mm, and 3 was given for large tumors of 41 mm or more in diameter.
- *Margin score.* A score of 1 was given for widely clear tumor-free margins of 10 mm or more. This was most commonly achieved by re-excision with the finding of no residual DCIS or only focal residual DCIS at the biopsy cavity. A score of 2 was given for intermediate margins of 1–9 mm, and a score of 3 for margins less than 1 mm.
- *Pathologic classification score.* A score of 3 was given for tumors classified as group 3 (all high nuclear grade lesions), 2 for tumors classified as group 2 (non-high nuclear grade lesion with comedo-type necrosis), and 1 for tumors classified as group 1 (non-high nuclear grade lesion without comedo-type necrosis).
- *Determining the Van Nuys Prognostic Index.* The initial VNPI formula was determined by using the beta values, obtained from the multivariate analysis, which show the relative contribution of each factor in the estimation of the likelihood of local recurrence.[93–95] Additional analyses revealed that the formula could be simplified, without compromising validity, by omitting the beta weighting suggested by the multivariate analysis, and by readjusting the numerical range for each of the three subgroups. The final formula for the Van Nuys Prognostic Index became:

$$\text{VNPI} = \text{pathologic classification score} + \text{margin score} + \text{size score.}$$

- This formula yielded seven groups with whole-number scores ranging from 3 to 9. The best possible VNPI score was 3, a score of 1 for each predictor (e.g., a 5-mm low-grade lesion with widely clear margins by re-excision would earn a score of 3). The worst possible score was 9, a score of 3 for each predictor (e.g., a 50-mm high-grade lesion with involved margins would earn a score of 9). Table 11.1 summarizes the scoring for the VNPI.

Results of analysis using the VNPI

The VNPI was initially evaluated on 254 breast conservation patients from The Van Nuys Breast Center (mastectomy patients were omitted from the analysis because they no longer had their ipsilateral breast at risk for local recurrence – the endpoint of this study). Following this, the VNPI was independently validated by analysing Lagios' series of 79 patients. Both groups use similar tissue

Table 11.1 *The Van Nuys Prognostic Index (VNPI) scoring system*

Score	1	2	3
Size (mm)	≤15	16–40	≥41
Margins (mm)	≥10	1–9	<1
Pathologic classification	Non-high grade without necrosis	Non-high grade with necrosis	High grade with or without necrosis

One to three points are awarded for each of three different predictors of local breast recurrence (size, margins, and pathologic classification). Scores for each of the predictors are totaled to yield a VNPI score ranging from a low of 3 to a high of 9.

processing and have consulted one another for more than 15 years. The disease-free survival curves for comparable patients in each group were almost identical, with no statistical differences found in any subgroup tested. The two groups of patients were therefore combined to yield a total of 333 patients with DCIS treated with breast preservation. These results were published in 1996.[93] For this chapter, we have updated the results through mid-1999 and included 515 breast conservation patients.

Treatment for these patients was highly selective. However, selection (treatment bias) is not an important bias in this series because we are testing a prognostic index rather than analysing treatment. Although the patient and her clinician control treatment selection, they cannot control final margins, tumor size, or pathologic classification. The fact that some patients opted for suboptimal treatments that were not recommended (e.g., 55 patients with VNPI scores of 8 or 9 who selected breast conservation treatment were all advised to undergo mastectomy) was actually helpful in developing and evaluating the VNPI.

The recurrence-free survival for all 515 patients is shown by tumor size in Figure 11.8, by margin width in Figure 11.9, and by pathologic classification in Figure 11.1. The differences between every survival curve for each of the three predictors that make up the VNPI are statistically significant.

Figure 11.10 groups patients with low (VNPI = 3 or 4), intermediate (VNPI = 5, 6, or 7), or high (VNPI = 8 or 9) recurrence rates together. These three groups are all statistically different from one another.

Patients with VNPI scores of 3 or 4 do not show a disease-free survival benefit from breast irradiation (Figure 11.11) ($p = 0.43$). Patients with an intermediate rate of local recurrence, VNPI 5, 6, or 7, benefit from irradiation (Figure 11.12). There is a statistically significant average 13% decrease in local recurrence rate in irradiated breasts compared to those treated by excision alone ($p = 0.02$). Figure 11.13 divides patients with a VNPI of 8 or 9 into those treated by excision plus irradiation and those treated by excision alone. Although the difference between the two groups is significant ($p = 0.03$),

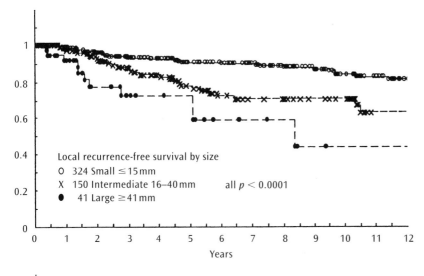

Figure 11.8 *The probability of local recurrence-free survival by tumor size for 515 breast conservation patients.*

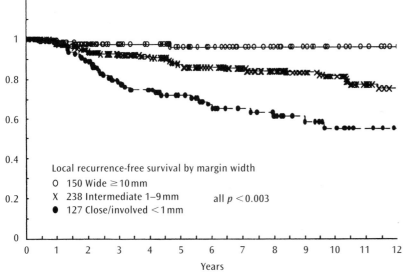

Figure 11.9 *The probability of local recurrence-free survival by margin width for 515 breast conservation patients.*

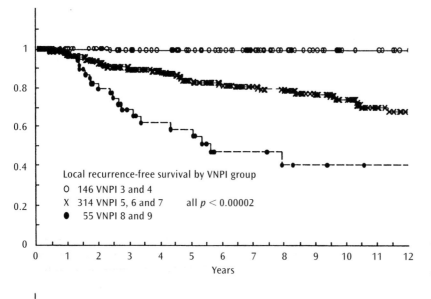

Figure 11.10 *The probability of local recurrence-free survival grouped by VNPI score for 515 breast conservation patients.*

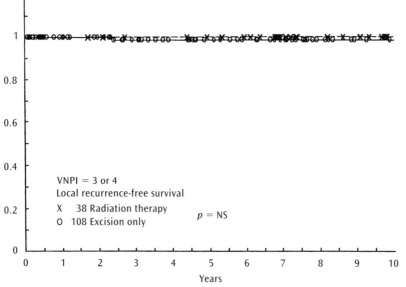

Figure 11.11 *The probability of local recurrence-free survival by treatment for 146 breast conservation patients with VNPI scores of 3 or 4.*

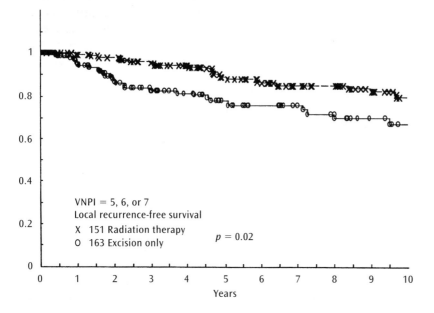

Figure 11.12 *The probability of local recurrence-free survival by treatment for 314 breast conservation patients with VNPI scores of 5, 6, or 7.*

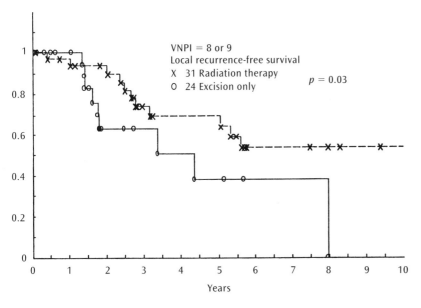

Figure 11.13 *The probability of local recurrence-free survival by treatment for 55 breast conservation patients with VNPI scores of 8 or 9.*

conservatively treated DCIS patients with a VNPI of 8 or 9 recur at an extremely high rate with or without radiation therapy.

Although mastectomy is curative for approximately 98–99% of patients with DCIS,[6,40,96–99] mastectomy represents significant over-treatment for the majority of cases detected by current methods. When breast conservation is elected rather than mastectomy, radiation therapy statistically decreases the likelihood of local recurrence when compared with excision alone;[61] but radiation therapy, like mastectomy, may also represent over-treatment for a significant number of patients who elect breast preservation.

Subsets of patients who are not likely to receive any significant benefit from radiation therapy can be identified, e.g., those with VNPI scores of 3 or 4 in the series presented here, low-grade lesions in the series of Lagios et al.,[34,66] small non-comedo lesions with uninvolved margins in the series of Schwartz et al.,[37] or the well-differentiated lesions of Zafrani et al.[91] Such patients may account for more than 30% of the total DCIS group.[34,37,38,66,91]

The broad recommendation by the NSABP that radiation therapy is appropriate for all patients with DCIS who are treated with breast preservation, while clearly correct based on their 1993 data, does not consider the histologic heterogeneity of DCIS or the differences in subsets demonstrated by our data,[38,40] their 1995 data,[83] and the data of others.[9,34,37–39,41,43,66,71,91]

Radiation therapy is not without side-effects. It changes the texture of the breast, makes subsequent mammography more difficult to interpret, and, perhaps most importantly, its use precludes additional radiation therapy and breast conservation should a metachronous invasive breast cancer develop. For these reasons, radiation therapy should only be offered to those patients with DCIS who are likely to obtain a benefit.

Patients in this series with VNPI scores of 8 or 9 present a different problem. Although these patients show the greatest relative benefit from post-excisional radiation therapy, their local recurrence rate continues to be unacceptably high, and a recommendation for mastectomy should be seriously considered.

Treatment recommendations for the intermediate group (patients with scores of 5, 6, or 7) are the most difficult. For patients with intermediate VNPI scores and margin scores of 2 or 3, re-excision may improve disease-free survival. If the score remains intermediate after re-excision, radiation therapy should be considered. However, some patients with scores of 7 may be better treated with mastectomy (e.g., a patient with a large nuclear grade 2 lesion without necrosis with less than 1 mm margins after re-excision), whereas some patients with scores of 5 (e.g., a patient with widely clear margins, small tumor size, but high nuclear grade) may elect no further treatment. These are independent judgments that must be made by the patient and her physician. We would hope that the VNPI would be a helpful adjunct as these difficult decisions are discussed.

Our work demonstrates that DCIS patients can be stratified into specific subsets based on the pathologic classification (using nuclear grade and necrosis), the size of the lesion, and the adequacy of surgical treatment as determined by pathologic margin assessment. If appropriate criteria are provided, pathologists should have little trouble making these determinations.

Counseling patients with DCIS in a rational manner can be extremely difficult when the range of treatment options is extreme. The VNPI allows a scientifically based discussion with the patient, using the parameters of the lesion obtained after an initial excision. Thus, in some cases, a patient can choose a re-excision in an effort to 'downscore' her lesion. Successful downscoring of a patient with a VNPI of 8 or 9 could result in substantial reduction in the risk of local recurrence, perhaps changing a recommendation from mastectomy to radiation therapy. Similarly, patients with close or involved margins, with VNPI scores of 5 or 6 after initial excision, could opt for re-excision. Successful downscoring by achieving widely clear margins could result in a final VNPI score sufficiently low to avoid breast irradiation.

Downscoring can be achieved only by re-excising patients with margin scores of 2 or 3. Re-excision will not lower the pathologic classification score, nor will it reduce the size of the tumor. In some cases, re-excision will 'upscore' the tumor, increasing the VNPI score by revealing a larger tumor size, a higher nuclear grade, the presence of previously undetected comedo necrosis, or an involved margin.

The proposed VNPI may be useful to clinicians because it divides DCIS into three groups with different risks for local recurrence after breast conservation therapy. Although there is an obvious treatment choice for each group – excision only for patients with scores of 3 or 4, excision plus radiation therapy for patients with scores of 5, 6, or 7, and mastectomy for patients with scores of 8 or 9 – the VNPI is offered only as a guideline, a starting place in the discussions with patients.

The VNPI was the first attempt to quantify known important prognostic factors in DCIS, making them clinically useful in the treatment decision-making process. Clearly, the validity of the VNPI must be independently confirmed by other groups with large series of DCIS patients and sufficient data to complete the subset analysis as outlined here. In the future, other factors, such as molecular markers, may be integrated into the VNPI or other prognostic indices when they are shown to statistically influence the likelihood of local recurrence after breast conservation therapy.

Case presentations using the VNPI to aid in treatment selection

1 *A 47-year-old woman with microcalcifications detected on screening mammography.* Wire-directed excision yielded a 10-mm, non-high-grade (cribriform) DCIS with comedo-type necrosis. The closest margin was less than 1 mm. VNPI score = 6 (size score = 1, pathologic classification score = 2, and margin score = 3). Re-excision was performed and no residual DCIS was found. This procedure downscored the lesion by converting her margin score to 1. The patient now has a VNPI of 4 and can be considered for careful clinical follow-up without additional radiation therapy.

2 *A 54-year-old woman with microcalcifications detected on screening mammography.* Wire-directed biopsy revealed a 10-mm (solid) DCIS of intermediate grade with focal comedo-type necrosis. The margins were involved. VNPI score = 6 (size score = 1, pathologic classification score = 2, and margin score = 3). This

score, of course, is inaccurate because the lesion was transected and the true size was not known. Re-excision was performed and extensive residual disease measuring 42 mm was found. In addition, foci of high-grade comedo DCIS were found. The closest margin was then 1 mm. VNPI score = 8 (size score = 3, pathologic classification score = 3, and margin score = 2). This procedure upscored the lesion by converting her size score to 3, her pathologic classification score to 3, and her margin score to 2. The patient then had a VNPI of 8 and would be best treated with mastectomy. An alternative would be to re-excise one more time in the hope of obtaining widely clear margins. If this were to happen, her margin score would become 1 and her VNPI would equal 7 and, at that point, radiation therapy would be an alternative to mastectomy.

3 *A 6-mm, low-grade (micropapillary) DCIS without necrosis was found inadvertently within a breast reduction specimen in a 44-year-old woman.* Because this was a reduction, tissue margins were not marked and tissue was not serially sectioned. All additional, previously unprocessed, formalin-fixed tissue was then processed, but no additional DCIS was found. Microscopically, the margins of the initial DCIS appeared widely clear, but we could not be certain. Pre-reduction mammography was negative. VNPI score = 3 or 4 (size score = 1, pathologic classification score = 1, and margin score = 1 or 2). A VNPI score of 3 or 4 is our best guess in this case. In the light of this, we would not treat this patient with radiation therapy. However, reduction mammoplasty causes scarring and this patient's future mammographic follow-up will not be optimal.

4 *A 74-year-old woman with a 5-mm area of microcalcifications detected on screening mammography.* Wire-directed breast biopsy revealed a 5-mm, high-grade (comedo) DCIS. The margins were widely clear (>10 mm in all directions). VNPI score = 5 (size score = 1, pathologic classification score = 3, and margin score = 1). Patients in the intermediate group (5, 6, or 7) generally require more thought and discussion. Some patients with scores of 5 may be better served by omitting radiation. Some patients with scores of 7 may be better served by mastectomy. In this particular case, we would not irradiate for the following reasons. The lesion was well marked by calcifications. It measured 5 mm on mammography and 5 mm on the microscopic slide – a good mammographic/pathologic correlation. Postoperative mammography showed no residual calcifications. The margins were widely clear. We prefer to omit radiation therapy in a patient of this age whenever possible. We would have no quarrel with the physician who elected to give radiation to this patient.

5 *A 47-year-old woman with a palpable upper outer quadrant thickening.* Mammography showed a non-diagnostic architectural distortion. FNA revealed

highly atypical cells. Core biopsy revealed a low-grade (micropapillary) DCIS without necrosis. The patient was strongly motivated for breast conservation. A four-wire bracketed upper outer quadrant segmental resection was done. A 6-cm DCIS identical to the core biopsy, extending tenuously close to three margins, was found. VNPI = 7 (size score = 3, pathologic classification score = 1, and margin score = 3). In this particular case, we would prefer skin-sparing mastectomy with immediate free TRAM reconstruction. We would choose this because the lesion was large and extended to three margins. Because it is not calcified, it is more difficult to excise completely and it would be more difficult to follow if this patient selected breast preservation. As an alternative, the wound could be allowed to heal for 3–6 months and a formal quadrantectomy performed. With low-grade lesions, there is little risk in delaying definitive treatment for 6 months. If the margins were widely clear (≥ 10 mm) after quadrantectomy, the VNPI score would then be 5 (size score = 3, pathologic classification score = 1, and margin score = 1) and consideration could be given to adding radiation therapy. However, data are weak regarding the benefits of radiation therapy for low-grade lesions and we would like to follow this patient closely without adding radiation therapy.

Margin width alone as a predictor of local recurrence

Margin width is the distance between DCIS and the closest inked or dyed margin and reflects the completeness of excision. Although the multivariate analysis used to derive

the VNPI suggests approximately equal importance for the three significant factors (margin width, tumor size, and biologic classification), the fact that DCIS can be thought of in Halstedian terms (it is a local disease and complete excision should cure it) suggests that margin width should be the single most important factor in terms of local recurrence.

Serial subgross evaluation of more than 100 breasts after mastectomy for DCIS suggests that when margin widths exceed 10 mm, the likelihood of residual disease is relatively small, in the range of 10–15%.[52,53,69] In May of 1999, we published data suggesting that there is little to be gained from postoperative radiation therapy if all margins are greater than 10 mm, regardless of nuclear grade, tumor size, or the presence of comedo-type necrosis (Table 11.2).[100]

We were recently asked by a colleague whether publication of these data in the *New England Journal of Medicine*[100] meant that we were abandoning the VNPI. Our answer was absolutely not. The VNPI is a superior tool because it takes into account not only margin width but tumor size and biologic classification. To score best (lowest) using the VNPI, one needs a small, well-excised, low-grade lesion. This type of lesion is not likely to recur, with or without radiation therapy. In our series, there are now 146 patients who scored 3 or 4 on the VNPI, only one of whom had recurred locally. In our recently published series using only margin width, there were three recurrences among 133 patients with margins of 10 mm or more; updated through mid-1999, there were four recurrences among 149 such patients. The VNPI is a slightly better predictor of local recurrence (and it should be), but clearly more difficult to use. It was not designed to be used without excellent support from both pathology and radiology.

Table 11.2 *Association of radiation therapy with recurrence after stratification according to the presence or absence of comedo necrosis, nuclear grade, and tumor size*

Margin width (mm)	Unadjusted analysis		Variable	Adjusted analysis	
	Relative risk (95% CI)[1]	p value[2]		Relative risk (95% CI)[1]	p value[3]
≥ 10	1.14 (0.10–12.64)	0.92	Comedo necrosis	1.22 (0.11–13.93)	0.87
			Nuclear grade	1.08 (0.09–12.70)	0.95
			Size	1.69 (0.15–18.79)	0.66
1 to <10	1.49 (0.76–2.90)	0.24	Comedo necrosis	1.84 (0.93–3.61)	0.08
			Nuclear grade	1.75 (0.87–3.56)	0.11
			Size	1.87 (0.93–3.78)	0.08
<1	2.54 (1.25–5.18)	0.01	Comedo necrosis	2.56 (1.25–5.26)	0.01
			Nuclear grade	2.30 (1.12–4.76)	0.03
			Size	2.52 (1.23–5.14)	0.02

[1]Values shown are the relative risks of recurrence in the group that did not receive radiation therapy as compared with the group that did.
[2]p values for the unadjusted analysis were calculated with the likelihood-ratio test of the Cox proportional-hazards model.
[3]p values for the adjusted analysis were calculated with the likelihood-ratio test of the Cox proportional-hazards model with stratification according to necrosis (present or absent), nuclear grade (1, 2, or 3), and tumor size (≤ 10 mm or >10 mm).
CI denotes confidence interval.
From Silverstein *et al.* N Engl J Med 1999; 340:1459.[100]

AXILLARY LYMPH NODE DISSECTION

In 1986, our group suggested that axillary lymph node dissection be abandoned for DCIS.[101,102] In 1987, the NSABP made axillary node dissection for patients with DCIS optional, at the discretion of the surgeon. Since that time, we have published a series of papers which continue to show that axillary node dissection is not indicated for patients with DCIS.[10,35,40,58,70] To date, our group have performed a total of 395 node dissections, 294 level I and II dissections and 101 samplings (fewer than 10 nodes). In two patients, a single positive node was found without evidence of invasion or microinvasion in the primary. Frykberg *et al.*, in their review of the management of DCIS, compiled the data of nine studies with a total of 754 patients.[103] The incidence of axillary lymph node metastasis for patients with DCIS was 1.7%. Despite these numbers, some authors continue to advocate removal of the axillary nodes in patients with palpable extensive DCIS who have a higher risk of occult invasion.[37,47,104]

Our current policy is as follows. In any patient with DCIS who is undergoing breast preservation, we do not remove any axillary nodes. In patients being treated with mastectomy, a thorough dissection of the axillary tail often yields one to ten nodes.[105] In addition, most of our current patients who undergo mastectomy are reconstructed with a free TRAM flap. This procedure requires dissection of the subscapular vessels. It is not uncommon to remove a few nodes during the dissection as the vessels are exposed. The final point revolves around the fact that most patients undergoing mastectomy have larger tumors, creating a greater possibility for occult invasion that is missed during routine histologic evaluation. In light of this, most patients are generally happy to have a few lower axillary nodes examined pathologically. A few negative nodes buy additional peace of mind for many patients.

There is now uniform agreement that, for patients with DCIS, the axilla does not need treatment.[58,102,106] For patients with DCIS undergoing breast conservation, the axilla should not be irradiated and no form of axillary sampling or dissection needs to be performed. For patients treated with excision plus postoperative radiation therapy, the lower axilla is included by the tangential fields to the breast.

For patients with DCIS lesions large enough to merit mastectomy, a sentinel node biopsy[106–109] using a vital blue dye or radioactive tracer, or both, can be performed at the time of mastectomy. This is done in the event that permanent sections of the mastectomy specimen reveal one or more foci of invasion. If invasion is documented, no matter how small, the lesion is no longer considered DCIS, but rather an invasive breast cancer. The sentinel node or nodes are evaluated by hematoxylin and eosin (H & E) staining followed by immunohistochemistry for cytokeratin when routine H & E stains are negative.

OUTCOME AFTER INVASIVE LOCAL RECURRENCE

Local recurrence after treatment for DCIS is demoralizing and, if invasive, it is a threat to life.[110] Approximately 50% of all local recurrences are invasive.[9,36,66,110] For the last decade, local recurrence (both invasive and non-invasive) has been used as the marker of treatment failure for patients with DCIS.

Through mid-1999, there were 821 patients in our series, with a total of 81 local recurrences, 40 invasive and 41 non-invasive. No patient with a non-invasive recurrence developed distant metastases and none died of breast cancer. For the 40 patients with invasive recurrences, 52% presented with stage IIa or more disease at the time of local recurrence, eight developed distant metastases, and five died of breast cancer. The breast cancer mortality rate at 10 years for the subgroup of patients with invasive local recurrences was 16%, and the distant disease rate for this subgroup was 23%, rates similar to those reported by others. Invasive recurrence after treatment for DCIS is a significant event, converting a patient with previous stage 0 disease to a patient, on average, with stage IIa breast cancer (range stage I–IV). Treatment for a patient with an invasive recurrence should be based on the stage of the recurrent disease.

Despite these five mortalities, one must not lose sight of the fact that, overall, DCIS is disease with a very favorable outcome. When the entire series of 821 patients is considered, the actuarial probability of an invasive recurrence at 10 years after mastectomy was less than 1%; after breast conservation, it was 13%. The probability of a breast cancer-specific mortality was only 1.4%. It is, however, a tragedy when a patient with DCIS recurs with invasive breast cancer and then goes on to die of metastatic disease.

PAGET'S DISEASE OF THE NIPPLE

Paget's disease presents with eczematoid changes of the nipple. In many cases, there is an underlying lesion that may or may not be palpable and may be invasive or non-invasive. After a complete mammographic work-up, we biopsy the nipple using local anesthesia and, if present, the underlying lesion. Treatment depends on many factors. If the underlying lesion is invasive, we excise it, along with the nipple areolar complex, do an axillary dissection, and treat the whole breast with radiation therapy. The cosmetic results for central lesions are generally quite good (Figure 11.14). Modified radical mastectomy can be performed if the patient chooses.

If the underlying lesion is DCIS, we generally excise the nipple areolar complex with a generous wedge of breast tissue which includes the underlying lesion. If the

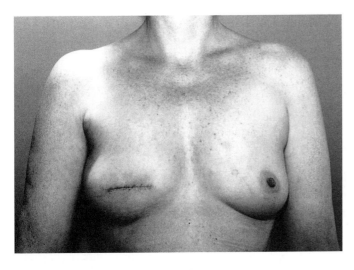

Figure 11.14 *The nipple areolar complex has been excised for Paget's disease.*

underlying lesion is marked with microcalcifications, we use wires to direct the wedge resection; if it is not calcified, the excision is done blindly. All edges of the resected specimen are color coded and the tissue is serially sectioned. If no underlying lesion is found, we do nothing further. If an underlying DCIS is found, we use the VNPI as a guideline for suggesting treatment. If histologic margins are involved, we either re-excise or perform a mastectomy with immediate reconstruction, depending on the size of the breast and the degree of margin involvement. We generally do not irradiate patients after complete excision with widely clear margins. Selected cases of Paget's disease can be treated with nipple preservation and radiation.[111] Node dissection is not indicated for Paget's disease unless an underlying invasive carcinoma is found. Nipple areolar reconstruction should be delayed until permanent sections are available that reveal clear histologic margins and a decision has been made about whether or not radiation therapy is going to be used.

OUR CURRENT TREATMENT PLAN FOR PATIENTS WITH DCIS

With the development of high-quality screening mammography, it has become common to see an asymptomatic patient in whom routine mammography has revealed an area of microcalcifications. During the 1980s, this patient would have had a wire-directed breast biopsy to make a diagnosis. During this time period, approximately 70–75% of biopsies for microcalcifications yielded benign lesions. In addition, surgeons did not fully appreciate the radial segmental distribution of most DCIS lesions or the importance of clear margins. During the 1980s, we irradiated all conservatively treated patients. We were not anxious to perform a wide segmental-type resection initially when the majority of lesions were benign, and we often accepted close or focally involved margins without suggesting re-excision.

Our thought was that radiation therapy would deal with any residual cancer cells.

Our approach changed in the late 1980s. We had a greater appreciation of the extent and distribution of DCIS. We were much more concerned with clear margins, and we lost our enthusiasm for radiation therapy for DCIS. The development of stereotactic core biopsy technology in the 1990s went hand in hand with our new thinking. It was now possible, using a specially designed table, with the patient in the prone position, to make a preoperative diagnosis with a 14-gauge core biopsy. This allowed preoperative consultation and planning and, for most patients, it meant only one trip to the operating room for definitive treatment. The main problem with the 14-gauge core biopsy was that, because of the relatively small sample size, the final diagnosis was upstaged about 20% of the time following surgery. In other words, one patient in five in whom the 14-gauge core diagnosis was DCIS actually had invasive breast cancer. This generally forced us back to the operating room on another day to dissect the axilla. We had the same problem with a 14-gauge core that yielded a diagnosis of atypical ductal hyperplasia. Again, about 20% of the time at definitive surgery, these lesions turned out to be DCIS. Because of this, we routinely recommended open biopsy following 14-gauge core biopsy with a diagnosis of atypical hyperplasia.

As mentioned above, by the late 1990s, this problem was remedied with the development of a number of new, larger core tissue acquisition systems for percutaneous minimally invasive breast biopsy. The 11-gauge vacuum-assisted Mammotome probe (Ethicon Endo-Surgery, Cincinnati, OH) takes significantly larger cores of tissue when compared with the 14-gauge needle and affords the ability to sample tissue contiguously. Upgrading or changing the diagnosis at the time of definitive surgery is far less frequent.

With this as a basis, we currently manage patients with suspicious, non-palpable mammographic lesions in the following manner. Our first step is to obtain an

11-gauge Mammotome biopsy. If the diagnosis of DCIS is made, we counsel the patient thoroughly about the nature of the disease, paying particular attention to the size and distribution of her disease as determined mammographically. If she is a good candidate for breast preservation (an area of DCIS that we think we can remove completely and with clear margins without dramatically deforming the breast) and she is anxious to preserve her breast, we generally perform a four-wire-directed segmental resection and commonly use a radial incision to take advantage of the radial distribution of DCIS. We often remove a small amount of overlying skin and dissect the entire segment down to and including the pectoralis major muscle fascia. This guarantees that the anterior and posterior margins will be clear. If widely clear margins, 10 mm or more in the other four directions (superior, inferior, medial, and lateral) are obtained, we do not recommend postoperative radiation therapy, regardless of nuclear grade, comedo necrosis or tumor size.[99] If the margins are 1 mm to less than 10 mm, we generally re-excise or add radiation therapy.

In patients whose lesions are too large mammographically to yield clear margins and an acceptable cosmetic result, we prefer to go directly to skin-sparing mastectomy and autologous reconstruction, generally with a TRAM flap. Having performed only a percutaneous minimally invasive breast biopsy in these patients, we are seldom faced with a skin incision in the wrong place or a biopsy scar that needs re-excision.

Some DCIS lesions are much larger than they appear mammographically, and may be extremely difficult to excise completely. These patients are probably better served with skin-sparing mastectomy and autologous reconstruction.

Patients with DCIS treated with breast preservation should be followed closely. Currently, at the Lee Breast Center within the USC/Norris Comprehensive Cancer Center, they are examined physically every 6 months forever. Mammography is performed every 6 months on the ipsilateral breast and yearly on the contralateral breast.

SUMMARY

DCIS is now relatively common and its frequency is increasing. Most of this is due to better mammographic detection. We are not sure whether there is a true increase in incidence.

Not all microscopic DCIS will progress to clinical cancer, but if a patient has DCIS and is not treated with a mastectomy, she is more likely to develop an ipsilateral invasive breast cancer than a woman without DCIS.

The comedo subtype of DCIS is more aggressive and malignant in its histologic appearance and is more likely to be associated with subsequent invasive cancer than the non-comedo subtypes. Comedo DCIS is more likely to

have a high S-phase, overexpress *HER2/neu*, and show increased thymidine labeling as compared to non-comedo DCIS. Comedo DCIS treated conservatively is also more likely to recur locally than non-comedo DCIS. However, separation of DCIS into two groups by architecture is an oversimplification and does not reflect the biologic potential of the lesion. Because many DCIS lesions are admixtures of multiple architectural types of DCIS, our group no longer stratifies DCIS by comedo versus non-comedo subtypes. Rather, we use nuclear grade and the presence or absence of comedo-type necrosis to classify lesions.[36]

Most DCIS detected today will be non-palpable. It will be detected by mammographic calcifications. It is not uncommon for DCIS to be larger than expected by mammography, to involve more than a quadrant of the breast, and to be unifocal in its distribution.

Preoperative evaluation should include film-screen mammography with compression magnification. The surgeon and the radiologist should plan the excision procedure carefully. The first attempt at excision is the best chance to get a complete excision with a good cosmetic result. Re-excisions often yield poor cosmetic results. In patients with lesions that look like DCIS, consideration should be given to stereotactic core biopsy to make a definitive diagnosis.

Following the establishment of the diagnosis, the patient can be counseled. If she is motivated for breast conservation, the surgeon and radiologist should plan the procedure carefully, using multiple wires to map out the extent of the lesion. Once the multiple-wire-directed excisional biopsy has been done, two factors can be evaluated: cosmesis and histopathology. If the cosmetic result is acceptable and the margins are clear, the patient can proceed with breast conservation. If she has a VNPI score of 3 or 4, no further therapy apart from very close clinical follow-up generally needs to be considered. If her score is 5 or above and initial margins are close or involved, re-excision can be considered. But, it may yield a poor cosmetic result if the breast is small and margins may continue to be involved.

At this point, patients with intermediate VNPI scores of 5, 6, or 7 should be considered for breast irradiation. Patients with high VNPI scores of 8 or 9 should be considered for mastectomy with or without immediate reconstruction. Skin-sparing mastectomy is appropriate for patients with DCIS because this lesion does not involve the skin.

Reconstruction can be accomplished with a variety of techniques, including expander, implant, TRAM flap, etc. In general, immediate reconstruction is preferred. It eliminates at least one surgical procedure in the future and usually results in a happier patient with a better cosmetic result.

The most controversial point in DCIS treatment is whether or not to add radiation therapy for a patient who has what appears to be a complete excision of her

DCIS. Much more information needs to be gathered on this subject. At the current time, we do not irradiate any patients with DCIS with a VNPI score of 3 or 4. For patients with scores of 5, 6, or 7, with margin scores of 2 or 3, re-excision is considered. If the score remains in the mid-range, radiation therapy is generally added to the patient's treatment plan. For patients with scores of 8 or 9, a mastectomy with immediate reconstruction is usually recommended.

For women with larger lesions (relative to breast size) that cannot be totally excised, mastectomy remains the treatment of choice. However, the results of NSABP B-24 suggest that positive margins and residual calcifications may be acceptable for breast preservation as long as the patient undergoes postoperative breast irradiation.

THE FUTURE

Our current treatment approach to DCIS is based on morphology rather than etiology, on phenotype rather than genotype. Future treatment will now be based on further fine tuning of known prognostic factors. For example, are 12-mm margins better than 10-mm margins? Genetic changes routinely precede morphologic evidence of malignant transformation. Using basic science, medicine must learn how to recognize these genetic changes, exploit them and, ultimately, prevent them. DCIS is a lesion in which the complete malignant phenotype of unlimited growth, angiogenesis, genomic elasticity, invasion, and metastasis has not been fully expressed. With sufficient time, most non-invasive lesions will learn how to invade and metastasize. We must learn how to prevent this.

REFERENCES

1. Silverstein MJ, Handel N, Hoffman RS, et al. The Breast Center – a multidisciplinary model. In Paterson AHG, Lees AW, eds. Fundamental problems in breast cancer. Boston, Martinus Nijhoff, 1987, 47–58.

2. Silverstein MJ. The Van Nuys Breast Center – the first free-standing multidisciplinary breast center. Surg Oncol Clin North Am 2000; 9:159–75.

3. Patchefsky AS, Schwartz GF, Finkelstein SD, et al. Heterogeneity of intraductal carcinoma of the breast. Cancer 1989; 63:731–41.

4. Lennington WJ, Jensen RA, Dalton LW, Page DL. Ductal carcinoma in situ of the breast. Heterogeneity of individual lesions. Cancer 1994; 73:118–24.

5. Silverstein MJ. Intraductal breast carcinoma: two decades of progress? Am J Clin Oncol 1991; 14(6):534–7.

6. Ashikari R, Hadju SI, Robbins GF. Intraductal carcinoma of the breast. Cancer 1971; 28:1182–7.

7. SEER cancer statistics review: 1973–1990. NIH Pub No. 93-2789. Bethesda, MD, National Cancer Institute, 1993.

8. Ernster VL, Barclay J, Kerlikowske K, et al. Incidence of and treatment for ductal carcinoma in situ of the breast. JAMA 1996; 275:913–18.

9. Lagios MD. Duct carcinoma in situ: pathology and treatment. Surg Clin North Am 1990; 70:853–71.

10. Silverstein MJ, Cohlan B, Gierson ED, et al. Duct carcinoma in situ: 227 cases without microinvasion. Eur J Cancer 1992; 28(2/3):630–4.

11. Landis SH, Murray T, Bolden S, Wingo PA. Cancer statistics, 1999. CA Cancer J Clinic 1999; 49:8–31.

12. Nielson M, Thomsen JL, Primdahl S, Dreyborg U, Anderson JA. Breast cancer and atypia among young and middle-aged women; a study of 110 medicolegal autopsies. Br J Cancer 1987; 56:814–19.

13. Page DL, Dupont WD, Roger LW, Landenberger M. Intraductal carcinoma of the breast: follow-up after biopsy only. Cancer 1982; 49:751–8.

14. Rosen PP, Braun DW, Kinne DE. The clinical significance of pre-invasive breast carcinoma. Cancer 1980; 46:919–25.

15. Alpers C, Wellings S. The prevalence of carcinoma in situ in normal and cancer-associated breast. Hum Pathol 1985; 16:796–807.

16. Page DL, Dupont WD, Rogers LW, Jensen RA, Schuyler PA. Continued local recurrence of carcinoma 15–25 years after a diagnosis of low grade ductal carcinoma in situ of the breast treated only by biopsy. Cancer 1995; 76:1197–200.

17. Cheatle GL. Early recognition of cancer of the breast. BMJ 1906; 1:1205–10.

18. Broders AC. Carcinoma in situ contrasted with benign penetrating epithelium. JAMA 1932; 99:1670–4.

19. Foote FW Jr, Stewart FW. A histologic classification of carcinoma of the breast. Surgery 1946; 19:74–99.

20. Schnitt SJ, Connolly JL, Tavassoli FA, et al. Interobserver reproducibility in the diagnosis of ductal proliferative breast lesions using standardized criteria. Am J Surg Pathol 1992; 16:133–43.

21. Rosai J. Borderline epithelial lesions of the breast. Am J Surg Pathol 1991; 15:209–21.

22. Page DL, Dupont WD, Rogers LW, Rados MS. Atypical hyperplastic lesions of the female breast. A long-term follow-up study. Cancer 1985; 55:2698–708.

23. Dupont WD, Page DL. Risk factors for women with proliferative breast disease. N Engl J Med 1985; 312:146–51.

24. Page DL, Anderson TJ. Diagnostic histopathology of the breast. New York, Churchill Livingstone, 1987, 157–74.

25. Tavassoli FA. Pathology of the breast. Norwalk, Appleton & Lange, 1992, 229–61.

26. Aasmundstad TA, Haugen OA. DNA ploidy in intraductal breast carcinomas. Eur J Cancer 1992; 26:956–9.

27. Meyer J. Cell kinetics of histologic variants of in situ breast carcinoma. Breast Cancer Res Treat 1986; 7:171–80.

28. Allred DC, Clark GM, Molin R, *et al.* Over-expression of progression of in situ to invasive breast cancer. Hum Pathol 1992; 23:974–9.

29. Liu E, Thor A, He M, Barcos M, Ljung BM, Benz C. The HER2 (c-erbB-2) oncogene is frequently amplified in in situ carcinomas of the breast. Oncogene 1992; 7:1027–32.

30. Barnes DM, Meyer JS, Gonzalez JG, Gullick WJ, Millis RR. Relationship between c-erbB-2 immunoreactivity and thymidine labelling index in breast carcinoma in situ. Breast Cancer Res Treat 1991; 18:11–17.

31. Bartkova J, Barnes DM, Millis RR, Gullick WJ. Immunohistochemical demonstration of c-erbB-2 protein in mammary ductal carcinoma in situ. Hum Pathol 1990; 21:1164–7.

32. Bobrow LG, Happerfield LC, Gregory WM, Springall RD, Millis RR. The classification of ductal carcinoma in situ and its association with biological markers. Semin Diagn Pathol 1994; 11:199–207.

33. van de Vijver MJ, Peterse JL, Mooi WJ, *et al.* Neu-protein over-expression in breast cancer: association with comedo-type ductal carcinoma in situ and limited prognostic value in stage II breast cancer. N Engl J Med 1988; 319:1239–45.

34. Lagios MD, Margolin FR, Westdahl PR, Rose NM. Mammographically detected duct carcinoma in situ. Frequency of local recurrence following tylectomy and prognostic effect of nuclear grade on local recurrence. Cancer 1989; 63:619–24.

35. Silverstein MJ, Waisman JR, Gierson ED, *et al.* Radiation therapy for intraductal carcinoma: is it an equal alternative? Arch Surg 1991; 126:424–8.

36. Solin LJ, Yet I-T, Kurtz J, *et al.* Ductal carcinoma in situ (intraductal carcinoma) of the breast treated with breast-conserving surgery and definitive irradiation. Correlation of pathologic parameters with outcome of treatment. Cancer 1993; 71:2532–42.

37. Schwartz GF, Finkel GC, Garcia JC, Patchefsky AS. Subclinical ductal carcinoma in situ of the breast. Cancer 1992; 70:2468–74.

38. Silverstein MJ, Poller DN, Waisman JR. Prognostic classification of breast ductal carcinoma in situ. Lancet 1995; 345:1154–7.

39. Lagios MD, Westdahl PR, Margolin FR, Rose MR. Duct carcinoma in situ: relationship of extent of noninvasive disease to the frequency of occult invasion, multicentricity, lymph node metastases, and short-term treatment failures. Cancer 1982; 50:1309–14.

40. Silverstein MJ, Barth A, Poller DN, *et al.* Ten-year results comparing mastectomy to excision and radiation therapy for ductal carcinoma in situ of the breast. Eur J Cancer 1995; 31A(9):1425–7.

41. Poller DN, Silverstein MJ, Galea M, *et al.* Ductal carcinoma in situ of the breast: a proposal for a new simplified histological classification association between cellular proliferation and c-erbB-2 protein expression. Mod Pathol 1994; 7:257–62.

42. Sloane JP, Ellman R, Anderson TJ, *et al.* Consistency of histopathological reporting of breast lesions detected by breast screening: findings of the UK national external quality assessment (EQA) scheme. Eur J Cancer 1994; 10:1414–19.

43. Bellamy COC, McDonald C, Salter DM, Chetty U, Anderson TJ. Noninvasive ductal carcinoma of the breast. The relevance of histologic categorization. Hum Pathol 1993; 24:16–23.

44. Lampejo OT, Barnes DM, Smith P, Millis RR. Evaluation of infiltrating ductal carcinomas with a DCIS component: correlation of the histologic type of the in situ component with grade of the infiltrating component. Semin Diagn Pathol 1994; 11:215–22.

45. Hermanek P, Hutter RVP, Sobin LH, Wagner G, Cittekind C. *Breast tumors in TNM atlas*, 4th edn. London, Springer, 1997, 201–12.

46. Schuh ME, Nemoto T, Penetrante RB, Rosner D, Dao TL. Intraductal carcinoma: analysis of presentation, pathologic findings, and outcome of disease. Arch Surg 1986; 121:1303–7.

47. Gump FR, Jicha DL, Ozzello L. Ductal carcinoma in situ (DCIS): a revised concept. Surgery 1987; 102:190–5.

48. Fisher ER, Sass R, Fisher B, *et al.* Pathologic findings from the National Surgical Adjuvant Breast Project (Protocol 6). i. Intraductal carcinoma (DCIS). Cancer 1986; 57:197–208.

49. Schwartz GF, Patchefsky AS, Finkelstein SD, *et al.* Nonpalpable in situ ductal carcinoma of the breast. Arch Surg 1989; 124:29–32.

50. Rosen PP, Senie R, Schottenfeld D, Ashikari R. Noninvasive breast carcinoma: frequency of unsuspected invasion and implications for treatment. Ann Surg 1979; 189:377–82.

51. Simpson T, Thirlby RC, Dail DH. Surgical treatment of ductal carcinoma in situ of the breast: 10 to 20 year follow-up. Arch Surg 1992; 127:468–72.

52. Holland R, Hendriks JHCL, Verbeek ALM, Mravunac M, Schuurmans SJH. Extent, distribution, and mammographic/histological correlations of breast ductal carcinoma in situ. Lancet 1990; 335:519–22.

53. Holland R. Whole organ studies. In Silverstein MJ, ed. *Ductal carcinoma in situ of the breast*. Baltimore: Williams and Wilkins, 1997; 233–40.

54. Noguchi S, Aihara T, Koyama H, Motomura K, Inaji H, Imaoka S. Discrimination between multicentric and

multifocal carcinomas of breast through clonal analysis. Cancer 1994; 74:872–7.

55. Tabar L, Dean PB. Basic principles of mammographic diagnosis. Diagn Imag Clin Med 1985; 54:146–57.

56. Silverstein MJ, Gierson ED, Waisman JR, Colburn WJ, Gamagami P. Predicting axillary node positivity in patients with invasive carcinoma of the breast by using a combination of T category and palpability. J Am Coll Surg 1995; 180:700–4.

57. Silverstein MJ, Gamagami P, Colburn WJ, et al. Nonpalpable breast lesions: diagnosis with slightly overpenetrated screen-film mammography and hook wire-directed breast biopsy in 1014 cases. Radiology 1989; 171:633–8.

58. Silverstein MJ. Noninvasive breast cancer: the dilemma of the 1990s. Obstet Gynecol Clin North Am 1994; 21(4):639–58.

59. Silverstein MJ. The first chance is the best chance. J Surg Oncol 1995; 58:229–30.

60. Fentiman IS, Fagg N, Millis RR, Haywood JL. In situ ductal carcinoma of the breast: Implications of disease pattern and treatment. Eur J Surg Oncol 1986; 12:261–6.

61. Fisher B, Costantino J, Redmond C, et al. Lumpectomy compared with lumpectomy and radiation therapy for the treatment of intraductal breast cancer. N Engl J Med 1993; 328:1581–6.

62. Swain SM. Ductal carcinoma in situ – incidence, presentation and guidelines to treatment. Oncology 1989; 3:25–42.

63. Fowble B. Intraductal noninvasive breast cancer: a comparison of three local treatments. Oncology 1989; 3:51–8.

64. Barth A, Brenner J, Giuliano AE. Current management of ductal carcinoma in situ. West J Med 1995; 163:360–6.

65. Jensen JA, Handel N, Silverstein MJ. Glandular replacement therapy (GRT) for intraductal breast carcinoma (DCIS). Proc Am Soc Clin Oncol 1995; 14:138.

66. Lagios MD. Ductal carcinoma in situ: controversies in diagnosis, biology, and treatment. Breast J 1995; 1:68–78.

67. Holland R, Veling SHJ, Mravunac M, Hendriks JHCL. Histologic multifocality of Tis, T1–2 breast carcinomas. Implications for clinical trials of breast conserving surgery. Cancer 1985; 56:979–90.

68. Sibbering DN, Blamey RW. Nottingham experience. In Silverstein MJ, ed. Ductal carcinoma in situ of the breast. Baltimore: Williams and Wilkins, 1997, 367–72.

69. Faverly DRG, Burgers L, Bult P, Holland R. Three dimensional imaging of mammary ductal carcinoma in situ: clinical implications. Semin Diagn Pathol 1995; 11(3):193–8.

70. Silverstein MJ, Gierson ED, Colburn WJ, et al. Can intraductal breast carcinoma be excised completely by local excision? Clinical and pathologic predictors. Cancer 1994; 73:2985–9.

71. Ottesen GL, Graversen HP, Blichert-Toft M, Zedeler K, Andersen JA. Ductal carcinoma in situ of the female breast. Short-term results of a prospective nationwide study. Am J Surg Pathol 1992; 16:1183–96.

72. Solin LJ, Recht A, Fourquet A, et al. Ten-year results of breast-conserving surgery and definitive irradiation for intraductal carcinoma of the breast. Cancer 1991; 68:2337–44.

73. McCormick B, Rosen PP, Kinne D, Cox L, Yahalom J. Duct carcinoma in situ of the breast: an analysis of local control after conservation surgery and radiotherapy. Int J Radiat Oncol Biol Phys 1991; 21:289–92.

74. Findlay P, Goodman R. Radiation therapy for treatment of intraductal carcinoma of the breast. Am J Clin Oncol 1983; 6:281–5.

75. Ray GR, Adelson J, Hayhurst E, et al. Ductal carcinoma in situ of the breast: results of treatment by conservative surgery and definitive radiation. Int J Radiat Oncol Biol Phys 1993; 28:105–11.

76. Recht A, Danoff B, Solin LJ, et al. Intraductal carcinoma of the breast: results of treatment with excisional biopsy and irradiation. J Clin Oncol 1985; 3:1339–43.

77. Zafrani B, Fourquet A, Vilcoq JR, Legal M, Calle R. Conservative management of intraductal breast carcinoma with tumorectomy and radiation therapy. Cancer 1986; 57:1299–301.

78. Kuske RR, Bean JM, Garcia DM, et al. Breast conservation therapy for intraductal carcinoma of the breast. Int J Radiat Oncol Biol Phys 1993; 26:391–6.

79. Bornstein BA, Recht A, Connolly JL, et al. Results of treating ductal carcinoma in situ of the breast with conservative surgery and radiation therapy. Cancer 1991; 67:7–13.

80. Solin L, Kurtz J, Fourquet A, et al. Fifteen year outcome for conservative surgery and radiotherapy for ductal carcinoma in situ (DCIS). Proc Am Soc Clin Oncol 1995; 14:107.

81. Lagios MD, Page DL. Radiation therapy for in situ or localized breast cancer (Letter). N Engl J Med 1993; 21:1577–8.

82. Page DL, Lagios MD. Pathologic analysis of the NSABP-B17 Trial. Cancer 1995; 75:1219–22.

83. Fisher ER, Costantino J, Fisher B, et al. Pathologic findings from the National Surgical Adjuvant Breast Project (NSABP) Protocol B-17. Cancer 1995; 75:1310–9.

84. Fisher ER, Dignam J, Tan-Chiu E, et al. Pathologic findings from the National Surgical Adjuvant Breast Project (NSABP) eight-year update of Protocol B-17: intraductal carcinoma. Cancer 1999; 86:429–38.

85. Fisher B, Dignam J, Wolmark N, *et al.* Lumpectomy and radiation therapy for the treatment of intraductal breast cancer: findings from National Surgical Adjuvant Breast and Bowel Project B-17. J Clin Oncol 1998; 16:441–52.

86. Fisher B, Dignam J, Wolmark N. Tamoxifen in treatment of intraductal breast cancer: National surgical adjuvant breast and bowel project B-24 randomized controlled trial. Lancet 1999; 353:1993–2000.

87. Fisher B, Costantino JP, Wickerham DL, *et al.* Tamoxifen for prevention of breast cancer: Report of the national surgical adjuvant breast and bowel project P-1 Study. J Natl Cancer Inst 1998; 90:1371–88.

88. Wolmark N. Tamoxifen after surgery/RT decreases local recurrence risk in DCIS patients. Oncol News Int 1999; 8(2) (Suppl. 2):12.

89. Julien J-P, Bijker N, Fentiman IS, *et al.* Radiotherapy in breast-conserving treatment for ductal carcinoma in situ: first results of the EORTC randomized phase III trial 10853. Lancet 2000; 355:528–33.

90. Recht A. Side effects of radiation therapy. In: Silverstein MJ, ed. *Ductal carcinoma in situ of the breast.* Baltimore: Williams and Wilkins, 1997, 347–52.

91. Zafrani B, Leroyer A, Fourquet A, *et al.* Mammographically-detected ductal carcinoma in situ of the breast analysed with a new classification. A study of 127 cases: correlation with estrogen and progesterone receptors, p53 and c-erbB-2 proteins and proliferative activity. Semin Diagn Pathol 1994; 11(3):208–13.

92. Lebow F. New prognostic index stratifies treatment for DCIS patients. Oncol Times 1995; 17(7):3–4.

93. Silverstein MJ, Poller DN, Craig PH, *et al.* A prognostic index for breast ductal carcinoma in situ. Breast Cancer Res Treat 1996; 37(Suppl.):34 (abstract).

94. Silverstein MJ, Poller DN, Craig PH, *et al.* A prognostic index for ductal carcinoma in situ of the breast. Cancer 1996; 77:2267–74.

95. The Van Nuys Prognostic Index for ductal carcinoma in situ. Breast J 1996; 2:38–40.

96. Silverstein MJ. Van Nuys Prognostic Index for DCIS. In Silverstein MJ, ed. *Ductal carcinoma in situ of the breast.* Baltimore: Williams and Wilkins, 1997, 491–504.

97. Fentiman IS, Fagg N, Millis RR, Hayward JL. In situ ductal carcinoma of the breast: implications of disease pattern and treatment. Eur J Surg Oncol 1986; 12:261–6.

98. Bradley SJ, Weaver DW, Bouwman DL. Alternative in the surgical management of in situ breast cancer. Am Surg 1990; 56:428–32.

99. Rosner D, Bedwani RN, Vana J, Baker HW, Murphy GP. Noninvasive breast carcinoma. Results of a national survey of the American College of Surgeons. Ann Surg 1980; 192:139–47.

100. Silverstein MJ, Lagios MD, Groshen S, *et al.* The influence of margin width on local control in patients with ductal carcinoma in situ (DCIS) of the breast. N Engl J Med 1999; 340:1455–61.

101. Silverstein MJ, Rosser RJ, Gierson ED, *et al.* Axillary lymph node dissection for intraductal carcinoma – is it indicated? Proc Am Soc Clin Oncol 1986; 5:265.

102. Silverstein MJ, Rosser RJ, Gierson ED, *et al.* Axillary lymph node dissection for intraductal carcinoma – is it indicated? Cancer 1987; 59:1819–24.

103. Frykberg ER, Masood S, Copeland EM, Bland KI. Duct carcinoma in situ of the breast. Surg Gynecol Obstet 1993; 177:425–40.

104. Balch CM, Singletary ES, Bland KI. Clinical decision-making in early breast cancer. Ann Surg 1993; 217:207–22.

105. Fisher B, Montague E, Redmond C, *et al.* Comparison of radical mastectomy with alternative treatments for primary breast cancer. Cancer 1977; 39:2827–39.

106. Hansen N, Giuliano A. Axillary dissection for ductal carcinoma in situ. In Silverstein MJ, ed. *Ductal carcinoma in situ of the breast.* Baltimore: Williams and Wilkins, 1997, 577–84.

107. Krag DN, Weaver DL, Alex JC, *et al.* Surgical resection and radiolocalization of sentinel lymph node in breast cancer using a gamma probe. Surg Oncol 1993; 2:335–40.

108. Giuliano AE, Dale PS, Turner RR, *et al.* Improved axillary staging of breast cancer with sentinel lymphadenectomy. Ann Surg 1995; 222:394–401.

109. Albertini JJ, Lyman GH, Cox C, *et al.* Lymphatic mapping and sentinel node biopsy in the patient with breast cancer. JAMA 1996; 276:1818–22.

110. Silverstein MJ, Lagios MD, Martino S, *et al.* Outcome after local recurrence in patients with ductal carcinoma in situ of the breast. J Clin Oncol 1998; 16:1367–73.

111. Stockdale AD, Brierley JD, Whire WF, Folkes A, Rostom AY. Radiotherapy for Paget's disease of the nipple: a conservative alternative. Lancet 1989; ii (8664):664–6.

ANNOTATED BIBLIOGRAPHY

Fisher ER, Costantino J, Fisher B, *et al.* Pathologic findings from the National Surgical Adjuvant Breast and Bowel Project (NSABP) Protocol B-17: intraductal carcinoma (ductal carcinoma in situ). Cancer 1995; 75:1310–19.
The NSABP performed a central slide review and reported outcome by nine histopathologic factors. Moderate to marked comedo necrosis and uncertain or involved excision margins were independent predictors of ipsilateral breast tumor recurrence.

Fisher B, Costantino J, Redmond C, et al. Lumpectomy compared with lumpectomy and radiation therapy for the treatment of intraductal breast cancer. N Engl J Med 1993; 328:1581–6.

The first published prospective randomized study (NSABP B Protocol B-17) comparing excision alone versus excision plus breast irradiation for patients with DCIS. At 5 years, there was a significant decrease in ipsilateral breast tumor recurrence for patients treated with post-excisional radiation therapy.

Fisher ER, Dignam J, Tan-Chiu E, et al. Pathologic findings from the National Surgical Adjuvant Breast and Bowel Project (NSABP) eight-year update of Protocol B-17: intraductal carcinoma. Cancer 1999; 86:429–38.

In this report, the NSABP's 8-year update of outcome based on histopathologic findings, only moderate to marked comedo necrosis was an independent predictor of ipsilateral breast tumor recurrence. As in all previous reports, the NSABP continued to recommend post-excisional radiation therapy for all subsets of patients with DCIS treated with breast preservation. Although ipsilateral breast tumor recurrence rates were higher after excision alone, there was no difference in breast cancer-specific survival, regardless of treatment.

Fisher B, Dignam J, Wolmark N, et al. Lumpectomy and radiation therapy for the treatment of intraductal breast cancer: findings from National Surgical Adjuvant Breast and Bowel Project B-17. J Clin Oncol 1998; 16:441–52.

In this report, the NSABP updated its 1993 paper. After 8 years of follow-up, all cohorts of patients who were treated with post-excisional breast irradiation continued to benefit, with a decreased rate of ipsilateral breast tumor recurrence.

Silverstein MJ, Lagios MD, Craig PH, et al. A prognostic index for ductal carcinoma in situ of the breast. Cancer 1996; 77:2267–74.

The Van Nuys groups introduced an algorithm as an aid to treatment selection. The Van Nuys Prognostic Index (VNPI) was based on biologic classification, margin width, and tumor size. The VNPI attempted to aid clinicians in selecting patients who could be treated safely by excision alone.

Silverstein MJ, Lagios MD, Groshen S, et al. The influence of margin width on local control in patients with ductal carcinoma in situ (DCIS) of the breast. N Engl J Med 1999; 340:1455–61.

Because of difficulty from laboratory to laboratory in reproducing tumor size and biologic classification, the Van Nuys group tested margin width alone as the sole predictor of local recurrence. Whereas not quite as good as the VNPI, it proved to be an excellent and reproducible surrogate.

Silverstein MJ, Lagios MD, Martino S, et al. Outcome after local recurrence in patients with ductal carcinoma in situ of the breast. J Clin Oncol 1998; 16:1367–73.

This paper looked at the most important outcome after treatment for DCIS: breast cancer-specific survival. Like the NSABP B-17 study, although ipsilateral breast tumor recurrence rates were higher after excision alone, there was no difference in breast cancer-specific survival, regardless of treatment.

Silverstein MJ, Poller DN, Waisman JR. Prognostic classification of breast ductal carcinoma in situ. Lancet 1995; 345:1154–7.

The Van Nuys group introduced a biologic DCIS classification based on nuclear grade and presence or absence of comedonecrosis.

Commentary

GORDON F SCHWARTZ

In the breast cancer spectrum, there may be no more currently contentious and controversial diagnosis than ductal carcinoma *in situ*. Both the diagnosis and the treatment of this particular breast lesion often provoke dogmatic, but unfortunately conflicting, opinions from renowned clinicians and pathologists. The options of therapy may be few – the treatment of the breast (and, infrequently, the axilla) – but the differences among these treatments are formidable to the patients who must make these decisions and live with them. Moreover, the dilemma about the treatment of DCIS became a matter of public debate in March 1996 with the publication of geographically related disparities in treatment for this disease.[1] Although treatment has generally shifted from mastectomy toward breast conservation, the increased detection of DCIS has led, at least until recently, to an actual increase in the number of mastectomies performed for this disease.

The contributions of Dr Silverstein and his associates to the knowledge about and treatment of DCIS are impressive and considerable. Therefore, the opinions expressed in the preceding chapter should be considered, at least from the clinical perspective, as knowledgeable and up to date. Dr Silverstein and I have shared our own information about DCIS since the early 1980s, so it is not surprising that our opinions are quite similar. Nevertheless, there are areas about which we have agreed to disagree. The organization of this commentary generally follows that of the preceding chapter wherever possible, to make it easier for the reader to appreciate the similarities and differences of opinions between us.

PATHOLOGY

Recognizing the lack of a universally accepted classification of DCIS, a consensus was held in Philadelphia in 1997 to address this very issue. From this conference emerged a consensus statement published later that year in three peer-review journals concurrently.[2–4] It was hoped that this report, representing the opinion of a group of recognized DCIS specialists in multiple disciplines, would help define classification so that DCIS encountered by one group of investigators would be classified in the same manner as that seen in another city or country. Because the endpoints of the treatment of DCIS include the probability of local recurrence, as further DCIS or as invasive carcinoma, and breast carcinoma-specific mortality, these factors were those considered by the consensus panelists, as well as the need for mastectomy following failed breast conservation.

The same architectural patterns were recognized as expressed in the preceding chapter (papillary, micropapillary, solid, cribriform, and comedo), and virtually the same comments about them were adopted in the consensus report. However, any system of classification must reflect the ability of the lesion to recur locally or progress to invasive cancer. Differences in architecture do not separate DCIS clearly enough in this regard; in general, the five subtypes have been divided into 'comedo' and 'non-comedo' types to try to reflect their biological differences. However, the term 'comedo' may be misleading because pathologists do not define the term alike. Because necrosis may occur with any of the architectural patterns, the term 'comedo' was used to refer specifically to solid intraepithelial growth within the basement membrane with central (zonal) necrosis. Such lesions are not invariably of high nuclear grade. For this reason, the Consensus Committee adopted clear definitions of the terms 'nuclear grade' and 'necrosis,' adding 'polarization' to the classification system. This last term is more often used in Europe than in the USA.

These definitions are summarized below, and their similarity to those expressed by Dr Silverstein *et al.* is obvious:

A. NUCLEAR GRADE

a. Low-grade nuclei (NG 1).

Appearance: monotonous (monomorphic).

Size: 1.5–2.0 normal red blood cell or duct epithelial cell nucleus dimensions.

Features: usually exhibit diffuse, finely dispersed chromatin, only occasional nucleoli and mitotic figures. Usually associated with polarization of constituent cells.

Caveat: the presence of nuclei that are of similar size but are pleomorphic precludes a low-grade classification.

b. High-grade nuclei (NG 3).

Appearance: markedly pleomorphic.

Size: nuclei usually > 2.5 red blood cell or duct epithelial cell nuclear dimensions.

Features: usually vesicular and exhibit irregular chromatin distribution and prominent, often multiple, nucleoli. Mitoses may be conspicuous.

c. Intermediate-grade nuclei (NG 2). Nuclei that are neither NG 1 nor NG 3.

B. NECROSIS. Definition of necrosis: the presence of ghost cells and karyorrhectic debris. These are important features, distinguishing necrotic debris from secretory material.

Necrosis quantification:

- Comedo necrosis: any central zone necrosis within a duct, usually exhibiting a linear pattern within ducts if sectioned longitudinally.
- Punctate: non-zonal-type necrosis (foci of necrosis that do not exhibit a linear pattern if longitudinally sectioned).

C. CELL POLARIZATION: polarization reflects the radial orientation of the apical portion of tumor cells toward intercellular (lumen-like) spaces, either larger lumina or minute 'microacinar' spaces that produce a rosette-like appearance. Such polarization is characteristic of lower grade DCIS with cribriform and solid architecture, but can also be recognized in epithelial protuberances, bridges, arcades and micropapillae of DCIS of lower grades with micropapillary architecture.

It is now accepted that the nuclear grade of DCIS is probably the single most important factor that determines its behavior. It is often difficult to assign a single nuclear grade to any specific lesion of DCIS because of the heterogeneity of nuclear grade often seen in the same specimen. Because it is unknown if the proportion of each affects outcome, it is probably safest if the pathology report reflects the highest nuclear grade but also cites the others and the proportions of each.

DETECTION AND DIAGNOSIS

The diagnosis of subclinical DCIS is almost always related to a mammographic finding, usually calcifications, that precipitates a recommendation for biopsy. Rarely, DCIS may be discovered by a pathologist as an incidental finding during review of a breast biopsy specimen that was excised for another reason. Occasionally, a non-palpable mass may prove to be DCIS, or DCIS may present as a subtle area of architectural distortion, without any mass or calcifications on the mammograms. These latter two presentations are uncommon, so that the vast majority of patients with DCIS have mammographically detected calcifications as the only finding.

The complete mammographic work-up of a patient whose calcifications are newly detected includes magnification films, even if a recommendation for biopsy may be made on the initial studies. It is most helpful if the full extent of the calcifications can be documented; faint, powdery calcifications may not be entirely imaged on the initial radiographs, and the overall area involved may influence the type of biopsy or the treatment recommended.

Once a biopsy recommendation has been made, the next question is 'What kind of biopsy?' Stereotactic fine-needle aspiration (FNA) is not usually useful in the diagnosis of DCIS. Although the 'tissue juice' obtained from FNA may indicate the presence of frankly malignant cells, invasion cannot be diagnosed without the ability to examine the cells in the context of their surroundings. Ultrasound-guided biopsy is usually not feasible because the lesions of DCIS are not often imaged by ultrasound. Therefore, the choices are stereotactic core biopsy versus open surgical needle-guided (wire-directed) biopsy.

Our first needle-guided biopsy for a non-palpable finding was performed in 1974; since that time we have performed more than 7000 such procedures, and it now represents the most common surgical breast biopsy procedure we perform. (Palpable masses are usually candidates for office FNA or core biopsy.) Nevertheless, despite our extensive experience with this technique, the use of an 11-gauge, vacuum-assisted biopsy device attached to a dedicated stereo table has made stereo-core biopsy an attractive first step in the diagnosis of DCIS.

The advantages of the initial stereo-core biopsy are several. If the diagnosis of DCIS can be made, and the volume of tissue removed is sufficient to be comfortable about the apparent absence of invasion, patient and physician can discuss further treatment much more precisely, especially if breast conservation is to be employed. If a needle-guided biopsy is the first step, the surgeon is confronted with an enigmatic decision – how much tissue to remove. There are two conflicting goals, namely, the wide excision of DCIS if present, but the least amount of tissue removal if the calcifications have a benign origin. If a wide local excision is performed and the lesion is found to be benign, too much tissue has been removed. If the first procedure is limited in extent and DCIS is the diagnosis, a re-excision is mandatory. The minimally invasive biopsy as the first step obviates this dilemma. When a core biopsy indicates DCIS, when breast conservation is the choice, plans for a wide excision may be made, at the same time confronting the concerns about cosmesis. For those patients who require or prefer mastectomy, this decision can be made without the need for an initial open surgical procedure.

Some areas of calcifications do not lend themselves well to stereo-core biopsy. If they are very powdery and faint, they may not be imaged on the stereo unit because its resolution is not as great as that of the best film-screen mammograms. Some calcifications may be too scattered to permit a substantive diagnosis using a needle-core biopsy, however well performed. Other patients' breasts may be too small to fit into the dedicated unit, or the

calcifications may be too far back in the breast to be approached by the stereo-guided needle.

In these cases, traditional needle-guided biopsy is the requisite first step. However, unlike Dr Silverstein et al., we do not believe that the first surgical procedure should be considered the most important time to achieve local excision with clear margins and optimal cosmesis, nor do we believe that multiple bracketing wires are necessary in each case. What is crucial is cooperation among the several members of the team – radiologist, surgeon, and pathologist. Whether one or more wires are used depends upon institutional experience, recognizing that the goal is the same – the removal of the area(s) of DCIS with negative margins. The orientation of the specimen for the specimen radiograph is more important than how many wires are in the field. We will usually ask the radiologist to clip the specimen if the calcifications are not centered. The radiograph of the specimen always accompanies the specimen to the pathologist. Frozen sections are never employed. These small specimens are entirely embedded and sectioned. Frozen sections require that a portion of the specimen be separated from the remainder; and, as the frozen sections are prepared, we fear the loss of important tissue on the floor of the cryostat.

The technique of tissue processing is another contentious point in determining the size of the area of DCIS and margin status. That the technique recommended by Dr Silverstein et al. is optimal is not questioned. Sequential step sections at 2–3-mm intervals do determine the size of the area of DCIS reliably and reproducibly. Unfortunately, most pathologists, even those at academic centers, have not adopted the technique because it is so time consuming and labor intensive. It is virtually impossible to perform truly serial sections of these specimens. To do so would require so many slides that pathologists would have little time to process other specimens.

Also, we do not ink margins, either for DCIS or for invasive cancers. Instead, we remove the area as indicated by the needle-guided procedure, with a wide rim of apparently normal-appearing breast tissue. We then shave the edges of the biopsy cavity, removing arcs of tissue, usually five, from medial, lateral, superior, and inferior margins, and from the base of the wound. Each of these is sent to the pathologist in a separate container, appropriately marked. If each is negative for tumor cells, we consider this equivalent to a 10-mm or greater clear margin. If any is even focally positive, it is considered an involved margin, and re-excision of that margin is performed if breast conservation is planned. Its location is precisely known, because the pathologist has separately accessed these marginal biopsy specimens. Additionally, when the margins are shaved, small metallic clips are placed at each margin, so that the site of the DCIS has been clearly marked for the radiologist or radiation oncologist. Our own pathologists have enthusiastically embraced this technique to assess margins, because coating the surface of the specimen with any type of ink, however carefully performed, is like trying to coat the surface of an English muffin, not the surface of a jelly bean. The ink runs into 'nooks and crannies' of the specimen surface, and the slides may still be misleading. Moreover, surgical specimens contract when they are excised from the contiguous tissue, and the actual distance from the edge of DCIS to true margin may be underestimated. If, however, the marginal biopsies are all negative, even though they are not truly 360 degrees around the biopsy cavity, we think they are more informative than the inked margins of an excised specimen.

The size question is more difficult to answer. Other than the technique espoused by Dr Silverstein *et al.*, there has been no general agreement among pathologists as to the best technique to estimate the size of the area of DCIS. The extent of the disease within the breast is invariably greater than the area of the calcifications seen on the mammograms. However, if this is a reasonably consistent observation (e.g., one can reasonably state that, if the calcifications are 2.0 cm in greatest diameter, the area of DCIS is not usually more than 3.0 cm in diameter, etc.), the size measurements for DCIS may underestimate the actual findings, but will do so in a reproducible manner. This would at least allow size comparisons measured in this way. (This technique of size measurement does not vitiate the need for clear margins, irrespective of the magnitude of this error.) Measuring the area of calcifications on the mammogram is reasonably easy to perform and is not as labor intensive as trying to cut slides at precisely stepped intervals.

In our own pathology laboratory, the entire specimen is embedded, and no tissue is discarded. Since 1992, when the techniques became more readily available, we have performed immunohistochemical marker determinations on our DCIS specimens. Initially, these included measurements of estrogen and progesterone receptors, Ki-67, p53, and c-erbB2. We have added p21 to this battery as well. We are currently retrieving the specimens from before 1992 to perform these determinations and add them to our database. As the tissues were formalin fixed and the blocks saved, we can always return to them again at a later date should other markers become identified as better predictors of recurrence. The limiting factor will be only the size of the area of DCIS.

TREATMENT

Recognizing the ongoing scientific debate concerning the appropriate treatment for DCIS, a second consensus conference was convened in April 1999, with a similar group of experts as in 1997 discussing current criteria for differing treatment recommendations. The consensus has been published again in three journals concurrently.[5–7] Many of the experts at the 1999 conference were at the 1997 conference as well. Because the 1999 conference was devoted to treatment, the high number of pathologists gave way to a greater number of clinicians – surgeons and radiation oncologists. The comments in this chapter in part reflect the discussion during this consensus conference as well as our own experience with DCIS over the past 20+ years.

Mastectomy

Breast conservation is the goal of treatment for DCIS; nevertheless, there is a group of patients still best served by mastectomy. There are no randomized clinical trials that compare total mastectomy with breast conservation; total ('simple') mastectomy remains the 'gold standard' against which any other treatment must be compared. There are ample data from retrospective studies of the treatment of DCIS and the treatment of invasive cancers to permit this extrapolation. Systemic failure after mastectomy implies the presence of undiagnosed (clinically occult) invasive carcinoma. Local failure after mastectomy, however, is rarely encountered.

Although the goal of treatment for DCIS is breast conservation, mastectomy is one of the acceptable treatment options for patients with DCIS. However, only a minority of patients with DCIS require mastectomy, probably less than 25% of patients with this diagnosis, but mastectomy could be performed if it were the patient's preference. There are specific circumstances that make mastectomy the preferable treatment option for DCIS. These include the following scenarios:

1 large areas of DCIS, of a size such that the lesion cannot undergo an oncologically acceptable excision while still conserving a cosmetically acceptable breast;
2 patients with multiple areas of DCIS in the same breast that cannot be encompassed through a single incision (there may be a highly selected subgroup of these patients, for example a patient with two, even three, very small areas of nuclear grade I DCIS, who might be treated by excision alone without radiation therapy, but as of this time, radiation therapists are uncomfortable treating patients with more than one site of DCIS in the breast);
3 patients who cannot undergo radiation therapy because of other medical problems, e.g., collagen vascular diseases, or prior therapeutic radiation to the chest for another illness, and for whom treatment by excision alone is not appropriate.

Mastectomy for DCIS mandates removal of all of the breast tissue, including the nipple and areola. So-called skin-sparing mastectomy is appropriate. This procedure is what Dr Silverstein *et al.* call 'glandular replacement therapy.' When the biopsy site can reasonably be included

Color plates

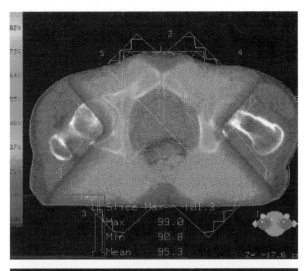

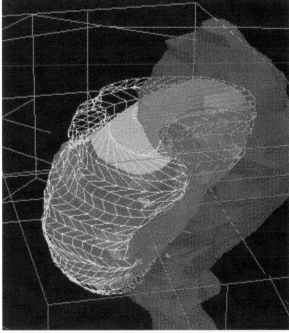

Plate 1 *Three-dimensional isodose curve conforming to the concave posterior shape of the prostate, thereby sparing rectum. Photograph courtesy of Varian Medical Systems, Palo Alto, CA.*

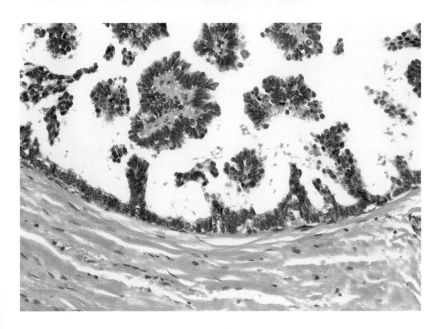

Plate 2 *Non-high-grade DCIS without necrosis (group 1).*

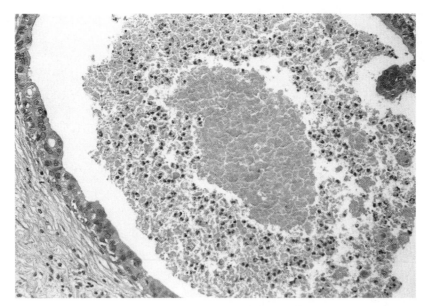

Plate 3 *Non-high-grade DCIS with central necrosis (group 2).*

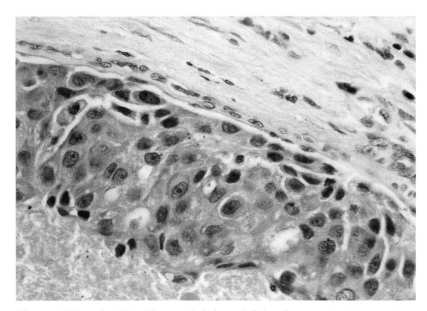

Plate 4 *High-grade DCIS with necrosis in lower left-hand corner.*

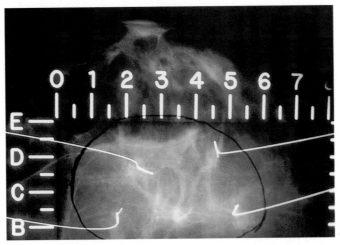

Plate 5 *Craniocaudal mammogram taken after insertion of four bracketing wires around an area of architectural distortion.*

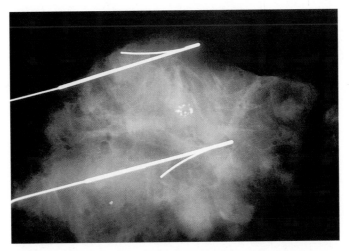

Plate 6 *Specimen radiograph of a double-wire-directed breast biopsy showing a cluster of microcalcifications excised with clear margins.*

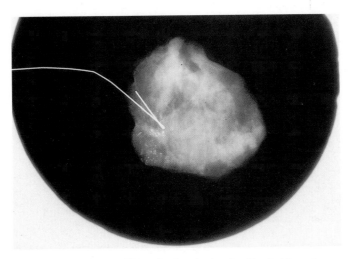

Plate 7 *A specimen radiograph of a single-wire-directed breast biopsy showing microcalcifications at the edge of the specimen.*

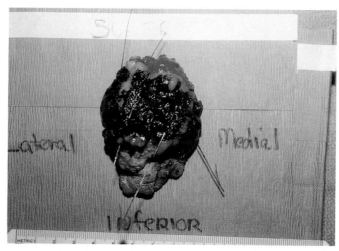

Plate 8 *The color-coded excision specimen with multiple wires in place.*

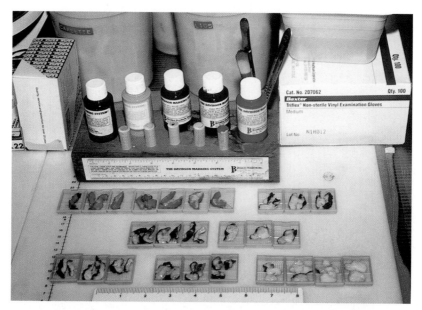

Plate 9 *The specimen has been color coded with dyes and serially sectioned.*

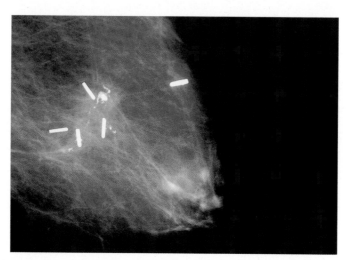

Plate 10 *A postoperative mediolateral mammogram. Metal clips mark the biopsy cavity.*

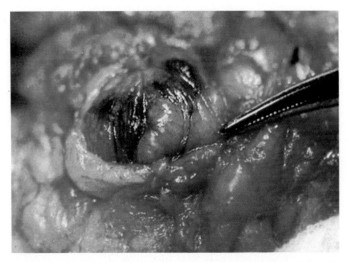

Plate 11 *Two side-by-side, blue-staining sentinel lymph nodes and lymphatic tracts in situ. (Reprinted with permission from Giuliano et al.[12])*

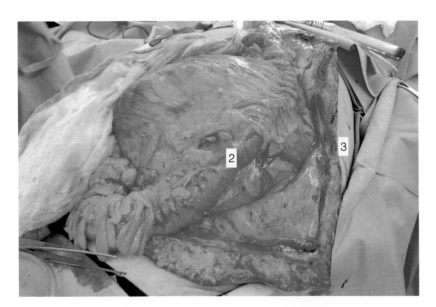

Plate 12 *Massive left-sided retroperitoneal liposarcoma. Intraoperative photograph prior to dissection demonstrating tumor with the left colon and its mesentery draped over the mass (2). T-extension off midline incision provides the required exposure (3).*

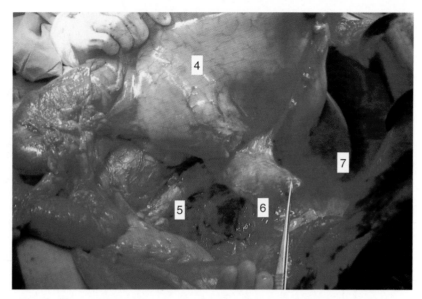

Plate 13 *Massive left-sided retroperitoneal liposarcoma. Retroperitoneum at the conclusion of resection. Resection of a portion of the left diaphragm, distal pancreatectomy, splenectomy, left adrenalectomy with uretero-nephrectomy, and left hemicolectomy along with portions of retroperitoneal musculature were required to remove the tumor mass. (4) Posterior wall of stomach; (5) aorta; (6) proximal pancreas; (7) lateral segment, left lobe liver.*

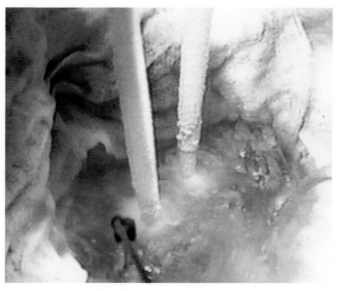

Plate 14 *Two cryoprobes in situ with propagating iceball. Note thermocouple in foreground.*

within the skin sacrificed, it should be removed with the nipple/areola and adjacent skin. When the biopsy site is at some distance from the central portion of the breast, if skin-sparing mastectomy is performed, separate excision of the biopsy site should be considered. This caveat should not apply for the site of a needle-core biopsy in DCIS. Reconstruction should be offered to each patient who chooses mastectomy. Women with DCIS who undergo mastectomy are ideal candidates for reconstruction, and there are few, if any, contraindications to an immediate reconstruction if the patient desires one. We also prefer a TRAM flap as the reconstruction, usually using a pedicle rather than a free flap. Skin-sparing mastectomy is not performed if the patient does not undergo an immediate reconstruction, because the wound closure would result in too much redundant skin. Leaving this redundant skin is not usually appropriate. We have done so only when the patient has chosen to have a delayed reconstruction, and she and the reconstructive surgeon have requested that we leave this skin, however 'wrinkled' it may look, to facilitate the later procedure.

There are situations in which the location or the extent of the DCIS within the breast brings it close to the posterior margin of the mastectomy specimen. The proximity of DCIS to this particular margin is not considered similar to its proximity to the other margins within the breast itself. There is no glandular breast tissue, i.e., ducts or lobules, deep to the deep layer of the superficial fascia of the breast. A so-called 'close' posterior margin following mastectomy for DCIS does not imply the need for adjuvant radiation therapy, as it might for an invasive cancer.

A formal dissection of the axilla is not part of the procedure for DCIS. However, it is virtually impossible to perform a total mastectomy without some lymph nodes in the axillary tail of the breast being part of the breast dissection. These are variable in number and location, and the pathologist will usually find several nodes in this portion of the breast as the specimen is dissected.

Breast conservation

The majority of women with DCIS are candidates for breast conservation. This implies wide local excision of the disease within the breast. Patients for whom breast conservation is anticipated should undergo a post-excision mammogram to ensure that all of the suspicious calcifications have been removed. If the specimen radiograph performed at the time of initial biopsy shows all of the suspicious calcifications to be well within the excised tissue and the margins are widely clear (≥ 10 mm) microscopically, this step might be avoided, but there is no harm done nor is it redundant if a post-biopsy mammogram is performed prior to a final recommendation about treatment. Because any residual calcifications must be imaged, the mammogram should not be performed until the

patient is comfortable enough to undergo the compression that is necessary to achieve a technically optimal mammogram. Magnification films of the biopsy site are also advisable. Therefore, for some patients, this post-biopsy mammogram may not be feasible for 2 or 3 months after the initial biopsy. Patients and physicians should not feel intimidated by any delay necessary to complete this important step, because the treatment of DCIS is not an emergency.

Whether radiation therapy, surveillance alone, or either of these plus tamoxifen is optimal treatment when breast conservation is employed is the current topic of greatest debate. Most investigators agree that there are groups of patients with DCIS who fall into each of these categories, but no one has yet defined the selection criteria for each of them precisely enough to make dogmatic recommendations. Clinical trials have shown that local excision and radiation therapy in patients with negative margins provide excellent rates of local control.[8,9] Patients treated by excision alone have a greater chance of local recurrence. There is evidence that recurrence is decreased with wider surgical margins around the area of DCIS. The available data indicate that the likelihood of developing *invasive* cancer of the breast following treatment by breast conservation with or without radiation therapy is about 1% or less per year following the initial diagnosis and treatment.

Although adding radiation therapy to wide local excision benefits all groups of DCIS patients who are candidates for breast conservation, the magnitude of that benefit may be small enough in some patient subgroups that radiation can be omitted. However, patients who may avoid radiation therapy have not been reproducibly and reliably identified by any clinical trials. There are institutional and individual reports of large series of such patients treated by wide excision alone who also achieve a 1% or less per year risk of invasive recurrence.

Wide excision only

We have been among the champions of wide excision and surveillance only as treatment for selected patients with DCIS. We agree with the preceding chapter that there are groups of patients for whom the addition of radiation therapy after adequate local excision provides only marginal protection against a second event. In general, these patients should fulfill the following criteria:

1 The size of the area of DCIS, whether measured by the pathologist or by measuring the area of calcifications on the mammogram, is less than 2–3 cm diameter. When size is based upon mammographic measurement of calcifications, if the area of calcifications on the mammogram is more quadrangular than round in shape, it should be less than approximately 6 cm^2 in area. Occasionally, somewhat larger areas of calcifications may be encountered that can be well excised

because the breast is large enough to accommodate the loss of a greater volume of tissue without significant deformity.

2 Margins around any site of DCIS should be 10 mm or greater.

3 The nuclear grade of the DCIS should be low or intermediate grade, as defined by the 1997 Consensus Conference, although we have also treated patients with nuclear grade 3 DCIS by local excision alone. This group of patients does have a higher likelihood of recurrence, but perhaps less so if margins wider than 10 mm can be achieved.

4 The aesthetic appearance of the breast following local excision should be appropriate. A well-performed mastectomy may be preferable to local excision that is so large with respect to the volume of the breast that the patient is unhappy with her appearance.

OUR OWN EXPERIENCE WITH EXCISION ALONE

Our own experience with the use of excision and surveillance alone for DCIS began in 1978, at which time we began to offer highly selected patients this option – local excision alone – with the caveat that perhaps as many as 30–40% (our initial estimates) of patients so treated would develop a subsequent invasive carcinoma of the same breast. Having championed the surveillance option for patients with lobular carcinoma *in situ* (LCIS) or lobular neoplasia (LN) from the inception, extrapolation from LCIS to DCIS was understandable if not accurate. The observations of Haagensen about LCIS afforded a more firm commitment to the surveillance option for LCIS. At the time this study was initiated, however, there was only a smattering of information available about patients with DCIS treated by local excision alone. In addition to the 79 initial patients reported by Lagios, however, there were both British and Swedish reports of patients with subclinical DCIS, detected by mammographic screening, treated by excision and surveillance alone.[10–12]

In 1992, we reported our own initial experience with 72 cases of subclinical DCIS in 70 patients, treated by local excision and surveillance alone.[13] The mean and median follow-ups of this group were 49 months and 47 months, respectively, with the longest follow-up being 168 months. Of this group, all were detected as calcifications on a screening mammogram, or as an incidental finding in a biopsy performed for another reason (60 and 12, respectively). Eleven breasts (15.3%) had recurrence, either further DCIS (8) or invasive duct carcinoma (3), the recurrence being detected from 8 to 85 months after initial diagnosis.

Encouraged by our initial success, we have continued to offer highly selected patients with DCIS the opportunity to be treated by local excision and surveillance alone. As of January 1999, we had treated 233 breasts in 224 women (nine bilateral) by local excision alone. The mean age of the group was 56, and they ranged in age from 29 to 87 years. The mean follow-up was 61 months, and the median was 52 months. The longest follow-up was 252 months (21 years).

Second events, either additional DCIS or invasive cancer, developed in 46 breasts (20%). Of these 46 events, 32 were as DCIS only (70%) and 14 (30%) were as microinvasive or frankly invasive cancer. One woman of those with invasive cancer had positive axillary lymph nodes. No patient thus far has developed metastases, and none has died of breast cancer. We would like to think it relevant that two of the women with an invasive recurrence had been followed elsewhere because of geographical constraints, and perhaps their recurrences might have been detected earlier had they been part of the same follow-up program as the other patients in the group.

Of the entire group of 233 breasts, therefore, only 6% developed a subsequent invasive cancer. These observations suggest that only a very small proportion of these carefully selected women with subclinical DCIS will develop a potentially life-threatening, i.e., frankly invasive, cancer, because we have not had any patient with microinvasive cancer develop subsequent systemic metastatic disease.

Another observation about recurrence in this group of women is the time from initial diagnosis until recurrence. Twenty-two of the 46 (48%) had recurrence within 2 years of the initial diagnosis; 30 (65%) by the end of 36 months; and 35 (76%) by the end of 48 months. Speculating about the growth rates of these and other cancers, it is tempting to suggest that these patients did not have recurrence, but *persistence* of incompletely excised DCIS in the same area of the breast. If these observations stand and can be confirmed, they provide clues to the natural history of this disease. Moreover, if the breast is not treated by more than a wide local excision at the site, that breast remains at the same risk of developing a new, *unrelated* cancer as the other breast. We should never expect 'recurrence' to be zero.

If our observations about recurrence are considered further, only 6% of these women with DCIS developed any form of invasive cancer following 'lumpectomy' alone. Should we be treating 100% of this group of women with radiation (or mastectomy) if only this small proportion will develop a theoretically life-threatening cancer subsequently? Additionally, because recurrence after radiation therapy usually implies mastectomy, does the use of radiation preclude an additional attempt at treatment by further local excision alone if all of these women undergo radiation the first time DCIS occurs? Of our patients who have had recurrence as DCIS alone, several have chosen to continue surveillance alone, without radiation or mastectomy. This includes one woman with bilateral DCIS with bilateral recurrence.

Documenting these observations about the nature of recurrence is crucial. If careful surveillance detects recurrence while it is still non-invasive, patients may be more enthusiastic about this alternative to mastectomy or irradiation, because of the implication that recurrence (as DCIS only) does not endanger the patient. However, if a sizable segment of the group treated by excision and surveillance does develop invasive carcinoma as the first sign of recurrence, there will be a small fraction of this group who will undoubtedly succumb to this disease and, for those women, however few, the price of surveillance was too high.

Therefore, the challenge to those of us who would advocate local excision and surveillance as an option for women whose subclinical DCIS is detected by screening mammography is to define precisely the ultimate risk of developing *invasive* cancer, not further DCIS – not only the likelihood that this unfortunate event might occur, but also within what period of time. We must try to develop biologic markers that predict who is at greatest risk.

Our own comparisons of the findings within biopsies and those within subsequent mastectomy specimens (when we used to treat all patients with DCIS this way) have helped to define the risks of multicentricity and microinvasion associated with these various subsets of subclinical DCIS.[14,15] For example, the incidental finding of DCIS in a specimen of tissue removed for another reason has not been associated with either microinvasion or multicentricity, and no patient with incidental DCIS treated by excision and surveillance has yet developed recurrence.

THE VAN NUYS PROGNOSTIC INDEX

As investigators wrestled with the quandary concerning the optimal treatment for DCIS, it became obvious that three variables – namely, size, biology (nuclear grade), and margin width – were the most significant factors that predicted the likelihood of local recurrence after treatment by breast conservation. Dr Silverstein et al. were the first to try to organize this information into a reproducible system that could be used to help categorize patients into different groups to guide clinicians toward one treatment path or another. After multivariate analysis of various parameters, they chose three predictors of recurrence – tumor size, margin width, and pathologic classification – and created a scoring system based upon these three variables, which they named the Van Nuys Prognostic Index (VNPI).[16,17] An eloquent description of this index is given in the preceding chapter, and needs no repetition here. The VNPI has not been universally accepted as gospel, but even its most severe critics must admit that it is the best attempt currently available to assign patients into different categories for treatment. One can criticize the selection of the different values within each category, i.e., whether size score 1 should be

< 1.0 cm instead of < 1.5 cm, or if margin width should be scored differently, but, overall, it is an excellent blueprint for predicting outcome and, therefore, helpful for recommending treatment.

We are currently trying to validate the VNPI in our own practice. Because we have accrued a large group of patients with DCIS, all of whom have undergone local excision by the same surgeon, followed by surveillance alone without supplemental irradiation, and whose slides and paraffin blocks have been studied by the same pathologists, criticisms about reproducibility may be mitigated. Thus far, we have calculated the VNPI for 152 of our cases of DCIS treated by local excision alone. They range between 3 and 8; but there is only one 8 and only four 7s. Like Dr Silverstein et al., we recognized the need for further treatment for those patients with large areas of DCIS, incompletely excised margins, and/or aggressive biologic features, and our patients who would have scored in the 7, 8, 9 category were offered mastectomy. Although not statistically significant, there is a trend toward recurrence as the VNPI escalates.

We are additionally adding the immunohistochemical determinations of hormone receptors, nuclear antigen Ki-67, and gene products p53, p21, and C-erbB2 to our database. Thus far, differences in hormone receptor values have not predicted recurrence. Elevations of Ki-67 or mutated p53 have been indicators of recurrence at a low *p*-value, but elevations of C-erbB2 and p21 have been statistically significant predictors of recurrence ($p < 0.01$). As they are not yet used to define treatment, what additional contributions these markers may offer to the DCIS treatment algorithm is currently only speculative.

WIDE LOCAL EXCISION PLUS RADIATION THERAPY

Candidates for breast conservation who do not fit the guidelines for breast conservation alone are best treated by the addition of radiation therapy after wide local excision. Most radiation therapists prefer that the size of the area of DCIS be < 5 cm in its greatest dimension. This is because of the difficulty in achieving a wide local excision with negative margins and an acceptable cosmetic result when the area is larger. Any grade or subtype of DCIS is appropriate for radiation therapy. Margins preferably should be 'clear,' but some radiation therapists will treat patients with what they call 'focally positive' margins. However, there has been no consistent definition of the term 'focally positive.'

MARGINS

We concur that clear surgical margins are a major criterion for treatment of DCIS by breast conservation; and the wider the margin, the lower the rate of local recurrence. Margin status is the one variable that the physician can control. The biological character, i.e., nuclear grade and architecture, and the size of the area of DCIS cannot be influenced by treatment. The margins can. A margin of 10 mm is the best compromise between removal of so much tissue that the cosmetic result would be less than desirable and the likelihood of local recurrence.

If an initial attempt is unsuccessful, re-excision to achieve clear margins is appropriate. We have, on several occasions, re-excised a single positive margin a third time. Our technique of marking margins provides precise information if one or more of them is positive, and those specific margins can be addressed at the second or subsequent surgery. At least in theory, whatever might be necessary to clear the margins is acceptable, consistent with the patient's desire for breast conservation and the final aesthetic result. However, we have recommended mastectomy if several margins remain positive after this second attempt at re-excision. We currently believe that the same local criteria, i.e., clear margins, should be used for both treatment decisions, i.e., excision alone or excision followed by radiation therapy. The choice between radiation and excision alone is usually made by using size and tumor biology as the discriminants. Although we have no clinical trial data to document our decision, we think that the measurements of prognostic markers, especially c-erbB2 and p21, and, to a slightly lesser degree, p53 and Ki-67, are helpful guides in making this recommendation (see above).

TREATMENT OF RECURRENCE AFTER BREAST CONSERVATION

Recurrence as invasive cancer is an endpoint that affects disease-specific survival. Evidence suggests that this event does increase the patient's risk of death from breast cancer, however 'early' the diagnosis is made. It also affects treatment recommendations, because attention to the axilla is usually mandated in invasive cancer. Although a 'censoring event' in the statistical analysis of the data, recurrence as DCIS alone may not be of this same significance.

If invasive cancer is the recurrence, its treatment should be as for any other invasive cancer of the same stage. The prognosis should be excellent, because most of these are detected as new areas of calcifications on follow-up mammograms and are often microinvasive in character (T1mic). However, a small number of these women are destined for metastasis, and this possibility is truly the crux of the treatment dilemma in breast conservation.

When DCIS only is the recurrence, a different question exists. When DCIS *only* (i.e., without invasive cancer) occurs after treatment by local excision alone, the usual treatment is radiation or mastectomy, based upon the same selection criteria as for DCIS treatment when it occurs for the first time. However, there are no data extant that address the likelihood of further recurrence, either DCIS or invasive cancer, if this second event is treated by local excision alone. Radiation therapy or mastectomy as a choice would be based upon the same criteria as noted at the time of initial diagnosis. Therefore, for the women who underwent local excision only as their first treatment, the subsequent treatment options include re-excision, re-excision and radiation therapy, or mastectomy. If the second event is entirely DCIS, highly motivated women may choose additional attempt(s) at local excision alone, recognizing the lack of information about their long-term outcome. Because radiation therapy to the same area cannot be undertaken safely, the recommendation for the treatment of recurrence in patients who underwent radiation at the time of the initial diagnosis must be mastectomy. There may be selected occasions when local excision alone may be employed; these infrequently encountered occasions do not diminish the consensus that mastectomy is the recommended treatment for the recurrence of DCIS after initial treatment by radiation therapy.

SUMMARY

Our current treatment for DCIS is based upon a little science and abundant speculation. In part, this has been because of our unwillingness to interfere less rather than more when it is detected, especially as tiny areas of calcification on a mammogram. The majority of the scientific community has adopted observation alone for LCIS, even though the long-term likelihood of developing an invasive cancer is similar. It is intriguing why we have been so reluctant to consider the same treatment for DCIS. The long-term chance of developing *invasive* carcinoma seems to be similar for both.

That the patient must recognize the limits of our current knowledge about this disease is implicit in the mutual agreement between patient and physician as they begin the dialogue about treatment when this disease is encountered. A clear understanding of the biology and natural history of the disease that we call subclinical DCIS still eludes us. As clinicians, we have been involved in the care of too many women with often lethal breast cancers, so that reluctance to abandon traditional treatment in favor of lesser options is understandable. Our respect for breast cancer is too great! 'Overkill' has always been assumed to be a more sound philosophy than 'underkill' when dealing with malignancy. If we could be convinced that certain diseases that we currently call malignant, such as DCIS, are not inevitably followed by invasive, life-threatening, cancers, and that, even if recurrence does occur, there is a second opportunity for successful interference, perhaps there would be greater enthusiasm for less, rather than for more, treatment.

REFERENCES

1. Ernster VL, Barclay J, Kerlikowske K, Grady D, Henderson C. Incidence of and treatment for ductal carcinoma in situ of the breast. JAMA 1996; 275(12):913–18.

2. The Consensus Conference Committee. Consensus Conference on the Classification of Ductal Carcinoma in situ, April 25–28, 1997. Cancer 1997; 80:1798–802.

3. The Consensus Conference Committee. Consensus Conference on the Classification of Ductal Carcinoma in situ (Editorial). Hum Pathol 1997; 28:1221–5.

4. Consensus Conference Committee. Consensus Conference on the Classification of Ductal Carcinoma in situ, April 25–28, 1997. Breast J 1997; 3:360–4.

5. Schwartz GF, Solin LJ, Olivotto IA, Ernster VL, Pressman PI, and the Consensus Conference Committee. The Consensus Conference on the Treatment of in situ Ductal Carcinoma of the Breast (Editorial). Hum Pathol 2000; 31:131–9.

6. Schwartz GF, Solin LJ, Olivotto IA, Ernster VL, Pressman PI, and the Consensus Conference Committee. Consensus Conference on the Treatment of in situ Ductal Carcinoma of the Breast. Cancer 2000; 88:946–54.

7. Schwartz GF, Solin LJ, Olivotto IA, Ernster VL, Pressman PI, and the Consensus Conference Committee. Consensus Conference on the Treatment of in situ Ductal Carcinoma of the Breast. Breast J 2000; 6:4–13.

8. Fisher B, Costantino J, Redmond C, et al. Lumpectomy compared with lumpectomy and radiation therapy for the treatment of intraductal breast cancer. N Engl J Med 1993; 328:1581–6.

9. Fisher ER, Dignam J, Wolmark N, et al. Lumpectomy and radiation therapy for the treatment of intraductal breast cancer: findings from NSABP Project B-17. J Clin Oncol 1998; 16:441–52.

10. Lagios MD, Westdahl PR, Margolin FR, et al. Duct carcinoma in situ: relationship of extent of noninvasive disease to the frequency of occult invasion, multicentricity, lymph node metastasis and 670 short-term treatment failures. Cancer 1982; 59:1309–14.

11. Carpenter R, Boulter PS, Cooke T, Gibbs NM. Management of screen detected ductal carcinoma in situ of the breast. Br J Surg 1989; 76:564–7.

12. Arnesson L-G, Smeds S, Fagerberg G, et al. Follow-up of two treatment modalities for ductal cancer in situ of the breast. Br J Surg 1989; 76:672–5.

13. Schwartz GF, Finkel GC, Garcia JC, Patchefsky AS. Subclinical ductal carcinoma in situ of the breast: treatment by local excision and surveillance alone. Cancer 1992; 70:2468–74.

14. Schwartz GF, Patchefsky AS, Finkelstein SD, et al. Nonpalpable in situ ductal carcinoma of the breast. Arch Surg 1989; 124:29–32.

15. Patchefsky AS, Schwartz GF, Finkelstein SD, et al. Heterogeneity of intraductal carcinoma of the breast. Cancer 1989; 63:731–41.

16. Silverstein MJ, Poller DN, Waisman JR, et al. Prognostic classification of breast ductal carcinoma-in situ. Lancet 1995; 345(8958):1154–7.

17. Silverstein MJ, Lagios MD, Craig PH, et al. A prognostic index for ductal carcinoma in situ of the breast. Cancer 1996; 77(11):2267–74.

Editors' selected abstracts

Genetic relation of lobular carcinoma in situ, ductal carcinoma in situ, and associated invasive carcinoma of the breast.

Buerger H, Simon R, Schafer KL, Diallo R, Littmann R, Poremba C, van Diest PJ, Dockhorn-Dworniczak B, Bocker W.

Gerhard-Domagk-Institute of Pathology, University of Munster, Germany.

Molecular Pathology 53(3):118–21, 2000, June.

Aims: The mutual relation of lobular carcinoma in situ (LCIS) and ductal carcinoma in situ (DCIS) of the breast, as accepted precursor lesions of invasive breast cancer, is controversial. Because they display genetic heterogeneity, it is not clear how genetically advanced these entities are and what causes the transition to an invasive carcinoma. Methods: Six cases of LCIS, four of them with associated lobular invasive carcinoma, four cases of intermediately differentiated DCIS with an associated invasive lobular carcinoma, and nine cases of intermediately and poorly differentiated DCIS with associated ductal invasive carcinoma were investigated by means of comparative genomic hybridisation (CGH) after microdissection and immunohisto-chemical staining of E-cadherin. Results: LCIS was characterised by a low average rate of copy number changes, no evidence of amplifications, and a high rate of gains and losses of chromosomal material at 1q and 16q, respectively. A high degree of genetic homology with well differentiated DCIS was obvious, as reported previously. The cases of intermediately differentiated DCIS with associated lobular invasive components and lobular differentiation revealed striking homologies, and a significant difference of E-cadherin expression. The comparison of preinvasive and invasive breast lesions, irrespective of differentiation within the same patient, revealed no specific alteration that might be associated with invasion. Genetic alterations seen in invasive carcinoma were not necessarily seen in the adjacent precursor lesions. *Conclusions:* These results provide strong evidence that invasive breast cancer is a disease with multiple cytogenetic subclones already present in preinvasive lesions. Moreover, specific CGH alterations associated with invasion were not observed. Furthermore, the close genetic association between well differentiated and a subgroup of intermediately differentiated DCIS and LCIS led to the hypothesis that LCIS and a subgroup of DCIS are different phenotypic forms of a common genotype.

Vacuum-assisted stereotactic breast biopsy: histologic underestimation of malignant lesions.

Burak WE Jr, Owens KE, Tighe MB, Kemp L, Dinges SA, Hitchcock CL, Olsen J.

Department of Surgery, James Cancer Hospital and Solove Research Institute, The Ohio State University, Columbus, OH, USA.

Archives of Surgery 135(6):700–3, 2000, June.

Hypothesis: The histopathologic correlation between stereotactic core needle biopsy and subsequent surgical excision of mammographically detected nonpalpable breast abnormalities is improved with a larger-core (11-gauge) device. *Design:* Retrospective medical record and histopathologic review. *Setting:* University-based academic practice setting. *Patients:* Two hundred one patients who underwent surgical excision of mammographic abnormalities that had undergone biopsy with an 11-gauge vacuum-assisted stereotactic core biopsy device. *Main outcome measure:* Correlation between stereotactic biopsy histologic results and the histologic results of subsequent surgical specimens. *Results:* Results of stereotactic biopsy performed on 851 patients revealed atypical hyperplasia in 46 lesions, ductal carcinoma in situ (DCIS) in 89 lesions, and invasive cancer in 73 mammographic abnormalities. Subsequent surgical excision of the 46 atypical lesions revealed 2 cases of DCIS (4.3%) and 4 cases of invasive carcinoma (8.7%). Lesions diagnosed as DCIS on stereotactic biopsy proved to be invasive carcinoma in 10 (11.2%) of 89 patients on subsequent excision. Stereotactic biopsy completely removed 21 (23.6%) of 89 DCIS lesions and 20 (27.4%) of 73 invasive carcinomas. *Conclusions:* In summary, 11-gauge vacuum-assisted core breast biopsy accurately predicts the degree of disease in the majority of malignant lesions; however, understaging still occurs in 11% to 13% of lesions showing atypical hyperplasia or DCIS.

Extent of excision margin width required in breast conserving surgery for ductal carcinoma in situ.

Chan KC, Knox WF, Sinha G, Gandhi A, Barr L, Baildam AD, Bundred NJ.

Department of Surgery, University Hospital of South Manchester, Manchester, UK.

Cancer 91(1):9–16, 2001, January 1.

Background: Breast conserving surgery (BCS) is common practice for unifocal ductal carcinoma in situ (DCIS) less than 4 cm in size, but the extent of tumor free margin width around DCIS necessary to minimize recurrence is unclear.

Methods: Clinical and pathologic details were recorded from all patients with pure DCIS <4 cm in size, treated with BCS between 1978 and 1997. Histologic margins were measured by using an ocular micrometer. Patients with clear margins (>1 mm) were divided up into 3 groups for analysis based on margin of normal tissue excised: 1.1–5 mm, 5.1–10 mm, and 10.1–40 mm. *Results:* There were 66 patients with close margins (≤1 mm), of which 25 cases (37.9%) recurred. The recurrence rates for the 3 clear margin groups ranged 4.5–7.1%. Median followup was 47 months (range 12–197 mos). Risk of recurrence in the group with close margins was greater than the subgroups with clear margins ($p < 0.001$); no differences in recurrence were seen between the individual subgroups with clear margins. Nuclear Grade 3 was predictive of recurrence ($p = 0.03$). Following excision alone, the recurrence rate was 18.6%, compared with 11.1% when radiotherapy was given as adjuvant therapy. Women with clear margins following excision had a recurrence rate of only 8.1%. *Conclusion:* After BCS for DCIS, close margins were associated with a high risk of local recurrence. Radiotherapy did not compensate for inadequate surgical clearance.

Intraductal carcinoma of the breast: pathologic features associated with local recurrence in patients treated with breast-conserving therapy.

Goldstein NS, Kestin L, Vicini F.

Department of Anatomic Pathology, William Beaumont Hospital, Royal Oak, MI, USA.

American Journal of Surgical Pathology 24(8):1058–67, 2000, August.

Local excision and radiation therapy is a standard treatment option for duct carcinoma in situ (DCIS) of the breast. There is no consensus regarding the significant histologic features associated with recurrence. The authors studied a large group of patients with mammographically detected DCIS treated with breast-conserving therapy to explore DCIS volume relationships, DCIS features, specimen characteristics, and the effect of patient age at diagnosis. Thirteen patients (10%) developed a recurrent carcinoma in the ipsilateral breast, resulting in 5- and 10-year actuarial recurrence rates of 8.9% and 10.3%, respectively. Local recurrences were identified as a true recurrence/marginal miss (TR/MM) in nine patients, and elsewhere in the breast in four patients. The notable features associated with TR/MM recurrences on univariate analysis included patient age less than 45 years old, six or more slides with DCIS, no microscopic calcifications within DCIS ducts, and five or more DCIS ducts or terminal duct lobular units (TDLUs) with cancerization of lobules (COL) within 0.42 cm of the final surgical margin. DCIS tumor size, nuclear grade, amount of central necrosis, and margin status were not associated with outcome. Multivariate analysis found that the absence of microcalcifications within DCIS ducts, patient age, number of slides with DCIS or TDLUs with COL, and the number of DCIS ducts or TDLUs with COL within 0.42 cm of the final margin were related significantly to TR/MM recurrence. Patients with a total of six or more slides with DCIS, or who have 11 or more DCIS ducts or TDLUs with COL near the final margin are at increased risk of having a substantial volume of residual

DCIS in the adjacent unexcised breast. These results suggest that the volume of DCIS in the specimen, and the volume of DCIS near the margin are associated with local recurrence. These features can be used to identify those patients with a higher chance of local recurrence.

Differences in the pathologic features of ductal carcinoma in situ of the breast based on patient age.

Goldstein NS, Vicini FA, Kestin LL, Thomas M.

Department of Anatomic Pathology, William Beaumont Hospital, Royal Oak, MI, USA.

Cancer 88(11):2553–60, 2000, June 1.

Background: Young patient age at diagnosis has been reported as a risk factor for recurrence in patients with ductal carcinoma in situ (DCIS) of the breast treated with breast-conserving therapy (BCT). The authors examined pathologic features of DCIS in three different age groups of patients to identify differences that might explain why young patient age at the time of diagnosis is a risk factor for recurrence. *Methods:* Excised specimens from 177 breasts of 172 patients with DCIS treated with BCT were studied. All slides from all specimens were reviewed. Patients were divided into 3 age groups: those aged <45 years, those aged 45–59 years, and those aged ≥60 years. The histologic features that were quantified included most common and highest nuclear grades, DCIS architectural pattern, amount of central necrosis (quartiles), calcifications, amount of DCIS, and number of terminal duct lobular units (TDLUs) with cancerization of lobules (COL) within 0.42 cm of the margin, margin status, and size and volume of excision specimens. *Results:* Patients aged <45 years at the time of diagnosis more frequently had higher nuclear grade DCIS (highest nuclear Grade 3: 69%, 60%, and 39%; $p = 0.003$), respectively and central necrosis (72%, 62%, and 44%; $p = 0.01$), respectively. Although not statistically significant, younger patients tended to have comedo subtype DCIS more often (31%, 23%, and 19%; $p = 0.35$), respectively. Younger patients also more often had smaller initial biopsy specimen maximum dimensions (4.3 cm, 5.2 cm, and 5.7 cm; $p = 0.004$), respectively, with close or positive margins (89%, 61%, and 64%; $p = 0.03$), and more TDLUs with COL in the 0.42-cm rim of tissue adjacent to the margin (5.2, 3.6, and 1.9; $p = 0.23$), respectively. No other features including the amount of DCIS when classified as >50% or >75% of ducts, calcifications within DCIS ducts, pattern of DCIS involvement, number of slides examined, number of slides with DCIS, and mean number of DCIS ducts near the margin were found to occur more frequently in younger patients. *Conclusions:* Younger patients with DCIS may have an increased risk of local recurrence when treated with BCT due to smaller initial excision volumes, a greater proportion of high nuclear grade DCIS, and central necrosis.

Radiotherapy in breast-conserving treatment for ductal carcinoma in situ: first results of the EORTC randomised phase III trial 10853. EORTC Breast Cancer Cooperative Group and EORTC Radiotherapy Group.

Julien JP, Bijker N, Fentiman IS, Peterse JL, Delledonne V, Rouanet P, Avril A, Sylvester R, Mignolet F, Bartelink H, Van Dongen JA.

Department of Surgery, Centre Henri Becquerel, Rouen, France.

Lancet 355(9203):528–33, 2000, February 12.

Background: Ductal carcinoma in situ (DCIS) of the breast is a disorder that has become more common since it may manifest as microcalcifications that can be detected by screening mammography. Since selected women with invasive cancer can be treated safely with breast conservation therapy it is paradoxical that total mastectomy has remained the standard treatment for DCIS. We did a randomised phase III clinical trial to investigate the role of radiotherapy after complete local excision of DCIS. *Methods:* Between 1986 and 1996, women with clinically or mammographically detected DCIS measuring less than or equal to 5 cm were treated by complete local excision of the lesion and then randomly assigned to either no further treatment ($n = 503$) or to radiotherapy ($n = 507$; 50 Gy in 5 weeks to the whole breast). The median duration of follow-up was 4.25 years (maximum 12.0 years). All analyses were by intention to treat. *Findings:* 500 patients were followed up in the no further treatment group and 502 in the radiotherapy group. In the no further treatment group 83 women had local recurrence (44 recurrences of DCIS, and 40 invasive breast cancer). In the radiotherapy group 53 women had local recurrences (29 recurrences of DCIS, and 24 invasive breast cancer). The 4-year local relapse-free was 84% in the group treated with local excision alone compared with 91% in the women treated by local excision plus radiotherapy (log rank $p = 0.005$; hazard ratio 0.62). Similar reductions in the risk of invasive (40%, $p = 0.04$) and non-invasive (35%, $p = 0.06$) local recurrence were seen. *Conclusions:* Radiotherapy after local excision for DCIS, as compared with local excision alone, reduced the overall number of both invasive and non-invasive recurrences in the ipsilateral breast at a median follow-up of 4.25 years.

Comments:
Comment in: *Lancet* 355(9203):510–12, 2000, February 12.
Comment in: *Lancet* 355(9220):2071; discussion 2072–3, 2000, June 10.
Comment in: *Lancet* 355(9220):2071–2; discussion 2072–3, 2000, June 10.
Comment in: *Lancet* 355(9220):2072; discussion 2072–3, 2000, June 10.

Mammographically detected ductal carcinoma in situ treated with conservative surgery with or without radiation therapy: patterns of failure and 10-year results.

Kestin LL, Goldstein NS, Martinez AA, Rebner M, Balasubramaniam M, Frazier RC, Register JT, Pettinga J, Vicini FA.

Department of Radiation Oncology, William Beaumont Hospital, Royal Oak, MI, USA.

Annals of Surgery 231(2):235–45, 2000, February.

Objective: The authors reviewed their institution's experience treating mammographically detected ductal carcinoma in situ (DCIS) of the breast with breast-conserving therapy (BCT) to determine 10-year rates of local control and survival, patterns of failure, and factors associated with outcome. *Summary background data:* From January 1980 to December 1993, 177 breasts in 172 patients were treated with BCT for mammographically detected DCIS of the breast at William Beaumont Hospital, Royal Oak, Michigan. *Methods:* All patients underwent an excisional biopsy, and 65% were reexcised. Thirty-one breasts (18%) were treated with excision alone, whereas 146 breasts (82%) received postoperative radiation therapy (RT). All patients undergoing RT received whole-breast irradiation to a median dose of 50.0 Gy. One hundred thirty-six (93%) received a boost to the tumor bed for a median total dose of 60.4 Gy. Median follow-up was 5.9 years for the lumpetomy alone group and 7.2 years for the lumpectomy + RT group. *Results:* In the entire population, 15 patients had an ipsilateral breast recurrence. The 5- and 10-year actuarial rates of ipsilateral breast recurrence were 7.8% and 7.8% for lumpectomy alone and 8.0% and 9.2% for lumpectomy + RT, respectively. Eleven of the 15 recurrences developed within or immediately adjacent to the lumpectomy cavity and were designated as true recurrences or marginal misses (TR/MM). Four recurred elsewhere in the breast. Eleven of the 15 recurrences were invasive, whereas 4 were pure DCIS. Only one patient died of disease, yielding 5- and 10-year actuarial cause-specific survival rates of 100% and 99.2%, respectively. Eleven patients were diagnosed with subsequent contralateral breast cancer, yielding 5- and 10-year actuarial rates of 5.1% and 8.3%, respectively. Clinical, pathologic, and treatment-related factors were analyzed for an association with ipsilateral breast failure or TR/MM. No factors were significantly associated with ipsilateral breast failure. In the entire population, the omission of RT and younger age at diagnosis were significantly associated with TR/MM. Patients younger than 45 years at diagnosis had a significantly higher rate of TR/MM in both the lumpectomy + RT and lumpectomy alone groups. None of the 37 patients who received a postexcisional mammogram had an ipsilateral breast failure versus 15 in the patients who did not receive a postexcisional mammogram. *Conclusions:* Patients diagnosed with mammographically detected DCIS of the breast appear to have excellent 10-year rates of local control and overall survival when treated with BCT. These results suggest that the use of RT reduces the risk of local recurrence and that patients diagnosed at a younger age have a higher rate of local recurrence with or without the use of postoperative RT.

Genetic abnormalities in mammary ductal intraepithelial neoplasia-flat type ('clinging ductal carcinoma in situ'): A simulator of normal mammary epithelium.

Moinfar F, Man YG, Bratthauer GL, Ratschek M, Tavassoli FA.

Department of Gynecologic and Breast Pathology, Armed Forces Institute of Pathology, Washington, DC, USA.

Cancer 88(9):2072–81, 2000, May 1.

Background: Mammary ductal intraepithelial neoplasia (DIN)-flat type ('clinging ductal carcinoma in situ [DCIS]') generally is a subtle epithelial alteration characterized by one or a few layer(s) of atypical cells replacing the native epithelium. The 'low power' appearance of DIN-flat type

can be misinterpreted easily as 'normal' because of the frequent absence of multilayered proliferation and often subtle cytologic atypia. Because it presents as an often unrecognized lesion or in association with tubular carcinoma, to the authors' knowledge the clinical and biologic significance of this lesion has not been well established. *Methods:* Using polymerase chain reaction, the authors examined DNA extracts from microdissected areas of 22 cases with extensive 'clinging DCIS,' including 13 cases associated with infiltrating ductal carcinoma as well as 5 cases associated with more conventional types of DCIS. Eight polymorphic DNA markers with a high rate of loss of heterozygosity (LOH) in classic types of DCIS were selected to identify possible genetic alterations on chromosomes 2p, 3p, 11q, 16q, and 17q. Two cases also were used for the assessment of clonality by means of X chromosome inactivation (methylation pattern of the human androgen receptor [HUMARA] gene). *Results:* LOH was detected in 17 of 22 lesions (77%), and monoclonality was established in the 2 cases analyzed. The most common genetic alterations were at chromosomes 11q21-23.2, 16q23.1-24.2, and 3p14.2 with LOH in 50%, 45%, and 41%, respectively, of informative cases. The DIN-flat type showed the same genetic alterations (LOH) identified in adjacent in situ and infiltrating ductal carcinoma. In contrast to the DIN-flat type, the perfectly normal mammary epthelium was associated very infrequently (1 of 16 cases; 6%) with LOH. *Conclusions:* The DIN-flat type represents one of the earliest, morphologically recognizable, neoplastic alterations of the breast. Recognition of the DIN-flat type is important not only for the early detection of intraductal neoplasia but also to prevent misinterpretation and utilization of this lesion as a normal control in studies. This distinctive lesion could be crucial as an explanation for at least part of the >20% reported incidence rate of breast carcinoma recurrence observed despite ostensibly 'negative' margins of breast biopsies.

Benefits of irradiation for DCIS: a Pyrrhic victory

Silverstein M, Lagios M.

Department of Surgery, University of Southern California, Los Angeles, CA, and the Breast Consultation Service, St Mary's Hospital, San Francisco, CA, USA.

Lancet 355:510–511, 2000, February 12.

The initial results of the National Surgical Adjuvant Breast and Bowel Project (NSABP B-17), in which excision alone was compared with excision plus radiotherapy for the treatment of ductal carcinoma in situ (DCIS), revealed a significant reduction in the 5-year rates of local recurrence for irradiated patients – from 10.4% to 7.5% for non-invasive recurrences and, more strikingly, from 10.5% to 2.9% for invasive recurrences. The investigators concluded that breast irradiation after excision was indicated for all women with localised DCIS, a position they have continued to support strongly in subsequent papers and at international meetings. Despite their data, there continued to be vigorous debate about whether or not all patients with DCIS require post-excisional radiotherapy.

The EORTC 10853 trial had a study design and definition of clear margin that were essentially the same as in the

B-17. The overall reductions in local recurrence are similar for the two trials, but there were differences in the rates of invasive local recurrence and contralateral breast cancer. The EORTC trial corroborates the main conclusion of the B-17 study: radiation therapy decreases rates of local recurrence of invasive and non-invasive disease in DCIS patients treated conservatively. The EORTC study, unfortunately, is open to the same criticism levelled at the initial B-17 report – that there was no subset analysis giving comparative rates of local recurrence for various subgroups, such as high-grade (nuclear grade 3) versus low-grade; wide excision margins versus narrow margins; or presence of comedonecrosis versus absence of this feature. So far there have been too few recurrences in the EORTC trial for such a subset analysis. However, the forthcoming central pathology review might yield some additional information.

A unique finding in the B-17 trial was the 3.5 fold reduction in invasive local recurrences after radiotherapy, an observation not found in the EORTC or any other study of breast conservation accompanied by radiotherapy. Although in B-17 DCIS recurrences were reduced by 47% in the radiotherapy group, invasive recurrences were reduced by 71%. By contrast, in the EORTC trial the reductions for in-situ and invasive local recurrences were similar. The NSABP investigators have used the marked decrease in invasive local recurrence as the main rationale for their recommendation that all patients with DCIS conservatively treated should receive postoperative breast irradiation.

The EORTC finding of an increased rate of contralateral breast cancer in irradiated patients is of especial interest. Although perhaps a chance finding, the difference reached statistical significance ($p = 0.01$). One possible cause for this difference was the EORTC requirement for a compensatory filter or wedge during breast radiotherapy. The use of a wedge or filter on the medial tangential field can increase the scatter dose to the contralateral breast.

Because of the higher rate of contralateral breast cancer in the EORTC study, there was no statistical difference between study groups in event-free survival rate. If the higher rate of contralateral breast cancer proves to be due to radiation scatter, it will decrease the relative value of a policy of radiotherapy for all patients with DCIS in favour of a policy only for those patients who stand to benefit substantially from breast irradiation.

Although radiotherapy reduced the rate of local recurrence, neither the EORTC nor the B-17 trial showed that irradiation had a beneficial effect on the most important outcome variables, distant recurrences and breast-cancer mortality. In both trials the rates for these variables were the same whether or not patients received radiotherapy. The investigators do point out that as the period of follow-up increases so does the potential for distant disease in patients with invasive local recurrence. Hence, the most important reason for radiotherapy would be prevention of invasive local recurrence. Of some concern is the fact that after only 4.25 years of follow-up, 24 patients in the EORTC trial had metastatic breast cancer, compared with only 15 after 8 years of follow-up in B-17.

Both the B-17 and EORTC trials did exactly what they were designed to do. They proved that, overall, radiotherapy was beneficial for patients with DCIS. Neither protocol, however, was designed to answer the questions that patients and their physicians ask today – namely, which subgroups will benefit from irradiation and by how much?

Impact of young age on outcome in patients with ductal carcinoma-in-situ treated with breast-conserving therapy.

Vicini FA, Kestin LL, Goldstein NS, Chen PY, Pettinga J, Frazier RC, Martinez AA.

Department of Radiation Oncology, William Beaumont Hospital, Royal Oak, MI, USA.

Journal of Clinical Oncology 18(2):296–306, 2000, January.

Purpose: We reviewed our institution's experience treating patients with ductal carcinoma-in-situ (DCIS) with breast-conserving therapy (BCT) to determine the impact of patient age on outcome. *Patients and methods:* From 1980 to 1993, 146 patients were treated with BCT for DCIS. All patients underwent excisional biopsy, and 64% underwent re-excision. All patients received whole-breast irradiation to a median dose of 45 Gy. Ninety-four percent of patients received a boost to the tumor bed, for a median total dose of 60.4 Gy. All slides on every patient were reviewed by one pathologist. The median follow-up period was 7.2 years. *Results:* Seventeen patients developed an ipsilateral local recurrence, for 5- and 10-year actuarial rates of 10.2% and 12.4%, respectively. The 10-year rate of ipsilateral failure was 26.1% in patients younger than 45 years of age versus 8.6% in older patients ($p = 0.03$). On multivariate analysis, young age was independently associated with recurrence of the index lesion (true recurrence/marginal miss TR/MM failures), regardless of how it was analyzed (e.g., <45 years of age or as a continuous variable). In addition, young patients had a dramatically higher 10-year rate of invasive TR/MM failures (19.9% v. 3.2%). In a separate multivariate analysis for the development of invasive TR/MM failures, only patient age and predominant nuclear grade were independently associated with recurrence. The relationship between excision volume and outcome was analyzed in the 95 patients who underwent re-excision. The 5-year actuarial rate of TR/MM failure was significantly worse only in young patients with smaller (<40 mL) re-excision volumes (33.3% v. 9.1%; $p = 0.02$). In a separate multivariate analysis of only these 95 patients (25 of whom were <45 years of age), the volume of re-excision had the strongest association with outcome ($p = 0.05$). Patient age was no longer associated with local recurrence. *Conclusion:* These findings suggest that young patients with DCIS have a significantly greater risk of local recurrence after BCT that is independent of other previously defined risk factors. Our data also suggest that the extent of resection may in part be related to the less optimal results that are observed in these patients.

Chromosomal alterations in ductal carcinomas in situ and their in situ recurrences.

Waldman FM, DeVries S, Chew KL, Moore DH 2nd, Kerlikowske K, Ljung BM.

Cancer Genetics Program, UCSF Cancer Center, University of California, San Francisco, CA, USA.

Journal of the National Cancer Institute 92(4):313–20, 2000, February 16.

Background: Ductal carcinoma in situ (DCIS) recurs in the same breast following breast-conserving surgery in 5–25% of patients, with the rate influenced by the presence or absence of involved surgical margins, tumor size and nuclear grade, and whether or not radiation therapy was performed. A recurrent lesion arising soon after excision of an initial DCIS may reflect residual disease, whereas in situ tumors arising after longer periods are sometimes considered to be second independent events. The purpose of this study was to determine the clonal relationship between initial DCIS lesions and their recurrences. *Methods:* Comparative genomic hybridization (CGH) was used to compare chromosomal alterations in 18 initial DCIS lesions (presenting in the absence of invasive disease) and in their subsequent ipsilateral DCIS recurrences (detected from 16 months to 9.3 years later). *Results:* Of the 18 tumor pairs, 17 showed a high concordance in their chromosomal alterations (median = 81%; range = 65–100%), while one case showed no agreement between the paired samples (having two and 20 alterations, respectively). Morphologic characterization of the DCIS pairs showed clear similarities. The mean number of CGH changes was greater in the recurrent tumors than in the initial lesions (10.7 versus 8.8; $p = 0.019$). The most common changes in both the initial and the recurrent in situ lesions were gains involving chromosome 17q and losses involving chromosomes 8p and 17p. The degree of concordance was independent of the time interval before recurrence and of the presence of positive surgical margins. *Conclusions:* In this study, DCIS recurrences were clonally related to their primary lesions in most cases. This finding is consistent with treatment paradigms requiring wide surgical margins and/or postoperative radiation therapy.

Pathologists' agreement with experts and reproducibility of breast ductal carcinoma-in-situ classification schemes.

Wells WA, Carney PA, Eliassen MS, Grove MR, Tosteson AN.

Department of Pathology, Dartmouth Medical School, Hanover, NH, USA.

American Journal of Surgical Pathology 24(5):651–9, 2000, May.

Several histologic classifications for breast ductal carcinoma in situ (DCIS) have been proposed. This study assessed the diagnostic agreement and reproducibility of three DCIS classifications (Holland [HL], modified Lagios [LA], and Van Nuys [VN]) by comparing the interpretations of pathologists without expertise in breast pathology with those of three breast pathology experts, each a proponent of one classification. Seven nonexpert pathologists in New Hampshire and three experts evaluated 40 slides of DCIS according to the three classifications. Twenty slides were reinterpreted by each nonexpert pathologist. Diagnostic accuracy (nonexperts compared with experts) and reproducibility were evaluated using inter- and intrarater techniques (kappa statistic). Final DCIS grade and nuclear grade were reported most accurately among nonexpert pathologists using HL (kappa = 0.53 and 0.49, respectively) compared with LA and VN (kappa = 0.29 and 0.35, respectively, for both classifications). An intermediate DCIS grade was assessed most accurately using HL and LA, and a high grade (group 3) was assessed most accurately using VN. Diagnostic reproducibility was highest using HL (kappa = 0.49). The VN interpretation of necrosis (present or absent) was reported more accurately than the LA criteria (extensive, focal, or absent; kappa = 0.59 and 0.45, respectively), but reproducibility of each was comparable (kappa = 0.48 and 0.46, respectively). Intrarater agreement was high overall. Comparing all three classifications, final DCIS grade was reported best using HL. Nuclear grade (cytodifferentiation) using HL and the presence or absence of necrosis were the criteria diagnosed most accurately and reproducibly. Establishing one internationally approved set of interpretive definitions, with acceptable accuracy and reproducibility among both pathologists with and without expertise in breast pathology interpretation, will assist researchers in evaluating treatment effectiveness and characterizing the natural history of DCIS breast lesions.

Outcomes and factors impacting local recurrence of ductal carcinoma in situ.

Weng EY, Juillard GJ, Parker RG, Chang HR, Gornbein JA.

Department of Radiation Oncology, University of California–Los Angeles, Los Angeles, CA, USA.

Cancer 88(7):1643–9, 2000, April 1.

Background: The optimal management of ductal carcinoma in situ (DCIS) remains controversial. Investigators have focused on identifying patients who are eligible for treatment by excision alone. A retrospective analysis of patients with DCIS treated by various modalities was conducted to compare outcomes and determine factors significant for local recurrence (LR). *Methods:* Between 1985–1992, 88 consecutive diagnoses of DCIS were identified in 85 patients. Seventy-four percent were detected mammographically. The most common histologic subtypes were comedo (54%) and cribriform (23%). Tumor sizes were <2.5 cm (49%), >2.5–5 cm (26%), >5 cm (23%), and unknown (2%). Final resection margins were tumor free (75%), close/positive (23%), and unknown (2%). Treatment methods included mastectomy (30%), localized surgery and radiation therapy (LSR) (43%), or wide localized surgery alone (LS) (27%). Radiation therapy (RT) was comprised of 50 grays to the breast, and 53% of treated patients received local 'boost' irradiation. *Results:* The median follow-up was 8.3 years. The overall recurrence rate was 13.6%, whereas the median time to LR was 27.8 months. Recurrence rates according to treatment modality were: LS: 25%; LSR: 13%; and mastectomy: 4%. However, if surgical margins were tumor free, LSR had a LR rate of 3.4%. After RT, no LR occurred prior to 15 months, and 4 of 5 tumors were noninvasive. Nine patients treated by excision alone conformed to the criteria of Lagios *et al.* criteria and LR occurred in three of nine tumors. Of the factors analyzed, margin status was found to be the best predictor for LR ($p = 0.05$). *Conclusions:* If surgical margins are tumor free, the LSR regimen is equivalent to mastectomy for local tumor control. Annual mammograms may be adequate for the follow-up of patients with irradiated breasts, but biannual studies still are recommended for patients treated with excision alone. Copyright 2000 American Cancer Society.

12

Surgical options for stage I and stage II breast cancer

VALERIE L STARADUB AND MONICA MORROW

INTRODUCTION

The local therapy of breast cancer has been a source of controversy for many years, with changes in the surgical approach to breast cancer reflecting changes in our understanding of the biology of the disease. Since the 1970s, modified radical mastectomy has been the most common operative treatment for patients with invasive breast cancer in the USA.[1–4] The term modified radical mastectomy encompasses a number of surgical procedures, all of which include complete removal of the breast and some of the axillary nodes. Although the modified radical mastectomy does not seem to differ significantly from the radical mastectomy, the procedure represents a major departure from the Halstedian principles of en bloc cancer surgery, and its widespread adoption in the 1970s signaled acceptance of the belief that treatment failure after breast cancer surgery was due to the systemic dissemination of tumor cells prior to surgery, and not to an inadequate surgical procedure. Clinical evidence supporting the idea that radical en bloc surgery is not necessary in breast cancer treatment comes from two prospective randomized trials,[5,6] as well as from several retrospective studies,[7,8] in which no survival differences were observed between women treated with modified radical and radical mastectomy.

Modified radical mastectomy is a treatment that is suitable for virtually all women with stage I and II breast carcinoma. The preservation of the pectoralis major muscle greatly facilitates the performance of breast reconstruction, and has made immediate breast reconstruction a clinical reality.

Some of the same principles that led to the use of modified radical mastectomy contributed to the development of breast-conserving therapy. These included the recognition that adherence to the principles of en bloc cancer surgery failed to cure many patients, the success of moderate-dose radiation therapy (RT) in eliminating microscopic foci of breast cancer after mastectomy, and the increasingly frequent identification of small breast cancers by mammography. Today, women with stage I and II breast cancer are candidates for treatment with modified radical mastectomy, modified radical mastectomy with immediate reconstruction, or breast-conserving therapy consisting of lumpectomy, axillary dissection, and RT. The identification of patterns of lymphatic drainage has led to the use of sentinel node biopsy in selected patients in place of a formal axillary dissection. In addition, the treatment of breast cancer has evolved from being the domain of the surgeon to a collaborative effort between surgeons, radiologists, pathologists, radiation oncologists, reconstructive surgeons, and medical oncologists. This chapter reviews the data on the outcome of local therapy with mastectomy, mastectomy and reconstruction, and breast-conserving therapy and addresses the issue of selection of local therapy for the individual patient.

BREAST-CONSERVING THERAPY

Clinical trials

In the past, a major objection to the use of breast-conserving therapy was the known multicentricity of breast cancer. The reported incidence of multicentricity ranged from 9% to 75%,[9–11] depending on the definition employed and the techniques of pathologic examination used. The likelihood of microscopic cancer at a distance from the primary tumor was used to argue against anything other than mastectomy as a treatment for breast cancer. Critical to an understanding of the role of surgery in breast-conserving treatment is the recognition that the surgical procedure will often not remove all of the tumor in the breast, and that moderate-dose radiation must be employed to eradicate any residual disease. The idea of surgery as a 'debulking' procedure was the antithesis of the Halstedian dogma, and a relatively large number of randomized clinical trials were conducted to determine if survival after breast-conserving treatment was equal to survival after mastectomy. Since 1970, there have been six prospective, randomized trials in which conservative surgery (CS) and RT have been compared with mastectomy (Table 12.1).[12-20] These studies differed widely in patient-selection criteria, the extent of the surgical procedure that was performed, and the techniques of irradiation used. For example, in the Milan trial,[12,13] only patients with clinical stage I breast cancer were eligible for entry (tumor size less than 2 cm, clinically negative nodes). Patients were treated with a formal quadrant resection, including skin and the underlying pectoral fascia. Radiation therapy to a dose of 50 Gy was given to the whole breast, and all patients received a 10-Gy boost to the tumor bed using orthovoltage radiation. In contrast, entry criteria for the National Surgical Adjuvant Breast and Bowel Project (NSABP) Protocol B06 were less restrictive, and the surgery was more limited.[14,15] Patients with tumors up to 4 cm in size were eligible for the study, and the surgical procedure was removal of the tumor with only enough grossly normal breast tissue to ensure that tumor cells did

not touch the inked margins of resection. A radiation boost was not required. Despite these differences in patient selection and treatment techniques, none of the randomized trials demonstrates a significant survival difference between patients treated by CS and RT or mastectomy.

As a result of these studies, the appropriateness of CS plus RT as a treatment for breast cancer is not in doubt. More recent trials have focused on refinements in the procedure, and an area of particular interest has been the identification of a subset of patients with invasive carcinoma who could undergo CS without RT. There are a number of benefits to eliminating RT as a part of breast-conserving therapy. Radiation therapy is time consuming and inconvenient, and patients often cite fear of radiation as a reason for choosing mastectomy.[21] In addition, radiation may compromise the cosmetic appearance of the breast and, although the incidence of complications is low, it is not zero. The use of radiation also significantly increases the cost of breast-conserving treatment.

Six prospective randomized trials have compared the results of CS alone to CS plus RT in the treatment of early-stage breast cancer.[14,15,22-28] Considerable variations in patient eligibility criteria and treatment techniques are present amongst trials (Table 12.2). The NSABP trial,[14,15] the Ontario study,[22,23] the Scottish trial,[27] and the English trial[28] were the most inclusive, with patients with tumors

Table 12.1 *Survival results in the modern randomized trials comparing conservative surgery (CS) and radiation therapy (RT) with mastectomy*

Trial	Patients	Follow-up (years)	Survival (%)	
			Mastectomy[a]	CS and RT
Institut Gustave-Roussy[19]	179	10	79	78
NCI, Milan[13]	701	13	69	71
NSABP trial B06[14,15]	1843	8	71	76
NCI, USA[18]	237	5	85	89
EORTC[16]	903	7	75	75
Danish Breast Cancer Group[17,20]	905	6	82	79

[a]None of the differences in survival was statistically significant.
EORTC, European Organization for Research and Treatment of Cancer; NCI, National Cancer Institute; NSABP, National Surgical Adjuvant Breast and Bowel Project.

Table 12.2 *Patient characteristics in the trials comparing conservative surgery with and without radiation therapy*

Trial	Number of patients	Tumor size (cm)	Lymph node status	Type of surgery	Final margins	Adjuvant therapy
NSABP B06[14,15]	1140	≤ 4	N+ or N−	Lumpectomy	Negative	Chemotherapy for N+ patients
Swedish[24,25]	381	≤ 2	N−	Sector resection	Negative	None
Ontario[22,23]	837	≤ 4	N−	Lumpectomy	Negative	None
Milan III[13,26]	567	≤ 2.5	N+ or N−	Quadrantectomy	Negative or positive	Chemotherapy for some N+ patients
Scottish[27]	585	≤ 4	N+ or N−	Lumpectomy	Negative	Chemotherapy
English[28]	418	≤ 5	N_0 or N_1	Wide local excision	Negative or positive	Chemotherapy

up to 4 cm in diameter eligible for entry, and limited surgical resections of normal breast tissue (lumpectomy) were employed. Both the Milan III study[13,26] and the Swedish trial[24,25] used larger surgical resections, termed 'quadrantectomy' and 'sector resection,' respectively. The patient population in the Swedish trial was the most highly selected and included only patients with mammographically detected T1 lesions. In addition, patients with histologic evidence of invasive or intraductal carcinoma at a distance greater than 2 cm from the primary tumor were excluded. These restrictive criteria resulted in only 51% of the patients with stage I breast cancer seen at participating hospitals being eligible for the study.

Despite the differences in eligibility criteria and treatment techniques amongst these studies, the results are very similar. The use of irradiation resulted in a large reduction in the rate of breast recurrences in all of the studies, with an average crude rate of reduction of 75% (range 63–89%, Table 12.3). One of the apparent advantages of treatment with excision alone is that recurrences can be salvaged with re-excision and irradiation. However, most of the women in these studies who developed breast recurrence either required or desired mastectomy. Only 30% of patients in the Swedish trial were salvaged with further breast preservation, a figure somewhat lower than the 43% and 57% rates seen in the Ontario and Scottish studies. In the Milan study, despite the fact that the initial breast resection was a quadrantectomy, 62% of patients with recurrence were treated with re-excision and radiotherapy. These data suggest that the expectation that most breast recurrences after conservative surgery alone can be salvaged with re-excision and irradiation is not true.[29]

Efforts have been made in the studies described above to identify subsets of patients with a low rate of recurrence after CS alone by using clinical and histologic features. Increasing patient age and small tumor size were the most commonly identified factors that predicted a low risk of breast recurrence, but these findings were not consistent from study to study. Additionally, no low-risk group could be identified in the Ontario and NSABP studies. A prospective, single-arm study from the Joint Center for Radiation Therapy (JCRT) attempted to identify a subset of women not requiring RT by using multiple clinical and pathologic variables.[30] Women with T1 tumors, histologically negative axillary lymph nodes, no evidence of lymphatic vessel invasion or an extensive intraductal component in the cancer, and no cancer cells within 1 cm of the inked margin were treated with CS alone. The median age of the patients was 67 years, and 76% of the tumors were detected by mammography alone. With a median follow-up of 56 months for surviving patients, recurrence in the breast was seen in 14 patients (16%). The average annual rate of local recurrence was 3.6%, and the 3-year crude rate of recurrence in the breast was 10.5%. Among a reference group of patients with similar characteristics who were treated with CS and RT, the 5-year rate of breast recurrence was 0%, suggesting that, when RT is omitted, there is a significant risk of early local recurrence, even in highly selected patients. In a similar prospective study of 23 highly selected patients treated with excision alone, Sauer et al. reported a 9.5% rate of breast recurrence after a median follow-up of 5 years.[31] The effect of adjuvant systemic therapy, either chemotherapy or tamoxifen, on local recurrence rates after CS alone has also been examined. The use of chemotherapy does not appear to have a major impact on the rate of breast recurrences.[29] The effect of tamoxifen is less clear, but most studies show a substantial reduction in the risk of breast recurrence with the addition of radiation to excision plus tamoxifen.[29]

A critical question regarding the use of radiotherapy after CS is its effect on survival. As shown in Table 12.3, none of the randomized trials demonstrates a statistically significant survival benefit for radiotheraphy. However, none of these studies has the statistical power to eliminate a 5–10% difference in survival should such a difference exist. The impact of local recurrence on the risk of mortality will vary with the patient population studied. In patients in whom the risk of breast cancer mortality at the time of diagnosis is substantial, such as those with positive axillary lymph nodes or larger, high-grade tumors, local recurrence is unlikely to influence survival. However, in non-randomized studies, the patients selected for CS alone have been those with a low risk of distant relapse (negative axillary nodes, small tumors). In this setting, the development of a breast recurrence of

Table 12.3 *Outcome in the trials comparing conservative surgery (CS) with and without radiation therapy (RT)*

Trial	Median follow-up (months)	Breast recurrences (%)		Overall survival (%)	
		CS	CS + RT	CS	CS + RT
NSABP B06[14,15]	144	35	10	58	62
Swedish[24,25]	64	18	2	90	91
Ontario[22,23]	91	35	11	76	79
Milan III[13,26]	52	18[a]	2[a]	No difference	
Scottish[27]	68	25	6	No difference	
English[28]	71	35	13	Not available	

[a]Estimated from curves.

larger size or higher histologic grade than the primary tumor may have the potential to increase the risk of breast cancer mortality. The available prospective studies have not reproducibly identified a subset of patients who will not benefit from RT, and at present RT should continue to be considered a standard part of breast-conserving therapy for invasive carcinoma.

Extent of surgery

A major unresolved question in breast-conserving surgery is how much normal breast tissue should be removed as part of a lumpectomy. In making this determination, the surgeon seeks to achieve a low rate of local recurrence in the breast while maintaining a good cosmetic outcome. An examination of the microscopic distribution of tumor in the breasts of patients with localized carcinoma is helpful in making a decision about the extent of resection. Holland *et al.* studied mastectomy specimens from 264 patients whose tumors were thought to be unicentric after standard clinical and mammographic evaluation.[32,33] A detailed evaluation of breast tissue using 5-mm sectioning of the mastectomy specimen, radiography of these thin slices, and extensive histologic sampling was carried out. This technique allowed precise mapping of the extent of residual carcinoma in relation to the primary, or reference, tumor. Only 39% of specimens showed no evidence of cancer beyond the reference tumor, and in 20% of cases additional cancer was confined to within 2 cm of the reference tumor. In 41% of cases residual cancer was present more than 2 cm from the reference tumor; of these, two-thirds had pure intraductal carcinoma and one-third had mixed intraductal and invasive carcinoma. Based on these findings, it is apparent that, if a small amount of normal breast tissue is resected with the primary tumor, the amount of residual microscopic disease which must be eradicated by radiation may be substantial, and the possibility of radioresistant cells is higher than when larger breast resections such as quadrantectomy are used (Figure 12.1). If the microscopic tumor detected in the studies of Holland *et al.*[32,33] is biologically significant, one would expect the incidence of breast recurrence after a limited lumpectomy to be higher than after a quadrantectomy. These principles were tested in a randomized trial by Veronesi *et al.*,[34,35] in which patients with tumors 2.5 cm or less in size were randomized to treatment with lumpectomy or quadrantectomy, followed by external-beam irradiation. Histologically negative margins were not required. Patients in the quadrantectomy group had a 5.3% incidence of breast recurrence at 7 years, compared to 13.3% in the lumpectomy group. These findings suggest that larger breast resections decrease the rate of breast recurrence by reducing the amount of microscopic residual disease that must be controlled by irradiation. However, a comparison of cosmetic outcome

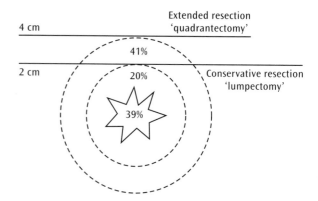

Figure 12.1 *Distribution of residual microscopic tumor in patients with clinically localized breast cancer based on the data of Holland et al.[32] When a limited resection of breast tissue is done, 41% of patients will have residual tumor, which must be eradicated by irradiation.*

between patients treated with quadrantectomy and lumpectomy showed that quadrantectomy was associated with a significantly poorer cosmetic result,[35] arguing against its routine use.

Ideally, the extent of breast resection should be individualized on the basis of the patient's tumor burden. Studies of magnetic resonance imaging suggest that this modality can detect microscopic tumor not seen with conventional imaging methods in 20–35% of cases,[36,37] but further data are needed before this technique is routinely employed. Conventional two-view mammography defines the extent of poorly differentiated ductal carcinoma *in situ* (DCIS) fairly accurately,[38] but underestimates the microscopic extent of well-differentiated DCIS by as much as 2 cm in 47% of cases.[39] The use of magnification mammography resolves much of this discrepancy. Morrow *et al.* examined the clinical utility of magnification mammography in identifying localized tumors suitable for breast preservation in 263 patients.[40] The extent of surgery was determined by the mammographic extent of disease, and breast preservation was successful in 97% of the 216 patients found to have localized tumors on magnification views.

Margin status and histologic tumor type are other parameters that are useful in determining the appropriate extent of breast resection. In general, the absence of tumor at surgical resection margins is associated with a lower incidence of breast recurrence than when tumor is present at the margin (Table 12.4).[34,41–46] However, as demonstrated in the studies of Solin *et al.*[46] and Wazer *et al.*,[44] the use of higher boost doses in patients with microscopic amounts of tumor at resection margins results in breast failure rates equal to those seen in patients with negative margins. These studies suggest that increased radiation doses (above 60 Gy) are needed in patients with positive margins, and a study to test this hypothesis is underway by the European Organization for Research and Treatment of Cancer (EORTC). In general, re-excision should be

Table 12.4 *Local recurrence rate and margin status*

Reference	Follow-up (years)	Margin status		
		Positive	Negative	Unknown
Anscher et al.[42]	5	15	2	2
Wazer et al.[44]	10	1.3	1.3	1.3
Schnitt et al.[45]	5	15	3	–
Solin et al.[46]	5	2	7	7
Van Dongen et al.[41]	8	20	9	–
Mariani et al.[34]	10	24.5	17.6	–

Table 12.5 *Residual carcinoma in relation to margins of initial biopsy specimen*

Reference	Initial positive margin (n)	Residual cancer (%)	Unknown margin (n)	Residual cancer (%)
Schnitt et al.[47]	29	69	33	64
Kearney and Morrow[48]	42	45	48	42
Gwin et al.[49]	54	65	100	45

undertaken in patients with gross or extensive microscopic disease at the margin after an initial conservative resection, as well as in patients whose margin status is unknown. Several studies have demonstrated that the likelihood of residual carcinoma does not differ between patients with positive and unknown margins, with residual tumor being present in about 50% of cases (Table 12.5).[47–49] The presence of residual tumor in the re-excision is not a contraindication to breast-conserving treatment. The status of the final margin should be used to determine the patient's suitability for the procedure. Kearney and Morrow found that 86 of 90 patients undergoing re-excision for positive or unknown margins were satisfactory candidates for breast-conserving treatment.[48] The need for re-excision in patients with focal microscopic disease at the margins is uncertain, and may be related to the histologic tumor type. Schnitt et al. observed a low rate of local recurrence (6%) in patients with focally positive margins whose tumor lacked an extensive intraductal component (EIC).[45] This observation is consistent with the findings of Schmidt-Ullrich et al. that the likelihood of residual carcinoma in a re-excision specimen with positive or unknown margins was related to the histologic type of the primary tumor.[43] Residual tumor was noted in only 37% of cases of infiltrating ductal carcinoma without an EIC, compared with 50% of infiltrating lobular carcinomas, and 67% of infiltrating ductal tumors with an EIC. Schnitt et al. also found that an EIC predicted a greater likelihood of residual tumor in re-excisions (88% EIC positive versus 48% EIC negative, $p = 0.002$).[47] These clinical observations are supported by the mapping studies of Holland et al.,[33] in which 30% of patients with EIC-positive tumors were found to have prominent residual tumor more than 2 cm from the primary tumor, compared to only 2% of patients with EIC-negative tumors ($p < 0.0001$, Figure 12.2).

The foregoing information suggests that the appropriate extent of lumpectomy can be determined using

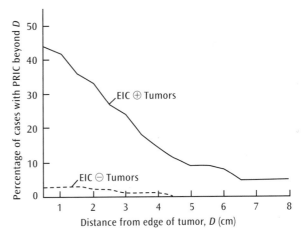

Figure 12.2 *Percentage of mastectomy specimens with prominent residual intraductal carcinoma (PRIC) ($\geqslant$6/low-power field) at or beyond certain distances from the edge of the primary tumor. EIC, extensive intraductal carcinoma. From Holland et al., J Clin Oncol 1990; 8:113–18.[33]*

magnification mammography, tumor histology, and the margin status of the initial excision. In patients with EIC-positive cancer or infiltrating lobular carcinoma, re-excision should be considered in those with close or focally positive margins. Tumors with an EIC adequately excised are at no increased risk for recurrence. For EIC-negative infiltrating ductal tumors with focally positive margins, cases should be assessed on an individual basis to determine whether re-excision or an increased radiation dose will best maintain the cosmetic appearance. When considering the issue of margin status, it is important to remember that 50% of patients with negative margins have residual tumor in the breast.[47,49] Thus, margin status is best regarded as a marker of the amount of residual tumor in the breast (not its presence or absence) and the likelihood of control with RT.

There is no consensus on the best technique for re-excision. Attempts to excise the entire biopsy cavity surrounded by normal breast tissue usually result in the sacrifice of unnecessary amounts of breast tissue unless the original biopsy cavity was extremely small, or enough time has elapsed that it is fibrosed and contracted. Our technique of re-excision is to excise each wall of the biopsy cavity separately, marking the new margin surface with a suture to orient the pathologist. If the initial specimen was marked with orienting sutures, re-excision is limited to the involved margins.

Cosmetic outcome

Maintaining a breast that is cosmetically acceptable to the patient is a major goal of breast-conserving surgery. A variety of patient, tumor, and treatment factors have been reported to influence the cosmetic result, but the major determinant of cosmetic outcome is the amount of breast tissue resected.[34,35,50–52] This is most convincingly demonstrated in the randomized trial from Milan comparing quadrantectomy to lumpectomy.[35] Of 148 patients in that study who participated in a cosmetic evaluation 18–24 months after RT, 21% of patients in the quadrantectomy group had a greater than 3 cm difference in nipple height, compared with 7% in the lumpectomy group. Similar differences in the distance from the midline to the nipple and in the inferior profile of the breast were observed. The technique of RT is also important in cosmetic outcome, with significantly greater amounts of retraction and fibrosis seen with whole-breast doses above 50 Gy, as well as with high boost doses.[52] However, in a small series reported by Matory et al. in which patients were evaluated both before and after RT, surgery was found to be the main contributor to cosmetic outcome.[53] Large breast size has also been reported to decrease cosmetic outcome. Clarke et al. reported excellent results in 100% of patients with an A bra cup, 84% with a B cup, 78% with a C cup, and 50% with a D cup ($p = 0.02$).[54] Dose inhomogeneity and increased fat content were postulated as the cause of the worse cosmetic results. Gray et al. also examined cosmetic outcome relative to breast size, comparing symmetry, edema, skin thickening, fibrosis, and retraction between women with large and average breasts.[55] At 3 and 5 years after treatment, only symmetry and retraction differed between the groups. Using a ten-point scale, patients with large breast size had a mean score of 7.69, compared to 8.45 for patients with average breast size. Thus, although cosmetic outcome was significantly worse in patients with large breasts, both groups had scores in a satisfactory range.

Tumor location and tumor size also influence the cosmetic result. Tumor size is important both in relation to the patient's breast size and because it determines the amount of breast tissue which must be resected. In addition, the depth of the tumor within the breast and the quadrant in which it is located will affect the cosmetic outcome. For example, distortion of the contour of the inferior breast which is visible only with the arms raised may be more acceptable to a patient than a similar degree of distortion in the upper inner quadrant which is visible in a variety of types of clothing.

The long-term outcome and stability of the cosmetic results after CS plus RT have been evaluated in a number of studies from the JCRT.[50,56–58] Cosmetic results were scored as excellent when the treated and untreated breast were identical, good when minimal treatment effect was apparent, fair when obvious changes due to treatment were present, and poor when severe alterations in the normal breast were evident. In addition, individual elements of cosmetic outcome such as breast edema, retraction, and telangiectasia were assessed. In a series of 593 patients treated between 1968 and 1981, the overall cosmetic result at 5 years was excellent in 65%, good in 25%, fair in 7%, and poor in 3%.[56] During the first 3 years after treatment, overall cosmetic results declined, paralleling the development of breast retraction, and then stabilized through 7 years of follow-up. Retraction was the major determinant of cosmetic outcome. Of the 36 patients with fair or poor results at 3 years, 78% had moderate or severe retraction, compared with only 6% of 266 patients with good or excellent scores.[57] In contrast, breast edema was most pronounced in the first year after treatment, with mild edema present in 33% of patients and moderate or severe edema in 6%. By 3 years, the incidence of mild edema had decreased to 20%, and moderate to severe edema to 1%. These findings suggest that edema is rarely the major determinant of long-term cosmetic outcome. The timing of adjuvant chemotherapy also influences cosmesis. Chemotherapy followed by radiation preserves cosmesis better than concurrent chemotherapy and radiation therapy.[58]

Local recurrence

Recurrent carcinoma in the breast after CS plus RT occurs in 4–20% of patients by 10 years after treatment.[12–20] In contrast to local failure after mastectomy, most of which occurs in the first 3 years after surgery, the time to local failure after CS plus RT may be quite prolonged.[59–61] Kurtz et al. observed the actuarial incidence of breast recurrence to increase from 7% at 5 years to 14% at 10 years and 20% at 20 years after treatment.[59] Recurrences at or near the primary tumor site are usually seen within the first 10 years post-treatment, whereas recurrences elsewhere in the breast occur later.[59,61] Kurtz et al. reported that 32% of breast recurrences seen after 5 years occurred at a distance from the primary tumor, compared with 14% of recurrences seen during the first 5 years.[59] After 5 years, the risk of recurrence elsewhere in the treated breast is remarkably similar to the risk of developing a contralateral breast carcinoma,[62] suggesting that whole-breast irradiation, while effective at eradicating microscopic multicentric disease, does not prevent the subsequent development of new carcinomas.

A great deal of attention has been devoted to the identification of factors associated with an increased risk of local recurrence. These factors can be divided into patient characteristics such as age or family history of breast cancer, tumor factors such as size and nodal status, and treatment factors. Young patient age, variously defined as under age 40, age 35, or age 30, has consistently been found to be associated with an increased risk of local recurrence.[63–66] Some of this increase in risk is due to an association between young age and pathologic features such as high histologic grade, the absence of estrogen receptors, lymphatic vessel invasion, and the presence of an extensive intraductal component. However, even after controlling for these factors, young patient age is still associated with an increased risk of breast failure in some studies.[66] Young patient age is also associated with an increased incidence of local recurrence after mastectomy.[65] These findings suggest that age should not be used as a selection factor for the type of local therapy, but is indicative of a poorer overall prognosis.

A family history of breast cancer has not been shown to increase the risk of local failure after breast-conserving surgery. Kurtz followed 905 patients with stage I and II cancer after breast-conserving therapy, and observed local recurrence in 15% of patients with a family history of breast cancer, compared to 12% in those who lacked such a history.[67] A similar study evaluated breast-conserving therapy in 201 patients aged 36 years or younger with a first-degree relative with ovarian cancer or premenopausal breast cancer, as these patients have a high probability of BRCA1 or BRCA2 gene mutation.[68] There was no increase in local recurrence between the groups. The group with the significant family history did, however, have an increased risk of developing a second, contralateral cancer. There is concern that women with genetically transmitted breast cancer may be poor candidates for breast conservation. No definitive studies in women documented to have genetic mutations are available, but Marcus et al. reported a study of mastectomy specimens from women with pedigrees consistent with genetically transmitted cancer.[69] No increase in the incidence of multicentric carcinomas or intraductal carcinoma associated with invasive tumors was identified. Although this is a subject for further study, at this time, a pedigree consistent with genetic breast cancer is not a contraindication to breast-conserving therapy.

Tumor factors such as size and nodal status are important predictors of the risk of distant relapse, but they are not major predictors of the risk of breast recurrence. In a study of 783 patients with stage I and II cancer treated with excision and RT including a boost to the tumor site, the rate of recurrence was 13% for T1 lesions and 12% for T2 lesions after a median follow-up of 91 months.[70] This observation is consistent with the findings of Holland et al. that the extent of residual tumor in the breast was not influenced by tumor size.[32] Histologic tumor type is also not a predictor of breast recurrence. Several studies have demonstrated that local failure rates for women with infiltrating lobular carcinoma are similar to those of women with infiltrating ductal carcinoma.[71] However, because the extent of infiltrating lobular carcinoma is often more difficult to assess, both mammographically and intraoperatively, it may be more difficult to obtain negative margins when excising lobular carcinomas.

Early studies in which tumors were grossly excised without attention to the inking of margins suggested that the presence of an EIC in association with the invasive carcinoma increased the risk of local recurrence.[71] More recent studies have indicated that when negative surgical margins are obtained, recurrence rates in these patients are similar to those in patients without an EIC.[14,42,45] As discussed previously, the presence of an EIC is often an indication that a wider surgical resection is needed to encompass the tumor. Some studies have identified lymphatic vessel invasion as a pathologic factor that predicts for an increased risk of local recurrence after breast-conserving therapy.[63,72] However, lymphatic vessel invasion is also known to be a risk factor for an increased incidence of local failure after mastectomy.[73]

This information suggests that there may be two types of local recurrence seen after breast-conserving therapy. The first type is indicative of biologically aggressive carcinoma, and is similar in behavior to the local recurrences seen after mastectomy. The second type of local recurrence is a reflection of a heavy tumor burden in the breast, and this type of recurrence is more likely to be impacted upon by alterations in therapy such as wider surgical resections and increased doses of RT. When considering mastectomy to avoid the problem of local recurrence after breast-conserving therapy, it is important to remember that, even in stage I and II cancer, mastectomy does not guarantee freedom from local failure. As illustrated in Table 12.6, the incidence of local failure after CS plus RT did not differ significantly from the incidence of local failure after mastectomy in five of the six randomized trials in which these treatments were compared.

MASTECTOMY AND IMMEDIATE RECONSTRUCTION

The switch from radical mastectomy to modified radical mastectomy and advances in plastic surgical technique have made immediate reconstruction an option for most patients who undergo mastectomy. Concerns about immediate reconstruction have included the possibility of an increased incidence of local failure, a delay in the diagnosis of local failure, or a delay in the administration of adjuvant therapy due to wound-healing problems.

There have been no prospective trials comparing mastectomy alone to mastectomy and immediate

Table 12.6 *Local recurrence rates in modern randomized trials comparing conservative surgery (CS) and radiation therapy (RT) with mastectomy*

Trial	Follow-up (years)	Local recurrence (%)		Type CS	Boost	Boost dose (Gy)
		Mastectomy	CS and RT			
Gustave-Roussy[19]	15	14	9	2 cm gross margin	Yes	15
NCI, Milan[13]	18	4	7	Quadrantectomy	Yes	10
NSABP B06[14,15]	12	8	10	Lumpectomy	No	
NCI, USA[18]	10	6	19	Gross tumor excision	Yes	15–20
EORTC[16]	8	9	13	1 cm gross margin	Yes	25
Danish Breast Cancer Group[17,20]	6	4	3	Wide excision	Yes	10–25

EORTC, European Organization for Research and Treatment of Cancer; NCI, National Cancer Institute; NSABP, National Surgical Adjuvant Breast and Bowel Project.

Table 12.7 *Types of reconstruction after mastectomy*

Type	Advantages	Disadvantages	Contraindications
Implant	One-stage procedure Short operative time Minimal prolongation of hospitalization and recovery Low cost	Capsular contracture Implant rupture or leakage Poor cosmetic outcome in very large ptotic breasts	Irradiated skin
Tissue expander	Short operative time Low cost Hospitalization, recovery not prolonged	Multiple physician visits Rupture of implant Implant leakage	Irradiated skin
Latissimus dorsi flap	Reliable flap Autogenous tissue Natural contour	Donor site scar Moderate prolongation of hospitalization and recovery Usually requires an implant	Major co-morbidities
Transverse rectus abdominis myocutaneous flap	Autogenous tissue Natural contour Abdominoplasty	Donor site scar Significant prolongation of hospitalization and recovery Partial flap loss Abdominal wall hernia	Major co-morbidities

reconstruction, but the available retrospective data do not support concerns about the incidence or detection of local recurrence in the reconstructed patient. Petit *et al.* compared 146 patients treated with both immediate and delayed silicone-gel implant reconstruction to a control group of patients treated with mastectomy alone.[74] The groups were matched for age, year of diagnosis, stage, histologic tumor type and grade, and nodal status. At 10 years, 8% of the reconstructed patients had experienced local recurrence, compared to 15% of the patients having mastectomy alone. In a similar study, Webster *et al.* compared 85 patients having immediate reconstruction using a variety of techniques to 85 controls undergoing mastectomy alone who were matched for age, stage nodal involvement, and receptor status.[75] At 30 months, the incidence of local and distant recurrence did not differ between groups.

The effect of reconstruction on the detection of local recurrence was studied by Noone and co-workers in 306

patients followed for a mean of 6.4 years.[76] Local recurrence as the first site of treatment failure occurred in 5.2% of the group. Fourteen of the 16 recurrences were in the skin or subcutaneous fat, so detection was not affected by the presence of the reconstruction. Noone *et al.*[76] observed no delay in the administration of chemotherapy in patients having reconstruction, a finding also reported by Eberlein and co-workers.[77]

In summary, immediate reconstruction has not been shown to alter the outcome of mastectomy or to delay the administration of systemic therapy. Immediate reconstruction has the advantages of avoiding the need for a second major operative procedure and the psychological morbidity of the loss of the breast. The two major reconstructive techniques involve the use of implants or of myocutaneous tissue flaps to create a new breast mound. The advantages and disadvantages of the techniques are summarized in Table 12.7. Implant reconstructions are most suitable for women with small to moderate size

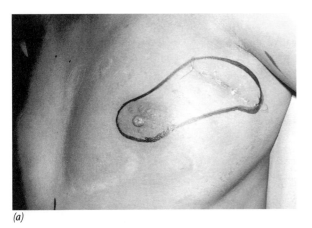
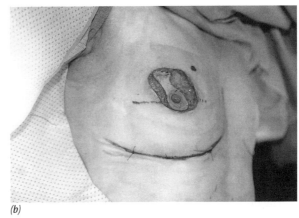

(a)   (b)

Figure 12.3 *Skin-sparing mastectomy incisions: (a) incorporating nipple areolar complex and upper outer quadrant biopsy scar; and (b) removing very small skin paddle including nipple areolar complex and biopsy scar. Horizontal lines mark potential sites of skin incision for additional exposure.*

breasts with minimal ptosis, whereas flap reconstructions allow more flexibility in the size and shape of the reconstructed breast. In the past, most breast implants were filled with silicone gel. However, after uncontrolled reports suggested an increased incidence of connective tissue disease in women with silicone implants,[78,79] the Food and Drug Administration (FDA) declared a moratorium on their use. Since that time, several epidemiological studies have failed to demonstrate an increased incidence of connective tissue disorders in women with implants compared to matched control populations.[80,81] Silicone implants are available for use in breast cancer patients, but many patients opt for saline implants or flap reconstructions as a result of the adverse publicity surrounding silicone implants.

Regardless of the reconstructive technique chosen, preservation of the skin envelope of the breast will aid the reconstructive surgeon in obtaining symmetry. From an oncologic point of view, the only skin that must be removed as part of mastectomy is the biopsy scar and the nipple areolar complex. Exposure for complete removal of the breast and axillary contents can be obtained by incision rather than excision of skin (Figure 12.3). Kroll *et al.* analysed 87 patients having 100 reconstructions using a skin-sparing technique who were followed for a mean of 23 months.[82] Two patients developed local recurrence, one of which was associated with wide-spread metastases. This low rate of local failure is consistent with prior observations that the extent of skin removal in patients treated with mastectomy alone is not a major determinant of the risk of chest-wall recurrence.[83]

AXILLARY DISSECTION

For many years, 'complete' axillary dissection was considered a critical component for the surgical cure of breast cancer, but by the 1970s there was increasing evidence that axillary dissection had a limited impact on survival.

This impression was confirmed by the results of NSABP Protocol B04, in which patients with clinically negative axillary nodes were randomized to treatment by radical mastectomy, total mastectomy with observation of the axillary nodes and delayed dissection if positive nodes developed, or total mastectomy plus RT to the regional lymphatics.[84] No statistically significant differences in survival were observed at 10 years, despite the fact that 40% of patients in the radical mastectomy group had positive nodes, and a similar percentage in the observation-only group were presumed to have positive nodes. This, coupled with the awareness that axillary node status was the primary predictor of prognosis after surgery, has led axillary dissection to be regarded primarily as a staging procedure which is also an excellent means of maintaining local control in the axilla. However, it is important to recognize that no studies have been done which have the statistical power to exclude a small (5%) but clinically significant survival benefit due to axillary dissection.

Extent of axillary dissection

A variety of surgical procedures ranging from an anatomic dissection of all visible axillary fat to attempts to identify and remove individual lymph nodes have been described. A number of studies have been undertaken to determine the extent of axillary surgery needed to determine if axillary nodes are positive or negative. Many of these studies examined the likelihood of 'skip metastases,' that is, involvement of the nodes in the upper axilla (level 3) in the absence of involvement of the lower axillary nodes.[85–91] As illustrated in Table 12.8, isolated metastases to level 3 are rare. This is not surprising as Veronesi *et al.* noted a mean of only 2.2 nodes per patient in level 3.[86] In contrast to the uniformly low level of skip metastases to level 3, there is considerable variability in the risk of skip metastases to level 2, probably due to differences in the definition of which nodal tissue constitutes level 1 and level 2.

Table 12.8 *Frequency of skip metastases*

Reference	Patients with axillary metastases	Negative levels 1/ positive level 2 (%)	Negative levels 1 and 2/ positive level 3 (%)
Rosen et al.[85]	429	2	0.2
Veronesi et al.[86]	539	1.5	0.4
Smith et al.[87]	309	16	10
Danforth et al.[88]	65	29	3.1
Chevinsky et al.[89]	93	7	2
Pigott et al.[90]	72	23.6	1.4
Boova et al.[91]	80	7.5	1.3

The procedures described as dissections are based on the removal of an anatomically defined volume of axillary tissue. Studies of axillary-sampling procedures have produced extremely variable results, depending on the extent of the sampling procedure employed. Kissin *et al.* observed a 24% error rate in staging with a sampling to the level of the intercostobrachial nerve.[92] In contrast, in a randomized study of 401 patients assigned to axillary dissection or axillary sampling, Steele *et al.* found no significant difference in the number of positive nodes between the two groups.[93]

A level 1 and 2 dissection is an effective means of maintaining local control in the axilla, with axillary recurrence rates of 3% or less reported in most studies.[94–96] With more limited sampling procedures, the likelihood of local control is related to the number of nodes that are removed. In the Danish Breast Cancer Group study of 3128 clinically node-negative patients, the 5-year probability of an axillary recurrence was 19% when no nodes were removed, 10% when one to two negative nodes were removed, 5% when three to four negative nodes were removed, and 3% when more than five negative nodes were sampled.[97] Fowble *et al.* noted a 21% failure rate for patients with fewer than three axillary nodes removed, compared to 5% when more than five nodes were removed.[98] The data suggest that a level 1 and 2 axillary dissection accurately stages patients and provides excellent local control. The formal identification of the neurovascular structures in the axillary triangle as part of an anatomic dissection allows them to be protected during the procedure, minimizing the risk of serious complications.

Elimination of axillary dissection in selected patients

Several developments in breast cancer therapy have prompted a re-evaluation of the need for axillary dissection in all cases of invasive carcinoma. These include the increased identification of very small breast cancers by mammography screening, the increasing use of breast-conserving therapy, the widespread use of adjuvant systemic therapy in both node-positive and node-negative patients, and a greater awareness of the morbidity of axillary dissection. Two general approaches to eliminating axillary dissection have been taken: first, to identify patients at a very low risk for nodal metastases and, second, to identify patients whose therapy would not be altered by axillary dissection. Elimination of axillary dissection should only be considered in clinically node-negative patients. In the presence of palpable axillary nodes, axillary dissection is mandatory to prevent the local complications of uncontrolled tumor growth.

The most common parameter used to identify patients at low risk for axillary metastases is tumor size. However, in reports of large, unselected patient populations, nodal metastases are present in 15–25% of patients with tumors measuring 1 cm or less in size and, even in tumors 0.5 cm or smaller, axillary metastases are reported in 3–28% of cases.[99–101] Elderly women with receptor-positive tumors are another subgroup for whom axillary dissection is unlikely to alter therapy. Avoiding axillary dissection when it will not alter therapy seems reasonable based on our current inability to tailor systemic therapy to the individual patient's risk of relapse, but there are a number of drawbacks to this approach. The presence of axillary nodal metastases remains the most important predictor of prognosis, and many patients want this information. If an axillary dissection is not done, maintaining local control in the axilla becomes an issue, and careful follow-up must be carried out to ensure that metastases are promptly detected. Finally, axillary dissection may have a therapeutic benefit for a small number of patients. This is suggested by the finding that 25–30% of the 20-year survivors in reports of patients treated by radical mastectomy alone had positive axillary nodes.[102–104] A prospective, randomized trial examining the value of axillary dissection has been reported.[105] In this study, 658 clinically node-negative patients were randomized to receive lumpectomy, axillary dissection, and breast irradiation, or lumpectomy alone with irradiation of the breast and the regional nodes. No significant difference in the incidence of axillary failure was observed between groups. The survival results are more difficult to evaluate because only patients in the axillary dissection arm received chemotherapy (when positive nodes were identified). However, at 5 years, a statistically significant survival advantage was observed in the patients having axillary dissection (97% versus 93%, $p = 0.01$), which was too large to be explained by the expected benefits for the subset of patients who received chemotherapy. Further support for the idea that local therapy may impact upon survival comes from studies demonstrating an improvement in survival for patients receiving post-mastectomy RT.[106,107] Taken together, this information suggests that the wholesale abandonment of axillary dissection is premature.

Sentinel lymph node biopsy

The technique of axillary sentinel lymph node biopsy allows the possibility of limiting full axillary dissection to those patients who will benefit most from the procedure. The sentinel node is defined as the first node that the lymphatics draining the cancer encounter. The sentinel node procedure was initially proposed for penile cancer in the 1970s,[108] popularized with melanoma,[109] and was adapted to breast cancer by Giuliano et al. in the mid-1990s.[110,111] This technique has been refined and can currently accurately stage 90% of patients,[112–122] but the identification of a sentinel node is associated with a significant learning curve. With experience, a sentinel node can be found in over 90% of patients.[112,113] Lymphatic mapping can be undertaken with blue dye (lymphazurin),[109,114] radiolabeled colloids,[110,115–117] or both.[118–120] Injection of the dye or radiolabeled colloid can be around the tumor site[110,118,121] or subdermal.[117]

Our preferred method involves using 5–7 mL of blue dye alone, injected into the breast parenchyma around the tumor in the majority of patients, reserving adjunctive radiolabeled colloid primarily for very medial lesions or patients with a large amount of axillary adipose tissue.[114] If the patient has had prior lumpectomy or excisional biopsy, the dye is instilled just outside the palpable edge of the cavity. For patients undergoing needle localization lumpectomy, a 23-gauge needle for injection of dye is inserted by the mammographer following the localization procedure. Four to 7 minutes of manual breast compression is then used, depending on the location of the injection site. The incision is placed at the inferior aspect of the hair-bearing portion of the axilla and continued down to the axillary fascia. It is essential that the most proximal blue-stained lymph node be identified as the sentinel node, as staining may have progressed into non-sentinel nodes by the time of identification. Attempts should also be made to identify a blue lymphatic leading to the sentinel node.

It is well known that there is a significant learning curve associated with the sentinel node procedure; however, the amount of experience necessary to master the technique remains controversial. Estimates between 10[122] and 80[123] cases have been reported. Different rates of mastery have been demonstrated among different surgeons.[114,115,120] Some studies suggest that incorporation of both blue dye and radioisotope can hasten the learning curve,[112] whereas others refute this idea.[114] Current guidelines recommend that completion axillary dissection be performed until the surgeon has demonstrated a

greater than 90% accuracy rate and < 5% false-negative rate with at least 30 sentinel node procedures.[112]

Several contraindications to sentinel lymph node biopsy have been identified. Patients with suspicious palpable axillary adenopathy should undergo a formal axillary dissection. Multicentric tumors or tumors larger than 5 cm may have more than one primary drainage pathway,[117] and therefore more than one sentinel node. Locally advanced tumors may cause plugging of lymphatics by tumor, thereby blocking access to the dye or tracer to the sentinel node. Preoperative chemotherapy can complicate lymphatic mapping because it is the original tumor site, often no longer identifiable after surgery, that must be mapped. Very large biopsy cavities also make it difficult to reliably assess the drainage from the primary tumor. Previous axillary surgery, for melanoma, hidradentitis, or other reason, may disrupt the native lymphatic channels and confound the sentinel lymph node technique. Finally, the safety of blue dye or radiolabeled colloid in pregnant or lactating women has not been established. If lymphatic mapping is attempted and it is not possible to identify the sentinel node, a full axillary dissection should be performed.

Once retrieved, the sentinel node can be subjected to much more detailed pathologic investigation than would be practical for the entire axillary contents. Examination of serial sections stained with hematoxylin and eosin, immunohistochemistry, or even reverse transcriptase–polymerase chain reaction (RT–PCR) methodology can identify tumor cells that would not have been visible by more limited methods.[124–128] Clare et al. demonstrated that serial sectioning may be as sensitive as immunohistochemistry for the demonstration of lymph node metastases.[128] The significance of these micrometastases in terms of prognostic implications, however, is not clear, especially those identified by RT–PCR.[114,127–131] Studies are ongoing to help define the answers to these questions.

Current standards of care dictate that a positive sentinel lymph node is an indication for completion axillary dissection to determine the status of the remainder of the axilla. It has, however, been observed that the sentinel lymph node is the only positive node 40–60% of the time.[110,111,115,117,118,121] This percentage may be even higher if the sentinel node contains only micrometastases.[132] The risk of axillary recurrence in these situations is unknown, as is the possibility of a survival advantage conferred by a completion axillary dissection. The question of whether completion axillary dissection is always necessary when the sentinel lymph node is positive is being addressed, and a prospective, randomized trial is currently being conducted by the American College of Surgeons Oncology Group.

SELECTION OF AN OPERATIVE PROCEDURE

Absolute and relative contraindications to breast-conserving therapy have been developed by a

Table 12.9 *Absolute and relative contraindications to breast-conserving treatment* [a]

Absolute contraindications
First or second trimester of pregnancy
Two or more gross tumors in separate quadrants of the breast
Diffuse indeterminate or malignant-appearing microcalcifications
History of therapeutic irradiation of the breast region
Persistent positive margins after reasonable attempt at breast-conserving treatment

Relative contraindications
Large tumor/breast ratio
History of collagen vascular (connective tissue) disease
Large breast size
Tumor location beneath the nipple

---

[a]Joint Committee of the American College of Surgeons, American College of Radiology,
College of American Pathologists, and Society of Surgical Oncology.

multidisciplinary committee of representatives from the American College of Surgeons, the American College of Radiology, the College of American Pathologists, and the Society of Surgical Oncology, and are listed in Table 12.9.[133] While there is little debate regarding the absolute contraindications, a number of the relative contraindications deserve comment. A history of collagen vascular disease is considered a contraindication on the basis of a number of anecdotal reports of severe fibrotic reactions to irradiation in patients with lupus or scleroderma.[134,135] The number of patients with these conditions who received RT and did not develop problems is unknown. In one study of patients with collagen vascular disease who received RT, no increase in the incidence of complications was observed.[136] Large breast size is considered a relative contraindication, but this is only true if there are insufficient technical resources to immobilize the breast and ensure dose homogeneity. In our opinion, tumor beneath the nipple, necessitating removal of the nipple, should not be considered a contraindication. Although removal of the nipple areolar complex worsens the cosmetic result, the patient still maintains a sensate breast mound, in contrast to mastectomy in which both the nipple and the breast are removed. A family history of breast cancer and *BRCA1* or *BRCA2* mutations are not considered contraindications to breast conservation, although the risk of recurrence in patients with genetically disposed breast cancer is currently under investigation.

The only real contraindication to immediate breast reconstruction for stage I and II cancer is the presence of co-morbid conditions that would make prolongation of the operative procedure unwise. Age, poor prognosis, and the need for chemotherapy are not contraindications to the procedure. In patients who have a high likelihood of needing postoperative RT (larger tumors with clinically suspicious nodes), implant reconstructions should be avoided because RT has been observed to increase the risk of both implant loss and capsular contracture.[137]

In the absence of medical contraindications, the choice between mastectomy alone, mastectomy with reconstruction, or breast-conserving therapy rests with the patient. Several studies indicate that more than 50% of women in the USA continue to be treated with mastectomy.[1–4] There is little evidence to suggest that medical contraindications to breast preservation or patient preference for mastectomy are responsible for high mastectomy rates. In a study of 456 unselected patients with DCIS and clinical stage I and II breast cancer evaluated by a multidisciplinary team, Morrow *et al.* found that medical contraindications to breast preservation were present in only 26% of patients, and 80% of eligible women opted for breast preservation.[138] Foster *et al.* found that 80% of patients with stage I and II cancer treated at the University of Vermont between 1989 and 1990 opted for breast-conserving treatment.[139]

Some studies suggest that physician bias or a misunderstanding of the contraindications to breast-conserving therapy is responsible for high mastectomy rates. Tarbox *et al.* surveyed 134 general surgeons in Colorado as to whether they believed that survival after mastectomy was equal to survival after breast-conserving surgery for T1 cancers.[140] Twenty-two percent of the surgeons surveyed felt that mastectomy was superior, and an additional 34% felt that, although the treatments were probably equal, they biased their presentations toward mastectomy. Surgeons in both of these groups performed mastectomy more often than breast preservation. Tate *et al.* studied factors influencing the choice of surgical therapy in a Kentucky community where only 10–20% of early-stage breast cancers were treated by breast preservation.[21] Reasons cited as contraindications to breast preservation included axillary adenopathy, dense fibrocystic disease, large breast size, and centrally located tumors. Eighty-two percent of medically eligible patients selected mastectomy, with fear of RT being the most common reason for this choice. This study suggests problems with the understanding of the contraindications to the breast-conserving treatment as well as with patient education.

In considering the choice between mastectomy alone or with immediate reconstruction and breast-conserving therapy, it is important to remember that there is no therapy that is 'right' for all women. Most studies comparing psychological distress between patients undergoing mastectomy and patients undergoing breast-conserving therapy have found no significant differences.[141–143]

The role of the surgeon in selecting a local therapy for breast cancer has changed from one of informing the patient of the treatment to one of assessing the presence of medical contraindications to any of the treatments, educating the patient as to the available treatments and what each entails, and providing her with access to multidisciplinary consultation and the time that she needs to make a treatment choice which meets her needs.

REFERENCES

1. Lazovich D, White E, Thomas D, et al. Underutilization of breast conserving surgery and radiation therapy among women with stage I and II breast cancer. JAMA 1991; 266:3433.

2. Samet J, Hunt W, Farrow D. Determinants of receiving breast conserving surgery: the surveillance, epidemiology and end results program, 1983–1986. Cancer 1994; 73:2344.

3. Nattinger A, Gottleib M, Veum J, et al. Geographic variation in the use of breast conserving treatment for breast cancer. N Engl J Med 1992; 126:1102.

4. Osteen RT, Winchester DP, Cunningham MP. Breast Cancer. In Steele GD, Jessup JM, Winchester DP, Menck HR, Murphy GP, eds. National Cancer Data Base annual review of patient care 1995. American Cancer Society, 1995, 12.

5. Turner L, Swindell R, Bell W. Radical versus modified radical mastectomy for breast cancer. Ann R Coll Surg Engl 1981; 63:239.

6. Maddox W, Carpenter J, Laws H, et al. A randomized prospective trial of radical (Halsted) mastectomy versus modified radical mastectomy in 311 breast cancer patients. Ann Surg 1983; 198:207.

7. Robinson D, Van Heerden J, Payne W, et al. The primary surgical treatment of carcinoma of the breast: a changing trend toward modified radical mastectomy. Mayo Clin Proc 1976; 51:433.

8. Baker R, Montague A, Childs J. A comparison of modified radical mastectomy to radical mastectomy in the treatment of operable breast cancer. Ann Surg 1979; 189:583.

9. Lagios MD, Westdahl P, Rose M. The concept and implications of multicentricity in breast carcinoma. In Sommers SG, ed. Pathology annual. New York, Appleton-Century-Crofts, 1981.

10. Qualheim R, Gall E. Breast carcinoma with multiple sites of origin. Cancer 1957; 10:460.

11. Rosen P, Fracchia A, Urban J, et al. 'Residual' mammary carcinoma following simulated partial mastectomy. Cancer 1975; 35:739.

12. Veronesi U, Luini A, Galimberti V, Zurrida S. Conservation approaches for the management of stage I/II carcinoma of the breast: Milan Cancer Institute trials. World J Surg 1994; 18:70.

13. Veronesi U, Salvadori B, Luini A, et al. Breast conservation is a safe method in patients with small cancer of the breast. Long-term results of three randomized trials on 1993 patients. Eur J Cancer 1995; 31A:1574.

14. Fisher B, Anderson S, Redmond CK, et al. Re-analysis and results after 12 years of follow-up in a randomized clinical trial comparing total mastectomy with lumpectomy with or without irradiation in the treatment of breast cancer. N Engl J Med 1995; 333:1456.

15. Fisher B, Redmond CK, Poisson R, et al. Eight-year results of a randomized clinical trial comparing total mastectomy and lumpectomy with or without irradiation in the treatment of breast cancer. N Engl J Med 1989; 320:822.

16. Van Dongen J, Bartelink H, Fentimen I, et al. Randomized clinical trial to assess the value of breast-conserving therapy in stage I and II breast cancer: EORTC 10801 trial. J Natl Cancer Inst Monogr 1992; 11:15.

17. Bilchert-Toft M, Brincker H, Anderson J, et al. A Danish randomized trial comparing breast preserving therapy with mastectomy in mammary carcinoma. Acta Oncol 1988; 27:671.

18. Jacobson JA, Danforth DN, Cown KH, et al. Ten-year results of a comparison of conservation with mastectomy in the treatment of stage I and II breast cancer. N Engl J Med 1995; 332:907.

19. Arriagada R, Le MG, Rochard F, Contesso G, for the Institute Gustave Roussy Breast Cancer Group. Conservative treatment to mastectomy in early breast cancer: patterns of failure with 15 years of follow-up data. J Clin Oncol 1996; 14:1558.

20. Blichert-Toft M, Rose C, Andersen J, et al. Danish randomized trial comparing breast conservation therapy with mastectomy: six years of life-table analysis. J Natl Cancer Inst Monogr 1992; 11:19.

21. Tate P, McGee E, Hopkins S, et al. Breast conservation versus mastectomy patient preferences in a community practice in Kentucky. Surg Oncol 1993; 52:213.

22. Clark RM, McCulloch PB, Levine MN, et al. Randomized clinical trial to assess the effectiveness of breast irradiation following lumpectomy and axillary dissection for node-negative breast cancer. J Natl Cancer Inst 1992; 84:683.

23. Clark R, Whelan T, Levine M, et al. Randomized clinical trial of breast irradiation following lumpectomy and axillary dissection for node-negative breast cancer: an update. Ontario Clinical Oncology Group. J Natl Cancer Inst 1996; 88:1659.

24. Sector resection with or without postoperative radiotherapy for stage I breast cancer: a randomized trial. Uppsala–Orebro Breast Cancer Study Group. J Natl Cancer Inst 1990; 82:277.

25. Liljegren G, Holmberg L, Adami H-O, Westman G, Graffman S, Bergh J. Sector resection with or without postoperative radiotherapy for stage I breast cancer: five-year results of a randomized trial. J Natl Cancer Inst 1994; 86:717.

26. Veronesi U, Luini A, Del Vecchio M, et al. Radiotherapy after breast preserving surgery in women with localized cancer of the breast. N Engl J Med 1993; 328:1587.

27. Forrest AP, Stewart HJ, Everington D, et al. Randomised controlled trial of conservation therapy for breast cancer: 6-year analysis of the Scottish trial. Scottish Cancer Trials Breast Group. Lancet 1996; 348:708.

28. Renton SC, Gazet JC, Ford HT, Corbishley C, Sutcliffe R. The importance of the resection margin in conservative surgery for breast cancer. Eur J Surg Oncol 1996; 22:17.

29. Morrow M, Harris Jr, Schnitt SJ. Local control following breast conserving surgery for invasive cancer: results of clinical trials. J Natl Cancer Inst 1995; 87:1671.

30. Schnitt S, Hayman J, Gelman R, et al. A prospective study of conservative surgery alone in the treatment of selected patients with stage I breast cancer. Cancer 1997; 77:1094.

31. Sauer R, Tulusan A, Lang N, Dunst J. Can breast irradiation be omitted in low-risk breast cancer patients after segmentectomy? First results of the Erlangen protocol. Int J Radiat Oncol Biol Phys 1993; 27(Suppl.):146.

32. Holland R, Veling S, Mravunac M, et al. Histologic multifocality of Tis, T1-2 breast carcinomas: implications for clinical trials of breast conserving treatment. Cancer 1985; 45:979.

33. Holland R, Connolly J, Gelman R, et al. The presence of an extensive intraductal component (EIC) following a limited excision correlates with prominent residual disease in the remainder of the breast. J Clin Oncol 1990; 8:113–18.

34. Mariani L, Salvadori B, Marubini E, et al. Ten year results of a randomised trial comparing two conservative treatment strategies for small size breast cancer. Eur J Cancer 1998; 34:1156.

35. Veronesi U, Luini A, Galmberti V, et al. Conservation approaches for the management of stage I/II carcinoma of the breast. Milan Cancer Institute trials. World J Surg 1994; 18:70.

36. Harms SE, Flamig DP, Helsey KL, et al. MR imaging of the breast with rotating delivery of excitation of resonance: clinical experience with pathologic correlation. Radiology 1993; 187:493.

37. Orel SG, Schnall MD, Powell CM, et al. Staging of suspected breast cancer: effect of MR imaging and MR guided biopsy. Radiology 1995; 196:115.

38. Holland R, Hendriks J, Verbeek A, et al. Extent, distribution, and mammographic/histological correlations of breast ductal carcinoma in situ. Lancet 1990; 335:519.

39. Holland R, Hendriks J. Microcalcifications associated with ductal carcinoma in situ: mammographic–pathologic correlation. Semin Diagn Pathol 1994; 11:181.

40. Morrow M, Schmidt R, Hassett C. Patient selection for breast conservation therapy with magnification mammography. Surgery 1995; 118:621.

41. Van Dongen J, Bartelink H, Fentiman I, et al. Factors influencing local relapse and survival and results of salvage treatment after breast conserving therapy in operable breast cancer: EORTC trial 10801, breast conservation compared with mastectomy in TNM stage I and II breast cancer. Eur J Cancer 1992; 28A:801.

42. Anscher M, Jones P, Prosnitz L, et al. Local failure and margin status in early stage breast carcinoma treated with conservative surgery and radiation therapy. Ann Surg 1993; 218:22.

43. Schmidt-Ullrich R, Wazer D, DiPetrillo T, et al. Breast conservation therapy for early stage breast carcinoma with outstanding local control rates: a case for aggressive therapy to the tumor bearing quadrant. Int J Radiat Oncol Biol Phys 1993; 27:545.

44. Wazer DE, Schmidt-Ullrich R, Ruthazer R, et al. Factors determining outcome for breast-conserving irradiation with margin-directed dose escalation to the tumor bed. Int J Radiat Oncol Biol Phys 1998; 40:851.

45. Schnitt S, Abner A, Gelman R, et al. The relationship between microscopic margins of resection and the risk of local recurrence in breast cancer patients treated with conservative surgery and radiation therapy. Cancer 1994; 74:1746.

46. Solin L, Fowble B, Schultz D, et al. The significance of the pathology margins of the tumor excision on the outcome of patients treated with definitive irradiation for early stage breast cancer. Int J Radiat Oncol Biol Phys 1991; 21:279.

47. Schnitt S, Connolly J, Khettry U, et al. Pathologic findings on re-excision of the primary site in breast cancer patients considered for treatment by primary radiation therapy. Cancer 1987; 59:675.

48. Kearney T, Morrow M. Effect of re-excision on the success of breast conserving surgery. Ann Surg Oncol 1995; 2:303.

49. Gwin J, Eisenberg B, Hoffman J, et al. Incidence of gross and microscopic carcinoma in specimens from patients with breast cancer after re-excision lumpectomy. Ann Surg 1993; 218:729.

50. de la Rochefordiere A, Abner A, Silver B, et al. Are cosmetic results following conservative surgery and radiation therapy for early breast cancer dependent on technique? Int J Radiat Oncol Biol Phys 1992; 23:925.

51. Pezner R, Patterson M, Lipsett J, *et al.* Factors affecting cosmetic outcome in breast conserving treatment-objective quantitative assessment. Breast Cancer Res Treat 1991; 29:85.

52. Wazer D, DiPetrillo T, Schmidt-Ullrich R, *et al.* Factors influencing cosmetic outcome and complication risk after conservative surgery and radiotherapy for early stage breast carcinoma. J Clin Oncol 1992; 10:356.

53. Matory WJ, Mertheimer M, Fitzgerald T, *et al.* Aesthetic results following partial mastectomy and radiation therapy. Plast Reconstr Surg 1990; 85:739.

54. Clarke D, Martinez A, Cox R. Analysis of cosmetic results and complications in patients with stage 1 and 2 breast cancer treated by biopsy and irradiation. Int J Radiat Oncol Biol Phys 1983; 9:1807.

55. Gray J, McCormick B, Cox L, *et al.* Primary breast irradiation in large breasted or heavy women: analysis of cosmetic outcome. Int J Radiat Oncol Biol Phys 1991; 21:347.

56. Rose M, Olivotto I, Cady B, *et al.* The long term results of conservative surgery and radiation therapy for early breast cancer. Arch Surg 1989; 124:153.

57. Olivotto I, Rose M, Silver B, *et al.* Late cosmetic outcome after conservative surgery and radiotherapy: analysis of causes of cosmetic failure. Int J Radiat Oncol Biol Phys 1989; 17:747.

58. Abner A, Recht A, Vicini F, *et al.* Cosmetic results after conservative surgery, chemotherapy, and radiation therapy for early breast cancer. Int J Radiat Oncol Biol Phys 1991; 21:331.

59. Kurtz J, Amalric R, Brandone H, *et al.* Local recurrence after breast conserving surgery and radiotherapy: frequency, time course, and prognosis. Cancer 1989; 63:1912.

60. Abner A, Recht A, Eberlein T, *et al.* Prognosis following salvage mastectomy for recurrence in the breast after conservative surgery and radiation therapy for early stage breast cancer. J Clin Oncol 1993; 11:44.

61. Vicini F, Recht A, Abner A, *et al.* Recurrence in the breast following conservative surgery and radiation therapy for early stage breast cancer. J Natl Cancer Inst Monogr 1992; 11:33.

62. Healey E, Cook E, Orav E, *et al.* Contralateral breast cancer: clinical characteristics and impact on prognosis. J Clin Oncol 1993; 11:1545.

63. de la Rochefordiere A, Asselain B, Campana G, *et al.* Age as a prognostic factor in premenopausal breast carcinoma. Lancet 1993; 341:1039.

64. Kurtz J, Spitalier J, Amalric R, *et al.* Mammary recurrences in women younger than forty. Int J Radiat Oncol Biol Phys 1988; 15:271.

65. Matthews K, McNeese M, Montague E, *et al.* Prognostic implications of age in breast cancer patients treated with tumorectomy and irradiation or mastectomy. Int J Radiat Oncol Biol Phys 1988; 14:659.

66. Nixon A, Neuberg D, Hayes D, *et al.* Relationship of patient age to pathologic features of the tumor and prognosis for patients with stage 1 or 2 breast cancer. J Clin Oncol 1994; 12:888.

67. Kurtz JM. Factors influencing the risk of local recurrence in the breast. Eur J Cancer 1992; 28:660.

68. Chabner E, Nixon A, Gelman R, *et al.* Family history and treatment outcome in young women after breast-conserving surgery and radiation therapy for early-stage breast cancer. J Clin Oncol 1998; 16:2045.

69. Marcus J, Watson P, Page D, *et al.* Hereditary breast cancer. Pathology, prognosis, and *BRCA1* and *BRCA2* gene linkage. Cancer 1996; 77:697.

70. Eberlein T, Connolly J, Schnitt S, *et al.* Predictors of local recurrence following conservative breast surgery and radiation therapy: the influence of tumor size. Arch Surg 1990; 125:771.

71. Harris JR, Morrow M. Local management of invasive breast cancer. In Harris JR, Lippman ME, Morrow M, Hellman S, eds. *Diseases of the breast.* Lippincott-Raven, 1996, 487.

72. Borger J, Kemperman H, Hart A, *et al.* Risk factors in breast conservation therapy. J Clin Oncol 1994;12:653.

73. Rosen P, Saigo P, Braun D, *et al.* Predictors of recurrence in stage 1 (T1N0M0) breast cancer. Ann Surg 1991; 193:15.

74. Petit J, Le M, Mouriesse H, *et al.* Can breast reconstruction with gel-filled silicone implants increase the risk of death and second primary cancer in patients treated by mastectomy for breast cancer? Plast Reconstr Surg 1994; 94:115.

75. Webster D, Mansel R, Hughes L. Immediate reconstruction of the breast after mastectomy: is it safe? Cancer 1984; 53:1416.

76. Noone R, Frazier T, Noone G, *et al.* Recurrence of breast carcinoma following immediate reconstruction: a 13 year review. Plast Reconstr Surg 1994; 90:96.

77. Eberlein T, Crespo L, Smith B, *et al.* Prospective evaluation of immediate reconstruction after mastectomy. Ann Surg 1993; 218:29.

78. Van Nunen S, Gatenby P, Basten A. Post mammoplasty connective tissue disease. Arthritis Rheum 1982; 26:694.

79. Byron M, Venning V, Mowat A. Post mammoplasty human adjuvant disease. Br J Rheumatol 1985; 23:227.

80. Gabriel S, O'Fallon WM, Kurland LT, *et al.* Risk of connective tissue disease and other disorders after breast implantation. N Engl J Med 1995; 330:1697.

81. Schusterman M, Kroll SS, Reece GP, *et al.* Incidence of autoimmune disease in patients after breast reconstruction with silicone gel implants versus

autogenous tissue. A preliminary report. Ann Plast Surg 1993; 31:1.

82. Kroll S, Ames F, Singletary S, *et al*. The oncologic risks of skin preservation at mastectomy when combined with immediate reconstruction of the breast. Surg Gynecol Obstet 1992; 172:17.

83. Dao T, Nemoto T. The clinical significance of skin recurrence after radical mastectomy in women with cancer of the breast. Surg Gynecol Obstet 1963; 117:447.

84. Fisher B, Redmond C, Fisher E, *et al*. Ten year results of a randomized clinical trial comparing radical mastectomy and total mastectomy with or without irradiation. N Engl J Med 1985; 312:674.

85. Rosen P, Martin M, Kinne D, *et al*. Discontinuous or skip metastases in breast carcinoma: analysis of 1228 axillary dissections. Ann Surg 1983; 197:276.

86. Veronesi U, Rilke F, Luini A, *et al*. Distribution of axillary node metastases by level of invasion. Cancer 1987; 59:682.

87. Smith J, Gamex A JJ, Gallager H, *et al*. Carcinoma of the breast: analysis of total lymph node involvement versus level of metastasis. Cancer 1977; 39:527.

88. Danforth D, Findlay P, McDonald H, *et al*. Complete axillary lymph node dissection for stage I–II carcinoma of the breast. J Clin Oncol 1986; 4:655.

89. Chevinsky A, Ferrara J, James A, *et al*. Prospective evaluation of clinical and pathologic detection of axillary metastases in patients with carcinoma of the breast. Surgery 1990; 108:612.

90. Pigott J, Nichols R, Maddox W, *et al*. Metastases to the upper levels of the axillary nodes in carcinoma of the breast and its implications for nodal sampling procedure. Surg Gynecol Obstet 1984; 158:255.

91. Boova R, Bonanni R, Rosat F. Patterns of axillary nodal involvement in breast cancer. Ann Surg 1982; 196:642.

92. Kissin M, Thompson E, Price A, *et al*. The inadequacy of axillary sampling in breast cancer. Lancet 1982; 1:1210.

93. Steele R, Forrest A, Gibson T, *et al*. The efficacy of lower axillary sampling in obtaining lymph node status in breast cancer: a controlled randomized trial. Br J Surg 1985; 72:368.

94. Halverson K, Taylor M, Perez C, *et al*. Regional nodal management and patterns of failure following conservative surgery and radiation therapy for stage I and II breast cancer. Int J Radiat Oncol Biol Phys 1993; 26:593.

95. Recht A, Pierce S, Abner A, *et al*. Regional node failure after conservative surgery and radiotherapy for early stage breast carcinoma. J Clin Oncol 1991; 9:988.

96. Siegel B, Mayzel K, Love S. Level I and II axillary dissection in the treatment of early stage breast cancer. Arch Surg 1990; 125:1144.

97. Axelsson C, Mouridsen H, Zedeler K, *et al*. Axillary dissections of level I and II lymph nodes is important in breast cancer classification. Eur J Cancer 1992; 28A:1415.

98. Fowble B, Solin L, Schultz D, *et al*. Frequency, sites of relapse, and outcome of regional node failures following surgery and radiation for early breast cancer. Int J Radiat Oncol Biol Phys 1989; 17:703.

99. Wilson R, Donegan W, Mettlin C, *et al*. The 1982 national survey of carcinoma of the breast in the United States by the American College of Surgeons. Surg Gynecol Obstet 1984; 159:309.

100. Baker L. Breast Cancer Detection Demonstration Project: five year summary report. Cancer 1982; 32:194.

101. Carter C, Allen C, Henson D. Relation of tumor size, lymph node status and survival in 24,740 breast cancer cases. Cancer 1989; 63:181.

102. Brinkley D, Haybittle J. The curability of breast cancer. Lancet 1975; 2:95.

103. Fentiman I, Cuzick J, Millis R. Which patients are cured of breast cancer? BMJ 1984; 289:1108.

104. Adair F, Berg J, Joubert L, *et al*. Long term follow-up of breast cancer patients: the 30 year report. Cancer 1974; 33:1145.

105. Cabanes P, Salmon R, Vilcoq J, *et al*. Value of axillary dissection in addition to lumpectomy and radiotherapy in early breast cancer. Lancet 1992; 339:1245.

106. Arriagada R, Rutqvist LE, Mattson A, Kramar A, Rotstein S. Adequate locoregional treatment for early breast cancer may prevent secondary dissemination. J Clin Oncol 1995; 13:2869.

107. Morrow M. Postmastectomy radiation therapy: a surgical perspective. Semin Radiat Oncol 1999; 9:269.

108. Cabanas R. An approach for the treatment of penile carcinoma. Cancer 1977; 39:456.

109. Morton DC, Duan-Ren W, Wong JH, *et al*. Technical details of intraoperative lymphatic mapping and sentinel node biopsy in the management of primary melanoma. Arch Surg 1992; 127:392.

110. Guiliano AE, Kirgan DM, Guenther JM, Morton DL. Lymphatic mapping and sentinel lymphadenectomy for breast cancer. Ann Surg 1994; 220:391.

111. Guiliano AE, Jones RC, Brennan M, Statman R. Sentinel lymphadenectomy in breast cancer. J Clin Oncol 1997; 15:2345.

112. Cody HS, Hill ADK, Tran KN, *et al*. Credentialing for breast lymphatic mapping: how many cases are enough? Ann Surg 1999; 229:723.

113. Cody HS. Sentinel lymph node mapping in breast cancer. Oncology 1999; 13:25.

114. Morrow M, Rademaker AW, Bethke KP, *et al*. Learning sentinel node biopsy: results of a

prospective randomized trial of two techniques. Surgery 1999; 126:714.

115. Krag D, Weaver D, Ashikaga T, *et al.* The sentinel node in breast cancer: a multicenter validation study. N Engl J Med 1998; 339:941.

116. Veronesi U, Paganelli G, Viale G, *et al.* Sentinel lymph node biopsy and axillary dissection in breast cancer: results of a large series. J Natl Cancer Inst 1999; 91:368.

117. Veronesi U, Paganelli G, Galimberti V, *et al.* Sentinel-node biopsy to avoid axillary dissection in breast cancer with clinically negative lymph-nodes. Lancet 1997; 349:1864.

118. Krag DN, Weaver OJ, Alex JC, Fairbank JT. Surgical resection and radiolocalization of the sentinel node in breast cancer using a gamma probe. Surg Oncol 1993; 2:332.

119. Cox CE, Pendas S, Cox JM, *et al.* Guidelines for sentinel node biopsy and lymphatic mapping of patients with breast cancer. Ann Surg 1998; 227:645.

120. Bass SS, Cox CE, Ku NN, *et al.* The role of sentinel lymph node biopsy in breast cancer. J Am Coll Surg 1999; 189:183.

121. Albertini JJ, Lyman GH, Cox C, *et al.* Lymphatic mapping and sentinel node biopsy in the patient with breast cancer. JAMA 1996; 276:1818.

122. Cox CE, Haddad F, Cox JM, *et al.* Lymphatic mapping in the treatment of breast cancer. Oncology 1998; 12:1283.

123. Morton DL. Intraoperative lymphatic mapping and sentinel lymphadenectomy: community standard care or clinical investigation? Cancer J Sci Am 1997; 3:328.

124. Saphir O, Amromin GD. Obscure axillary lymph node metastases in carcinoma of the breast. Cancer 1949; 1:238.

125. Pickren JW. Significance of occult metastases. A study of breast cancer. Cancer 1961; 14:1266.

126. Fisher ER, Swamidoss S, Lee CH, *et al.* Detection and significance of occult axillary node metastases in patients with invasive breast cancer. Cancer 1978; 42:2025.

127. International (Ludwig) Breast Cancer Study Group. Prognostic importance of occult axillary lymph node micrometastases from breast cancer. Lancet 1990; 335:1565.

128. Clare SE, Sener SF, Wilkens W, *et al.* Prognostic significance of occult lymph node metastases in node-negative breast cancer. Ann Surg Oncol 1997; 4:447.

129. Lockett MA, Baron PL, O'Brien PH, *et al.* Detection of occult breast cancer micrometastases in axillary lymph nodes using a multimarker reverse transcriptase–polymerase chain reaction panel. J Am Coll Surg 1998; 187:9.

130. Mori M, Mimori K, Inoue M, *et al.* Detection of cancer micrometastases in lymph nodes by reverse transcriptase–polymerase chain reaction. Cancer Res 1995; 55:3417.

131. Siziopikou KP, Schnitt SJ, Connolly JL, Hayes DF. Detection and significance of occult axillary metastatic disease in breast cancer patients. Breast J 1999; 5:221.

132. Chu KU, Turner RR, Hansen NM, *et al.* Do all patients with sentinel node metastasis from breast cancer need complete axillary node dissection? Ann Surg 1999; 229:536.

133. American College of Radiology, American College of Surgeons, College of American Pathologists, and the Society of Surgical Oncology. Standards for diagnosis and management of invasive breast carcinomas. CA Cancer J Clin 1998; 48:83.

134. Robertson J, Clarke D, Pezner M, *et al.* Breast conservation therapy: severe fibrosis after radiation therapy in patients with collagen vascular disease. Cancer 1991; 68:502.

135. Fleck R, McNeese M, Ellerbroek N, *et al.* Consequences of breast irradiation in patients with pre-existing collagen vascular disease. Int J Radiat Oncol Biol Phys 1989; 17:829.

136. Ross J, Hussey D, Mayr N, *et al.* Acute and late reactions to radiation therapy in patients with collagen vascular disease. Cancer 1993; 71:3744.

137. Barreau-Pouhaer L, Le M, Rietjens M, *et al.* Risk factors for failure of immediate breast reconstruction with prostheses after total mastectomy for breast cancer. Cancer 1992; 70:1145.

138. Morrow M, Quiet C, Hellman S, *et al.* Treatment selection for breast cancer: are our biases correct? Proc Am Soc Clin Oncol 1994; 13:99.

139. Foster R, Farwell M, Costanza M. Breast conserving surgery for invasive breast cancer: patterns of care in a geographic region and estimation of potential applicability. Ann Surg Oncol 1995; 2:275.

140. Tarbox B, Rockwood J, Abernathy C. Are modified radical mastectomies done for T1 breast cancer because of surgeon's advice or patient's choice? Am J Surg 1992; 164:417.

141. Holmberg L, Omne-Ponte M, Burns T, *et al.* Psychosocial adjustment after mastectomy and breast conserving treatment. Cancer 1989; 64:969.

142. Wolberg W, Romsaas E, Tanner M, *et al.* Psychosexual adaptation to breast cancer surgery. Cancer 1989; 63:1645.

143. Baider L, Rizel S, Kaplan De-Nour A. Comparison of couples' adjustment to lumpectomy and mastectomy. Gen Hosp Psychiatry 1986; 8:251.

Commentary

JOHN A BUTLER

The surgical treatment of early stage I and stage II breast cancer has undergone considerable change in the last 25 years. Long-term data gathered from the pathologic staging of Halsted radical mastectomies allowed surgeons to challenge his theory of the orderly progression of breast cancer which provided the theoretical basis for the en bloc resection which he championed. Beginning in the late 1970s, a number of well-designed prospective, randomized trials demonstrated that overall survival was not reduced when lumpectomy and radiation therapy were substituted for mastectomy as the primary surgical procedure. Additional studies have refined the calculation of risk of recurrence associated with these lesser procedures, and the preponderance of evidence strongly suggests that minor variations in the local recurrence rate have no significant impact on overall survival. A second area of evolution in the management of early breast cancer which has taken place over the past decade concerns the management of the axilla. While adaptation of sentinel lymph node sampling will occur at a much more rapid pace than that observed for breast conservation therapy, long-term follow-up will be required to validate the use of this technique from the standpoint of its efficacy in determining the lymph node status of the patient, the risk of subsequent relapse in the axilla, and the validity of various management options in those patients with microscopic disease identified by multiple sectioning and/or immunohistochemical staining of the sentinel lymph node. With the increasing application of screening mammography and the development of other non-invasive techniques for the early detection of breast cancer, the answers to the clinical questions posed in the management of early breast cancer will become of increasing importance. The number of new breast cancers projected for the USA in the year 2001 is approximately 194 000, the median size of newly diagnosed breast cancers currently approaches 1.5 cm, and two-thirds to three-quarters of the patients will be diagnosed with node-negative disease.[1]

In this chapter, Dr Staradub and Dr Morrow provide an overview of the recent changes in the surgical management of stage I and II breast cancer as well as the outcome data for the various surgical procedures employed which led to these changes. The six prospective randomized trials, designed to answer the question of whether breast conservation therapy would achieve results similar to those of mastectomy, were remarkable in the consistency of the data supporting the equivalency of these treatment options, despite rather wide variations in patient eligibility, extent of surgery, and radiation treatment techniques. On the basis of these results, the 1992

National Institutes of Health Consensus Development Conference stated that breast conservation treatment was preferable in women with stage I and II breast cancer 'because it provides survival equivalent to total mastectomy and axillary dissection while preserving the breast.'[2]

It is important to realize that the most important factor in making that recommendation was the equivalent survival provided by both techniques despite some variation in local recurrence rates. The largest of the six trials, NSABP Trial B06, included a third treatment arm, which involved lumpectomy and axillary dissection without radiation therapy. All patients with tumors less than or equal to 4 cm in size were considered eligible for this trial. With an average follow-up of 144 months, the lumpectomy-alone group had a 35% local recurrence rate, in comparison to a 10% recurrence rate for the lumpectomy and radiation therapy group.[3] The most provocative finding of this trial was that, despite this major discrepancy in local recurrence, there was no difference in overall survival between these two groups. While a 35% recurrence rate would argue for the necessity of radiation therapy, the more important point is that this high incidence of local recurrence had no adverse impact on survival.

A major factor for patients who choose mastectomy over breast conservation therapy involves the fear and/or time constraints required for a 6-week course of radiation therapy. The B06 data cited above suggest the possibility that radiation therapy could be omitted in a highly select group of patients with early breast cancer.

Five additional randomized studies comparing conservative surgery with and without radiation therapy all demonstrated no difference in overall survival, despite a local recurrence rate as high as 35% (NSABP) in those patients treated with surgery alone. The authors cite two prospective single-arm studies in which conservative surgery alone was employed in patients with small tumors, negative margins, and favorable prognostic factors such as lack of lymphatic vessel invasion or extensive intraductal component in the cancer. With a median follow-up of 5 years, the recurrence rates in the two studies were 9.5% and 16%, respectively.[4,5] Similar to the experience with local recurrence following mastectomy, where the majority of events occurred in the first 3–5 years following surgery, these numbers should reflect the vast majority of all expected recurrences in the absence of radiation therapy. Although the recurrence rate for a similar group of patients treated with radiation therapy would be expected to be quite low (less than 5%), it must be remembered that a local recurrence of 10–15% had been felt to be quite acceptable for the initial trials of mastectomy versus lumpectomy and radiation therapy, provided that local recurrence did not negatively impact survival. The ability to salvage patients with local recurrence with a re-excision and radiation therapy has also been questioned on the basis of prior studies which show that less than 50% of patients with recurrence actually are treated with something less than mastectomy. Those numbers, however, come from trials in which patients with tumors up to 5 cm in size were initially included and also reflect the hesitancy on the part of patients confronted with recurrence to have a second limited resection. As the median size of newly diagnosed breast cancers approaches 1.5 cm, the extent of the initial lumpectomy should make re-excision a viable option in an increasing proportion of patients, particularly in light of the fact that radiation therapy would be employed in the majority of these cases to prevent a subsequent recurrence. For patients with estrogen and progesterone receptor-positive tumors who choose lumpectomy without radiation therapy as the initial treatment of their breast cancer, the addition of tamoxifen should substantially reduce the risk of local recurrence by approximately 50%, although this has not been rigorously tested in trials to date.

Another alternative to lumpectomy and radiation as is currently practiced would be to restrict the radiation field to the area immediately surrounding the lumpectomy site. The study by Holland of mastectomy specimens from T1–T2 breast carcinomas, which documented the presence of tumor foci separate from the primary lesion in 63% of the patients, also showed that less than 10% of tumors will have multifocal disease beyond 3–4 cm from the primary lesion.[6] Imaging techniques such as magnetic resonance imaging and magnification mammography, as suggested by the authors, may be helpful in identifying that percentage of patients who would be at risk for local recurrence with radiation therapy targeted only to the lumpectomy site. Radiation therapy to the remainder of the breast is not effective in preventing the development of new primaries as the risk of recurrence in the other quadrants of the treated breast is very similar to that of developing a contralateral breast carcinoma.

There are several potential advantages to a reduced field of radiation therapy. The possibility of alterations in the treatment fractions and/or the use of brachytherapy techniques could shorten the time period for which radiation therapy would have to be administered. Restriction of radiation fields to the lumpectomy site should obviate the risk of excess mortality associated with radiation which continues to be a source of considerable controversy.[7] Its effect on cosmesis, however, particularly in the case of using increased fractions, would require careful evaluation.

The chapter section on local recurrence is a cogent analysis of the available data by the authors. Whereas margin status and its effect on local recurrence have received enormous attention with respect to ductal carcinoma *in situ*, this also remains an area of controversy in the treatment of infiltrating disease, particularly with respect to what constitutes an adequate lumpectomy. It would seem surprising that tumor size and axillary status would not have an effect on breast recurrence, but this does reflect the findings of Holland, who showed that the presence of multifocal disease is not influenced by the size of the primary lesion. The authors also make the point that pathologic features such as lobular histology and an extensive intraductal component to the tumor are also not predictors of increased risk of recurrence. It is critical to realize, however, that this is only true when taken in the context of final margin status. As the authors point out, these two pathologic entities usually require more extensive lumpectomy to achieve a negative margin status. The majority of these patients, nevertheless, are candidates for breast conservation therapy. Even in the case of an initial positive margin, re-excision should be offered with the expectation that negative margins can be achieved in these patients. The impact of factors such as young age at diagnosis, inherited breast cancer, and pathologic characteristics such as lympho/vascular invasion require additional study in terms of their impact on local recurrence rates and suitability for conservation therapy. At the present time, however, tumor size in relation to the size of the breast is the primary determinant of the applicability of breast conservation therapy.

A final area that requires further clarification concerns the impact of a boost dose of radiation to the lumpectomy site and its subsequent influence on local recurrence. Whereas a boost dose to the tumor bed does not appear to reduce the risk of recurrence in patients with clear margins, data from Joint Center for Radiation Therapy in Boston would indicate that focally positive margins, defined as tumor at the margin in three or fewer low-power fields, have a low (6%) incidence of local recurrence at 5 years when treated with a radiation dose of 60 Gy or greater to the surgical site.[8]

The aspect of the surgical management of early-stage breast cancer that has undergone the most recent and rapid changes concerns the identification and treatment of axillary disease. Clinical assessment of axillary disease is inaccurate in approximately 30% of cases, evenly distributed between false positives and false negatives. In the past, the risks associated with the significant morbidity of axillary dissection were felt to be outweighed by the benefits of local control of axillary disease, identification of patients at high risk for subsequent relapse, and a possible survival benefit given that 20–30% of patients with axillary metastasis are long-term survivors following surgical procedures which include removal of the axillary disease.

As is noted by the authors, the results of the NSABP B04 Protocol provided the initial data that challenged the theory that axillary dissection had a significant impact on survival.[9] For patients with clinically node-negative disease, no differences in survival were noted between those treated by radical mastectomy, total mastectomy with axillary observation, or total mastectomy plus radiation therapy to the regional lymphatics. Another study from England involving an even larger number of patients compared total mastectomy with or without radiation therapy to the axilla.[10] This study also showed no adverse impact on survival if axillary treatment was restricted to those who subsequently developed evidence of clinical disease. However, there are several trials that do demonstrate an impact on survival associated with immediate axillary treatment,[11,12] but, overall, these trials involve smaller numbers of patients and improved survival due, at least in part, to the additional therapy given to the patient with clinically negative but histologically positive lymph nodes. Whereas the majority of the evidence argues against an improvement in survival associated with axillary dissection, the authors correctly point out that no study has sufficient power to rule out the possibility of a small survival advantage.

Whereas axillary lymph node dissection is a highly effective means of attaining local control in patients with positive lymph nodes, the salient factor in the current management of early breast cancer is that anywhere from 65% to 75% of newly diagnosed breast cancers in the USA now present with node-negative disease. Sentinel lymph node biopsy is a technique that, in the hands of experienced surgeons, can provide accurate staging of the axilla in more than 95% of cases.[13] Although the absolute risk of local recurrence is unknown at the present time, extrapolation of the more mature melanoma data would suggest that it will be no more than 3% or 4%. This compares favorably with results achieved by radiation therapy as the primary treatment of the axilla and is just slightly higher than an expected 1–2% recurrence rate associated with surgical treatment of the axilla. The more important question is whether an erroneous downstaging on the basis of a false-negative sentinel node biopsy would deny that patient the benefits of adjuvant therapy. The argument most often used for abandoning axillary dissection, that the vast majority of patients will be treated with adjuvant therapy anyway, can successfully be used to negate this risk. The only patients who would be negatively impacted would be those with receptor-negative tumors that are less than 1 cm in size, where tamoxifen would be ineffective and the risk of relapse too small to justify the application of adjuvant chemotherapy. The combination of the low false-negative rate associated with sentinel node sampling and the restricted subset of patients who would be at risk of being undertreated strongly argues for the routine utilization of sentinel node biopsy in the staging of patients with early breast cancer.

There are many variations in the technique of lymphatic mapping, ranging from the site of injection to the tracing materials used. As is common with many surgeons, the authors reserve the use of radiolabeled colloid for patients with medially placed lesions or a large amount of axillary adipose tissue. Although the routine use of radiolabeled colloid with lymphoscintigraphy does add some complexity to the scheduling of surgery, it does have some significant advantages. On multiple occasions, a blue node with appropriately stained afferent lymphatics was found early in the course of an axillary exploration. It was only the finding of a second hotspot on preoperative lymphoscintigraphy that dictated further dissection to retrieve a second sentinel lymph node which, on these occasions, was both blue and hot. In all cases, the pathology was congruent in both specimens, but these instances do raise the possibility of a false-negative result associated with the use of blue dye alone. This would be particularly relevant in patients who had a prior excisional biopsy, for whom the primary lymphatic drainage may be in question due to the relatively large area encompassed by the biopsy cavity.

The authors raise the question of both the clinical significance of micrometastatic disease identified in the sentinel lymph node and the necessity of further axillary dissection in patients who have a positive sentinel node biopsy. As they state, these questions will be answered in the course of clinical trials which are already underway. Outside of these trials, however, an axillary dissection should be considered the standard of care for those with a histologically positive sentinel lymph node. For patients with a sentinel node demonstrating micrometastatic disease, a limited level 1 dissection or close follow-up would be appropriate alternatives.

Dr Staradub and Dr Morrow end the chapter by stating that there is no therapy that is 'right' for all women, and that the role of the surgeon has changed from deciding the best treatment option to providing the patient with access to the information necessary for her to make a choice appropriate for her needs. This could not be better stated. While one could argue that we were initially slow to change, over the past 25 years surgeons have been in the forefront of modifying their operative approach to reflect both the evolving understanding of how breast cancer spreads and the improvements in stage of diagnosis associated with screening techniques. As these trends continue, a similar evolution will be required in the field of medical oncology from the standpoint of shifting the focus of adjuvant therapy toward identifying the increasing number of patients who require no additional therapy following their surgical procedure. For surgeons, however, the next decade will bring a shift in focus from the en-bloc lumpectomy excision, which is currently practiced, to newer methods of ablating the tumor *in situ* through a percutaneous approach, utilizing rapidly evolving technologies such as cryosurgery, radiofrequency ablation, and laser photocoagulation.[14–16]

REFERENCES

1. Smith B. Approaches to breast-cancer staging. N Engl J Med 2000; 342:580.

2. National Institute of Health Consensus Development Conference. Consensus statement: treatment of early-stage breast cancer. J Natl Cancer Inst Monogr 1992; 11:105.

3. Fisher B, Anderson S, Redmond CK, *et al.* Re-analysis and results after 12 years of follow-up in a randomized clinical trial comparing total mastectomy with lumpectomy with or without irradiation in the treatment of breast cancer. N Engl J Med 1999; 333:1456.

4. Schnitt S, Hayman J, Gelman R, *et al.* A prospective study of conservative surgery alone in the treatment of selected patients with stage 1 breast cancer. Cancer 1997; 77:1094.

5. Sauer R, Tulusan A, Lang N, Dunst J. Can breast irradiation be omitted in low-risk breast cancer patients after segmentectomy? First results of the Erlangen protocol. Int J Radiat Oncol Biol Phys 1993; 27(Suppl.):146.

6. Holland R, Veling S, Mravunac M, *et al.* Histologic multifocality of Tis, T1–2 breast carcinomas: implications for clinical trials of breast conserving treatment. Cancer 1985; 45:979.

7. Early Breast Cancer Trialists' Collaborative Group. Favourable and unfavourable effects on long-term survival of radiotherapy for early breast cancer: an overview of the randomized trials. Lancet 2000; 355:1757.

8. Abner A, Gelman R, Connolly J, *et al.* The relationship between microscopic margins of resection and the risk of local recurrence in patients with breast cancer treated with breast-conserving surgery and radiation therapy. Cancer 1994; 74:1746.

9. Fisher B, Redmond C, Fisher E, *et al.* Ten year results of a randomized clinical trial comparing radical mastectomy and total mastectomy with or without irradiation. N Engl J Med 1985; 312:674.

10. CRC Working Party (King's/Cambridge) trial for early breast cancer. A detailed update at the tenth year. Lancet 1980; 2:55.

11. Hayward J. The surgeon's role in primary breast cancer. Breast Cancer Res Treat 1981; 1:27.

12. White RE, Vezeridis MP, Konstadoulakis M, *et al.* Therapeutic options and results for the management of minimally invasive carcinoma of the breast: influence of axillary dissection for treatment of T1a and T1b lesions. JACS 1996; 183:575.

13. Cody H. Sentinel lymph node mapping in breast cancer. Oncology 1999; 13:25.

14. Jeffrey S, Birdwell R, Ikeda D, *et al.* Radiofrequency ablation of breast cancer. Arch Surg 1999; 134:1064.

15. Staren ED, Sabel M, Gianakakis LM, *et al.* Cryosurgery of breast cancer. Arch Surg 1997; 132:28.

16. Mumtaz H, Hall-Craggs MA, Wotherspoon A, *et al.* Laser therapy for breast cancer: MR imaging and histopathologic correlation. Radiology 1996; 200:651.

Editors' selected abstracts

The relation between the presence and extent of lobular carcinoma in situ and the risk of local recurrence for patients with infiltrating carcinoma of the breast treated with conservative surgery and radiation therapy.

Abner AL, Connolly JL, Recht A, Bornstein B, Nixon A, Hetelekidis S, Silver B, Harris JR, Schnitt SJ.

Joint Center for Radiation Therapy, Harvard Medical School, Boston, MA, USA.

Cancer 88(5):1072–7, 2000, March 1.

Background: When found in an otherwise benign biopsy, lobular carcinoma in situ (LCIS) has been associated with an increased risk of development of a subsequent invasive breast carcinoma. However, the association between LCIS and the risk of subsequent local recurrence in patients with infiltrating carcinoma treated with conservative surgery and radiation therapy has received relatively little attention. *Methods:* Between 1968 and 1986, 1625 patients with clinical Stage I–II invasive breast carcinoma were treated at the Joint Center for Radiation Therapy at Harvard Medical School with breast-conserving surgery (CS) and radiation therapy (RT) to a total dose to the primary site of ⩾ 60 grays. Analysis was limited to 1181 patients with infiltrating ductal carcinoma, infiltrating lobular carcinoma, or infiltrating carcinoma with mixed ductal and lobular features who, on review of their histologic slides, had sufficient normal tissue adjacent to the tumor to evaluate for the presence of LCIS and also had a minimum potential follow-up time of 8 years. The median follow-up time was 161 months. *Results:* One hundred thirty-seven patients (12%) had LCIS either within the tumor or in the macroscopically normal adjacent tissue. The 8-year crude risk of recurrence was not significantly increased for patients with LCIS associated with invasive ductal, invasive lobular, or mixed ductal and lobular carcinoma. Among the 119 patients with associated LCIS adjacent to the tumor, the 8-year rate of local recurrence was 13%, compared with 12% for the 1062 patients without associated LCIS. For the 70 patients with moderate or marked LCIS adjacent to the tumor, the 8-year rate of local recurrence was 13%. The extent of LCIS did not affect the risk of recurrence. The risks of contralateral disease and of distant failure were similarly not affected by the presence or extent of LCIS. *Conclusions:* Breast-conserving therapy involving limited surgery and radiation therapy is an appropriate method of treating patients with invasive breast carcinoma with or without associated LCIS. Neither the presence nor the extent of LCIS should influence management decisions regarding patients with invasive breast carcinoma. [See editorial counterpoint and reply to counterpoint on pages 978–81 and 982–3, this issue.]

Saline-enhanced radiofrequency ablation of breast tissue: an in vitro feasibility study.

Bohm T, Hilger I, Muller W, Reichenbach JR, Fleck M, Kaiser WA.

Institut fur Diagnostische und Interventionelle Radiologie, Friedrich-Schiller-Universitat, Jena, Germany.

Investigative Radiology 35(3):149–57, 2000, March.

Rationale and objectives: The feasibility of radiofrequency (RF) ablation for the treatment of breast tumors was investigated in vitro. The best parameters for ablation of breast tissue were chosen. *Methods:* Saline-enhanced RF ablation was performed in human breast tissue specimens and cow udder tissue. Temperature profiles were measured depending on RF power (20, 28, 36 W) and NaCl infusion rate (15, 30, 60 mL/h) using eight thermocouples. Lesion development was monitored by ultrasound. Thermolysis efficiency was measured by tissue weight determinations before and after ablation. *Results:* After RF ablation of tissue samples, 73.6% turned into a fat/saline emulsion. Ultrasound monitoring showed a cone-shaped hyperechoic area during the first 2 minutes of RF ablation, followed by an irregular expansion of the area. Time-dependent spatial temperature curves were more homogeneous at low infusion rates (15 mL/h). Peak temperatures up to 160 °C were measured. *Conclusions:* Controlled RF ablation of breast tissue is feasible. The irregular expansion of RF lesions in fatty breast tissue is due to liquefied fat. Low saline interstitial infusion rates result in better control of lesioning.

Breast reconstruction by tissue expansion. A retrospective technical review of 197 two-stage delayed reconstructions following mastectomy for malignant breast disease in 189 patients.

Collis N, Sharpe DT.

Department of Plastic Surgery, Bradford Royal Infirmary, Bradford, West Yorkshire, UK.

British Journal of Plastic Surgery 53(1):37–41, 2000, January.

Despite the advent of free tissue transfer, breast reconstruction by tissue expansion is an important technique in the armamentarium of the reconstructive breast surgeon. The concept is deceptively simple and yet in reality can produce difficult complications and poor results. A database was compiled of all the patients receiving tissue expanders and/or implants for cosmetic, congenital and reconstructive purposes between 1986 and 1998. 189 patients had 197 delayed two-stage tissue expansion breast reconstructions following mastectomies for malignant breast disease between 1986 and 1997. 103 breasts (52%) had two uncomplicated stages. The remainder had one or more complications, revisional procedures for complications or alterations to the reconstruction for size, position or shape. Overall each breast reconstruction required 2.9 procedures (range 2–9). The complications and additional procedures are discussed. In particular, capsular contracture of the definitive implant (12%) was related to implant type and not to the speed of tissue expansion or the degree or duration of overexpansion. Although 17% of patients received radiotherapy,

none of those who developed contracture around the definitive implant had this adjuvant therapy, $p < 0.05$. Twelve reconstructions (6%) totally failed due to complications of which six underwent secondary flap reconstruction. Twenty-one patients have subsequently developed metastatic disease of which 15 have died to date. Breast reconstruction by tissue expansion is still an important technique. It should be used carefully and thoughtfully by surgeons trained to deal with any complications. Patients need to be carefully selected and counselled prior to undertaking this process.

Adjuvant radiation after modified radical mastectomy for breast cancer fails to prolong survival.

Geisler DP, Boyle MJ, Malnar KF, Melichar RM, McGee JM, Nolen MG, Broughan TA.

Department of Surgery, University of Oklahoma Health Sciences Center–Tulsa, OK, USA.

American Surgeon 66(5):452–8; discussion 458–9, 2000, May.

Recent literature has reported improved local disease control and overall survival in premenopausal node-positive (stage II and III) breast cancer patients undergoing modified radical mastectomy (MRM) using radiation therapy (RT) combined with chemotherapy. To assess the efficacy of postoperative RT in our own community, we analyzed all patients undergoing MRM for carcinoma utilizing an extensive database from the three major teaching hospitals in Tulsa, OK, between 1965 and 1993. A total of 5257 patients underwent MRM during this time period. One hundred thirty-seven patients were excluded for insufficient data or because they were found to be at stage IV, leaving a total study population of 5125. Overall survival (OS), overall mean survival (MS), disease-free survival (DFS), and locoregional DFS (LRDFS) were analyzed for all patients and were further analyzed according to stage, lymph node involvement, and menopausal status. Median follow-up was 103 months. Statistical analysis was performed using Kaplan–Meier and t-tests. The DFS at 10 years was 65 per cent in the RT group and 80 per cent in the patients who did not receive RT ($p = 0.00$). No improved DFS was obtained in the radiation-treated patients, regardless of stage, lymph node involvement, or menopausal status. Similarly, the LRDFS at 10 years was 91 per cent in the RT group and 96 per cent in the patients who did not receive RT ($p = 0.00$). No improved LRDFS was obtained in the radiation-treated patients, regardless of stage, lymph node involvement, or menopausal status. The overall MS was 97 months in the RT group and 104 months in the patients who did not receive RT ($p = 0.00$). Comparisons of overall MS rates revealed apparent survival benefits from RT in the premenopausal node-negative group, postmenopausal one to four-positive-node group, and all stage I patients. This apparent survival advantage was not confirmed by Kaplan–Meier curves of OS. No other overall MS differences were detected according to stage, lymph node, or menopausal status. Using Kaplan–Meier survival curves, the OS in the RT group at 10 years was 46 per cent, and 63 per cent in the patients who did not receive RT ($p = 0.00$). No improved OS was obtained in the radiation-treated patients, regardless of stage, lymph node involvement, or menopausal status. These findings from a large breast cancer database failed to demonstrate any meaningful benefit from RT after MRM and serve to further question the efficacy of this treatment modality in post-mastectomy breast cancer patients.

Antibiotic prophylaxis for post-operative wound infection in clean elective breast surgery.

Gupta R, Sinnett D, Carpenter R, Preece PE, Royle GT.

Department of Surgery, Royal South Hants Hospital, Southampton, UK.

European Journal of Surgical Oncology 26(4):363–6, 2000, June.

Antibiotic prophylaxis has been used to good effect in the prevention of post-operative wound infections in patients undergoing gastrointestinal operations. We have assessed the use of a single dose of intravenous antibiotic (Augmentin 1.2 g), given with induction of anaesthesia as prophylaxis, against post-operative wound infection in women undergoing clean, elective breast surgery. Three hundred and thirty-four patients were recruited. Of the 164 receiving antibiotic prophylaxis 29 (17.7%) had wound infections compared with 32 (18.8%) in the placebo group ($p = 0.79$). There were no significant differences in any other post-operative infective complications. Antibiotic prophylaxis is probably not required in clean, elective breast surgery.

Relationship between tumor location and relapse in 6,781 women with early invasive breast cancer.

Lohrisch C, Jackson J, Jones A, Mates D, Olivotto IA.

Breast Cancer Outcomes Unit and Systemic and Radiation Therapy Programs of the British Columbia Cancer Agency, and Fraser Valley Cancer Centers and the Faculty of Medicine, University of British Columbia, Vancouver, Canada.

Journal of Clinical Oncology 18(15):2828–35, 2000, August.

Purpose: To explore the independent prognostic impact of medial hemisphere tumor location in early breast cancer. Patients and methods: A comprehensive database was used to review patients referred to the British Columbia Cancer Agency from 1989 to 1995 with early breast cancer. Patients were grouped according to relapse risk (high or nonhigh) and adjuvant systemic therapy received. Multiple regression analysis was used to determine whether the significance of primary tumor location (medial v lateral hemisphere) was independent of known prognostic factors and treatment. Results: In the adjuvant systemic therapy groups, medial location was associated with a 50% excess risk of systemic relapse and breast cancer death compared with lateral location. Five-year systemic disease-free survival rates were 66.3% and 74.2% for high-risk medial and lateral lesions, respectively ($p < 0.005$). Corresponding 5-year disease-specific survival rates were 75.7% and 80.8%, respectively ($p < 0.03$). No significant differences were observed between medial and lateral location for low-risk disease regardless of adjuvant therapy or for high-risk disease with no adjuvant therapy. Local recurrence rates were similar for all risk and therapy groups. Conclusion: The two-fold risk of relapse and breast cancer death associated with

high-risk medial breast tumors may be due to occult spread to internal mammary nodes (IMNs). Enhanced local control, such as with irradiation of the IMN chain, may be one way to reduce the excess risk. Ongoing randomized controlled trials may provide prospective answers to the question of the optimal volume of radiotherapy.

Development of stereotactically guided laser interstitial thermotherapy of breast cancer: in situ measurement and analysis of the temperature field in ex vivo and in vivo adipose tissue.

Milne PJ, Parel JM, Manns F, Denham DB, Gonzalez-Cirre X, Robinson DS.

Ophthalmic Biophysics Center, Bascom Palmer Eye Institute, University of Miami School of Medicine, Miami, FL, USA.

Lasers in Surgery & Medicine 26(1):67–75, 2000.

Background and objective: The size (0.5–1.0 cm) of early nonpalpable breast tumors currently detected by mammography and confirmed by stereotactic core biopsy is of the order of the penetration depth of near infrared photons in breast tissue. In principle, stereotactically biopsied tumors, therefore, could be safely and efficiently treated with laser thermotherapy. The aim of the current study is to confirm the controlled heating produced by clinically relevant power levels delivered with an interstitial laser fiber optic probe adapted for use with stereotactic mammography and biopsy procedures. Study design/materials and methods: Temperature increases and the resultant thermal field produced by the irradiation of ex vivo (porcine and human) and in vivo (porcine) tissue models appropriate to the treatment of human breast tissue by using cw Nd:YAG laser radiation delivered with a interstitial fiber optic probe with a quartz diffusing tip, were recorded with an array of fifteen 23-gauge needle thermocouple probes connected to a laboratory computer-based data acquisition system. Results: By using a stepwise decreasing power cycle to avoid tissue charring, acceptably symmetric thermal fields of repeatable volumetric dimensions were obtained. Reproducible thermal gradients and predictable tissue necrosis without carbonization could be induced in a 3-cm-diameter region around the fiber probe during a single treatment lasting only 3 minutes. The time-dependences of the temperature rise of the thermocouples surrounding the LITT probe were quantitatively modeled with simple linear functions during the applied laser heating cycles. Conclusion: Analysis of our experimental results show that reproducible, symmetric and predictable volumetric temperature increases in time can be reliably produced by interstitial laser thermotherapy.

MR imaging-guided sonography followed by fine-needle aspiration cytology in occult carcinoma of the breast.

Obdeijn IM, Brouwers-Kuyper EM, Tilanus-Linthorst MM, Wiggers T, Oudkerk M.

Department of Radiology, Dr Daniel den Hoed Cancer Center, University Hospital Rotterdam, The Netherlands.

American Journal of Roentgenology 174(4):1079–84, 2000, April.

Objective: In patients with axillary metastases as clinical evidence of possible occult breast cancer, a combined approach of MR imaging, sonography, and aspiration biopsy cytology was evaluated. *Subjects and methods:* Thirty-one women with metastatic adenocarcinoma in their axillary lymph nodes originating from an unknown primary site underwent MR imaging of the breast because physical examination and mammography findings were normal. Twenty of the 31 women had no history of malignancy, 10 had been previously treated for contralateral breast cancer, and one patient had nodal metastases in the contralateral axilla at the time breast cancer was detected. When a contrast-enhancing lesion was revealed on MR imaging of the breast, sonography and fine-needle aspiration cytology were also performed. *Results:* MR imaging revealed the primary breast cancer in eight (40%) of the 20 patients without a history of malignancy. MR imaging of the breast revealed a second primary cancer in three (27%) of the 11 patients with previous or simultaneous breast cancer. All lesions were identified with sonography and verified by cytology and histology. *Conclusion:* In women with axillary lymph node metastases from adenocarcinoma, MR imaging of the breast should be added to clinical examination and mammography before defining the breast cancer as occult. The combined approach of MR imaging, sonography, and aspiration fine-needle cytology is a good alternative to the MR imaging-guided biopsy.

Second malignancies after treatment of early-stage breast cancer: lumpectomy and radiation therapy versus mastectomy.

Obedian E, Fischer DB, Haffty BG.

Department of Therapeutic Radiology, Yale University School of Medicine, New Haven, CT, USA.

Journal of Clinical Oncology 18(12):2406–12, 2000, June.

Purpose: To determine the risk of second malignancies after lumpectomy and radiation therapy (LRT), and to compare it with that in a similar cohort of early-stage breast cancer patients undergoing mastectomy without radiation (MAST). *Patients and methods:* Between January 1970 and December 1990, 1,029 breast cancer patients at our institution underwent LRT. A cohort of 1,387 breast cancer patients who underwent surgical treatment by mastectomy (MAST), and who did not receive postoperative radiation during the same time period, served as a comparison group. Second malignancies were categorized as contralateral breast versus nonbreast. In the cohort of patients undergoing LRT, a detailed analysis was carried out with respect to age, disease stage, smoking history, radiation therapy technique, dose, the use of chemotherapy or hormone therapy, and other clinical and/or pathologic characteristics. *Results:* As of March 1999, the median follow-up was 14.6 years for the LRT group and 16 years for the MAST group. The 15-year risk of any second malignancy was nearly identical for both cohorts (17.5% v 19%, respectively). The second breast malignancy rate at 15 years was 10% for both the MAST and LRT groups. The 15-year risk of a second nonbreast malignancy was 11% for the LRT and 10% for the MAST group. In the subset of patients 45 years

of age or younger at the time of treatment, the second breast and nonbreast malignancy rates at 15 years were 10% and 5% for patients undergoing LRT versus 7% and 4% for patients undergoing mastectomy (*p*, not statistically significant). In the detailed analysis of LRT patients, second lung malignancies were associated with a history of tobacco use. There were fewer contralateral breast tumors in patients undergoing adjuvant hormone therapy, although this did not reach statistical significance. The adjuvant use of chemotherapy did not significantly affect the risk of second malignancies. *Conclusion:* There seems to be no increased risk of second malignancies in patients undergoing LRT using modern techniques, compared with MAST. Continued monitoring of these patient cohorts will be required in order to document that these findings are maintained with even longer follow-up periods. With nearly 15 years median follow-up periods, however, these data should be reassuring to women who are considering LRT as a treatment option.

Breast conserving therapy in breast cancer patients presenting with nipple discharge.

Obedian E, Haffty BG.

Department of Therapeutic Radiology, Yale University School of Medicine, New Haven, CT, USA.

International Journal of Radiation Oncology, Biology, Physics 47:137–42, 2000, April 1.

Purpose: To retrospectively review the outcome of conservatively treated breast cancer patients who present with nipple discharge at initial diagnosis. *Methods and materials:* The charts of 1097 patients undergoing conservative surgery and radiation therapy between January 1970 and December 1990 were reviewed. All patient data, including clinical, pathologic, treatment, and outcome variables were entered onto a computerized database. For the current study, specific attention was directed to the initial presenting symptoms and patients were divided into two groups: those presenting at initial diagnosis with nipple discharge (D/C–YES, *n* = 17), and those presenting without nipple discharge (D/C–NO, *n* = 1080). *Results:* As of August 1998, with a median follow-up of 12 years, the 10-year actuarial survival, distant metastasis-free survival, and breast relapse-free survival rates for the overall population were 73%, 78%, and 83%, respectively. Although the D/C–YES and D/C–NO groups were well balanced with respect to the majority of clinical factors, the D/C–YES patients had a higher percentage of DCIS histology (7.3% vs 1.2%, *p* < 0.01), were less likely to undergo reexcision (12% vs 35%), and were more frequently under age 40 (35% vs 12%) than the D/C–NO patients. Over the time span of this study, status of the final surgical margin was indeterminate in the majority of cases. Local relapses occurred in 6 of the 17 patients in the D/C–YES group, resulting in a 10-year actuarial breast relapse-free survival rate of 50%, which was significantly lower than the 10-year breast relapse-free survival rate of 86% in the D/C–NO population. Among the patients presenting with nipple discharge, those with sacrifice of the nipple areolar complex had a lower local relapse rate than those patients who had conservation of the nipple areolar complex (20% vs 42%), although this difference did not reach statistical significance. *Conclusions:* Although patients presenting with nipple discharge may be suitable candidates for radiation therapy, local relapse rates were higher than those presenting without nipple discharge. The limitations of the study and implications regarding breast conserving management in patients presenting with nipple discharge are discussed.

The influence of infiltrating lobular carcinoma on the outcome of patients treated with breast-conserving surgery and radiation therapy.

Peiro G, Bornstein BA, Connolly JL, Gelman R, Hetelekidis S, Nixon AJ, Recht A, Silver B, Harris JR, Schnitt SJ.

Department of Pathology, Beth Israel Deaconess Medical Center and Harvard Medical School, Boston, MA, USA.

Breast Cancer Research & Treatment 59(1):49–54, 2000, January.

Background: The role of conservative surgery and radiation therapy (CS and RT) in the treatment of patients with infiltrating ductal carcinoma is well established. However, the efficacy of CS and RT for patients with infiltrating lobular carcinoma is less well documented. The goal of this study was to examine treatment outcome after CS and RT for patients with infiltrating lobular carcinoma and to compare the results to those of patients with infiltrating ductal carcinoma and patients with mixed ductal–lobular histology. *Methods:* Between 1970 and 1986, 1624 patients with Stage I or II invasive breast cancer were treated with CS and RT consisting of a complete gross excision of the tumor and $\geqslant 6000$ cGy to the primary site. Slides were available for review for 1337 of these patients (82%). Of these, 93 had infiltrating lobular carcinoma, 1089 had infiltrating ductal carcinoma, and 59 had tumors with mixed ductal and lobular features; these patients constitute the study population. The median follow-up time for surviving patients was 133 months. A comprehensive list of clinical and pathologic features was evaluated for all patients. Additional histologic features assessed for patients with infiltrating lobular carcinoma included histologic subtype, multifocal invasion, stromal desmoplasia, and the presence of signet ring cells. *Results:* Five and 10-year crude results by site of first failure were similar for patients with infiltrating lobular, infiltrating ductal, and mixed histology. In particular, the 10-year crude local recurrence rates were 15%, 13% and 13% for patients with infiltrating lobular, infiltrating ductal, and mixed histology, respectively. Ten-year distant/regional recurrence rates were 22%, 23%, and 20% for the three groups, respectively. In addition, the 10-year crude contralateral breast cancer rates were 4%, 13% and 6% for patients with infiltrating lobular, infiltrating ductal and mixed histology, respectively. In a multiple regression analysis which included established prognostic factors, histologic type was not significantly associated with either survival or time to recurrence. *Conclusions:* Patients with infiltrating lobular carcinoma have a similar outcome following CS and RT to patients with infiltrating ductal carcinoma and to patients with tumors that have mixed ductal and lobular features. We conclude that the presence of infiltrating lobular histology should not influence decisions regarding local therapy in patients with Stage I and II breast cancer.

Ultra-conservative skin-sparing 'keyhole' mastectomy and immediate breast and areola reconstruction.

Peyser PM, Abel JA, Straker VF, Hall VL, Rainsbury RM.

Breast Unit, Royal Hampshire County Hospital, Winchester, UK.

Annals of the Royal College of Surgeons of England 82(4):227–35, 2000, July.

The popularity of skin-sparing mastectomy (SSM) which preserves the breast skin envelope is increasing, but the risks and benefits of this approach are only beginning to emerge. A technique involving ultra-conservative SSM and immediate breast reconstruction (IBR) has been evaluated to establish the surgical and oncological sequelae of skin conservation. Between 1994–1998, 67 consecutive patients underwent 71 SSM and expander-assisted immediate latissimus dorsi (LD) breast reconstructions (follow up, 24.1 months; range, 2–52 months). Breast resection, axillary dissection and reconstruction were performed through a 5–6 cm circular peri-areolar 'keyhole' incision. Patients were discharged 6.5 days (range, 5–15 days) after the 3.9 h (range, 3.0–5.5 h) procedure, and expansion was completed by 4.0 months (range, 0–10 months). Local recurrence occurred in 3% of breasts at risk, skin envelope necrosis occurred in 10%, and contralateral surgery was required to achieve symmetry in 14%. SSM and IBR is an oncologically safe, minimal-scar procedure which can be performed by surgeons trained in 'oncoplastic' techniques. It results in low rates of local recurrence and complication, and reduces the need for contralateral surgery.

Role of axillary surgery in early breast cancer: review of the current evidence.

Spillane AJ, Sacks NP.

Breast Unit, Royal Marsden Hospital, London, UK.

Australian & New Zealand Journal of Surgery 70(7):515–24, 2000, July.

Background: Controversy continues to surround the best practice for management of the axilla in patients with early breast cancer (EBC), particularly the clinically negative axilla. The balance between therapeutic and staging roles of axillary surgery (with the consequent morbidity of the procedures utilized) has altered. This is due to the increasing frequency of women presenting with early stage disease, the more widespread utilization of adjuvant chemoendocrine therapy and, more recently, the advent of alternative staging procedures, principally sentinel node biopsy (SNB). The aim of the present review is to critically analyse the current literature concerning the preferred management of the axilla in early breast cancer and make evidence-based recommendations on current management. *Methods:* A review was undertaken of the English language medical literature, using MEDLINE database software and cross-referencing major articles on the subject, focusing on the last 10 years. The following combinations of key words have been searched: breast neoplasms, axilla, axillary dissection, survival, prognosis, and sentinel node biopsy. *Results:* Despite the trend to more frequent earlier stage diagnosis, levels I and II axillary dissection remain the treatment of choice in the majority of women with EBC and a clinically negative axilla. *Conclusions:* Sentinel node biopsy has no proven superiority over axillary dissection because no randomized controlled trials have been completed to date. Despite this, SNB will become increasingly utilized due to encouraging results from major centres responsible for its development, and patient demand. Therefore if patients are not being enrolled in clinical trials strict quality controls need to be established at a local level before SNB is allowed to replace standard treatment of the axilla. Unless this is strictly adhered to there is a significant risk of an increase in the frequency of axillary relapse and possible increased understaging and resultant inadequate treatment of patients.

Radiation therapy after immediate breast reconstruction with implants.

Vandeweyer E, Deraemaecker R.

Department of Plastic and Reconstructive Surgery, Bordet Institute, Tumor Center of the Universite Libre de Bruxelles, Brussels, Belgium.

Plastic & Reconstructive Surgery 106(1):56–8; discussion 59–60, 2000, July.

The use of implants in immediate breast reconstruction is presently a common option. However, the practice should be evaluated in consideration of possible adjuvant therapies needed to control disease and to rule out negative interactions. This article discusses the effects of radiotherapy on breast implants with regard to the final cosmetic result. Six out of 124 cases of immediate breast reconstruction with implants were followed and evaluated in terms of capsular contracture and final aesthetic result after adjuvant radiotherapy and compared with the results of 118 patients who did not require irradiation. All of the patients who received irradiation demonstrated poor to fair results, with grade III to IV capsular contracture. Two patients received radiation therapy for local recurrences, which worsened their capsular contracture, emphasizing the deleterious effect of irradiation on breast implants. Statistical analysis of the results demonstrated a significant difference between the two groups in terms of capsular contracture and breast symmetry. In the selection of patient candidates

for immediate breast reconstruction with implants, adjuvant radiation therapy must be considered as a contraindication, at least from an aesthetic point of view.

Long-term results of a randomized trial comparing breast-conserving therapy with mastectomy: European Organization for Research and Treatment of Cancer 10801 trial.

van Dongen JA, Voogd AC, Fentiman IS, Legrand C, Sylvester RJ, Tong D, van der Schueren E, Helle PA, van Zijl K, Bartelink H.

Journal of the National Cancer Institute 92(14):1143–50, 2000, July 19.

Background: Breast-conserving therapy (BCT) has been shown to be as effective as mastectomy in the treatment of tumors 2 cm or smaller. However, evidence of its efficacy, over the long term, in patients with tumors larger than 2 cm is limited. From May 1980 to May 1986, the European Organization for Research and Treatment of Cancer carried out a randomized, multicenter trial comparing BCT with modified radical mastectomy for patients with tumors up to 5 cm. In this analysis, we investigated whether the treatments resulted in different overall survival, time to distant metastasis, or time to locoregional recurrence. *Methods:* Of 868 eligible breast cancer patients randomly assigned to the BCT arm or to the modified radical mastectomy arm, 80% had a tumor of 2.1–5 cm. BCT comprised lumpectomy with an attempted margin of 1 cm of healthy tissue and complete axillary clearance, followed by radiotherapy to the breast and a supplementary dose to the tumor bed. The median follow-up was 13.4 years. All *p* values are two-sided. *Results:* At 10 years, there was no difference between the two groups in overall survival (66% for the mastectomy patients and 65% for the BCT patients; $p = 0.11$) or in their distant metastasis-free rates (66% for the mastectomy patients and 61% for the BCT patients; $p = 0.24$). The rate of locoregional recurrence (occurring before or at the same time as distant metastasis) at 10 years did show a statistically significant difference (12% of the mastectomy and 20% of the BCT patients; $p = 0.01$). *Conclusions:* BCT and mastectomy demonstrate similar survival rates in a trial in which the great majority of the patients had stage II breast cancer.

13

The role of adjuvant therapy in node-negative breast cancer patients

CHRISTY A RUSSELL AND EDMUND S LEE

INTRODUCTION

Providing a standard of care for the systemic management of early-stage breast cancer patients has been elusive. A large number of prospective, randomized trials and recent international overviews or meta-analyses of all available randomized trials of adjuvant systemic therapy have determined that both chemotherapy and hormonal therapy reduce the odds of recurrence and cancer-related deaths in patients with primary breast cancer. The decision making used in offering adjuvant systemic therapy requires balancing many factors learned from the anatomic and biologic aspects of the tumor as well as the patient's age, menopausal status, and general health. The proper decision maximizes the patient's chances of avoiding a recurrence and possible death, but with the price of a temporary impact on quality of life and possible drug toxicity.

For the clinician, the first step is to estimate recurrence based on established prognostic factors. In general, a patient's risk of recurrence and survival is based upon the axillary lymph node status, the size of the tumor, and the hormone receptor status of the tumor. Other prognostic factors are currently being defined, mostly through retrospective analyses of large, randomized trials. A large meta-analysis of randomized trials suggests that the relative reduction in the risk of recurrence and death with systemic therapy is similar for patients with node-positive and node-negative breast cancer. However, absolute reductions in recurrence are quite different depending upon the initial risk. Expressed differently, there was no subgroup of patients with breast cancer who did not have a reduction in the odds of recurrence or death from adjuvant systemic therapy. More simply stated, a woman may receive a 30% reduction in the risk of recurrence of metastatic breast cancer with a particular chemotherapy regimen. If her risk

of recurrence is 100%, the risk will be reduced from 100% to 70% (a 30% decrease). A risk of recurrence of 50% will be reduced to 35%, and a risk of recurrence of 10% will be reduced to 7%. For those patients with a low risk of recurrence, it may be reasonable to be spared adjuvant therapy because the absolute risk reduction will be so small that the toxicity and expense of treatment are not justified. This chapter attempts to elucidate the prognostic factors that allow us to identify this low-risk group, and the predictive factors that allow us to choose specific forms of systemic therapy to maximize a reduction in recurrence and an improvement in survival from breast cancer.

For many years, axillary dissection has been standard management for patients with invasive breast cancer undergoing either mastectomy or lumpectomy followed by radiation. As dictated by the Halstedian concept of breast cancer spread, axillary dissection was considered a critical component of the surgical cure of the disease. The axillary nodes had been presumed to filter and hold cancer cells before spread to distant sites could occur. Although it has since been shown to provide no proven survival benefit, axillary dissection has become accepted as useful in assessing prognosis and in assuring local tumor control in the axilla for those shown to have axillary lymph node involvement.

Given that the majority of breast cancer patients found to be lymph node negative will probably be cured by local surgical therapy alone, the approximately 30–40% of node-negative patients who will eventually develop and succumb to metastatic disease must be identified. Many lymph node-negative studies have been designed and performed in order to determine whether or not chemotherapy and/or hormonal therapy can prolong disease-free survival in these patients following surgery for breast cancer. However, until recently, these had been difficult to interpret, given that, in general, it is necessary to study large populations of similar patients and to establish a long follow-up, as node-negative patients have a lower relapse rate and a longer time to relapse than a similar population of node-positive patients. Given the difficulty in predicting who may fail, the specific role of adjuvant systemic therapy in node-negative breast cancer is being increasingly defined, and it is becoming widely accepted that the majority of node-negative breast cancer patients may benefit from adjuvant systemic therapy to prevent recurrent disease.

CLINICAL TRIALS

The modern era of clinical trials of systemic adjuvant therapy for lymph node-negative breast cancer began in the 1980s. Prior to that time, trials were not conducted because of the mistaken belief that women with lymph node-negative breast cancer had an excellent prognosis after local management of their cancer, and that it would be harmful to expose these women to systemic chemotherapy because of a concern regarding secondary malignancies. In 1989, three major trials were completed, and data were published which have had a permanent impact on our standard of care for women with lymph node-negative breast cancer.[1-4]

NSABP B-13

In August 1981, the National Surgical Adjuvant Breast and Bowel Project (NSABP) conducted a randomized trial to determine the value of chemotherapy in women with lymph node-negative, *estrogen receptor-negative* early breast cancer. The regimen selected was M → F, two antimetabolites given sequentially, followed by leucovorin; 760 women who met the criteria for the study were randomly assigned to no systemic therapy versus methotrexate (M) 100 mg/m^2 and 5-fluorouracil (F) 600 mg/m^2 intravenously on days 1 and 8. Leucovorin was administered at 10 mg/m^2 every 6 h for six consecutive doses, beginning 24 h after M administration. Therapy was administered every 4 weeks for 12 cycles. An update of these data was published in 1996.[5] A significant benefit was seen for disease-free survival (DFS) (74% versus 59%) and distant disease-free survival (DDFS) (76% versus 69%) at 8 years of follow-up for those receiving chemotherapy (Figure 13.1). This represents a 37% reduction in treatment failure. Older women had a larger benefit for DFS than younger women (50% versus 30%, respectively). Overall survival (OS) was improved by 22% at 8 years, which was of borderline statistical significance ($p = 0.06$).

NSABP B-14

Between 1982 and 1987, 2844 women with lymph node-negative and *estrogen receptor-positive* breast cancer were

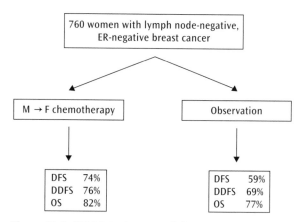

Figure 13.1 *NSABP B-13: 8-year follow-up. (ER, estrogen receptor; DFS, disease-free survival; DDFS, distant disease-free survival; OS, overall survival.)*

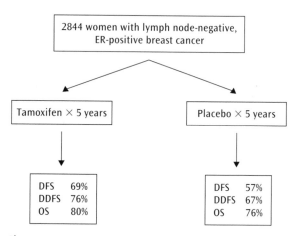

Figure 13.2 *NSABP B-14: 10-year follow-up. (For abbreviations, see Figure 13.1.)*

randomly assigned to placebo versus tamoxifen for 5 years. The publication in 1989 presented a significant prolongation of DFS among women taking tamoxifen versus placebo (83% versus 77%).[2] This advantage was seen regardless of age or size of the tumor. Updated data from this trial show a highly significant improvement in both DFS and OS for those women randomly assigned to tamoxifen ($p < 0.0001$ and $p = 0.02$, respectively) (Figure 13.2).[6] The advantage was seen regardless of age. Toxicities reported from tamoxifen that were significantly different from placebo included hot flushes, vaginal discharge, irregular menses, thromboembolic events, and endometrial cancer.

Intergroup node-negative trial

Between 1981 and 1988, 536 women with lymph node-negative breast cancer were enrolled in an intergroup trial comparing no systemic therapy with chemotherapy using cyclophosphamide, methotrexate, fluorouracil, and prednisone (CMFP). The treatment group received six cycles

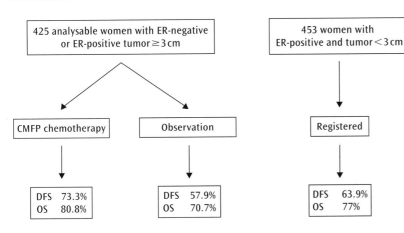

Figure 13.3 *Intergroup node-negative study: 10-year follow-up. (For chemotherapy regimens, see text; for other abbreviations, see Figure 13.1.)*

of cyclophosphamide ($100 \, mg/m^2$ orally, days 1–14), methotrexate ($40 \, mg/m^2$ intravenously, days 1 and 8), fluorouracil ($600 \, mg/m^2$ intravenously, days 1 and 8), and prednisone ($40 \, mg/m^2$ orally, days 1–14). Cycles were administered every 4 weeks. The patients enrolled were women with tumors of any size with negative estrogen receptors (ER), or women with tumors ≥ 3 cm with positive ER. Women with tumors under 3 cm with positive ER were registered and observed without systemic chemotherapy. At 3 years of follow-up, there was a statistically significant advantage in DFS for those with systemic treatment (84% versus 69%). These data have been recently updated with a 10-year analysis.[7] At 10 years, DFS was 73% versus 58% (chemotherapy versus none) and OS was 81% versus 71%. Both the DFS and OS are statistically significant, with a 37% reduction in risk of recurrence and a 34% reduction in mortality risk. For those patients who were considered low risk (ER positive and tumor < 3 cm) and were observed, only 64% continue to be disease free and 77% are alive at 10 years of follow-up (Figure 13.3).

NIH Consensus Conference

Based on the data from these three powerful trials, the NIH held a Consensus Conference in 1990 to address five questions:[8]

1 What are the roles of mastectomy versus breast conservation in the treatment of early-stage breast cancer?
2 What are the optimal techniques for breast conservation?
3 What is the role of adjuvant therapy for patients with node-negative breast cancer?
4 How should prognostic factors be used to manage node-negative breast cancer?
5 What are the directions for future research?

The consensus panel stated that, for all lymph node-negative breast cancer patients who were ineligible for or refused entry into clinical trials, information should be provided regarding the benefits and risks of systemic therapy. Adjuvant therapy should consist of either combination chemotherapy or tamoxifen. At that time, there

were no completed studies comparing tamoxifen with chemotherapy or comparing combination chemohormonal therapy with either therapy alone, and no recommendations could be given regarding these options.

The consensus panel suggested eight directions for future research:

1 Refine prognostic factors by reassessing the TNM staging system, standardizing a nuclear grading system, exploring the relationships between individual prognostic factors and resistance to therapy, and developing tissue banks for studying prognostic factors.
2 Develop risk factor profile systems that might accurately identify those patients who require no systemic therapy, do not require axillary lymph node dissection, and do not require radiation therapy after lumpectomy.
3 Improve chemotherapy regimens through investigation of dose intensity, timing, and duration, and evaluate new agents and chemohormonal combinations.
4 Gather further information regarding the safety, toxicity, and efficacy of tamoxifen.
5 Assess quality-of-life parameters in future clinical trials.
6 Determine optimal margins for local primary excision with or without extensive intraductal component.
7 Determine the benefit of boost irradiation.
8 Determine the optimal sequence of radiation and systemic adjuvant chemotherapy.

Although none of these research questions has been completely answered, recently published randomized trials have moved us closer toward this mandate from the NIH Consensus Conference in 1990.

Early Breast Cancer Trialists' Collaborative Group

In 1998, the Early Breast Cancer Trialists' Collaborative Group published their updated results from an overview of data from multiple randomized trials performed throughout the world.[9,10] In 1995, they sought information on each woman enrolled in any randomized clinical trial that began before 1990 and either differed with respect to *chemotherapy* regimens being utilized, or which investigated the use of *tamoxifen* versus no tamoxifen prior to breast cancer recurrence in the adjuvant setting. The overview analysis involved 18 000 women in 47 trials of *prolonged chemotherapy* versus no chemotherapy, about 6000 women in 11 trials of *longer* versus shorter chemotherapy, and about 6000 women in 11 trials of *anthracycline*-containing regimens versus CMF-type regimens. An additional approximately 37 000 women were analysed in 55 *tamoxifen*-based trials, comprising about 87% of the worldwide evidence of benefit of tamoxifen.

Analysis of data

Figures 13.4–13.9 reflect recurrence and mortality curves for women evaluated in the Early Breast Cancer Trialists' Collaborative Group 1998 publication. Recurrence and mortality reductions may be expressed in one of two ways.

1 *Absolute reductions* reflect a simple mathematical subtraction. If 50% of patients who get no therapy live for 5 years and 70% of patients who get a therapy live for 5 years, then there is a 20% absolute reduction in mortality as a result of the therapy.

2 *Proportional reductions* in mortality use a different formula. If 50% of patients who get no therapy live for 5 years, then the proportional reduction in death is reflected only in those patients with a chance of dying, not the proportion who may be cured (the other 50%). Therefore the mathematical formula used is to take the difference between the two values (in this case 70% minus 50% = 20%) and divide the difference by the lowest of the values (50%). Twenty percent divided by 50% is equal to 40%. Therefore, there is a 40% proportional reduction in mortality over 5 years.

Polychemotherapy overview

The overview of the polychemotherapy trials found that, for tumor recurrence, there was a 23.5% reduction in the annual hazard of recurrence. The reductions were seen in women under the age of 50 (35% reduction) (Figure 13.4) and for women aged 50–69 (20% reduction) (Figure 13.5). For mortality, chemotherapy produced a 15.3% reduction in the annual hazard, with the benefit being larger in women under 50 (27% reduction) compared to women aged 50–69 (11% reduction) (Figures 13.6 and 13.7). The proportional reductions for recurrence and survival were similar regardless of lymph node status. The authors noted that the age-specific benefits of chemotherapy were evident regardless of the ER status of the tumor and whether tamoxifen was taken. For women under the age of 50, the reductions in recurrence were

40% and 33% for those with ER-poor tumors and ER-positive tumors, respectively. For women aged 50–69, the proportional reduction in recurrence was 30% versus 18% for ER-poor versus ER-positive tumors.

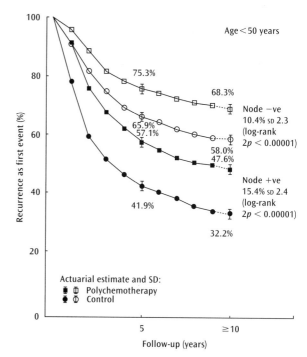

Figure 13.4 *Polychemotherapy effect for recurrence in node-negative and node-positive patients, age <50. From* Lancet *1998; 352:930–42.[10]*

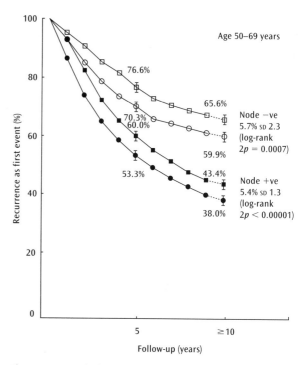

Figure 13.5 *Polychemotherapy effect for recurrence in node-negative and node-positive patients, age 50–69. From* Lancet *1998; 352:930–42.[10]*

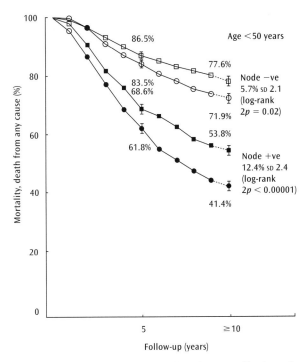

Figure 13.6 *Polychemotherapy effect for mortality in node-negative and node-positive patients, age <50. From* Lancet *1998; 352:930–42.*[10]

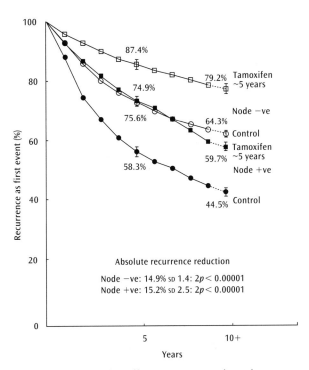

Figure 13.8 *Tamoxifen effect on recurrence in node-negative and node-positive patients. From* Lancet *1998; 351:1451–67.*[9]

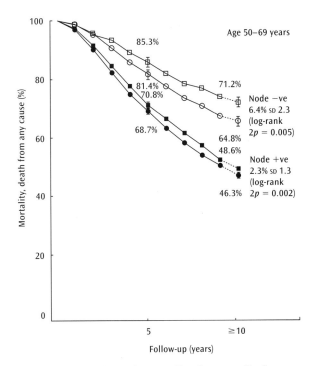

Figure 13.7 *Polychemotherapy effect for mortality in node-negative and node-positive patients, age 50–69. From* Lancet *1998; 352:930–42.*[10]

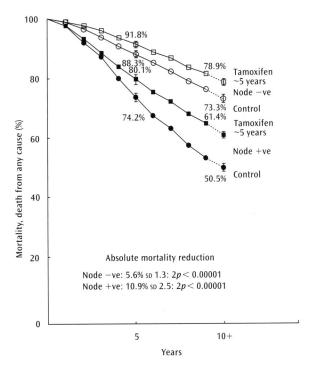

Figure 13.9 *Tamoxifen effect on mortality in node-negative and node-positive patients. From* Lancet *1998; 351:1451–67.*[9]

Effects of different polychemotherapy regimens

There were 11 trials in which chemotherapy for at least 6 months was compared to longer regimens and others where a minimum of 6 months of chemotherapy was compared to less than 6 months of therapy. There was a slight (7%) but non-significant difference among these groups. There were 11 randomized trials in which an anthracycline regimen was compared to CMF chemotherapy. For recurrence, the anthracycline regimens delivered an additional 12% proportional reduction in recurrence and an 11% additional reduction in mortality compared to the CMF regimens. The majority (70%) of women in these trials were under the age of 50.

Effects of chemotherapy on other outcomes

Contralateral breast cancer occurrence was reduced by 20% with polychemotherapy. Age did not influence these findings. There was no effect on the risk of death from other malignancies or from vascular disease secondary to chemotherapy.

Tamoxifen randomized trials

Among the 37 000 women on randomized tamoxifen trials, approximately 8000 had very low or zero levels of ER protein. The effect of tamoxifen was negligible in these women. Therefore, the overview analysis is limited to 18 000 women with ER-positive tumors and 12 000 women with ER-unknown tumors (of which about 8000 would be expected to be positive). Trials that were included in the analysis used 1, 2, or about 5 years of tamoxifen. For these groups, there were 21%, 29%, and 47% proportional reductions in the risk of recurrence, respectively, with a marked trend toward a greater effect related to the length of tamoxifen therapy. The corresponding proportional reductions in mortality were 12%, 17%, and 26%. The proportional reductions in recurrence and mortality were similar for lymph node-positive and lymph node-negative patients (Figures 13.8 and 13.9). The benefits were found to be irrespective of age, menopausal status, or addition of chemotherapy.

Other outcomes of tamoxifen trials

Again, when comparing tamoxifen trial durations of 1, 2, or 5 years, there were proportional reductions of contralateral breast cancers by 13%, 26%, and 47%. The incidence of endometrial cancer was doubled in exposures of 1 or 2 years of tamoxifen and there was an approximately fourfold increase in women exposed to about 5 years of tamoxifen. There was no tamoxifen effect on the incidence of colorectal cancer or on any other cause of death, including death from cardiovascular disease.

Although the polychemotherapy and tamoxifen overviews do not deal only with lymph node-negative breast cancers, the proportional benefits of the multiple therapies are the same regardless of lymph node status and provide substantial data with which to educate women regarding their expected benefit from these various treatments.

Second-generation systemic therapy trials for lymph node-negative breast cancer

As the first-generation trials really only investigated single-modality systemic therapy (chemotherapy or tamoxifen) for lymph node-negative breast cancer patients, the second generation of studies has been performed to further elucidate whether a combination of these modalities is superior to any single modality, and to evaluate the most efficacious form of chemotherapy to be used.

NSABP B-19

NSABP B-19 was initiated in 1988 to compare the benefit and toxicity of either M → F or conventional CMF chemotherapy in women with lymph node-negative, ER-negative primary breast cancer.[5] This trial was performed because the NSABP had been using M → F and other investigators had been using conventional CMF in this setting, both of which had been shown to be of benefit. As they had not previously been compared to one another for either efficacy or toxicity, this randomized trial of 1095 women was undertaken.

Results

The published report was based on 1074 eligible women with a mean follow-up of 61 months. Through 5 years of follow-up, an overall DFS advantage (82% versus 73%) and a borderline significant OS advantage (88% versus 85%) were seen with CMF when compared to M → F (Figure 13.10). The DFS and OS advantages of CMF were most marked in women aged ≤ 49 years. Thus, although there was an advantage to either chemotherapy used, there did prove to be a therapeutic advantage of CMF over M → F, especially for young women.

NSABP B-20

NSABP B-20, also initiated in 1988, was designed to test the hypothesis that the *addition* of chemotherapy to tamoxifen would improve the recurrence-free and OS seen in those women given tamoxifen alone.[11] Because the optimal chemotherapy regimen in lymph node-negative women had yet to be determined, women who were randomly assigned to chemotherapy with tamoxifen received either the regimen CMF or M → F (the chemotherapy regimen used in the B-13 trial). A

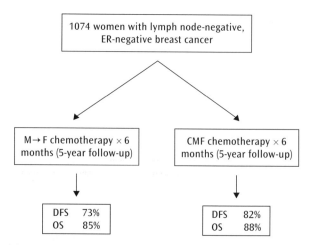

Figure 13.10 *NSABP B-19: 5-year follow-up. (For chemotherapy regimens, see text; for other abbreviations, see Figure 13.1.)*

total of 2363 women with histologically node-negative, *estrogen receptor-positive* breast cancer were randomly assigned to tamoxifen (788), sequential methotrexate and 5-fluorouracil plus tamoxifen (786), or CMF plus tamoxifen (CMFT; 789). All groups of women received tamoxifen for a 5-year interval and the tamoxifen was initiated simultaneously with the chemotherapy. Both $M \rightarrow F$ and CMF were delivered every 4 weeks for six cycles.

Results

Women who were assigned to one of the two chemotherapy groups plus tamoxifen were found to have a significantly better DFS (90% versus 85%), DDFS (92% and 91% versus 87%), and OS (97% and 96% versus 94%) when considering MFT, CMFT versus tamoxifen alone, respectively, through 5 years of follow-up (Figure 13.11). Benefit was seen regardless of the type of chemotherapy, tumor size, hormone receptor level, or age. The reduction was greatest in women who were ≤ 49 years of age. The authors concluded that there was no subgroup of patients who failed to benefit from the addition of chemotherapy to tamoxifen, and suggested that any woman with lymph node-negative breast cancer who meets the criteria for this study is a candidate for both tamoxifen and chemotherapy.

Two studies were subsequently initiated to compare anthracycline-based regimens versus conventional CMF in women with lymph node-negative breast cancer. As the meta-analysis has suggested a small benefit of anthracycline-based regimens over CMF, this question was specifically addressed in lymph node-negative patients.

NSABP B-23

NSABP B-23 has been completed, but the findings have not yet been reported. This trial compares AC (adriamycin 60 mg/m^2 and cyclophosphamide 600 mg/m^2 intravenously) with conventional CMF, and then either regimen with or without tamoxifen for women with lymph node-negative, ER-negative breast cancer (Figure 13.12). (See abstract by Fisher, Anderson, *et al.*, page 351.)

Intergroup Trial 0102

A second study (Intergroup Trial 0102) has been published in abstract form, which investigates a similar

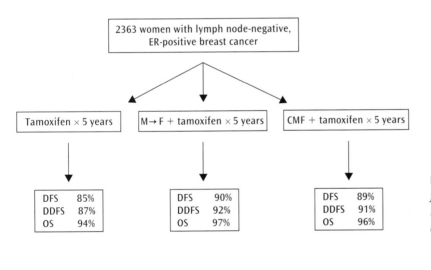

Figure 13.11 *NSABP B-20: 5-year follow-up. (For chemotherapy regimens, see text; for other abbreviations, see Figure 13.1.)*

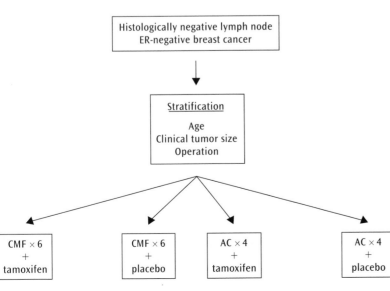

Figure 13.12 *NSABP B-23. (For chemotherapy regimens, see text, for other abbreviations, see Figure 13.1.)*

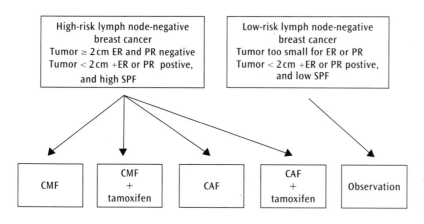

Figure 13.13 *Intergroup Trial 0102: 5-year follow-up. (SPF, S-phase fraction; for chemotherapy regimens, see text; for other abbreviations, see Figure 13.1.)*

group of women.[12] Between 1989 and 1993, 4406 women were registered to this trial, which initially stratified women into risk groups based on tumor size, ER or progesterone-receptor (PgR) status, and S-phase fraction (SPF). Women classified as low risk had either a tumor too small for biochemical RE/PgR assay, or had tumors <2 cm, were ER or PgR positive, and had a low SPF. High-risk women were those with any of the following: tumor ≥2 cm, ER and PgR negative, or tumors <2 cm with positive ER or PgR and a *high* SPF. All high-risk women were randomly assigned to CMF or CAF chemotherapy (for 6 months), either with or without tamoxifen (for 5 years). All low-risk women were followed without systemic therapy. There were 2691 high-risk women and 1208 low-risk women evaluated in the trial (Figure 13.13).

Results

CAF was found to be marginally, but significantly, superior to CMF when considering either DFS or OS ($p = 0.03$). DFS on CAF versus CMF was 86% versus 84%. OS was 92% versus 91%, respectively. The use of tamoxifen resulted in a significant benefit for women with hormone receptor-positive tumors compared to those women not given tamoxifen (DFS 88% versus 82%). Postmenopausal women benefited more than premenopausal women from tamoxifen. Surprisingly, there appeared to be a DFS detriment for those women with ER-negative tumors who were given tamoxifen. The benefit of CAF chemotherapy came at a cost of increased toxicity. For the low-risk group of women (who received no adjuvant chemotherapy), there was no difference in outcome for those women with tumors which were too small for biochemical hormone receptor testing and those with all of the following factors: tumors <2 cm, ER-positive, and low SPF. Five-year DFS and OS were 89% and 96%, respectively, for these low-risk patients.

CURRENT TRIALS

Current cooperative group trials for lymph node-negative breast cancer have been designed to determine

whether the addition of a taxane (either paclitaxel or docetaxel) to the anthracycline adriamycin results in a better DFS or OS for 'high-risk' breast cancer patients. These trials are underway based on data from women with lymph node-positive breast cancer, which suggest that the addition of a taxane in the adjuvant setting provides a superior outcome. Neoadjuvant trials are also underway for those women with clinically negative axillae to determine the best timing of surgery around adjuvant therapies, and which regimen is superior when evaluating toxicity, DFS, and OS. Because women are not surgically staged prior to systemic therapy in the neoadjuvant trials, there will be a mix of lymph node-positive and lymph node-negative patients in these groupings. Specific recommendations with regard to the management of lymph node-negative patients will not be possible from these trials.

PROGNOSTIC VERSUS PREDICTIVE FACTORS

Prognostic factors have been described as those factors that give information on clinical outcome.[13] The best example of this in breast cancer is lymph node involvement. Having lymph node involvement is an independent prognostic marker for poor outcome, and the delivery of systemic therapy does not alter the significance of this marker. A *predictive factor* is described as being able to predict which tumors will respond or benefit from a specific type of systemic therapy. The most commonly cited predictive factor is hormone receptor status. Those breast cancers with positive ERs respond to hormonal therapy and those with negative receptors do not. Some markers have both predictive and prognostic significance.

Prognostic factors

Once axillary node status has been eliminated as the primary prognostic factor, secondary prognostic factors become essential to identify those patients at great risk for recurrence. Secondary prognostic factors include tumor size, histologic grade and subtype, ER/PgR expression, DNA ploidy and SPF measurement, and oncogene expression.[14]

Tumor size

Tumor size has become the most important single prognostic factor to determine the risk of recurrence and benefit from therapy in axillary node-negative breast cancer. The clear relationship between the size of the primary tumor, recurrence, and survival rates has been demonstrated in studies by Rosen et al.[15] Seven hundred and sixty-seven women with T1-2, N0, M0 breast cancer treated consecutively from 1964 through 1970 by modified radical mastectomy and no systemic therapy were analysed for recurrence and death with a median duration of follow-up of 18 years. Size and special histologic subtypes defined the prognostic groupings. No other prognostic testing was done on these tumors. Tumor size of 1 cm or less or special tumor types ≤ 3.0 cm were associated with a very favorable prognosis (13% recurrence rate at 20 years of follow-up), whereas those larger than 1 cm or those of special subtype >3.0 cm had a rapidly rising recurrence risk based purely on the size of the tumor, with 32% recurrence rate at 20 years of follow-up. Special tumor histologic types were identified as follows: medullary, mucinous, papillary, and tubular.

In a second retrospective review of prognostic factors, investigators from the University of Chicago reported on 826 women with node-negative breast cancer who were treated at the University of Chicago from 1927 to 1984.[16] Patients underwent either a radical or extended radical mastectomy (83%) or a modified radical mastectomy (13%). Follow-up evaluation ranged from 9 to 523 months (43.6 years); the mean follow-up period of survivors is 162 months (13.5 years). On multivariate analysis, the strongest predictor of outcome and time to relapse was pathologic tumor size. Patients with tumors less than 2 cm had a 20-year DFS rate of 79% and a median time to recurrence of 48 months. Those patients with tumors greater than 2 cm had a survival rate of 64% ($p < 0.001$) and a median time to recurrence of 37 months ($p = 0.01$). The authors suggested that, with extended follow-up evaluation, node-negative breast cancer can be a curable disease, with size proving to be a strong predictor of dissemination and rate of relapse.

Tumor grade and histologic type

Several histologic grading systems have been described that have prognostic value in the evaluation of breast carcinoma. The most frequently used is that of the Modified Scarff–Bloom–Richardson (SBR) Scale.[17] This system evaluates the extent of tubular formation, nuclear pleomorphism, and the extent of mitoses.

Alternatively, Fisher et al. have found that, upon retrospective review of 950 women with node-negative, stage I breast cancer enrolled in NSABP B-06, there were only two histologic factors which, on multivariate analysis, had prognostic implications.[18] The first of these was nuclear grade, which was scored as good versus poor, and the second was special histologic type, which included mucinous, tubular, or papillary cancers. Unfortunately, histologic grading has never been incorporated into a prospective, randomized trial for the purpose of stratification for therapy. There continues to be a question as to whether there is acceptable interobserver agreement and reproducibility. However, two groups of investigators have found that, when specific and strict guidelines for grading are followed, interobserver agreement is clinically acceptable.[19,20]

Hormone receptor status

The measurement of ER has become standard practice in the evaluation of patients with primary breast cancer. Most large studies have not shown ER and/or PgR to strongly distinguish patients with favorable and unfavorable outcomes. However, studies have consistently shown a trend for better DFS and OS for patients who are ER+ or PR+. However, the majority of these studies have found the hormone receptor status falls out as an independent prognostic variable when other histologic and biologic features are considered. An example for such a trend was seen in NSABP B-06, where there were 825 node-negative patients with known ER. The risk of systemic relapse at 5 years was 28% in the ER-negative subset and 20% in the ER-positive subset. The risks of death at 5 years were 18% and 8%, respectively.[21]

DNA flow cytometry/S phase

The proliferative rate of breast cancer can be determined by studying the percentage of cells in the DNA synthetic phase of the cell cycle (S phase). It does not require fresh tissue and can be performed on frozen or formalin-fixed, paraffin-embedded material. Reports have demonstrated that increased percent S phase predicts for early recurrence or poor survival in both axillary node-negative and node-positive breast cancer patients. Ploidy can be determined by DNA flow cytometry. The majority of breast tumors are aneuploid, having an abnormal DNA content. Although ploidy is not an independent prognostic variable, there are different 'cut points' for the SPF prognosis depending upon whether the tumor is aneuploid or diploid.[22,23] Unfortunately, there is a marked lack of standardization for the measurement of SPF. Different laboratories have established different cut points for 'low' SPFs, with the clinicians being unable to tell whether these cut points carry any validity. One randomized trial (Intergroup 0102) has been completed using SPF as a stratification factor for treatment or nontreatment arms. All ploidy and SPF measurements were performed in the same laboratory as part of the study. Clinicians should continue to view SPF results with caution.

HER-2/*neu* oncogene expression

The HER-2/*neu* (c-erbB-2) gene codes for a transmembrane receptor protein that is homologous to, but distinct from, the epidermal growth factor receptor. Slamon *et al.* first published a pilot study in 1987 of 86 node-positive breast cancer patients that correlated HER-2/*neu* oncogene amplification with recurrence and shortened survival.[24] There appeared to be no prognostic significance for HER-2/*neu* in 101 node-negative patients in the same study. In 1993, Press and colleagues reported on 210 node-negative patients who by univariate analysis had an inferior DFS with HER-2/*neu* amplification.[25] Many additional studies have failed to show consistently the prognostic significance of HER-2/*neu* for lymph node-negative breast cancer. Press *et al.* have suggested that this lack of consistent prognostic significance may be for two reasons: there is not enough statistical power in the studies to show a clinical outcome difference; and methodological problems are significant in the testing of this gene.[26] This same group recently reported on 324 lymph node-negative breast cancer patients who had undergone only surgical therapy for their malignancy. Archival specimens were obtained for these women and HER-2/*neu* gene amplification was assessed by fluorescence *in situ* hybridization (FISH) technique. Among these surgically treated patients, the relative risks of early recurrence, recurrence at any time, and disease-related death were statistically significantly associated with HER-2/*neu* amplification. Paik *et al.*[27] published a retrospective study of 292 axillary node-negative patients and found an association of HER-2/*neu* overexpression and decreased survival among women with tumors with a favorable nuclear grade. In this subgroup, HER-2/*neu* overexpression was associated with an approximately fivefold increase in mortality rate.

Predictive factors

Evidence is growing that there is a multitude of potential predictive markers for malignancies. They include levels of thymidylate synthase, topisomerase I and II enzyme levels, p53 mutant protein expression, and many more. For the most part, these markers are still investigational and there is not a large enough body of evidence to show that they play a consistent role in breast cancer. However, there are two predictive markers that have been defined in breast cancer: hormone receptor status, and HER-2/*neu* amplification.

HER-2/*neu*

There is growing evidence that high levels of c-erbB-2 expression do correlate with resistance to certain types and sensitivity to other forms of adjuvant therapy. This observation was first noted in two separate clinical trials in which the chemotherapy regimen CMF was used in comparison to very short-course (i.e., 1 month) or no

chemotherapy. Both observed a significant benefit for improved DFS and OS in favor of the prolonged CMF arm. The one subset of patients who did not benefit comprised those patients who were retrospectively found to have overexpression of HER-2/*neu*.[28,29] These data suggested that HER-2/*neu* gene amplification or protein overexpression predicted for resistance to CMF chemotherapy. In a separate body of data, several studies have now been published suggesting a relative sensitivity to anthracycline-based chemotherapy when this gene is amplified. The original observation by Muss *et al.* in 1994 suggested that the benefits from adjuvant CAF chemotherapy in lymph node-positive breast cancer patients were similar when three different dose levels of the chemotherapy were delivered: low, moderate, and high (standard) dose.[30] Those tumors with gene amplification showed a differential response to the three doses of chemotherapy, with the highest dose resulting in best outcome. This same conclusion has been reached by other investigators who have retrospectively re-analysed their data for the correlation of response in gene-amplified tumors to adriamycin versus non-adriamycin regimens (NSABP B-11 and SWOG 9445 trials).

This lack of sensitivity to non-anthracycline regimens may also extend to hormonal therapies. In 1996, Carlomagno *et al.* published data showing an inferior outcome in women given adjuvant tamoxifen for their hormone-receptor positive, lymph node-negative breast cancer when there was amplification of HER-2/*neu*.[31] These data suggesting a relative resistance to tamoxifen in the setting of gene amplification allowed other groups to retrospectively analyse their results for women being randomly assigned to tamoxifen versus no systemic therapy. In 1998, data were presented from the GUN-1 trial, which began in the 1970s and randomized about 433 women between tamoxifen and no further therapy.[32] HER-2/*neu* expression was determined in 245 of the 433 women. HER-2/*neu* overexpression was found to be an independent predictor of tamoxifen failure. Further data are expected to be forthcoming from several other cooperative-group trials with regard to the predictive nature of HER-2/*neu* gene amplification.

Because there continue to be significant methodological and standardization issues with regard to HER-2/*neu* tissue evaluation, to date, the American Society of Clinical Oncology has not supported the use of this gene amplification for the selection of therapy.[33] However, as these data mature, it is likely that there will be a reversal of this opinion.

Having noted the multitude of clinical trials that have been performed and reported on since the 1980s, our understanding of the optimal use of systemic therapy in women with lymph node-negative breast cancer is maturing. However, there is considerable progress to be made. All women who have been diagnosed with early breast cancer should be considered for eligibility in

Table 13.1 *Risk categories for patients with node-negative breast cancer*

Factors	Minimal/low risk (has all listed factors)	Intermediate risk	High risk
Tumor size (cm)	≤1	>1–2	>2
ER or PgR	Positive	Positive	Negative
Grade	1	1–2	2–3
Age (years)	≥35	–	<35

ER, estrogen receptor; PgR, progesterone receptor.

Table 13.2 *Adjuvant treatment recommendations*

Patient group	Minimal/low risk	Intermediate risk	High risk
Premenopausal, ER or PgR positive	**None or tamoxifen**	**Tamoxifen ± chemotherapy** Ovarian ablation GnRH analogue	**Chemotherapy + tamoxifen** Ovarian ablation GnRH analogue **Chemotherapy**
Premenopausal ER and Pgr negative			
Postmenopausal, ER or PgR positive	**None or tamoxifen**	**Tamoxifen ± chemotherapy**	**Tamoxifen + chemotherapy**
Postmenopausal, ER and PgR negative			**Chemotherapy**
Elderly	**None or tamoxifen**	**Tamoxifen ± chemotherapy**	**Tamoxifen** **If negative ER and PgR: chemotherapy**

ER, estrogen receptor; PgR, progesterone receptor; GnRH, gonadotropin releasing hormone. Bold entries are treatments accepted for routine use or baseline in clinical trials. Non-bold treatments are still being tested in randomized clinical trials.

clinical trials. For those women who choose not to participate in such trials, guidelines have been suggested for the standards of treatment for both early and advanced breast cancers.

INTERNATIONAL CONSENSUS PANEL ON THE TREATMENT OF PRIMARY BREAST CANCER

Every 2–3 years, a scientific conference is held in St Gallen, Switzerland, to update the world's experience in clinical trials of women with primary breast cancer. At the conclusion of these conferences, a consensus panel has convened and subsequently published a series of guidelines and recommendations for the selection of adjuvant systemic treatments for specific groups of women with breast cancer.[34,35] The conference last met in February 1998, and the guidelines were published in November 1998.

The group established risk categories for patients with node-negative breast cancer, as shown in Table 13.1. Adjuvant treatment recommendations have thus been made with these risk factor categories (Table 13.2).

Tamoxifen is given for a 5-year interval for these different risk groups. The specific types of chemotherapy to be given were not addressed by this consensus statement.

CONCLUSIONS

As we approach a new era in the treatment of breast cancer, we will witness the increasing use of agents designed to apply the lessons learned from our study of tumor biology. Progress in this field will require a better understanding of the process of metastasis, the resistance to local and systemic therapies, and the development of more active cytotoxic and hormonal therapies. These therapies will probably include agents that interfere with tumor growth mechanisms by delivering growth factor receptor-directed therapy, treat tumor invasive capacity with matrix metalloproteinase inhibition, and alter tumor angiogenesis with angiogenesis inhibitors. The future of adjuvant therapy may involve the use of many combinations of these agents in addition to chemotherapy and/or hormone therapy that blocks the progression of the tumor from the micrometastatic to the overt metastatic in addition to attempting to eradicate every last micrometastatic cell.

REFERENCES

1. Fisher B, Redmond C, Dimitrov NV, *et al*. A randomized clinical trial evaluating sequential methotrexate and

fluorouracil in the treatment of patients with node-negative breast cancer who have estrogen receptor-negative tumors. N Engl J Med 1989; 320:473–8.

2. Fisher B, Costantino J, Redmond C, *et al*. A randomized clinical trial evaluating tamoxifen in the treatment of patients with node-negative breast cancer who have estrogen receptor-positive tumors. N Engl J Med 1989; 320:479–84.

3. Mansour EG, Gray R, Shatila AH, *et al*. Efficacy of adjuvant chemotherapy in high-risk node-negative breast cancer. An Intergroup study. N Engl J Med 1989; 320:485–90.

4. Fisher B, Redmond C, Wickerham L, *et al*. Systemic therapy in patients with node-negative breast cancer. Ann Int Med 1989; 111:703–12.

5. Fisher B, Dignam J, Eleftherios P, *et al*. Sequential methotrexate and fluorouracil for the treatment of node-negative breast cancer patients with estrogen receptor-negative tumors: eight-year results from National Surgical Adjuvant Breast and Bowel Project (NSABP) B-13 and first report of findings from NSABP B-19 comparing methotrexate and fluorouracil with conventional cyclophosphamide, methotrexate, and fluorouracil. J Clin Oncol 1996; 14:1982–92.

6. Fisher B, Dignam J, Bryant J, *et al*. Five versus more than five years of tamoxifen therapy for breast cancer patients with negative lymph nodes and estrogen receptor-positive tumors. J Natl Cancer Inst 1996; 88:1529–42.

7. Mansour EG, Gray R, Shatila AH, *et al*. Survival advantage of adjuvant chemotherapy in high-risk node-negative breast cancer: ten-year analysis – an Intergroup study. J Clin Oncol 1998; 16:3486–92.

8. NIH Consensus Conference. Treatment of early-stage breast cancer. JAMA 1991; 265(3):391–5.

9. Early Breast Cancer Trialists' Collaborative Group. Tamoxifen for early breast cancer: an overview of the randomised trials. Lancet 1998; 351:1451–67.

10. Early Breast Cancer Trialists' Collaborative Group. Polychemotherapy for early breast cancer: an overview of the randomised trials. Lancet 1998; 352:930–42.

11. Fisher B, Dignam J, Wolmark N, *et al*. Tamoxifen and chemotherapy for lymph node-negative, estrogen receptor-positive breast cancer. J Natl Cancer Inst 1997; 89(22):1673–82.

12. Hutchins L, Green S, Ravdin P, *et al*. CMF versus CAF with and without tamoxifen in high-risk node-negative breast cancer patients with a natural history follow-up study in low-risk node-negative patients: first results of Intergroup Trial INT 0102. *Proceedings of ASCO* (Abstract 2), 1998.

13. Gasparini G, Pozza F, Harris AL. Evaluating the potential usefulness of new prognostic and predictive indicators in node-negative breast cancer patients. J Natl Cancer Inst 1993; 85:1206–19.

14. Ravdin PM. A practical view of prognostic factors for staging, adjuvant treatment planning, and as baseline studies for possible future therapy. Hematol/Oncol Clin North Am 1994; 8(1):197–211.

15. Rosen PP, Groshen S, Kinne DW, Norton L. Factors influencing prognosis in node-negative breast carcinoma: analysis of 767 T1N0M0/T2N0M0 patients with long-term follow-up. J Clin Oncol 1993; 11:2090–100.

16. Quiet CA, Ferguson DJ, Weichselbaum RR, *et al*. Natural history of node-negative breast cancer: a study of 826 patients with long-term follow-up. J Clin Oncol 1995; 13:1144–51.

17. Le Doussal V, Tubiana-Hulin M, Friedman S, *et al*. Prognostic value of histologic grade nuclear components of Scarff–Bloom–Richardson (SBR). Cancer 1989; 64:1914–21.

18. Fisher ER, Redmond C, Fisher B, *et al*. Pathologic findings from the National Surgical Adjuvant Breast and Bowel Projects (NSABP). Prognostic discriminants for 8-year survival for node-negative invasive breast cancer. Cancer 1990; 65:2121–8.

19. Dalton LW, Page DL, Dupont WD. Histologic grading of breast carcinomas. A reproducibility study. Cancer 1994; 73:2765–70.

20. Robbins P, Pinder S, deKlerk N, *et al*. Histologic grading of breast carcinomas: a study of interobserver agreement. Hum Pathol 1995; 26:873–9.

21. Fisher B, Redmond C, Fisher ER, *et al*. Relative worth of estrogen or progesterone receptor and pathologic characteristics of differentiation as indicators of prognosis in node negative breast cancer patients: findings from National Surgical Adjuvant Breast and Bowel Project Protocol B-06. J Clin Oncol 1988; 6:1076–87.

22. Clark GM, Dressler LG, Owens MA, *et al*. Prediction of relapse or survival in patients with node-negative breast cancer by DNA flow cytometry. N Engl J Med 1989; 320:627–33.

23. Clark G, Mathieu M-C, Owens M, *et al*. Prognostic significance of S-phase fraction in good-risk, node-negative breast cancer patients. J Clin Oncol 1992; 10:428–32.

24. Slamon DJ, Clark GM, Wong SG, *et al*. Human breast cancer: correlation of relapse and survival with amplification of the Her-2/*neu* oncogene. Science 1987; 235:177–82.

25. Press MF, Pike MC, Chazin VR, *et al*. Her-2/*neu* expression in node-negative breast cancer: direct tissue quantitation by computerized image analysis and association of overexpression with increased risk of recurrent disease. Cancer Res 1993; 53:4960–70.

26. Press MF, Bernstein L, Thomas PA, *et al*. HER-2/*neu* gene amplification characterized by fluorescence *in situ* hybridization: poor prognosis in node-negative breast carcinomas. J Clin Oncol 1997; 15(8):2894–904.

27. Paik S, Hazen R, Fisher ER, *et al*. Pathologic findings from the National Surgical Adjuvant Breast and Bowel Project: prognostic significance of small erbB-2

protein overexpression in primary breast cancer. J Clin Oncol 1990; 8(1):103–12.

28. Allred DC, Clark GM, Tandon AK, *et al.* HER-2/*neu* in node-negative breast cancer: prognostic significance of overexpression influenced by the presence of *in situ* carcinoma. J Clin Oncol 1992; 10:599–605.

29. Gusterson BA, Gelber RD, Goldhirsch A, *et al.* Prognostic importance of c-erbB-2 expression in breast cancer. *J Clin Oncol* 1992; 10:1049–56.

30. Muss HB, Thor AD, Berry DA, *et al.* C-erbB-2 expression and response to adjuvant therapy in women with node positive early breast cancer. N Engl J Med 1994; 330:1260–6.

31. Carlomagno C, Perrone F, Gallo C, *et al.* C-erbB-2 overexpression decreases the benefit of adjuvant tamoxifen in early-stage breast cancer without axillary lymph node metastases. J Clin Oncol 1996; 14:2702–8.

32. Bianco AR, DeLaurentis M, Carlomagno C, *et al.* 20-year update of the Naples GUN trial of adjuvant breast cancer therapy: evidence of interaction between c-erbB-2 expression and tamoxifen efficacy. *Proceedings of ASCO* (Abstract 373), 1998.

33. Clinical practice guidelines of the use of tumor markers in breast and colorectal cancer. J Clin Oncol 1996; 14:2843–77.

34. Goldhirsch A, Wood WC, Senn HJ, Glick JH, Gelber RD. Meeting highlights: International Consensus Panel on the Treatment of Primary Breast Cancer. J Natl Cancer Inst 1995; 87(19):1441–5.

35. Goldhirsch A, Glick JH, Gelber RD, Senn H-J. Meeting highlights: International Consensus Panel on the Treatment of Primary Breast Cancer. J Natl Cancer Inst 1998; 90(21):1601–8.

Commentary

EDWARD M WOLIN

We live in an era when the detection of breast cancer in an early stage can be accomplished quite routinely. Screening mammography and careful self-examination, in addition to physician examination, have resulted in 40–50% of all newly diagnosed breast cancer patients having node-negative disease. Although prognosis is certainly better when lymph nodes are not involved, there is still a mortality risk for node-negative breast cancer that can range up to 30% or 40%, depending on the status of prognostic risk indicators. Although the initial trials which proved the benefit of adjuvant chemotherapy were conducted in women with positive lymph nodes, it is now clear that a similar percentage reduction in risk can be accomplished when chemotherapy is used with node-negative patients. This has resulted in a new generation of clinical trials, which are now in progress, intended to optimize the adjuvant chemotherapy strategies for these node-negative patients.

In order to determine whether adjuvant chemotherapy would be useful in a particular patient and to optimize the choice of chemotherapy program, all known predictive and prognostic markers are taken into consideration in treatment planning. However, this strategy is only useful in planning the treatment of a node-negative breast cancer if the axillary staging can be verified and there is sufficient certainty that the axillary lymph nodes are truly negative for metastatic malignancy. An accurate determination of 'node-negative' status requires a proper level I and level II surgical dissection of the axilla, with examination of at least ten axillary lymph nodes.[1] Risk assessment is more difficult when axillary staging is performed by sentinel lymph node biopsy or after neoadjuvant chemotherapy, because long-term follow-up in these situations is not available and both of these treatment strategies could result in understaging of the axilla. In addition, there is variability between pathology departments in the thoroughness of lymph node examination, with immunostaining for cytokeratin or obtaining multiple sections through each lymph node being techniques that yield a higher rate of lymph node positivity but are not universally applied.

Expression of estrogen and progesterone receptors in tumors is a major factor predicting the response to tamoxifen and other hormone therapies. However, the change in measurement technique to the use of an immunohistochemical assay has recently occurred, and the cut-off points to define endocrine responsiveness are still being defined[2] when immunostains for estrogen receptor and progesterone receptor are used.

For patients not being treated in a clinical trial, the consensus recommendations of the February 1998 6th International Conference on Adjuvant Therapy of Primary Breast Cancer, held at St Gallen, Switzerland, would appear to be the best course of action.[3] For those stage I patients with a chance of relapse estimated to be < 10% in 10 years, no adjuvant chemotherapy program would be recommended. This low-risk category is defined as patients with an invasive tumor ≤ 1 cm, positive estrogen and/or progesterone receptor, age ≥ 35, and grade 1 histology (probably any grade of tumor would still be low risk if the invasive component was ≤ 1 cm). For high-risk, node-negative patients (patients who have at least one high-risk feature: tumor > 2 cm, negative hormone receptors, grade 2–3, or age less than 35 years old), chemotherapy would usually be recommended for reduction of the risk of relapse, except in the elderly and for those women who could not medically or psychologically tolerate chemotherapy. Tamoxifen would be used for 5 years in addition to chemotherapy in all patients who are estrogen-receptor or progesterone-receptor positive, and could be used by itself in the elderly and in those unable to tolerate chemotherapy. Patients who have an intermediate risk of relapse (defined as falling between the low-risk category and high-risk category) would generally receive tamoxifen with or without chemotherapy.

The aggressiveness of the chemotherapy approach depends upon the estimated risk of recurrence without chemotherapy, considering all available prognostic factors, the age of the patient, and comorbid conditions. To choose between the multiple potentially effective chemotherapy regimens for a specific patient also requires a detailed discussion between the physician and patient regarding the potential risks and benefits of cyclophosphamide, methotrexate, fluorouracil (CMF)-type regimens versus anthracycline-containing regimens. If CMF is used, the 'classical' regimen, with oral cyclophosphamide on days 1–14, and intravenous methotrexate and 5-fluorouracil on days 1 and 8, repeated every 28 days, appears to be more effective than the intravenous CMF variance.[4] The meta-analysis of the Early Breast Trialists' Collaborative Group, published in 1998,[5] demonstrated that anthracycline-containing regimens (such as the combination of adriamycin plus cyclophosphamide) resulted in a 12% proportional reduction in recurrence risk compared with CMF, and appear to be superior regimens, although at a cost of some increased toxicity. Patients who overexpress Her-2/neu can be predicted to have a better outcome with anthracycline-based chemotherapy than with CMF.[6]

Adjuvant chemotherapy is certainly playing a major role in preventing relapse in women with node-negative breast cancer. However, the results are not yet good enough, because death from breast cancer is the usual outcome of systemic relapse after primary therapy, even though the disease may have started out as an early-stage disease with negative lymph nodes. Approaches now being investigated to improve the results of adjuvant chemotherapy in node-negative breast cancer include the integration of taxanes (docetaxel and paclitaxel) into adjuvant chemotherapy programs, and the use of the recombinant humanized anti-Her-2 monoclonal antibody known as trastuzumab (Herceptin[R]). It is expected that, as other novel approaches of antineoplastic therapy prove useful in the setting of metastatic disease, they will also be investigated in the adjuvant setting to advance the goal of curing all women with breast cancer using low-toxicity programs.

REFERENCES

1. Axelsdon CK, Mouridsen HT, Zedeler K. Axillary dissection of Level I and Level II lymph nodes is important in breast cancer classification. The Danish Breast Cancer Cooperative Group (DBCG). Eur J Cancer 1992; 28A:1415–18.

2. Clark GM, Harvey JM, Osborne CK, Allred DC. Estrogen receptor status (ER) determined by immunohistochemistry (IHC) is superior to biochemical ligand-binding (LB) assay for evaluating breast cancer patients [abstract 454]. Proc ASCO 1997; 16:129a.

3. Goldhirsch A, Glick JH, Gelber RD, Senn H-J. Meeting highlights: International Consensus Panel on the Treatment of Primary Breast Cancer. J Natl Cancer Inst 1998; 90(21):1601–8.

4. Fisher B, Dignam J, Wolmark N, et al. Tamoxifen and chemotherapy for lymph node negative, estrogen receptor positive breast cancer. J Natl Cancer Inst 1997; 89:1673–82.

5. Early Breast Cancer Trialists' Collaborative Group. Polychemotherapy for early breast cancer: an overview of the randomised trials. Lancet 1998; 352:930–42.

6. Andrulis IL, Bull SB, Blackstein ME, et al. neu/erbB-2 amplification identifies a poor prognosis group of women with node negative breast cancer. J Clin Oncol 1998; 16:1340–9.

Editors' selected abstracts

Local and distant failures after limited surgery with positive margins and radiotherapy for node-negative breast cancer.

Cowen D, Houvenaeghel G, Bardou V, Jacquemier J, Bautrant E, Conte M, Viens P, Largillier R, Puig B, Resbeut M, Maraninchi D.

Department of Radiation Oncology, Institut Paoli-Calmettes Cancer Center and Reseau Convergence Cancer (R2C), Marseille, France.

International Journal of Radiation Oncology, Biology, Physics 47:305–12, 2000, May 1.

Purpose: To determine the outcome of patients with positive margins after lumpectomy for breast cancer and to address the issue of the relationship between local recurrences and distant metastasis in the absence of chemotherapy. Methods and materials: Among 3697 patients with primary breast cancer, we retrospectively analyzed 152 patients who had undergone conservative surgery with axillary dissection, had infiltrating carcinomas with positive margins, were node-negative, and received radiotherapy without chemotherapy. One-third received hormonal therapy. Endpoints were local failure and distant metastasis. Median follow-up was 72 months. Results: Five- and 10-year recurrence-free survival were 0.80 and 0.71 respectively for local recurrences, and 0.85 and 0.73 respectively for metastasis. Infiltrating carcinoma on the margins was associated with early local relapse as opposed to intraductal carcinoma. Local and distant recurrences had similar patterns of yearly-event probabilities. Hazard of relapsing from metastasis was 2.5 times higher after a local recurrence. In the multivariate analysis, negative estrogen receptors (ER−) ($p = 0.0012$), histologic multifocality ($p = 0.0028$), and no hormonal therapy ($p = 0.017$) predicted local relapses, while ER− ($p = 0.004$) and pathologic grade ($p = 0.009$) predicted metastasis. Hormonal therapy did not prevent early local recurrences. *Conclusion*: In this population, reexcision is advisable for local purposes and because the data support the hypothesis that local and distant recurrences are tightly connected.

High local recurrence risk after breast-conserving therapy in node-negative premenopausal breast cancer patients is greatly reduced by one course of perioperative chemotherapy: a European Organization for Research and Treatment of Cancer Breast Cancer Cooperative Group Study.

Elkhuizen PH, van Slooten HJ, Clahsen PC, Hermans J, van de Velde CJ, van den Broek LC, van de Vijver MJ.

Departments of Clinical Oncology, Leiden University Medical Center, Leiden, The Netherlands.

Journal of Clinical Oncology 18(5):1075–83, 2000, March.

Purpose: Patients with invasive breast cancer may develop a local recurrence (LR) after breast-conserving therapy (BCT). Younger age has been found to be an independent risk factor for LR. Within a group of premenopausal node-negative breast cancer patients, we studied risk factors for LR and the effect of perioperative chemotherapy (PeCT) on LR. *Patients and methods:* The European Organization for Research and Treatment of Cancer (EORTC) conducted a randomized trial (EORTC 10854) to compare surgery followed by one course of PeCT (fluorouracil, doxorubicin, and cyclophosphamide) with surgery alone. From patients treated on this trial, we selected premenopausal patients with node-negative breast cancer who were treated with BCT to examine whether histologic characteristics and the expression of various proteins (estrogen receptor, progesterone receptor, p53, Ki-67, bcl-2, CD31, c-erbB-2/*neu*) are risk factors for subsequent LR. Also, the effect of one course of PeCT on the LR risk (LRR) was studied. *Results:* Using multivariate analysis, age younger than 43 years (relative risk [RR], 2.75; 95% confidence interval [CI], 1.46 to 5.18; $p = 0.002$), multifocal growth (RR, 3.34; 95% CI, 1.27 to 8.77; $p = 0.014$), and elevated levels of p53 (RR, 2.14; 95% CI, 1.13 to 4.05; $p = 0.02$) were associated with higher LRR. Also, PeCT was found to reduce LRR by more than 50% (RR, 0.47; 95% CI, 0.25 to 0.86; $p = 0.02$). Patients younger than 43 years who received PeCT achieved similar LR rates as those of patients younger than 43 years who were treated with BCT alone. *Conclusion:* In premenopausal node-negative patients, age younger than 43 years is the most important risk factor for LR after BCT; this risk is greatly reduced by one course of PeCT. The main reason for administering systemic adjuvant treatment is to improve overall survival. The important reduction of LR after BCT is an additional reason for considering systemic treatment in young node-negative patients with breast cancer.

Tamoxifen and chemotherapy for axillary node-negative, estrogen receptor-negative breast cancer: findings from national surgical adjuvant breast and bowel project B-23.

Fisher B, Anderson S, Tan-Chiu E, Wolmark N, Wickerham DL, Fisher ER, Dimitrov NV, Atkins JN, Abramson N, Merajver S, Romond EH, Kardinal CG, Shibata HR, Margolese RG, Farrar WB.

National Surgical Adjuvant Breast and Bowel Project, 4 Allegheny Center, Suite 602, Pittsburgh, PA, USA

Journal of Clinical Oncology 19(4):931–42, 2001, February 15.

Purpose: Uncertainty about the relative worth of doxorubicin/cyclophosphamide (AC) and cyclophosphamide/methotrexate/fluorouracil (CMF), as well as doubt about the propriety of giving tamoxifen (TAM) with chemotherapy to patients with estrogen receptor-negative tumors and negative axillary nodes, prompted the National Surgical Adjuvant and Breast and Bowel Project to initiate the B-23 study. *Patients and methods:* Patients ($n = 2,008$) were randomly assigned to CMF plus placebo, CMF plus TAM, AC plus placebo, or AC plus TAM. Six cycles of CMF were given for 6 months; four cycles of AC were administered for 63 days. TAM was given daily for 5 years. Relapse-free survival (RFS), event-free survival (EFS), and survival (S) were determined by using life-table estimates. Tests for heterogeneity of outcome used log-rank statistics and Cox proportional hazards models to detect differences across all groups and according to chemotherapy and hormonal therapy status. *Results:* No significant difference in RFS, EFS, or S was observed among the four groups through 5 years ($p = 0.96$, 0.8, and 0.8, respectively), for those aged ≤49 years ($p = 0.97$, 0.5, and 0.9, respectively), or for those aged ≥50 years ($p = 0.7$, 0.6, and 0.6, respectively). A comparison between all CMF- and all AC-treated patients demonstrated no significant differences in RFS (87% at 5 years in both groups, $p = 0.9$), EFS (83% and 82%, $p = 0.6$), or S (89% and 90%, $p = 0.4$). There were no significant differences in RFS, EFS, or S between CMF and AC in patients aged ≤49 or ≥50 years. No significant difference in any outcome was observed when chemotherapy-treated patients who received placebo were compared with those given TAM. RFS in both groups was 87% ($p = 0.6$), 87% in patients aged ≤49 ($p = 0.9$), and 88% and 87%, respectively ($p = 0.4$), in those aged ≥50 years. *Conclusion:* There was no significant difference in the outcome of patients who received AC or CMF. TAM with either regimen resulted in no significant advantage over that achieved from chemotherapy alone.

Prognosis and treatment of patients with breast tumors of one centimeter or less and negative axillary lymph nodes.

Fisher B, Dignam J, Tan-Chiu E, Anderson S, Fisher ER, Wittliff JL, Wolmark N.

National Surgical Adjuvant Breast and Bowel Project, 4 Allegheny Center, Suite 602, Pittsburgh, PA, USA.

Journal of the National Cancer Institute 93(2):112–20, 2001, January 17.

Background: Uncertainty about prognosis and treatment of axillary lymph node-negative patients with estrogen receptor (ER)-negative or ER-positive invasive breast tumors of 1 cm or less prompted the analysis of data from five

National Surgical Adjuvant Breast and Bowel Project randomized clinical trials. *Methods:* Two hundred thirty-five patients with ER-negative tumors and 1024 patients with ER-positive tumors were identified in these trials. Patients with ER-negative tumors received surgery alone or surgery and chemotherapy. Patients with ER-positive tumors received surgery alone; surgery and tamoxifen; or surgery, tamoxifen, and chemotherapy. End points were relapse-free survival (RFS), event-free survival, and overall survival. A result was considered to be statistically significant with a p value of 0.05 or less; all statistical tests were two-sided. *Results:* The 8-year RFS of women with ER-negative tumors who received surgery alone or with chemotherapy was 81% and 90%, respectively ($p = 0.06$). Survival was similar in both groups (93% and 91%; $p = 0.65$). The 8-year RFS of women with ER-positive tumors was 86% after surgery alone, 93% when tamoxifen was added ($p = 0.01$), and 95% after the addition of tamoxifen and chemotherapy ($p = 0.07$ compared with tamoxifen). Survival in the three groups was 90%, 92% ($p = 0.41$), and 97%, respectively. The difference between the latter two groups was significant ($p = 0.01$). Regardless of ER status or treatment, overall mortality was 8%; one half of the deaths were related to breast cancer. Several covariates affected the risk of recurrence in ER-negative and ER-positive patients. Risk was greater in women with tumors of 1 cm than in those with tumors of less than 1 cm, in women aged 49 years or younger than in those aged 50 years or older, and in women with infiltrating ductal or lobular carcinoma than in those with other histologic tumor types. *Conclusions:* Chemotherapy and/or tamoxifen should be considered for the treatment of women with ER-negative or ER-positive tumors of 1 cm or less and negative axillary lymph nodes.

Primary node negative breast cancer in *BRCA1* mutation carriers has a poor outcome.

Foulkes WD, Chappuis PO, Wong N, Brunet JS, Vesprini D, Rozen F, Yuan ZQ, Pollak MN, Kuperstein G, Narod SA, Begin LR.

Department of Medicine, Sir M.B. Davis–Jewish General Hospital, Montreal, Quebec, Canada.

Annals of Oncology 11(3):307–13, 2000, March.

Background: The association between *BRCA1* germ-line mutations and breast cancer prognosis is controversial. A historical cohort study was designed to determine the prognosis for women with axillary lymph node negative hereditary breast cancer. *Patients and methods:* We tested pathology blocks from 118 Ashkenazi Jewish women with axillary lymph node negative breast cancer for the presence of the two common *BRCA1* founder mutations, 185delAG and 5382insC. Patients were followed up for a median of 76 months. Somatic *TP53* mutations were screened for by immunohistochemistry, and direct sequencing was performed in the *BRCA1*-positive tumours. *Results:* Sixteen breast cancer blocks (13.6%) carried a *BRCA1* mutation. Young age of onset, high nuclear grade, negative estrogen receptor status and over-expression of *p53* were highly associated with *BRCA1*-positive status (*p*-values all < 0.01). *BRCA1* mutation carriers had a higher mortality than non-carriers (five-year overall survival, 50% and 89.6%, respectively,

$p = 0.0001$). Young age of onset, estrogen receptor negative status, nuclear grade 3, and over-expression of *p53* also predicted a poor outcome. Cox multivariate analyses showed that only germ-line *BRCA1* mutation status was an independent prognostic factor for overall survival ($p = 0.01$). Among nuclear grade 3 tumours, the *BRCA1* mutation carrier status was a significant prognostic factor of death (risk ratio 5.8, 95% confidence interval: 1.5–22, $p = 0.009$). Sequencing of *BRCA1*-related breast cancers revealed one *TP53* missense mutation not previously reported in breast cancer. *Conclusions:* Using a historical cohort approach, we have identified *BRCA1* mutation status as an independent prognostic factor for node negative breast cancer among the Ashkenazi Jewish women. Those managing women carrying a *BRCA1* mutation may need to take these findings into consideration. Additionally, our preliminary results, taken together with the work of others, suggest a different carcinogenic pathway in *BRCA1*-related breast cancer, compared to non-hereditary cases.

Cathepsin B, a prognostic indicator in lymph node-negative breast carcinoma patients: comparison with cathepsin D, cathepsin L, and other clinical indicators.

Lah TT, Cercek M, Blejec A, Kos J, Gorodetsky E, Somers R, Daskal I.

Department of Genetic Toxicology and Cancer Biology, National Institute of Biology, Ljubljana, Slovenia.

Clinical Cancer Research 6(2):578–84, 2000, February.

New prognosticators are needed for breast cancer patients after the initial surgical treatment to make therapeutic decisions that ultimately will affect their DFS. These consist of specific proteolytic enzymes including lysosomal endopeptidases. In this study, the activity and protein concentrations of cathepsins (Cats) D, B, and L were measured in 282 invasive breast tumor cytosols. These potential biological prognostic indicators were compared with other histopathological parameters, such as tumor size, lymph node involvement, tumor-node-metastasis stage, histological grade, DNA analysis, and steroid receptors. CatD protein concentration correlated with lymph node involvement. CatB and CatL levels correlated significantly with Scarf–Bloom–Richardson histological grade and were also higher in estrogen-negative tumors, and CatB was higher in larger tumors. As prognostic markers, CatB concentration was significant for increased risk for recurrence in the entire patient population and specifically also in lymph node-negative patients as follows: high CatB concentration (above 371 micrograms/g) in tumor cytosols was significant ($p < 0.00$) for high risk of recurrence but was of only borderline prognostic significance ($p < 0.06$) for overall survival of all patients. In lymph node-negative patients, CatB (above 240 micrograms/g, $p < 0.003$) was highly significant for recurrence-free survival, followed by CatL (above 20 micrograms/g, $p < 0.049$) and CatD (above 45 nmol/g, $p < 0.044$) concentrations. For overall survival of node-negative patients, only CatB was a significant ($p < 0.014$) prognosticator. We conclude that CatB is useful as a prognostic indicator in lymph node-negative patients. This suggests that selective adjuvant therapy should be applied in this lower risk group of patients when high levels of CatB are determined.

14

Neoadjuvant therapy in the treatment of breast cancer

LESLIE MEMSIC

INTRODUCTION

The benefits of chemotherapy in preventing recurrence and metastases and in prolonging survival in patients with breast cancer have long been established. Long-term results of randomized, controlled studies by the NSABP,[1] National Cancer Institute of Italy,[2] and the Dana–Farber Cancer Institute[3] all confirm the statistical improvement in relapse-free and absolute survival in those breast cancer patients with positive nodes treated with chemotherapy. The best drug regimen and optimal treatment duration remain under investigation, but clearly combination chemotherapy makes a significant difference in the treatment of node-positive breast cancer and is the standard of care. Traditionally, chemotherapy is given as adjuvant therapy after local treatment, such as surgery, in those patients at high risk for systemic disease.

As chemotherapeutic agents have improved in efficacy, and side-effects have been minimized by both antiemetic pretreatment and rescue therapy with bone marrow stimulators, the indications for chemotherapy have broadened to incorporate more and more women with breast cancer.

Initially reserved for patients with node-positive disease, recent data from the NSABP and others[4–7] demonstrate the value of adjuvant chemotherapy in the treatment of node-negative breast cancer patients as well. Combination chemotherapy reduces the annual odds of recurrence by at least 30% in patients with node-negative breast cancer. A specific individual's benefit from chemotherapy depends upon how likely it is that her cancer will recur. The more aggressive features a tumor displays, based on size, histological grade, hormone receptor status, proliferative rate, and the expression of the HER-2/neu gene, the more likely it is that she will benefit from adjuvant chemotherapy.

RATIONALE FOR NEOADJUVANT THERAPY

Neoadjuvant chemotherapy, also known as preoperative, primary, or induction chemotherapy, is defined as the use of systemic chemotherapy before local treatment of the primary lesion with surgery and/or irradiation. The concept of neoadjuvant chemotherapy derives from pre-clinical and clinical evidence which collectively suggests that, in women who have a high risk of harboring micrometastatic disease, early and effective treatment by systemic chemotherapy may be necessary to improve the clinical outcome of locoregional therapy.

The biologic rationale for this approach is based on a variety of observations. Studies in animal models have demonstrated that the removal of a primary tumor may accelerate the rate of growth of micrometastases. Fisher et al. proposed the existence of a serum growth factor and showed that the antitumor efficacy of cyclophosphamide was greater in preventing distant metastases when administered preoperatively rather than postoperatively.[8,9]

More recent evidence points toward production of angiogenesis inhibitors by the primary tumor, the removal of which before effective systemic chemotherapy may allow neovascularization and result in the growth of micrometastases.[10,11] Goldie and Coldman proposed that, as the number of tumor cells increases, the likelihood of the development of chemoresistant clones also increases.[12] According to their hypothesis, the proliferation of these clones, which may be a critical reason for the failure of adjuvant chemotherapy of cancer, may be minimized by the early administration of chemotherapy. Thus, the use of neoadjuvant chemotherapy has the potential clinical advantages of treating metastases at the earliest possible time and avoiding accelerated growth of micrometastases after resection of the primary tumor (via the release of serum growth factors or loss of angiostatic control), thereby preventing the development of chemoresistant tumor clones.

In addition, decreasing the size of the primary may transform unresectable tumors into resectable ones, allow breast conservation in those patients initially candidates for mastectomy only, and improve local control. In contrast to the standard use of adjuvant chemotherapy to treat occult disease that may or may not be present, primary chemotherapy allows for immediate objective assessment of response. This may be an important prognosticator for the ultimate outcome for the patient. Response or the lack of a response by the primary tumor may also be used to alter therapy. Patients with breast cancer who have had significant residual disease after chemotherapy have very poor prognoses, and subsequent treatment has not had much impact.[13,14] However, with the advent of new chemotherapeutic agents, including the taxanes and monoclonal antibodies, alternative treatments may be devised with potentially better outcomes in these patients.[15,16,17]

Perhaps more importantly for long-term progress in cancer treatment, the response of the primary tumor can be used to test new drugs and regimens more rapidly than is possible for standard adjuvant strategies. Primary chemotherapy allows for important detailed studies of the relationship of different pathologic and molecular markers to responsiveness, which can advance our understanding of cancer biology and chemoresistance.

NEOADJUVANT THERAPY FOR LOCALLY ADVANCED BREAST CANCER

Neoadjuvant chemotherapy for breast cancer was first proposed for use in patients with locally advanced or inoperable breast cancer. The designation of locally advanced breast carcinoma (LABC) is a heterogeneous group of tumors ranging from neglected, relatively slow growing, large, primary tumors to small breast tumors presenting with extensive nodal metastases. LABC corresponds to stage III as defined by the International Union Against Cancer–American Joint Committee on Cancer (UICC–AJCC) system. Inflammatory carcinoma characterized by diffuse edema and erythema of the breast, and defined pathologically by the presence of tumor emboli in the dermal lymphatics, is a particularly virulent form of an LABC. The biologic diversity seen in LABC makes the comparison of different treatment results and the formation of a single treatment recommendation for all women difficult.

Despite increasing recognition by physicians and the public of the importance of screening and early detection to decrease breast cancer mortality, 10–20% of women with breast cancer have locally advanced disease at diagnosis,[18,19] and its prevalence worldwide has been estimated to be as high as 70%. Although clinical features

at presentation and prognosis among women with LABC vary, there are two common problems in the treatment of these patients: achieving local control, and prolonging survival by preventing or delaying distant metastases.

Historically, the treatment of LABC was surgical, with dismal results. In 1942, Haagensen and Stout developed the Columbia Clinical Classification of Breast Cancer, based on 1135 carcinomas treated at Columbia Presbyterian Hospital from 1915 through 1942.[20] This classification identified clinical features associated with a high local recurrence rate and poor survival after surgery. Radical mastectomy in these patients was associated with a 53% local failure rate and 0% 5-year disease-free survival. Haagensen identified five grave signs denoting inoperability, including edema, ulceration of the skin overlying the breast, tumor fixed to the chest wall, fixed axillary lymph nodes, or axillary lymph nodes greater than 2.5 cm.

The first non-operative therapy utilized in patients with LABC was irradiation. Early studies demonstrated a dose-dependent relationship between radiation and local control. Increasing the dose of radiation increased the likelihood of local tumor control, but, at the same time, increased the risk of debilitating complications, including fibrosis, necrosis, and arm edema. More importantly, in patients with LABC, radiation, like surgery, resulted in unsatisfactory local control, and the majority of patients continued to die of distant metastatic disease. Bedwinek et al. observed that 65% of 43 women with non-inflammatory T4 lesions failed locally after treatment doses of 4000–7000 cGy.[21] Rubens et al. reported that the treatment of inoperable stage III cancer with radiotherapy alone resulted in poor local control (28% at 5 years) and very low overall survival (13% at 5 years).[22] Similarly, Zucali et al. reported that median survival among 454 T3 and T4 patients treated with radiation therapy alone was only 2.1 years. When surgery could be performed after radiation therapy, median survival was improved to 13.9 years. However, surgery was only undertaken in a small number of patients who had a complete response to radiation.[23]

Terz et al. prospectively planned preoperative radiation therapy followed by surgery for patients with 'borderline operable' stage III breast cancer. Median survival in these patients was 55 months, but the 5-year disease-free survival rate was only 17%.[24]

With the development of effective chemotherapy for breast cancer and response rates greater or equal to 50% in patients with metastatic disease, several groups in the 1970s and 1980s began using primary neoadjuvant chemotherapy for patients with inoperable breast cancer or LABC. De Lena et al. reported a prospective, randomized study including 132 women with LABC. A response rate of 85% was noted for patients treated with doxorubicin and vincristine.[25] Similarly high response rates were noted in subsequent studies using a variety of agents.

In 1983 Hortobagyi et al., at M.D. Anderson, reported their results for non-inflammatory inoperable breast cancer using chemotherapy – 5-fluorouracil (5-FU), adriamycin, cytoxan (FAC) – as the first treatment modality. With selective use of surgery, local control was 79%, and overall survival at 5 years was 55%.[26] Multiple groups confirmed the improvement in outcomes in patients with LABC and inflammatory cancer with the addition of neoadjuvant chemotherapy.

In reviewing the literature, however, it is not clear that the benefit is dependent so much on chemotherapy given preoperatively as it is on the use of any systemic chemotherapy rather than local treatment alone. Because of the historic development of this approach with a subset of patients deemed inoperable, it was generally assumed that giving primary chemotherapy was the key to improved outcomes. However, multiple studies suggest that adjuvant chemotherapy results in survival that is similar to that with neoadjuvant chemotherapy for LABC. In fact, one of the few trials specifically addressing this showed no differences in survival, but there were only 12 patients in each group.[27]

While the available data do not prove conclusively that LABC or inoperable breast cancer necessarily constitutes an absolute indication for primary chemotherapy, for those patients with LABC, particularly those with T4 tumors, inflammatory cancer, or N2 or N3 nodal disease, primary surgery is not a realistic option, and primary radiotherapy for bulky disease is often suboptimal. The radiation doses needed to treat such patients primarily, even with hyperfractionation, are frequently associated with significant morbidity and poor cosmesis. Surgical intervention after high-dose radiation therapy may also be more complex and morbid. Therefore, in most patients with LABC, neoadjuvant chemotherapy is strongly preferred. Whether or not it is associated with a clear-cut survival advantage, primary chemotherapy may make unresectable cancers resectable and may reduce the scope and difficulty of surgery. Its use will make it less likely that skin grafts or complex reconstruction will be required, and it may also avoid the need for surgery in a previously irradiated field.[28] Chemotherapy may also decrease the intensity and morbidity of the irradiation needed to treat the breast and chest wall. Furthermore, the presence of residual disease in the breast or lymph nodes may indicate the need for further and/or different systemic treatment postoperatively. Neoadjuvant chemotherapy may also improve survival in subsets of patients and may allow breast conservation therapy in patients who previously could not be made disease free, even with radical surgery. In 1986, Hery et al. reported on 25 patients with LABC treated with primary chemotherapy.[29] Treatment comprised radiation therapy after three cycles of doxorubicin, vincristine, cyclophosphamide, and 5-FU, followed by a second course of chemotherapy upon completion of radiation. Local control was achieved in 76% of these patients, and overall survival

was 56% at 5 years. Jacquillat et al. reported a series of 98 patients with stage IIIA and IIIB disease treated with induction chemotherapy using four to six cycles of vinblastine, thiotepa, methotrexate, 5-FU, doxorubicin, and prednisone, followed by radiation, followed by 24 more cycles of chemotherapy.[30] The early results of this intensive approach demonstrated the achievement of disease-free states, without mastectomy, and overall survival rates at 3 years of 75%.

Other investigators have proven the feasibility of breast conservation therapy in patients with LABC treated with neoadjuvant chemotherapy. Of importance, however, is adhering to the basic surgical oncologic principle of obtaining clear margins. Merajver et al. demonstrated 61% of patients with an apparent complete clinical response were found to have cancer present on histological examination.[31] Patients with a clinically apparent complete clinical response should undergo biopsy or surgical resection to confirm this finding. The presence of occult residual cancer is of particular concern for regimens that eliminate surgical excision of the primary site after chemotherapy, depending on radiation therapy to control residual local disease. Patients who respond dramatically to induction chemotherapy, but cannot be cleared pathologically by lumpectomy, require mastectomy.

Neoadjuvant chemotherapy has become established as the preferred treatment approach for patients with LABC, particularly stage IIIB breast cancer, but a number of questions remain to be answered. Investigations are ongoing to determine the optimal agents and regimens. The relative merits of using alternative sequential or combined drug strategies with non-cross-resistant drugs (such as doxorubicin and the taxanes) have not been defined, nor has the role of high-dose chemotherapy, which has not been proven to improve survival over more standard regimens to date. In fact, it is not clear that additional chemotherapy is always needed after a good response to neoadjuvant therapy and local treatment. Nor has it been demonstrated that additional systemic treatment will benefit patients who have had a poor or incomplete response to preoperative chemotherapy. If additional adjuvant chemotherapy would be beneficial, would the complete or partial responders benefit most? The optimal duration of chemotherapy before and after locoregional therapy is also undefined.

NEOADJUVANT THERAPY IN OPERABLE BREAST CANCER

The high response rates seen with neoadjuvant chemotherapy in the treatment of LABC and inoperable breast cancers prompted oncologists to consider its use in patients with operable breast cancers, particularly those with larger lesions. The use of primary chemotherapy in these patients has definite potential benefits.

Clinically, neoadjuvant chemotherapy allows for the assessment of tumor response to treatment. If a tumor does not respond, appropriate changes in therapeutic regimen can be made. In addition, the reduction of tumor size may downstage the patient such that breast conservation surgery may be undertaken in higher percentages. The theoretical advantages of neoadjuvant chemotherapy in LABC also apply to operable breast cancer. Primary chemotherapy may treat undetected micrometastases promptly and prevent the accelerated growth of metastases through angiogenetic and serum growth factors stimulated by tumor resection, thereby decreasing the likelihood of developing chemoresistant tumor cell clones.

Bonadonna et al. first reported the use of neoadjuvant chemotherapy for the treatment of operable breast cancer in 1990.[32] They concluded that neoadjuvant chemotherapy resulted in significant downstaging, allowing for breast conservation in 127 of 161 women who would otherwise have undergone mastectomy. Guidelines for breast conservation therapy in Italy at the time of the study dictated mastectomy for tumors $\geqslant 3$ cm. Using current guidelines for breast conservation therapy, it is unclear what percentage of these patients could have had breast conservation therapy at the time of initial presentation.

Calais et al. reported 158 patients with operable breast cancer > 3 cm treated with neoadjuvant chemotherapy.[33] The mean tumor size was 5.6 cm. Patients were treated with three courses of two different chemotherapeutic agents. The overall response rate was 60.8%, with 20.2% of patients achieving complete clinical response. After undergoing neoadjuvant chemotherapy, 48% of patients were successfully treated with breast conservation surgery. Age, tumor stage, histology, menopausal status, and hormone receptor status were found to have no predictive value for tumor response.

These and multiple studies confirm the high response rate of primary operative breast cancer to neoadjuvant chemotherapy similar to that seen in LABC. However, even with the treatment of smaller tumors, complete response was rare. Breast conservation rates appear to be increased, but survival benefits could not be assessed.

A number of randomized trials addressing the issue of neoadjuvant chemotherapy for operable breast cancer have also been performed. Mauriac et al. randomly allocated 272 women with tumors > 3 cm either to primary chemotherapy with epirubicin, vincristine, and methotrexate for three cycles, and mitomycin C, thiotepa, and vindesine for three cycles, followed by local treatment, or to primary modified radical mastectomy followed by chemotherapy in patients with positive nodes or receptor-negative tumors.[34] In the neoadjuvant chemotherapy group, 84 of 134 patients had breast conservation therapy, including 44 patients who were treated with radiation therapy alone and no surgery. Not surprisingly, in view of the incomplete pathological responses seen in other trials, the neoadjuvant chemotherapy group had a higher local recurrence rate, which may have been a result of inadequate treatment of the primary without surgery in those patients with apparent, but not pathologic, complete clinical responses. The group treated with preoperative chemotherapy did have a higher rate of survival. However, while this may have resulted from the sequence of treatments, it can also be explained by the fact that all the patients in the primary group received chemotherapy, whereas only 104 of 138 in the primary surgery group received adjuvant chemotherapy. By current standards, all these patients may have received adjuvant chemotherapy regardless of nodal status. In the UK, Powles et al. conducted a prospective, randomized trial in 212 patients with operable breast cancer diagnosed by fine-needle aspirate.[35] More than 50% of patients had tumors > 3 cm in diameter. Standard adjuvant chemotherapy with mitoxantrone, methotrexate, mitomycin C, and tamoxifen, for eight cycles following surgery was compared with neoadjuvant chemotherapy with four cycles of chemotherapy given before surgery and four cycles given after surgery. The combined complete clinical response and partial response rate for the neoadjuvant chemotherapy group was 85%; 10% of patients had pathological complete clinical responses. The rate of mastectomy was decreased by neoadjuvant chemotherapy from 28% to 13% ($p < 0.005$), but the small size of the study makes any meaningful survival comparison impossible. In Paris, Scholl et al. studied 414 women with T3 or T4 breast cancers with N0 or N1 nodal disease.[36] These patients were randomized either to four cycles of neoadjuvant chemotherapy (FAC) followed by radiation therapy or to primary radiotherapy followed by four cycles of FAC. In both arms of the study, surgery was used only if there was a persistent mass after chemotherapy and radiation. Overall survival was statistically significantly greater with primary chemotherapy (86% versus 78%) at 5 years, and the breast conservation rate was higher in the primary chemotherapy group compared to those who received chemotherapy as an adjuvant (82% versus 77%). The difference in disease-free survival was not statistically significant (59% versus 55%).

The improved survival with chemotherapy may have resulted from the sequence of treatments or may simply reflect the fact that the neoadjuvant chemotherapy group was able to receive a higher dose-intensity treatment, but this may be an additional advantage of primary chemotherapy. The National Surgical Adjuvant Breast and Bowel Project (NSABP) completed a randomized trial of 1523 patients, comparing four cycles of preoperative chemotherapy (adriamycin and cytoxan) with the same treatment given after surgery for patients with operable breast cancer.[37] Analysis of this trial (B-18) indicates that preoperative chemotherapy downstages disease at the primary site and nodes and increases the use of breast-conserving therapy with overall survival that is at least equal to that achieved with standard adjuvant chemotherapy.

Neoadjuvant chemotherapy for patients with operable breast cancer has both real and theoretical advantages over traditional therapy. The main disadvantages associated with this approach are related to a lack of preoperative prognostic information and the risk of overtreatment or undertreatment. Pretreatment pathologic axillary lymph node status is unknown. Posttreatment axillary lymph node downstaging can result in undertreatment of patients who would have otherwise had large numbers of positive lymph nodes. This depends, of course, on accepting the still unproven premise that more aggressive chemotherapy (i.e., high-dose chemotherapy with stem-cell support) results in improved survival for a subset of high-risk patients (i.e., women with more than six to ten positive lymph nodes). It also assumes that patients who have been downstaged require more aggressive therapy than they have already received with good response. Overtreatment of patients with gross ductal carcinoma *in situ* or tumors with favorable histology might result from the incomplete sampling of the primary lesion provided by fine-needle aspirate or core-needle biopsy. Four percent of patients in the adjuvant arm of Powles *et al.*'s study were found to have gross ductal carcinoma *in situ* (DCIS), and presumably a similar number of these patients had been overtreated by the neoadjuvant arm. Precise histological grading of a small biopsy sample is difficult. The identification of accurate markers of prognosis that can be detected in the limited biopsy material provided by fine-needle aspirate or core-needle biopsy may allow chemotherapy treatment to be individualized and minimize overtreatment and undertreatment problems associated with neoadjuvant chemotherapy. Alternatively, as new chemotherapeutic agents become available with added efficacy and fewer side-effects, and indications for chemotherapy in patients with breast cancer (including DCIS) broaden and become standardized across the board, these issues may become moot.

The objective evaluation of a patient's response to neoadjuvant chemotherapy poses another problem in utilizing this treatment regimen. Chemotherapy-induced fibrosis may be confused with residual tumor, and clinical measurement can be inaccurate. Segel *et al.* concluded that mammography is complementary to clinical examination in the assessment of the response to neoadjuvant chemotherapy.[38] Other investigators have shown mammography to be inaccurate in differentiating residual disease from chemotherapy-induced fibrosis.[39–42] Magnetic resonance imaging (MRI) can distinguish between fibrosis and tumor and is the best method currently available for this task. Ultrasound, positron emission tomography (PET), and 2-methoxy isobutyl isonitrite (MIBI) scanning have all been utilized less successfully. Abraham *et al.* reported on 39 patients with stage II, III, or IV breast cancer who were prospectively evaluated before and after neoadjuvant chemotherapy, using MRI, physical examination, and

mammography. Detailed pathologic correlation of residual disease was obtained. The clinical evaluation of tumor response was made by both surgical and medical oncologists. Abraham *et al.* found that MRI accurately predicted the pathologic determination of residual disease in 97% of cases. The medical and surgical oncologists' clinical assessment of response agreed with the MRI results in 55% and 52% of cases, respectively. Mammography correlated with the MRI response in 52% of cases.[41]

SURGICAL TREATMENT AFTER NEOADJUVANT THERAPY

Surgical treatment following neoadjuvant therapy raises several issues. Multiple studies confirm the equivalence of modified radical mastectomy and lumpectomy, axillary dissection and radiation therapy in patients with tumor/breast ratios amenable to breast conservation therapy at diagnosis. Can these results be applied to those patients who became breast conservation therapy candidates after neoadjuvant chemotherapy? How extensive must resection be post-chemotherapy, and what should be excised in patients with a complete response? Do these patients require surgery at all? Several trials studying neoadjuvant chemotherapy did not include surgery for all patients. Scholl *et al.* included surgery only if a mass persisted after primary chemotherapy and radiotherapy or radiotherapy alone. The trial of Calais *et al.* omitted surgery for patients with clinical and mammographic complete tumor regression following neoadjuvant therapy, treating them with radiation alone. Neither study compared local recurrence rates for patients with neoadjuvant chemotherapy, followed by breast irradiation alone, with those for patients given neoadjuvant therapy followed by surgery with or without radiation therapy (breast conservation therapy patients). Previous studies have shown local recurrence rates to be high in patients treated with radiotherapy alone.[43] Neoadjuvant chemotherapy followed by breast irradiation alone for LABC has also resulted in high locoregional failure rates.[44] The efficacy of neoadjuvant chemotherapy followed by breast irradiation alone in providing adequate local control for patients with operable breast cancer remains to be determined, but it is likely to be inadequate, except perhaps in patients who exhibit a complete pathologic response to chemotherapy. This is difficult to determine definitively without resection. Brenin and Morrow note that the method of tumor shrinkage in response to chemotherapy may be variable.[45] The tumor may shrink concentrically to a smaller but discrete mass, or cell death may occur randomly throughout the tumor, resulting in fibrosis and nests of viable tumor cells left behind throughout the initial tumor volume. Singletary *et al.* reported on 143 patients with LABC who responded to induction chemotherapy and then underwent mastectomy. Pathological examination of the mastectomy specimens revealed tumor in more than one quadrant of the breast in 38% of patients. Patients with larger residual tumors ($>4\,cm$), persistent skin edema, lymphatic invasion, and multicentric lesions evident on mammography were more likely to have multiquadrant disease at the time of mastectomy.[46] In multiple trials, complete clinical and radiologic response did not translate into complete pathologic remissions for the majority of patients. Residual gross and/or microscopic disease was found at surgery in more than two-thirds of patients who were reported to have had a complete response.[35,37] At this time, the extent of surgery required to provide local control following neoadjuvant chemotherapy is unclear. In patients found to have multifocal disease in a lumpectomy specimen not encompassing the entire volume of the initial tumor, consideration should be given to the resection of additional tissue, even when margins are clear. Only controlled trials evaluating pathological margin status, local recurrence, and cosmesis will define optimal treatment in this group of patients.

A major impetus for neoadjuvant chemotherapy is the increased number of patients who may become candidates for breast preservation who would otherwise require mastectomy. This impact, however, may be minimal. At present, despite the NSABP and other studies, which clearly show that lumpectomy, axillary dissection, and radiation therapy are equivalent to modified radical mastectomy in terms of disease-free and absolute survival, nationwide statistics for the USA place breast conservation therapy at around 50%. This is far below the $70+\%$ of patients predicted to be candidates for this procedure. This discrepancy appears to be more of a misunderstanding among physicians and patients rather than due to technical or scientific considerations. Morrow *et al.* reviewed the medical contraindications to breast conservation therapy in 336 patients with stage I and stage II breast cancer treated by a multidisciplinary team between 1988 and 1993.[47] The technical contraindications of a large tumor to breast-size ratio was identified in 20 (6%) of patients. Morrow argues that if these 20 candidates for downstaging received neoadjuvant chemotherapy and obtained an 80% response rate, an additional 16 patients would have been able to undergo breast conservation therapy. Based on this study, the addition of neoadjuvant chemotherapy in the treatment of patients with stage I and stage II breast cancer may increase the optimal breast conservation rate from 77.5% to 81%. Similarly, in the NSABP B-18 trial,[37] the breast conservation therapy rate was increased by only 8% in the neoadjuvant therapy group. Of course, this does translate into a fair number of women who, on an individual basis, would benefit substantially more than statistics imply. It may also help that subset of patients who appear to be breast conservation therapy candidates at diagnosis but, upon resection, prove to have more

extensive disease than expected (invasive or DCIS) and ultimately require re-excision and/or mastectomy. It is not clear just how to identify this subset of patients preoperatively, however.

Bear noted that, with regard to the incorporation of neoadjuvant chemotherapy into the treatment of operable breast cancer, some of the same questions that apply to LABC remain to be answered here, too.[28] How and when should the response to initial therapy be used to modify subsequent treatment? What is the role of combined versus alternating versus sequential therapy with non-cross-resistant agents (adriamycin and taxane)? It is also not clear whether patients should get additional chemotherapy after locoregional treatment. If so, do all patients need more chemotherapy or just a certain subset (i.e., node-positive patients)? Should chemotherapy after surgery with or without radiation be the same agents as given initially, or should different agents be used, or should it depend upon the response of the primary to the preoperative chemotherapy? Some of these questions are being addressed by the successor trial to the NSABP B-18: NSABP B-27. In this trial, patients with operable breast cancer diagnosed with needle biopsy are all treated initially with four cycles of adriamycin, cytoxan (AC), and tamoxifen. One group then goes directly to surgery (modified radical mastectomy) or surgery and radiation (breast conservation therapy); a second group receives four additional cycles of chemotherapy with docetaxel before surgery; and a third group receives four cycles of docetaxel after surgery. All patients continue tamoxifen for 5 years. A comparison of the first and second groups will indicate whether the addition of docetaxel before surgery increases the clinical and histological responses and improves survival. A comparison of the first and third groups will determine whether the addition of docetaxel to the AC combination improves survival, and may also indicate whether this benefit is greater in patients who respond well to AC or in those who respond incompletely to AC. Perhaps more importantly, a companion study will assess the relationship of a variety of tumor markers with the response to chemotherapy. In the future, B-18, B-27, and subsequent trials will tell us whether response of the primary tumor is an indication for systemic response. If so, we can anticipate much more rapid progress in evaluating new chemotherapeutic strategies in the treatment of breast cancer.

The addition of new agents in the chemotherapeutic armamentarium, such as monoclonal antibodies (c-erb B2), protein kinase inhibitors, angiogenesis inhibitors, signal transduction inhibitors, and retinoids, may alter our whole approach to therapy.

The technique of sentinel node-guided axillary dissection is currently under investigation. Pretreatment with chemotherapy that may downstage or sterilize the axilla in selected patients may broaden the application of this surgical option, as well.

CONCLUSION

Whether there are absolute indications for neoadjuvant chemotherapy can be argued, but this approach is the standard of care in the treatment of patients with inoperable LABC (stage IIIA and IIIB) and inflammatory carcinoma. The use of neoadjuvant chemotherapy to treat patients with operable breast cancer remains controversial. Neoadjuvant chemotherapy is highly effective in achieving significant tumor regression. However, the primary goal of improved survival has yet to be demonstrated. Thus, utilizing primary chemotherapy in patients with operable breast cancer should be considered investigational, especially in those women who are breast conservation therapy candidates at diagnosis. Neoadjuvant chemotherapy is an option in all patients with operable breast cancer that would otherwise require mastectomy. This approach mandates strict adherence to the policy of obtaining clear histological surgical margins and lifelong follow-up, as the long-term local recurrence rate, risk of metastatic spread, and survival statistics for those patients with neoadjuvant therapy-induced downstaging followed by breast conservation therapy are not yet available.

The definitive application of neoadjuvant chemotherapy to patients with operable breast cancer awaits the results of ongoing clinical trials.

REFERENCES

1. Fisher B, Carbone P, Economou SG. L-phenylalanine mustard (L-PAM) in the management of primary breast cancer: a report of early findings. N Engl J Med 1975; 292:117–22.

2. Bonadonna G, Brusamolino E, Valagussa P. Combination chemotherapy as an adjuvant treatment in operable breast cancer. N Engl J Med 1976; 294:405–10.

3. Shapiro CL, Henderson IC, Gelman RS. A randomized trial of 15 vs 30 weeks of adjuvant chemotherapy in high risk breast cancer patients: results after a median follow up of 9.1 years. Proc Am Soc Clin Oncol (Abstract) 1991; 10:44.

4. Fisher B, Redmond C, Dimetrov N, et al. A randomized clinical trial evaluating sequential methotrexate and fluorouracil in the treatment of patients with node negative breast cancer who have estrogen receptor negative tumors. N Engl J Med 1989; 320:473–8.

5. Bonadonna G. Evolving concepts in the systemic adjuvant treatment of breast cancer. Cancer Res 1992; 52(8):2127–37.

6. Zambetti M, Bonadonna G, Valagussa P. CMF for node negative and estrogen receptor negative breast cancer. J Natl Cancer Inst Monogr 1992; 11:77–83.

7. Mansour EG, Eudey L, Shatila AH. Adjuvant therapy in node negative breast cancer: is it necessary for all patients? An Intergroup study. In Salman SE, ed. Adjuvant therapy of cancer VI. Philadelphia, WB Saunders, 1990, 174–89.

8. Fisher B, Gundez N, Saffer EA. Influence of the interval between primary tumor removal and chemotherapy on kinetics and growth of metastases. Cancer Res 1983; 43:1488–92.

9. Gundez N, Fisher B, Saffer EA. Effect of surgical removal on growth and kinetics of residual tumor. Cancer Res 1979; 39:3861–5.

10. O'Reilly MS, Holmgren L, Shing Y, et al. Angiostatin: a circulating endothelial cell inhibitor that suppresses angiogenesis and tumor growth. Cold Spring Harbor Symp Quant Biol 1994; 59:471–82.

11. O'Reilly MS, Holmgren L, Chen C, et al. Angiostatin induces and sustains dormancy of human primary tumors in mice. Nat Med 1996; 2:689–92.

12. Goldie JH, Coldman AJ. A mathematical model for relating the drug sensitivity of tumors to their spontaneous mutation rate. Cancer Treat Rep 1979; 63:1729–33.

13. Skipper HE. Kinetics of mammary tumor cell growth and implications for therapy. Cancer 1971; 28:1479–99.

14. McCready DR, Hortobagyi GN, Kau SW, et al. The prognostic significance of lymph node metastasis after preoperative chemotherapy for locally advanced breast cancer. Arch Surg 1989; 124:21–5.

15. Seidman AD, Reickman BS, Crown JPA, et al. Paclitaxel as second and subsequent therapy for metastatic breast cancer: activity independent of prior anthracycline-resistant or anthracenedione-resistant breast cancer. J Clin Oncol 1995; 13:1152–9.

16. Ravdin PM, Burns HA III, Cook G, et al. Phase II trials of docetaxel in advanced anthramycin-resistant or anthracenedione-resistant breast cancer. J Clin Oncol 1995; 13:2879–85.

17. Vallero N, Holmes FA, Walters RS, et al. Phase II trial of docetaxel: a new highly effective antineoplastic agent in the management of patients with anthracycline-resistant metastatic breast cancer. J Clin Oncol 1995; 13:2886–94.

18. Donegan W. Cancer of the breast, 3rd edn. Philadelphia, WB Saunders, 1988.

19. Swain MS. Selection of therapy for Stage III breast cancer. Surg Clin North Am 1990; 70:1061–80.

20. Haagensen C, Stout A. Carcinoma of the breast: criteria of operability. Ann Surg 1943; 118:859–70.

21. Bedwinek J, Rao D, Perez C. Stage III and localized Stage IV breast cancer: irradiation alone vs irradiation plus surgery. Int J Radiat Oncol Biol Phys 1982; 8:31–6.

22. Rubens RD, Armitage P, Winter PJ, et al. Prognosis in inoperable Stage III carcinoma of the breast. Eur J Cancer 1977; 13:805–11.

23. Zucali R, Uslenghi C, Kenda R, *et al.* Natural history and survival of inoperable breast cancer treated with radiotherapy and radiotherapy followed by radical mastectomy. Cancer 1976; 37:1422–31.

24. Terz JJ, Romero CA, Kay S, *et al.* Preoperative radiotherapy for stage III carcinoma of the breast. Surg Gynecol Obstet 1978; 147:497–502.

25. De Lena M, Varini M, Zucali R, *et al.* Multimodal treatment for locally advanced breast cancer: results of chemotherapy–radiotherapy versus chemotherapy–surgery. Cancer Clin Trials 1981; 4:229–36.

26. Hortobagyi GN. Multimodal treatment of locoregionally advanced breast cancer. Cancer 1983; 51:763–8.

27. Rubens RD, Sexton S, Jong D, *et al.* Combined chemotherapy and radiotherapy for locally advanced breast cancer. Eur J Cancer 1980; 16:351–6.

28. Bear HD. Indications for neoadjuvant chemotherapy for breast cancer. Semin Oncol 1998; 2(Suppl. 3):3–12.

29. Hery M, Namer M, Moro M, *et al.* Conservative treatment (chemotherapy/radiotherapy) of locally advanced breast cancer. Cancer 1986; 57:1744–9.

30. Jacquillat C, Baillet F, Weil M, *et al.* Results of a conservative treatment combining induction (neoadjuvant) and consolidation chemotherapy, hormonotherapy, and external and interstitial irradiation in 98 patients with locally advanced breast cancer (IIIA–IIIB). Cancer 1988; 61:1977–82.

31. Merajver SD, Weber BL, Cody R, *et al.* Breast conservation and prolonged chemotherapy for locally advanced breast cancer: the University of Michigan experience. J Clin Oncol 1997; 15:2873–81.

32. Bonadonna G, Veronesi U, Brambula C, *et al.* Primary chemotherapy to avoid mastectomy in tumors with diameters of three centimeters or more. J Natl Cancer Inst 1990; 82:1539–45.

33. Calais G, Berger C, Descamps P, *et al.* Conservative treatment feasibility with induction chemotherapy, surgery and radiotherapy for patients with breast carcinoma larger than 3 cm. Cancer 1994; 74:1283–8.

34. Mauriac L, Durand M, Avril A, *et al.* Effects of primary chemotherapy in conservative treatment of breast cancer patients with operable tumors larger than 3 cm: results of a randomized trial in a single centre. Ann Oncol 1991; 2:347–54.

35. Powles JJ, Hickish TF, Makris A, *et al.* Randomized trial of chemoendocrine therapy started before or after surgery for treatment of primary breast cancer. J Clin Oncol 1995; 13:547–52.

36. Scholl SM, Fourquet A, Asselain B, *et al.* Neoadjuvant versus adjuvant chemotherapy in premenopausal patients with tumor considered too large for breast conserving surgery: preliminary results of a randomized trial. Eur J Cancer 1994; 30A:645–52.

37. Fisher B, Brown A, Mamounas E, *et al.* Effect of preoperative chemotherapy on locoregional disease in women with operable breast cancer: findings from NSABP B-18. J Clin Oncol 1997; 15(7):2483–93.

38. Segel M, Paulus D, Hortobagyi G. Advanced primary breast cancer: assessment of mammography to response of induction chemotherapy. Radiology 1988; 169:49–54.

39. Cocconi G, Del Blasto B, Alberti G, *et al.* Pathologic assessment of response to induction chemotherapy in breast cancer. Cancer Res 1986; 46:8578–81.

40. Gilles R, Guinebretiere JM, Toussaint C, *et al.* Locally advanced breast cancer: contrast-enhanced subtraction magnetic resonance imaging of response to preoperative chemotherapy. Radiology 1994; 191:633–8.

41. Abraham DC, Jones RC, Jones SE, *et al.* Evaluation of neoadjuvant chemotherapeutic response of locally advanced breast cancer by MRI. Cancer 1996; 78:91–100.

42. Bossa P, Kim FE, Inoue J, *et al.* Evaluation of preoperative chemotherapy using PET with fluorene-18-fluorodeoxyglucose in breast cancer. J Nucl Med 1996; 37:931–8.

43. Limbergen EV, Van der Schueren E, Van den Bogaert W, *et al.* Local control of operable breast cancer after radiotherapy alone. Eur J Cancer 1990; 26:671–9.

44. Pierce LJ, Lippman M, Ben-Baruch N, *et al.* The effect of systemic therapy on local–regional control in locally advanced breast cancer. Int J Radiat Oncol Biol Phys 1992; 23:949–60.

45. Brenin DR, Morrow M. Breast conserving surgery in the neoadjuvant setting. Semin Oncol 1998; 2(Suppl. 3):13–18.

46. Singletary S, McNeese MD, Hortobagyi GN. Feasibility of breast conservation surgery after induction chemotherapy for locally advanced breast cancer. Cancer 1992; 69:2049–52.

47. Morrow M, Bucci C, Rademaker A. Medical contraindications are not a major factor in the underutilization of breast conserving therapy. J Am Coll Surg 1998; 186:269–74.

ANNOTATED BIBLIOGRAPHY

Bear HD. Indications for neoadjuvant chemotherapy for breast cancer. Semin Oncol 1998; 25(2):3–12.
A good review of the literature regarding rationale and clinical investigations of neoadjuvant therapy in the treatment of breast cancer.

Fisher B, Brown A, Mamounas E, *et al.* Effect of preoperative chemotherapy on locoregional disease in women with operable breast cancer: findings from NSABP B-18. J Clin Oncol 1997; 15(7):2483–93.
1523 women were randomized to either preoperative chemotherapy (AC) followed by surgery or surgery followed by postoperative chemotherapy (AC). Preoperative therapy

reduced the size of most tumors (80%) and decreased the incidence of positive nodes (by 37%), with an overall increase by 12% of lumpectomies, with the greatest increase in women with tumor greater than 5 cm, in which a 175% increase in breast preservation was achieved. This is the largest study to date of neoadjuvant chemotherapy in breast cancer.

Fisher B, Gundez N, Saffer EA. Influence of the interval between primary tumor removal and chemotherapy on kinetics and growth of metastases. Cancer Res 1983; 43:1488–92.

The original paper investigating the phenomenon by which removal of the primary tumor in animals may increase the growth rate of micrometastases via a 'serum growth factor.' The finding that preoperative cyclophosphamide prevented this growth was strong evidence to proceed with neoadjuvant treatment in humans.

Kuerer HM, Hunt KK, Newman LA, *et al.* Neoadjuvant chemotherapy in women with invasive breast carcinoma: conceptual basis and fundamental surgical issues. J Am Coll Surg 2000; 190(3):350–63.

An excellent review of the current status of neoadjuvant chemotherapy.

Commentary

STEVEN J TUCKER AND JOHN A GLASPY

Systemic chemotherapy for breast cancer has evolved over the last 30 years from palliative therapy for metastatic disease to adjuvant therapy for node-positive and node-negative disease and is progressing to neoadjuvant therapy for operable breast cancer. Historically, single doses of perioperative chemotherapy demonstrated a decrease in breast cancer recurrences and death in women receiving mastectomies, as reported by Scandinavian researchers and by the NSABP.[1,2] This was followed by reports from Greenspan[3] and Cooper,[4] who showed a 50% response rate to combination chemotherapy in metastatic breast cancer and that responders had improved overall survival (OS) compared to non-responders. The Ludwig Breast Cancer Study Group demonstrated that a single cycle of perioperative combination chemotherapy improves disease-free survival (DFS) in all patients and OS in women with estrogen receptor (ER)-negative tumors.[5,6] Numerous randomized clinical trials of adjuvant combination chemotherapy, in both node-positive and node-negative disease, have shown improved DFS and OS.[7–9] Finally, the Oxford overview analysis of polychemotherapy for breast cancer demonstrated that adjuvant chemotherapy improves both DFS and OS in all women with invasive breast cancer larger than 1.0 cm, regardless of nodal, menopausal, and ER status.[10]

Current concepts regarding neoadjuvant chemotherapy for breast cancer arise from the successful treatment of locally advanced breast cancer (LABC) (stage IIIA–B) with combination chemotherapy. One practical and well-accepted advantage of this approach is the ability to convert inoperable breast cancer to operable breast cancer, as well as to perform more frequent breast conservation therapy (BCT) in lesions that would traditionally require mastectomy. Bonadonna *et al.* achieved BCT in

85% of 536 patients with tumors greater than 3 cm after neoadjuvant combination chemotherapy,[11] and surgeons at M.D. Anderson Cancer Center were able to perform BCT in 30% of 372 patients with tumors greater than 4 cm.[12] However, selection bias is evident in this group, as demonstrated by a significantly improved survival advantage for the BCT patients (82% versus 66%, $p < 0.01$). Patients in the M.D. Anderson series who received BCT were more likely to have stage IIA, IIB, or IIIA disease and more likely to have had a complete clinical response to neoadjuvant chemotherapy. The magnitude of benefit of BCT may be overstated by these single-institution, non-randomized studies, and the benefits of BCT may not extend to palpable operable breast cancer. The NSABP protocol B-18 randomized over 1500 women with palpable, operable breast cancer to preoperative or postoperative adriamycin and cytoxan for four cycles of chemotherapy. Although the study did demonstrate that more BCT was performed in the neoadjuvant arm, the magnitude of difference between the two arms was only 7% (67% versus 60%, $p < 0.002$).[13]

To date, numerous randomized, clinical trials of neoadjuvant chemotherapy have been performed in operable breast cancer and none has demonstrated any superiority over postoperative chemotherapy in DFS or OS. However, and of importance, none of these trials has shown that neoadjuvant chemotherapy has in any way compromised the beneficial effects of adjuvant combination chemotherapy.[13–15] Apart from the modest improvement in BCT, neoadjuvant chemotherapy can provide an *in-vivo* tumor sensitivity assay and allow optimization of chemotherapy treatment. Theoretically, this should minimize micrometastatic disease, decrease *de novo* drug resistance, and improve cell-cycle kinetics that may be altered at sites of micrometastatic disease.

These theoretical advantages originate in the work of Fisher *et al.* and Skipper, who suggest that removal of a primary tumor increases the proliferative rate at sites of metastatic disease.[16,17]

Despite no observable difference in DFS and OS, response to neoadjuvant chemotherapy is a powerful prognostic factor. Clinical and pathological responses to neoadjuvant chemotherapy correlate with clinical outcome and are a surrogate for treatment effectiveness. Data from the M.D. Anderson Cancer Center show that patients who achieve a pathological complete response have a significantly improved 5-year DFS (87% versus 58%) and OS (89% versus 64%).[12] Additionally, other studies have shown that failure to respond to neoadjuvant chemotherapy is indicative of poor survival.[15] In the NSABP study, outcome was tied to both the clinical response rate (36%) and pathological response rate (9%), with the best DFS and OS being in patients who achieved both (83% and 87%, respectively).[13] Current clinical trials aim to improve the clinical and pathological response rate, while identifying non-responders earlier by either biological or imaging studies.

Biological markers that have preliminary utility include Ki-67, Bcl-2, HER-2/*neu*, and apoptotic index. Decreases in proliferation as measured by Ki-67 or increases in the apoptotic index may be associated with improved responses.[18] Increased expression of the anti-apoptotic molecule Bcl-2 may also be a surrogate marker of poor response to neoadjuvant chemotherapy.[19] Overexpression of the proto-oncogene HER-2/*neu* has also been correlated with poor response to chemotherapy and decreased survival in patients treated with neoadjuvant chemotherapy.[20,21] Recently, mismatch repair proteins such as MLH1 have been proposed as molecular markers of drug resistance and decreased survival in breast cancer patients treated with primary chemotherapy. Persistent expression of MLH1 by immunohistochemistry after neoadjuvant therapy predicts for poor DFS, implicating its role in drug resistance.[22]

Imaging studies such as magnetic resonance imaging (MRI) and positron emission tomography (PET) are now sufficiently sensitive to assist in the diagnosis and evaluation of breast cancer. Preliminary studies show that MRI results can be accurately correlated with pathological results in patients receiving neoadjuvant chemotherapy.[23,24] Scans are performed as a baseline and after the first and fourth cycles of neoadjuvant therapy. MRI response has been highly correlated with both complete and partial pathological response. PET scans using radiolabeled fluorodeoxyglucose have been able to predict complete pathologic response with a sensitivity of 90% and specificity of 74% after a single cycle of chemotherapy.[25] Additional studies have been able to identify responders to neoadjuvant chemotherapy with 100% sensitivity and pathologic response with greater than 90% accuracy.[26] Ideally, these studies will be integrated into randomized clinical trials and use algorithms to predict responders and non-responders. Ultimately, these trials would allow non-responders to participate in novel therapies without requiring surgical evaluation of response.

In summary, neoadjuvant chemotherapy for operable breast cancer provides a modest improvement in BCT without compromising DFS and OS in comparable women treated with standard adjuvant chemotherapy. Neoadjuvant chemotherapy can be safely recommended in any patient with palpable breast cancer without significant compromise of traditional prognostic information. Additional prognostic information can be gathered by pretreatment tumor molecular characteristics, imaging response to therapy, and pathological response to therapy. Neoadjuvant chemotherapy of breast cancer presents an excellent opportunity to design clinical trials of novel therapies in patients unresponsive to current treatment.

REFERENCES

1. Nissen-Meyer R, Kjellgren K, Mansson B. Preliminary report from the Scandinavian Adjuvant Chemotherapy Study Group. Cancer Chemother Rep 1971; 55:561–6.
2. Fisher B, Ravdin RG, Ausman RK, et al. Surgical adjuvant chemotherapy in cancer of the breast: results of a decade of cooperative investigation. Ann Surg 1968; 168:337–56.
3. Greenspan EM. Chemotherapy of cancer. N Engl J Med 1973; 289:271.
4. Cooper RG. Combination chemotherapy of breast cancer. Mt Sinai J Med 1985; 52:443–6.
5. Goldhirsch A, Castiglione M, Gelber RD. A single perioperative adjuvant chemotherapy course for node-negative breast cancer: five-year results of trial V. International Breast Cancer Study Group (formerly Ludwig Group). J Natl Cancer Inst Monogr 1992; 11:89–96.
6. Prolonged disease-free survival after one course of perioperative adjuvant chemotherapy for node-negative breast cancer. The Ludwig Breast Cancer Study Group. N Engl J Med 1989; 320:491–6.
7. Bonadonna G, Valagussa P, Moliterni A, et al. Adjuvant cyclophosphamide, methotrexate, and fluorouracil in node-positive breast cancer: the results of 20 years of follow-up [see comments]. N Engl J Med 1995; 332:901–6.
8. Fisher B, Redmond C, Dimitrov NV, et al. A randomized clinical trial evaluating sequential methotrexate and fluorouracil in the treatment of patients with node-negative breast cancer who have estrogen-receptor-negative tumors. N Engl J Med 1989; 320:473–8.
9. Mansour EG, Gray R, Shatila AH, et al. Survival advantage of adjuvant chemotherapy in high-risk

node-negative breast cancer: ten-year analysis – an Intergroup study. J Clin Oncol 1998; 16:3486–92.

10. Polychemotherapy for early breast cancer: an overview of the randomised trials. Early Breast Cancer Trialists' Collaborative Group [see comments]. Lancet 1998; 352:930–42.

11. Bonadonna G, Valagussa P, Brambilla C, *et al*. Primary chemotherapy in operable breast cancer: eight-year experience at the Milan Cancer Institute. J Clin Oncol 1998; 16:93–100.

12. Kuerer HM, Newman LA, Smith TL, *et al*. Clinical course of breast cancer patients with complete pathologic primary tumor and axillary lymph node response to doxorubicin-based neoadjuvant chemotherapy [see comments]. J Clin Oncol 1999; 17:460–9.

13. Fisher B, Bryant J, Wolmark N, *et al*. Effect of preoperative chemotherapy on the outcome of women with operable breast cancer. J Clin Oncol 1998; 16:2672–85.

14. Makris A, Powles TJ, Ashley SE, *et al*. A reduction in the requirements for mastectomy in a randomized trial of neoadjuvant chemoendocrine therapy in primary breast cancer [see comments]. Ann Oncol 1998; 9:1179–84.

15. Scholl SM, Fourquet A, Asselain B, *et al*. Neoadjuvant versus adjuvant chemotherapy in premenopausal patients with tumours considered too large for breast conserving surgery: preliminary results of a randomised trial: S6. Eur J Cancer 1994; 5:645–52.

16. Skipper HE. Kinetics of mammary tumor cell growth and implications for therapy. Cancer 1971; 28:1479–99.

17. Fisher B, Gunduz N, Coyle J, *et al*. Presence of a growth-stimulating factor in serum following primary tumor removal in mice. Cancer Res 1989; 49:1996–2001.

18. Ellis PA, Smith IE, Detre S, *et al*. Reduced apoptosis and proliferation and increased Bcl-2 in residual breast cancer following preoperative chemotherapy. Breast Cancer Res Treat 1998; 48:107–16.

19. Jalava PJ, Collan YU, Kuopio T, *et al*. Bcl-2 immunostaining: a way to finding unresponsive postmenopausal N+ breast cancer patients. Anticancer Res 2000; 20:1213–19.

20. MacGrogan G, Mauriac L, Durand M, *et al*. Primary chemotherapy in breast invasive carcinoma: predictive value of the immunohistochemical detection of hormonal receptors, p53, c-erbB-2, MiB1, pS2 and GST pi. Br J Cancer 1996; 74:1458–65.

21. Gregory RK, Powles TJ, Salter J, *et al*. Prognostic relevance of cerbB2 expression following neoadjuvant chemotherapy in patients in a randomised trial of neoadjuvant versus adjuvant chemoendocrine therapy. Breast Cancer Res Treat 2000; 59:171–5.

22. Mackay HJ, Cameron D, Rahilly M, *et al*. Reduced MLH1 expression in breast tumors after primary chemotherapy predicts disease-free survival [published erratum appears in J Clin Oncol 2000; 18(4):944]. J Clin Oncol 2000; 18:87–93.

23. Abraham DC, Jones RC, Jones SE, *et al*. Evaluation of neoadjuvant chemotherapeutic response of locally advanced breast cancer by magnetic resonance imaging. Cancer 1996; 78:91–100.

24. Esserman L, Hylton N, Yassa L, *et al*. Utility of magnetic resonance imaging in the management of breast cancer: evidence for improved preoperative staging. J Clin Oncol 1999; 17:110–19.

25. Smith IC, Welch AE, Hutcheon AW, *et al*. Positron emission tomography using [(18)F]-fluorodeoxy-D-glucose to predict the pathologic response of breast cancer to primary chemotherapy. J Clin Oncol 2000; 18:1676–88.

26. Schelling M, Avril N, Nahrig J, *et al*. Positron emission tomography using [(18) F]fluorodeoxyglucose for monitoring primary chemotherapy in breast cancer. J Clin Oncol 2000; 18:1689–95.

Editors' selected abstracts

Accelerated superfractionated radiotherapy for inflammatory breast carcinoma: complete response predicts outcome and allows for breast conservation.

Arthur DW, Schmidt-Ullrich RK, Friedman RB, Wazer DE, Kachnic LA, Amir C, Bear HD, Hackney MH, Smith TJ, Lawrence W Jr.

Department of Radiation Oncology, Medical College of Virginia Hospitals of Virginia Commonwealth University (VCU), Richmond, VA, USA.

International Journal of Radiation Oncology, Biology, Physics 44(2):289–96, 1999, May 1.

Purpose: Chemotherapy and accelerated superfractionated radiotherapy were prospectively applied for inflammatory breast carcinoma with the intent of breast conservation. The efficacy, failure patterns, and patient tolerance utilizing this approach were analyzed. *Methods and materials:* Between 1983 and 1996, 52 patients with inflammatory breast carcinoma presented to the Medical College of Virginia Hospitals of VCU and the New England Medical Center. Thirty-eight of these patients were jointly evaluated in multidisciplinary breast clinics and managed according to a defined prospectively applied treatment policy. Patients received induction chemotherapy, accelerated superfractionated radiotherapy selected use of mastectomy, and concluded with additional chemotherapy. The majority were treated with 1.5 Gy twice daily to field arrangements covering the entire breast and regional lymphatics. An additional 18–21 Gy was then delivered to the breast and clinically involved nodal regions. Total dose to clinically involved areas was 63–66 Gy. Following chemoradiotherapy, patients were evaluated with physical examination, mammogram, and fine needle aspiration × 3. Mastectomy was reserved for those patients with evidence of persistent or progressive disease in the involved breast. All patients received additional chemotherapy. *Results:* Median age was 51 years. Median follow-up was 23.9 months (6–86 months). The breast preservation rate at the time of last follow-up was 74%. The treated breast or chest wall as the first site of failure occurred in only in 13%, and the ultimate local control rate with the selected use of mastectomy was 74%. Ten patients underwent mastectomy, 2 of which had pathologically negative specimens despite a clinically palpable residual mass. Response to chemotherapy was predictive of treatment outcome. Of the 15 patients achieving a complete response, 87% remain locoregionally controlled without the use of mastectomy. Five-year overall survival for complete responders was 68%. This is in contrast to the 14% 5-year overall survival observed with incomplete responders. The 5-year actuarial disease-free survival and overall survival for the entire patient cohort was 11% and 33%, respectively. All patients tolerated irradiation with limited acute effects, of which all were managed conservatively. *Conclusion:* Our experience demonstrates that induction chemotherapy, accelerated superfractionated radiotherapy, and the selected use of mastectomy results in excellent locoregional control rates, is well tolerated, and optimizes breast preservation. Based on our present results, we recommend that a patient's response to induction chemotherapy guide the treatment approach used for locoregional disease, such that mastectomy be reserved for incomplete responders and avoided in those achieving a complete response.

Three new active cisplatin-containing combinations in the neoadjuvant treatment of locally advanced and locally recurrent breast carcinoma: a randomized phase II trial.

Cocconi G, Bisagni G, Ceci G, Di Blasio B, De Lisi V, Passalacqua R, Zadro A, Boni C, Morandi P, Savoldi L.

Medical Oncology Institution of Parma, Italian Oncology Group for Clinical Research (GOIRC), Italy.

Breast Cancer Research & Treatment 56(2):125–32, 1999, July.

We designed three new four-drug cisplatin-containing combinations and evaluated their activity in a randomized phase II study including patients with locally advanced (stage III) and locally recurrent breast carcinoma. All combinations included methotrexate (M) on day 1 and cisplatin (P) on day 2 (MVAC-like combinations) and differed from one another by the addition of Epirubicin (Epi), Vincristine (V), Etoposide (E), Mitomycin (Mi). Based on the administered agents, they were named MPEMi, MPEpiE, MPEpiV. The combinations were randomly assigned to 101 patients, 57 with locally advanced and 44 with locally recurrent breast carcinoma. Response was evaluated after 4 cycles. The complete response (CR) rates were 7% and 43% and the CR plus partial response (PR) rates were 84% and 89% in locally advanced and in locally recurrent disease, respectively. In locally advanced disease, a pathologic CR (pCR)

was assessed in seven of 57 patients (12%). There were no significant differences among the three combinations. The toxicities were at times severe, but generally tolerable, as demonstrated by the high cumulative doses of the drugs received by the patients. In conclusion, these three innovative chemotherapy regimens induced high CR plus PR rates in the neoadjuvant treatment of stage III and of locally recurrent breast carcinoma, and a high rate of pCR in stage III disease. These regimens warrant testing in phase III trials.

Identification and evaluation of axillary sentinel lymph nodes in patients with breast carcinoma treated with neoadjuvant chemotherapy.

Cohen LF, Breslin TM, Kuerer HM, Ross MI, Hunt KK, Sahin AA.

Department of Pathology, The University of Texas M.D. Anderson Cancer Center, Houston, TX, USA.

American Journal of Surgical Pathology 24(9):1266–72, 2000, September.

Sentinel lymph node (SLN) biopsy has been shown to predict axillary metastases accurately in early stage breast cancer. Some patients with locally advanced breast cancer receive preoperative (neoadjuvant) chemotherapy, which may alter lymphatic drainage and lymph node structure. In this study, we examined the feasibility and accuracy of SLN mapping in these patients and whether serial sectioning and keratin immunohistochemical (IHC) staining would improve the identification of metastases in lymph nodes with chemotherapy-induced changes. Thirty-eight patients with stage II or III breast cancer treated with neoadjuvant chemotherapy were included. In all patients, SLN biopsy was attempted, and immediately afterward, axillary lymph node dissection was performed. If the result of the SLN biopsy was negative on initial hematoxylin and eosin-stained sections, all axillary nodes were examined with three additional hematoxylin and eosin sections and one keratin IHC stain. SLNs were identified in 31 (82%) of 38 patients. The SLN accurately predicted axillary status in 28 (90%) of 31 patients (three false negatives). On examination of the original hematoxylin and eosin-stained sections, 20 patients were found to have tumor-free SLNs. With the additional sections, 4 (20%) of these 20 patients were found to have occult lymph node metastases. These metastatic foci were seen on the hematoxylin and eosin staining and keratin IHC staining. Our findings indicate that lymph node mapping in patients with breast cancer treated with neoadjuvant chemotherapy can identify the SLN, and SLN biopsy in this group accurately predicts axillary nodal status in most patients. Furthermore, serial sectioning and IHC staining aid in the identification of occult micrometastases in lymph nodes with chemotherapy-induced changes.

US-guided implantation of metallic markers for permanent localization of the tumor bed in patients with breast cancer who undergo preoperative chemotherapy.

Edeiken BS, Fornage BD, Bedi DG, Singletary SE, Ibrahim NK, Strom EA, Holmes F.

Department of Diagnostic Radiology, University of Texas M.D. Anderson Cancer Center, Houston, TX, USA.

Radiology 213(3):895–900, 1999, December.

Metallic markers were implanted with ultrasonographic guidance in 51 malignant breast tumors in 49 patients to tag the tumor bed in anticipation of complete or almost complete response to preoperative neoadjuvant induction chemotherapy before breast-conservation surgery. The markers were the only remaining evidence of the original tumor site in 47% (23 of 49) of the patients preoperatively. This technique effectively addresses the problem of preoperative localization of the tumor bed in complete or nearly complete response of breast cancer to neoadjuvant chemotherapy.

Original *p53* status predicts for pathological response in locally advanced breast cancer patients treated preoperatively with continuous infusion 5-fluorouracil and radiation therapy.

Formenti SC, Dunnington G, Uzieli B, Lenz H, Keren-Rosenberg S, Silberman H, Spicer D, Denk M, Leichman G, Groshen S, Watkins K, Muggia F, Florentine B, Press M, Danenberg K, Danenberg P.

Department of Radiation Oncology, University of Southern California School of Medicine, Los Angeles, CA, USA.

International Journal of Radiation Oncology, Biology, Physics 39(5):1059–68, 1997, December 1.

Purpose/objective: 1) To test feasibility of preoperative continuous infusion (c.i.) 5-fluorouracil (5-FU) and radiation (RT) in locally advanced breast cancer. 2) To study clinical and pathological response rates of 5-FU and radiation. 3) To attempt preliminary correlations between biological probes and pathological response. *Methods and materials:* Previously untreated, locally advanced breast cancer patients were eligible: only patients who presented with T3/T4 tumors that could not be resected with primary wound closure were eligible, while inflammatory breast cancer patients were excluded. The protocol consisted of preoperative c.i. infusion 5-FU, 200 mg/m^2/day with radiotherapy, 50 Gy at 2 Gy fractions to the breast and regional nodes. At mastectomy, pathological findings were classified based on persistence of invasive cancer: pathological complete response (pCR) = no residual invasive cells in the breast and axillary contents; pathological partial response (pPR) = presence of microscopic foci of invasive cells in either the breast or nodal specimens; no pathological response (pNR) = pathololgical persistence of tumor. For each patient pretreatment breast cancer biopsies were analyzed by immunohistochemistry for nuclear grade, ER/PR hormonal receptors, HER2/*neu* and *p53* overexpression. *Results:* Thirty-five women have completed the protocol and are available for analysis. 5-FU was interrupted during radiation in 10 of 35 patients because of oral mucositis in 8 patients, cellulitis in 1, and patient choice in another. Objective clinical response rate before mastectomy was 71% (25 of 35 patients): 4 CR, 21 PR. However, in all 35 patients tumor response was sufficient to make them resectable with primary wound closure. Accordingly, all patients underwent modified radical mastectomy: primary wound closure was achieved in all patients. At mastectomy there were 7 pCR (20%), 5 pPR (14%) and the remaining 23 patients (66%) had pathological persistence of cancer (pNR).

Variables analyzed as potential predictors for pathological response (pPR and pCR) were: initial TNM clinical stage, clinical response, nuclear grade, hormonal receptor status, *p53* overexpression, and HER2/*neu* overexpression in the pretreatment tumor biopsy. Only initial *p53* status (lack of overexpression at immunohistochemistry) significantly correlated with achievement of a pathological response to this regimen ($p = 0.010$). *Conclusion:* The combination of c.i. 5-FU and radiation was well tolerated and generated objective clinical responses in 71% of the patients. With the limitation of the small sample size, the complete pathological response achieved (20%) compares favorably with that reported in other series of neoadjuvant therapy for similar stage breast cancer. These preliminary data suggest that initial *p53* status predicts for pathological response (pPR and pCR) to the combination of c.i. 5-FU and radiotherapy in locally advanced breast cancer.

Combined modality treatment of locally advanced breast carcinoma in elderly patients or patients with severe comorbid conditions using tamoxifen as the primary therapy.

Hoff PM, Valero V, Buzdar AU, Singletary SE, Theriault RL, Booser D, Asmar L, Frye D, McNeese MD, Hortobagyi GN.

Department of Breast Medical Oncology, The University of Texas M.D. Anderson Cancer Center, Houston, TX, USA.

Cancer 88(9):2054–60, 2000, May 1.

Background: The purpose of the current study was to evaluate the objective response rate and possibility of breast-conserving surgery using neoadjuvant tamoxifen in the multimodality treatment, including surgery and radiotherapy, of elderly or frail patients with locally advanced breast carcinoma. *Methods:* Forty-seven patients age > 75 years or age < 75 years with comorbid conditions and locally advanced breast carcinoma were treated with neoadjuvant tamoxifen (20 mg/day) for 3–6 months. This was followed by surgery and radiotherapy when feasible and adjuvant tamoxifen for 5 years or until disease recurrence. *Results:* The median age of the patients was 72 years (range, 48–86 years). Approximately 22% had T3 lesions, 57% had T4 lesions, 22% were stage II (AJCC *Manual for staging cancer*, 3rd edition), and 78% were stage III. Eighty percent were estrogen receptor positive. After 6 months of treatment with neoadjuvant tamoxifen, a response rate of 47% was observed, including a complete response rate of 6%. Twenty-nine patients (62%) were rendered free of disease by surgery, including 5 with breast-conserving procedures. After a median follow-up of 40 months, 23 patients (49%) remained disease free. The median survival time had not been reached at the time of last follow-up. No major toxicity was observed, with the exception of one patient who developed a possible tamoxifen-related stage I endometrial carcinoma. The estimated 2-year and 5-year progression free and overall survival rates were 50% and 41%, and 83% and 59%, respectively. *Conclusions:* The results of the current study show that neoadjuvant tamoxifen was effective in the treatment of elderly or frail patients with locally advanced breast carcinoma with estrogen receptor positive tumors, and resulted in a reasonable response rate, including complete responses and good overall survival.

Clinical course of breast cancer patients with complete pathologic primary tumor and axillary lymph node response to doxorubicin-based neoadjuvant chemotherapy.

Kuerer HM, Newman LA, Smith TL, Ames FC, Hunt KK, Dhingra K, Theriault RL, Singh G, Binkley SM, Sneige N, Buchholz TA, Ross MI, McNeese MD, Buzdar AU, Hortobagyi GN, Singletary SE.

Department of Surgical Oncology, University of Texas M.D. Anderson Cancer Center, Houston, TX, USA.

Journal of Clinical Oncology 17(2):460–9, 1999, February.

Purpose: To assess patient and tumor characteristics associated with a complete pathologic response (pCR) in both the breast and axillary lymph node specimens and the outcome of patients found to have a pCR after neoadjuvant chemotherapy for locally advanced breast cancer (LABC). *Patients and methods:* Three hundred seventy-two LABC patients received treatment in two prospective neoadjuvant trials using four cycles of doxorubicin-containing chemotherapy. Patients had a total mastectomy with axillary dissection or segmental mastectomy and axillary dissection followed by four or more cycles of additional chemotherapy. Patients then received irradiation treatment of the chest-wall or breast and regional lymphatics. Median follow-up was 58 months (range, 8 to 99 months). *Results:* The initial nodal status, age, and stage distribution of patients with a pCR were not significantly different from those of patients with less than a pCR ($p > 0.05$). Patients with a pCR had initial tumors that were more likely to be estrogen receptor (ER)-negative ($p < 0.01$), and anaplastic ($p = 0.01$) but of smaller size ($p < 0.01$) than those of patients with less than a pCR. Upon multivariate analysis, the effects of ER status and nuclear grade were independent of initial tumor size. Sixteen percent of the patients in this study ($n = 60$) had a pathologic complete primary tumor response. Twelve percent of patients ($n = 43$) had no microscopic evidence of invasive cancer in their breast and axillary specimens. A pathologic complete primary tumor response was predictive of a complete axillary lymph node response ($p < 0.01$). The 5-year overall and disease-free survival rates were significantly higher in the group who had a pCR (89% and 87%, respectively) than in the group who had less than a pCR (64% and 58%, respectively; $p < 0.01$). *Conclusion:* Neoadjuvant chemotherapy has the capacity to completely clear the breast and axillary lymph nodes of invasive tumor before surgery. Patients with LABC who have a pCR in the breast and axillary nodes have a significantly improved disease-free survival rate. However, a pCR does not entirely eliminate recurrence. Further efforts should focus on elucidating the molecular mechanisms associated with this response.

Incidence and impact of documented eradication of breast cancer axillary lymph node metastases before surgery in patients treated with neoadjuvant chemotherapy.

Kuerer HM, Sahin AA, Hunt KK, Newman LA, Breslin TM, Ames FC, Ross MI, Buzdar AU, Hortobagyi GN, Singletary SE.

Department of Surgical Oncology, The University of Texas M.D. Anderson Cancer Center, Houston, TX, USA.

Annals of Surgery 230(1):72–8, 1999, July.

Objective: To determine the incidence and prognostic significance of documented eradication of breast cancer axillary lymph node (ALN) metastases after neoadjuvant chemotherapy. *Summary background data:* Neoadjuvant chemotherapy is the standard of care for patients with locally advanced breast cancer and is being evaluated in patients with earlier-stage operable disease. *Methods:* One hundred ninety-one patients with locally advanced breast cancer and cytologically documented ALN metastases were treated in two prospective trials of doxorubicin-based neoadjuvant chemotherapy. Patients had breast surgery with level I and II axillary dissection followed by additional chemotherapy and radiation treatment. Nodal sections from 43 patients who were originally identified as having negative ALNs at surgery were reevaluated and histologically confirmed to be without metastases. An additional 1112 sections from these lymph node blocks were obtained; half were stained with an anticytokeratin antibody cocktail and analyzed. Survival was calculated using the Kaplan–Meier method. *Results:* Of 191 patients with positive ALNs at diagnosis, 23% (43 patients) were converted to a negative axillary nodal status on histologic examination (median number of nodes removed = 16). Of the 43 patients with complete axillary conversion, 26% ($n = 11$) had N1 disease and 74% ($n = 32$) had N2 disease. On univariate analysis, patients with complete versus incomplete histologic axillary conversion were more likely to have initial estrogen-receptor-negative tumors, smaller primary tumors, and a complete pathologic response in the primary tumor. The 5-year disease-free survival rates were 87% in patients with preoperative eradication of axillary metastases and 51% for patients with residual nodal disease after neoadjuvant chemotherapy. Of the 39 patients with complete histologic conversion for whom nodal blocks were available, occult nodal metastases were found in additional nodal sections in 4 patients (10%). At a median follow-up of 61 months, the 5-year disease-free survival rates were 87% in patients without occult nodal metastases and 75% in patients with occult nodal metastases. *Conclusions:* Neoadjuvant chemotherapy can completely clear the axilla of microscopic disease before surgery, and occult metastases are found in only 10% of patients with a histologically negative axilla. The results of this study have implications for the potential use of sentinel lymph node biopsy as an alternative to axillary dissection in patients treated with neoadjuvant chemotherapy.

Primary tumor response to induction chemotherapy as a predictor of histological status of axillary nodes in operable breast cancer patients.

Lenert JT, Vlastos G, Mirza NQ, Winchester DJ, Binkley SM, Ames FC, Ross MI, Feig BW, Hunt KK, Strom E, Buzdar AU, Hortobagyi GN, Singletary SE.

Department of Surgical Oncology, The University of Texas M.D. Anderson Cancer Center, Houston, TX, USA.

Annals of Surgical Oncology 6(8):762–7, 1999, December.

Background: Routine use of axillary lymph node dissection is being questioned, especially in clinically N0 patients. The goal of this study was to determine whether primary tumor response to induction chemotherapy (IC) can predict the histological volume of residual axillary disease in patients who were candidates for breast conservation surgery after IC. *Methods:* Forty-seven patients with stage II or IIIA breast cancer who received breast conservation surgery were selected from a population of patients randomized to received four cycles of IC. Largest clinical tumor size before and after IC was determined by physical examination, mammography, and breast ultrasound. Clinical nodal status was determined by physical examination and axillary ultrasound and compared with histological findings. *Results:* In patients with at least 50% reduction in primary tumor size after IC, 12 of 14 (86%) N0 patients and 11 of 17 (65%) N1 patients were histologically negative. In patients with a less than 50% reduction, 0 of 3 N0 patients and 2 of 13 (15%) N1 patients were histologically negative. *Conclusions:* There is significantly less axillary disease in responders than in nonresponders after IC. For N0 responders, axillary irradiation may be an acceptable alternative to axillary lymph node dissection, and could easily be incorporated into the postsurgical radiotherapy that is standard protocol for breast conservation therapy. The more aggressive disease in nonresponders is best treated by axillary lymph node dissection, pending further study.

Locoregional irradiation for inflammatory breast cancer: effectiveness of dose escalation in decreasing recurrence.

Liao Z, Strom EA, Buzdar AU, Singletary SE, Hunt K, Allen PK, McNeese MD.

Department of Radiation Oncology, The University of Texas M.D. Anderson Cancer Center, Houston, TX, USA.

International Journal of Radiation Oncology, Biology, Physics 47(5):1191–200, 2000, July 15.

Purpose: To evaluate the effect of radiation dose escalation on locoregional control, overall survival, and long-term complication in patients with inflammatory breast cancer. *Patients and methods:* From September 1977 to December 1993, 115 patients with nonmetastatic inflammatory breast cancer were treated with curative intent at The University of Texas M.D. Anderson Cancer Center. The usual sequence of multimodal treatment consisted of induction FAC or FACVP chemotherapy, mastectomy (if the tumor was operable), further chemotherapy, and radiation therapy to the chest wall and draining lymphatics. Sixty-one patients treated from September 1977 to September 1985 received a maximal radiation dose of 60 Gy to the chest wall and 45–50 Gy to the regional lymph nodes, 22 treated once a day at 2 Gy per fraction, and 35 were treated b.i.d. (32 after mastectomy and all chemotherapy was completed, and 2 immediately after mastectomy; one patient had distant metastases discovered during b.i.d. irradiation, and treatment was stopped). Four additional patients received preoperative radiation with standard fractionation. Based on the analysis of the failure patterns of the patients, the dose was increased for the b.i.d. patients in the new series, with 51 Gy delivered to the chest wall and regional nodes, followed by a 15-Gy boost to the chest wall with electrons. From January 1986 to December 1993, 39 patients were treated b.i.d. to this higher dose after mastectomy and all the chemotherapy was completed; and 8 additional patients received preoperative irradiation with b.i.d. fractionation to 51 Gy. During this period, another 7 patients were treated using standard daily doses of 2 Gy per fraction to a total of 60 Gy, either because they had a complete response or minimal residual disease at mastectomy or because their work schedule did not permit the b.i.d. regimen. Comparison was made between the groups for locoregional control, disease-free and overall survival, and complication rates. *Results:* The median follow-up time was 5.7 years (range, 1.8–17.6 years). For the entire patient group, the 5- and 10-year local control rates were 73.2% and 67.1%, respectively. The 5- and 10-year disease-free survival rates were 32.0% and 28.8%, respectively, and the overall survival rates for the entire group were 40.5% and 31.3%, respectively. To evaluate the effectiveness of dose escalation, a specific comparison of patients who received b.i.d. radiation after mastectomy and completion of adjuvant chemotherapy was performed. There were 32 patients treated b.i.d. to 60 Gy in the old series versus 39 patients treated b.i.d. to 66 Gy in the new series. There was a significant improvement in the rate of locoregional control for the b.i.d. patients for the old versus new series, from 57.8% to 84.3% and from 57.8% to 77.0% ($p = 0.028$) at 5 and 10 years, respectively. Chemotherapy regimens did not change significantly during this time period. Long-term complications of radiation, such as arm edema more than 3 cm (7 patients), rib fracture (10 patients), severe chest wall fibrosis (4 patients), and symptomatic pneumonitis (5 patients), were comparable in the two groups, indicating that the dose escalation did not result in increased morbidity. Significant differences in the rates of locoregional control ($p = 0.03$) and overall survival ($p = 0.03$), and a trend of better disease-free survival ($p = 0.06$) were also observed that favored the recently treated patients receiving the higher doses of irradiation. *Conclusion:* Twice-daily postmastectomy radiation to a total of 66 Gy for patients with inflammatory breast cancer resulted in improved locoregional control, disease free survival, and overall survival, and was well tolerated.

Reduction in angiogenesis after neoadjuvant chemoendocrine therapy in patients with operable breast carcinoma.

Makris A, Powles TJ, Kakolyris S, Dowsett M, Ashley SE, Harris AL.

Breast Unit, Royal Marsden Hospital, Sutton, Surrey, UK.

Cancer 85(9):1996–2000, 1999, May 1.

Background: The intensity of angiogenesis, as measured by microvessel density, is a strong independent predictor of survival in breast carcinoma patients. The impact of chemotherapy and/or endocrine therapy on this process is unknown. *Methods:* Histologic samples from patients randomized to a trial of neoadjuvant (NEO) versus adjuvant (ADJ) chemoendocrine therapy for operable breast carcinoma were obtained. Samples from 195 patients (90 NEO samples and 105 ADJ samples) were analyzed. Immunostaining was performed with the CD34 monoclonal antibody and the scoring of microvessels was performed using the Chalkley method. *Results:* The median score of the NEO patients was 5.7 (95% confidence interval [CI], 5.3–6.0) and the median score of the ADJ patients was 6.3 (95% CI, 6–6.7) ($p = 0.025$). Using previously validated scoring categories, there were fewer samples with a poor prognosis (score $\geqslant 7$) in the NEO group (26%) compared with the ADJ group (32%) ($p = 0.04$). *Conclusions:* The results of the current study suggest that NEO chemoendocrine therapy causes a reduction in microvessel density in primary breast carcinomas, which could be secondary to tumor regression or due to a direct effect on angiogenesis.

Neoadjuvant chemotherapy for breast cancer.

Sapunar F, Smith IE.

Breast Unit, Royal Marsden Hospital, London, UK.

Annals of Medicine 32(1):43–50, 2000, February.

Primary or neoadjuvant chemotherapy in early breast cancer offers the chance to use the tumor as an *in vivo* measure of response, with the additional possibility of downstaging and avoidance of mastectomy. Tumor response to preoperative chemotherapy correlates with the outcome and could be a surrogate for evaluating the effect of chemotherapy on micrometastases. Randomized studies have shown that preoperative chemotherapy is as effective as postoperative chemotherapy, but there has not been a significant increase in the disease-free survival or overall survival in the groups studied. The overall response rates reported have varied between 60% and 100% with complete clinical responses from 10% to almost 50%, avoiding mastectomy in most cases. Clinical responders have a better prognosis than nonresponders; pathological complete remissions at present offer the best prediction of good long-term outcome, but occur in less than 20% of patients. Biological predictors reflecting changes in apoptosis and/or proliferation may in the future offer the best surrogate markers for long-term outcome, and trials have recently begun in this area.

Preoperative paclitaxel and radiotherapy for locally advanced breast cancer: surgical aspects.

Skinner KA, Silberman H, Florentine B, Lomis TJ, Corso F, Spicer D, Formenti SC.

Department of Surgery, Kenneth Norris Comprehensive Cancer Center, and the University of Southern California, Los Angeles, CA, USA.

Annals of Surgical Oncology 7(2):145–9, 2000, March.

Introduction: Approximately 15% of breast cancer patients present with large tumors that involve the skin, the chest wall, or the regional lymph nodes. Multimodality therapy is required, to provide the best chance for long-term survival. We have developed a regimen of paclitaxel, with concomitant radiation, as a primary therapy in patients with locally advanced breast cancer. *Methods:* Eligible patients had locally advanced breast cancer (stage IIB or III). After obtaining informed consent, patients received paclitaxel ($30 \, mg/m^2$ during 1 hour) twice per week for 8 weeks and radiotherapy to 45 Gy (25 fractions, at 180 cGy/fraction, to the breast and regional nodes). Patients then underwent modified radical mastectomy followed by postoperative polychemotherapy. *Results:* Twenty-nine patients were enrolled. Of these, 28 were assessable for clinical response and toxicity, and 27 were assessable for pathological response. Objective clinical response was achieved in 89%. At the time of surgery, 33% had no or minimal microscopic residual disease. Chemoradiation-related acute toxicity was limited; however, surgical complications occurred in 41% of patients. *Conclusions:* Preoperative paclitaxel with radiotherapy is well tolerated and provides significant pathological response, in up to 33% of patients with locally advanced breast cancer, but with a significant postoperative morbidity rate.

The feasibility of minimally invasive surgery for stage IIA, IIB, and IIIA breast carcinoma patients after tumor downstaging with induction chemotherapy.

Vlastos G, Mirza NQ, Lenert JT, Hunt KK, Ames FC, Feig BW, Ross MI, Buzdar AU, Singletary SE.

Department of Surgical Oncology, The University of Texas M.D. Anderson Cancer Center, Houston, TX, USA.

Cancer 88(6):1417–24, 2000, March 15.

Background: Induction chemotherapy (IC) has become the standard of care of locally advanced breast carcinoma, frequently downstaging both the primary tumor and the axilla, and making patients eligible for less invasive surgical procedures. The usefulness of IC in earlier stage operable breast carcinoma is now being considered. *Methods:* This study involved a subset of 129 patients from a series of 174 with T2-3, N0-1, M0 or T1, N1, M0 breast carcinoma (stage IIA, IIB, or IIIA) who were registered in a prospective IC trial using paclitaxel or a combination of fluorouracil, doxorubicin, and cyclophosphamide (FAC). The subset included patients who had received no preoperative radiation therapy but had completed 3–5 cycles of induction chemotherapy and had undergone a level I–II axillary lymph node dissection. The objective was to evaluate the effectiveness of induction chemotherapy with paclitaxel or FAC in downstaging the primary tumor and axillary metastases in these early stage breast carcinoma patients. *Results:* The median initial tumor size was 4 cm (range, 0.6–10.0); after IC, tumor size was downstaged to 1.6 cm (range, 0.0–7.0) ($p < 0.0001$). Clinical response to IC was complete in 24% of patients and partial in 36%. Primary tumor shrinkage was similar with paclitaxel and FAC. Among patients clinically classified as N1, 34% became histologically negative and 38% had only 1–3 positive lymph nodes after induction chemotherapy. *Conclusions:* IC with paclitaxel or FAC resulted in effective downstaging of primary tumors and axillary metastases in patients with stage IIA, IIB, and IIIA breast carcinoma. However, a significant proportion of patients still had residual but low volume microscopic disease; such disease status may allow minimally invasive surgical approaches to locoregional therapy.

15

Axillary lymphadenectomy for breast cancer: *impact on survival*

HOWARD SILBERMAN

Over the past century, the natural history of breast cancer has been formulated in three successive theoretical models (Table 15.1).[1] The *Halstedian Model*[2] perceives breast cancer as a disease that spreads exclusively via the lymphatic system. The primary tumor infiltrates adjacent lymphatic channels, thereby reaching regional lymph nodes, from which systemic dissemination subsequently occurs by contiguous extention to distant sites. This concept logically led to the view that, for a period of time, prior to systemic spread, breast cancer could be cured by regional surgical extirpation sufficiently extensive to encompass all of the potentially involved tissues, including the entire breast and its overlying skin, the underlying pectoral muscles, and all of the ipsilateral axillary lymph nodes – the *radical mastectomy* of Meyer and Halsted.[2,3] This approach was subsequently extended by Urban[4] to the super-radical mastectomy, a procedure that also encompassed the internal mammary lymph nodes.

High rates of systemic failure despite satisfactory local control by surgical resection led to the *Systemic Model* of

Table 15.1 *Various models of breast cancer spread*

Halsted	Systemic	Spectrum
Tumor spreads in an orderly manner based on mechanical considerations	There is no orderly pattern of tumor cell dissemination	In most patients, axillary nodal involvement precedes distant metastases
The positive lymph node is an indicator of tumor spread and is the instigator of distant metastases	The positive lymph node is an indicator of a host–tumor relationship that permits development of metastases, rather than the instigator of distant metastases	The positive lymph node is an indicator of a host–tumor relationship that is correlated with the subsequent appearance of distant disease
RLNs are barriers to passage of tumor cells	RLNs are ineffective as barriers to tumor cell spread	RLNs are ineffective as barriers to tumor spread, but involvement of RLNs is not always associated with distant metastases
The bloodstream is of little significance as a route of tumor dissemination	The bloodstream is of considerable importance in tumor dissemination	The bloodstream is of considerable importance in tumor dissemination
Operable breast cancer is a local–regional disease	Operable breast cancer is a systemic disease	Operable breast cancer is a systemic disease in many but not all cases
The extent and nuances of the operations are the dominant factors influencing a patient's outcome	Variations in local–regional therapy are unlikely to affect survival	Variations in local–regional therapy are unlikely to have a major influence on survival but are of significance in some patients

RLNs, regional lymph nodes.
From Hellman, Harris. In Harris *et al. Diseases of the breast.* Lippincott Williams & Wilkins, 2000; 419.

breast cancer spread. This paradigm, now widely adopted and promulgated primarily by Fisher and his associates,[5–7] envisions two types of breast cancer. One type is a local neoplasm with little propensity to spread distantly, whereas in the second type systemic dissemination is already present at the time of clinical diagnosis. In the first type, adequate local treatment to the breast is curative. In the second type, local therapy is seen as useful in dealing with the primary tumor and in controlling locoregional recurrence; but local treatment, no matter how radical, can have no impact on cure because distant disease, the determinant of survival, already exists at the time of diagnosis. The most important scientific support for this theoretical concept of breast cancer biology derives from the work of Fisher et al.,[5] under the auspices of the National Surgical Adjuvant Breast and Bowel Project (NSABP). The major influence on therapy deriving from NSABP randomized trial B-04 is that axillary lymphadenectomy, heretofore regarded as an inherent component of the curative approach to breast cancer, in fact, accords no improvement in the cure rate of breast cancer.

More recently, an intermediate theoretical model of breast cancer spread has emerged, the *Spectrum Model*,[8,9] in which the disease is viewed as systemic in many but not all cases, and, therefore, in some patients early diagnosis and effective regional treatment can improve survival.[1]

It is widely accepted that axillary dissection is of value in preventing the local recurrence of tumor in the axilla, in evaluating prognosis, and in influencing the decision for adjuvant therapy. The issue, intensely discussed and controversial, is whether partial or complete axillary lymphadenectomy has an important, clinically applicable, impact on survival and quality of life in any subset of patients. The resolution of this issue requires careful assessment of past and current data because of critical reviews of the NSABP trial[1,10] and new technological and scientific developments (such as advances in the biology of tumor dissemination, high-resolution screening mammography, sentinel node analysis, and immunohistochemical detection of nodal micrometastases). Also necessary is a re-evaluation of the morbidity of axillary dissection in modern practice in relation to any potential benefit.

Conceptually, removing axillary lymph nodes can affect survival only if the lymph nodes removed contain metastatic deposits, if these nodal metastases can themselves metastasize to distant sites, and if nodal involvement, at least sometimes, precedes incurable systemic dissemination. In assessing the therapeutic value of axillary lymphadenectomy, the specific relevant issues to be considered include the following:

1 Can lymph node metastases spread to distant sites?
2 Are there problems or concerns in the conduct of the NSABP trial[5] which are sufficient to weaken the strength of its conclusions or their applicability in current practice?

3 What are the data from other studies that may reasonably reflect on the value of treating axillary metastases?
4 Does *complete* axillary clearance, including level III lymph nodes, contribute to the benefit, if any, of lymphadenectomy?
5 What is the morbidity of axillary dissection in relation to any benefit observed?

DISSEMINATION OF AXILLARY METASTASES

Considerable evidence exists that metastases can, in fact, metastasize,[11] and, further, that the microenvironment within lymph nodes appears suitable for dissemination of nodal metastases.[12]

Zeidman and Buss demonstrated in a rabbit model that lymph nodes initially formed an effective barrier to further spread of metastatic carcinoma, but metastases to more distant lymph nodes and viscera developed when nodal resection was delayed beyond a certain point.[13]

In a series of experiments using parabiotic mice, Hoover and Ketcham demonstrated that, for several different tumor lines, including a mammary adenocarcinoma, tumor present only in lung metastases could spread from one animal to another when the primary tumor had been removed before joining the circulation of the metastases-bearing animal to that of its syngeneic counterpart.[14]

Recent data have established that tumor progression is critically dependent on the ability of the tumor to induce a neovascular stroma.[12,15,16] Moreover, after tumor cells spread to distant sites, the metastatic deposits must then induce their own vascular stroma in order to grow and, potentially, give rise to secondary metastases.[17] Guidi and associates assessed the extent of this process of angiogenesis in the primary tumors and axillary nodes containing metastases from patients with breast cancer.[12] The primary tumor and the tumor-bearing lymph nodes were examined for the presence or absence of focal areas of relatively intense neovascularization (vascular 'hot spots'), and a quantitative assessment of intratumoral microvessel density was performed. Patients who had increased neovascularization by these markers of angiogenesis in their axillary lymph node metastases (but not in the primary tumor) experienced a statistically significant decrease in overall and disease-free survival. These data strongly support the concept that, in the presence of the requisite microenvironment, lymph node metastases from human breast cancer can produce secondary metastatic deposits, evidently accounting for the adverse effect on survival observed by Guidi and associates.

ANALYSIS OF NSABP PROTOCOL B-04

In 1971, Fisher and associates began a prospective clinical trial to compare the value of variations in locoregional treatment on the survival of patients with clinically evident, operable breast cancer.[5] Patients judged to have clinically negative axillary nodes were randomly assigned to be treated by radical mastectomy, total mastectomy and regional irradiation, or total mastectomy alone. The impact of axillary lymphadenectomy was assessed by comparing outcome in the groups treated by radical mastectomy ($n = 362$) or total mastectomy alone ($n = 365$). The results at 10 years indicated a survival rate of 58% for the radical mastectomy group, compared with 54% for the total mastectomy group, a difference that was not statistically significant. These findings led to the widely accepted conclusion that axillary lymphadenectomy does not alter the incidence of systemic recurrence or patient survival and, furthermore, lymph node metastases are 'indicators rather than instigators' of distant disease. The results of this trial are also offered as validating the *Systemic Model* of breast cancer spread (Table 15.1), wherein survival-determining systemic metastases are perceived as already present at the time of the clinical diagnosis of the primary tumor.

Critical reviews of this historic study suggest that a survival benefit attributable to axillary dissection may have been masked by several problematic clinical, pathologic, and statistical features of the protocol design:[1,10,18]

1 Among the 365 patients assigned to receive *total mastectomy alone*, 129 patients (35%) inadvertently had a limited axillary dissection, undoubtedly because of the anatomic interdigitation of breast tissue in the axillary tail with level I lympho-adipose tissue. In fact, up to five lymph nodes were removed in 23% of the patients; six to ten nodes in 6%; and more than ten nodes in 7%, including several patients with more than 20 nodes removed.[18–20]

2 The trial protocol allowed for salvage surgery for postoperative axillary failure, so that, by 10 years' follow-up, 18% of the *total mastectomy-only* group developed clinically evident nodal metastases which were treated by delayed axillary dissection. Such delayed nodal involvement was not considered a treatment failure and was not included in the determination of disease-free survival.[5] The impact of salvage lymphadenectomy on the survival of those patients is unknown.[1,10]

3 It is clear that axillary lymphadenectomy cannot improve the survival of patients free of nodal metastases, yet 60% of the patients in each arm of the study were estimated to be free of axillary disease. Consequently, only about 40% of the patients, who had axillary involvement, comprised the true critical population to whom benefit could possibly accrue from axillary dissection. Taking this fact into account and, further, by estimating the likelihood of occult distant disease (which would preclude benefit from locoregional treatment) and considering the potential curative benefit of delayed salvage node dissection,

Harris and Osteen determined that only 9% of the total group could potentially benefit from initial axillary treatment.[1,10] This analysis led the authors to conclude that the B-04 trial did not have the statistical power to prove or disprove the efficacy of axillary dissection, because they calculated that approximately 1000 patients in each arm would be required to have a 90% chance of detecting a 9% difference between two treatment arms in a clinical trial at a statistically significant level of $p = 0.05$.

4 Even if the conclusions of the B-04 trial were rigorously validated and true, new developments in diagnosis and treatment since the accrual of patients into that study may alter the impact of axillary lymphadenectomy and unmask a survival benefit. Thus, patients entered into the B-04 trial had *clinically evident* primary tumors. With current screening programs employing vastly improved, high-resolution imaging techniques, primary breast cancer is often diagnosed in a *preclinical*, even *microscopic*, phase in which regional lymph nodes may be involved *prior* to systemic dissemination. This concept, consistent with the *Spectrum Model* of breast cancer spread rather than the *Systemic Model* (Table 15.1), is supported by several lines of evidence. Modern mammographic screening of asymptomatic women, presumably resulting in earlier diagnoses, is associated with a decrease in breast cancer mortality of at least 50%.[21–23] If metastases always occur at the inception of breast cancer (*Systemic Model*), early detection could not be effective in preventing metastases or decreasing breast cancer mortality. Additional evidence supporting the *Spectrum Model* and, inferentially, the potential therapeutic benefit of axillary dissection, comes from the older literature, wherein 26–50% of the long-term survivors of radical mastectomy alone had positive lymph nodes. Evidently, these surviving patients received effective regional treatment prior to systemic spread of their disease.[20,24–27]

5 The advent of effective adjuvant chemotherapy is another advance that appears to alter the applicability of the B-04 data. Systemic occult metastases that were assumed to be survival limiting in the population of patients studied in the NSABP trial and which, therefore, precluded any benefit from lymphadenectomy, are now amenable to eradication by such adjuvant therapy.[28,29] Current adjuvant chemotherapy regimens are evidently less effective against locoregional disease than systemic micrometastases,[30] thereby raising the possibility of improving survival with regional treatment even in patients with occult systemic disease. Support for this concept comes from reports of Overgaard and Ragaz and their associates[31,32] (see below).

6 Finally, the sentinel node hypothesis is a new concept which, if confirmed by currently ongoing clinical trials, may also affect the interpretation of the B-04 data.

In relation to breast cancer, this hypothesis holds that the presence or absence of metastatic disease in the first one or two axillary nodes (the *sentinel nodes*) that receive drainage from a primary breast cancer accurately reflects the presence or absence of metastatic disease in all of the remaining axillary lymph nodes (see Chapter 16). Consequently, sentinel node analysis could be used to restrict axillary lymphadenectomy to only those patients with a very high likelihood of bearing metastatic disease in the remaining non-sentinel nodes. Thus, axillary clearance would be withheld from patients with negative sentinel nodes. In addition, according to data from the John Wayne Cancer Institute at Saint John's Hospital and Health Center, Santa Monica, CA, lymphadenectomy may be omitted in patients with a sentinel node containing only a micrometastasis (≤ 2 mm) or in patients with a sentinel node metastasis that is associated with a T1a breast tumor, because, in these two subsets of patients, non-sentinel node involvement is rare.[33] Evaluating the therapeutic efficacy of axillary dissection only in patients highly likely to have residual axillary metastases may well reveal a benefit masked in the B-04 series where, as Harris and Osteen pointed out,[10] any favorable effect was diluted by including patients of whom the majority had no axillary disease.

EFFECT OF RADIATION ON SURVIVAL AFTER LIMITED AXILLARY DISSECTION

Recently, results have been published from two prospective, randomized trials designed to determine the worth of postoperative locoregional radiation therapy in patients treated with modified radical mastectomy and adjuvant chemotherapy.[31,32] The survival benefit that was observed in both studies might suggest that adjuvant radiation is routinely indicated after modified radical mastectomy for patients with high-risk breast cancer.[30] Such a conclusion, however, is questionable, because very limited axillary dissections were performed, and the radiotherapy appears only to be a surrogate for more adequate surgical dissection. Paradoxically, however, the results of radiation after limited axillary clearance derived from these trials provide important information concerning the worth of treating axillary metastases.

In the Danish Breast Cancer Cooperative Group Trial,[31] 1708 premenopausal women who had undergone mastectomy for pathologic stage II or III breast cancer and who were to have adjuvant chemotherapy with cyclophosphamide, methotrexate, and fluorouracil (CMF) were randomly assigned to receive or not receive irradiation of the chest wall and regional lymph nodes. The axillary dissections performed were limited to level I and part of level II. A median of seven lymph nodes was removed; moreover, in 15% of the patients, only zero to three nodes were retrieved, and in 76% nine or fewer lymph nodes were removed. Axillary metastases were documented in 92% of the patients. Disease-free survival and overall survival at 10 years were significantly improved ($p < 0.001$) in the cohort of patients receiving adjuvant radiation.

Ragaz and associates conducted a similar trial in Vancouver, British Columbia.[32] Three hundred and eighteen premenopausal women with node-positive breast cancer were randomly assigned, after modified radical mastectomy, to receive CMF chemotherapy plus radiotherapy or chemotherapy alone. Axillary dissection yielded a median of only 11 lymph nodes. Mortality from breast cancer was reduced by 29% in the group receiving radiotherapy ($p = 0.05$).

Silberman and associates analysed the two trials in relation to their own experience.[34] In 131 modified radical mastectomies performed in their series, a mean of 25 lymph nodes were removed in an operation designed to provide complete axillary clearance. These authors suggest that the radiotherapy employed in the Danish and Canadian trials merely compensated for inadequate axillary surgery that resulted in a group of patients highly likely to have residual nodal disease (see below).[35] Thus, they believe that the results do not support the routine use of adjuvant postmastectomy radiotherapy when complete lymph node dissections are performed. Nevertheless, these two trials lend strong scientific support to the notion that the obliteration of axillary metastases has a salutary effect on survival. This conclusion is further strengthened by the fact that, in the NSABP randomized trial of adjuvant radiation therapy after radical mastectomy with *complete* axillary dissection, the radiation therapy did not confer a survival advantage.[36] Probable residual axillary metastases appears to be the only important variable between the two current studies and the NSABP trial. Therefore, obliteration of the remaining axillary disease by radiation in the two current reports is the likely basis for the favorable impact on survival that was observed. The addition of adjuvant chemotherapy in the two recent trials cannot be responsible for the improvement in survival noted between the irradiated and non-irradiated groups, because the patients in both study groups received this therapy. However, the *magnitude* of the potential survival benefit attributable to axillary treatment may well be enhanced by adjuvant chemotherapy, because survival-limiting occult systemic micrometastases can now be cured in a significant proportion of patients who receive such systemic drug therapy, as discussed above.

OTHER STUDIES EXAMINING THE WORTH OF AXILLARY LYMPHADENECTOMY

Various additional studies examining the impact of axillary lymphadenectomy on survival have been published,

Table 15.2 *Meta-analysis of axillary dissection*

Trial	Number of patients	Follow-up (years)	Survival (%)		Difference (%)	Reduction (%)	*p*-value
			Control	Treated			
Copenhagen	425	10	46	50	4	7.4	NS
Guy's I	370	10	43.6	51.6	8	14.2	NS
SES	498	10	51.5	61	9.5	19.6	0.04
B-04	727	10	54	58	4	8.7	NS
Guy's II	258	10	57	73	16	37.2	0.01
Curie	658	5	92.6	96.6	4	45.9	0.03

NS, not significant.
From Orr, Ann Surg Oncol 1999; 6:109.

but most, unfortunately, have methodological, design, or clinical features which tend to hinder definitive interpretation.

Recently, Orr performed a meta-analysis of published trials in which standard treatment for breast cancer (mastectomy with axillary dissection or segmental mastectomy, breast radiation, and axillary dissection) was compared to standard treatment without axillary node dissection (Table 15.2).[37] Orr excluded from his analysis trials that referred to stage II patients only, but included trials with mixtures of stage I and II patients. Six randomized controlled trials, consisting of nearly 3000 patients and spanning four decades, were identified for inclusion in the meta-analysis. The trials included were those from Copenhagen,[38,39] the south-east Scotland (SES) trial,[40–42] the NSABP B-04 trial,[5] two trials from Guy's Hospital in London,[43–46] and the Institut Curie trial.[47] All six trials showed that prophylactic axillary node dissection improved survival, ranging from 4% to 16%, corresponding to a risk reduction of 7–46%. Combining the six trials showed an average survival benefit of 5.4% (95% confidence interval = 2.7–8.0%, probability of survival benefit >99.5%). Adjusting for biases in the individual studies did not alter the conclusions, nor did subset analysis of stage I patients. The author concluded that axillary node dissection improves survival in women with operable breast cancer. However, he identified two important limitations of the analysis. First, few of the patients in the six trials had T1a tumors, so extrapolation of these results to this subset (and to those with non-palpable tumors) may be inappropriate. Second, essentially no patients in the six trials were treated with adjuvant therapy, as contrasted to current clinical practice, so that it is possible that the risk reduction seen in this meta-analysis may be altered in patients receiving adjuvant chemotherapy.

In an editorial critique of Orr's meta-analysis, Morrow identified several additional limitations.[48] The Guy's Hospital trials contributed 21% of the patients analysed. These studies compared patients treated by radical mastectomy to those treated by wide local resection and a dose of breast irradiation deemed to be inadequate, so that the absence of axillary clearance may not have been the only factor contributing to the survival differences observed. Similarly, some patients included in the meta-analysis underwent extended radical mastectomies, with resection of internal mammary nodes.

THE ARGUMENT FOR COMPLETE AXILLARY CLEARANCE

In current practice, patients with invasive breast cancer generally undergo an axillary dissection which encompasses the lymph nodes lateral to and deep to the pectoralis minor muscle (levels I and II), with the primary goals of achieving regional control and of providing staging information relevant to the decision for adjuvant therapy.

In contrast, for clinicians who perceive lymphadenectomy as potentially therapeutic, a strong case can be made for complete axillary clearance, including the apical lymph nodes medial to the pectoralis minor (level III nodes) and Rotter's interpectoral nodes. This recommendation is based on the fact that, among patients with axillary metastases, a significant proportion will harbor metastatic tumor in the apical nodes. In a report from the National Cancer Institute, Danforth and associates analysed the distribution of nodal metastases from breast cancer according to their anatomic location (Table 15.3).[49] Among patients with axillary nodes found to be positive on pathologic examination but which were deemed negative on physical examination, 17% had level III metastases; among clinically and pathologically node-positive women, 45.8% had apical involvement. Overall, 27.7% of the 65 node-positive patients analysed had level III nodal involvement.

In a review of published series,[35,50–57] Moffat and associates found that, among women with pathologically involved axillary nodes, apical metastases were present in 18.9–58.1%, and up to 15% had involvement of Rotter's nodes (Table 15.4).[58] Senofsky *et al.* reported that, when axillary metastases are present in level I and II lymph nodes, apical or Rotter's nodes are also involved in about one-third of patients.[50] Similarly, Veronesi and associates

Table 15.3 *Distribution of nodal metastases in patients with pathologically positive nodes*

Axillary level	All patients (%)	Clinically node-negative patients (%)	Clinically node-positive patients (%)
N[a]	65	41	24
Level I only	20 (30.8)	15 (36.6)	5 (20.8)
Level II only	14 (21.5)	13 (31.7)	1 (4.2)
Level III only	2 (3.1)	1 (2.4)	1 (4.2)
Level I, II	13 (20.0)	6 (14.6)	7 (29.2)
Level I, III	1 (1.5)	0 (0.0)	1 (4.2)
Level II, III	3 (4.6)	1 (2.4)	2 (8.3)
Level I, II, III	12 (18.5)	5 (12.2)	7 (29.2)

[a]Number of patients with pathologically positive lymph nodes.
Modified after Danforth *et al.* J Clin Oncol 1986; 4:655–62.

Table 15.4 *Incidence of apical (level III) and Rotter's (interpectoral) nodal metastases in patients with pathologically positive nodes*

Reference	Number of cases	Number of pN+ cases	Number with apical metastases (%)	Number with Rotter's metastases (%)	Number with 'skip' metastases[a] (%)
Senofsky *et al.*[50]	278	92	24 (26.1)	14 (15.2)	5 (5.4)
Rosen *et al.*[51]	933	429	104 (24.2)	1 (0.2)	2 (0.5)
Schwartz *et al.*[52]	277	127	— —	— —	4 (3.1)
Pigott *et al.*[53]	146	72[b]	30 (41.7)	— —	3 (4.2)
Attiyeh *et al.*[54]	—	105	61 (58.1)	— —	12 (11.4)
Smith *et al.*[55]	408	304	136 (44.7)	— —	30 (9.9)
Veronesi *et al.*[35]	—	539	102 (18.9)	— —	2 (0.4)
Boova *et al.*[56]	200	80	17 (21.3)	— —	1 (1.3)
Cody *et al.*[57]	500	134	— —	13 (9.7)	— —

Percentages in parentheses pertain to pN+ patients.
[a] For purposes of this discussion, 'skip' metastases are defined as tumor in apical and/or Rotter's nodes in the absence of metastases in level I and II nodes.
[b] Seventy-two evaluable patients of 80 pN+ patients in this series.
Modified after Moffat *et al.* J Surg Oncol 1992; 51:8.

found that the risk of level III metastases was 35% in women with tumors ≤2 cm in size when levels I and II were involved.[59]

Consequently, a common clinical scenario is one in which a woman with an invasive breast tumor undergoes partial lymphadenectomy (usually levels I–II) in connection with either a mastectomy alone or a segmental mastectomy with planned postoperative breast irradiation. Several days after surgery, the pathologist reports that the lymph nodes sampled contain metastatic disease. Based on the data presented above, a significant number of these women will have tumor present in the remaining axillary nodes. The common and perhaps prevailing view in such a scenario is that the remaining tumor has no impact on survival because outcome is determined by already existing systemic metastatic disease, of which the positive lymph nodes are merely indicators. If this *systemic* view of breast cancer were established beyond doubt, there would be no concern about leaving tumor behind in the axilla, the local treatment provided initially would be considered sufficient, and no further treatment

to the axilla (such as additional surgical dissection or axillary radiotherapy) would be indicated to improve the cure rate. On the other hand, if the *spectrum model* were perceived as possibly valid or applicable at least in a subset of patients, then complete lymphadenectomy would be more commonly offered, except for the prevailing fear of severe morbidity thought to accompany this procedure, primarily arm lymphedema.[60,61]

In fact, many reports indicate that there is little increase in the incidence of lymphedema with extension of the surgical dissection to encompass the apical lymph nodes. In a review of collected series analysing the incidence of lymphedema in relation to the extent of axillary dissection and the effect of concomitant axillary irradiation, Moffat and associates at the University of Miami[58] reported that lymphedema developed in 0–2.8% of patients undergoing axillary sampling procedures;[62,63] in 2.7–7.4% of patients treated by partial (level I and II) axillary dissection;[62–64] and in 3.1–8.0% of patients in whom complete axillary lymphadenectomy was performed.[50,65,66] Axillary irradiation alone was associated

Table 15.5 *Incidence of lymphedema following treatment of the axilla in breast cancer patients*

	Number of patients	Number with lymphedema (%)	Follow-up
Axillary sampling			
Benson and Thorogood[62]	463	13 (2.8)	2–7 years
Larson *et al.*[68]	191[a]	12 (6.3)	45 months
Carabell *et al.*[70]	84[a]	0 (0)	Minimum 1 year
Kissin *et al.*[63]	17	0 (0)	Minimum 1 year
	22[a]	2 (9.1)	Minimum 1 year
Partial axillary lymphadenectomy			
Benson and Thorogood[62]	497	25 (5.0)	2–7 years
Siegel *et al.*[64]	259	7 (2.7)	27 months
Larson *et al.*[68]	49[a]	18 (36.7)	45 months
Kissin *et al.*[63]	94	7 (7.4)	Minimum 1 year
	47[a]	18 (38.3)	Minimum 1 year
Beadle *et al.*[69]	109[a]	13 (11.9)	30 months
Total axillary lymphadenectomy			
Kissin *et al.*[65]	50	4 (8.0)	5 years
Senofsky *et al.*[50]	217	13 (6.0)	50 months
	61[a]	13 (21.3)	50 months
Veronesi *et al.*[66]	352[b]	11 (3.1)	7 years
	349[c]	23 (6.6)	7 years
Radiotherapy only			
Delouche *et al.*[67]	294	10 (3.4)	11 years
Larson *et al.*[68]	235	10 (4.3)	45 months
Kissin *et al.*[63]	12	1 (8.3)	Minimum 1 year
Beadle *et al.*[69]	96	2 (2.1)	30 months

[a] These patients received postoperative adjuvant axillary radiotherapy (XRT).
[b] Treated with conservative surgery, total axillary lymphadenectomy, and XRT.
[c] Treated by radical mastectomy.
Modified after Moffat *et al.* J Surg Oncol 1992; 51:8.

with an incidence of lymphedema of 2.1–8.3%.[63,67–69] Combined axillary dissection and irradiation[50,63,68–70] were synergistic in their effect on the development of lymphedema, resulting in a threefold to sevenfold increase in incidence (Table 15.5).

Veronesi *et al.* reported an overall incidence of lymphedema of 5% following complete axillary clearance.[66] Using a water-displacement technique to compare the volume of the two arms, Hoe *et al.* determined that 7.6% of their patients developed lymphedema after full axillary dissection.[71] Finally, in a study of lymphedema performed at the Memorial Sloan-Kettering Cancer Center, Werner and associates reported that the level of node dissection was not statistically related to the development of arm edema;[72] the only factor that was significantly associated was obesity, manifest as a high body mass index (BMI). Moreover, the higher the BMI, the greater was the frequency of lymphedema.

that would preclude any survival benefit from lymphadenectomy, it is likely that there are some patients who develop axillary disease prior to systemic dissemination or who have coexisting distant micrometastases that can be eradicated by modern adjuvant chemotherapy. Many data support the therapeutic benefit of axillary clearance in this latter group of patients. Among the population of women with invasive breast cancer, the overall value of lymphadenectomy would be considerably enhanced and the overall incidence of morbidity would be considerably reduced if the application of the procedure could be limited to the subset of patients known to have positive axillary nodes. Thus, sentinel node analysis appears to be an extremely promising method of identifying those patients most likely to benefit from axillary dissection, which, when done with the hope of improving survival, should logically encompass all three anatomic levels of the axilla.

SUMMARY AND CONCLUSIONS

Whereas patients with axillary metastases from breast cancer may have incurable synchronous systemic metastases

REFERENCES

1. Hellman S, Harris JR. Natural history of breast cancer. In Harris JR, Lippman ME, Morrow M, Osborne CK, eds.

Diseases of the breast, 2nd edn. Philadelphia, Lippincott Williams & Wilkins, 2000, 407–23.

2. Halsted W. The results of operations for the cure of cancer of the breast performed at the Johns Hopkins Hospital from June 1889 to January 1984. Johns Hopkins Hosp Bull 1895; 4:297–350.

3. Meyer W. An improved method of the radical operation for carcinoma of the breast. Med Rec 1894; 46:746–9.

4. Urban JA. Clinical experience and results of excision of the internal mammary lymph node chain in primary operable breast cancer. Cancer 1959; 12:14–22.

5. Fisher B, Redmond C, Fisher ER, *et al.* Ten-year results of a randomized clinical trial comparing radical mastectomy and total mastectomy with or without radiation. N Engl J Med 1985; 312:674–81.

6. Fisher B. Breast cancer management: alternatives to radical mastectomy. N Engl J Med 1979; 310:326–8.

7. Fisher B. A commentary on the role of the surgeon in primary breast cancer. Breast Cancer Res Treat 1981; 1:17–26.

8. Hellman S. The natural history of small breast cancers. J Clin Oncol 1994; 12:2229–34.

9. Hellman S, Harris J. The appropriate breast carcinoma paradigm. Cancer Res 1987; 2:339–42.

10. Harris JR, Osteen RT. Patients with early breast cancer benefit from effective axillary treatment. Breast Cancer Res Treat 1985; 5:17–21.

11. Fidler IJ. Molecular biology of cancer: invasion and metastasis. In DeVita VT Jr, Hellman S, Rosenberg SA, eds. *Cancer: principles and practice of oncology*, 5th edn. Philadelphia, Lippincott–Raven Publishers, 1997; 135–52.

12. Guidi AJ, Berry DA, Broadwater G, *et al.* Association of angiogenesis in lymph node metastases with outcome of breast cancer. J Natl Cancer Inst 2000; 92:486–92.

13. Zeidman I, Buss JM. Experimental studies on the spread of cancer in the lymphatic system. I. Effectiveness of the lymph node as a barrier to the passage of embolic tumor cells. Cancer Res 1954; 14:403–5.

14. Hoover HC, Ketcham AS. Metastasis of metastases. Am J Surg 1975; 130:405–11.

15. Folkman J. What is the evidence that tumors are angiogenesis dependent? J Natl Cancer Inst 1990; 82:4–6.

16. Blood CH, Zetter BR. Tumor interactions with the vasculature: angiogenesis and tumor metastasis. Biochim Biophys Acta 1990; 1032:89–118.

17. Folkman J. Angiogenesis and breast cancer. J Clin Oncol 1994; 21:441–3.

18. Cody HS, III, Urban JA. The role of axillary dissection in managing patients with breast cancer: the case for complete axillary clearance. In Wise L, Johnson H Jr, eds. *Breast cancer: controversies in management.*

Armonk, NY, Futura Publishing Company, Inc., 1994, 69–176.

19. Fisher B, Wolmark N, Bauer M, *et al.* The accuracy of clinical nodal staging and of limited axillary dissection as a determinant of histologic nodal status in carcinoma of the breast. Surg Gynecol Obstet 1981; 152:765–72.

20. Kinne DW. Axillary clearance in operable breast cancer: still a necessity? Recent Results Cancer Res 1998; 152:161–9.

21. Cady B, Michaelson JS. The life-sparing potential of mammographic screening. Cancer 2001; 91:1699–703.

22. Tabar L, Fagerberg C, Duffy S, *et al.* Update of the Swedish two county program of mammographic screening for breast cancer. Radiol Clin North Am 1992; 30:187–210.

23. Tabar L, Vitak B, Chen H-HT, *et al.* Beyond randomized controlled trials: organized mammographic screening substantially reduces breast carcinoma mortality. Cancer 2001; 91:1724–31.

24. Morrow M, Harris JR. Primary treatment of invasive breast cancer. In Harris JR, Lippman ME, Morrow M, Osborne CK, eds. *Diseases of the breast*, 2nd edn. Philadelphia, Lippincott Wilkins & Williams, 2000, 515–60.

25. Adair F, Berg J, Joubert L, Robbins GF. Long term follow up of breast cancer patients: the 30 year report. Cancer 1974; 33:1145–50.

26. Brinkley D, Haybittle JL. The curability of breast cancer. Lancet 1975; 2:95–7.

27. Rosen PP, Groshen S, Saigo PE, *et al.* A long-term follow-up study of survival in stage I (T1N0M0) and stage II (T1N1M0) breast carcinoma. J Clin Oncol 1989; 7:355–66.

28. Bonadonna G, Brusamolino E, Valagussa P, *et al.* Combination chemotherapy as an adjuvant treatment in operable breast cancer. N Engl J Med 1976; 294:405–10.

29. McCarthy NJ, Swain SM. Update on adjuvant chemotherapy for early breast cancer. Oncology 2000; 14:1267–80.

30. Hellman S. Stopping metastases at their source. N Engl J Med 1997; 337:996–7.

31. Overgaard M, Hansen PS, Overgaard J, *et al.* Postoperative radiotherapy in high-risk premenopausal women with breast cancer who receive adjuvant therapy. N Engl J Med 1997; 337:949–55.

32. Ragaz J, Jackson SM, Nhu L, *et al.* Adjuvant radiotherapy and chemotherapy in node-positive premenopausal women with breast cancer. N Engl J Med 1997; 337:956–62.

33. Chu KU, Turner RR, Hansen NM, *et al.* Do all patients with sentinel node metastasis from breast carcinoma need complete axillary node dissection? Ann Surg 1999; 229:536–41.

34. Silberman AW, Sarna GP, Palmer D. Adjuvant radiation trials for high-risk breast cancer patients: adequacy of lymphadenectomy. Ann Surg Oncol 2000; 7:357–60.

35. Veronesi U, Rilke F, Luini A, *et al.* Distribution of axillary node metastases by level of invasion. An analysis of 539 cases. Cancer 1987; 59:682–7.

36. Fisher B, Slack NH, Cavanaugh PJ, *et al.* Postoperative radiotherapy in the treatment of breast cancer: results of the NSABP clinical trial. Ann Surg 1970; 172:711–32.

37. Orr RK. The impact of prophylactic node dissection on breast cancer survival – a Bayesian meta-analysis. Ann Surg Oncol 1999; 6:109–16.

38. Johansen H, Kaae S, Schiodt T. Simple mastectomy with postoperative irradiation versus extended radical mastectomy in breast cancer: a twenty-five year follow-up of a randomized trial. Acta Oncol 1990; 29:709–15.

39. Kaae S, Johansen H. Does simple mastectomy followed by irradiation offer survival comparable to radical procedures? Int J Radiat Oncol Biophys 1977; 2:1163–6.

40. Bruce J. Operable cancer of the breast – a controlled clinical trial. Cancer 1971; 28:1443–52.

41. Hamilton T, Langlands AO, Prescott RJ. The treatment of operable cancer of the breast: a clinical trial in the south-east region of Scotland. Br J Surg 1974; 61:758–61.

42. Langlands AO, Prescott RJ, Hamilton T. A clinical trial in the management of operable cancer of the breast. Br J Surg 1980; 67:170–4.

43. Hayward J, Caleffi M. The significance of local control in the primary treatment of breast cancer. Arch Surg 1987; 122:1244–7.

44. Atkins H, Hayward JL, Klugman DJ, Wayte AB. Treatment of early breast cancer: a report after ten years of a clinical trial. BMJ 1972; 2:423–9.

45. Hayward JL. The Guy's trial of treatments of 'early' breast cancer. World J Surg 1977; 1:314–16.

46. Hayward JL. The Guy's Hospital trials on breast conservation. In Harris JR, Hellman S, Silen W, eds. *Conservative management of breast cancer: new surgical and radiotherapeutic techniques.* Philadelphia, JB Lippincott, 1983, 77–90.

47. Cabanes PA, Salmon RJ, Vilcoq JR, *et al.* Value of axillary dissection in addition to lumpectomy and radiotherapy in early breast cancer. Lancet 1992; 339:1245–8.

48. Morrow M. A survival benefit from axillary dissection: was Halsted correct? Ann Surg Oncol 1999; 6:17–18.

49. Danforth DN, Findlay PA, McDonald HD, *et al.* Complete axillary lymph node dissection for stage I–II carcinoma of the breast. J Clin Oncol 1986; 4:655–62.

50. Senofsky GM, Moffat FL, Davis K, *et al.* Total axillary lymphadenectomy in the management of breast cancer. Arch Surg 1991; 126:1336–42.

51. Rosen PP, Lesser ML, Kinne DW, Beattie EJ. Discontinuous or 'skip' metastases in breast carcinoma. Analysis of 1228 axillary dissections. Ann Surg 1983; 197:276–83.

52. Schwartz GF, D'Ugo DM, Rosenberg AL. Extent of axillary dissection preceding irradiation for carcinoma of the breast. Arch Surg 1986; 121:1395–8.

53. Pigott J, Nichols R, Maddox WA, Balch CM. Metastases to the upper level of the axillary nodes in carcinoma of the breast and implications for nodal sampling procedures. Surg Gynecol Obstet 1984; 158:255–9.

54. Attiyeh FF, Jensen M, Huvos AG, Fracchia A. Axillary micrometastasis and macrometastasis in carcinoma of the breast. Gynecol Obstet 1977; 144:839–42.

55. Smith JA, Gamez-Araujo JJ, Gallager HS, *et al.* Carcinoma of the breast. Analysis of total lymph node involvement versus level of metastasis. Cancer 1977; 39:527–32.

56. Boova RS, Bonanni R, Rosato FE. Patterns of axillary node involvement in breast cancer. Predictability of level one dissection. Ann Surg 1982; 196:642–4.

57. Cody HS III, Egeli RA, Urban JA. Rotter's node metastases. Therapeutic and prognostic considerations in early breast cancer. Ann Surg 1984; 199:266–70.

58. Moffat FL, Senofsky GM, Davis K, *et al.* Axillary node dissection for early breast cancer: some is good but all is better. J Surg Oncol 1992; 51:8–13.

59. Veronesi U, Luini A, Galimberti V, *et al.* Extent of metastatic axillary involvement in 1446 cases of breast cancer. Eur J Surg Oncol 1990; 16:127–33.

60. Recht A, Houlihan MJ. Axillary lymph nodes and breast cancer: a review. Cancer 1995; 76:1491–512.

61. Petrek JA, Lerner R. Lymphedema. In Harris JR, Lippman ME, Morrow M, Osborne CK, eds. *Diseases of the breast*, 2nd edn. Philadelphia, Lippincott Williams & Wilkins, 2000, 1033–40.

62. Benson EA, Thorogood J. The effect of surgical technique on local recurrence rates following mastectomy. Eur J Surg Oncol 1986; 12:267–71.

63. Kissin MW, Querci della Rovere G, Easton D, Westbury G. Risk of lymphoedema following the treatment of breast cancer. Br J Surg 1986; 73:580–4.

64. Siegel BM, Mayzel KA, Love SM. Level I and II axillary dissection in the treatment of early-stage breast cancer. An analysis of 259 consecutive patients. Arch Surg 1990; 125:1144–7.

65. Kissin MW, Thompson EM, Price AB, *et al.* The inadequacy of axillary sampling in breast cancer. Lancet 1982; 2:1210–12.

66. Veronesi U, Saccozzi R, Del Vecchio M, *et al.* Comparing radical mastectomy with quadrantectomy, axillary dissection and radiotherapy in patients with small cancers of the breast. N Engl J Med 1981; 305:6–11.

67. Delouche G, Bachelot F, Premont M, Kurtz JM. Conservation treatment of early breast cancer: long term results and complications. Int J Radiat Oncol Biophys 1987; 13:29–34.

68. Larson D, Weinstein M, Goldberg I, *et al.* Edema of the arm as a function of the extent of axillary surgery in

patients in stage I–II carcinoma of the breast treated with primary radiotherapy. Int J Radiat Oncol Biophys 1986; 12:1575–82.

69. Beadle GF, Silver B, Botnick L, *et al.* Cosmetic results following primary radiation therapy for early breast cancer. Cancer 1984; 54:2911–18.

70. Carabell SC, Richter MP, Bryan JH, *et al.* Radiation therapy as an alternative to mastectomy for breast cancer – the role of axillary sampling. Int J Radiat Oncol Biophys 1981; 7:31–2.

71. Hoe AL, Iven D, Royle GT, Taylor I. Incidence of arm swelling following axillary clearance for breast cancer. Br J Surg 1992; 79:261–2.

72. Werner RS, McCormick B, Petrek JA, *et al.* Arm edema in conservatively managed breast cancer: obesity is a major predictive factor. Radiology 1991; 180:177–84.

Commentary

BLAKE CADY

This chapter by Dr Silberman on the potential therapeutic benefit of axillary dissection summarizes a traditional view of the role of lymph node metastases in the survival of patients with cancer. Unfortunately, his review is limited to breast cancer, but a good deal of the literature regarding the value of regional node dissection in cancer has been obtained from other cancer sites, which also bear on the issues.[1,2] The argument he sets out can be defined by the basic biological theories in breast cancer applicable to other cancers also. The original Halsted theory was that the lymphatic system was dominant in cancer spread; visceral metastases occurred by direct or indirect lymphatic vessel connections between the breast and the liver, for instance. This concept was called into question by many studies indicating the absence of benefit of nodal resections on the outcome in a variety of cancers, but particularly breast cancer. The 'systemic from onset' theory of Fisher was based on his animal experimental work as well as on the early randomized trials of the NSABP and dominated biological thinking for a number of years.[3] Fisher postulated that survival is dependent on systemic metastases and their response to treatment, not on nodal metastatic involvement, because survival was equivalent whether lymph nodes were treated or not treated in breast and other cancers. The biological theory most applicable today, however, is based on data from screening, particularly in breast cancer, but also in gastric cancer, and indicates that the majority of patients develop cancers that change their biological behavior as they progress and increase in size. This has been called the spectrum model or biological theory.[4] It is based on the fact that most cancers arise as small lesions of low biological potential, low virulence,[5] and low metastagenicity.[6] As they increase in size, their genetically unstable cells continue to evolve; further genetic events occur and the tumor grade, predominantly low or intermediate when very small, shifts or dedifferentiates and becomes predominantly high when they exceed 2 cm in diameter (T2; T3). Thus, outcome in cancer clearly depends on the time at which the clinical or biologic progression is interrupted. Because population screening reduces the size of lesions to 1 cm or less in the majority of breast cancers,[7] early biological features are predominant, the biological progression is interrupted early, and the cure rate is high. Increasing virulence and metastagenicity accompany the dedifferentiation with increase in size. Although this progression pattern is not universal, it is dominant in early cancers. There is still a subset of 'systemic from origin' cancers as occasional small cancers are seen with poorly differentiated histology and the presence of lymph vessel invasion or lymph node metastases,[8] and, of course, most definitively, a few deaths from breast cancer do occur. However, with small cancers up to 14 mm in diameter detected on mammographic screening, 75% of the uncommon mortality is restricted to about 14% of such cases that have unique biological and mammographic features.[9] Thus, the vast majority of such small (≤ 14 mm) cancers, (± 86%) have a 15-year disease-specific survival of approximately 98%. Other cancers of progressive nature also include some that have no capacity to metastasize at all and have only local growth capacity, even when large. Patients with these T3 cancers without node metastases have a good long-term survival, even in the absence of systemic therapy. The allocation of cases into these three biologic categories probably involves two-thirds of the progressive type fitting the spectrum model, perhaps 10–15% in the 'systemic from origin' category, and the residual 15% or 20% displaying local growth characteristics only. Lymph node metastases (beyond one or two node metastases, particularly micrometastases) may be manifestations of the 'systemic' type or components of progression in the spectrum model, but none of these three models recognizes lymph node metastases as the causative elements of survival – mortality is governed exclusively by distant metastases.[2]

In breast cancer, numerous surgical trials show no survival advantage for nodal dissection, whether of the internal mammary nodes, the axillary apex (level III), or the lower axilla.[10] If one looks beyond breast cancer into the impact of node metastases in other human cancers, such as melanoma and cancers of the stomach, esophagus, colon, rectum, thyroid, and head and neck, one can flesh out the biological implications of the major randomized trials regarding lymph node metastases in breast cancer.[2,10] Thus, prospective randomized trials in melanoma[11] and gastric cancer[12,13] show no overall advantage for lymph node dissection or variations in nodal resection. In melanoma, only through retrospective subset analysis do individual subcategories of patients, amounting to, at most, 10% or 15% of patients, indicate some advantage for nodal dissection. Of course, such retrospective subset analysis is not an appropriate interpretation of patient data in trials when the characteristics analysed are not initially stratified. Node dissection in any cancer does increase the accuracy of staging and may result in stage shifting, which in turn may lead to the increased use of systemic therapy that is perhaps not otherwise indicated. This systemic treatment is likely to be the vehicle for any altered survival results.

A recent comprehensive analysis of the literature on the lymphatic system and variations in lymphatic surgery came to the conclusion that no survival benefit accrued from performance or modifications of lymphatic resection.[10] This conclusion is emphasized by the fact that, when studying long-term survivors at either at 5 years or 10 years, one notes few 10-year survivors of cancers of the breast, lung, colon and rectum, or stomach with more than three node metastases.[14] These results have been borne out by the recent publication of the American College of Surgeons' Gastric Cancer Report, which also revealed rare survivors if multiple lymph node metastases were present.[15]

All these data fit with the comprehensive understanding of the anatomy, embryology, physiology, and function of the lymphatic system.[2,10] The lymphatic system has only two original purposes: to return interstitial fluid to the vascular space and nutrients from the digestive tract to the circulation. In later evolutionary development, collections of lymphocytes in lymph nodes interspersed in the lymphatic system developed for the sole purposes of antigen recognition and humoral and cytotoxic antibody production. Lymph nodes are clearly not millipore filters and do not fulfill that role. Labeled tumor cells injected into the nodal afferent lymphatics are rapidly detected in the efferent nodal lymphatics and the thoracic duct. As a matter of fact, whenever regional lymphatic structures are destroyed by surgery, radiation therapy, parasitic infestation, or tumors, regional edema is almost universal. Mammals, such as pigs, have extremely numerous, large and active regional lymph nodes because of their constant exposure to an environment with copious quantities of bacteria, parasites, and viruses, yet do not display limb edema. Lymph flow is not impeded by the lymph nodes, clearly demonstrating that lymph nodes are a unique porous, filtering organ, but not millipore filters. Indeed, the discovery of a few cells by immunohistochemical staining in sentinel lymph nodes merely indicates the frequency with which foreign material or normal or cancer cells are temporarily held up but then allowed continued passage without impact on survival. Indeed, bone marrow epithelial cells (metastatic cells) are an indicator of metastatic disease but in no data published so far[16,17] do they demonstrate the inevitability of such metastatic disease. Interestingly, in the published trials of bone marrow examination[16,17] in breast cancer patients, the survival impact of bone marrow epithelial cells is exactly equivalent to that of lymph node metastases, suggesting their similar roles as markers or indicators of the risk of metastatic disease, but not a controlling or causative function.

The unique feature of the recent trials reported by Overgaard[18,19] and Ragaz[20] that distinguishes them from all previous trials, which revealed no survival difference by the addition of radiation to surgical therapy for breast cancer, is the uniform use of systemic adjuvant chemotherapy. Failures or recurrences following systemic adjuvant chemotherapy, by definition, are caused by chemoresistant cells, which were not an aspect of previous trials that did not utilize systemic therapy initially. Recent studies on neoadjuvant chemotherapy emphasize this aspect of chemosensitivity or resistance in that even advanced clinical presentation of breast cancer with multiple node metastases or large inflammatory primary cancers can be cured in a high proportion of cases if there is a complete clinical, or especially a complete pathological, response.[21] These studies clearly display the controlling influence of chemosensitivity on the outcome of breast cancer, not the initial presentation of disease, whether indicated by an advanced primary, multiple node metastases, or other poor prognostic features. These neoadjuvant trials display the overriding importance of sensitivity to hormonal or chemotherapy systemic treatments as the *sine qua non* of curability and survivability in breast cancer. Because breast cancer survival is related only to the presence and growth of systemic metastases, the particular features of the primary cancer or the lymph node metastases are relegated to an indicator role. Survivability in small, screen-detected cancers is still related to the absence of clinical distant metastases, even though sentinel node or even bone marrow micrometastases are frequent. Breast cancer patients never die of the local breast disease, its recurrence, or lymph node metastases in the axilla or their recurrence. Because women do not die of the axillary metastases themselves, by definition, the axillary metastases are indicators of the outcome determined by distant metastases: node metastases are statistically linked to the probability of the controlling distant metastases but do not cause them.[2]

The biological explanation of this indicator function has been found in recent research regarding the cell and organ specificity of distant metastatic disease.[22] While this is observed in human models of isolated distant metastases that can be cured by resection, such as liver metastases following colorectal carcinoma,[23] or pulmonary metastases in sarcoma,[24] a similar biological feature applies to lymph node metastases.[25] Thus, Brodt and colleagues[25] have amply displayed the unique cell and lymph node stroma features that govern the presence of lymph node metastases: a cell that grows in a lymph node may have little or no capacity to grow in other organs. Similarly, patients with liver metastases who survive following hepatic resection clearly had circulating metastatic cells that had no capacity to lodge and grow elsewhere in the body. An obvious example of this feature can be seen in differentiated thyroid cancer in young patients in whom the presence of multiple lymph node metastases occurs in at least 75% of patients who have routine node dissections, yet distant metastases are rare.[26] Here, obviously, cells that have the capacity to spread to, lodge in, and grow in lymph nodes have no such capacity in other organs. Contrariwise, sarcoma patients who frequently develop pulmonary metastases seldom have lymph node metastases. These lymph node metastases fill only an indicator function, as sarcoma patients with lymph node metastases indeed have a poor prognosis, but survival is governed entirely by the distant metastases.

These arguments regarding the indicator, but not governing, role of lymph node metastases are emphasized by lymph node recurrence in breast cancer: survival is better if there is longer delay before recurrent lymph node metastases. If lymph node metastases themselves had the capacity to cause distant metastases, then the longer they were present or the longer the disease-free interval, the worse should be the survival – the exact opposite of what occurs. The longer the disease-free interval the better the outcome, the higher the survival rate, and the higher the proportion of patients cured. Indeed, if one looks at lymph node recurrences (or local recurrences), they may appear prior to, simultaneous with, or after distant metastases, or independently without metastatic disease, in approximately equal proportions.[2] Yet the causative role of lymph node metastases in survival could only be postulated if they appeared first and distant metastases appeared subsequently, the situation in only a minority of nodal recurrences. Indeed, when lymph nodes are not dissected initially, but only at the time of recurrence, the number and location of such node metastases are approximately the same as in prophylactic removal, and equivalent curability is achieved, even though the lymph node metastases were present for long periods of time and only removed late in their clinical course. The similar survival comparing initial prophylactic to later therapeutic nodal dissection as seen in breast cancer and melanoma trials emphasizes the indicator, not governing, role of such lymph node metastases.

Thus, a critical review of the role of lymph node metastases has to conclude that they perform an indicator role, not a controlling or causative function in the outcome for patients. As a result, whether they are resected initially or not will have no impact on survival.

Our task should be to detect the presence of lymph node metastases, to aid in systemic therapy choice, in the least morbid fashion. Sentinel lymph node biopsy fulfills that role and can be performed under minimal anesthesia. Only in the case of gross nodal involvement of sentinel nodes in larger primary cancers will subsequent axillary dissection help to prevent regional recurrence.

For several decades we have ignored internal mammary lymph node dissection or sampling and we need not do it now in the era of sentinel node biopsy; it seldom provides critical information.

REFERENCES

1. Cady B. Is axillary lymph node dissection necessary in routine management of breast cancer? Cancer – Principles & Practice of Oncology (PPO Updates) 1998; 12(7):1–12.
2. Cady B. Oncology lecture. Fundamentals of contemporary surgical oncology: biological principles and the threshold concept govern treatment and outcome. J Am Coll Surg 2001; 192(6):777–92.
3. Fisher B. Laboratory and clinical research in breast cancer – a personal adventure: the David A. Karnovsky Memorial Lecture. Cancer Res 1980; 40:3863–74.
4. Hellman S. Karnovsky Memorial Lecture. Natural history of small breast cancers. J Clin Oncol 1994; 12(10):2229–34.
5. Heimann R, Ferguson D, Recant WM, Hellman S. Breast cancer metastatic phenotype as predicted by histologic tumor markers. Cancer J Sci Am 1997; 3:224–9.
6. Heimann R, Hellman S. Aging, progression, and phenotype in breast cancer. J Clin Oncol 1998; 16:2686–92.
7. Cady B, Stone MD, Schuler JG, Thakur R, Wanner MA, Lavin PT. The new era in breast cancer: invasion, size, and nodal involvement dramatically decreasing as a result of mammographic screening. Arch Surg 1996; 131:301–8.
8. Leitner SP, Swern AS, Weinberger D, *et al.* Predictors of recurrence for patients with small (one centimeter or less) localized breast cancer (T1a, N0, M0). Cancer 1995; 76(11):2266–74.
9. Tabar L, Chen HH, Duffy S, *et al.* A novel method for prediction of long-term outcome of women with T1a, T1b, and 10–14 mm invasive breast cancers: a prospective study. Lancet 2000; 355(9202):429–33.
10. Gervasoni JE, Taneja C, Chung MA, Cady B. Biologic and clinical significance of lymphadenectomy. Surg Oncol Clin North Am 2000; 80(6):1631–73.
11. Balch CM, Soong SJ, Bartolucci AA, *et al.* Efficacy of elective regional lymph node dissection of 1 to 4 mm thick melanomas for patients 60 years and younger. Ann Surg 1996; 224:255–63.

12. Bonenkamp JJ, Hermans J, Sasako M, van de Velde CJH. Extended lymph node dissection for gastric cancer. N Engl J Med 1999; 340:908–14.

13. Cuschieri A, Weeden S, Fielding J, *et al.* Patient survival after D-1 and D-2 resections for gastric cancer: long-term results of the MRC randomized surgical trial. Br J Cancer 1999; 79:1522–30.

14. Cady B. Basic principles in surgical oncology. Presidential Address. Arch Surg 1997; 132:338–46.

15. Hundahl SA, Phillips JL, Mench HR. The National Cancer Data Base Report on poor survival of U.S. gastric carcinoma patients treated with gastrectomy: Fifth Edition American Joint Committee on Cancer staging, proximal disease, and the 'difference disease' hypothesis. Cancer 2000; 88(4):921–32.

16. Diel IJ, Kaufmann M, Costa SD, *et al.* Micrometastatic breast cancer cells in bone marrow at primary surgery: prognostic value in comparison with nodal status. J Natl Cancer Inst 1996; 88:1652–8.

17. Braun S, Pantel K, Muller P, *et al.* Cytokeratin-positive cells in the bone marrow and survival of patients with Stage I, II, or III breast cancer. N Engl J Med 2000; 342(8):525–33.

18. Overgaard M, Hansen PR, Overgaard J, *et al.* Postoperative radiotherapy in high-risk premenopausal women with breast cancer who receive adjuvant chemotherapy. N Engl J Med 1997; 337(14):949–55.

19. Overgaard M, Jensen MB, Overgaard J, *et al.* Postoperative radiotherapy in high-risk postmenopausal breast-cancer patients given adjuvant tamoxifen: Danish Breast Cancer Cooperative Group DBCG 82c randomised trial. Lancet 1999; 353:1641–8.

20. Ragaz J, Jackson SM, Le N, *et al.* Adjuvant radiotherapy and chemotherapy in node-positive premenopausal women with breast cancer. N Engl J Med 1997; 337:956–62.

21. Fisher B, Bryant J, Wolmark N, *et al.* Effect of preoperative chemotherapy on the outcome of women with operable breast cancer. J Clin Oncol 1998; 16:2672–85.

22. Chambers AF, Naumov GN, Varghese HJ, *et al.* Critical steps in hematogenous metastasis – an overview. Surg Oncol Clin North Am 2001; 10:243–55.

23. Cady B, Jenkins RL, Steele GD, *et al.* Surgical margin in hepatic resection for colorectal metastasis. Ann Surg 1998; 227(4):566–71.

24. Vezeridis MP, Moore R, Karakousis CP. Metastatic patterns in soft-tissue sarcomas. Arch Surg 1983; 118:915.

25. Brodt P, Reich R, Moroz LA, *et al.* Differences in the repertoires of basement membrane degrading enzymes in two carcinoma sublines with distinct patterns of site-selective metastasis. Biochem Biophys Acta 1992; 77:1139.

26. Cady B. Presidential address: Beyond risk groups: a new look at differentiated thyroid cancer. Surgery 1998; 124(6):947–57.

Editors' selected abstracts

Impact of axillary dissection on staging and regional control in breast tumors ≤10 mm – the DBCG experience. The Danish Breast Cancer Cooperative Group (DBCG), Rigshisoutalet, Copenhagen, Denmark.

Axelsson CK, Rank F, Blichert-Toft M, Mouridsen HT, Jensen MB.

Surgical Department A, Odense University Hospital, Denmark.

Acta Oncologica 39(3):283–9, 2000.

Data from 4771 patients with tumor diameters ≤10 mm were analyzed. Results of surgery and pathoanatomical examinations indicated that nodal status was related to diameter, but not to number of nodes removed. More axillary metastases were found in group T1b tumors than in T1a. In 8% of tumors, at least 4 positive nodes were identified. Mean number of positive nodes was related to number of nodes removed, and when 10 or more nodes were removed a significantly lower axillary recurrence rate and better recurrence-free survival were demonstrated, confirming that axillary surgery has two goals: staging and regional disease control. Age, receptor status, grade and histological type, but not tumor location, were related to prognosis. In accordance with the classical prognostic factors, it was not possible to define a patient group where axillary surgery was superfluous. We conclude that proper staging and regional control renders a full axillary level I–II dissection necessary.

Axillary dissection in breast-conserving surgery for Stage I and II breast cancer: a National Cancer Data Base study of patterns of omission and implications for survival.

Bland KI, Scott-Conner CE, Menck H, Winchester DP.

Department of Surgery, Brown University, Providence, RI, USA.

Journal of the American College of Surgeons 188(6):586–95, 1999, June.

Background: Breast conservation (partial mastectomy, axillary node dissection or sampling, and radiotherapy) is the current standard of care for eligible patients with Stages I and II breast cancer. Because axillary node dissection (AND) has a low yield, some have argued for its omission. The present study was undertaken to determine factors that correlated with omission of AND, and the impact of the decision to omit AND on 10-year relative survival. *Study design:* A retrospective review of National Cancer Data Base (NCDB) data for 547 847 women with Stage I and Stage II breast cancer treated in US hospitals from 1985 to 1995 was undertaken. A subset of 47 944 Stage I and 23 283 Stage II women treated with breast-conserving surgery (BCS) was identified. Cross-tab analysis was used to compare patterns of surgical care within this subset. Relative survival was calculated as the ratio of observed survival to the expected survival for women of the same age and racial/ethnic background. *Results:* The rate of BCS with and without AND increased steadily from 17.6% and 6.4% of patients from 1985–1989, to 36.6% and 10.6% of patients from 1993–1995 respectively. AND was more likely to be omitted in women with Stage I than women with Stage II disease (14.5% versus 5.5%). Similarly, AND was omitted more frequently in women with Grade 1 than women with higher grades (Grade 1, 14.9%; Grade 2, 10.1%; Grade 3, 7.1%; Grade 4, 7%). Although the rate of BCS with AND varied considerably according to location in the breast, the overall rate of BCS without AND appeared independent of site of lesion. Women over the age of 70 years were more than twice as likely to have AND omitted from BCS than their younger counterparts. Women with lower incomes, women treated in the Northeast, or at hospitals with annual caseloads <150 were all less likely to undergo AND than their corresponding counterparts. Ten-year relative survival for Stage I women treated with partial mastectomy and AND was 85% ($n = 1242$) versus 66% ($n = 1684$) for comparable women in whom AND was omitted. BCS with AND followed by radiation therapy for Stage I disease resulted in 94% ($n = 5469$) 10-year relative survival, compared with 85% ($n = 1284$) without AND. Addition of both radiation and chemotherapy to BCS with AND for Stage I disease resulted in 86% ($n = 2800$) versus 58% ($n = 512$) without AND. In contrast, Stage II women treated with BCS with AND followed by radiation and chemotherapy experienced a 72% 10-year relative survival. *Conclusions:* A significant number of women with Stage I breast cancer do not undergo AND as part of BCS. The trend is most pronounced for the elderly, but significant fractions of women of all ages are also being undertreated by current standards. Ten-year survival is significantly worse when AND is omitted. This adverse survival effect is not solely from understaging.

Axillary lymphadenectomy for breast cancer: paradigm shifts and pragmatic surgeons.

Dent DM.

Department of Surgery, University of Cape Town, Cape Town, South Africa.

Archives of Surgery 131(11):1125–7, 1996, November.

The debate has proceeded to whether there is a survival advantage to axillary lymphadenectomy. Many surgeons hold a lingering remnant of the Halstedian concept that involvement of the lymph nodes precedes systemic metastases, a concept that must include the notion that lymph node metastases may themselves systemically metastasize and their removal may prevent such dissemination. This paradigm underwent the rigorous test of randomized clinical trials to test its veracity. I am aware of 3 prospective randomized trials that compared mastectomy with axillary clearance with mastectomy without it and avoided the confounding additions of radiotherapy or systemic treatment

(although these were used on relapse): the NSABP (B04) trial, the Cancer Research Campaign (Kings and Cambridge hospitals) trial and the small Groote Schuur Hospital trial. None showed a significant survival advantage to axillary lymphadenectomy, although axillary relapse was more frequent in the groups with untreated axillae. Further, the meta-analytic verdict of the Early Breast Cancer Trialists' Collaborative Group was that axillary lymphadenectomy conferred no survival advantage. They used data from 58 randomized trials involving 12 000 deaths among 28 405 women with early breast cancer, and recognized that either clearance of or radiotherapy to the axilla, when used as an adjunct to mastectomy, yielded equivalent 10-year survival rates. Equivalent survival was also found in patients with undissected axillae when compared with those who had undergone axillary dissection. Survival in each of the comparisons appeared to be determined by whether the glands were involved and not by the treatment options. This lack of survival advantage supports Devitt's prescient observation over 30 years ago that 'axillary lymph node metastases are an expression of a bad prognosis rather than a determinant,' as have the consistent and weighty views of, among others, Fisher, Baum, and Cady. The staging of intramammary nodes has fallen away from routine practice, although they are known to be involved in 22% of centromedial tumors and after mastectomy are unlikely to be irradiated prophylactically. This avoidance of treatment after mastectomy constitutes tacit agreement with the lack of importance of management of these potentially involved nodes. It is difficult to conceive how intramammary node involvement would differ from that of the axilla for pathological behavior, treatment, and survival.

Mastectomy with axillary clearance versus mastectomy without it. Late results of a trial in which patients had no adjuvant chemo-, radio- or endocrine therapy.

Dent DM, Gudgeon CA, Murray EM.

Department of Surgery, University of Cape Town, Cape Town, South Africa.

South African Medical Journal 86(6):670–1, 1996, June.

Objective: Long-term outcome of comparison of mastectomy with axillary clearance to mastectomy without it. *Design:* Second analysis of a terminated prospective randomised trial. *Setting:* The Breast Clinic, Groote Schuur Hospital, Cape Town. *Patients:* Ninety-five women aged under 76 years with stages 1 and 2 (T1–2 N0–1 M0) breast cancer. *Interventions:* Radical mastectomy (mastectomy and formal axillary dissection with pectoral muscle excision) or simple mastectomy (mastectomy without axillary dissection if nodes were not clinically palpable, or local excision of the nodes if they were). *Outcome measures:* Loco-regional recurrence and survival. *Results:* Whereas initial analysis at 40 months had showed more axillary recurrences ($p = 0.056$) in the simple mastectomy group (leading to the termination of the trial), this difference has disappeared at 10 years ($p = 0.113$). There was no difference in rate of recurrence at all other sites, time to recurrence, or survival rates at 40 months or at 10 or 25 years. *Conclusions:* Full axillary clearance offered no better long-term loco-regional control or survival. Early analysis and marginally significant differences in axillary recurrence prompted premature termination of this trial.

Is radiation alone adequate treatment to the axilla for patients with limited axillary surgery? Implications for treatment after a positive sentinel node biopsy.

Galper S, Recht A, Silver B, Bernardo MV, Gelman R, Wong J, Schnitt SJ, Connolly JL, Harris JR.

Joint Center for Radiation Therapy, Boston, MA, USA.

International Journal of Radiation Oncology, Biology, Physics 48(1):125–32, 2000, August 1.

Purpose: To estimate the possible efficacy of axillary radiation therapy (AXRT) following a positive sentinel node biopsy (SNB), we evaluated the risk of regional nodal failure (RNF) for patients with clinical Stage I or II, clinically node-negative invasive breast cancer treated with either no dissection or a limited dissection (LD) defined as removal of 5 nodes or less followed by AXRT. *Materials and methods:* From 1978 to 1987, 292 patients underwent AXRT in the absence of axillary dissection; 126 underwent AXRT following LD. The median dose to the axilla was 46 Gy. The median dose to the supraclavicular fossa was 45 Gy. Among patients found to have positive nodes on LD, adjuvant chemotherapy and tamoxifen were administered to 81% and 7% of subjects, respectively. All patients had potential 8-year follow-up. *Results:* Six of the 418 patients (1.4%) developed RNF as a first site of failure within 8 years. Among these 6 patients (1.4%) with RNF as a first site of failure, 4 had simultaneous distant and regional recurrences; and 2 had isolated axillary failures. Three of the 292 patients (1%) with no axillary dissection, none of 84 patients with pathologically negative nodes and 3 of 42 patients (7%) with pathologically involved nodes had RNF as a first site of failure. Radiation pneumonitis developed in 5 patients (1.2%), brachial plexopathy in 5 (1.2%) and arm edema in 4 (1.2%). In all cases, radiation pneumonitis and brachial plexopathy were transient. *Conclusion:* These results imply that AXRT may be an effective and safe alternative to completion dissection for treatment of the axilla following a positive SNB. Further studies comparing these two options in specific patient subgroups are needed.

Breast cancer patients treated without axillary surgery: clinical implications and biologic analysis.

Greco M, Agresti R, Cascinelli N, Casalini P, Giovanazzi R, Maucione A, Tomasic G, Ferraris C, Ammatuna M, Pilotti S, Menard S.

General Surgery B-Breast Unit, National Cancer Institute, Milan, Italy.

Annals of Surgery 232(1):1–7, 2000, July.

Objective: To evaluate the impact of breast carcinoma (T1–2N0) surgery without axillary dissection on axillary and distant relapses, and to evaluate the usefulness of a panel of pathobiologic parameters determined from the primary tumor, independent of axillary nodal status, in planning adjuvant treatment. *Methods:* In a prospective nonrandomized pilot study, 401 breast cancer patients who underwent breast surgery without axillary dissection were accrued from January 1986 to June 1994. At surgery, all patients were clinically node-negative and lacked evidence of distant metastases after clinical or radiologic examination. A precise 4-month clinical and radiologic follow-up was performed to detect axillary or distant metastases. Patients with clinical evidence of axillary nodal relapse were considered for surgery as salvage treatment. Biologic characteristics of primary carcinomas were investigated by immunohistochemistry, and four pathologic and biologic parameters (size, grading, laminin receptor, and c-erbB-2 receptor) were analyzed to determine a prognostic score. *Results:* The 5-year follow-up of these patients revealed a low rate of nodal relapses (6.7%), particularly for T1a and T1b patients (2% and 1.7%, respectively), whereas T1c and T2 patients showed a 10% and 18% relapse rate, respectively. Surgery was a safe and feasible salvage treatment without technical problems in all 19 cases of progressive disease at the axillary level. The low rate of distant metastases in T1a and T1b groups ($<$ 6%) increased to 15% in T1c and 34% in T2 patients. Analyzing the primary tumor with respect to the panel of pathologic and biologic parameters was predictive of metastatic spread and therefore can replace nodal status information for planning adjuvant treatment. *Conclusions:* Middle-term follow-up shows that the rate of axillary relapse in this patient population is lower than expected, suggesting that only a minimal number of microembolic nodal metastases become clinically evident. Avoidance of axillary dissection has a negligible effect on the outcome of T1 patients, particularly in T1a and T1b tumors with no palpable nodes, because the rate of axillary node relapse is very low for both. In T1 breast carcinoma, postsurgical therapy should be considered on the basis of biologic characteristics rather than nodal involvement. The authors' prognostic score based on the primary tumor identified patients who required postsurgical treatment, providing a practical alternative to axillary status for deciding on adjuvant treatment. Conversely, in the T2 group, the high rate of salvage surgery for axillary relapses, which is expected in tumors larger than 2.5 cm or 3.0 cm, represents a limit for avoiding axillary dissection. Preoperative evaluation of axillary nodes for modification of surgical dissection in this subgroup would be more useful than in T1 breast cancer because of the high risk. Complete dissection is feasible without technical problems if precise follow-up detects progressive axillary disease.

Sentinel lymphadenectomy accurately predicts nodal status in T2 breast cancer.

Olson JA Jr, Fey J, Winawer J, Borgen PI, Cody HS 3rd, Van Zee KJ, Petrek J, Heerdt AS.

Department of Surgery, Memorial Sloan-Kettering Cancer Center, New York, NY, USA.

Journal of the American College of Surgeons 191(6):593–9, 2000, December.

Background: Sentinel lymph node biopsy (SLNB) has emerged as a reliable, accurate method of staging the axilla for early breast cancer. Although widely accepted for T1 lesions, its use in larger tumors remains controversial. This study was undertaken to define the role of SLNB for T2 breast cancer. *Study design:* From a prospective breast sentinel lymph node database of 1,627 patients accrued between September 1996 and November 1999, we identified 223 patients with clinical T1–2N0 breast cancer who underwent 224 lymphatic mapping procedures and SLNB followed by a standard axillary lymph node dissection (ALND). Preoperative lymphatic mapping was performed by injection of unfiltered technetium 99 sulfur colloid and isosulfan blue dye. Data about patient and tumor characteristics and the status of the sentinel lymph nodes and the axillary nodes were analyzed. Statistics were performed using Fisher's exact test. *Results:* Two hundred four of 224 sentinel lymph node mapping procedures (91%) were successful. Median tumor size was 2.0 cm (range 0.2 to 4.8 cm). One hundred forty-five of the 204 patients had T1 lesions and 59 patients had T2 lesions. There were 92 pathologically positive axillae, 5 (5%) of which were not evident either by SLNB or by intraoperative clinical examination. The false-negative rate and accuracy were not significantly different between the two groups, but axillary node metastases were observed more frequently with T2 than with T1 tumors ($p = 0.005$); other factors, including patient age, prior surgical biopsy, upper-outer quadrant tumor location, and tumor lymphovascular invasion were not associated with a higher incidence of false-negative SLNB in either T1 or T2 tumors. *Conclusions:* SLNB is as accurate for T2 tumors as it is for T1 tumors. Because no tumor or patient characteristics predict a high false-negative rate, all patients with T1–2N0 breast cancer should be considered candidates for the procedure. Complete clinical examination of the axilla should be undertaken to avoid missing palpable axillary nodal metastases.

Sentinel lymph node biopsy with metastasis: can axillary dissection be avoided in some patients with breast cancer?

Reynolds C, Mick R, Donohue JH, Grant CS, Farley DR, Callans LS, Orel SG, Keeney GL, Lawton TJ, Czerniecki BJ.

Departments of Laboratory Medicine and Pathology, and Surgery, Mayo Clinic, Rochester, MN, USA.

Journal of Clinical Oncology 17(6):1720–6, 1999, June.

Purpose: Recent studies have suggested that the sentinel lymph node (SLN) biopsy is an accurate alternative staging procedure for women with breast cancer. The goal of this study was to identify a subset of breast cancer patients in whom metastatic disease was confined only to the SLN. *Materials and methods:* From two institutions, we recruited 222 women with breast cancer for SLN biopsy. A SLN biopsy was performed in each patient, followed by an axillary dissection in 182 patients. Histologic and immunohistochemical cytokeratin stains were used on all SLNs. *Results:* The SLN was identified in 220 (97.8%) of the 225 biopsies. Evidence of metastatic breast cancer in the SLN was found in 60 (27.0%) of the 222 patients. Of these patients, 32 (53.3%) had evidence of tumor in the SLN only. By multivariate analysis, two factors were found to be significantly associated with a higher likelihood of tumor involvement in the non-SLNs: primary tumor size larger than 2.0 cm ($p = 0.0004$) and macrometastasis (>2.0 mm) in the SLN ($p = 0.002$). Additional analysis revealed that none (0%; 95% confidence interval, 0% to 18.5%) of the 18 patients with primary tumors $\leqslant 2.0$ cm and micrometastasis to the

SLN had remaining axillary lymph node involvement. *Conclusion:* The primary tumor size and metastasis size in the SLN are independent factors in predicting the incidence of tumor in the non-SLNs. Therefore, the SLN biopsy alone may be adequate for staging and/or therapy decision making in patients with primary breast tumors $\leqslant 2.0$ cm and micrometastasis in the SLN.

Association between extent of axillary lymph node dissection and survival in patients with stage I breast cancer.

Sosa JA, Diener-West M, Gusev Y, Choti MA, Lange JR, Dooley WC, Zeiger MA.

Department of Surgery, The Johns Hopkins University School of Medicine, Baltimore, MD, USA.

Annals of Surgical Oncology 5(2):140–9, 1998, March.

Background: The role of axillary lymph node dissection for stage I (T1N0) breast cancer remains controversial because patients can receive adjuvant chemotherapy regardless of their nodal status and because its therapeutic benefit is in question. The purpose of this study was to determine whether extent of axillary dissection in patients with T1N0 disease is associated with survival. *Methods:* Data from 464 patients with T1N0 breast cancer who underwent axillary dissection from 1973 to 1994 were examined retrospectively. Kaplan–Meier estimates of overall survival, disease-free survival, and recurrence were calculated for patients according to the number of lymph nodes removed (<10 or $\geqslant 10$; <15 or $\geqslant 15$), and survival curves compared using the Wilcoxon–Gehan statistic. Cox proportional hazards regression modelling was used to adjust for confounding prognostic variables. *Results:* Median follow-up time was 6.4 years. Patient groups were similar in age, menopausal status, tumor size, hormonal receptor status, type of surgery, and adjuvant therapy. There was a statistically significant improvement in disease-free survival in the $\geqslant 10$ versus <10 nodal groups ($p < 0.01$). Five-year estimates of survival were 75.7% and 86.2% for <10 nodes and $\geqslant 10$ nodes, respectively; 10-year estimates were 66.1% and 74.3%. There also was a notable improvement in the survival comparison of patients with <15 versus $\geqslant 15$ nodes ($p \leqslant 0.05$). These findings were confirmed in the multivariate analysis. *Conclusions:* These results may reflect a potential for misclassification of tumor stage among patients who had fewer nodes removed. The data, however, suggest that in patients with stage I breast cancer, improved survival is associated with a more complete axillary lymph node dissection.

Do cytokeratin-positive-only sentinel lymph nodes warrant complete axillary lymph node dissection in patients with invasive breast cancer?

Teng S, Dupont E, McCann C, Wang J, Bolano M, Durand K, Peltz E, Bass SS, Cantor A, Ku NN, Cox CE.

H. Lee Moffitt Cancer Center at the University of South Florida, Tampa, FL, USA.

American Surgeon 66(6):574–8, 2000, June.

The small number of nodes harvested with lymphatic mapping and sentinel lymph node (SLN) biopsy has allowed a more detailed pathologic examination of those nodes. Immunohistochemical stains for cytokeratin (CK-IHC) have been used in an attempt to minimize the false negative rate for SLN mapping. This study examines the value of CK-IHC positivity in predicting further lymph node involvement in the axillary basin. From April 1998 through May 1999, 519 lymphatic mappings and SLN biopsies were performed for invasive breast cancer. SLNs were examined by imprint cytology, hematoxylin and eosin (H & E), and CK-IHC. Patients with evidence of metastatic disease by any of the above techniques were eligible for complete axillary node dissection (CAND). The frequency with which these modalities predicted further lymph node involvement in the axillary basin was compared. Of the 519 lymphatic mappings, 39 patients (7.5%) had a CK-IHC-positive-only SLN. Five (12.8%) of these 39 patients had at least 2 SLNs positive by CK-IHC. Twenty-six of the CK-IHC-positive-only patients underwent CAND. Three of these 26 patients (11.5%) had additional metastases identified after CAND. The sensitivity levels with which each modality detected further axillary lymph node involvement were as follows: CK-IHC, 98 per cent; H & E, 94 per cent; and imprint cytology, 87 per cent. A logistic regression to compare the prognostic value of the three modalities were performed. All were significant, with odd ratios of 19.1 for CK-IHC ($p = 0.015$), 5.3 for H & E ($p = 0.033$), and 3.86 for imprint cytology ($p = 0.0059$). These data validate the enhanced detection of CK-IHC for the evaluation of SLNs. Detection of CK-IHC-positive SLNs appears to warrant CAND in patients with invasive breast cancer. However, the therapeutic value of CAND or adjuvant therapies based on CK-IHC-positive SLNs would be best answered by prospective randomized trials.

The relationship between lymphatic vessel invasion, tumor size, and pathologic nodal status: can we predict who can avoid a third field in the absence of axillary dissection?

Wong JS, O'Neill A, Recht A, Schnitt SJ, Connolly JL, Silver B, Harris JR.

Joint Center for Radiation Therapy, Boston, MA, USA.

International Journal of Radiation Oncology, Biology, Physics 48(1):133–7, 2000, August 1.

Purpose: Tangential (2-field) radiation therapy to the breast and lower axilla is typically used in our institution for treating patients with early-stage breast cancer who have 0–3 positive axillary nodes, as determined by axillary dissection, whereas a third supraclavicular/axillary field is added for patients with 4 or more positive nodes. However, dissection may result in complications and added expense. We, therefore, assessed whether clinical or pathologic factors of the primary tumor could reliably predict, in the absence of an axillary dissection, which patients with clinically negative axillary nodes have such limited pathologic nodal involvement that they might be effectively treated with only tangential fields. This would eliminate both the complications of axillary dissection and the added complexity and potential morbidity of a supraclavicular/axillary field. *Methods and materials:* In this study, 722 women with clinical Stage I or II unilateral invasive breast cancer of infiltrating ductal histology, with clinically negative axillary nodes, at least 6 lymph nodes recovered on axillary dissection, and central pathology review were treated with breast-conserving therapy from 1968 to 1987. Pathologic nodal status was assessed in relation to clinical T stage, the presence of lymphatic vessel invasion (LVI), age, histologic grade, and the location of the primary tumor. *Results:* LVI, T stage, and tumor location were each significantly correlated with nodal status on univariate analysis. Ninety-seven percent of LVI-negative patients had 0–3 positive axillary nodes compared to 87% of LVI-positive patients. There was no association between T stage and extent of axillary involvement within LVI-negative and LVI-positive subgroups. In a logistic regression model, only LVI remained a significant predictor of having 4 or more positive nodes, although tumor size was of borderline significance. The odds ratio for LVI (positive vs. negative) as a predictor of having 4 or more positive nodes was 3.9 (95% CI, 2.0–7.6). *Conclusion:* For patients with clinical T1–2, N0, infiltrating ductal carcinomas, the presence of LVI is predictive of having 4 or more positive axillary nodes. Only 3% of patients with clinical T1–2, N0, LVI-negative breast cancers had 4 or more positive nodes on axillary dissection. Such patients may be reasonable candidates for treatment with tangential radiation fields in the absence of axillary dissection.

16

Concepts and development of sentinel lymph node techniques for the management of melanoma and breast cancer

RALPH C JONES, JAMES E DUNCAN, AND ARMANDO E GIULIANO

INTRODUCTION

The most powerful prognosticator of survival for patients with a wide variety of solid tumors is the status of regional lymph nodes. This is reflected in staging schemes and often conveys a change in the treatment required if lymph node metastases are identified. Nuances specific to the origin of the primary are relevant to interpretation of the impact of lymph node involvement. These nuances target our understanding of the disease-specific metastatic process and must be evaluated for each neoplasm individually.

Of the many promising developments in the realm of oncology, the concept of intraoperative lymphatic mapping (LM) and sentinel lymphadenectomy (SLND) is revolutionizing staging schemes, treatment protocols, and surgical management for some solid tumors. LM/SLND is undertaken to identify and excise the lymph node(s) most likely to contain any tumor cells that have metastasized from the primary tumor. Prior to the surgical procedure, lymphoscintigraphy may be used to identify at-risk lymphatic basins, lymphatic drainage pathways, and lymph nodes in aberrant locations. At the start of the surgical procedure, a vital dye is injected at the site of the primary tumor. Intraoperative visualization of the dye, combined with intraoperative measurement of the radiotracer injected during preoperative lymphoscintigraphy, enables the surgeon to identify the first or 'sentinel' lymph nodes draining a specific patient's tumor (Plate 11). Lymph nodes that primarily drain the site of a malignancy are more likely to receive metastasizing tumor cells than lymph nodes that do not drain the primary site – or do so only after receiving lymph from the sentinel node. Although LM/SLND may potentially be beneficial for the evaluation of a wide variety of neoplasms, it is most commonly used in melanoma and, with increasing frequency, in breast cancer.[1–30] To appreciate fully the impact of sentinel node technology, the underlying issues for these two specific malignancies must be elucidated.

MELANOMA

Elective lymph node dissection

Standard treatment for patients with melanoma metastatic to regional lymph nodes is radical lymph node dissection. If performed for confirmed disease, it is a therapeutic lymphadenectomy. In this case, radical lymphadenectomy is the principal treatment, with an anticipated 10-year survival rate of approximately 25–40%, depending on the number of tumor-involved nodes.[31–33] Elective lymph node dissection (ELND) may be performed in a patient who has no clinically evident nodal disease but whose primary melanoma is associated with an increased risk of nodal metastasis. Despite innumerable retrospective analyses and several prospective trials, the role of ELND remains a source of considerable controversy.[34–40] If ELND is not used, i.e., if nodal disease is permitted to progress until clinically evident, then perhaps for some patients the chance for cure may be sacrificed. Conversely, if ELND is routinely used, the majority of patients would undergo radical lymphadenectomy for non-involved nodes – a disfiguring and often debilitating surgery without any derived therapeutic benefit. Long-term results from the Intergroup Melanoma Surgical Trial, the largest randomized, prospective evaluation of ELND with 740 patients, did not show a 10-year overall survival benefit for the entire group that received ELND versus nodal observation (77% versus 73%, $p = 0.12$).[41] Subgroup analysis did identify some variables that favored ELND, with a 10-year overall survival benefit versus nodal observation. Mortality was also lower when ELND was undertaken in patients with non-ulcerated melanomas (30%, $p = 0.03$), Breslow tumor thickness of 1.0–2.0 mm (30%, $p = 0.03$), limb melanomas (27%, $p = 0.05$), and age no greater than 60 years (27%, $p = 0.03$). Despite these important data, the pathologic assessment of lymph node involvement is becoming increasingly desirable to stratify patients for consideration of interferon alfa-2b (IFNα-2b)[42] or investigational adjuvant therapies. Also, early lymphadenectomy for melanoma reduces the frequency and mortality of late melanoma recurrences after 10-year disease-free intervals.[43]

The sentinel node concept

One solution to the dilemma is a less invasive means to identify individuals who have clinically occult nodal metastases. This would target patients who could benefit from radical lymphadenectomy and subsequent treatment, while sparing those patients without nodal involvement the morbidity of surgery and adjuvant therapy. Morton and associates[1,2] have championed just such a technique: their procedure of SLND is a selective sampling technique that is followed by radical lymphadenectomy only if nodal metastases are confirmed. Selective excision and analysis of the sentinel node could render the practice of ELND obsolete and eliminate much of its attendant controversy.

Evolution of LM/SLND

The concept of LM for cutaneous malignancy as developed by Morton's group can be traced back to their experience with cutaneous lymphoscintigraphy using colloidal gold.[44–46] Even then, the ambiguous lymphatic drainage from cutaneous sites was well recognized. ELND opponents cite the complexity of drainage patterns and occasional multiple drainage routes to various regional lymph node basins as reason to 'watch and wait.' Continued reassessment for optimal radionuclides and increasing experience with cutaneous lymphoscintigraphy in melanoma patients helped to determine lymph node regions at risk for potential metastases.[10,47–55] However, cutaneous lymphoscintigraphy reveals lymph *flow*, not lymph node metastases. Thus, it may not be helpful in patients with clinically inapparent nodal disease and concomitant lymphostasis in the path of a tumor-involved sentinel node.[49,53,56,57] Because of this inherent problem, Morton and associates evaluated vital dyes for intraoperative assessment of sentinel nodes, to allow the operating surgeon to reconfirm that the lymph node identified was indeed the first node to receive lymph flow and dye from the primary melanoma.

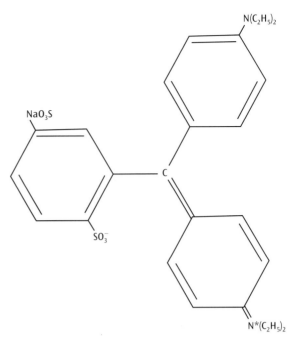

Figure 16.1 *Structural formula of isosulfan blue dye, a monosodium salt of a 2,5-disulfonated triphenylmethane, used in lymphatic mapping.*

The foundation for LM/SLND was assessed in a feline model by Wong *et al.*[58] Although a variety of vital dyes were evaluated, isosulfan blue emerged as the dye that predictably demonstrated lymphatic channels and isolated sentinel nodes (Figure 16.1). In human use, isosulfan blue (1%) is safe, efficacious in delineating lymphatic anatomy, and Food and Drug Administration (FDA)-approved.[59] Technical details of LM/SLND for melanoma were developed in conjunction with preoperative lymphoscintigraphy. The development and institution of hand-held gamma detection devices (gamma probes) have further changed the landscape of SLND. These devices use the radioactive tracer injected for preoperative lymphoscintigraphy to facilitate sentinel node localization in conjunction with the dye. Thus, most groups concur that visualization of the blue dye and gamma-probe measurement of radioactivity are complementary for sentinel node identification. As currently practiced, there are three stages to the technique: preoperative lymphoscintigraphy, intraoperative LM/SLND, and pathologic assessment of the sentinel node specimen. Successful completion of all three stages requires multidisciplinary cooperation between nuclear medicine physicians, pathologists, and operating surgeons.

Patient selection and preoperative lymphoscintigraphy

For biopsy-proven melanoma, patients undergo cutaneous lymphoscintigraphy to evaluate lymph node regions at risk for metastases and isolate potential sentinel nodes.

Prior to study, patients are evaluated to exclude clinical evidence of satellite lesions, intransit metastases, and regional nodal or distant metastases. Cutaneous lymphoscintigraphy is used to analyse at-risk lymph regions in those patients without suspicion for metastatic disease. Most of these patients have intermediate-thickness primary melanomas, but lymphoscintigraphy may also be undertaken to identify drainage patterns from superficial melanomas that have regression, melanomas that have been incompletely biopsied (shave biopsy), and lesions whose depth is unknown because of specimen mishandling or the presence of vertical growth.[60]

LM/SLND has been performed in patients with deep melanomas and in those who have undergone prior wide excision,[61] but there is no consensus in these situations.[62] Thus, patients whose primary melanomas have been excised with wide margins (excision diameter ≥ 3.0 cm and shortest margin from tumor edge to excision edge ≥ 1.5 cm), and patients who have undergone any geometric excision with more than a 1.5-cm margin beyond the tumor edge, or flap rotation closure, should be counseled appropriately. These patients may not be candidates for SLND because the dye/tracer would be injected too far from the primary site or lymphatics could be disrupted. The argument for SLND in deep melanomas is entertained eloquently by Gershenwald et al.,[63] who evaluated 131 patients with melanomas ≥ 4.0 mm in thickness. Median follow-up was 3 years. Patients with positive sentinel nodes underwent lymph node dissection; those with negative sentinel nodes were observed. Although ulceration was an independent important prognosticator, sentinel node status was the most powerful indicator of overall and disease-free survival by both univariate and multivariate analyses. This finding awaits confirmation by other centers before widespread application.

Because lymphoscintigraphy is linked with probe-guided LM/SLND, a variety of radionuclides have been reported for both melanoma and breast cancer. In the USA, the most common agents are unfiltered and filtered technetium-labeled sulfur colloid. Other technetium-labeled agents, such as human serum albumin, dextran, or albumin colloid, are equally effective in isolating sentinel nodes during preoperative lymphoscintigraphy, but may be less helpful in discriminating sentinel nodes from non-sentinel nodes during probe-guided LM/SLND. A consensus on the best radionuclide is unlikely because success has been widely reported with a variety of agents. Comparable results are more likely to be a function of experience and familiarity with a specific agent.

The study is initiated with intradermal injection of the radionuclide at the primary malignancy or biopsy site. Using a scintillation camera via computer interface, real-time images are interpreted to map lymphatic vessel routes and distinguish sentinel nodes from non-sentinel nodes. During preoperative lymphoscintigraphy, the location of each drainage basin and its sentinel node(s) is marked on the overlying skin, to assist the surgeon in planning the operative approach.

Study times vary widely, depending on the location of the primary, the distance from the primary to the nodal basins, the volume and type of agent used, the amount of specific radioactivity, and other intrinsic patient factors.[51–53] Generally, technetium-labeled sulfur colloid isolates sentinel nodes within 5–30 min, but occasionally imaging requires several hours.[50] Accurate marking of sentinel node locations on the skin surface is facilitated by an experienced nuclear medicine physician capable of reducing parallax errors by cross-imaging at several angles[53] or concurrent use of hand-held gamma probes. Uniformity in positioning patients for skin marking cannot be overstressed. This is particularly important in lymph regions with considerable overlying skin mobility, such as the axilla. Collaboration between surgeons and nuclear medicine physicians is paramount so that the external dye marks overlie sentinel nodes at the start of the surgical procedure. Remember that the patient's position during preoperative lymphoscintigraphy will not match his or her position on the operating room table. Skin movement is of particular concern in elderly and obese patients.

Intraoperative LM/SLND

After induction of local/regional or general anesthesia, 0.5–1.0 mL of isosulfan blue (1%) vital dye is injected with a 25-gauge needle at the primary or previous biopsy site. Extreme care is exercised so that dye is delivered only intradermally. This prevents dye uptake by deeper lymphatic vessels that might drain to lymph nodes that do not drain the primary malignancy. Local massage at the injection site may be helpful in facilitating dye transit. Repeat injection of 0.5 mL of dye every 15–20 min is recommended to ensure that sentinel nodes remain identifiable during difficult dissections. The hand-held gamma-probe is used to localize 'hot' (radioactive) spots overlying sentinel nodes. These hot spots should approximate the skin sites marked during preoperative lymphoscintigraphy. Prior to incising the skin, radioactivity is measured over the injection site, over the lymphatic drainage basin(s), and over remote soft tissue. The last reading serves as a background measurement.

A small incision is made proximal to the sentinel node location. This incision would be incorporated in a larger incision if a radical lymphadenectomy is indicated. Skin flaps are developed approximately 5 min after dye injection, without disrupting the dye-stained afferent lymphatic vessels. Blue-stained sentinel nodes are confirmed by tracing lymphatics proximal to the limit of exposure. In most cases, the blue sentinel node is also hot. Unfortunately, there is no uniform definition of a hot sentinel node; radioactive nodes are identified by average counts *ex vivo*, signal-to-background ratios, or percentage comparison to the hottest node *ex vivo*. After the removal of all hot nodes (and, of course, all blue-stained nodes), lymphatic basin counts should return to average background counts or <10% of the hottest node.

Some surgeons rely on the radioisotope more than the dye; others vary the delivery of the agents and/or alter the timing of lymphoscintigraphy from 1 to 4 h or even longer. In any case, success of a specific LM/SLND technique assumes periodic review for quality assessment. We stress that *only the sentinel nodes, i.e., those nodes that are the first to absorb the dye and confirmed by a gamma-probe, should be biopsied*. Sampling non-sentinel second-echelon nodes or randomly selecting additional nodes destroys the value of the sentinel node concept by increasing sample size and thereby decreasing the practicality of meticulous pathologic exam using molecular biologic techniques such as immunohistochemistry. This issue cannot be overemphasized because the sentinel node concept is based on the *non-random* involvement of regional lymph nodes during metastasis of tumor cells from primary melanoma or breast cancer.[1,3,4]

Pathologic evaluation

Freshly excised sentinel nodes are delivered to a pathologist familiar with sentinel node concepts. The first goal is to confirm lymph node retrieval, because lymphatic lakes, dilated lymphatic vessels, or adipose tissue that contains radioactivity or dye from transected lymphatics may be misconstrued as sentinel nodes. When lymph node tissue is confirmed, evaluation for metastatic disease is completed by standard hematoxylin and eosin (H & E) staining of sentinel nodes. Surgeons may then elect to close the wound without considering immediate radical lymphadenectomy; if H & E and immunohistochemical staining of permanent sections subsequently reveals tumor cells, then radical lymphadenectomy is undertaken as a second procedure. Other surgeons may decide for or against immediate radical lymphadenectomy based on frozen-section demonstration of metastases, recognizing that secondary lymphadenectomy will be necessary if the permanent section subsequently reveals tumor cells. Although either course is acceptable, the latter course has the added dimension of the control and safe handling of radioactive material/specimens which is governed by local, state, and federal guidelines.

Permanent pathologic specimens are evaluated by H & E staining of bivalved lymph nodes. When results are negative for tumor, the analysis of additional levels by H & E staining and immunohistochemical analysis reduces the cost for standard extensive analyses applied to all sentinel nodes. Murine monoclonal antibodies to S-100 and HMB45 increase the sensitivity for the detection of occult metastases.[64–66] Although immunohistochemical techniques may be performed on frozen section, their most cost-effective application

is on permanent section, where false-negative results are minimized. In Morton's initial experience of 194 procedures yielding sentinel node biopsy specimens, metastases were identified in 40 cases, 23/40 (57%) by H & E staining alone and 17/40 (43%) by immunohistochemistry.[1] These observations have been confirmed by others.

More sophisticated molecular biologic techniques for the identification of occult metastases are on the horizon. Reverse transcriptase–polymerase chain reaction (RT–PCR) can recognize specific gene sequences, such as tyrosinase, that may detect so-called 'submicroscopic' metastases.[3,67] Although intriguing, the clinical significance of RT–PCR analysis for melanoma is not well established and may require comparison with the clinical significance of immunohistochemical analysis before the molecular technique is incorporated in routine pathologic assessment. The value of detecting occult metastases by special pathologic techniques, the clinical implications, and the impact of stage migration (Will Roger's effect) are important considerations that are currently under scrutiny in large, international, multi-institutional trials.

Results and developments

In April 1992, Morton *et al.*[1] published their results of LM/SLND in 237 lymph node dissections of patients with clinical stage I melanoma. At least one sentinel node was identified in 82% of cases. As expected, the surgeon performing most procedures had the highest rate of success (96%). In all cases, LM/SLND was followed by ELND to evaluate the pathologic status of non-sentinel nodes. Notably, 259 nodes in 194 lymphadenectomy specimens (1.34 sentinel nodes/specimen) were identified as sentinel nodes. Forty-seven (18%) of these sentinel nodes contained metastases, compared with only 2 (0.06%) of 3079 non-sentinel nodes. The false-negative rate of metastases based on sentinel node examination was <1%. Thus, these results offered the first evidence that lymph node metastasis in melanoma patients is a non-random process.

Morton and colleagues[2,55] subsequently reported their experience with LM/SLND for cervical node basins, and then truncal and lower extremity early-stage melanomas. Successful localization of sentinel nodes was 90% and 98%, respectively, with false negatives less than 0.1%. Reports of the technique's reproducibility and acceptance soon followed from several institutions.[68,69] Although early studies described difficulty in acquiring the skills and 'steep' learning curves, subsequent entry-level success rates for the identification of sentinel nodes exceeded expectations. Thompson and colleagues,[69] from the Sydney Melanoma Unit, reported an entry-level accuracy of 75% for axillary basins and 86% for cervical/inguinal basins in 102 patients. At the University of South Florida,

Miliotes *et al.*[3] studied 132 patients, 23 (17%) of whom had evidence of regional nodal metastases. In the 23 patients with metastatic disease, 30/35 (86%) sentinel nodes contained metastases, whereas 25/357 (7%) of non-sentinel nodes had metastases ($p < 0.001$). Eighteen of the 23 patients had metastases only in sentinel lymph nodes. This study's statistical analysis and conclusions validated the observations of Morton's group: metastasis to sentinel nodes is a non-random process.

Currently, the concept of sentinel lymphadenectomy for early-stage melanoma is being validated by international, multicenter, randomized trials. Interim results from the Multicenter Selective Lymphadenectomy Trial (MSLT) of LM/SLND and selective complete lymph node dissection have confirmed that LM/SLND performed using blue dye and radioactive tracer is more successful than LM/SLND performed using dye alone (99.1% versus 95.2%, $p = 0.014$) (Figure 16.2).[7] After completion of the 30-case learning curve, subsequent success was independent of case volume or expertise. Other large studies reporting similar success and experience are the World Health Organization Melanoma Group and the Sunbelt Melanoma Trial (www.sunbeltmelanoma.com). Thus, it is widely accepted that SLND is superior to routine ELND for clinically localized melanoma, because ELND would subject approximately 80% of patients, those without lymph node metastases, to potentially unnecessary surgical morbidity at considerable cost. However, follow-up of patients with tumor-negative sentinel nodes suggests that there are recurrences.[7,67,70] Therefore, patients should be aware of this risk, and they should be prepared to undergo ELND if they fit the appropriate subgroup versus observation if sentinel node localization fails.

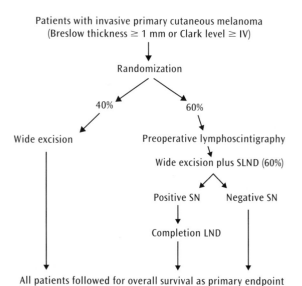

Figure 16.2 *The design of the ongoing Multicenter Selective Lymphadenectomy Trial (MSLT) of sentinel lymphadenectomy (SLND) in patients undergoing wide excision of a primary melanoma. SN, sentinel node.*

Perhaps the greatest future benefit of LM/SLND is the early identification of patients with nodal metastases, who could receive early definitive lymphadenectomy and adjuvant therapy. Results from these large studies should define the role of SLND in patients with prior wide excision and adjuvant treatment with IFNα-2b, identify subgroups of node-positive patients who may not require adjuvant treatment or further lymph node dissection, define the role of advanced pathological assessment with RT–PCR, and bring consensus to the application of radio-guided techniques. In an age of cost-consciousness and patient advocacy, SLND has tremendous appeal and is well positioned for a lasting impact in the management of melanoma.

BREAST CANCER

Historical concepts

The concepts behind the primary surgical management of breast cancer have evolved rapidly over the last century. An early theory offered by Samson Handley and later championed by William Halstead was that breast cancer spread through direct extension of the primary in a sequential process (permeation theory).[71,72] Pathologic support for this theory was largely acquired by the review of mastectomy specimens from patients with advanced disease. Radical mastectomy was then justified based on the prevailing evidence of the time. This must be viewed in context, because optimal adjuvant regimens were not well characterized and surgery offered the only chance for cure. The permeation theory gave way to the tumor embolic theory when pathologists of the 1930s identified tumor emboli in lymphatic vessels or in regional nodes.[72] Thus, it was suggested that tumors spread locoregionally in an embolic fashion. Proponents of radical mastectomy still justified the procedure, despite the change of theories. In time, breast cancer was diagnosed earlier and general awareness prompted directed research with the hope of developing a lasting cure. The theories of the past were gradually replaced by the pioneering work of Bernard Fisher.[73–75] His concepts suggested the early systemic nature of breast cancer but did not fully explain surgical cures of more advanced disease. Radical operations were abandoned for more cosmetic procedures, with equivalent locoregional control facilitated by advances in radiotherapy. At the same time, chemotherapeutic and hormonal agents became available, offering improved survival.

Currently, our understanding of breast cancer incorporates the salient features of preceding theories, describing a spectrum of disease. Women with occult primary cancer may have extensive nodal involvement and progress rapidly to disseminated disease, whereas some women with large primaries and no nodal involvement may be cured by surgery alone. How to stage all breast cancers accurately and determine the appropriate degree of surgical and/or adjuvant intervention is a current dilemma.

Axillary dissection: current issues

Axillary nodal status remains the most significant prognostic factor for patients with early breast cancer. In a multivariate analysis based on 30 years of follow-up, Adair et al.[76] demonstrated that axillary node status most closely correlated with the overall survival of patients undergoing mastectomy. Additionally, Nemoto et al.[77] reported that the risk of tumor recurrence was a continuum correlating with the number of tumor-involved axillary nodes. A trial conducted by the National Surgical Adjuvant Breast and Bowel Project (NSABP) confirmed that increasing numbers of tumor-involved lymph nodes increased the incidence of treatment failure.[78,79] In this study, survival dropped markedly when more than three nodes were involved, and then again when more than ten nodes were involved. Because of this, many oncologists will recommend clinical trials of high-dose chemotherapy with autologous peripheral blood progenitor cell support for patients with numerous tumor-involved nodes.[80]

Routine axillary lymph node dissection (ALND) has been used to identify breast cancer patients who would benefit from adjuvant treatment or a more aggressive adjuvant regimen. However, as the call for more conservative breast cancer therapy continues, surgical treatment of the axilla has been scrutinized for some patients. This trend started in the mid-1980s with a recommendation to eliminate ALND for ductal carcinoma in situ.[81] This recommendation was extended to microinvasive carcinoma[82] and, more recently, to T1a (<0.5 cm) breast cancer.[83] Some ruefully predict that routine adjuvant treatment may replace axillary surgery in patients who are clinically node negative. This 'watch and wait approach'[84–87] might also be used for elderly or infirm postmenopausal women with significant comorbidity, in whom hormonal therapy would be used regardless of the results of axillary dissection.

As adjuvant therapy for node-negative patients becomes common practice,[88–95] the population of patients undergoing ALND for primary breast carcinoma could diminish substantially. However, oncologists should not forget that the effectiveness of adjuvant therapy might correlate with optimal locoregional control. In previous studies of patients receiving substandard axillary surgery or no axillary surgery, the incidence of axillary failure in clinically node-negative patients ranged from 13% to 37%.[96–99] The Christie Hospital (Manchester, UK) experience reported by Gately et al.[100] revealed that 11% (126/1137) of patients treated by segmental resection or simple mastectomy without ALND or radiotherapy developed uncontrollable axillary disease, compared with only 3% of patients (18/544) who had a Patey mastectomy. This may suggest that ALND is not as efficacious when it is not part of the initial definitive treatment.

Patients with tumors < 1.0 cm have a 10-year disease-free survival rate exceeding 90%.[101,102] In 1991, the National Institutes of Health (NIH) Breast Cancer Consensus Conference recommended that these patients should rarely receive systemic adjuvant therapy if their ALND specimen is negative for tumor.[103] However, chemotherapy could be offered if their tumors expressed a high mitotic rate or were of high histologic grade.[80] Additionally, for node-negative patients with tumors 1.0–2.0 cm in diameter, adjuvant therapy would be recommended if a patient had one or more unfavorable prognostic factors. A meta-analysis from the Early Breast Cancer Trialists Collaborative Group demonstrated a survival advantage for node-negative patients treated with systemic therapy.[95] If these findings are used to justify adjuvant therapy for all patients whose axillary status is unknown, then a large population of patients will be receiving treatment in which no benefit may be realized. More importantly, standard therapy has had little effect on the high (approximately 70–90%) 10-year recurrence rate among patients with ten or more tumor-involved nodes. For this group, elimination of ALND would delay entry into more aggressive treatment protocols and may have grave consequences in dealing with uncontrolled axillary disease.

The complexity of the underlying issues will certainly fuel controversy well into the next century.[104,105] Although prognostic models hold some promise for evaluating patients with breast carcinoma, they are far from eliminating the need for axillary assessment.[106] Currently, the addition of adjuvant radiation to the treatment plan for some patients with node-positive disease,[107,108] the use of adjuvant chemotherapy/hormonal therapy to treat ever-smaller primary lesions in premenopausal patients, and the emerging promise of the addition of taxanes to the treatment of node-positive breast cancer present even more compelling evidence that axillary assessment is required.[80] Our goal is to set the stage for a discussion of alternatives to 'blind' ALND (which is unlikely to benefit node-negative patients) and 'blind' adjuvant therapy (which may not be the optimal approach in patients whose axillary nodal status is unknown). In addition, we wish to emphasize the importance of identifying patients with tumor-positive axillary nodes because as many as 30% of these patients might have the same prognosis as patients with local disease, if their regional disease is resected at the time of initial definitive surgery.[109] When compared with complete response rates for accepted adjuvant regimens, the effectiveness of ALND in this group cannot be dismissed. Thus, instead of debating the pros and cons of ALND versus adjuvant therapy, we should focus on techniques to evaluate axillary status, so that treatment can be adjusted according to the presence and extent of nodal involvement.

Axillary dissection and alternatives

Several methods have been evaluated to identify breast cancer patients at risk of nodal metastases. Fisher *et al.*[110] demonstrated that approximately 35% of nodes considered normal on physical examination contained carcinoma, and 25% of enlarged lymph nodes contained no evidence of malignancy; therefore, clinical exam alone is poorly predictive of axillary status. Computerized tomography, magnetic resonance imaging, and mammography present similar difficulties with respect to determining the tumor status of lymph nodes. Positron emission tomography can identify nodal metastases larger than 1 cm, but its use would have limited value in the majority of patients.[111] Similar arguments hold for the application of other nuclear medicine techniques, such as sestamibi scanning.

Haagensen[112] credits Berg with popularizing the anatomic subdivision of the axillary nodes into three functional levels related to the pectoralis minor muscle. Lymph nodes lateral and inferior to pectoralis minor are level I nodes, those located behind this muscle are level II nodes, and nodes superio-medial to pectoralis minor are termed level III nodes. Thus, several types of axillary dissections are defined by the permutations of Berg levels included. A low ALND removes Berg level I nodes, partial ALND removes Berg levels I and II, and total ALND removes all three Berg level nodes. Lesser procedures termed axillary sampling refer to the random biopsy of low axillary nodes without anatomic reference.[79]

As a result of recommendations from the NIH Consensus Conference of 1991,[103] most breast surgeons perform partial ALND. Lymphedema for this procedure is reportedly low (2.7–9.4%), and skip metastases to Berg level III or other sites should understage approximately 3% of patients.[113–117] Total ALND, rarely used, is associated with significantly increased lymphedema (37%),[118] but it may have value for node-positive patients by significantly reducing axillary recurrence rates.[119,120] Because most patients do not require intraoperative pathologic assessment, its practice is limited. Attempts to reduce the morbidity of partial ALND with lesser procedures such as low ALND[110,118] or axillary sampling[110,121–125] were abandoned due to false-negative rates of approximately 20% and 42%, respectively. Motivated by the success of SLND in melanoma, and the need for more accurate, less-invasive axillary assessment, SLND was investigated in breast cancer.

Adaptation of LM/SLND for breast cancer

In October 1991, Giuliano's group[12] began a feasibility study of LM/SLND adapted for the detection of sentinel nodes in the axillary lymphatic basin draining a primary breast carcinoma. The modified technique involves injection of 3–5 mL of 1% isosulfan blue dye into the breast tissue at the site of the malignancy. This site varies depending on whether the lesion is palpable, mammographically/ultrasonographically detected, or already removed by open excisional biopsy. Dye is injected adjacent to the palpable tumor, through mammographic/ultrasonographic-assisted needle placement, or into the wall of the biopsy cavity.

For the first 20 cases in the feasibility study, the interval between the injection of dye and commencement of LM/SLND was varied to evaluate dye transit time. In subsequent cases, a 5-min interval was used to allow dye to adequately stain lymphatic vessels and lymph nodes. The axillary incision was made inferior to the hair-bearing region. Dissection proceeded to the interface of subcutaneous adipose tissue with the axillary lymphatic tissue. In this plane of dissection, but anterior, the tail of the breast was encountered as it entered the axilla. Dye-stained lymphatic vessels were identified at the tail of the breast and followed to the sentinel node. On occasion, a dye-stained node was immediately obvious; however, the afferent lymphatic vessels were traced back to the tail of the breast to ensure that this node was the most proximal node and that there was no bifurcation that could lead to dual sentinel nodes. After confirmation of the sentinel nodes, SLND was completed and the specimen sent separately for pathologic evaluation. Patients then underwent partial ALND and segmental resection or modified radical mastectomy, as indicated.

In the initial study, 172 patients were accrued; because two patients had synchronous bilateral breast carcinoma, there were 174 LM/SLND procedures.[12] Sentinel nodes were located in 66% (114/174) of procedures overall; however, the detection rate improved to 78% in the last 50 cases. Axillary nodal status was correctly predicted by sentinel node pathology in 109/114 (96%) specimens. The five remaining cases were falsely negative and occurred in the first 87 procedures. Retrospective evaluation of falsely negative sentinel node specimens revealed that three were dye-stained adipose tissue; the subsequent addition of intraoperative sentinel node analysis by frozen section eliminated false-negative results due to misidentification of tissues. The fourth falsely negative sentinel node proved to be tumor positive by immunohistochemical analysis for cytokeratin. Only the fifth was a true false-negative lymph node, indicating that in this single case tumor cells had spread to non-sentinel nodes rather than sentinel nodes. The sensitivity and specificity of the technique were 88% and 100%, respectively, including the five false-negative specimens.

Thus, this analysis indicated that metastases in breast cancer occur in a non-random manner. Notably, 34 patients had clinically negative/histologically positive axillae. Of 751 lymph nodes removed, 63 (8.3%) were sentinel nodes. Of the 63 sentinel nodes, 39 (62%) contained tumor. Of the 688 (91.7%) non-sentinel nodes, only 93 (13.5%) contained tumor ($p < 0.0001$). This confirmed in breast cancer what had been demonstrated in melanoma: if axillary metastases are present, they are significantly more likely to be found in sentinel nodes than in non-sentinel nodes.[12]

Probe-guided LM in breast cancer

Adaptation of probe-guided LM to identify the sentinel node draining a primary breast cancer was first reported by Krag and coworkers[126] in 22 patients. Peritumoral or pericavitary injections of unfiltered technetium-labeled sulfur colloid were used in concert with a hand-held gamma-probe. Sentinel nodes were identified in 18 of 22 patients (82%). No false negatives were reported. Adaptation and successful incorporation of the gamma-probe during LM/SLND for breast cancer became prolific. The tenets of this technique regarding the localization of hot spots, *in-vivo* averaged counts, background counting, *ex-vivo* counting, and definition of a hot sentinel node are similar to those for probe-guided surgery in melanoma. At the completion of SLND using the probe, axillary counts should return to near background levels. As in melanoma, there is no consensus on the type of radiopharmaceutical, on its volume, timing, or site of injection, or on the specific radioactivity that defines a sentinel node. In addition, breast cancer presents unique technical considerations when the primary is close to or overlying the drainage site.

Despite these obstacles, successful sentinel node programs flourish. Veronesi *et al.*[19] used technetium-labeled albumin colloid with subdermal injections over the primary site in 163 breast cancer patients. They were successful in 98% of cases, with a false-negative rate of 5%. Other technetium-labeled agents, such as human serum albumin, dextran, or albumin colloid, are equally effective in isolating sentinel nodes and have similar reported success rates. More recently, surgeons have combined the use of isosulfan blue dye (1%) and radioisotope during breast cancer SLND. Albertini *et al.*[16] first reported a 92% rate of successful localization of sentinel nodes in 62 breast cancer patients, with no false negatives. Other centers confirmed this experience. Hill *et al.*[29] consolidated lessons learned from 500 procedures and observed that their 93% success rate was independent of tumor size, histologic type, location, nuclear grade, or prior biopsy technique. Further, the use of dye and radioactive tracers was complementary. In all of the published series,[12–29] the false-negative rates ranged from zero to 15%. False-negative rates for breast cancer LM/SLND should be balanced against partial ALND's 3% expected rate of understaging due to skip metastases[103] and against the 30% rate of misdiagnosis (false negatives) with standard pathologic assessment of a nodal specimen.[127–130]

Pathologic assessment

Tedious dissection and specialized clearing techniques have increased the number of lymph nodes identified in an axillary specimen, but neither approach has substantially improved the assessment of axillary node status. The rate of tumor detection can be increased by using serial sectioning at multiple levels rather than bivalve techniques to examine axillary nodes. When 'tumor-negative' bivalved nodes are subjected to additional serial sectioning, nearly 30% are found to contain metastases.[127–130] Special immunohistochemical staining techniques against specific epithelial cell markers for breast carcinoma, such as milk fat globulin, mucin, low/intermediate molecular weight cytokeratin or pancytokeratin, have increased the rate of tumor detection in axillary lymph nodes further than step sectioning at multiple levels.[129–133] However, serial sectioning and immunohistochemical staining techniques are labor intensive, costly, and still require the large population of node-negative patients to submit to ALND in order to identify the subgroup of patients who would be upstaged by more sophisticated pathologic methods.

Giuliano's group[13] therefore used sentinel node technology to evaluate *focused* histopathologic study of axillary nodes. LM/SLND identifies axillary lymph nodes that have the greatest potential for harboring metastases from a primary breast carcinoma. Thus, what may be cost prohibitive and impractical for the pathologic assessment of the entire axillary contents could be extremely efficacious when applied to the one or two nodes (sentinel nodes) most likely to harbor metastases. Two groups of patients equivalent with respect to age (median 55 versus 54 years), size of primary tumor (median 1.5 cm in both groups), clinically suspicious axillary disease (5% versus 7%), and number of axillary nodes excised (median 19 versus 21) were studied. The ALND group underwent excision of Berg levels I and II nodes (partial ALND) without LM/SLND. The SLND group underwent LM/SLND followed by partial ALND. In the ALND group, axillary contents were examined without clearing techniques. Lymph nodes were embedded in paraffin blocks and, depending on specimen size, one or two levels per block were evaluated by H & E staining for all nodes (standard practice in the community). In the SLND group, sentinel nodes were confirmed by intraoperative frozen section and then bivalved to yield two paraffin-block specimens. One or two permanent section levels per block were reviewed with H & E staining. If these were negative for metastases, immunohistochemical stains were performed with an antibody cocktail directed to low/intermediate molecular weight cytokeratin on six to eight levels of each sentinel node. The remainder of the axillary contents were processed and evaluated as in the ALND group. Axillary metastases were identified in 39/134 (29%) patients in the ALND group: 35/39 (90%) patients had metastases >2 mm (macrometastases) and 4/39 (10%) patients had metastases <2 mm (micrometastases). In the SLND group, 68/162 (42%) patients had axillary metastases: 42/68 (62%) had macrometastases identified by H & E staining,

15/68 (22%) had micrometastases identified by H & E staining, and 11/68 (16%) had micrometastases identified solely by immunohistochemical staining. The yield of metastases and micrometastases was significantly higher ($p < 0.03$ and $p < 0.0005$, respectively) in the SLND group than the ALND group.[13] This finding has been confirmed at other centers.

As a result of these data, we recommend that the pathologist receive the sentinel nodes immediately to assess the retrieval of lymph node tissue, examine an intraoperative frozen section to confirm nodal tissue if in doubt, stain permanent sections with H & E, and undertake immunohistochemical analysis of multiple sections of each node that stains negative by H & E. Our application of this protocol in 100 patients resulted in a 93% rate of successful sentinel node identification.[134] There were no false negatives, and the pathologic status of the sentinel node correctly reflected overall axillary status in all 93 patients.

Validation studies of SLND for breast cancer

After successful feasibility studies, Giuliano et al.[14] reported on 107 patients using the mature technique of LM/SLND. One hundred patients underwent successful mapping (93%), with no false negatives. Sentinel node status invariably predicted the axillary status. A more comprehensive analysis of the histopathologic validation of the sentinel node hypothesis was performed by this group.[135] One hundred and three patients underwent SLND followed by partial ALND. A mean of two sentinel nodes (range one to eight) and 18.9 non-sentinel nodes (range 7–37) was removed. Thirty-three patients had positive sentinel nodes on H & E stains, and immunohistochemistry to cytokeratin at multiple levels identified ten more patients with positive nodes. In the 60 remaining sentinel node-negative patients, 1087 non-sentinel lymph nodes were examined at additional levels with immunohistochemistry for cytokeratin. Only one lymph node was found to harbor metastases, for a conversion rate of 0.09% ($1/1087$, $p < 0.0001$) and a false-negative rate of 1.7% ($1/60$, $p < 0.0001$).

Multicenter validation of probe-guided LM/SLND followed by partial ALND was conducted by Krag and colleagues.[28] Eleven centers participated after completing a prerequisite five-case training phase. Sentinel nodes were identified in 91% of cases (405/443 patients). The accuracy of the sentinel node as a predictor of axillary status was 97% (392/405 patients). The false-negative rate was 11%. Interestingly, all false negatives were in the outer quadrants, where hot-spot identification is hampered by the short distance between the primary injection site and the axilla. Medial lesions, prior excisional biopsy, and age > 50 years were associated with failure to localize a hot spot. These investigators suggest that successful SLND is feasible in a variety of practice settings.

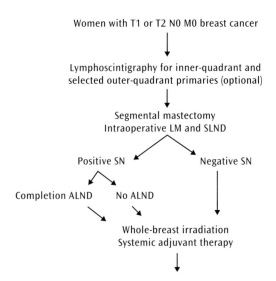

Figure 16.3 *The design of the ongoing American College of Surgeons Oncology Group (ACOSOG) Trial of intraoperative lymphatic mapping (LM) and sentinel lymphadenectomy (SLND) in patients with primary breast carcinoma. SN, sentinel node; ALND, axillary lymph node dissection.*

These studies and the plethora of single-institution studies have led to large multicenter trials evaluating SLND. In the USA, the American College of Surgeons Oncology Group (ACOSOG) Trial (www.acosog.org) (Figure 16.3) and the NSABP B-32 Trial (www.nsabp.pitt.edu/b-32.htm) are poised to answer questions regarding observation in sentinel node-negative patients, and SLND alone for patients whose axillary disease is limited to a micrometastatic deposit in a single sentinel node.

Micrometastases and SLND in early breast cancer

The clinical relevance of highly sensitive pathologic techniques for the analysis of axillary nodes from breast cancer patients depends largely on whether occult axillary metastases increase the risk of recurrence and/or decrease overall survival. Numerous studies demonstrate a higher disease recurrence and a lower overall survival, approximately 10–20%, in patients with confirmed occult metastases.[129,130,136–139] The International Breast Cancer Study Group used multilevel sectioning and immunohistochemical staining to identify micrometastases in 83 of 921 (9%) patients with tumor-negative H & E results.[129] These 83 patients had a significantly lower 5-year disease-free survival rate (58% versus 74%, respectively, $p = 0.002$). More recently, Clare et al.[130] used multilevel sectioning, H & E stains, and immunohistochemistry against low molecular weight cytokeratin to identify occult metastases in 11 of 86 (13%) patients with previously reported histologic node-negative breast cancer.

During a median follow-up of 80 months, distant metastases occurred in 45% (5/11) of node-positive patients, compared with only 17% (13/75) of node-negative patients ($p = 0.048$). Although Rosen et al.[101] demonstrated that patients with T1 tumors and micrometastatic axillary disease had a 12-year survival equal to that of patients with macrometastases, their 6-year observations showed better survival for patients with micrometastases.

Community screening programs, patient education, and increased physician awareness have cultivated a shift in detection to smaller primary malignancies. Concurrently, the utilization of breast conservation together with the selective elimination of ALND has been advocated for patients whose small breast carcinomas are associated with a relatively low risk of axillary metastases.[81–83] Of course, this approach is not optimum for patients with occult lymph node disease, who would not receive the benefit of partial ALND and/or timely adjuvant therapy appropriate for node-positive patients. LM/SLND could have tremendous impact as a selection tool in these patients with breast carcinomas. Patients with tumor-positive sentinel nodes could be treated with partial ALND and adjuvant therapy at the time of definitive treatment, whereas those with tumor-negative sentinel nodes could be followed without further surgery and selective application of adjuvant treatment.

To evaluate this concept, Giuliano's group[30] studied 259 patients with T1 breast cancer. Of these, 69 had axillary metastases by H & E alone. Seven additional patients had axillary metastases identified by immunohistochemistry for cytokeratin. Although a variety of prognostic factors (age, hormone receptor status, presence of ductal carcinoma in situ, histology, DNA ploidy, and S-phase) were evaluated, only tumor size held significant value in predicting nodal metastases ($p = 0.001$). The incidence of axillary metastases in this study was 29% overall and 33%, 15%, and 15% for T1c, T1b, and T1a tumors, respectively. Because of the significant incidence of axillary metastases, even in tumors < 10 mm, the elimination of partial ALND may be premature. Consequently, LM/SLND may be a suitable alternative for discriminating node-positive from node-negative patients, with SLND used as the sole staging procedure for node-negative patients.[140] An even more provocative report by Chu et al.[141] suggests that certain patients with tumor-positive sentinel nodes might be adequately staged and treated with SLND only.

Limitations and pitfalls

The large experience with isosulfan blue as an agent for LM can be traced back to 1982, when it became commercially available.[59] For both melanoma and breast cancer mapping, we recommend a 1% solution, largely because of a previous study showing no local toxicity for 1% solutions of triphenylmethane dyes but widespread tissue necrosis for solutions > 3%. As may be expected

from any drug, there have been reports of mild hypersensitivity reactions, with a probable incidence of 1/1000 patients. These are self-limited and may be reduced with SLND due to removal of the bulk of the injected dye during wide excision (melanoma) or segmental resection (breast cancer). Most of the residual systemic dye is excreted via the biliary system; approximately 10% is via renal excretion. Blue discoloration of urine persists for < 24 h and can alarm the patient if not forewarned. Residual deep tissue staining is rare if dye injection is limited to those tissues intended for resection. Superficial contact of isosulfan blue 1% with the skin will impart a transient blue coloration, but this does not occur when dye volume is controlled and extraneous dye is promptly removed.

The success of LM with vital dyes has prompted the adaptation of sentinel node technology for use with radionuclides. Investigators are attempting to identify the most efficacious technetium-labeled vehicle, the appropriate lag time between injection and surgery (reported range 2–24 h), and the definition of a radiolabeled sentinel node (e.g., 15 counts/10 s, ratio three times background, 30 counts/10 s prior to incision versus 25 counts/10 s ex vivo or 10% of the hottest node). Results are promising, but a definitive assessment is not likely because similar success rates are being reported with a wide array of closely related procedures. As with any technology-based procedures, systems do fail, batteries malfunction, and equipment can lose calibration. Contingency planning and knowledge of LM can salvage minor disasters.

Likewise, the incorporation of recent advances in detecting 'submicroscopic' metastases by RT–PCR in breast cancer is promising; however, the ideal marker (mRNA transcript) or combination of markers has not been established.[142,143] The clinical significance of metastases discovered by RT–PCR is a source of controversy that will require closer scrutiny, particularly for patients whose axillary nodes are tumor negative by H & E and immunohistochemical staining but tumor positive by RT–PCR. Until these issues are resolved, this special technique will remain the interest of research centers and is not recommended for routine sentinel node assessment.

Metastatic involvement of internal mammary nodes is an independent negative prognostic factor in patients with breast cancer.[144] These nodes may be involved in 5–10% of patients with inner quadrant malignancies and tumor-negative axillae.[145–147] Although routine internal mammary lymphadenectomy is not recommended,[148] many centers are evaluating the application of sentinel node technology in patients with inner quadrant lesions and tumor-negative axillary nodes or in those patients with hot spots in internal mammary nodes. Preoperative lymphoscintigraphy identifies those patients with internal mammary node lymph flow. If axillary assessment is negative and the patient agrees to internal mammary assessment, the internal mammary sentinel node is biopsied. If this node contains tumor, then adjuvant treatment may be changed. However, we can make no firm recommendations concerning internal mammary LM/SLND until we have determined its clinical relevance by studying a larger patient population.

In some cases, a sentinel node cannot be found. The reasons for this may be multifactorial. Egress of dye from the primary site may be impeded by edema, infection, or tumor. Injection into a previous biopsy cavity or injection into large tumors may retard the flow of dye or radioactive tracer. Drainage to high Berg level II or Berg level III nodes may follow routes undetectable by present methods. Patients may have internal mammary node lymph flow, unusual lymph patterns to deep lymphatics, and/or direct supraclavicular lymph drainage; lymphoscintigraphy may elucidate these unusual lymphatic pathways. Another possibility is that lymphatic vessels may be transected before adequate localization with vital dye or may increase the background radioactivity, reducing the discrimination between sentinel nodes and non-sentinel nodes. Proximity of primary tumors to lymph node regions at risk and inappropriate injection of tissues other than the breast may impair LM. Thus, the possibility of non-localization of the sentinel node together with an appropriate contingency plan should be discussed with the patient.[103] In any event, non-localization of sentinel nodes should not exceed 15% in experienced hands. Furthermore, before sentinel node biopsy is undertaken as a sole discriminating procedure, we encourage surgeons to prospectively evaluate this technique in conjunction with partial ALND to confirm mastery of the skills and to establish their own success rates in breast cancer patients.

Guidelines

The American Society of Breast Surgeons assembled a panel of experts to review the status of SLND for breast cancer (www.breastsurgeons.org/pr01.htm). Their recommendations, which were released in November 1998, serve as guidelines but do not usurp local requirements and institutional review board approval.

According to the society's guidelines, the following criteria contraindicate SLND for breast cancer:

clinically positive axillary nodes,

multifocal malignancies,

primary tumor >5 cm, history of previous chemotherapy or radiation therapy for breast cancer (ipsilateral),

history of extensive breast/axillary surgery.

Each surgeon at a collaborating institution should document individual experience as surgeon or first assistant of ≥30 cases with LM/SLND followed by completion ALND, regardless of the tumor status of the sentinel node. This experience should yield a sentinel node identification rate ≥85% and a false-negative rate ≤5%, or a single falsely negative case in the series.

SLND when performed by experienced surgeons is sufficient in lieu of ALND if sentinel nodes are negative for tumor. However, if SLND is the only staging procedure, axillary recurrence rates should be <5%. Completion ALND should be undertaken in any patient with tumor-positive sentinel nodes.

CONCLUSIONS

The concept and practice of LM/SLND have been validated by surgeons throughout the world for both melanoma and breast cancer. Despite different techniques and procedures, the resultant sentinel lymph node information has tremendous impact on recommendations for further surgical intervention, adjuvant therapy, and staging schemes. The technique of LM/SLND was pioneered as a rational alternative to ELND or 'watch and wait' philosophies for clinically localized cutaneous melanoma. Technological advances provided gamma-probes adaptable to the operating theater. Consequently, surgeons entered the nuclear age of probe-guided surgery in conjunction with established dye-guided LM techniques. Dye and probe techniques are complementary, not competitive, for both melanoma and breast cancer.

Successful programs require cooperative innovation. Centers should have a nuclear medicine staff familiar with preoperative lymphoscintigraphy and probe-guided surgery, pathologists versed in the techniques of immunohistochemistry, support staff to assist in quality-control issues, and surgeons versed in the multidisciplinary constructs of oncology. All members of the team should have sufficient training in sentinel node concepts, basic knowledge of radiation physics, and firm understanding of radiation safety according to local, state, and federal requirements. The multidisciplinary requirements for LM/SLND cannot be overstressed. Only with strict attention and uniform adherence to these prerequisites can the value of LM/SLND for melanoma and breast cancer be confirmed in a controlled trial setting. When possible, we strongly support entry into these ongoing multicenter studies. If this is not possible, surgeons are encouraged to enter into national registries, or at a minimum their own tumor registry.

Each surgeon and/or institution must prospectively evaluate LM/SLND in conjunction with planned partial ALND for breast cancer or with ELND in the appropriate subgroup for melanoma to establish mastery and demonstrate accuracy in approximately 30 cases. Another acceptable process is acquiring the necessary skills under the direct instruction or supervision of an accomplished sentinel node surgeon acting as first assistant or primary surgeon.

Finally, the sentinel node concept focuses on the ability of a tumor to spread in a non-random process to the associated regional lymph nodes. Therefore, it does not detract or defend other theories of sequential dissemination from primary locations to regional nodes, or the more contemporary view that regional lymph node involvement is an indicator of potential disseminated disease.

Sentinel lymph node technology is well positioned to revolutionize the staging, surgical treatment, and subsequent adjuvant therapy of patients with clinically localized melanoma and breast cancer. Adaptation for other solid neoplasms is almost a certainty. If ongoing trials validate the ramifications of this technique, we may relieve a generation of patients of the morbidity of routine regional lymphadenectomy, without sacrificing early intervention for those with regional lymph node metastases.

NOTE

The views expressed herein are those of the authors and do not necessarily reflect the views of the US Army, US Navy, National Naval Medical Center, Uniformed Services University of the Health Sciences, or the Department of Defense.

REFERENCES

1. Morton DL, Wen D-R, Wong JH, *et al*. Technical details of intraoperative lymphatic mapping for early stage melanoma. Arch Surg 1992; 127:392–9.
2. Morton DL, Wen D-R, Foshag LJ, Essner R, Cochran AJ. Intraoperative lymphatic mapping and selective cervical lymphadenectomy for early-stage melanomas of the head and neck. J Clin Oncol 1993; 11:1751–6.
3. Miliotes G, Albertini J, Berman C, *et al*. The tumor biology of melanoma nodal metastases. Am Surg 1996; 62:81–8.
4. Albertini J, Cruse W, Rapaport D, *et al*. Intraoperative radiolymphoscintigraphy improves sentinel lymph node identification for patients with melanoma. Ann Surg 1996; 223:217–24.
5. Krag D, Meijer S, Weaver D, *et al*. Minimal-access surgery for staging of malignant melanoma. Arch Surg 1995; 130:654–8.
6. Pijpers R, Borgenstein P, Meijer S, *et al*. Sentinel node biopsy in melanoma patients: dynamic lymphoscintigraphy followed by intraoperative gamma probe and vital dye guidance. World J Surg 1997; 21:788–93.
7. Morton D, Thompson J, Essner R, *et al*. Validation of the accuracy of intraoperative lymphatic mapping and sentinel lymphadenectomy for early-stage melanoma. A multicenter trial (MSLT). Ann Surg 1999; 230:453–65.
8. Reintgen D, Albertini J, Milliotes G, *et al*. The orderly progression of melanoma metastases. Ann Surg 1994; 220:759–67.
9. Ross M, Reintgen D, Balch C. Selective lymphadenectomy: emerging role for lymphatic mapping and sentinel node biopsy in the management of early stage melanoma. Semin Surg Oncol 1993; 9:219–23.
10. Thompson J, Uren R, Shaw H, *et al*. Location of sentinel lymph nodes in patients with cutaneous melanoma: new insights into lymphatic anatomy. J Am Coll Surg 1999; 189:195–206.
11. Leong S, Steinmetz I, Habib F, *et al*. Optimal selective sentinel lymph node dissection in primary malignant melanoma. Arch Surg 1997; 132:666–73.
12. Giuliano AE, Kirgan DM, Guenther JM, *et al*. Lymphatic mapping and sentinel lymphadenectomy for breast cancer. Ann Surg 1994; 220:391–401.
13. Giuliano AE, Dale PS, Turner RR, *et al*. Improved axillary staging of breast cancer with sentinel lymphadenectomy. Ann Surg 1995; 222:394–401.
14. Giuliano AE, Jones RC, Brennan M, *et al*. Sentinel lymphadenectomy in breast cancer. J Clin Oncol 1997; 15:2345–50.
15. O'Hea B, Hill A, El-Shirbiny A, *et al*. Sentinel lymph node biopsy in breast cancer: initial experience at Memorial Sloan-Kettering Cancer Center. J Am Coll Surg 1998; 186:423–7.
16. Albertini J, Lyman G, Cox C, *et al*. Lymphatic mapping and sentinel node biopsy in the patient with breast cancer. JAMA 1996; 276:1818–22.
17. Offodile R, Hoh C, Barsky S, *et al*. Minimally invasive breast carcinoma staging using lymphatic mapping with radiolabeled dextran. Cancer 1998; 82:1704–8.
18. Cox C, Pendas S, Cox J, *et al*. Guidelines for sentinel node biopsy and lymphatic mapping of patients with breast cancer. Ann Surg 1998; 227:645–53.
19. Veronesi U, Paganelli G, Galimberti V, *et al*. Sentinel-node biopsy to avoid axillary dissection in breast cancer with clinically negative lymph-nodes. Lancet 1997; 349:1864–7.
20. Borgstein P, Pijpers R, Comans E, *et al*. Sentinel lymph node biopsy in breast cancer: guidelines and pitfalls of lymphoscintigraphy and gamma probe detection. J Am Coll Surg 1998; 186:275–83.
21. Guenther J, Krishnamoorthy M, Tan L. Sentinel lymphadenectomy for breast cancer in a community managed care setting. Cancer J Sci Am 1997; 3:336–40.
22. Dale P, Williams J. Axillary staging utilizing selective sentinel lymphadenectomy for patients with invasive breast carcinoma. Am Surg 1998; 64:28–32.
23. Koller M, Barsuk D, Zippel D, *et al*. Sentinel lymph node involvement – a predictor for axillary node status with breast cancer – has the time come? Eur J Surg Oncol 1998; 24:166–8.

24. Flett M, Going J, Stanton P, *et al.* Sentinel node localization in patients with breast cancer. Br J Surg 1998; 85:991–3.

25. Miner T, Shriver C, Jaques D, *et al.* Ultrasonographically guided injection improves localization of the radiolabeled sentinel lymph node in breast cancer. Ann Surg Oncol 1998; 5:315–21.

26. Pijpers R, Meijer S, Hoekstra O, *et al.* Impact of lymphoscintigraphy on sentinel node identification with technetium-99m-colloidal albumin in breast cancer. J Nucl Med 1997; 38:366–8.

27. Barnwell J, Arredondo M, Kollmorgen D, *et al.* Sentinel node biopsy in breast cancer. Ann Surg Oncol 1998; 5:126–30.

28. Krag D, Weaver D, Ashikaga T, *et al.* The sentinel node in breast cancer: a multicenter validation study. N Engl J Med 1998; 339:941–6.

29. Hill A, Tran K, Akhurst T, *et al.* Lessons learned from 500 cases of lymphatic mapping for breast cancer. Ann Surg 1999; 229:528–35.

30. Giuliano AE, Barth AM, Spivack B, Beitsch PD, Evans SW. Incidence and predictors of axillary metastasis in T1 breast cancer. J Am Coll Surg 1996; 183:185–9.

31. Callery C, Cochran AJ, Roe RJ, *et al.* Factors prognostic in patients with malignant melanoma spread to the regional lymph nodes. Ann Surg 1982; 196:69–75.

32. Das Gupta TK. Results of treatment of 265 patients with primary cutaneous melanoma: a five-year prospective study. Ann Surg 1977; 186:201–9.

33. Morton DL, Wanek L, Nizze JA, *et al.* Improved long-term survival after lymphadenectomy of melanoma metastatic to regional nodes. Ann Surg 1991; 214:491–9.

34. Milton GW, Shaw HM, McCarthy WH, *et al.* Prophylactic lymph node dissection in clinical stage I cutaneous malignant melanoma: results of surgical treatment in 1,319 patients. Br J Surg 1982; 69:108–11.

35. Reintgen DS, Cox EB, McCarty KJ Jr, *et al.* Efficacy of elective lymph node dissection in patients with intermediate thickness primary melanoma. Ann Surg 1983; 198:379–85.

36. McCarthy WH, Shaw HM, Milton GW. Efficacy of elective lymph node dissection in 2,347 patients with clinical stage I malignant melanoma. Surg Gynecol Obstet 1985; 161:575–80.

37. Urist MM, Balch CM, Soong S-J, *et al.* Head and neck melanoma in 534 clinical stage I patients. A prognostic factors analysis and results of surgical treatment. Ann Surg 1984; 200:769–75.

38. Veronesi U, Adamus J, Bandiera DC, *et al.* Stage I melanoma of the limbs. Intermediate versus delayed node dissection. Tumori 1980; 66:373–96.

39. Veronesi U, Adamus J, Bandiera DC, *et al.* Inefficacy of immediate node dissection in stage I melanoma of the limbs. N Engl J Med 1977; 297:627–30.

40. Sim FH, Taylor WF, Pritchard DJ, *et al.* Lymphadenectomy in the management of stage I malignant melanoma: a prospective randomized study. Mayo Clin Proc 1986; 61:697–705.

41. Balch C, Soong S-J, Ross M, *et al.* Long-term results of a multi-institutional randomized trial comparing prognostic factors and surgical results for intermediate thickness melanomas (1.0–4.0 mm). Ann Surg Oncol 2000; 7:87–97.

42. Kirkwood JM, Strawderman MH, Ernstoff MS, Smith TJ, Borden EC, Blum RH. Interferon alfa-2b adjuvant therapy of high-risk resected cutaneous melanoma: the Eastern Cooperative Oncology Group Trial EST 1684. J Clin Oncol 1996; 14:7–17.

43. Shen P, Guenther JM, Wanek LA, Morton DL. Can elective complete lymph node dissection decrease the incidence and mortality of late melanoma recurrences? Ann Surg Oncol 2000; 7:114–19.

44. Fee HJ, Robinson DS, Sample WF, *et al.* The determination of lymph shed by colloidal gold scanning in patients with malignant melanoma: a preliminary study. Surgery 1978; 84:626–32.

45. Holmes EC, Moseley HS, Morton DL, *et al.* A rational approach to the surgical management of melanoma. Ann Surg 1977; 186:481–9.

46. Robinson DS, Sample WF, Fee HJ, *et al.* Regional lymphatic drainage in primary malignant melanoma of the trunk determined by colloidal gold scanning. Surg Forum 1977; 28:147–8.

47. Nathanson S, Anaya P, Avery M, *et al.* Sentinel lymph node metastases in experimental melanoma: relationships among primary tumor size, lymphatic vessel diameter, and 99m-Tc-labeled human serum albumin clearance. Ann Surg Oncol 1997; 4:161–8.

48. Lamki LM, Logic JR. Defining lymphatic drainage patterns with cutaneous lymphoscintigraphy. In Balch CM, Houghton AN, Milton GW, *et al.*, eds. *Cutaneous melanoma,* 2nd edn. Philadelphia, JB Lippincott, 1992, 367–75.

49. Norman J, Cruse CW, Espinosa C, *et al.* Redefinition of cutaneous lymphatic drainage with the use of lymphoscintigraphy for malignant melanoma. Am J Surg 1991; 162:432–7.

50. Glass EC, Essner R, Giuliano A, Morton DL. Comparative efficacy of three lymphoscintigraphic agents. J Nucl Med 1995; 36(5):199P.

51. O'Brien CJ, Uren RF, Thompson JF, *et al.* Prediction of potential metastatic sites in cutaneous head and neck melanoma using lymphoscintigraphy. Am J Surg 1995; 170:461–6.

52. Wanebo HJ, Harpole D, Teates CD. Radionuclide lymphoscintigraphy with technetium 99m antimony sulfide colloid to identify lymphatic drainage of cutaneous melanoma at ambiguous sites in the head and neck and trunk. Cancer 1985; 55:1403–13.

53. Uren RF, Howman-Giles RB, Shaw HM, Thompson JF, McCarthy WH. Lymphoscintigraphy in high-risk

melanoma of the trunk: predicting draining node groups, defining lymphatic channels and locating the sentinel node. J Nucl Med 1993; 34:1435–40.

54. Krag DN, Meijer SJ, Weaver DL, *et al.* Minimal-access surgery for staging of malignant melanoma. Arch Surg 1995; 130:654–8.

55. Essner R, Wen DR, Cochran AJ, Morton DL, Ramming KP. Lymphatic mapping and selective lymph node biopsy: an alternative to elective lymphadenectomy for early-stage melanomas of the trunk and lower extremities. Proc Am Soc Clin Oncol 1993; 12:391.

56. Uren RF, Howman-Giles R, Thompson JF, *et al.* Lymphoscintigraphy to identify sentinel lymph nodes in patients with melanoma. Melanoma Res 1994; 4:395–9.

57. Schneebaum S, Stadler Y, Cohen M, Baron J, Skornik Y. Gamma probe-guided sentinel node biopsy – optimal timing for injection. Eur J Surg Oncol 1998; 24:515–19.

58. Wong JH, Cagle LA, Morton DL. Lymphatic drainage of skin to a sentinel lymph node in a feline model. Ann Surg 1991; 214:637–41.

59. Hirsch JI, Tisnado J, Cho S-R, Beachley MC. Use of isosulfan blue for identification of lymphatic vessels: experimental and clinical evaluation. Am J Roentgenol 1982; 139:1061–4.

60. Bedrosian I, Faries M, Guerry D IV, *et al.* Incidence of sentinel node metastases in patients with thin primary melanoma ($\leqslant$ 1 mm) with vertical growth phase. Ann Surg Oncol 2000; 7:262–7.

61. Kelemen PR, Essner R, Foshag LJ, Morton DL. Lymphatic mapping and sentinel lymphadenectomy after wide local excision of primary melanoma. J Am Coll Surg 1999; 189:247–52.

62. Karakousis C, Grigoropoulos P. Sentinel node biopsy before and after wide excision of the primary melanoma. Ann Surg Oncol 1999; 6:785–9.

63. Gershenwald J, Mansfield P, Lee J, Ross M. Role for lymphatic mapping and sentinel lymph node biopsy in patients with thick ($\geqslant$4 mm) primary melanoma. Ann Surg Oncol 2000; 7:160–5.

64. Cochran AJ, Wen DR, Morton DL. Occult tumor cells in the lymph nodes of patients with pathological stage I malignant melanoma: an immunohistological study. Am J Surg Pathol 1988; 12:612–18.

65. Cochran AJ, Wen DR, Herschman HR. Occult melanoma cells in lymph nodes detected by antiserum to S-100 protein. Int J Cancer 1984; 34:159–63.

66. Gibbs J, Huang P, Zhang P, *et al.* Accuracy of pathologic techniques for the diagnosis of metastatic melanoma in sentinel lymph nodes. Ann Surg Oncol 1999; 6:699–704.

67. Shivers S, Wang X, Li W, *et al.* Molecular staging of malignant melanoma. JAMA 1998; 280:1410–15.

68. Ross MI, Reintgen D, Balch CM. Selective lymphadenectomy: emerging role for lymphatic mapping and sentinel node biopsy in the management of early stage melanoma. Semin Surg Oncol 1993; 9:219–23.

69. Thompson J, McCarthy W, Robinson E, *et al.* Sentinel lymph node biopsy in 102 patients with clinical stage I melanoma undergoing elective lymph node dissection. Presented at the 47th Annual Cancer Symposium, Society of Surgical Oncology, March 17–20, 1994, Houston, Texas.

70. Gadd M, Cosimi B, Yu J, *et al.* Outcome of patients with melanoma and histologically negative sentinel lymph nodes. Arch Surg 1999; 134:381–7.

71. Halsted WS. The results of radical operations for cancer of the breast. Ann Surg 1967; 46:1–19.

72. Harris JR, Osteen RT. Patients with early breast cancer benefit from effective axillary treatment. Breast Cancer Res Treat 1985; 5:17–21.

73. Fisher B, Fisher ER. Transmigration of lymph nodes by tumor cells. Science 1966; 152:1397–8.

74. Fisher B, Fisher ER. Barrier function of lymph node to tumor cells and erythrocytes. I. Normal nodes. Cancer 1967; 20:1907–13.

75. Fisher B, Fisher ER. The interrelationship of hematogenous and lymphatic tumor cell dissemination. Surg Gynecol Obstet 1966; 122:791–8.

76. Adair F, Berg J, Joubert L, *et al.* Long-term follow-up of breast cancer patients: the 30-year report. Cancer 1974; 33:1145–50.

77. Nemoto T, Vana J, Bedwani RN, Baker HW, McGreger FH, Murphy GP. Management and survival of female breast cancer: results of a national survey by the American College of Surgery. Cancer 1980; 45:2917–24.

78. Fisher B, Ravdin RG, Ausman RK, *et al.* Surgical adjuvant chemotherapy in cancer of the breast: results of a decade of cooperative investigation. Ann Surg 1968; 168:337–56.

79. Kinne DW. Controversies in primary breast cancer management. Am J Surg 1993; 166:502–8.

80. Carlson R, *et al.* Update: NCCN Practice Guidelines for the Treatment of Breast Cancer. Oncology 1999; 13 (Suppl. 5A):41–66.

81. Silverstein MJ, Rosser RJ, Gierson ED, *et al.* Axillary lymph node dissection for intraductal carcinoma: is it indicated? Cancer 1987; 59:1819–24.

82. Wong JH, Kopald KH, Morton DL. The impact of microinvasion on axillary node metastases and survival in patients with intraductal breast cancer. Arch Surg 1990; 125:1298–302.

83. Silverstein MJ, Gierson ED, Waisman JR, *et al.* Axillary lymph node dissection for T1a breast carcinoma: is it indicated? Cancer 1994; 73:664–7.

84. Lin PP, Allison DC, Wainstock J, *et al.* Impact of axillary lymph node dissection on the therapy of breast cancer patients. J Clin Oncol 1993; 11:1536–44.

85. Recht A. Commentary. Nodal treatment for patients with early breast cancer. Radiother Oncol 1992; 25:79–82.

86. Fentiman IS, Chetly U. Axillary surgery in breast cancer – is there still debate? Eur J Cancer 1992; 28A:1013–14.

87. Ruffin WK, Stacey-Clear A, Younger J, Hoover HC. Rationale for routine axillary dissection in carcinoma of the breast. J Am Coll Surg 1995; 180:245–51.

88. Adjuvant chemotherapy for breast cancer. NIH Consensus Conference. JAMA 1985; 254:3461–3.

89. Fisher B, Redmond C, Dimitrov NV, et al. A randomized clinical trial evaluating sequential methotrexate and fluorouracil in the treatment of patients with node-negative breast cancer who have estrogen receptor-negative tumors. N Engl J Med 1989; 320:473–8.

90. Fisher B, Costantino J, Redmond C, et al. A randomized clinical trial evaluating tamoxifen in the treatment of patients with node-negative breast cancer who have estrogen receptor-positive tumors. N Engl J Med 1989; 320:479–84.

91. Bonadonna G, Valagussa P, Zambetti M, et al. Milan adjuvant trials for stage I–II breast cancer. In Salmon SE, ed. Adjuvant therapy of cancer V. New York, Grune & Stratton Inc., 1987, 211–21.

92. Nolvadex Adjuvant Trial Organization (NATO). Controlled trial of tamoxifen as single adjuvant agent in management of early breast cancer. Analysis at 6 years by NATO. Lancet 1985; 2:836–40.

93. Adjuvant tamoxifen in the management of operable breast cancer: the Scottish Trial. Report from the Breast Cancer Trials Committee, Scottish Cancer Trials Office (MCR), Edinburgh. Lancet 1987; 2:171–5.

94. Henderson IC. Adjuvant systemic therapy for early breast cancer. Cancer 1994; 74(s):401–9.

95. Early Breast Cancer Trialists Collaborative Group. Systemic treatment of early breast cancer by hormonal, cytotoxic, or immune therapy. Lancet 1992; 339:1–15, 71–85.

96. Fisher B, Redmond C, Fisher ER, et al. Ten-year results of a randomized clinical trial comparing radical mastectomy and total mastectomy with or without radiation. N Engl J Med 1985; 312:674–81.

97. Graversen HP, Blichert-Toft M, Andersen JA, Zedeler K. Breast cancer: risk of axillary recurrence in node-negative patients following partial dissection of the axilla. Eur J Surg Oncol 1988; 14:407–12.

98. Lythgoe JP, Palmer MK. Manchester Regional Breast Study – 5 and 10 year results. Br J Surg 1982; 69:693–6.

99. Ribeiro GG, Dunn G, Swindell R, Harris M, Banerjee SS. Conservation of the breast using two different radiotherapy techniques: interim report of a clinical trial. Clin Oncol 1990; 2:27–34.

100. Gately CA, Mansel RE, Owen A, Redford J, Sellwood RA, Howell A. Treatment of the axilla in operable breast cancer (Abstract). Br J Surg 1991; 78:750.

101. Rosen PP, Groshen S, Kinne DW, Norton L. Factors influencing prognosis in node-negative breast carcinoma: analysis of 767 T1N0M0/T2N0M0 patients with long-term follow-up. J Clin Oncol 1993; 11:2090–100.

102. Tabar L, Fagerberg G, Day NE, et al. Breast cancer treatment and natural history: new insights from results of screening. Lancet 1992; 339:412–14.

103. National Institutes of Health Consensus Conference. Treatment of early-stage breast cancer. JAMA 1991; 265:391–5.

104. Mueller CB. The case against the use of adjuvant chemotherapy in breast cancer. Am Coll Surg Bull 1993; 78(6):25–31.

105. Foster RS. Adjuvant chemotherapy for breast cancer: modest but clinically important benefits. Am Coll Surg Bull 1993; 78(6):18–24.

106. Osborne CK. Prognostic factors for breast cancer: have they met their promise? J Clin Oncol 1992; 10:679–82.

107. Ragaz J, Jackson S, Le N, et al. Adjuvant radiotherapy and chemotherapy in node positive premenopausal women with breast cancer. N Engl J Med 1997; 337:956–62.

108. Overgaard M, Hansen P, Overgaard J, et al. Postoperative radiotherapy in high risk premenopausal women with breast cancer who receive adjuvant chemotherapy. N Engl J Med 1997; 337:949–55.

109. Gardner B, Feldman J. Are positive axillary nodes in breast cancer markers for incurable disease? Ann Surg 1993; 218:270–8.

110. Fisher B, Wolmark N, Bauer M, et al. The accuracy of clinical nodal staging and of limited axillary dissection as a determinant of histologic nodal status in carcinoma of the breast. Surg Gynecol Obstet 1981; 152:765–72.

111. Nieweg O, Kim E, Wong W, et al. Positron emission tomography with fluorine-18-deoxyglucose in the detection and staging of breast cancer. Cancer 1993; 71:3920–5.

112. Haagensen CD. Lymphatics of the breast. In Diseases of the breast, 3rd edn. Philadelphia, WB Saunders, 1986, 300–21.

113. Seigel BM, Mayzel KA, Love SM. Level I and II axillary dissection in the treatment of early-stage breast cancer. An analysis of 259 consecutive patients. Arch Surg 1990; 125:1144–7.

114. Benson EA, Thorogood J. The effect of surgical technique on local recurrence rates following mastectomy. Eur J Surg Oncol 1986; 12:267–71.

115. Delouche G, Bachelot F, Premont M, et al. Conservation treatment of early breast cancer: long term results and complications. Int J Radiat Oncol Biol Phys 1987; 13:29–34.

116. Kissin MW, Querci della Rovere G, Easton D, et al. Risk of lymphoedema following the treatment of breast cancer. Br J Surg 1986; 73:580–4.

117. Rosen PP, Lesser ML, Kinne DW, *et al.* Discontinuous or 'skip' metastases in breast carcinoma. Analysis of 1228 axillary dissections. Ann Surg 1983; 197:276–83.

118. Larson D, Weinstein M, Goldberg I, *et al.* Edema of the arm as a function of the extent of axillary surgery in patients with stage I–II carcinoma of the breast treated with primary radiotherapy. Int J Radiat Oncol Biol Phys 1986; 12:1575–82.

119. Ball A, Waters R, Fish S, *et al.* Radical axillary dissection in the staging and treatment of breast cancer. Ann R Coll Surg 1992; 74:126–9.

120. Cabanes P, Salmon R, Vilcoq J, *et al.* Value of axillary dissection in addition to lumpectomy and radiotherapy in early breast cancer. Lancet 1992; 74:126–9.

121. Forrest A, Stewart H, Roberts M, *et al.* Simple mastectomy and axillary node sampling (pectoral node biopsy) in the management of primary breast cancer. Ann Surg 1982; 196:371–8.

122. Forrest A, Roberts M, Cant E, *et al.* Simple mastectomy and pectoral node biopsy. Br J Surg 1976; 63:569–75.

123. Boova R, Bonanni R, Rosato F. Patterns of axillary nodal involvement in breast cancer; predictability of level one dissection. Ann Surg 1982; 196:642–4.

124. Fisher C, Boyle S, Burke M, *et al.* Intraoperative assessment of nodal status in the selection of patients with breast cancer for axillary clearance. Br J Surg 1993; 80:457–8.

125. Steele R, Forrest A, Gibson T, *et al.* The efficacy of lower axillary sampling in obtaining lymph node status in breast cancer: a controlled randomized trial. Br J Surg 1985; 72:368–9.

126. Krag DN, Weaver DL, Alex JC, Fairbank JT. Surgical resection and radiolocalization of the sentinel lymph node in breast cancer using a gamma probe. Surg Oncol 1993; 2:335–40.

127. Saphir O, Amromin GD. Obscure axillary lymph node metastases in carcinoma of breast. Cancer 1948; 1:238.

128. Kingsley WB, Peters GN, Cheek JH. What constitutes adequate study of axillary lymph nodes in breast cancer? Ann Surg 1985; 201:311–14.

129. International (Ludwig) Breast Cancer Study Group. Prognostic importance of occult axillary lymph node micrometastases from breast cancers. Lancet 1990; 335:1565–8.

130. Clare S, Sener SF, Wilkens W, Goldschmidt R, Merkel D, Winchester DJ. Prognostic significance of occult metastases in node-negative breast cancer. Ann Surg Oncol 1997; 4:447–51.

131. Fisher ER, Swamidoss S, Lee CH, *et al.* Detection and significance of occult axillary node metastases in patients with invasive breast cancer. Cancer 1978; 42:2025–31.

132. Neville AM. Are breast cancer axillary node micrometastases worth detecting? [Editorial] J Pathol 1990; 161:283–4.

133. Hainsworth PJ, Tjandra JJ, Stillwell RG, *et al.* Detection and significance of occult metastases in node-negative breast cancer. Br J Surg 1993; 80:459–63.

134. Statman RC, Jones RC, Cabot MC, Giuliano AE. Sentinel lymphadenectomy. A technique to eliminate axillary dissection in node-negative breast cancer. Proc Am Assoc Clin Oncol 1996; 15:125.

135. Turner R, Ollila D, Krasne D, Giuliano A. Histopathologic validation of the sentinel lymph node hypothesis for breast carcinoma. Ann Surg 1997; 226:271–8.

136. Trojani M, de Mascarel I, Bonichon F, *et al.* Micrometastases to axillary lymph nodes from carcinoma of breast: detection by immunohistochemistry and prognostic significance. Br J Cancer 1987; 55:303–6.

137. Sedmak DD, Meineke TA, Knechtges DS, Anderson J. Prognostic significance of cytokeratin-positive breast cancer metastases. Mod Pathol 1989; 2:516–20.

138. Chen Z-L, Wen D-R, Coulson WF, *et al.* Occult metastases in the axillary lymph nodes of patients with breast cancer node negative by clinical and histologic examination and conventional histology. Dis Markers 1991; 9:239–48.

139. de Mascarel I, Bonichon F, Coindre JM, Trojani M. Prognostic significance of breast cancer axillary lymph node micrometastases assessed by two special techniques: reevaluation with longer follow-up. Br J Cancer 1992; 66:523–7.

140. Giuliano AE, Haigh PI, Brennan MB, *et al.* A prospective observational study of sentinel lymphadenectomy without further axillary dissection in patients with sentinel node-negative breast cancer. J Clin Oncol 2000; 18:2553–9.

141. Chu K, Turner R, Hansen N, *et al.* Do all patients with sentinel node metastasis from breast carcinoma need complete axillary node dissection? Ann Surg 1999; 229:536–41.

142. Noguchi S, Aihara T, Nakamori S, *et al.* The detection of breast carcinoma micrometastases in axillary lymph nodes by means of reverse transcriptase–polymerase chain reaction. Cancer 1994; 74:1595–600.

143. Mori M, Mimori K, Inoue H, *et al.* Detection of cancer micrometastases in lymph nodes by reverse transcriptase–polymerase chain reaction. Cancer Res 1995; 55:3417–20.

144. Noguchi M, Nagayoshi O, Koyasaki N, *et al.* Reappraisal of internal mammary node metastases as a prognostic factor in patients with breast cancer. Cancer 1991; 68:1918–24.

145. Veronesi U, Cascinelli N, Greco M, *et al.* Prognosis of breast cancer patients after mastectomy and

dissection of internal mammary nodes. Ann Surg 1985; 202:702–7.

146. Morrow M, Foster RS. Staging of breast cancer. Arch Surg 1981; 116:748–51.

147. Veronesi U, Cascinelli N, Bufalino R, *et al.* Risk of internal mammary lymph node metastases and its relevance on prognosis of breast cancer patients. Ann Surg 1983; 198:681–4.

148. Veronesi U, Valagussa P. Inefficacy of internal mammary nodes dissection in breast cancer surgery. Cancer 1981; 47:170–5.

Commentary

SETH P HARLOW AND DAVID N KRAG

The surgical management of regional lymph nodes has long been an integral component of the treatment of most adult solid malignancies. Two such malignancies for which this dictum has recently been questioned are breast cancer and melanoma. The controversies concerning these diseases have occurred largely due to the morbidity associated with the surgical removal of the affected regional lymph nodes. The original hypothesis dictating en-bloc resection of the regional nodes in solid tumors, the classic model being breast cancer, was that the cancer progressed in a centrifugal fashion with direct extension from the primary tumor site to the draining lymph nodes. This hypothesis was later changed when it was realized that tumor cells actually embolize to the regional nodes and do not progress by direct extension. Regional lymph node dissections persisted, however, as it was thought that all nodes in the regional basin were at risk for the development of metastatic disease. It was not until the 1960s that surgeons treating testicular carcinoma began to believe that there might be a limited number of lymph nodes that receive the primary lymphatic drainage from a specific tumor site.[1,2] It was the work of Cabanas in 1977 that first demonstrated that selective biopsy of a 'sentinel', or primary, draining lymph node could predict the presence or absence of metastatic disease in a regional lymph node basin.[3] The patient population studied consisted of men with squamous cell carcinoma of the penis. Cabanas' technique was to perform direct lymphography, in which lymphatic channels leading out from the tumor site were cannulated and injected with x-ray contrast. The sentinel nodes, as he called them, were identified by subsequent x-rays and selectively removed. This was followed by a completion lymph node dissection. His results showed a 100% accuracy rate of the sentinel node predicting the presence of metastatic disease in the regional basin. Thus, the sentinel node concept was born. Sentinel node localization, for whatever reasons, did not gain favor in the surgical community until the early 1990s. It was then that the work of Morton *et al.*[4] in developing the sentinel node biopsy technique in melanoma utilizing vital blue dye brought attention to this procedure. Their results

showed a similarly high rate (99%) of concordance of the sentinel node status with that of the regional lymph node basin. This remarkable success led to an explosion of interest in these techniques for the management of solid malignancies from a variety of tumor sites. Further developments in sentinel node identification occurred in 1993 when Alex and Krag introduced the use of radiolabeled tracers for localizing sentinel lymph nodes.[5] Following injection of the radioactive tracer around a tumor site, a surgeon could use a hand-held gamma detector probe to identify precisely the location of the sentinel node(s) before an incision was ever made. This technique allowed for sentinel node localization and removal with a minimum of tissue dissection and for localization of sentinel nodes in locations outside of the expected lymph node drainage basins.

In the year 2000, virtually all sentinel node procedures use one or both of these basic methods (vital blue dye or radiolabeled tracer) for sentinel node identification. Proponents of each method point out certain advantages that each technique has over the other. The blue-dye technique has the advantages of not requiring the use of radioactive tracers, which necessitate specific handling procedures, or the purchase of specialized equipment such as a gamma detector. The blue-dye method also avoids the problem of 'shine through', which can occur when radioactive tracer at the injection site interferes with sentinel node localization if it is close to the lymph node drainage site. The radiolabeled technique, however, has a distinct advantage in that a sentinel node site can be precisely localized prior to an incision being made, allowing optimal placement and the potential to avoid excessive tissue dissection. This technique allows the surgeon to confirm complete removal of all sentinel nodes by measuring the residual radioactivity in the surgical bed without the need for tissue dissection to visualize those nodes. The radiolabeled technique also provides an easy method for surveying all potential lymph node drainage sites, including those in unexpected locations. A combination of the two techniques has been advocated by many to combine the advantages of each to increase the likelihood of a successful procedure. This combination strategy is rapidly becoming the most accepted method of sentinel node identification.

A word of caution: when using these agents for sentinel node identification there is a risk of adverse reactions to these compounds. Allergic reactions ranging from urticaria to profound anaphylaxis have been reported with the use of isosulfan blue dye and patent blue violet, the two most commonly used blue dyes for sentinel node procedures. The risk has recently been reported to be significantly higher than previously thought, with reactions occurring in up to 1% of patients injected with these agents.[6] Mild allergic reactions can occur with the most commonly used radiolabeled agent, technetium sulfur colloid, although at a much lower frequency.

SENTINEL NODE LOCALIZATION IN MELANOMA

The use of sentinel node biopsy techniques in melanoma has become widespread in the past decade. The accuracy of the procedure for identifying the presence of regional lymph node metastases was demonstrated by Morton et al.[4] and confirmed by other investigators.[7–9] The sentinel node procedure has gained rapid popularity because it offers an alternative to elective lymph node dissection, which has not been found to provide significant improvement in survival in prospective, randomized trials in this disease.[10,11] Prior to sentinel node biopsy, simple observation of the regional nodes was an accepted, and often argued, preferred management for the regional nodes in patients with melanoma. However, the prospect of a minimally invasive procedure that could accurately stage patients without the associated morbidity of an elective node dissection led to its rapid acceptance. This popularity was further enhanced by the results of the Eastern Cooperative Oncology Group (ECOG) EST 1684 Trial[12] evaluating the efficacy of adjuvant interferon alfa-2B for the treatment of high-risk (node-positive or thick primary) melanoma. This trial was the first prospective, randomized trial to show a survival benefit for patients who received an adjuvant treatment for melanoma. Therefore, without clear evidence that surgical treatment of the regional nodes might impact patient survival in this disease, from a staging perspective, sentinel node biopsy could now possibly impact survival by indicating those patients who may benefit most from adjuvant therapy.

The actual method a surgeon uses for sentinel node biopsy in melanoma is probably less important than the surgeon performing that chosen method well. Similar success rates and accuracy rates have been found when using either the blue-dye or radiolabeled method alone or in combination.[4,7–9] Our preference is to use the radiolabeled method either alone or with blue dye for the previously stated advantages gained by the radiolabeled

technique. Our current technique is to inject a small volume, 0.5–2.0 mL, of unfiltered technetium-99m-sulfur colloid (TSC) (0.4–1.0 mCi) into the dermis around the melanoma, biopsy site, or prior excision site. Because of the rich lymphatic network in the dermis, there is rapid uptake and transit of the agent to the sentinel nodes, reaching those nodes in most cases in between 5 and 30 min. The TSC we inject is not filtered, as is done for lymphoscintigraphy, and consists primarily of larger particles. These larger particles are more effectively trapped in the sentinel nodes, with fewer escaping to travel to second-echelon nodes, making the intraoperative localization of sentinel nodes easier. We have found that preoperative lymphoscintigraphy may be helpful but is not always required, as sentinel nodes may not be localized by the scan. This is probably due to the larger particle size of the unfiltered TSC having a slower transit time, making it a poorer agent for imaging purposes. Rather, we rely on a careful systematic evaluation of all potential node-bearing sites by the surgeon in the operating room with a hand-held gamma detector. The surgeon performing a careful survey in this fashion will be more sensitive than a lymphoscintigram, and will often find hot-spot locations that were not identified on the scanned images. The sentinel node location is identified as a discrete area of increased radioactivity that is identified by the audio feedback of the probe. The hot spot will have a 10-s count, which is greater than the counts obtained from the tissue immediately between it and the injection site (background count). The actual number of counts at the hot spot is not important as long as those counts are greater than that of the background. This relationship of hot-spot counts to background holds true because radioactive counts will steadily decrease as one travels away from the injection site. When there is a lymph node present which is sequestering the radiolabeled agent, this steady decline is interrupted by a sudden rise in the audible count rate. We have employed the use of a lower count limit for defining a hot spot of 15 counts per 10 s. This is the level at which one can confidently use the audio feedback of the probe to identify a true hot spot over low background. Based on the precise localization with the probe, a small incision is made over the hot spot and, with minimal dissection, the radiolabeled node(s) are removed. The probe is used to confirm that all sentinel nodes have been removed by measuring the residual counts in the surgical bed. Any node containing 10% or more of the counts of the hottest removed sentinel node is also removed and treated as a sentinel node. When the blue-dye technique is combined with the radiolabeled technique, we still use the gamma-probe to identify the hot spot and center the incision over that spot to minimize tissue dissection. The blue dye will almost always trace to the same nodes as the radiolabeled tracer. However, if a node is blue and not radiolabeled, or *vice versa*, it is removed and considered to be a sentinel node as well.

Most recent series have shown success rates of identifying and removing sentinel nodes in melanoma to be in the 95–100% range.[4,7–9] The accuracy rates of sentinel nodes in reflecting the true pathologic status of the regional node basin come from three clinical studies in which sentinel node biopsy was followed by a completion lymph node dissection.[4,7,8] The combined number of patients in these studies was 383; sentinel nodes were identified and removed in 325 (85% success rate). The sentinel node status correctly predicted the regional node status in 98.8% of these patients. The false-negative rate, a more precise measurement to assess the true utility of the procedure, was 6% (4 of 68 node-positive patients). These results demonstrate that, for melanoma, sentinel node biopsy procedures are both highly successful and highly accurate in staging this disease. However, the impact of sentinel node biopsy in improving disease recurrence rates and overall survival have not yet been quantified and are the objectives of ongoing multicenter randomized trials (the Multicenter Selective Lymphadenectomy Trial and the Sunbelt Melanoma Trial).

Whereas the effectiveness of sentinel node biopsy in melanoma is rarely disputed, some controversy exists over which patients should have sentinel node procedures performed and which should not. Any patient with invasive melanoma (Clark level 2 or higher) is at theoretical risk for developing lymph node metastases. This risk is clearly related to the depth of invasion of the primary tumor as measured by the Clark[13] or Breslow[14] method. Patients with thin melanomas (< 1 mm depth) are at low risk for lymph node metastases, whereas patients with deep lesions (> 4 mm depth) are at high risk, but also have a high risk for concurrent systemic micrometastases. In the era of elective lymph node dissections, these findings were used to stratify patients into groups based on those who were most likely to benefit from these relatively morbid procedures, offering them primarily to patients with intermediate-thickness melanomas (1–4 mm deep).[15] Many surgeons have adopted these same criteria for determining which patients should have sentinel node biopsy procedures performed. The sentinel node biopsy procedure, however, may provide important staging information that could alter subsequent treatment plans but, unlike elective node dissection, does so in a minimally morbid fashion. An example of how extending these indications may prove useful is a report of Gershenwald et al. of patients with deep melanomas who were treated with sentinel node biopsy.[16] These investigators found that patients who were sentinel node negative had surprisingly high survival rates and that, in multivariate analysis, sentinel node status was the most important predictor of survival. Therefore, in this group of patients, the sentinel node biopsy not only provides important prognostic information, but may also identify a patient population that may not be at as high a risk for recurrence as previously thought and may not benefit

as much from available systemic adjuvant therapies. Conversely, patients with thin melanomas are known to be at very low risk for lymph node metastases; however, this risk is still present. With sentinel node techniques, these patients can now have accurate pathologic staging while exposing the entire group to minimal morbidity. This allows the chance to impact positively on the outcome for the occasional patient with nodal metastases with thin melanomas. The group of patients with thin melanomas at greatest risk for nodal disease are those with Clark level 3 or 4 primaries,[17] whereas the risk may be essentially zero for Clark level 2 lesions.[18] Anecdotally, we have found positive sentinel nodes in patients with lesions as thin as 0.54 mm deep, Clark level 3. Our recommendation, therefore, is that, rather than setting rigid guidelines about who should or should not have these procedures, the surgeon should discuss the pros and cons of the procedure with the patient. This discussion should include the risk of finding lymph node metastases and the possible complications of the procedure so that a joint decision can be made in this regard.

SENTINEL LYMPH NODE BIOPSY IN BREAST CANCER

Breast cancer is another disease in which there has been debate as to the benefit of elective regional lymph node dissection. Axillary lymph node dissection has long been the standard procedure for managing these patients and is the only treatment that fulfills the three goals of regional node management; pathologic staging, regional disease control, and maximal opportunity for survival advantage. Unlike melanoma, in which nodal observation was the recommended management prior to sentinel node biopsy, the recommended management of invasive breast cancer was and remains a level 1 and 2 axillary lymph node dissection.[19]

From the staging perspective, axillary node dissection provides important prognostic information that has been found to be the most important predictor of patient survival in patients with early breast cancer.[20] This staging information is used to determine the best options for systemic adjuvant treatment. Systemic adjuvant treatments have clearly shown an improvement in survival rates in patients with node-positive disease.[21]

From the regional disease-control standpoint, axillary dissection alone achieves excellent long-term regional control rates of 98–99% in patients who are clinically node negative before surgery.[22]

From the overall survival perspective, debate arises as to the impact that axillary node dissection has on patient survival from breast cancer. The largest prospective, randomized study comparing axillary node dissection to axillary observation, The National Surgical Adjuvant Breast and Bowel Project (NSABP) B-04 study, demonstrated a small but statistically non-significant survival improvement for patients treated with axillary dissection versus observation.[22] Criticisms of this trial were that a substantial number of patients in the observation arm in fact had tumor-containing lymph nodes removed at the time of simple mastectomy, potentially improving the survival for that group. Other concerns were that the number of patients enrolled on this study did not have the power to demonstrate statistical significance for the modest survival differences seen on the study, and that the study was performed prior to the use of adjuvant systemic treatments for breast cancer. Some researchers have hypothesized that current systemic adjuvant therapies perform best when there is optimal control of local–regional disease. This theory has recently been supported by the findings of improved patient survival in patients receiving post-mastectomy radiation to the chest wall.[23,24]

Despite fulfilling the three objectives of regional treatment, the routine use of axillary dissection has been questioned by some, primarily because of the morbidity associated with the procedure. Improved screening for breast cancer has led to an increased incidence of small (<1 cm) invasive cancers, with lower rates of axillary nodal metastases, while patients with tumors >1 cm are frequently given adjuvant systemic treatments, even if their nodes are negative, further eroding support for routine surgical staging. There was little surprise that the successes of sentinel node biopsy in melanoma quickly led to trials of these techniques in breast cancer. However, some distinct differences exist in performing sentinel node biopsies in breast cancer as compared to melanoma. First, the breast is a subcutaneous structure that is comprised predominantly of fibroglandular tissue and fat. Unlike the dermis, which has a rich lymphatic network, the lymphatic network in the breast is largely confined to the fibroglandular tissue. In the population in which breast cancer is most commonly found, postmenopausal women, there tends to be an increase in the proportional amount of fat tissue in the breast. This can lead to wide variations in the rate of flow of sentinel node-targeting agents when the injections are made into the breast parenchyma adjacent to a tumor. In addition, the primary lymph node basins in breast cancer are located in close proximity to the primary tumor site, unlike most melanomas. This can lead to challenging cases with the radiolabeled techniques due to overlap of the injection site background levels with the lymph node basins. Despite these obstacles, highly successful methods for sentinel node biopsy in breast cancer have been developed. The technique of lymphatic mapping with vital blue dye was developed by Guiliano et al.[25,26] and is nicely described in the chapter by Dr Jones et al. The technique of radiolabeled biopsy in breast cancer was developed by Krag et al. at the University of Vermont.[27] The development phase of this technique evaluated a number of different parameters to determine the most optimal method of radioguided sentinel lymph node biopsy. Parameters evaluated

included a variety of different tracers, tracer doses, and dilution volumes. The best results were obtained when unfiltered TSC, 1 mCi in 8 mL saline, was injected in four quadrants around the tumor into the breast parenchyma and allowed a minimum of 30 min to migrate to the sentinel nodes. It is not uncommon, however, for some patients, particularly those with fatty replaced breasts, to require 2–3 h or more for sufficient tracer to migrate to the sentinel nodes, which would allow sentinel node localization. Variations of the injection location have been tested with the goal of improving the ease of the procedure. Injections into the dermis above the tumor or in a subareolar location have shown greater counts in the axillary sentinel nodes than are typically found if a straight parenchymal injection is used. The nodes that are isolated using these skin injections appear to be the same nodes that are identified with parenchymal injections, based on pathologic correlation studies compared to completion axillary dissection.[28,29] A combination of parenchymal injection with injection into the skin may be ideal for increasing axillary sentinel node counts, thereby making localization easier, but also preserves the potential for labeling of nodal sites that may be outside the axilla and that are best identified after a parenchymal injection.

Lymphoscintigrams need not be routinely performed as part of the sentinel node procedure for breast cancer. These scans are less helpful than in melanoma and are often difficult to perform due to overlap of the injection site with the nodal basins. The use of unfiltered TSC also limits the scan because of the slow migration of this agent. As in melanoma, it is the trained surgeon equipped with a hand-held gamma detector that is the most accurate and sensitive method for identifying sentinel nodes. The surgeon performs a careful survey of all potential lymph node drainage areas with the probe. This survey includes nodal sites outside the axilla (internal mammary, supraclavicular, and intramammary), which may be locations of sentinel nodes as well. Similar to melanoma, a sentinel node is localized beneath a discrete hot spot on the skin where the underlying counts are greater than the background counts between the hot spot and the injection site. If a combination technique of blue dye plus radiolabeled tracer is used, we inject the blue dye after this survey is completed. We inject 5 mL of isosulfan blue dye in four locations around the tumor and gently massage the breast for 5–10 min. The incision placement for the sentinel node is guided by the probe localization, but is usually placed into the site where a completion axillary dissection incision would be made. The probe is inserted intermittently into the incision to guide the dissection toward the sentinel node(s); this helps to decrease tissue dissection. The hottest radiolabeled nodes are removed and a 10-s 'ex-vivo' count of each node is recorded. The probe is re-inserted and, by carefully angling it to different areas of the axilla, any additional radiolabeled nodes can be identified without further dissection. We have found that intact nodes with less than 10% of the counts of the hottest node removed have minimal risk of containing metastatic disease if the radioactive sentinel nodes are found to be free of tumor, therefore these nodes are left in place. When the blue dye is simultaneously used, any node with blue dye in it, or a blue lymphatic channel leading to it, is removed as a sentinel node. In almost all cases, these nodes are also radiolabeled. We have also found that the risk of false-negative sentinel node biopsy may be reduced if the remaining axillary nodes are palpated at the time of surgery. We have found that some nodes are completely replaced with tumor that seems to divert all lymphatic flow to an adjacent node without metastatic disease. These tumor-replaced nodes may therefore be missed by either sentinel node localizing method and may only be detected by palpation of a round, hard node. The role of extra-axillary sentinel node biopsy has not yet been completely defined. Direct lymphatic drainage to the internal mammary nodes, supraclavicular nodes, or intramammary nodes is a known clinical reality. Tumor metastases to these nodes carry the same, or worse, prognostic significance as axillary nodal metastases. Therefore, evaluation of these nodes has potential clinical importance. Studies of lymphatic drainage patterns in normal breast tissue performed in the 1970s demonstrated significant lymphatic flow to the internal mammary nodes occurring in 20–86% of patients, depending on the site in the breast that was injected.[30] A retrospective clinical review of internal mammary node metastases by Morrow and Foster looked at several reported studies, which included 7070 patients treated with axillary dissection and internal mammary biopsy or dissection.[31] They found a 22.4% incidence of internal mammary node metastases and, in 4.9% of patients, the only positive lymph node was an internal mammary node, highlighting the potential importance of these sites. The beauty of the radiolabeled sentinel node procedure is that these sites can be evaluated in each patient and, in those in whom this pattern of lymphatic drainage is found, the extra-axillary nodes can be removed in a minimally invasive fashion. In this way, optimal nodal staging can be accomplished for each patient. A recent review of our experience with sentinel node biopsy for breast cancer found the overall rate of extra-axillary sentinel nodes identified was 6.5%.[32] This rate increased to 14.8% when an injection volume of 8 mL TSC was used. Metastatic disease was found in the extra-axillary lymph nodes in 6.8% of patients, in whom these nodes were removed, with 4.5% of patients having metastatic disease only in the extra-axillary nodes.

Sentinel node procedures in breast cancer have demonstrated very good results in preliminary studies looking at pathologic correlation to axillary dissection. The success rates for identifying sentinel nodes, using a variety of different methods, have generally been greater than 90%, with pathologic accuracy rates of 95–100%. False-negative rates have ranged from zero to 15%.[25–28,33,34]

The multicenter study of Krag et al.[35] gave insight into how successful these procedures may be in the general practicing surgical community. In this study, surgeons from 11 different sites participated, including surgeons from a number of different practice patterns. There was an overall success rate of sentinel node identification and removal of 91%, a pathologic accuracy rate of 97%, and a false-negative rate of 11.4%. These results were obtained with a procedure using only a radiolabeled tracer. It is hoped that further refinements in the radiolabeled technique as well as the combination of this technique with the blue dye lymphatic mapping will further improve these results and make this procedure even easier to perform.

The practicing surgeon, however, should be cautious about replacing a well-defined surgical procedure with a known track record for a new procedure, especially in the management of malignant disease. Sentinel node procedures certainly add information to the results of axillary lymph node dissection, but there is a paucity of clinical data currently available to conclude that these procedures alone can replace axillary dissection at this time. There are currently two large, prospective, randomized clinical trials being performed to answer these questions. The NSABP B-32 study was designed to answer the question: is sentinel node biopsy alone the equivalent of sentinel node biopsy plus axillary node dissection in the sentinel node-negative patient? In this study, there is a straight randomization for patients who are sentinel node negative to either completion axillary dissection or observation. All patients with pathologically positive nodes in this study will have a completion axillary dissection. Patients will be followed for disease-free and overall survival as well as for differences in functional measures of the affected extremity. The American College of Surgeons Oncology Group Trial Z0011 will attempt to answer a similar question of the need for completion axillary dissection in the sentinel node-positive patient. Accrual to and completion of these studies are imperative if we wish to continue to use these procedures based on sound scientific evidence of their efficacy.

The final issue with sentinel node procedures is that of pathologic evaluation of the sentinel nodes. It is well known that the more lymph node specimens are scrutinized, the greater the likelihood that small foci of disease may be identified. With sentinel node biopsy procedures, we are now able to hand over a small number of nodes which have the greatest likelihood of containing metastatic disease to our pathologists. How these nodes should best be handled is controversial and is the subject of ongoing research. With currently available techniques of immunohistochemistry and reverse transcriptase–polymerase chain reaction, it is now possible to detect as few as one tumor cell in one million normal cells. The question that needs to be answered with these techniques is: what are the clinical implications of a positive finding with these studies, if any at all? It has been well documented that tumor cells are shed into the blood-stream at an early stage in their development and can be identified circulating in the blood in a surprisingly high percentage of patients with early cancers.[36,37] The majority of these patients do not succumb to metastatic disease, because these circulating cells, for the most part, are not capable of forming independent metastatic colonies. It is reasonable to assume that these same cells are capable of embolizing into the lymphatics just as well as the blood and may be trapped in the first draining lymph nodes. Detecting individual or small numbers of tumor cells in these nodes may therefore not have the same significance as detecting a viable focus of established metastatic disease in that node. The latter would indicate that, not only had tumor embolization occurred, but a clone of cells capable of establishing a viable metastatic colony had embolized. Therefore, an overly sensitive technique capable of detecting tumor cells that may lack the potential to form metastatic colonies may lead to over-staging of those patients. Clearly, additional longitudinal studies are needed to assess the clinical relevance of such findings on patient survival before they should be considered standard studies in the pathologic staging of malignant disease. The College of American Pathologists has recently addressed this debate and has issued a consensus statement indicating that the pathologic staging of sentinel lymph nodes should be based on routine histologic evaluation throughout the nodes at approximately 2-mm intervals. The routine use of immuno-histochemistry for cytokeratin should not be considered standard until clinical trials demonstrate its clinical significance.[38]

SUMMARY

In summary, sentinel node techniques have advanced considerably since they were first performed by Cabanas in the 1970s. Clearly, these techniques will alter the way that solid malignancies are surgically managed and pathologically staged in the future. As responsible physicians and scientists, we should confirm our hypotheses regarding these techniques by completing properly performed, randomized, clinical trials so that we have a solid basis for their continued use in the future.

REFERENCES

1. Busch FM, Sayeh ES, Chenault OW. Some uses of lymphangiography in the management of testicular tumors. J Urol 1964; 93:490–3.

2. Chiappa S, Uselenghi C, Bonnadonna G, et al. Combined testicular and foot lymphangiography in testicular carcinoma. Surg Gynecol Obstet 1966; 13:10–14.

3. Cabanas RM. An approach to the treatment of penile carcinoma. Cancer 1977; 39:456–66.

4. Morton DL, Wen D-R, Wong JH, et al. Technical details of intraoperative lymphatic mapping for early stage melanoma. Arch Surg 1992; 127:392–9.

5. Alex JC, Krag DN. Gamma probe guided localization of lymph nodes. Surg Oncol 1993; 2:137–43.

6. Leong SP, Donegan E, Heffernon W. Adverse reaction to isosulfan blue during sentinel lymph node dissection in melanoma. Ann Surg Oncol 2000; 7:361–6.

7. Thompson JF, McCarthy WH, Bosch CMJ, et al. Sentinel lymph node status as an indicator of the presence of metastatic melanoma in regional lymph nodes. Melanoma Res 1995; 5:255–60.

8. Reintgen D, Cruise CW, Wells K, et al. The orderly progression of melanoma nodal metastases. Ann Surg 1994; 220:759–67.

9. Krag DN, Meijer SJ, Weaver DL, et al. Minimal access surgery for staging of malignant melanoma. Arch Surg 1995; 130:654–8.

10. Veronesi U, Adamus J, Bandiera DC, et al. Inefficacy of immediate node dissection in stage I melanoma of the limbs. N Engl J Med 1977; 297:627–30.

11. Sim FH, Taylor WF, Pritchard DJ, et al. Lymphadenectomy in the management of stage I malignant melanoma: a prospective randomized study. Mayo Clin Proc 1986; 61:697–705.

12. Kirkwood JM, Strawderman MH, Ernstoff MS, et al. Interferon alfa-2b adjuvant therapy of high risk resected cutaneous melanoma: the Eastern Cooperative Oncology Group Trial EST 1684. J Clin Oncol 1996; 149(1):7–17.

13. Clark WH Jr. The histogenesis and biological behavior of primary malignant melanoma of the skin. Cancer Res 1969; 29:705–27.

14. Breslow A. Thickness, cross sectional areas and depth of invasion in the prognosis of cutaneous melanoma. Ann Surg 1970; 1970:902–8.

15. Balch CM, Soong SJ, Murad TM, et al. A multifactorial analysis of melanoma. II. Prognostic factors in patients with stage I (localized) melanoma. Surgery 1979; 86:343–51.

16. Gershenwald J, Mansfield P, Lee J, Ross M. Role for lymphatic mapping and sentinel lymph node biopsy in patients with thick (≥4 mm) primary melanoma. Ann Surg Oncol 2000; 7:160–5.

17. Corsetti RL, Allen HM, Wanebo HJ. Thin < or =1 mm level III and IV melanomas are high risk lesions for regional failure and warrant sentinel lymph node biopsy. Ann Surg Oncol 2000; 7:456–60.

18. Harlow SP, Krag DN, Ashikaga T, et al. Gamma probe guided biopsy of the sentinel node in malignant melanoma: a multicenter study. Melanoma Res 2001; 11:45–55.

19. Treatment of early stage breast cancer. NIH Consensus Statement 1990; 8:1–19.

20. Adair F, Berg J, Joubert L, *et al.* Long term follow-up of breast cancer patients: the 30 year report. Cancer 1974; 33:1145–50.

21. Early Breast Cancer Trialists Collaborative Group. Systemic treatment of early breast cancer by hormonal, cytotoxic or immune therapy. Lancet 1992; 339:1–15, 71–85.

22. Fisher B, Montague E, Redmond C, *et al.* Comparison of radical mastectomy with alternative treatments for primary breast cancer: a first report of results from a prospective randomized clinical trial. Cancer 1977; 39:2827–39.

23. Ragaz J, Jackson S, Le N, *et al.* Adjuvant radiotherapy and chemotherapy in node positive premenopausal women with breast cancer. N Engl J Med 1997; 337:956–62.

24. Overgaard M, Hansen P, Overgaard J, *et al.* Postoperative radiotherapy in high risk premenopausal women with breast cancer who receive adjuvant chemotherapy. N Engl J Med 1997; 337:949–55.

25. Guiliano AE, Kirgan DM, Guenther JM, *et al.* Lymphatic mapping and sentinel lymphadenectomy for breast cancer. Ann Surg 1994; 220:391–401.

26. Guiliano AE, Jones RC, Brennan M, *et al.* Sentinel lymphadenectomy in breast cancer. J Clin Oncol 1997; 15:2345–50.

27. Krag DN, Ashikaga T, Harlow SP, Weaver DL. Development of sentinel node targeting technique in breast cancer patients. Breast J 1998; 4:67–74.

28. Veronesi U, Paganelli G, Viale G, *et al.* Sentinel lymph node biopsy and axillary dissection in breast cancer: results in a large series. J Natl Cancer Inst 1999; 91:368–72.

29. Klimberg VS, Rubio IT, Henry R, *et al.* Subareolar versus peritumoral injection for location of the sentinel lymph node. Ann Surg 1999; 229:860–5.

30. Vendrell-Trone E, Setoain-Quinquer J, Domenech-Torne F. Study of normal mammary lymphatic drainage using radioactive isotopes. J Nucl Med 1972; 13:801–5.

31. Morrow M, Foster R Jr. Staging of breast cancer: a new rationale for internal mammary node biopsy. Arch Surg 1981; 116:748–51.

32. Harlow SP, Krag DN, Weaver DL, Ashikaga T. Extra-axillary sentinel lymph nodes in breast cancer. Breast Cancer 1999; 6:159–65.

33. Albertini J, Lyman G, Cox C, *et al.* Lymphatic mapping and sentinel node biopsy in the patient with breast cancer. JAMA 1996; 276:1818–22.

34. Linehan DL, Hill ADK, Akhurst T, *et al.* Intradermal radiocolloid and intraparenchymal blue dye injection optimize sentinel node identification in breast cancer patients. Ann Surg Oncol 1999; 6:450–4.

35. Krag DN, Weaver DL, Ashikaga T, *et al.* The sentinel node in breast cancer: a multicenter validation study. N Engl J Med 1998; 339:941–6.

36. Racila E, Euhus D, Weiss AJ, *et al.* Detection and characterization of carcinoma cells in the blood. Proc Natl Acad Sci USA 1998; 95:4589–94.

37. Krag DN, Ashikaga T, Moss TJ, *et al.* Breast cancer cells in blood: a pilot study. Breast J 1999; 5:354–8.

38. Fitzgibbons PL, Page DL, Weaver D, *et al.* Prognostic factors in breast cancer: College of American Pathologists Consensus Statement 1999. Arch Pathol Lab Med 2000; 124:966–78.

Editors' selected abstracts

The effects of postinjection massage on the sensitivity of lymphatic mapping in breast cancer.

Bass SS, Cox CE, Salud CJ, Lyman GH, McCann C, Dupont E, Berman C, Reintgen DS.

Department of Surgery, H. Lee Moffitt Cancer Center and Research Institute, University of South Florida, Tampa, FL, USA.

Journal of the American College of Surgeons 192:9–16, 2001.

Background: The technique of lymphatic mapping and sentinel lymph node (SLN) biopsy is rapidly becoming the preferred method of staging the axilla of the breast cancer patient. This report describes the impact of postinjection massage on the sensitivity of this surgical technique. *Study design:* Lymphatic mapping at the H Lee Moffitt Cancer Center is performed using a combination of isosulfan blue dye and Tc^{99m} labeled sulfur colloid. Data describing the rate of SLN identification and the node characteristics from 594 consecutive patients were calculated. Patients who received a 5-minute massage after injection of blue dye and radiocolloid were compared with a control group in which the patients did not receive a postinjection massage. *Results:* When compared with controls, the proportion of patients who had their SLN identified using blue dye after massage increased from 73.0% to 88.3%, and the proportion of patients who had their SLN identified using radiocolloid after massage increased from 81.7% to 91.3%. The overall rate of SLN identification increased from 93.5% to 97.8%. The proportion of nodes that were stained blue among those removed increased from 73.4% to 79.7% after massage. *Conclusions:* As experience increases with this new procedure, the surgical technique of lymphatic mapping continues to evolve. The addition of a postinjection massage significantly improves the uptake of blue dye by SLNs and may also aid in the accumulation of radioactivity in the SLNs, further increasing the sensitivity of this procedure.

Incidence of sentinel node metastasis in patients with thin primary melanoma (≤ 1 mm) with vertical growth phase.

Bedrosian I, Faries MB, Guerry D 4th, Elenitsas R, Schuchter L, Mick R, Spitz FR, Bucky LP, Alavi A, Elder DE, Fraker DL, Czerniecki BJ.

Department of Surgery, University of Pennsylvania, Philadelphia, PA, USA.

Annals of Surgical Oncology 7(4):262–7, 2000, May.

Background: Patients with thin primary melanomas (≤ 1 mm) generally have an excellent prognosis. However, the presence of a vertical growth phase (VGP) adversely impacts the survival rate. We report on the rate of occurrence of nodal metastasis in patients with thin primary melanomas with a VGP who are offered sentinel lymph node (SLN) biopsy. Methods: Among 235 patients with clinically localized cutaneous melanomas who underwent successful SLN biopsy, 71 had lesions 1 mm or smaller with a VGP. The SLN was localized by using blue dye and a radiotracer. If negative for tumor by using hematoxylin and eosin staining, the SLN was further examined by immunohistochemistry. Results: The rate of occurrence of SLN metastasis was 15.2% in patients with melanomas deeper than 1 mm and 5.6% in patients with thin melanomas. Three patients with thin melanomas and a positive SLN had low-risk lesions, based on a highly accurate six-variable multivariate logistic regression model for predicting 8-year survival in stage I/II melanomas. The fourth patient had a low- to intermediate-risk lesion based on this model. At the time of the lymphadenectomy, one patient had two additional nodes with metastasis. Conclusions: VGP in a melanoma 1 mm or smaller seems to be a risk factor for nodal metastasis. The risk of nodal disease may not be accurately predicted by the use of a multivariate logistic regression model that incorporates thickness, mitotic rate, regression, tumor-infiltrating lymphocytes, sex, and anatomical site. Patients with thin lesions having VGP should be evaluated for SLN biopsy and trials of adjuvant therapy when stage III disease is found.

Functional lymphatic anatomy for sentinel node biopsy in breast cancer: echoes from the past and the periareolar blue method.

Borgstein PJ, Meijer S, Pijpers RJ, van Diest PJ.

Department of Surgical Oncology, Nuclear Medicine, and Pathology, Academic Hospital of the Vrije Universiteit, Amsterdam, The Netherlands.

Annals of Surgery 232(1):81–9, 2000, July.

Objective: To simplify and improve the technique of axillary sentinel node biopsy, based on a concept of functional lymphatic anatomy of the breast. Summary background data: Because of their common origin, the mammary gland and its skin envelope share the same lymph drainage pathways. The breast is essentially a single unit and has a specialized lymphatic system with preferential drainage, through select channels, to designated (sentinel) lymph nodes in the lower axilla. Methods: These hypotheses were studied by comparing axillary lymph node targeting after intraparenchymal peritumoral radiocolloid (detected by a gamma probe) with the visible staining after an intradermal blue dye injection, either over the primary tumor site (90 procedures) or in the periareolar area (130 procedures). The radioactive content, blue coloring, and histopathology of the individual lymph nodes harvested during each procedure were analyzed. Results: Radiolabeled axillary nodes were identified in 210 procedures, and these were colored blue in 200 cases (94%). The targeting concordance between peritumoral radiocolloid and intradermal blue dye was unrelated to the breast tumor location or the site of dye injection. Radioactive sentinel nodes were not stained blue in 10 procedures (5%), but this mismatching could be explained by technical problems in all cases. In two cases (1%), the (pathologic) sentinel node was blue but had no detectable radiocolloid uptake. Conclusions: The lessons learned from this study provide a functional concept of the breast lymphatic system and its role in metastasis. Anatomical and clinical investigations from the past strongly support these views, as do recent sentinel node studies. Periareolar blue dye injection appears ideally suited to identify the principal (axillary) metastasis route in early breast cancer. Awareness of the targeting mechanism and inherent technical restrictions remain crucial to the ultimate success of sentinel node biopsy and may prevent disaster.

Do all patients with sentinel node metastasis from breast carcinoma need complete axillary node dissection?

Chu KU, Turner RR, Hansen NM, Brennan MB, Bilchik A, Giuliano AE.

Joyce Eisenberg Keefer Breast Center, John Wayne Cancer Institute at Saint John's Health Center, Santa Monica, CA, USA.

Annals of Surgery 229(4):536–41, 1999, April.

Objective: To determine the likelihood of nonsentinel axillary metastasis in the presence of sentinel node metastasis from a primary breast carcinoma. Summary background data: Sentinel lymphadenectomy is a highly accurate technique for identifying axillary metastasis from a primary breast carcinoma. Our group has shown that nonsentinel axillary lymph nodes are unlikely to contain tumor cells if the axillary sentinel node is tumor-free, but as yet no study has examined the risk of nonsentinel nodal involvement when the sentinel node contains tumor cells. Methods: Between 1991 and 1997, axillary lymphadenectomy was performed in 157 women with a tumor-involved sentinel node. Fifty-three axillae (33.5%) had at least one tumor-involved nonsentinel node. The authors analyzed the incidence of nonsentinel node involvement according to clinical and tumor characteristics. Results: Only two variables had a significant impact on the likelihood of nonsentinel node metastasis: the size of the sentinel node metastasis and the size of the primary tumor. The rate of nonsentinel node involvement was 7% when the sentinel node had a micrometastasis (≤ 2 mm), compared with 55% when the sentinel node had a macrometastasis (> 2 mm). In addition, the rate of nonsentinel node tumor involvement increased with the size of the primary tumor. Conclusions: If a primary breast tumor is small and if sentinel node involvement is micrometastatic, then tumor cells are unlikely to be found in other axillary lymph nodes. This suggests that axillary lymph node dissection may not be necessary in patients with sentinel node micrometastases from T1/T2 lesions, or in patients with sentinel node metastases from T1a lesions.

Prospective observational study of sentinel lymphadenectomy without further axillary dissection in patients with sentinel node-negative breast cancer.

Giuliano AE, Haigh PI, Brennan MB, Hansen NM, Kelley MC, Ye W, Glass EC, Turner RR.

Joyce Eisenberg-Keefer Breast Center, Division of Surgical Oncology, Statistical Coordinating Unit, Department of Nuclear Medicine, Santa Monica, CA, USA.

Journal of Clinical Oncology 18(13):2553–9, 2000, July.

Purpose: Immediate complete axillary lymphadenectomy (ALND) after sentinel lymphadenectomy (SLND) has confirmed that tumor-negative sentinel nodes accurately predict tumor-free axillary nodes in breast cancer. Therefore, we hypothesized that SLND alone in patients with tumor-negative sentinel nodes would achieve axillary control, with minimal complications. *Patients and methods:* Between October 1995 and July 1997, 133 consecutive women who had primary invasive breast tumors clinically Sentinel nodes were examined by standard microscopy or immunohistochemistry. SLND was the only axillary surgery if sentinel nodes were tumor-free. Completion ALND was performed only if sentinel nodes contained metastases or if they were not identified. Excluded from subsequent analysis were patients with unsuspected multifocal carcinoma and those who refused completion ALND. The complication and axillary recurrence rates after SLND without ALND were determined. *Results:* Sentinel nodes were identified in 132 (99%) of 133 patients. Eight patients were excluded from further analysis. Of the 125 assessable patients, 57 had tumor-positive sentinel nodes and one had an unsuccessful mapping procedure; these patients underwent completion ALND. In the remaining 67 patients (54%), SLND was the only axillary procedure. Complications occurred in 20 patients (35%) undergoing ALND after SLND but in only two patients (3%) undergoing SLND alone ($p = 0.001$). There were no local or axillary recurrences at a median follow-up of 39 months. *Conclusion:* Complication rates are negligible after SLND alone. An absence of axillary recurrences supports SLND as an accurate staging alternative for breast cancer and suggests that routine ALND can be eliminated for patients with histopathologically negative sentinel nodes.

Biopsy method and excision volume do not affect success rate of subsequent sentinel lymph node dissection in breast cancer.

Haigh PI, Hansen NM, Qi K, Giuliano AE.

Division of Surgical Oncology, John Wayne Cancer Institute at Saint John's Health Center, Santa Monica, CA, USA.

Annals of Surgical Oncology 7(1):21–7, 2000, January–February.

Introduction: Sentinel lymph node dissection (SLND) is becoming a recognized technique for accurately staging patients with breast cancer. Its success in patients with large tumors or prior excisions has been questioned. The purpose of this study was to evaluate the effect of biopsy method, excision volume, interval from biopsy to SLND, tumor size, and tumor location on SLND success rate. *Methods:* Consecutive patients who underwent SLND followed by completion axillary lymph node dissection from October 1991 to December 1995 were analyzed. Included were cases performed early in the series before the technique was adequately developed. Excision volume was derived from the product of three dimensions as measured by the pathologist. Two end points were analyzed: sentinel node identification rate and accuracy of SLND in predicting axillary status. Univariate analyses using chi2 or Fisher's exact test for categorical variables and Wilcoxon rank sums for continuous variables were performed. Multivariate analysis was performed using logistic regression. *Results:* There were 284 SLND procedures performed on 283 patients. Median age was 55 years. The most recent biopsy method used before SLND was stereotactic core biopsy in 41 (14%), fine-needle aspiration in 62 (22%), and excision in 181 (64%) procedures. The mean excision volume was 32 ml with a range of 0.3–169 ml. The mean time from biopsy to SLND was 17 days with a range of 0–140 days. The mean tumor size was 2.0 cm (15 Tis [5%], 184 T1 [65%], 72 T2 [25%], and 13 T3 [5%]). Tumors were located in the outer quadrants in 74%, the inner quadrants in 18%, and subareolar region in 8%. The sentinel node was identified in 81%, and 39% had metastases. There were three false-negative cases early in the series. Sensitivity was 97%, and accuracy was 99%. Negative predictive value was 98% in cases in which the sentinel node was identified. On the basis of biopsy method, excisional volume, time from biopsy to SLND, tumor size, and tumor location, there was no statistically significant difference ($p > 0.05$) in sentinel node identification rate or accuracy of SLND. *Conclusions:* SLND has a high success rate in breast cancer patients regardless of the biopsy method or the excision volume removed before SLND. In addition, the interval from biopsy to SLND, tumor size, and tumor location have no effect on the success rate of SLND, even in this series which included patients operated on before the technique was adequately defined. Patients with breast cancers located in any quadrant and diagnosed either with a needle or excisional biopsy could be evaluated for trials of SLND.

Lessons learned from 500 cases of lymphatic mapping for breast cancer.

Hill AD, Tran KN, Akhurst T, Yeung H, Yeh SD, Rosen PP, Borgen PI, Cody HS 3rd.

Department of Surgery, Memorial Sloan-Kettering Cancer Center, New York City, NY, USA.

Annals of Surgery 229(4):528–35, 1999, April.

Objective: To evaluate the factors affecting the identification and accuracy of the sentinel node in breast cancer in a single institutional experience. *Summary background data:* Few of the many published feasibility studies of lymphatic mapping for breast cancer have adequate numbers to assess in detail the factors affecting failed and falsely negative mapping procedures. *Methods:* Five hundred consecutive sentinel lymph node biopsies were performed using isosulfan blue dye and technetium-labeled sulfur colloid. A planned conventional axillary dissection was performed in 104 cases. *Results:* Sentinel nodes were identified in 458 of 492 (92%) evaluable cases. The mean number of sentinel nodes removed was 2.1. The sentinel node was successfully identified by blue dye in 80% (393/492), by isotope in 85% (419/492), and by the combination of blue dye and isotope in 93% (458/492) of patients. Success in locating the sentinel node was unrelated to tumor size, type, location, or multicentricity; the presence of lymphovascular invasion; histologic or nuclear grade; or a previous surgical biopsy. The false-negative rate of 10.6% (5/47) was calculated using only those 104 cases where a conventional axillary dissection was planned before surgery. *Conclusions:* Sentinel node biopsy in patients with early breast cancer is a safe and effective alternative to routine axillary dissection for patients with negative nodes. Because of a small but definite rate of false-negative results, this procedure is most valuable in patients with a low risk of axillary nodal metastases. Both blue dye and radioisotope should be used to maximize the yield and accuracy of successful localizations.

Sentinel lymph node mapping in breast cancer using subareolar injection of blue dye.

Kern KA.

Department of Surgery, Hartford Hospital and University of Connecticut School of Medicine, Farmington, CT, USA.

Journal of the American College of Surgeons 189(6):539–45, 1999, December.

Background: Lymphatic mapping in breast cancer performed solely by intraparenchymal injections of blue dye remains an accepted method of identifying sentinel nodes, largely because of its simplicity. As currently practiced, the technique is associated with a marked learning curve, variable identification rates of sentinel nodes, and high false-negative rates. The purpose of this study is to improve dye-only lymphatic mapping of the breast by using an alternative site for injection of blue dye: the subareolar lymphatic plexus. *Study design:* In the 10 months between August 1998 and May 1999, 40 women with operable breast cancer in stages I and II underwent lymphatic mapping and sentinel node biopsy performed solely by subareolar injections of blue dye, followed by complete axillary node dissection. The technique involved the injection of 5 mL of 1% isosulfan blue into the subareolar plexus, which consists of breast tissue located immediately beneath the areola. No peritumoral injections of blue dye were performed. The ability of subareolar dye injections to identify sentinel nodes and accurately predict the pathologic status of the axilla was determined and compared with published results for dye-only lymphatic mapping using intraparenchymal injections. *Results:* The identification rate of sentinel nodes was 98% (in 39 of 40 patients). Axillary basins harboring positive lymph nodes were found in 15 of these 39 patients (38.5%). Sentinel nodes correctly predicted the status of these 15 positive axillary basins in 100% of the patients. There were no false-negative sentinel node biopsies, indicating a false-negative rate of 0 (in 0 of 15). The overall accuracy, sensitivity, and specificity were 100%. *Conclusions:* Compared with other series of dye-directed lymphatic mapping, the present study of dye-only injections into the subareolar plexus demonstrates a high sentinel node identification rate, absent false-negative rate, and rapid learning curve. On the basis of these findings, we propose that injections into the subareolar lymphatic plexus are the optimal way to perform dye-only lymphatic mapping of the breast.

Subareolar versus peritumoral injection for location of the sentinel lymph node.

Klimberg VS, Rubio IT, Henry R, Cowan C, Colvert M, Korourian S.

Department of Surgery, University of Arkansas for Medical Sciences, Arkansas Cancer Research Center, John L. McClellan Veterans Administration Hospital, Little Rock, AR, USA.

Annals of Surgery 229(6):860–4; discussion 864–5, 1999, June.

Background: Sentinel lymph node (SLN) biopsy is fast becoming the standard for testing lymph node involvement in many institutions. However, questions remain as to the best method of injection. The authors hypothesized that a subareolar injection of material would drain to the same lymph node as a peritumoral injection, regardless of the location of the tumor. *Methods:* To test this theory, 68 patients with 69 operable invasive breast carcinomas and clinically node-negative disease were enrolled in this single-institution Institutional Review Board-approved trial. Patients were injected with 1.0 mCi of technetium-99 sulfur colloid (unfiltered) in the subareolar area of the tumor-bearing breast. Each patient received an injection of 2 to 5 cc of isosulfan blue around the tumor. Radioactive SLNs were identified using a hand-held gamma detector probe. *Results:* The average age of patients entered into this trial was 55.2 ± 13.4 years. The average size of the tumors was 1.48 ± 1.0 cm. Thirty-two percent of the patients had undergone previous excisional breast biopsies. Of the 69 lesions, 62 (89.9%) had SLNs located with the blue dye and 65 (94.2%) with the technetium. In four patients, the SLN was not located with either method. All blue SLNs were also radioactive. All located SLNs were in the axilla. Of the 62 patients in which the SLNs were located with both methods, an average of 1.5 ± 0.7 SLNs were found per patient, of which 23.2% had metastatic disease. All four patients in which no SLN was located with either method had undergone prior excisional biopsies. *Conclusions:* The results of this study suggest that subareolar injection of technetium is as accurate as peritumoral injection of blue dye. Central injection is easy and avoids the necessity for image-guided injection of nonpalpable breast lesions. Finally, subareolar injection of technetium avoids the problem of overlap of the radioactive zone of diffusion of the injection site with the radioactive sentinel lymph node, particularly in medial and upper outer quadrant lesions.

Adverse reactions to isosulfan blue during selective sentinel lymph node dissection in melanoma.

Leong SPL, Donegan E, Heffernon W, Dean S, Katz JA.

University of California/Mount Zion Medical Center, San Francisco, CA, USA.

Annals of Surgical Oncology 5:361–6, 2000, June.

Background: Selective sentinel lymph node (SLN) dissection can spare about 80% of patients with primary melanoma from radical lymph node dissection. This procedure identifies the SLN either visually by injecting isosulfan blue dye around the primary melanoma site or by handheld gamma probe after radiocolloid injection. *Methods:* During selective SLN mapping, 1 to 5 ml of isosulfan blue was injected intradermally around the primary melanoma. From November 1993 to August 1998, 406 patients underwent intraoperative lymphatic mapping with the use of both isosulfan blue and radiocolloid injection. Three cases of selective SLN dissection, in which adverse reactions to isosulfan blue occurred, were reviewed. *Results:* We report three cases of anaphylaxis after intradermal injection with isosulfan blue of 406 patients who underwent intraoperative lymphatic mapping by using the procedure as described above. The three cases we report vary in severity from treatable hypotension with urticaria and erythema to severe cardiovascular collapse with or without bronchospasm or urticaria. *Conclusions:* In our series, the incidence of anaphylaxis to isosulfan blue was approximately 1%. Anaphylaxis can be fatal if not recognized and treated rapidly. Operating room personnel who participate in intraoperative lymphatic mapping where isosulfan blue is used must be aware of the potential consequences and be prepared to treat anaphylaxis.

Practical guidelines for optimal gamma probe detection of sentinel lymph nodes in breast cancer: results of a multi-institutional study. For the University of Louisville Breast Cancer Study Group.

Martin RC 2nd, Edwards MJ, Wong SL, Tuttle TM, Carlson DJ, Brown CM, Noyes RD, Glaser RL, Vennekotter DJ, Turk PS, Tate PS, Sardi A, Cerrito PB, McMasters KM.

Department of Surgery, Division of Surgical Oncology, James Graham Brown Cancer Center, and the Department of Mathematics, University of Louisville, KY, USA.

Surgery 128(2):139–44, 2000, August.

Introduction: Multiple radioactive lymph nodes are often removed during the course of sentinel lymph node (SLN) biopsy for breast cancer when both blue dye and radioactive colloid injection are used. Some of the less radioactive lymph nodes are second echelon nodes, not true SLNs. The purpose of this analysis was to determine whether harvesting these less radioactive nodes, in addition to the 'hottest' SLNs, reduces the false-negative rate. *Methods:* Patients were enrolled in this multicenter (121 surgeons) prospective, Institutional Review Board-approved study after informed consent was obtained. Patients with clinical stage TI–II, N0, M0 invasive breast cancer were eligible. This analysis includes all patients who underwent axillary SLN biopsy with the use of an injection of both isosulfan blue dye and radioactive colloid. The protocol specified that all blue nodes and all nodes with 10% or more of the ex vivo count of the hottest node should be removed and designated SLNs. All patients underwent completion level I/II axillary dissection. *Results:* SLNs were identified in 672 of 758 patients (89%). Of the patients with SLNs identified, 403 patients (60%) had more than 1 SLN removed (mean, 1.96 SLN/patient) and 207 patients (31%) had nodal metastases. The use of filtered or unfiltered technetium sulfur colloid had no impact on the number of SLNs identified. Overall, 33% of histologically positive SLNs had no evidence of blue dye staining. Of those patients with multiple SLNs removed, histologically positive SLNs were found in 130 patients. In 15 of these 130 patients (11.5%), the hottest SLN was negative when a less radioactive node was positive for tumor. If only the hottest node had been removed, the false-negative rate would have been 13.0% versus 5.8% when all nodes with 10% or more of the ex vivo count of the hottest node were removed ($p = 0.01$). *Conclusions:* These data support the policy that all blue nodes and all nodes with 10% or more of the ex vivo count of the hottest SLN should be harvested for optimal nodal staging.

Sentinel lymph node biopsy for breast cancer: a suitable alternative to routine axillary dissection in multi-institutional practice when optimal technique is used.

McMasters KM, Tuttle TM, Carlson DJ, Brown CM, Noyes RD, Glaser RL, Vennekotter DJ, Turk PS, Tate PS, Sardi A, Cerrito PB, Edwards MJ.

Department of Surgery, Division of Surgical Oncology, J. Graham Brown Cancer Center, University of Louisville, Louisville, KY, USA.

Journal of Clinical Oncology 18(13):2560–6, 2000, July.

Purpose: Previous studies have demonstrated the feasibility of sentinel lymph node (SLN) biopsy for nodal staging of patients with breast cancer. However, unacceptably high false-negative rates have been reported in several studies, raising doubt about the applicability of this technique in widespread surgical practice. Controversy persists regarding the optimal technique for correctly identifying the SLN. Some investigators advocate SLN biopsy using injection of a vital blue dye, others recommend radioactive colloid, and still others recommend the use of both agents together. *Patients and methods:* A total of 806 patients were enrolled by 99 surgeons. SLN biopsy was performed by single-agent (blue dye alone or radioactive colloid alone) or dual-agent injection at the discretion of the operating surgeon. All patients underwent attempted SLN biopsy followed by completion level I/II axillary lymph node dissection to determine the false-negative rate. *Results:* There was no significant difference (86% v 90%) in the SLN identification rate among patients who underwent single- versus dual-agent injection. The false-negative rates were 11.8% and 5.8% for single- versus dual-agent injection, respectively ($p < 0.05$). Dual-agent injection resulted in a greater mean number of SLNs identified per patient (2.1 v 1.5; $p < 0.0001$). The SLN identification rate was significantly less for patients older than 50 years as compared with that of younger patients (87.6% v 92.6%; $p = 0.03$). Upper-outer quadrant tumor location was associated with an increased likelihood of a false-negative result compared with all other locations (11.2% v 3.9%; $p < 0.05$). *Conclusion:* In multi-institutional practice, SLN biopsy using dual-agent injection provides optimal sensitivity for detection of nodal metastases. The acceptable SLN identification and false-negative rates associated with the dual-agent injection technique indicate that this procedure is a suitable alternative to routine axillary dissection across a wide spectrum of surgical practice and hospital environments.

Increased false negative sentinel node biopsy rates after preoperative chemotherapy for invasive breast carcinoma.

Nason KS, Anderson BO, Byrd DR, Dunnwald LK, Eary JF, Mankoff DA, Livingston R, Schmidt RA, Jewell KD, Yeung RS, Moe RE.

Department of Surgery, University of Washington, Seattle, WA, USA.

Cancer 89(11):2187–94, 2000, December 1.

Background: Sentinel lymph node dissection (SLND) has been a promising new technique in breast carcinoma staging, but could be unreliable in certain patient subsets. The current study assessed whether age, preoperative chemotherapy, tumor size, and/or previous excisional biopsy influenced the identification of sentinel nodes (SLNs) or the reliability of a node-negative SLND in predicting a node negative axilla. Methods: Eighty-two patients who had clinically negative axillae underwent SLND followed by Level I/II axillary lymph node dissection (ALND). SLNDs were performed using both technetium-99m (Tc-99m) labeled colloid and isosulfan blue dye. SLNs were analyzed by hematoxylin and eosin and immunocytochemical techniques. Results: SLNs were successfully identified in 80% of patients. Mapping success was decreased among postmenopausal women but was not influenced by preoperative chemotherapy, large tumor size, or previous excisional biopsy. Of the 31 successfully mapped, node positive patients, 5 had false negative (FN) SLNDs (overall FN rate = 16%). Of the 9 successfully mapped patients who had received preoperative chemotherapy and had positive axillary nodes, 3 had FN SLND (FN rate = 33%). The presence of clinically positive lymph nodes before chemotherapy did not predict which patients would have a subsequent FN SLND. T3 tumor size, but not previous excision, was associated significantly with increased FN rate, although the FN rate for previous excision was 11%. No FN SLND occurred with T1/T2 tumors that were not excised previously and had not received preoperative chemotherapy. Conclusions: Preoperative chemotherapy was associated with an unacceptably high FN rate for SLND. While larger tumor size also was associated with FN SLND, this effect might have been due to preoperative chemotherapy use in these patients. Small sample size precluded determining whether excisional biopsy before mapping increased FN SLND rates independently.

Sentinel node biopsy in ductal carcinoma in situ patients.

Pendas S, Dauway E, Giuliano R, Ku N, Cox CE, Reintgen DS.

Comprehensive Breast Cancer Program, H. Lee Moffitt Cancer Center, University of South Florida, Tampa, FL, USA.

Annals of Surgical Oncology 7(1):15–20, 2000, January–February.

Background: Sentinel lymph node (SLN) mapping is an effective and accurate method of evaluating the regional lymph nodes in breast cancer patients. The SLN is the first node that receives lymphatic drainage from the primary tumor. Patients with micrometastatic disease, previously undetected by routine hematoxylin and eosin (H & E) stains, are now being detected with the new technology of SLN biopsy, followed by a more detailed examination of the SLN that includes serial sectioning and cytokeratin immunohistochemical (CK IHC) staining of the nodes. Methods: At Moffitt Cancer Center, 87 patients with newly diagnosed pure ductal carcinoma in situ (DCIS) lesions were evaluated by using CK IHC staining of the SLN. Patients with any focus of microinvasive disease, detected on diagnostic breast biopsy by routine H & E, were excluded from this study. DCIS patients, with biopsy-proven in situ tumor by routine H & E stains, underwent intraoperative lymphatic mapping, using a combination of vital blue dye and technetium-labeled sulfur colloid. The excised SLNs were examined grossly, by imprint cytology, by standard H & E histology, and by IHC stains for CK. All SLNs that had only CK-positive cells were subsequently confirmed malignant by a more detailed histological examination of the nodes. Results: CK IHC staining was performed on 177 SLNs in 87 DCIS breast cancer patients. Five of the 87 DCIS patients (6%) had positive SLNs. Three of these patients were only CK positive and two were both H & E and CK positive. Therefore, routine H & E staining missed microinvasive disease in three of five DCIS patients with positive SLNs. In addition, DCIS patients with occult micrometastatic disease to the SLN underwent a complete axillary lymph node dissection, and the SLNs were the only nodes found to have metastatic disease. Of interest, four of the five node-positive patients had comedo carcinoma associated with the DCIS lesion, and one patient had a large 9.5-cm low grade cribriform and micropapillary type of DCIS. Conclusions: This study confirms that lymphatic mapping in breast cancer patients with DCIS lesions is a technically feasible and a highly accurate method of staging patients with undetected micrometastatic disease to the regional lymphatic basin. This procedure can be performed with minimal morbidity, because only one or two SLNs, which are at highest risk for containing metastatic disease, are removed. This allows the pathologist to examine the one or two lymph nodes with greater detail by using serial sectioning and CK IHC staining of the SLNs. Because most patients with DCIS lesions detected by routine H & E stains do not have regional lymph node metastases, these patients can safely avoid the complications associated with a complete axillary lymph node dissection and systemic chemotherapy. However, DCIS patients with occult micrometastases of the regional lymphatic basin can be staged with higher accuracy and treated in a more selective fashion.

Multicenter trial of sentinel node biopsy for breast cancer using both technetium sulfur colloid and isosulfan blue dye.

Tafra L, Lannin DR, Swanson MS, Van Eyk JJ, Verbanac KM, Chua AN, Ng PC, Edwards MS, Halliday BE, Henry CA, Sommers LM, Carman CM, Molin MR, Yurko JE, Perry RR, Williams AR.

Breast Center, Anne Arundel Medical Center, Annapolis, MD, and the Department of Surgery, Leo Jenkins Cancer Center, East Carolina University, Greenville, NC; Breast Care Center of the Blue Ridge, Roanoke, VA (Henry); Martha Jefferson Hospital, Charlottesville, VA (Sommers); Breast Care Specialists, PC, Norfolk, VA (Carman); Mercy Hospital, Portland, ME (Molin); Carteret General Hospital, Morehead City, NC (Yurko); Eastern Virginia Medical

School, Norfolk, VA (Perry); and Lewis-Gale Medical Center, Salem, VA (Williams), USA.

Annals of Surgery 233(1):51–9, 2001, January.

Objective: To determine the factors associated with false-negative results on sentinel node biopsy and sentinel node localization (identification rate) in patients with breast cancer enrolled in a multicenter trial using a combination technique of isosulfan blue with technetium sulfur colloid (Tc99). *Summary background data:* Sentinel node biopsy is a diagnostic test used to detect breast cancer metastases. To test the reliability of this method, a complete lymph node dissection must be performed to determine the false-negative rate. Single-institution series have reported excellent results, although one multicenter trial reported a false-negative rate as high as 29% using radioisotope alone. A multicenter trial was initiated to test combined use of Tc99 and isosulfan blue. *Methods:* Investigators (both private-practice and academic surgeons) were recruited after attending a course on the technique of sentinel node biopsy. No investigator participated in a learning trial before entering patients. Tc99 and isosulfan blue were injected into the peritumoral region. *Results:* Five hundred twenty-nine patients underwent 535 sentinel node biopsy procedures for an overall identification rate in finding a sentinel node of 87% and a false-negative rate of 13%. The identification rate increased and the false-negative rate decreased to 90% and 4.3%, respectively, after investigators had performed more than 30 cases. Univariate analysis of tumor showed the poorest success rate with older patients and inexperienced surgeons. Multivariate analysis identified both age and experience as independent predictors of failure. However, with older patients, inexperienced surgeons, and patients with five or more metastatic axillary nodes, the false-negative rate was consistently greater. *Conclusions:* This multicenter trial, from both private practice and academic institutions, is an excellent indicator of the general utility of sentinel node biopsy. It establishes the factors that play an important role (patient age, surgical experience, tumor location) and those that are irrelevant (prior surgery, tumor size, Tc99 timing). This widens the applicability of the technique and identifies factors that require further investigation.

Optimal histopathologic examination of the sentinel lymph node for breast carcinoma staging.

Turner RR, Ollila DW, Stern S, Giuliano AE.

Department of Pathology, Saint John's Health Center, Santa Monica, CA, USA.

American Journal of Surgical Pathology 23(3):263–7, 1999, March.

Sentinel lymph node dissection is a minimally invasive surgical technique for staging of breast carcinoma. The optimal pathologic examination of the sentinel node (SN) has not yet been determined. Our standard protocol for evaluation of the SN in patients with breast cancer included frozen section at one level, plus paraffin sections at two levels, separated by 40 microm, and stained with hematoxylin and eosin and cytokeratin immunohistochemistry (IHC) at each paraffin section level. In the current study, we

evaluated the use of step sections and cytokeratin IHC in 60 SNs (42 consecutive patients) that were tumor-negative on frozen section and hematoxylin and eosin staining at permanent section levels 1 and 2. The SNs were reexamined with cytokeratin IHC at eight additional levels (levels 3–10) of the paraffin block, each separated by 40 microm. Previous IHC sections from levels 1 and 2 had shown micrometastases in nine SNs (eight patients) and no tumor cells in the remaining 51 SNs (34 patients). Of the 51 previously negative SNs, only two (4%) SNs from one (3%) patient had metastatic carcinoma cells in levels 3–10. Thus, the additional step sections with cytokeratin IHC did not significantly increase the number of patients with tumor-positive SNs. We currently recommend that the SN be examined with cytokeratin IHC at two levels of the paraffin block. This should optimize sentinel lymph node dissection as a staging technique and minimize the labor and financial burden associated with multiple step sections and IHC stains.

Sentinel lymph node biopsy for melanoma: experience with 234 consecutive procedures.

Wagner JD, Corbett L, Park HM, Davidson D, Coleman JJ, Havlik RJ, Hayes JT 2nd.

Department of Surgery, Indiana University School of Medicine at Indiana University Purdue University at Indianapolis, IN, USA.

Plastic & Reconstructive Surgery 105(6):1956–66, 2000, May.

Sentinel lymph node biopsy is increasingly used to identify occult metastases in regional lymph nodes of patients with melanoma. Selection of patients for sentinel lymph node biopsy and subsequent lymphadenectomy is an area of debate. The purpose of this study was to describe a large clinical series of these biopsies for cutaneous melanoma and to identify patients most likely to gain useful clinical information from sentinel lymph node biopsy. The Indiana University Melanoma Program computerized database was queried to identify all patients who underwent this procedure for clinically localized cutaneous melanoma. It was performed using preoperative technetium Tc 99m lymphoscintigraphy and isosulfan blue dye. Pertinent demographic, surgical, and histopathologic data were recorded. Univariate and multivariate logistic regression and classification table analyses were performed to identify clinical variables associated with sentinel node and nonsentinel node positivity. In total, 234 biopsy procedures were performed to stage 291 nonpalpable regional lymph node basins. Mean Breslow's thickness was 2.30 mm (2.08 mm for negative sentinel lymph node biopsy, 3.18 mm for positive). The mean number of sentinel nodes removed was 2.17 nodes per basin (range, 1 to 8). Forty-seven of 234 melanomas (20.1 percent) and 50 of 291 basins (17.2 percent) had a positive biopsy. Positivity correlated with AJCC tumor stage: T1, 3.6 percent; T2, 8.1 percent; T3, 27.4 percent; T4, 44 percent. By univariate logistic regression, Breslow's thickness ($p = 0.003$, continuous variable), ulceration ($p = 0.003$), mitotic index $\geqslant 6$ mitoses per high power field ($p = 0.008$), and Clark's level ($p = 0.04$) were significantly associated with sentinel lymph node biopsy result. By multivariate analysis, only Breslow's thickness ($p = 0.02$), tumor ulceration ($p = 0.02$), and mitotic index ($p = 0.02$) were significant predictors of biopsy positivity. Classification table analysis showed the Breslow cutpoint of 1.2 mm to be the most efficient cutpoint for sentinel lymph node biopsy result ($p = 0.0004$). Completion lymphadenectomy was performed in 46 sentinel node-positive patients; 12 (26.1 percent) had at least one additional positive nonsentinel node. Nonsentinel node positivity was marginally associated with the presence of multiple positive sentinel nodes ($p = 0.07$). At mean follow-up of 13.8 months, four of 241 sentinel node-negative basins demonstrated same-basin recurrence (1.7%). Sentinel lymph node biopsy is highly reliable in experienced hands but is a low-yield procedure in most thin melanomas. Patients with melanomas thicker than 1.2 mm or with ulcerated or high mitotic index lesions are most likely to have occult lymph node metastases by sentinel lymph node biopsy. Completion therapeutic lymphadenectomy is recommended after positive biopsy because it is difficult to predict the presence of positive nonsentinel nodes.

17

Management of regional lymph nodes in patients with cutaneous melanoma

DANIEL F ROSES

INTRODUCTION

The issue of whether the ablation of clinically occult, regional nodal metastases improves survival is certainly the longest standing controversy in the surgical management of cutaneous malignant melanoma. The dramatic rise in the incidence of malignant melanoma over the past two decades has, fortunately, been accompanied by an increasing proportion of patients with lesions diagnosed early in their evolution[1] and without clinical evidence of regional lymph node metastases. This has further heightened the controversy surrounding the appropriateness of elective regional lymph node dissection.

Arguments by proponents of elective regional lymph node dissection have traditionally been countered by those who believe that any form of regional lymphadenectomy might be more appropriately reserved only for patients whose nodes become clinically palpable. Exhaustive debate on this issue has led to varied practices among major institutions with great experience in the treatment of cutaneous malignant melanoma.[2] Even with the broad acceptance of highly selective sentinel lymphadenectomy, the therapeutic impact of any elective surgical approach to the nodal drainage of a primary melanoma remains uncertain. Furthermore, the basic question of the impact of regional lymph node metastases on the pathophysiology of melanoma has been recast by even greater refinement in the histologic assessment of regional nodes. What might have been previously undetected micrometastases are now being diagnosed by advanced histochemical technology.

This review considers the evolution of surgical approaches to the regional nodal basin(s) draining a melanoma, the sources of surgical controversy, and the recent experience directed at making surgery more specific and consistent with a greater biologic understanding of the disease.

EVOLUTION OF ELECTIVE REGIONAL LYMPH NODE DISSECTION FOR CUTANEOUS MELANOMA

The concept that regional lymph nodes provide an early barrier to systemic dissemination was empirically embraced as early as the eighteenth century. It was granted scientific legitimacy, however, in the nineteenth century by the development of microscopic pathology. Rudolph Virchow, discussing breast cancer in his 1858 volume *Cellular pathology,* stated that axillary lymph nodes served as a temporary barrier and provided a period of protection from the spread of malignant disease. Eventually, the nodes themselves became an independent source for further dissemination.[3] In 1892, this concept was applied to the treatment of melanoma by H.L. Snow. He proposed wide excision and elective lymph node dissection, noting that the initial spread of melanoma was always to the regional lymph nodes. Reflecting an approach which echoed the contemporary approach to breast cancer as most forcefully advocated by W.S. Halsted, Snow wrote of the nodal metastases from melanoma:[4]

Eventually they pass beyond such 'traps' into the blood current; then death with multiple visceral metastases ensues. Palpable enlargement of these glands is unfortunately but a late symptom of deposit therein; by the time it occurs there is almost always implication of deeper organs or tissues ... We further see the paramount importance of securing, whenever possible, the perfect eradication of those lymph glands which will necessarily be first infected; before enlargement takes place radical removal of such organs in the axilla, groin, surface regions of the neck ... is a safe and easy measure which, under the conditions indicated, should never be neglected.

This view was endorsed in 1903 by Frederic Eve, who, in reviewing the experience at the London Hospital, found regional lymph node involvement to be present in the great majority of cases, whether palpable or not.[5]

The most important advocate of surgical treatment based upon a presumed sequential process of early lymphatic permeation was the highly influential British surgeon W. Sampson Handley, who applied his experience with breast cancer to a consideration of melanoma. In two Hunterian lectures published in 1907 in the *Lancet,* Handley asserted that the 'growth of tendril-like cylinders of cells along the finer lymphatics that surround the primary growth' was the major mechanism of metastasis from melanoma, and that 'embolic spread by way of the blood stream is a later event, dependent on the infiltration and invasion of the veins and arteries from concomitant permeated lymphatics.'[6] It is curious that his point of reference for these concepts of dissemination of melanoma was his autopsy study of a single patient who had died with widely disseminated disease.

Handley advocated that the surgical treatment of a primary malignant melanoma should be its excision with a margin of skin by 'what is judged by present standards to be a safe and practicable distance.'[6] He also advised excising the deep fascia and even a portion of muscle subjacent to the lesion as well as the regional lymph nodes as part of the first operation. If two regional drainage basins were involved, he advocated dissection of both. Handley's contemporary, J.H. Pringle, further elaborated upon the surgical treatment of malignant melanoma in an article the following year advising that the operation be extended beyond the local skin, subcutaneous tissue, and fascia by an en-bloc resection of the areas of 'lymphatic permeation' between the primary neoplasm and the regional lymph nodes.[7] Inherent in all of these surgical approaches was the concept that permeation of malignant melanocytes within regional lymphatics might serve to seed further local or distant metastases, a concept reinforced by the development and wide acceptance of contemporaneous en-bloc radical resections for a variety of other solid malignant neoplasms.

These traditional concepts were accepted with little challenge for most of the twentieth century. Over the past three decades, however, the underlying biologic premise of elective regional lymph node dissection for many solid malignant neoplasms, including melanoma, has been met with increasing skepticism. Critics point out that tumor cells may bypass nodes through alternate lymphatico-venous channels.[8] Even tumor cells that are proliferating in regional lymph nodes may be biologically selected and, rather than being initiators of further dissemination, more likely reflect tumor growth potential elsewhere. Furthermore, there may be instances in which micrometastatic disease in lymph nodes may be destined for tumor destruction rather than tumor proliferation. The growing recognition of the heterogeneity of tumor cells within a given neoplasm, their varied metastatic potential, and even their varied predilection for specific metastatic locations has further eroded the concept of an orderly progression of dissemination whereby regional lymph nodes serve as the first metastatic site.[9]

Perhaps the most important stimulus to the reassessment of surgical therapy for melanoma was the recognition that primary cutaneous melanoma represented a wide spectrum of disease. Microstaging of primary cutaneous melanoma was most clearly validated and enunciated by Clark, whose histopathologic studies made clear that the potential for metastatic spread was related to the depth of invasion of the melanoma from its origin in the epidermis.[10] This concept was refined by Breslow, who related prognosis inversely to the thickness of the lesion as measured by an ocular micrometer from the top of the granular zone of the epidermis to the base of the neoplasm.[11] Thickness has certainly supplanted level of invasion as the major prognostic variable in the histologic staging of cutaneous melanoma, to which has also been added ulceration as an adverse determinant of survival. It should always be emphasized that, to utilize such important histopathologic prognostic information in surgical practice, a properly performed and serially sectioned biopsy specimen, preferably by total excision, is required.

Such precise assessment of prognosis from the histopathologic evaluation of the primary lesion made clear that, at least for 'thin' melanomas (generally < 1.0 mm in thickness, although some investigators set the threshold at 0.75 mm), elective regional lymph node dissection was unlikely to have any impact on survival.[12–14] In a study of 119 patients from New York University with stage I primary cutaneous malignant melanoma undergoing regional lymph node dissection, each of the lymph nodes in the dissection specimen was evaluated by serial sections, and micrometastases were correlated with primary tumor thickness. None of the patients with lesions < 1.0 mm in thickness had nodal micrometastases.[15] Data from major centers, as reported by such investigators as Balch[16] and Essner and Morton,[17] have correlated thickness with nodal micrometastases and survival, and have made clear that microstaging of the primary lesion is critical in considering the issue of elective lymph node dissection and in assessing any data purporting to show a survival benefit from such procedures.

MORBIDITY OF ELECTIVE LYMPH NODE DISSECTION

Any discussion of regional lymph node dissection for melanoma must consider the potential morbidity of such procedures. To demonstrate the efficacy of surgical ablation of regional nodes requires proof that there is an improvement in survival, either directly realized from the procedure itself or from the prognostic information that can be used to initiate effective adjuvant therapy. Until this can be convincingly demonstrated, the potential morbidity of such procedures, and even their economic impact, will have heightened significance.

Complication rates for regional lymph node dissection approaching or even exceeding 50% have been reported.[18,19] Such rates are dependent on how stringent the criteria are for defining morbidity, as well as on such patient characteristics as age, obesity,[20] and the specific types of nodal dissections that are considered.[21–23] Indeed, most complications associated with elective lymph node dissections are in the early postoperative period and related to wound infection, flap necrosis, seroma, and temporary nerve dysfunction.[24–31]

Many reports on the complications of node dissection combine the elective dissections of non-palpable nodes with therapeutic dissections for palpable disease, the latter having a greater potential for local complications. Even prior biopsy of a palpable lymph node may negatively impact on a subsequent lymph node dissection.[32] Coit et al. found that other factors increasing the risk of complications in patients undergoing either groin or axillary dissection included obesity, age greater than 60 years, and a history of smoking, hypertension, or diabetes. Multiple risk factors were found to be additive in predisposing to complications.[33] Less definable and difficult to assess is the experience of the surgeon and the impact of appropriate surgical technique in decreasing morbidity.

The greatest source of long-term morbidity has been persistent extremity lymphedema after axillary or inguinal node dissection. In the axilla, this has been infrequent, with a reported incidence of 2% or less in most series,[20,23,34] although a rate of 10% has been reported.[21] A lack of objective reporting criteria may be responsible for such variations. Groin dissections may, however, produce significant edema, particularly when a deep iliac and obturator dissection is performed along with a superficial inguinal dissection.[19,21,35] Urist and associates reported that 26% of patients experienced leg edema for 6 months or longer following dissection of inguinal nodes, but that only 8% suffered significant functional deficit.[20] Usually, edema is confined to the thigh[20,23,29] and is relatively asymptomatic; however, up to 10% of patients may have long-term edema that impairs function.[20,23] Edema may occur less frequently in patients undergoing groin dissection for primary melanoma of the trunk rather than extremities, as scars from wide excisions on the lower extremity may further impair lymphatic flow. Prophylactic measures such as elastic stockings and elevation[21,36] may decrease the incidence, but the effect of these measures is difficult to define.

Long-term numbness or paresthesias may result from the division of cutaneous sensory nerves such as branches of the femoral nerve, the lateral cutaneous nerve in the groin, the intercostobrachial in the axilla, and the rich distribution of sensory nerves in the head and neck. Although elective radical neck dissection has been supplanted by selective and modified procedures that preserve the spinal accessory nerve, any dissection of the posterior cervical triangle risks limitation in shoulder function. The facial nerve and its branches are at risk in superficial parotid resections for melanomas with drainage pathways to the preauricular nodes or to submandibular or facial nodes in the vicinity of the marginal mandibular nerve. In the head and neck region in particular, even limited dissections having no definable functional morbidity may carry a cosmetic morbidity that is difficult to define objectively, but which is a potential source of concern to the patient.

Clearly, arguments against elective lymph node dissection that cite such morbidity, or even that cite cost issues, should be countered by data that demonstrate their therapeutic efficacy. Citing a low rate of morbidity in the effort to contain a potentially lethal neoplasm as an acceptable rationale to justify elective lymph node dissection without such data has become unacceptable. How has the issue of whether there is a survival advantage for patients having elective regional lymph node dissections been addressed to date? The consideration of this issue has served as a focal point for defining the surgical treatment of melanoma for the second half of the last century, first in retrospective analyses and then, more importantly, in prospective trials.

RETROSPECTIVE AND NON-RANDOMIZED SERIES OF ELECTIVE LYMPH NODE DISSECTION

The justification for elective lymph node dissection prior to microstaging was primarily derived from comparing the survival of patients with micrometastases in elective regional lymphadenectomy specimens to those having therapeutic lymph node dissection for clinically palpable disease. Pack et al., in 1952, reported a 27% improvement in 5-year survival for patients having elective regional lymphadenectomy.[37] Several studies since, including several in which patients' primary lesions were microstaged, have substantiated a comparable improvement in survival[38–43] for patients with nodal micrometastases in elective regional lymphadenectomy specimens compared to those with clinically palpable macrometastases in therapeutic lymph node dissection specimens (Table 17.1). The conclusion of such analyses was that most, if not all, micrometastatic nodal disease was a harbinger of more extensive and ultimately clinically palpable disease which, if allowed to progress, would lead to further disease progression. Even allowing for the often suboptimal assessment of what are now regarded as identifiable prognostic factors, most importantly

Table 17.1 *Survival of patients with regional node metastases on pathological examination in relation to clinical status of regional nodes*

Source	Long-term survival		
	CS-I (%)	CS-II (%)	Difference (%)
McNeer and Das Gupta (1964)[39]	52	19	33
Cohen et al. (1977)[40]	55	38	17
Das Gupta (1977)[41]	69	20[a]	49
Balch et al. (1981)[38]	48	24	24
Callery et al. (1982)[42]	48	36	12
Roses et al. (1985)[43]	44	20	24
Average	53	26	27

CS-I = clinical stage I: regional lymph nodes not palpable or suspicious.
CS-II = clinical stage II: regional lymph nodes enlarged by palpation and suspicious for metastases.
All data are for 5-year survival rates, except in Cohen et al., which are 10-year results.
[a] Patients with Clark's levels III and IV.
From Morton DL, Wen D-R, Wong JH, et al.; *Archives of Surgery* 1992; 127:392–9.[89]

thickness (Breslow),[38,43–51] such retrospective analyses were inherently flawed by possible selection bias and, as a result, the validity of any conclusions was compromised. The possibility also exists that patients with nodal macrometastases may be biologically dissimilar to patients with micrometastases. Even if similar, a lead-time bias favoring the micrometastatic group would require prolonged follow-up and closely matched groups prognostically to make comparisons meaningful. This is not achievable in a retrospectively analysed database.

One means of overcoming inherent flaws in such analyses was to perform multivariate analyses, comparing large groups of patients without clinically palpable nodes, who either did or did not have elective regional lymphadenectomy, and matching them by prognostic indicators. The most significant study in this regard came from a combined series from the University of Alabama and the Melanoma Unit in Sydney, Australia, as reported by Balch and Milton. The major prognostic determinants supported by their analysis were tumor thickness and ulceration. An analysis of their experiences,[13,45–47] as well as that of more limited series,[48,49] supported a survival benefit from elective lymph node dissection for patients with a primary tumor between 0.76 mm and 4.0 mm in thickness ('intermediate thickness'). At 8 years, the survival advantage for patients who had elective lymph node dissections with a primary lesion between 1.5 mm and 4.0 mm in thickness was sustained in rates as high as 20–40%.[2,13,45,49] The benefit was more modest for patients with a primary tumor between 0.76 mm and 1.5 mm in thickness. The apparent failure of elective regional lymphadenectomy to improve survival for patients with a thicker primary tumor in these studies was attributed to the probable high frequency of occult distant metastases at the time of initial surgical treatment if nodal metastases were already present. In contrast, the great majority of patients with a thin

primary tumor would have minimal potential benefit from elective regional lymphadenectomy because of a low incidence of both occult nodal metastases and distant metastases and would therefore accrue no survival advantage.

From such retrospective analyses, thickness emerged as a significant prognostic determinant in patients with nodal micrometastases in several series.[42,52–54] Our own data at New York University were consistent with this observation.[43] In a review of the prognostic relevance of the extent of nodal metastases, lesion thickness, level of invasion, site of lesion, satellitosis, age, sex, and year of diagnosis and treatment in 213 consecutive patients with regional nodal metastases (157 with clinically negative/histologically positive disease and 56 with clinically positive/histologically positive disease), the difference in survival between patients with clinically negative/histologically positive nodes and clinically positive/histologically positive nodes was apparent throughout the follow-up period, as had been observed by others. In particular, a 10-year survival rate of 65% was achieved for the clinically negative patients having primary lesions of <2.0 mm in thickness, while it was 19% for patients having primary lesions of 5.0 mm or more in thickness. This was consistent with the retrospective analyses showing that thickness impacted on a survival advantage for patients having elective regional lymphadenectomy, favoring those with thinner lesions even if they had nodal micrometastases. Balch and associates[55] were also able to show ulceration to be a significant adverse prognostic determinant in node-positive patients. Indeed, it was the only tumor-related adverse determinant in their node-positive patients.

In 1991, Morton and associates at the John Wayne Cancer Institute (Santa Monica, CA) reviewed their experience with 1134 melanoma patients whose disease had spread to regional lymph nodes.[54] Univariate analysis indicated that the number of involved nodes, gender, site of the primary (extremity versus trunk), and depth could be used to determine a patient's prognosis. Elective regional lymphadenectomy was performed in those patients with primary lesions thicker than 0.65 mm. As with previous studies, survival rates at 5 and 10 years were significantly better for those patients who underwent elective regional lymphadenectomy for occult metastases than for those undergoing therapeutic regional lymphadenectomy for clinically evident disease. Likewise, a retrospective review of 3616 patients from nine centers in Germany demonstrated a 5-year survival advantage of 20% for male patients with axial and acral melanomas with thicknesses of greater than 1.5–4.5 mm and a 5–10% improvement for women with melanomas with thicknesses of 2.5–5.0 mm.[56]

Despite the breadth of experience represented by such large retrospective studies, which employed multivariate analyses to adjust for multiple prognostic determinants and which supported the efficacy of elective lymph node dissection, other retrospective studies reached different conclusions. Elder and associates reviewed their experience with 72 patients with a minimum of 5 years' follow-up and reported statistically equivalent survival at both 5 and 10 years for patients having wide excision alone or wide excision with elective lymphadenectomy.[57] Binder and associates[58] and Bagley and associates[59] similarly found equivalent 5-year survival in a review of 168 patients having wide excision alone and 147 patients having wide excision and elective lymphadenectomy. A review of the Duke University Melanoma Clinic experience with 910 patients having wide excision and elective lymphadenectomy and 2023 patients having wide excision alone failed to demonstrate a survival difference at 5 and 10 years.[60] Equivalent survival was demonstrated as well when these groups were analysed by increasing Breslow thickness range (0.75–1.50 mm, 1.51–2.99 mm, and 3.0–3.99 mm). This experience was further analysed in a review of 4682 patients by Singluff and associates,[50] which again failed to demonstrate an advantage to elective lymphadenectomy. A large review from the Sydney Melanoma Unit (which had previously reported a survival advantage for elective lymphadenectomy for intermediate-thickness melanoma) of 1278 patients with melanomas of the trunk or limbs exceeding 1.5 mm thickness, treated from 1960 to 1991, also failed to demonstrate a survival advantage for patients having elective lymphadenectomy (Figure 17.1).[51] This study differed from previous studies from the same institution in that it excluded patients referred after definitive local treatment elsewhere, as inclusion of such patients, whose first evidence of failure was regional and who were then referred to the Sydney Melanoma Unit, may have created a bias favoring elective lymphadenectomy in the earlier studies.

Whereas the largest experience in reported series has been with melanomas of the trunk and limbs, the reported experience with melanomas of the head and

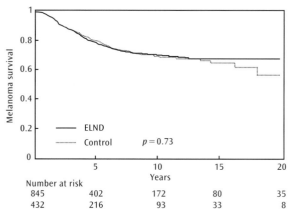

Figure 17.1 *Melanoma-specific survival by treatment for all patients. ELND, elective lymph node dissection. From Coates* et al.[51]

neck has been more limited, and also associated with controversy relating to the issue of elective lymphadenectomy. In a series of 206 patients with head and neck melanomas from New York University,[61] 90 of whom had regional lymph node dissections, the dominant prognostic determinant was the presence of nodal metastases. Twenty-nine of 31 patients with nodal metastases followed for more than 5 years developed systemic metastases. Although some patients were treated prior to microstaging, elective lymph node dissection clearly did not offer any advantage for those 15 patients who had micrometastases when compared to the 16 who had clinically palpable disease. A report by Belli and associates[62] on their experience with 93 patients with regional node metastases for melanoma in the head and neck region reached a similar conclusion. O'Brien *et al.* reporting from the Sydney Melanoma Unit, noted that an improvement in survival could be seen for patients who had elective lymph node dissection with lesions in the 1.5–3.9 mm thickness range using a univariate analysis, but the benefit was lost when the data were assessed by multivariate analysis that adjusted for differences in prognostic variables.[63]

Of note in the New York University study on head and neck melanoma was the presence of metastases in the group of lymph nodes adjacent to the primary melanoma site, extending beyond that site in some instances but never skipping over the initial draining nodal depot. This suggested an anatomic progression of regional nodal metastases. When these data were considered together with our data on serially sectioned elective nodal dissection specimens from all anatomic regions demonstrating the absence of metastases with lesions < 1.0 mm in thickness,[16] a policy limiting elective lymph node dissections both anatomically and for lesions > 1.0 mm was adopted. Radical neck and modified radical neck dissections were abandoned, and selective nodal dissections to include the nodal group or groups subjacent or adjacent to the anatomic site of the primary lesion were adopted. For example, for a lesion of the forehead, the lymphadenectomy would include a superficial parotidectomy; for a lesion in the region of the mandible, it would include a supraomohyoid dissection; and for a lesion of the posterior scalp, it would include an occipital and posterior cervical triangle dissection with preservation of the spinal accessory nerve. The rationale of such limited dissections was to allow any potential benefits of elective lymphadenectomy to be achieved for patients with lesions >1.0 mm thick in whom there was an immediately subjacent or adjacent nodal drainage basin that could optimally be dissected at the time of treatment of the primary lesion. This would circumvent the need for subsequent surgery if nodal recurrence were to develop, as such procedures might then require more extensive surgical considerations if the metastases were subjacent or adjacent to the site of initial primary excision.

In looking at retrospective analyses from this era, therefore, it was apparent that divergent conclusions were often reached, and that certainly a definitive case for elective node dissection had not been made. There did emerge, however, the suggestion that, if a benefit were to be realized, it would probably be for patients with disease that had selectively spread to regional nodes but not distant sites, and that, based on microstaging criteria, these would probably be patients with 'intermediate-thickness' lesions. This emerging hypothesis was compelling enough to justify its evaluation in more stringently controlled prospective trials. Notably, some prospective trials had already been conducted before the universal application of microstaging criteria, and this provided a framework and stimulus for the next stage in the study of elective lymph node dissection.

PROSPECTIVE RANDOMIZED STUDIES OF ELECTIVE LYMPH NODE DISSECTION

Prospective, randomized trials, carefully controlling for prognostic variables, should provide the most reliable data to assess the efficacy of elective lymph node dissection. Even before microstaging had become standardized for prognostic assessment, two prospective, randomized trials had been conducted to address this issue. In both, patients with malignant melanomas of the extremities were randomized to either wide excision alone or wide excision and elective lymph node dissection. Both studies failed to show a statistically significant benefit to elective lymphadenectomy. The earlier of these two studies, performed at the Mayo Clinic and reported by Sim and associates,[64] randomized 171 patients to wide excision alone (reserving lymph node dissection only if nodes became clinically positive), to wide excision and immediate elective lymph node dissection, or to wide excision and elective lymph node dissection 1–3 months after wide excision. A larger, multicenter study in Europe of extremity melanomas, under the auspices of the World Health

Organization (WHO) and reported by Veronesi and associates,[65] had two randomization arms: wide excision and elective lymph node dissection, or wide excision alone, reserving lymph node dissection only if the nodes became clinically positive. As both trials were begun before the microstaging systems of Clark or Breslow had come into general use, patients were not always prospectively stratified for these variables. There was also a predominance of lesions in women, who usually demonstrate favored survival compared to men.

In these studies, 5-year survival was not statistically different in any treatment group. In the WHO study, survival in patients with occult microscopic disease who had elective lymph node dissection was not significantly different from survival amongst those who had wide excisions alone, reserving therapeutic node dissection if they developed clinically positive nodes during observation (36.8% versus 30.2%). These studies became the most frequently cited data to counter the arguments of the proponents of elective lymph node dissection.

There were reservations, however, about the Mayo and WHO studies. Following the publication of the data of Balch and associates supporting a survival advantage of elective lymphadenectomy for patients with intermediate-thickness melanoma,[13] it was noted that the percentage of patients with melanomas in the 1.5–4.0 mm thickness range in the WHO study was 34%, whereas it was 61% for patients entered into the much smaller Mayo Clinic study. These were the patients for whom the greatest potential benefit from elective lymph node dissection might be realized. Furthermore, there was a difference in the WHO study, although not statistically significant, in the 5-year survival of patients with melanomas of 1.6–4.5 mm thickness, favoring wide excision and elective lymphadenectomy compared to wide excision alone (78.5% versus 69.7%). The possibility existed that, with much larger numbers of patients with malignant melanomas in this thickness range, a statistically significant benefit for elective lymph node dissection might have been demonstrated.

Because subgroups of patients may have benefited from elective lymph node dissection, Cascinelli and associates[66] evaluated survival 15 years after the original publication of the WHO study, according to prognostic criteria: sex, tumor thickness, Clark levels III and IV, and ulceration. No significant survival differences were noted in any of these subgroups. Of the 286 patients who had wide excision alone, 75 (26%) went on to develop nodal metastases requiring regional node dissection; survival in this group at 10 years was not statistically different from survival in the 54 patients who had been randomized to have elective lymphadenectomy and in whom nodal micrometastases had been diagnosed histologically in the lymph node dissection specimens (Figure 17.2). In response to the study of Balch and associates[13] demonstrating a survival advantage for patients with intermediate tumor thickness (between 1.5 mm and 4.0 mm),

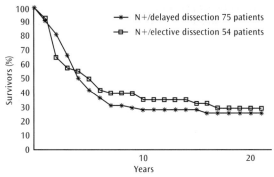

Figure 17.2 *Survival of 129 patients from the WHO trial with node metastases according to clinical status (elective node dissection versus delayed therapeutic node dissection). The elective node dissection group had occult micrometastases, and the delayed dissection group developed palpable nodal metastases during follow-up. Survival has been evaluated from the time of surgery for primary melanoma (p = 0.74). From Cascinelli et al.*[66]

a multivariate analysis was performed on the subgroup of 185 melanoma patients with primary tumor thicknesses between 1.5 mm and 4.0 mm, and this also failed to show a benefit for elective lymph node dissection.[66] Ulceration of the melanoma, as defined by histologic rather than clinical evaluation, was the only prognostic factor in addition to thickness that impacted on survival. Other factors, including initial surgical treatment (wide local excision with or without elective lymph node dissection), sex, age, and maximal tumor diameter failed to correlate with survival.

Because the first WHO trial was limited to lesions on the extremities and was initiated before the widespread adoption of the Breslow thickness microstaging, and before the availability of retrospective data on the potential value of elective node dissection for intermediate-thickness lesions, another trial was initiated for melanomas thicker than 1.5 mm located on the trunk. Patients were randomized to receive wide excision alone or wide excision and elective lymph node dissection.[67] Of the 252 patients entered in the study, 21% were found to have nodal micrometastases, and 26% in the wide excision group developed clinically detectable regional nodal metastases during follow-up. The overall survivals of the two groups of patients were statistically equivalent. Survival according to type of treatment was also evaluated in two subgroups of patients: those with tumor thickness between 1.5 mm and 4.0 mm, and those with tumor thickness >4.0 mm. The observed differences in the intermediate-thickness subgroup were statistically significant, favoring the elective lymph node dissection group (p = 0.03). There was no difference for lesions greater than 4.0 mm in thickness. In an analysis at 8 years of follow-up, patients with micrometastases in elective lymph node dissection specimens had a 5-year survival rate of 48.2%, versus 26.6% for patients having a delayed dissection when clinically palpable nodal metastases were detected.[68,69]

The reservations regarding several of these studies, as well as the retrospective data supporting a significant survival advantage for elective lymph node dissection for intermediate-thickness melanomas, led to the Intergroup Melanoma Surgical Trial, directed by Balch and supported by the National Cancer Institute, to evaluate elective lymph node dissection for patients with intermediate-thickness melanomas (1.0–4.0 mm).[70] Also included in the study was the prospective assessment of differing margins of excision around the primary lesion, the other important surgical issue for primary melanoma requiring prospective study. After randomization to either 2.0-cm or 4.0-cm margins of excision, patients with melanomas of the trunk or proximal extremities were randomized to have or not to have elective lymph node dissection. Patients with head and neck and distal extremity melanomas were also included if a 2.0-cm-margin excision could be achieved and then also randomized to have or not have an elective lymph node dissection. Patients were stratified according to:

1 melanoma thickness (1.0–2.0 mm, 2.0–3.0 mm, 3.0–4.0 mm),
2 location of the primary melanoma (proximal extremity versus trunk, or distal extremity versus head and neck),
3 ulceration of the epidermis overlying the melanoma on microscopic sections, ulceration having repeatedly been demonstrated in prior studies to be a highly significant adverse prognostic indicator.

The Intergroup Melanoma Surgical Trial prerandomized 786 patients, of whom 740 were eligible and evaluable for study. The average follow-up when reported in 1996 was 7.4 years. Adverse prognostic indicators were greater tumor thickness, ulceration, site of the primary melanoma on the trunk, and patient age, particularly over 60 years. There was no statistically significant difference between patients having or not having elective lymph node dissection at 5 years (64% versus 82%, p = 0.25). However, subset analysis did demonstrate a survival advantage for elective lymph node dissection in two groups: a trend for patients with melanoma between 1.0 mm and 2.0 mm in thickness (p = 0.08), the trend achieving statistical significance when the survival rates were based on actual treatment received (p = 0.031); and those patients aged 60 years or younger compared to older patients, with survival rates of 88% versus 81% (p = 0.04). The most significant improvement was seen in the younger group compared to the older group for melanomas between 1.0 mm and 2.0 mm with no tumor ulceration, the survival difference for elective lymph node dissection compared to observation of the regional nodes being 97% compared to 87% (p = 0.005). This improvement in survival achieved even

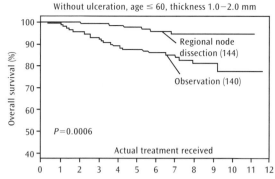

Figure 17.3 *The most significant improvement in survival in the Intergroup Melanoma Surgical Trial was for those patients having elective lymph node dissection if less than 60 years of age and with melanomas between 1.0 mm and 2.0 mm in thickness (p = 0.0006). From Balch et al.[70]*

greater significance if analysed by actual treatment received (Figure 17.3). This was the first prospectively randomized study that showed a survival advantage for elective lymph node dissection for some subsets of patients.

ELECTIVE 'SELECTIVE' REGIONAL LYMPHADENECTOMY

If elective lymph node dissection did provide patients with a survival advantage, it should be most compellingly demonstrated in patients proven to have nodal micrometastases, for whom the rationale of regional lymphadenectomy would be most applicable. Optimally, these patients would be those who have nodal metastases but no evolving metastases at other sites. As most series report an incidence of nodal metastases in elective lymph node dissection specimens of approximately 25%, the number who would theoretically be in this group would be even smaller. Even allowing for the one prospective study to demonstrate an advantage for subsets of patients less than 60 years of age and having lesions of 1.0–2.0 mm in thickness, arguably most clinical stage I melanoma patients will not benefit from elective regional lymphadenectomy, based on the collective experiences to date. However, if only those patients who have micrometastases to regional lymph nodes and who therefore might benefit from elective lymph node dissection could be identified, studies could then be designed to focus with statistical magnitude on the fundamental biologic significance of nodal micrometastases and whether their ablation does, in fact, affect survival. This is the basis of the current phase of studying the issue of regional lymphadenectomy. It has been made possible by the application of advances in nuclear imaging, lymphatic mapping, and histopathology.

LYMPHATIC MAPPING

The understanding of cutaneous lymphatic drainage for most of the twentieth century has been grounded in the classic nineteenth-century studies of Sappey,[71] in which the lymphatics were mapped using cutaneous red oxide of mercury injections. Such studies were adapted to delineate the presumed potential pathway of lymphatic dissemination, information of particular relevance for patients with malignant melanoma, a cutaneous neoplasm with a propensity for dermal lymphatic invasion. Our own studies on lymph node metastases from head and neck melanoma found the closest echelon of nodes to be always involved, occasionally extending to more distal nodes, but never skipping over the first nodal group. This suggested an orderly progression of lymph node metastases within a drainage basin.[61] Lymphatic mapping became of particular importance to several investigators concerned with the direction of nodal drainage from lesions in areas with potentially ambiguous drainage pathways, such as many sites on the trunk and the head and neck.

Following the work of several investigators, including Sherman and Ter-Pogossian[72] using radioactive colloidal gold ([198]Au) to demonstrate cutaneous lymphatic flow, Fee and associates[73] applied this technique for the determination of lymphatic pathways from specific cutaneous melanoma sites. Because of the high radiation exposure from [198]Au, other tracers were evaluated, among which were ^{99m}Tc-labeled sulfur colloid (Tc-SC),[74] ^{99m}Tc-labeled antimony sulfide, and ^{99m}Tc-labeled human serum albumin (Tc-HSA).[75]

Whereas nodal drainage pathways from the extremities are invariably directed to the ipsilateral axilla or groin and uncommonly directed to epitrochlear or popliteal nodes, data accumulated from several studies have demonstrated that drainage pathways from primary lesions on the trunk and the head and neck are less predictable and do not conform in many instances to the guidelines originally provided from Sappey's studies. In particular, Sappey established a dividing line on the trunk from the second lumbar vertebra to the umbilicus, with lesions above going to the ipsilateral axilla, those below to the ipsilateral groin, with the exception of a zone surrounding both Sappey's line and the midline for a distance of 2.5 cm, from which drainage could be bidirectional. In a lymphoscintigraphic study by Norman and associates,[76] it was noted that up to 59% of elective regional lymphadenectomies directed by such guidelines might have resulted in the ablation of the wrong nodal group or a failure to dissect one of multiple groups to which the truncal sites drained. As many as 50% of melanoma sites will drain to multiple lymphatic basins or have pathways that are not predictable by Sappey's studies.[76–78] For head and neck sites, Wanebo and associates[79] also reported that the predictability of cutaneous lymphatic flow may be less certain than believed by strict anatomic criteria. This has also been substantiated by other reports demonstrating a discordance of one-third from lymphoscintigraphic findings and anatomically predicted pathways.[80–84] Data from the Moffitt Cancer Center (Tampa, FL) of 212 patients who were candidates for elective lymph node dissection and had preoperative lymphoscintigraphy showed a discordance rate in the head and neck for lymphoscintigraphic pattern compared to predicted anatomic pathways of 63%. For truncal lesions, the discordance rate was 32%. Lymphoscintigraphy changed the plan of operative intervention in 47%, with 19% having a basin dissected that would have been unpredicted by classical criteria and 28% not having a dissection because of failure of the lymphoscintigram to indicate a predominant drainage basin or a pattern of multiple drainage basins.[85]

A formidable experience with lymphoscintigraphy, as reported by Thompson and associates,[86] has provided a particularly compelling argument for delineating the lymphatic flow from cutaneous sites, which they also found to not infrequently differ from classical teaching. In their study of 1759 patients with primary cutaneous melanoma, 1089 had drainage to one nodal field, 491 to two nodal fields, 134 to three nodal fields, and 6 to five nodal fields. In many instances, the pathways were at variance with traditional precepts. Interval nodes outside drainage basins and to nodal fields on opposite sides of the body were also observed. Studies such as these clearly weaken the assumptions of many previous studies on elective lymph node dissection in which lymphoscintigraphy was not utilized, particularly those with large numbers of patients having truncal and head and neck melanomas.

Lymphoscintigraphy requires that the skin surrounding the primary melanoma site be injected with radiocolloid intradermally. Care is taken to raise a wheal to insure intradermal entry of the radiocolloid into the dermal lymphatics. Images are then obtained at approximately 15–20-min intervals. It should be noted that, of the prospective trials of elective lymph node dissection, only the Intergroup Melanoma Trial required lymphoscintigraphy to identify the nodal basin(s) at risk for truncal melanomas. It should also be emphasized that lymphoscintigraphy is useful only if the primary melanoma is intact or has been excised conservatively, as with an excisional biopsy. If, however, the primary melanoma has been widely excised, disruption of the inceptive lymphatic drainage significantly compromises the reliability of lymphoscintigraphy for demonstrating the direction of regional lymphatic flow.

Lymphoscintigraphy demonstrated the feasibility of clinical lymphatic mapping, but in itself did not allow the extent of elective node dissection to be contained. For this to be achieved, techniques for intraoperative lymphatic mapping were required to provide a means of testing the hypothesis that lymphatic metastases progress in a predictable pattern. Investigations by Kinmonth,[87] using patent blue V dye to demonstrate the regional lymphatics in preparation for lymphangiography, established that agent as well suited for intraoperative lymphatic mapping. Wong and associates,[88] of the John Wayne Cancer Institute, compared patent blue V, methylene blue, isosulfan blue, and Evans blue dyes in cats to determine which agent appeared to be optimal for the staining of draining lymph nodes. Patent blue V and isosulfan blue were demonstrated to be the most consistent and useful. They then proceeded to apply lymphatic mapping clinically in melanoma patients. As first reported by Morton and associates,[89] patent blue V or isosulfan blue was injected intradermally at the primary melanoma site in 223 consecutive patients as a means of mapping the sentinel node(s). By 'sentinel' was meant the node or nodes which drained the specific cutaneous sites and were presumed to be the initial potential site of regional nodal micrometastases. The technique was found to be effective for sites draining to the neck, axilla, and groin. A standardized technique was utilized in conjunction with preoperative lymphoscintigraphy, and the 'blue' nodes with their blue-stained afferent lymphatics were identified. To test the hypothesis that a specific site would preferentially lead to metastasis to a draining sentinel node, the incidence of micrometastases in the sentinel node was correlated with the remaining nodes in a completed lymph node dissection specimen. Morton et al. reported on their initial 4-year experience, demonstrating the successful identification in 194 of 237 (82%) regional lymph node dissection specimens. Micrometastases were demonstrated in 47 (18%) of 259 sentinel nodes, and non-sentinel nodes were the sole site of metastases in two (0.06%) of 3079 non-sentinel nodes from 194 lymphadenectomy specimens that had an identifiable sentinel node. This supported a predictable pattern of initial sentinel regional node metastases.

Soon after the introduction of sentinel lymphadenectomy using dye, an additional technique was introduced that enabled the experience gained with lymphoscintigraphy to be utilized intraoperatively. Following radioisotopic lymphoscintigraphy or preoperative re-injection of radioisotope, a gamma-probe was used as a primary means of identifying the sentinel node(s). Alex and associates[90] first reported on this technique with their early experience using a hand-held gamma-probe alone. A report by Krag and associates followed.[91] Thereafter, several investigators added this approach to the dye technique to direct the incision and dissection and to augment the visual identification allowed by blue dye (Figure 17.4).[92–97] As currently used, a radioisotope, most commonly ^{99m}Tc sulfur colloid, is injected at least 1 hour prior to surgery. The sentinel node will concentrate the radioisotope and become a 'hot' node with in-vivo counts in ratios in excess of at least 2:1, usually much higher, over background or non-sentinel nodes, with higher ratios ex-vivo. The reliable ratios to confirm

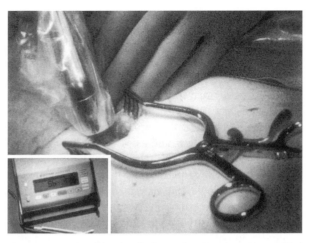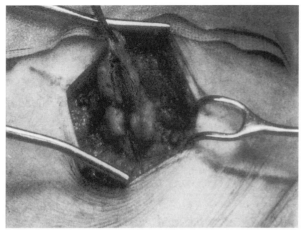

Figure 17.4 *Combined technique of technetium-99 m sulfur colloid with gamma-probe and isosulfan blue dye to identify the inguinal sentinel node.*

identification of a sentinel node remain to be precisely defined and validated.

Successful sentinel node identification has been verified in several large series from numerous centers, most confirming the optimal efficacy of a combined technique, with the gamma-probe facilitating limited surgery to rapidly identify the blue-stained node(s). A secondary benefit of radiocolloid-directed surgery is the identification of additional sentinel nodes when the level of background activity does not return. Additional 'hot' nodes might not be identified after the blue-stained node has been removed. The significance of sentinel nodes that show discordance between radioisotopic uptake and blue dye is uncertain at the present time. The ratio of radioactive counts to background to verify a sentinel node is also unclear. A blue-stained node with a feeding blue-stained lymphatic is clearly verifiable and must be considered the standard for positive identification at this time, with radioisotopic-directed gamma-probe location a valuable adjunct. The optimal radioisotope and the timing of injection to allow surgical identification remain issues that require further clarification. Isosulfan blue dye itself has a rapid transit time and should allow identification of the sentinel node within 20 min, with variations depending on the primary site in relation to the regional nodal basin.

Intraoperative lymphatic mapping with sentinel lymphadenectomy has now been validated as a technique that can be successfully learned and applied in a standardized fashion. A success rate of 97% was achieved by a Multicenter Selective Lymphadenectomy Trial Group study directed from the John Wayne Cancer Institute. As reported by Morton *et al.*,[98] 551 patients accrued from 16 international centers participating in a learning phase were compared to 584 patients from the organizing group at the John Wayne Cancer Institute. In both groups, blue dye plus radiocolloid was more successful (99.1%) than blue dye alone (95.2%, $p = 0.014$). In a learning phase of 30 cases in which a completion lymph

node dissection was performed to assess the accuracy of sentinel node identification, a 97% identification rate was achieved by the participating centers, with an incidence of nodal metastases approaching that reported by the organizing center. A recent review of the reported experience of lymphatic mapping and sentinel lymphadenectomy from ten clinical trials[99] using dye or radioisotopes or a combination has further confirmed a high sentinel node identification rate of 82–100%, with a micrometastasis detection rate of 15–26%.

It should be emphasized that, if a sentinel node is negative for micrometastatic disease, it does not abrogate the need for future surveillance of the regional nodal basin from which it has been harvested. The John Wayne Cancer Institute reported a 4.8% incidence of same-basin recurrence at a median follow-up of 45 months.[98]

Recurrences may represent pathologic failure to identify micrometastases due to sampling error or failure to utilize immunohistochemical staining techniques, or may be due to technical errors at surgery, with a resulting misidentification of the true sentinel node(s). Gershenwald and associates[100] reported on ten first recurrences in a previously mapped nodal basin from which a sentinel node that was negative by H & E staining had been harvested. This was from a series of 243 sentinel lymphadenectomies. Re-evaluation by immunohistochemical staining of the sentinel node revealed previously undetected metastases in seven. These reports from experienced groups also support the importance of an institutional learning phase of sentinel lymphadenectomy with completion regional node dissection to validate the capability, not only of the surgical team, but also of the nuclear imaging and pathology contributors and their effective coordination to achieve reproducible and accurate results. Sentinel lymphadenectomy is obviously dependent on accurate lymphatic mapping and a reproducible surgical technique, but has also focused attention on the importance of detailed and highly sensitive nodal histopathology.

HISTOPATHOLOGY OF REGIONAL LYMPH NODES

As early as 1958, Lane and associates[101] demonstrated that the survival rate for patients with melanoma and metastatic nodal involvement was highest for those with a single microscopic focus within a lymph node, and that, whereas regional lymph nodes might be pronounced normal after thorough but routine pathologic examination, serial sections of the same nodes often demonstrated the presence of microscopic melanoma. In our study of regional nodal micrometastases, we trisected each node and step-sectioned each segment.[15] Micrometastases were demonstrated in 28% of patients with melanomas 1.0–2.0 mm in thickness and in 50% of patients with melanoma > 4.0 mm in thickness. Whereas routine H & E staining identifies most nodal micrometastases and has traditionally been the basis of assessing trials of elective regional lymphadenectomy, the identification and ability to stain for melanoma markers, including S-100 protein and HMB-45, have added to the sensitivity of detecting nodal disease.

Immunohistochemical staining with antibody to S-100 protein has demonstrated it to be present in primary and metastatic melanoma cells, as well as in normal melanocytes and non-melanocytic cell types, including neurons, pituicytes, Langerhans' cells, dendritic cells, and macrophages. Anti-S-100 antibody staining has been used as an adjunct in the diagnosis of histologically ambiguous primary melanoma, including amelanotic lesions and desmoplastic melanomas, and for diagnosing metastatic melanomas which are histopathologically undifferentiated, particularly in the absence of a definable primary lesion. Anti-S-100 antibody staining is quite sensitive, because most reports show that more than 90% of primary and metastatic lesions are positive, including clinically occult foci of metastaic melanoma in lymph nodes.[102–105]

Staining for the HMB-45 antigen has demonstrated its presence in the junctional component of melanocytic nevi and primary and metastatic melanoma cells. Expression of HMB-45 appears to be a more specific marker for melanoma than does expression of S-100 and is also more sensitive for metastatic lesions.[106–108] Goscin et al. have indicated, however, that it may have a sensitivity of only 50% for micrometastatic melanoma in lymph nodes.[109] Staining for other melanoma-associated antigens, such as NKI/C3, has been used to augment the diagnosis of primary and metastatic melanoma.

It has long been suggested that even those patients without histologically documented regional node involvement may benefit from elective regional lymphadenectomy, because removed nodes may, in fact, harbor micrometastases which are undetected by standard pathologic sectioning and H & E staining. Cochran and colleagues reported that the rate of detecting micrometastases rose 14% in regional lymph nodes examined by immunohistological techniques, as compared to routine staining methods.[103,104] Reverse transcriptase–polymerase chain reaction (RT–PCR) to detect tyrosinase mRNA, a product of melanin-producing cells, allows the detection of melanoma cells in lymph nodes with great sensitivity and has been the focus of study to even further upstage the histologic assessment of nodal metastases.[110] Reintgen and associates[111] have reported on the use of this assay for evaluating the lymph nodes of 29 patients with intermediate-thickness melanoma. Standard pathologic staining was compared to RT–PCR. Eleven (38%) were pathologically positive, and 19 (66%) were RT–PCR positive. In a study by Goydos and associates,[112] 50 patients had sentinel nodes evaluated after sectioning along their long axes, one-half of the node by H & E and immunohistochemical staining 'when appropriate' and the other half frozen in liquid nitrogen for RT–PCR for tyrosinase and MART-1 (melanoma-antigen recognized by T-cells). Ten patients had nodes positive by routine histopathology, and an additional three patients had positive nodes detected by RT–PCR. The sensitivity of this assay is clearly increased compared to previous techniques and highlights the probable inadequacy of traditional approaches to assessing the efficacy of elective regional lymphadenectomy based on routine histopathologic assessment. However, the prognostic significance of RT–PCR-detected tumor-positive nodes that are otherwise undetectable by other histopathologic techniques remains to be established in long-term follow-up. It is possible that it may allow further stratification of patients who previously would have been considered node negative into favorable groups if RT–PCR negative and higher risk groups if RT–PCR positive. Other markers, such as MART-1 and GalNAc-T, may further amplify the sensitivity of nodal staging.[113,114] This, in turn, may lower the risk of future regional nodal basin recurrences that might result from the failure to identify patients with micrometastatic nodal disease for whom completion lymphadenectomy would otherwise not be performed.

MULTICENTER SELECTIVE LYMPHADENECTOMY TRIAL

The development of intraoperative lymphatic mapping and immunohistochemical staining to detect nodal metastases with great sensitivity made the design of trials to incorporate these advances of obvious importance. As already noted, Morton and colleagues at the John Wayne Cancer Institute organized the Multicenter Selective Lymphadenectomy Trial with other institutions having a documented breadth of experience in the treatment of cutaneous malignant melanoma.[115] The study was designed to determine whether intraoperative lymphatic

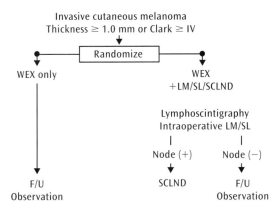

Figure 17.5 *Study design of the Multicenter Selective Lymphadenectomy Trial comparing wide excision (WEX) and lymphatic mapping (LM), sentinel lymphadenectomy and selective complete lymph node dissection (SL/SCLND) for patients having proven sentinel node micrometastases, to wide excision alone. From Morton et al.[98]*

mapping, selective lymphadenectomy, and completion lymphadenectomy when sentinel node metastases were detected, along with wide excision of the primary site provided a survival advantage over wide excision alone (Figure 17.5).

The randomization scheme essentially selects patients with melanomas of 1.0 mm or greater thickness to either wide excision alone or wide excision with preoperative lymphoscintigraphy, intraoperative lymphatic mapping and sentinel lymphadenectomy. A complete lymph node dissection is performed if sentinel node micrometastases are demonstrated histologically. This trial offers the opportunity to sensitively test the efficacy of elective lymph node dissection by optimally determining the nodal site(s) at risk and selecting only those patients with nodal micrometastases for regional lymphadenectomy. Until this trial is completed, the value of such a 'selective' elective lymph node dissection remains unproven. Despite this, sentinel lymphadenectomy has been broadly adopted as a staging procedure, independently of its possible inherent surgical therapeutic value. The therapeutic extension of this staging information is to identify patients at high risk of recurrence and thereby direct efforts at adjuvant systemic therapy.

REGIONAL LYMPH NODES IN THE ASSESSMENT OF PROGNOSIS AND ADJUVANT THERAPY

The prognostic assessment of a primary cutaneous malignant melanoma is more precisely defined than with any other solid malignant neoplasm, thickness being the foundation of this evaluation. Within any thickness range, however, the presence or absence of regional lymph node metastases remains the most powerful predictor of survival, altering survival statistics in the range of 50%.[116] Prognostic assessment by histologic examination of regional lymph nodes has therefore been advanced as a major reason to perform elective regional lymphadenectomy. Clearly, this argument hinges on the ability to translate such prognostic information into an effective systemic adjuvant strategy to improve the survival of patients at the greatest risk of recurrence, thereby enabling the clearest evaluation of the impact of treatment as well as sparing others the potential toxicity of such therapies.

Efforts to alter the course for high-risk patients have been ongoing for more than two decades, involving a variety of chemotherapeutic and immunotherapeutic approaches. The earliest efforts which showed the promise of prolonging survival used *Bacillus Calmette–Guérin* (BCG). A survival advantage was not sustained when randomized trials were conducted,[117,118] an experience that was repeated with levamisole[119,120] and transfer factor.[121] Results with *C. parvum*, when compared to BCG in patients with resected regional node metastases, showed a prolongation in disease-free interval, although a statistically significant improvement in survival could not be demonstrated.[122] Likewise, randomized adjuvant chemotherapy trials using single agents (most commonly dacarbazine), combination regimens, or chemoimmunotherapy regimens have failed to demonstrate a benefit in high-risk patients to date.[117,123–125]

Non-specific immunotherapeutic approaches have given way to specific immunotherapy programs, most commonly with a variety of vaccines using irradiated melanoma cells, shed antigens from melanoma cells maintained in cell culture or cell lysates, often in conjunction with other immunologic adjuvants. Data from randomized trials to date in node-positive patients have failed to demonstrate an improvement in survival.[126–130]

Trials using interferon-α (IFN-α) in patients with advanced melanoma have demonstrated partial or complete responses in approximately 15–20%.[131] In keeping with other immunotherapy regimens, patients free of disease but at high risk of recurrence have been the focus of efforts to improve survival using IFN. The Eastern Cooperative Oncology Group (ECOG) conducted a randomized, controlled study (Trial 1684) of 1 year of high-dose IFN-α-2b ($n = 143$) versus observation ($n = 137$), which has generated great interest. As reported by Kirkwood and associates,[131] a statistically significant prolongation of relapse-free and overall survival for treated patients was observed. At 5 years, the estimated survival in the treated group was 46%, compared to 37% in the untreated group. The survival benefit was greatest in node-positive patients. Hepatotoxicity was noted, with two patients dying of this complication early in the study. A WHO study of 444 patients, with resected-node-positive patients randomized to receive low-dose IFN-α-2a versus observation, failed to demonstrate an advantage in disease-free or overall survival.[132] Other studies of IFN-α-2a,[133–135] using different dosages and schedules, failed to show a statistically significant advantage in disease-free or overall survival. Dosage would therefore seem to be a crucial issue if benefits are to be realized, but the issue of toxicity with high-dose INF-α will require careful scrutiny and the benefits will require confirmation if use as an adjuvant in high-risk patients is to gain wide acceptance. A confirmatory trial by ECOG (1690) has been conducted and final reporting is awaited. Preliminary results, however, have been reported to show a significant improvement in disease-free survival, but not in overall survival compared to the control arm.[136]

Stratification for adjuvant therapy trials most optimally uses the status of regional lymph nodes, the dominant prognostic indicator. This provides great incentive for performing selective ('sentinel') lymphadenectomy as a staging procedure. However, the issue of lymphadenectomy as a staging procedure does not address the fundamental biologic issue of whether surgical ablation of micrometastases has an independent impact on survival. This issue may remain unresolved unless appropriate trials, using all means of identifying and studying those regional lymph nodes at risk of harboring micrometastases, are conducted and brought to completion. In addition to the Multicenter Selective Lymphadenectomy Trial, a Sunbelt Melanoma Trial randomizes patients with melanomas ≥1.0 mm thick and histologically negative but RT–PCR-positive sentinel lymph nodes to observation, completion lymph node dissection, or completion lymph node dissection and 1 month of high-dose adjuvant IFN-α-2b. For patients with histologically positive sentinel node(s), a completion lymph node dissection is performed. If found to have no additional positive nodes, they are randomly assigned to observation or adjuvant IFN-α-2b. If there are additional positive nodes or extracapsular extension of the single positive node, they receive IFN.

CONCLUSION

The application of lymphatic mapping, selective lymphadenectomy, and histologic assessment requires sound techniques in surgery, nuclear imaging, and histopathology. Most importantly, it requires validation in appropriate trials before it is adopted with the same untested enthusiasm that elective lymph node dissection was at the beginning of the twentieth century. It is clear, however, that lymphoscintigraphy, intraoperative lymphatic mapping, and sentinel lymphadenectomy have dramatically altered the surgical approach to malignant melanoma and, if not changing the biologic controversy on the value of ablating nodal micrometastases, have made the study of the issue far more sensitive and focused.

Sentinel node identification is a reproducible and validated technique. It would appear that, with some specific exceptions, the performance of an elective axillary, inguinal, or selective neck dissection without a properly performed sentinel lymphadenectomy to confirm the presence of regional nodal micrometastases may no longer be appropriate. The success of sentinel node identification should exceed 95% with appropriate quality control of lymphoscintigraphy, surgery, and pathologic evaluation. Whether sentinel lymphadenectomy is sustained as a therapeutically valid procedure remains to be proven. Pursuing this issue, however, will undoubtedly bring us closer to an understanding of the pathophysiology of lymph node metastases, as we enter a new century of study of cutaneous malignant melanoma.

REFERENCES

1. Kosary CL, Ries LAG, Miller BA, *et al. SEER cancer statistics review*, 1973–1992. Tables and graphs (abstract). National Cancer Institute. NIH Publication No. 96-2789, Bethesda, MD, National Cancer Institute, 1995.
2. McCarthy WH, Shaw HM, Cascinelli N, *et al.* Elective lymph node dissection for melanoma: two perspectives. World J Surg 1992; 16:203–13.
3. Virchow R. *Cellular pathology*, translated by F Chance. London, J. Churchill, 1860, p.187.
4. Snow HL. Melanotic cancerous disease. Lancet 1892; 2:872–4.
5. Eve F. A lecture on melanoma. The Practitioner 1903; 70:165–74.
6. Handley WS. The pathology of melanotic growths in relation to their operative treatment: lecture I & II. Lancet 1907; 1:927–35, 996–1003.
7. Pringle JH. A method of operation in cases of melanotic tumours of the skin. Edinburgh Med J 1908; 23:496–9.
8. Edwards JM, Kinmouth JB. Lymphovenous shunts in man. BMJ 1969; 4:579–84.
9. Weiss L. Site-associated differences in cancer cell populations. Clin Exp Metastasis 1991; 9:193–7.
10. Clark WH, From L, Bernardino EH, Mihm MC. The histogenesis and biologic behavior of primary human malignant melanomas of the skin. Cancer Res 1969; 29:705–27.
11. Breslow A. Thickness, cross-sectional areas, and depth of invasion in the prognosis of cutaneous melanoma. Ann Surg 1970; 172:902–8.
12. Balch CM, Soong SJ, Murad TM, *et al.* A multifactorial analysis of melanoma. II: Prognostic factors in patients with stage I (localized) melanoma. Ann Surg 1979; 86:343–51.
13. Balch CM, Soong SJ, Milton GW, *et al.* A comparison of prognostic factors and surgical results in 1,786 patients with localized (stage I) melanoma treated in Alabama, USA, and New South Wales, Australia. Ann Surg 1982; 196:677–84.

14. Balch CM, Milton GW, Cascinelli N, Sim FH. Elective lymph node dissection: pros and cons. In: Balch CM, Houghton AN, Milton GW, *et al.*, eds. *Cutaneous melanoma*, 2nd edn. Philadelphia: JB Lippincott, 1992, 345–66.

15. Roses DF, Harris MN, Hidalgo D, *et al.* Correlation of the thickness of melanoma and regional lymph node metastases. Arch Surg 1982; 117:921–5.

16. Balch CM, Murad TM, Soong S, *et al.* Tumor thickness as a guide to surgical management of clinical stage I melanoma patients. Cancer 1979; 43:883–8.

17. Essner R, Morton DL. Elective lymph node dissection. In: Lejeune FJ, Chaudhar AK, DasGupta TK, eds. *Malignant melanoma*. New York, McGraw-Hill, Inc., 1994, 207.

18. Polk HC Jr, Bland KI. Routine elective lymph node dissection in melanoma: unnecessary treatment? In: O'Connell TX, ed. *Surgical oncology: controversies in cancer treatment*. Boston, GK Hall, 1981; 122–36.

19. McCarthy JG, Haagenson CD, Herter FP. The role of groin dissection in the management of melanoma of the lower extremity. Ann Surg 1972; 179:156–9.

20. Urist MM, Maddox WA, Kennedy JE, *et al.* Patient risk factors and surgical morbidity after regional lymphadenectomy in 204 melanoma patients. Cancer 1983; 51:2152–6.

21. Ingvar C, Erichsen C, Johnsson P. Morbidity following prophylactic and therapeutic lymph node dissection: a comparison. Tumori 1984; 70:529–33.

22. Bowsher WG, Taylor BA, Hughes LE. Morbidity, mortality, and local recurrence following regional node dissection for melanoma. Br J Surg 1986; 73:906–8.

23. Holmes EC, Moseley HS, Morton DL, *et al.* A rational approach to the surgical management of melanoma. Ann Surg 1977; 186:481–90.

24. Karakousis CP, Goumas W, Rao U, Driscoll DI. Axillary node dissection in malignant melanoma. Am J Surg 1991; 162:202–7.

25. Gumport SL, Harris MN. Results of regional lymph node dissection for melanoma. Ann Surg 1974; 179:105–8.

26. Coit DG, Brennan MF. Extent of lymph node dissection in melanoma of the trunk or lower extremity. Arch Surg 1989; 124:162–6.

27. Baas PC, Koops HS, Hoekstra JH, *et al.* Groin dissection in the treatment of lower extremity melanoma, short-term and long-term morbidity. Arch Surg 1992; 127:281–6.

28. Finck SJ, Giuliano AE, Mann BD, Morton DL. Results of ilioinguinal dissection for stage II melanoma. Ann Surg 1982; 196:180–6.

29. Karakousis CP, Heiser MA, Moore RH. Lymphedema after groin dissection. Am J Surg 1983; 145:205–8.

30. Karakousis CP, Driscoll DL, Rose B, Walsh DL. Groin dissection in malignant melanoma. Ann Surg Oncol 1994; 1:271–7.

31. Shaw JHF, Rumball EM. Complications and local recurrence following lymphadenectomy. Br J Surg 1990; 77:760–4.

32. Shaw JH, Koea J. Morbidity of lymphadenectomy for melanoma. Surg Oncol Clin North Am 1992; 1(2):195–203.

33. Coit DG, Peters M, Brennan MF. A prospective randomized trial of perioperative Cefazolin treatment in axillary and groin dissection. Arch Surg 1991; 126:1366–9.

34. Silberman AW. Malignant melanoma: practical considerations concerning regional lymph node dissection. Ann Surg 1987; 206:206–9.

35. Karakousis CP, Emrich LJ, Rao U. Groin dissection in malignant melanoma. Am J Surg 1985; 152:491–5.

36. Harris MN, Gump SL, Berman IR, *et al.* Ilio-inguinal lymph node dissection for melanoma. Surg Gynecol Obstet 1973; 136:33–9.

37. Pack GT, Gerber DM, Scharnagel IM. End results in the treatment of malignant melanoma. A report of 1190 cases. Ann Surg 1952; 136:905–11.

38. Balch CM, Soong S, Murad TM, *et al.* Multifactorial analysis of melanoma. III: prognostic factors in patients with regional lymph node metastases (stage II). Ann Surg 1981; 193:377–88.

39. McNeer G, Das Gupta TK. Prognosis in malignant melanoma. Surgery 1964; 56:512–18.

40. Cohen MH, Ketcham AS, Felix EL, *et al.* Prognostic factors in patients undergoing lymphadenectomy for malignant melanoma. Ann Surg 1977; 186:635–42.

41. Das Gupta TK. Results of treatment of 269 patients with primary cutaneous melanoma: a five-year prospective study. Ann Surg 1977; 186:201–9.

42. Callery C, Cochran AJ, Roe DJ, *et al.* Factors prognostic for survival in patients with malignant melanoma spread to the regional lymph nodes. Ann Surg 1982; 196:69–75.

43. Roses DF, Provet JA, Harris MN, Gumport SL, Dubin N. Prognosis of patients with pathologic stage II cutaneous malignant melanoma. Ann Surg 1985; 201:103–7.

44. Wanebo JH, Fortner JG, Woodruff J, *et al.* Selection of the optimum surgical treatment of stage I melanoma by depth of microinvasion: use of the combined microstage technique (Clark–Breslow). Ann Surg 1975; 182:302–15.

45. Balch CM, Murad TQ, Soong S, *et al.* Tumor thickness as a guide to surgical management of clinical stage I melanoma patients. Cancer 1979; 43:883–8.

46. Milton GW, Shaw HM, McCarthy WH, *et al.* Prophylactic lymph node dissection in clinical stage I cutaneous malignant melanoma: results of surgical treatment in 1319 patients. Br J Surg 1982; 69:108–11.

47. McCarthy WH, Shaw HM, Milton GW. Efficacy of elective lymph node dissection in 2,347 patients with

clinical stage I malignant melanoma. Surg Gynecol Obstet 1985; 161:575–80.

48. Biess B, Broker EB, Drepper H, et al. Should elective lymph node dissection be used for treatment of primary melanoma? J Cancer Res Clin Oncol 1989; 115:470–3.

49. Reintgen DC, Cox EB, McCarty KS, et al. Efficacy of elective lymph node dissection in patients with intermediate thickness primary melanoma. Ann Surg 1983; 198:379–85.

50. Singluff EL, Stidham KR, Ricci WM, et al. Surgical management of regional lymph nodes in patients with melanoma. Experience with 4,682 patients. Ann Surg 1994; 219:120–30.

51. Coates AS, Ingvar CI, Petersen-Schaefer K, et al. Elective lymph node dissection in patients with primary melanoma of the trunk and limbs treated at the Sydney Melanoma Unit from 1960 to 1991. J Am Coll Surg 1995; 180:402–9.

52. Day CL, Sober SJ, Lew RA, et al. Malignant melanoma patients with positive nodes and relatively good prognosis: microstaging retains prognostic significance in clinical stage I patients with metastases to regional nodes. Cancer 1981; 47:955–62.

53. Slingluff CL, Vollmer R, Seigler HF. Stage II malignant melanoma: presentation of a prognostic model and an assessment of specific active immunotherapy in 1273 patients. Surg Oncol 1988; 39:139–47.

54. Morton DL, Wanek L, Nizze JA, et al. Improved long-term survival after lymphadenectomy of melanoma metastatic to regional nodes; analysis of prognostic factors in 1134 patients from the John Wayne Cancer Clinic. Ann Surg 1991; 214:491–9.

55. Balch CM, Soong SJ, Murad TM, et al. A multifactorial analysis of melanoma. III. Prognostic factors in patients with lymph node metastases (stage II). Ann Surg 1981; 193:377–85.

56. Drepper H, Kohler CO, Bastian B, et al. Benefit of elective lymph node dissection in subgroups of melanoma patients. Cancer 1993; 72:741–9.

57. Elder DE, Guerry D, VanHorn M, et al. The role of lymph node dissection for clinical stage I malignant melanoma of intermediate thickness (1.51–3.99 mm). Cancer 1985; 56:413–18.

58. Binder M, Pehamberger H, Steiner A, et al. Elective regional node dissection in malignant melanoma. Eur J Cancer 1990; 26:871–3.

59. Bagley FH, Cady B, Lee A, et al. Changes in clinical presentation and management of malignant melanoma. Cancer 1981; 47:2126–34.

60. Crowley NJ. The case against elective lymphadenectomy. Surg Oncol Clin North Am 1992; 1(2):223–46.

61. Roses DR, Harris MN, Grunberger I, et al. Selective surgical management of cutaneous melanoma of the head and neck. Ann Surg 1980; 192:629–32.

62. Belli F, Nova M, Santinami M, et al. Management of nodal metastases from head and neck melanoma. J Surg Oncol 1989; 42:47–53.

63. O'Brien CJ, Gianoutsos MP, Morgan MJ. Neck dissection for cutaneous malignant melanoma. World J Surg 1992; 16:222–6.

64. Sim FH, Taylor WF, Ivins JC, et al. A prospective randomized study of the efficacy of routine prophylactic lymphadenectomy in management of malignant melanoma: preliminary results. Cancer 1978; 41:946–56.

65. Veronesi U, Adamus J, Bandierra DC, et al. Inefficacy of immediate node dissection on stage I melanoma of the limbs. N Engl J Med 1977; 297:627–30.

66. Cascinelli N, Santinami M, Belli I. The case against elective lymph node dissection. World J Surg 1992; 16:206–13.

67. Cascinelli N. The role of clinical trials in assessing optimal treatment of cutaneous melanoma not extending beyond the regional nodes. Eur J Surg Oncol 1996; 22:123–35.

68. Cascinelli N, Morabito A, Santinami M, et al. Immediate or delayed dissection of regional nodes in patients with melanoma of the trunk: a randomized trial. Lancet 1998; 351:783–96.

69. Balch CM, Cascinelli N, Sim FH, et al. Elective lymph node dissection: results of prospective randomized surgical trials. In: Balch CM et al., eds. Cutaneous melanoma, 3rd edn. St Louis, MI, Quality Medical Publishing Inc., 1998; 209–25.

70. Balch CM, Soong S-J, Bertolucci AA, et al. Efficacy of an elective regional lymph node dissection of 1.0 to 4.0 mm-thick melanomas for patients 60 years of age and younger. Ann Surg 1996; 224:255–66.

71. Sappey MPC. Injection preparation et conservation des vaisseau lymphatiques. Thèse pour le doctorate en medecine, N. 241. Paris Rignoux Imprimerie de la faculte de Medecine, Paris, 1843.

72. Sherman A, Ter-Pogossian M. Lymph node concentration of radioactive colloid gold following interstitial injection. Cancer 1953; 6:1238–40.

73. Fee HJ, Robinson DS, Sample WF, et al. The determination of lymph shed by colloidal gold scanning patients with malignant melanoma: a preliminary study. Surgery 1978; 84:626–32.

74. Sullivan DC, Croker BP Jr, Harris CC, Deery P, Seigler HF. Lymphoscintigraphy in malignant melanoma: ^{99m}Tc-antimony sulfur colloid. Am J Roentgenol 1981; 137:847–51.

75. Lamki LM, Haynie TP, Balch CM, et al. Lymphoscintigraphy in the surgical management of patients with truncal melanoma: comparison of Tc sulfur colloid with Tc human serum albumin (abstract). J Nucl Med 1989; 30:844.

76. Norman J, Cruse CW, Espinosa C, et al. Redefinition of cutaneous lymphatic drainage with the use of

lymphoscintigraphy for malignant melanoma. Am J Surg 1991; 162:432–7.

77. Lamki LM, Logic JR. Defining lymphatic drainage patterns with cutaneous lymphoscintigraphy. In Balch CM, Houghton AN, Milton GW et al. eds. *Cutaneous melanoma*, 2nd edn. Philadelphia, JB Lippincott, 1992; 367–75.

78. Reintgen DS, Cruse CW, Wells K, et al. The orderly progression of melanoma nodal metastases. Ann Surg 1994; 220:759–67.

79. Wanebo HJ, Harpole D, Teates CD. Radionuclide lymphoscintigraphy with technetium ^{99m}antimony sulfide colloid to identify lymphatic drainage of cutaneous melanoma at ambiguous sites in the head and neck and trunk. Cancer 1985; 55:1403–13.

80. Uren RF, Howman-Giles RB, Shaw HM, et al. Lymphoscintigraphy in high risk melanoma of the trunk: predicting draining node groups, defining lymphatic channels, and locating the sentinel node. J Nucl Med 1993; 34:1435–40.

81. Berman DG, Norman J, Cruse CW, et al. Lymphoscintigraphy in malignant melanoma. Ann Plast Surg 1992; 28:29–32.

82. Berger DH, Feig B, Podoloff D, et al. Lymphoscintigraphy as a predictor of lymphatic drainage from cutaneous melanoma. Ann Surg Oncol 1997; 4:247–251.

83. Wells RE, Cruse CW, Daniels S, et al. The use of lymphoscintigraphy in melanoma of the head and neck. Plast Reconstr Surg 1994; 93:757–61.

84. O'Brien CJ, Uren RF, Thompson JF, et al. Prediction of potential metastatic sites in cutaneous head and neck melanoma using lymphoscintigraphy. Am J Surg 1995; 170:461–6.

85. Reintgen DS, Rapaport DP, Tanabe K, et al. Lymphatic mapping and sentinel lymphadenectomy. In Balch CM et al., eds. *Cutaneous melanoma*. St Louis, MI, Quality Medical Publishing Inc., 1998; 227–44.

86. Thompson JF, Uren RF, Shaw HM, et al. Location of sentinel lymph nodes in patients with cutaneous melanoma; new insights into lymphatic anatomy. J Am Coll Surg 1999; 189:195–206.

87. Kinmonth JB. *The lymphatics: diseases, lymphography, and surgery*. Baltimore, Williams and Wilkins, 1972.

88. Wong JH, Cagle LH, Morton DL. Lymphatic drainage of skin to a sentinel lymph node in a feline model. Ann Surg 1991; 214:637–41.

89. Morton DL, Wen D-R, Wong JH, et al. Technical details of intraoperative lymphatic mapping for early stage melanoma. Arch Surg 1992; 127:392–9.

90. Alex JC, Weaver DL, Fairbank JJ, et al. Gamma-probe-guided lymph node localization in malignant melanoma. Surg Oncol 1993; 2:303–8.

91. Krag DN, Meijer ST, Weaver DL, et al. Minimal-access surgery for staging of malignant melanoma. Arch Surg 1995; 130:654–8.

92. Albertini JJ, Cruse CW, Rapaport D, et al. Intraoperative radiolymphoscintigraphy improves sentinel lymph node identification for patients with melanoma. Ann Surg 1996; 223:217–24.

93. Leong SP, Steinmetz I, Habib FA, et al. Optimal selective sentinel lymph node dissection in primary malignant melanoma. Arch Surg 1997; 132:666–73.

94. Thompson JF, McCarthy WH, Bosch CM, et al. Sentinel lymph node status as an indicator of the presence of metastatic melanoma in regional lymph nodes. Melanoma Res 1995; 5:255–60.

95. Lingam MK, Mackie RM, McKay AJ. Intraoperative identification of sentinel lymph node in patients with malignant melanoma. Br J Cancer 1997; 75:1505–8.

96. Bostick P, Essner R, Glass E, et al. Comparison of blue dye and probe-assisted intraoperative lymphatic mapping in melanoma to identify sentinel nodes in 100 lymphatic basins. Arch Surg 1999; 134:43–9.

97. Gershenwald JE, Thompson W, Mansfield PF, et al. Multi-institutional melanoma lymphatic mapping experience: the prognostic value of sentinel lymph node status in 612 stage I or II melanoma patients. J Clin Oncol 1999; 17:976–83.

98. Morton DL, Thompson JF, Essner R, et al. Validation of the accuracy of intraoperative lymphatic mapping and sentinel lymphadenectomy for early stage melanoma: a multicenter trial. Ann Surg 1999; 23:453–65.

99. Morton DL, Chan AD. Current status of intraoperative lymphatic mapping and sentinel lymphadenectomy for melanoma: is it standard of care? J Am Coll Surg 1999; 189:214–23.

100. Gershenwald JE, Colome MI, Lee JE, et al. Patterns of recurrence following a negative sentinel lymph node biopsy in 243 patients with stage I or II melanoma. J Clin Oncol 1998; 16:2253–60.

101. Lane N, Lattes R, Malm J. Clinico-pathological correlation in a series of 117 malignant melanomas of the skin of adults. Cancer 1958; 11:1025–43.

102. Ordonez NG, Ji XL, Hickey RC. Comparison of HMB-45 monoclonal antibody and S-100 protein in the immunohistochemical diagnosis of melanoma. Am J Clin Pathol 1988; 90:385–90.

103. Cochran AJ, Wen D-R, Herschman HR. Occult melanoma in lymph nodes detected by antiserum to S-100 protein. Int J Cancer 1984; 34:159–63.

104. Cochran AJ, Wen D-R, Morton DL. Occult tumor cells in the lymph nodes of patients with pathological stage I malignant melanoma. Am J Surg Pathol 1988; 12:612–18.

105. Cochran AJ, Lu HF, Li PX, et al. S-100 protein remains a practical marker for melanocytic and other tumours. Melanoma Res 1993; 3:325–30.

106. Wick MR, Swanson PE. Recognition of malignant melanoma by monoclonal antibody HMB-45: an immunohistochemical study of 200 paraffin-embedded cutaneous tumors. J Cutan Pathol 1988; 15:201–7.

107. Fernando SS, Johnson S, Bate J. Immunohistochemical analysis of cutaneous malignant melanoma: comparison of S-100 protein, HMB-45 monoclonal antibody and NKI/C3 monoclonal antibody. Pathology 1994; 26:16–19.

108. Balch CM, Houghton AN. Diagnosis of metastatic melanoma at distant sites. In Balch CM, Houghton AN, Milton CW, et al., eds. Cutaneous melanoma, 2nd edn. Philadelphia, J.B. Lippincott, 1992, 441–5.

109. Goscin C, Glass F, Messina JL. Pathologic examination of the sentinel lymph node in melanoma. Surg Oncol Clin North Am 1999; 8:427–34.

110. Wang X, Heller R, VanVoorhis N, et al. Detection of sub-microscopic lymph node metastases with polymerase chain reaction in patients with malignant melanoma. Ann Surg 1994; 220:768–74.

111. Reintgen D, Albertini J, Miliotes G, et al. The accurate staging and modern-day treatment of malignant melanoma. Cancer Res Therapy Control 1995; 4:183–97.

112. Goydes JS, Ravikumar TS, Germino FJ, et al. Minimally invasive staging in patients with melanoma: sentinel lymphadenectomy and detection of the melanoma-specific proteins MART-1 and tyrosinase by reverse transcriptase polymerase chain. J Am Coll Surg 1998; 187:182–90.

113. Sarantou T, Chi DD, Garrison DA, et al. Melanoma associated antigens as messenger RNA detection markers for melanoma. Cancer Res 1997; 57:1371–6.

114. Kuo CT, Bostick PJ, Irie RF, et al. Assessment of messenger RNA of β14→ N-acetylgalactosaminyl-transferase as a molecular marker for metastatic melanoma. Clin Cancer Res 1998; 4:411–18.

115. Morton DL. Sentinel lymphadenectomy for patients with clinical stage I melanoma. J Surg Oncol 1997; 66:267–9.

116. Coit DG. Prognostic factors in patients with melanoma to regional lymph nodes. Surg Oncol Clin North Am 1992; 1(2):281–95.

117. Cunningham TJ, Schoenfeld D, Nathanson L, et al. A controlled ECOG study of adjuvant therapy with BCG or BCG plus DTIC in patients with stage I and II malignant melanoma. In Terry WD, Rosenberg SA, eds. Immunotherapy of human cancer. Amsterdam, Elsevier North Holland, 1982; 271–7.

118. Morton DL, Holmes EC, Eilber FR, et al. Adjuvant immunotherapy of malignant melanoma: results of a randomized trial in patients with lymph node metastases. In Terry WD, Rosenberg SA, eds. Immunotherapy of human cancer. Amsterdam, Elsevier North Holland, 1982; 245–9.

119. Quirt IC, Shelley WE, Pater JL, et al. Improved survival in patients with poor-prognosis malignant melanoma treated with adjuvant levamisole: a phase III study by the National Cancer Institute of Canada Clinical Trials Group. J Clin Oncol 1991; 9:729–35.

120. Spitler LE. A randomized trial of levamisole versus placebo as adjuvant therapy in malignant melanoma. J Clin Oncol 1991; 9:736–40.

121. Miller LL, Spitler LE, Allen RE, et al. A randomized, double-blind, placebo-controlled trial of transfer factor as adjuvant therapy for malignant melanoma. Cancer 1988; 61:1543–9.

122. Lipton A, Harvey HA, Balch CM, et al. Corynebacterium parvum versus Bacille Calmette–Guérin adjuvant immunotherapy of stage II malignant melanoma. J Clin Oncol 1991; 9:1151–6.

123. Karakousis CP, Didolkar MS, Lopez R, et al. Chemoimmunotherapy (DTIC and Corynebacterium parvum) as adjuvant treatment in malignant melanoma. Cancer Treat Rep 1979; 63:1739.

124. Veronesi U, Adamus J, Aubert C, et al. A randomized trial of adjuvant chemotherapy and immunotherapy in cutaneous melanoma. N Engl J Med 1982; 307:913–16.

125. Misset JL, Mathe G, Cupissol D, et al. Eight-year update on the Oncofrance Melanoma Adjuvant Trial. In Salmon SE, Jones SE, eds. Adjuvant therapy of cancer IV. New York, Grune & Stratton, 1984, 557.

126. McIllmurray MB, Embleton MJ, Reeves WG, et al. Controlled trial of active immunotherapy in management of stage IIB malignant melanoma. BMJ 1977; 1:540–2.

127. Morton DL. Adjuvant immunotherapy of malignant melanoma: status of clinical trials at UCLA. Int J Immunother 1986; 2:31.

128. Terry WD, Hodes RJ, Rosenberg SA, et al. Treatment of stage I and II malignant melanoma with adjuvant immunotherapy or chemotherapy: preliminary analysis of a prospective randomized trial. In Terry WD, Rosenberg SA, eds. Immunotherapy of human cancer. Amsterdam, Elsevier North Holland, 1982; 251–7.

129. Steffens TA, Livingston PO. Status of adjuvant therapy of melanoma. Surg Oncol Clin North Am 1992; 1(2):307–33.

130. Kirkwood JM, Agarwala S. Systemic cytotoxic and biologic therapy of melanoma. PPO Updates 1993; 7:1–16.

131. Kirkwood JM, Strawdrerman MH, Ernstoff MS, et al. Interferon alpha-2b adjuvant therapy of high-risk resected cutaneous melanoma: the Eastern Cooperative Oncology Group Trial 5T 1684. J Clin Oncol 1996; 14:7–17.

132. Cascinelli N. Evaluation of efficacy of adjuvant IFN-α-2a in melanoma patients with regional node

metastases. Proc Am Soc Clin Oncol 1995; 14:410 (abstract).

133. Grob J, Dreno B, Delauney M, *et al.* Results of the French multicenter trial on adjuvant therapy with interferon-α-2a in resected primary melanoma (1.5 mm). Proc Am Soc Clin Oncol 1996; 15:437.

134. Pehamberger H, Soyer P, Steiner A, *et al.* Adjuvant interferon α-2a treatment in resected primary cutaneous melanoma. Melanoma Res 1997; 7(Suppl. 1):S31.

135. Creagan E, Dalton R, Ahmann D, *et al.* Randomized, surgical adjuvant clinical trial of recombinant interferon α-2a in selected patients with malignant melanoma. J Clin Oncol 1995; 13:2776–83.

136. Kirkwood J, Ibrahim J, Sondak V, *et al.* Role of high-dose IFN in high-risk melanoma: preliminary results of the E1690/S9111/C9190 U.S. Intergroup Postoperative Adjuvant Trial of high- and low-dose IFNα2b (HDI and LDI) in resected high-risk primary or regionally lymph node metastatic melanoma in relation to 10-year updated results of E1684. Symposium on Advances in Biology and Treatment of Cutaneous Melanoma, November 7, 1998, Boston.

ANNOTATED BIBLIOGRAPHY

Balch CM, Soong SW, Bartolucci AA, *et al.* Efficacy of an elective regional lymph-node dissection of 1.0 to 4.0 mm thick melanomas for patients 60 years of age and younger. Ann Surg 1996; 224:255–66.

The Intergroup Melanoma Surgical Trial report on a major study to determine if clinical and pathologic prognostic determinants could identify subgroups of patients at higher risk for occult regional micrometastases and whether elective lymph node dissection improves survival. Seven hundred and forty patients were eligible and evaluable for study, and the average length of follow-up was 7.4 years. Whereas overall survival at 5 years was no different whether or not ELND was performed, subgroup analysis demonstrated a statistically significant benefit for ELND in patients aged 60 years or under whose melanomas were 1.0–2.0 mm thick without ulceration.

Balch CM, Soong SJ, Milton GW, *et al.* A comparison of prognostic factors and surgical results in 1786 patients with localized (stage I) melanoma treated in Alabama, USA, and New South Wales, Australia. Ann Surg 1982; 196:677–84.

This is the major retrospective study of patients treated by either wide excision alone or wide excision and elective regional lymphadenectomy. The benefit of elective regional lymphadenectomy was greatest in patients with lesion thickness of 1.50–3.99 mm. For lesions 0.76–1.49 mm in thickness, the benefit was more modest; there was no benefit of elective regional lymphadenectomy for patients with thin lesions (<0.76 mm) or thick lesions (⩾4.00 mm).

Coates AS, Ingvar CI, Petersen-Schaefer K, *et al.* Elective lymph node dissection in patients with primary melanoma of the trunk and limbs treated at the Sydney Melanoma Unit from 1960 to 1991. J Am Coll Surg 1995; 180:403–9.

A retrospective analysis of 1278 clinical stage I patients with melanomas of the trunks or limbs measuring 1.5 mm or more in thickness: 845 (66%) were treated with elective regional lymphadenectomy, the remainder with wide excision alone. No benefit was demonstrated for patients having elective regional lymphadenectomy compared to wide excision alone.

Morton DL, Thompson JF, Essner R, *et al.* Validation of the accuracy of intraoperative lymphatic mapping and sentinel lymphadenectomy for early stage melanoma: a multicenter trial. Ann Surg 1999; 230:453–65.

Report of the International Multicenter Selective Lymphadenectomy Trial (MSLT) examined the accuracy of the technique of sentinel node identification using the experience of the organizing center (John Wayne Cancer Institute), by which to compare the experiences at the other participating centers. There were 551 patients in the multicenter group and 584 patients in the organizing center group. In both groups, blue dye plus a radiocolloid was more successful (99.1%) than blue dye alone (95.2%). After a center had completed the 30-case learning phase, the success was independent of the center's case volume or experience. This validated the technique when a multidisciplinary approach (surgery, nuclear medicine, and pathology) and a learning phase of ⩾30 consecutive cases in which sentinel lymphadenectomy was followed by completion lymphadenectomy were utilized.

Morton DL, Wen DR, Wong JH, *et al.* Technical details of intraoperative lymphatic mapping for early stage melanoma. Arch Surg 1992; 127:392–9.

This initial major report presented a new procedure for identifying the specific lymph node(s) within the regional nodal drainage basin(s) draining the primary melanoma cutaneous site and therefore most likely to be the site of micrometastases ('sentinel node'). The reliability of this technique was assessed by following with a completion regional lymphadenectomy. In 194 lymphadenectomy specimens with an identifiable sentinel lymph node, skip metastases in non-sentinel nodes without sentinel node metastases were present in only 1% of instances.

Roses DF, Provet JA, Harris MN, Gumport SL, Dubin N. Prognosis of patients with pathologic stage II cutaneous malignant melanoma. Ann Surg 1985; 201:103–7.

Traditional analyses of regional lymph node dissections have compared patients with micrometastases (clinical stage I) to those with clinically palpable disease (clinical stage II). In this study, the 5-year and 10-year survival rates for clinical stage I patients were 44% and 28%, respectively, and for clinical stage II patients, 21% and 12%, respectively ($p < 0.0001$). A 5-year cumulative survival rate of 65% was achieved for clinical stage I patients having primary lesions of < 2.0 mm in thickness, whereas it was 19% for patients having primary lesions of 5.0 mm or more.

Veronesi U, Adamus J, Bandierra DC, *et al*. Delayed regional lymph node dissection in stage I malignant melanoma of the skin of the lower extremities. Cancer 1982; 49:2420–30.

The WHO Melanoma Group randomized study compared patients with extremity melanoma having wide excision and elective regional lymphadenectomy (267 patients) to those having wide excision alone followed by lymph node dissection only if clinical nodal metastases developed on follow-up observation (286 patients). There was no statistically significant difference in survival between the two groups. Subsequent retrospective microstaging and re-analysis by major prognostic variables (World J Surg 1992; 16:206–13) demonstrated no difference in survival in the two groups by sex, thickness, or by the presence of micrometastases in the elective node group compared to those developing clinical nodal metastases on follow-up.

Commentary

CHARLES M BALCH

The chapter by Dr Roses is an excellent review of the controversies surrounding the role of elective node dissection in melanoma. In my view, much of the debate at this point has subsided for two reasons:

1 The technological advance of sentinel lymphadenectomy has supplanted, for the most part, the decision making which was previously based upon the statistical probability of clinically occult nodal metastases.

2 The long-term results of the Intergroup Surgical Trial have now been published (since the submission of Dr Roses' chapter) and demonstrate even more definitively than before that intermediate-thickness, non-ulcerated melanoma patients have a statistically improved survival rate with elective node dissection. This means that surgeons who substitute a sentinel lymphadenectomy (with complete node dissection for histologically demonstrated nodal metastases) must be careful to avoid a false-negative result in their patients, or they may miss an opportunity to maximize their chance for cure.

Thus, research into the prognostic factors predicting the risk of nodal metastases and survival outcome has reached a point of agreement that has fostered a major revision of the melanoma staging classification.[1,2]

This commentary summarizes four areas pertaining to this important subject:

1 the rationale for lymph node dissection in melanoma,
2 the new staging system for melanoma,
3 updated information from the Intergroup Melanoma Surgical Trial with regard to elective node dissection,
4 the role of intraoperative lymphatic mapping and sentinel lymphadenectomy.

RATIONALE FOR LYMPH NODE DISSECTION IN MELANOMA

There are three major goals of cancer surgery: staging, cure, and palliation. Surgical excision of metastatic melanoma in the regional lymph nodes is one of the few clinical situations in which all three goals are a central part of the treatment, including a curative benefit in some patients with metastatic nodal disease, especially when the tumor burden is microscopic. Naturally, the earlier the surgeon removes nodal metastases (as a potential source of life-threatening distant metastases), the greater the likelihood of cure for an individual patient. However, even in a non-curative situation, surgery is the most effective treatment for removing or preventing disabling symptoms from the local growth of metastasis while the patient is dying from metastatic growth in a distant vital organ.

Decisions regarding node dissection for clinically occult disease are so much better today because of improved staging techniques and the technology associated with intraoperative lymphatic mapping and sentinel lymphadenectomy. Microstaging of a primary melanoma, with the combined use of tumor thickness and ulceration, can now provide an accurate statistical probability of a patient having clinically occult nodal metastases. Over the past few years, there has been a worldwide validation of the staging accuracy and reproducibility of intraoperative lymphatic mapping and sentinel lymphadenectomy, pioneered by Dr Donald Morton at the John Wayne Cancer Center in Santa Monica, California.[3] This surgical technique has provided the surgeon with a precise tool that, when properly used, can stage for the presence or absence of a metastatic tumor down to a threshold of 10^5 to 10^6 cells with an accuracy of 95%. In fact, the technique has proved so reproducible and valuable as a staging procedure that the American Joint Committee on Cancer (AJCC) Melanoma Committee has recommended that *all* patients with T2, T3, and T4 melanomas should have a sentinel lymphadenectomy, both to improve their cure rates (for T2 and T3 lesions) and for staging prior to entry into a melanoma clinical trial (for T2, T3, and T4 lesions).

The rationale for a node dissection (either electively or via sentinel lymphadenectomy) is to remove microscopic nodal metastases before they can disseminate to distant sites. On the other hand, if the patient already has distant microscopic metastases, then there will surely be no survival benefit from removing regional nodal metastases at that point. But which patients fit in this theoretical category? Results from the Intergroup Melanoma Surgical Trial demonstrate that prognostic factors (especially tumor thickness and ulceration) can prospectively identify melanoma patients at a sufficiently high risk for occult regional metastases to justify surgical excision of their regional lymph nodes, and at a sufficiently low risk for distant occult metastases to have a therapeutic benefit.[4] The window of time during which early surgical intervention halts the further dissemination of melanoma metastases from regional to distant sites is estimated at 16 months, which is the average relapse time for patients who had a primary excision and nodal observation, and whose original nodal micrometastases evolved into clinically detectable disease. The results are summarized below.

There is also a very compelling rationale for the pathological staging of regional lymph nodes for patients prior to entry into adjuvant systemic therapy trials. Differences in 2-year and 5-year survival for patients with and without clinically occult nodal metastases can vary by as much as 20–25%. Indeed, some of the problems in interpreting and comparing past clinical trials involving melanoma have concerned the inability to account fully for the pathological differences in nodal status in a heterogeneous group of T3 and T4 patients, some of whom had pathological assessment of their regional nodes, whereas others had only clinical assessment.

STAGING OF MELANOMA

The summary here focuses on those prognostic factors that predict the risk of nodal metastases and survival of stage III patients. The reader is referred to the complete staging information for further details.[1] The AJCC has now approved major revisions of the melanoma TNM and stage grouping criteria for melanoma that will become official with the publication of the sixth edition of the staging manual in 2002. The proposed TNM classifications are shown in Table 1 and the proposed stage groupings are shown in Table 2.

Major revisions in melanoma staging include:

1 melanoma thickness and ulceration to be used in the T classification,
2 the number of metastatic lymph nodes, rather than their gross dimensions, and the delineation of microscopic versus macroscopic nodal metastases to be used in the N classification,
3 an upstaging of all patients with stage I, II, and III disease when a primary melanoma is ulcerated,
4 a new convention for defining clinical and pathological staging so as to take into account the new staging information gained from intraoperative lymphatic mapping and sentinel node biopsy.

For stage III melanoma, in almost all studies analysing prognosis using Cox regression analysis, either the number or the percentage of metastatic lymph nodes was the strongest predictor of outcome.[2,5–7] This was true regardless of whether the patient presentation involved microscopic or macroscopic nodal metastases. In all studies that have examined prognosis based upon the number of metastatic nodes, patients with one metastatic node did better than those with any combination of two or more metastatic nodes.

The AJCC Melanoma Staging Committee concluded that it was important to identify patients with clinically occult (microscopic) separately from those with clinically apparent (macroscopic) nodal metastases in the staging classification. This is because of data demonstrating that patients with microscopic nodal involvement fare better compared to those who have a therapeutic node dissection for clinically evident nodal metastases.[8] The staging convention will use the designation 'clinical stage' or 'pathological stage' to make such a delineation.

Clinical staging is defined when the available information comprises microstaging of the primary melanoma, and clinical/radiological evaluation for metastases. By convention, it would be used after complete excision of the primary melanoma with clinical assessment for regional and distant metastases.

Pathological staging is defined when the available information comprises microstaging of the primary melanoma and pathological information about the regional lymph nodes after partial or complete lymphadenectomy, except that pathological stage 0 or stage IA patients do not need pathological evaluation of their lymph nodes.

The convention for defining microscopic disease is somewhat arbitrary because occasional patients may have a substantial tumor burden that is still 'clinically occult' (e.g., an obese patient or a deep-seated axillary metastasis).

Tumor thickness and ulceration are the two independent prognostic factors that predict the risk of occult or microscopic nodal metastases.[9–12] Using a melanoma database from the University of Alabama at Birmingham and the Sydney Melanoma Unit, we had first demonstrated the

Table 1 *Proposed TNM classification*

T classification	Thickness (mm)	Ulceration status
T1	≤1.0	a: without ulceration
T1		b: with ulceration
T2	1.1–2.0	a: without ulceration
T2		b: with ulceration
T3	2.1–4.0	a: without ulceration
T3		b: with ulceration
T4	>4.0	a: without ulceration
T4		b: with ulceration

N classification	Number of metastatic nodes	Nodal metastatic mass
N1	1 node	a: micrometastasis[1] b: macrometastasis[2]
N2	2–3 nodes	a: micrometastasis[1] b: macrometastasis[2] c: in-transit metastasis(es)/ satellite(s) without metastatic nodes
N3	≥4 metastatic nodes or matted nodes or in-transit metastasis(es)/ satellite(s) and metastatic nodes	

M classification	Site	Serum LDH
M1a	Distant skin, SQ or nodal metastases	Normal
M1b	Lung metastases	Normal
M1c	All other visceral metastases or any distant metastasis	Normal Elevated

[1] Micrometastases are diagnosed after elective or sentinel lymphadenectomy and are metastases confined within an intact capsule of a normal-sized lymph node.
[2] Macrometastases are defined as clinically detectable nodal metastases confirmed by therapeutic lymphadenectomy or when any nodal metastasis exhibits extracapsular extension.

correlation of melanoma thickness and ulceration (on histopathological sections) and the incidence of nodal metastases in a series of papers published between 1978 and 1982.[9,10,13,14] More recently, in a definitive prognostic factors analysis from MD Anderson Cancer Center, melanoma thickness and ulceration were the two most powerful predictors of finding a microscopic nodal metastasis by sentinel lymphadenectomy. Once the nodal status was known, the presence or absence of nodal metastasis was the most powerful predictor of survival.[11,15]

Stage grouping for regional metastases (stage III)

In patients with metastatic regional metastases after sentinel or elective lymphadenectomy, the new stage grouping for pathological stage III melanoma uses the number and clinical status of metastatic regional disease as well as the presence or absence of ulceration of the primary melanoma (Table 2). The presence of one to three microscopic (i.e., clinically occult) nodal metastasis (N1a and N2a) identified after sentinel or elective

lymphadenectomy in patients with a non-ulcerated primary melanoma (T1–4a) is associated with a 5-year survival of 63–69% (unpublished data). This is such an excellent prognostic group that the AJCC Melanoma Committee put them in a separate stage group designated as pathological stage IIIA. Patients with one to three microscopic (clinically occult) nodes (N2a) arising from an ulcerated primary melanoma (T1–4b) are equivalent prognostically to patients with one to three macroscopic metastatic node (N1b and N2b) arising from a non-ulcerated primary melanoma (T1–4a) and are grouped together as pathological stage IIIB. All patients with four or more macroscopic nodes (N3) or those with any nodal disease in the presence of satellites/in transit metastases are at especially high risk for systemic metastases and are grouped as pathological stage IIIC (Table 2).

ELECTIVE NODE DISSECTION

The long-term results of the Intergroup Melanoma Surgical Trial have recently been published.[4] This randomized

Table 2 *Proposed stage groupings for cutaneous melanoma*

Clinical staging[1]				Pathologic staging[2]			
0	Tis	N0	M0	0	Tis	N0	M0
IA	T1a	N0	M0	IA	T1a	N0	M0
IB	T1b	N0	M0	IB	T1b	N0	M0
	T2a	N0	M0		T2a	N0	M0
IIA	T2b	N0	M0	IIA	T2b	N0	M0
	T3a	N0	M0		T3a	N0	M0
IIB	T3b	N0	M0	IIB	T3b	N0	M0
	T4a	N0	M0		T4a	N0	M0
IIC	T4b	N0	M0	IIC	T4b	N0	M0
III	Any T	Any N	M0	IIIA	T1–4a	N1a	M0
					T1–4a	N2a	M0
				IIIB	T1–4b	N1a	M0
					T1–4b	N2a	M0
					T1–4a	N1b	M0
					T1–4a	N2b	M0
					T1–4a	N2c	M0
				IIIC	T1–4b	N1b	M0
					T1–4b	N2b	M0
					T1–4b	N2c	M0
					Any T	N3	M0
IV	Any T	Any N	Any M	IV	Any T	Any N	Any M

[1] Clinical staging includes microstaging of the primary melanoma, and clinical/radiological evaluation for metastases. By convention, it should be used after complete excision of the primary melanoma with clinical assessment for regional and distant metastases.
[2] Pathological staging includes microstaging of the primary melanoma and pathological information about the regional lymph nodes after partial or complete lymphadenectomy. Pathological stage 0 or stage IA patients are the exception; they do not need pathological evaluation of their lymph nodes.

surgical trial demonstrated, for the first time, that prospectively defined groups of melanoma patients have a significant reduction of mortality if they have an elective node dissection compared to those whose initial management was clinical observation of the nodal basin and a later therapeutic lymphadenectomy for clinically apparent nodal metastases, an event that took place on an average of 16 months after the diagnosis. Presumably, this delay in treating established metastases allowed further growth and dissemination at distant sites during that average 16-month delay.

The Intergroup Melanoma Surgical Trial has been conducted since 1983 to prospectively determine:

1 whether early intervention with elective or immediate regional node dissection would have a therapeutic benefit;
2 whether currently available prognostic factors could identify subgroups of patients with intermediate-thickness melanomas who had a high risk for clinically occult regional node metastases.

This is the largest randomized surgical trial ever conducted to address the surgical management of regional lymph nodes for melanoma and to confirm the validity of prognostic factors to define risk groups. The stated objective of the trial was to test whether any combination of clinical and pathological factors could be used to predict a high-risk subgroup for which elective lymph node dissection (ELND) would improve survival rates.

Ten-year to 15-year survival results were analysed from a prospective, multi-institutional, randomized surgical trial involving 740 stage I and II melanoma patients with intermediate-thickness melanomas (1.0–4.0 mm), comparing (immediate) ELND to clinical observation of the lymph nodes as well as prognostic factors independently predicting outcomes. Using Cox stepwise multivariate regression analysis, the independent predictors of outcome were tumor thickness ($p < 0.001$), the presence of tumor ulceration ($p < 0.001$), trunk site ($p = 0.003$) and patient age >60 years ($p = 0.01$). Overall 10-year survival was not significantly different for patients who received ELND or nodal observation (77% versus 73%, $p = 0.12$). Among the prospectively stratified subgroups of patients, 10-year survival rates favored those patients with ELND, with a 30% mortality reduction for the 543 patients with non-ulcerated melanomas (84% versus 77%, $p = 0.03$), a 30% mortality reduction for the 446 patients with tumor thickness of 1.0–2.0 mm (86% versus 80%, $p = 0.03$) and a 27% reduction in mortality for 385 patients with extremity melanomas (84% versus 78%, $p = 0.05$). Of these subgroups, the presence or absence of ulceration should be the key factor for making treatment recommendations with regard to ELND for patients with intermediate-thickness melanomas.

When designing this trial, we anticipated that not all patients with intermediate-thickness melanoma would benefit from ELND. We therefore prospectively defined subgroups of patients based upon the available data at that time. Even though the overall results did not demonstrate a survival benefit, there was a 25–30% relative reduction in mortality in three prospectively defined subgroups: those without tumor ulceration, those with tumor thickness of 1.0–2.0 mm, and those with extremity melanomas. Of these three groups, we believe the most significant for clinical decision making is the presence or absence of melanoma ulceration. Indeed, it appears likely that the reason thicker melanomas and trunk melanomas did not have a survival benefit is because of the higher incidence of ulcerated melanomas among these other subgroups of patients.

The Intergroup Melanoma Trial is therefore the only randomized surgical trial designed at the outset to examine any benefit of ELND in a prospectively defined subgroup known to have a potential survival benefit based on prior retrospective studies. The survival benefit demonstrated in this trial is entirely consistent with what is predicted from previous studies describing the natural history of metastatic melanoma based on prognostic factors,[5,9–11,13] with the results of non-randomized surgical studies showing a therapeutic benefit for patients with intermediate-thickness melanomas,[10,16] and with the negative results of the prior three randomized ELND trials which were not designed to address a potential benefit in this specific subgroup of patients.[17]

Our results from a mature database demonstrate that prognostic factors (especially tumor thickness and ulceration) can prospectively identify melanoma patients at a sufficiently high risk for occult regional metastases to justify surgical excision of their regional lymph nodes, and at a sufficiently low risk for distant occult metastases to have a therapeutic benefit. The window of time during which early surgical intervention halts the further dissemination of melanoma metastases from regional to distant sites is estimated at 16 months, which is the average relapse time for patients who had wide excision only, and whose original micrometastases subsequently evolved into clinically detectable disease.

SENTINEL NODE DISSECTION

Intralymphatic mapping and sentinel lymphadenectomy (SLND) comprise a major technological advance, pioneered by Dr Donald Morton and colleagues after the Intergroup Melanoma Surgical Trial was completed.[3,12] The use of SLND has two inherent advantages over ELND:

1 The indications for a complete lymph node dissection with SLND are based upon a pathological documentation of nodal metastasis, whereas with ELND the decision for performing a complete node dissection is based upon the mathematical probability of a patient harboring occult nodal metastasis.

2 The SLND procedure provides the pathologist with a limited amount of lymph node tissue which is most likely to contain metastases and for which a more detailed examination, with serial sectioning and immunohistochemical staining looking for micrometastases, is better justified.

The survival benefit of the ELND surgical trial described above provides an underpinning of data supporting the survival advantage of early surgical intervention to remove regional micrometastases. It is important for surgeons to minimize their false-negative rate when substituting SLND for ELND in those patients defined by this trial who might otherwise develop a later recurrence and have missed their opportunity for a curative intervention. ELND should be considered with curative intent in the subgroups described above (i.e., intermediate-thickness melanomas without ulceration) in those circumstances in which SLND is not available, when a patient has already had a wide excision (which negates the accuracy of the mapping procedure), or if the mapping is not technically feasible.

It is important to emphasize that the sentinel lymph node is anatomically defined as the first lymph node receiving afferent lymphatic drainage from a primary melanoma site. It would therefore probably contain micrometastases if they were present. The sentinel node is not a 'blue node' or a 'hot node' – which are simply reflections of the technology that is applied to identify the biological event of nodal metastases. If the technique is not performed correctly, the true sentinel lymph node may not be identified, leading to a false-negative result and a clinical relapse months later. It is therefore vitally important that surgeons using SLND engage a coordinated team of surgeons, nuclear medicine physicians, and surgical pathologists. If the technique of intradermal injections of the tracer material and the pathological review of the specimen is relegated to less experienced individuals, the false-negative rate may exceed those already published by experienced centers. In our opinion, this false-negative rate should not exceed 5%, especially in view of the recent evidence from the randomized ELND surgical trial demonstrating the benefit in nonulcerative melanomas of intermediate thickness.

In a recent paper, Drs Essner, Morton, and colleagues from the John Wayne Cancer Institute found that the actuarial 5-year survival rates were essentially equivalent in those patients undergoing SLND (with complete lymph node dissection if pathologically indicated) and ELND.[12] In addition, the incidence of metastatic nodes in SLND specimens was twice that of ELND specimens (24% versus 12%) for the 1.5–4.0 mm subgroup. These confirm prior results from other institutions where the yield of documenting micrometastases in serially sectioned lymph nodes was twice that for an ELND surgical pathology specimen of the entire nodal basin using conventional pathological processing (i.e., hematoxylin and eosin staining of a bivalved nodal specimen). Results from the MD Anderson Cancer Center have also shown that the incidence of nodal metastases is approximately the same for SLND and ELND when comparing pathological yield using routine pathological processing.[11] The increased incidence of nodal metastases described by Essner et al. is likely to be due to 'stage migration' because of more rigorous examination of the nodal specimen (i.e., using serial sectioning and immunohistochemical staining) and to imbalances of prognostic factors, such as tumor ulceration, that could not be accounted for in a retrospective matched-pair analysis. Nevertheless, the true incidence of nodal micrometastases is substantially greater than that identified in ELND specimens, as demonstrated in the 1.0–4.0 mm thickness subgroup followed prospectively in the Intergroup Melanoma Surgery Trial.[4]

Unquestionably, the SLND technique facilitates a more accurate pathological staging and, as a consequence, contributes to a significant 'upstaging' of patients to stage III melanoma who previously would otherwise be designated as node-negative or stage I or II melanoma. It also creates a more homogeneous group of node-negative melanoma patients for entry into clinical trials. Such accurately staged melanoma patients at high risk for systemic micrometastases should be considered for clinical trials involving adjuvant systemic therapy.

Dr Morton and his colleagues have made a major contribution to surgical oncology with the sentinel lymphadenectomy technique. Their procedure contributes to more accurate staging of melanoma patients and will probably improve the cure rates of patients with clinically occult metastatic nodal disease, both by better staging and by surgical removal of micrometastases before they disseminate further.

Dr Roses is to be commended for providing a lucid and comprehensive review of elective node dissection, which has been one of the most controversial surgical management issues for over 30 years. Thankfully, advances in our understanding of prognosis, clinical trials, and sentinel node technology now enable surgeons to better stage melanoma patients and to recommend a treatment plan that is more precisely and individually tailored to the biology and natural history of their disease presentation. However, there is still much research to do, especially in the area of molecular staging and effective adjuvant system therapy. Advances in these two areas are paramount to further improving cure rates for this increasingly common cancer.

REFERENCES

1. Balch CM, Buzaid AC, Atkins MB, et al. A New American Joint Committee on Cancer staging system for cutaneous melanoma. Cancer 2000; 88:1484–91.

2. Buzaid AC, Ross MI, Balch CM, et al. Critical analysis of the current American Joint Committee on Cancer staging system for cutaneous melanoma and proposal of a new staging system. J Clin Oncol, 1997; 15: 1039–51.

3. Morton DL, Wen D-R, Wong JH, et al. Technical details of intraoperative lymphatic mapping for early stage melanoma. Arch Surg, 1992; 127:392–9.

4. Balch CM, Soong S-J, Ross MI, et al. Long-term results of a multi-institutional randomized trial comparing prognostic factors and surgical results for intermediate thickness melanomas (1.0 to 4.0 mm). Ann Surg Oncol 2000; 7:87–97.

5. Balch CM. Cutaneous melanoma: prognosis and treatment results worldwide. Semin Surg Oncol, 1992; 8:400–14.

6. Balch CM, Soong SJ, Murad TM, et al. A multifactorial analysis of melanoma: III. Prognostic factors in melanoma patients with lymph node metastases (stage II). Ann Surg, 1981; 193:377–88.

7. Morton DL, Wanek L, Nizze JA, et al. Improved long-term survival after lymphadenectomy of melanoma metastatic to regional nodes. Ann Surg 1991; 214:491–9.

8. Cascinelli N, Morabito A, Santinami M, et al. Immediate or delayed dissection of regional nodes in patients with melanoma of the trunk: a randomised trial. Lancet 1998; 351:793–6.

9. Balch CM, Murad TM, Soong SJ, et al. A multifactorial analysis of melanoma: prognostic histopathological features comparing Clark's and Breslow's staging methods. Ann Surg 1978; 188:732–42.

10. Balch CM, Soong SJ, Murad TM, et al. A multifactorial analysis of melanoma. II. Prognostic factors in patients with stage I (localized) melanoma. Surgery 1979; 86:343–51.

11. Gershenwald JE, Colome MI, Lee JE, et al. Patterns of recurrence following a negative sentinel lymph node biopsy in 243 patients with stage I or II melanoma. J Clin Oncol 1998; 16:2253–60.

12. Essner R, Conforti A, Kelley MC, et al. Efficacy of lymphadenectomy and selective complete lymph node dissection as a therapeutic procedure for early-stage melanoma. Ann Surg Oncol 1999; 6:442–9.

13. Balch CM, Soong SJ, Milton GW, et al. A comparison of prognostic factors and surgical results in 1,786 patients with localized (stage I) melanoma treated in Alabama, USA, and New South Wales, Australia. Ann Surg 1982; 196:677–84.

14. Balch CM, Wilkerson JA, Murad TM, et al. The prognostic significance of ulceration of cutaneous melanoma. Cancer 1980; 45:3012–17.

15. Gershenwald JE, Thompson W, Mansfield PF, *et al*. Multi-institutional melanoma lymphatic mapping experience: the prognostic value of sentinel lymph node status in 612 stage I or II melanoma patients. J Clin Oncol 1999; 17:976–83.

16. Balch CM. The role of elective lymph node dissection in melanoma: rationale, results, and controversies. J Clin Oncol 1988; 6:163–72.

17. Balch CM. Surgical management of melanoma: results of prospective randomized trials. Ann Surg Oncol 1998; 5:301–9.

Editors' selected abstracts

HMB-45 immunohistochemical staining of sentinel lymph nodes: a specific method for enhancing detection of micrometastases in patients with melanoma.

Baisden BL, Askin FB, Lange JR, Westra WH.

Department of Pathology, The Johns Hopkins Medical Institutions, Baltimore, MD, USA.

American Journal of Surgical Pathology 24(8):1140–6, 2000, August.

Despite the profound therapeutic and prognostic implications of nodal metastases in patients with melanoma, there is no consensus strategy for the optimal detection of metastases in sentinel lymph node biopsies. Traditional microscopic examination may be too crude to detect scattered, individual tumor cells. Conversely, molecular genetic techniques are prone to false-positive results. The authors evaluated the ability of HMB-45 immunohistochemistry to enhance detection of melanoma cells in histologically negative sentinel lymph nodes. Ninety-six sentinel lymph nodes, collected over a 25-month period from 66 consecutive patients with melanoma, were processed routinely and sectioned serially. Slides 1, 3, and 5 were stained with hematoxylin and eosin. HMB-45 staining was performed on an intervening slide in histologically negative nodes. To assess the background incidence of HMB-45-positive cells in lymph nodes draining the skin, the authors stained 244 cervical and axillary lymph nodes from patients without melanoma. Metastases were apparent microscopically in 12 (18%) of the 66 patients with melanoma. Of the remaining 54 patients, four patients (7%) had lymph nodes harboring individual, scattered HMB-45-positive cells. Benign nevocellular aggregates were present in four of the 96 sentinel lymph nodes (4% nodal incidence), but they were HMB-45-negative. The authors did not observe a single HMB-45-positive cell in the 244 lymph nodes from patients without melanoma. Immunohistochemistry appears to represent a specific means of enhancing tumor detection in sentinel lymph nodes from patients with melanoma.

Incidence of sentinel node metastasis in patients with thin primary melanoma (≤1 mm) with vertical growth phase.

Bedrosian I, Faries MB, Guerry D 4th, Elenitsas R, Schuchter L, Mick R, Spitz FR, Bucky LP, Alavi A, Elder DE, Fraker DL, Czerniecki BJ.

Department of Surgery, University of Pennsylvania, Philadelphia, PA, USA.

Annals of Surgical Oncology 7(4):262–7, 2000, May.

Background: Patients with thin primary melanomas (≤1 mm) generally have an excellent prognosis. However, the presence of a vertical growth phase (VGP) adversely impacts the survival rate. We report on the rate of occurrence of nodal metastasis in patients with thin primary melanomas with a VGP who are offered sentinel lymph node (SLN) biopsy. *Methods:* Among 235 patients with clinically localized cutaneous melanomas who underwent successful SLN biopsy, 71 had lesions 1 mm or smaller with a VGP. The SLN was localized by using blue dye and a radiotracer. If negative for tumor by using hematoxylin and eosin staining, the SLN was further examined by immunohistochemistry. *Results:* The rate of occurrence of SLN metastasis was 15.2% in patients with melanomas deeper than 1 mm and 5.6% in patients with thin melanomas. Three patients with thin melanomas and a positive SLN had low-risk lesions, based on a highly accurate six-variable multivariate logistic regression model for predicting 8-year survival in stage I/II melanomas. The fourth patient had a low- to intermediate-risk lesion based on this model. At the time of the lymphadenectomy, one patient had two additional nodes with metastasis. *Conclusions:* VGP in a melanoma 1 mm or smaller seems to be a risk factor for nodal metastasis. The risk of nodal disease may not be accurately predicted by the use of a multivariate logistic regression model that incorporates thickness, mitotic rate, regression, tumor-infiltrating lymphocytes, sex, and anatomical site. Patients with thin lesions having VGP should be evaluated for SLN biopsy and trials of adjuvant therapy when stage III disease is found.

Examination of regional lymph nodes by sentinel node biopsy and molecular analysis provides new staging facilities in primary cutaneous melanoma.

Blaheta HJ, Ellwanger U, Schittek B, Sotlar K, MacZey E, Breuninger H, Thelen MH, Bueltmann B, Rassner G, Garbe C.

Department of Dermatology, Skin Cancer Program, Eberhard-Karls-University, Tuebingen, Germany.

Journal of Investigative Dermatology 114(4):637–42, 2000, April.

Histopathologic parameters of the primary tumor, such as Breslow's tumor thickness and Clark's level of invasion are the current basis for prognostic classifications of primary cutaneous melanoma. Once patients develop regional node metastasis, histopathologic features of the primary melanoma no longer contribute significantly to survival prediction. In this tumor stage, the extent of lymph node involvement is the main prognostic factor. This study addresses the question whether application of a highly sensitive molecular biology assay for detection of submicroscopic melanoma cells in sentinel lymph nodes may be suitable to improve melanoma staging. One hundred and sixteen patients with primary cutaneous melanoma with a total of 214 sentinel lymph nodes were enrolled. Sentinel lymph nodes were analyzed by histopathology including immunohistochemistry and by reverse transcription–polymerase chain reaction for tyrosinase. Patients were examined for tumor recurrences during a follow-up period of 19 mo (median). Disease-free survival probabilities were calculated and independent prognostic factors were determined by multivariate analysis. Using histopathology, micrometastatic nodal involvement was detected in 15 patients (13%). Of the 101 patients with histopathologically negative sentinel lymph nodes, 36 were reclassified by positive tyrosinase reverse transcription–polymerase chain reaction and 65 patients were still negative by reverse transcription–polymerase chain reaction. Recurrences were observed in 23 (20%) of 116 patients. These tumor recurrences were demonstrated in 10 patients (67%) with histopathologically positive sentinel lymph nodes, in nine patients (25%) with submicroscopic tumor cells detected by reverse transcription–polymerase chain reaction, and in four patients (6%) negative by both methods. The differences in recurrence rates were statistically significant ($p = 0.01$). In a multivariate analysis, histopathologic and reverse transcription–polymerase chain reaction status of the sentinel lymph node were demonstrated to be the only significant prognostic factors for predicting disease-free survival. Tyrosinase reverse transcription–polymerase chain reaction for the detection of minimal residual melanoma in sentinel lymph nodes is a powerful tool to determine patients who are at increased risk for subsequent metastasis. Moreover, a group of patients with high tumor thickness was identified by negative reverse transcription–polymerase chain reaction to be at low risk for recurrent disease. These data may have an impact on future tumor classifications of primary cutaneous melanoma.

Prognostic significance of occult metastases detected by sentinel lymphadenectomy and reverse transcriptase–polymerase chain reaction in early-stage melanoma patients.

Bostick PJ, Morton DL, Turner RR, Huynh KT, Wang HJ, Elashoff R, Essner R, Hoon DS.

Department of Molecular Oncology, John Wayne Cancer Institute, Santa Monica, CA, USA.

Journal of Clinical Oncology 17(10):3238–44, 1999, October.

Purpose: Detection of micrometastases in the regional tumor-draining lymph nodes is critical for accurate staging and prognosis in melanoma patients. We hypothesized that a multiple-mRNA marker (MM) reverse transcriptase–polymerase chain reaction (RT–PCR) assay would improve the detection of occult metastases in the sentinel node (SN), compared with hematoxylin and eosin (H & E) staining and immunohistochemistry (IHC), and that MM expression is predictive of disease relapse. *Patients and methods:* Seventy-two consecutive patients with clinical early-stage melanoma underwent sentinel lymphadenectomy (SLND). Their SNs were serially sectioned and assessed for MAGE-3, MART-1, and tyrosinase mRNA expression by RT–PCR, in parallel with H & E staining and IHC, for melanoma metastases. MM expression in the SNs was correlated with H & E and IHC assay results, standard prognostic factors, and disease-free survival. *Results:* In 17 patients with H & E- and/or IHC-positive SNs, 16 (94%) expressed two or more mRNA markers. Twenty (36%) of 55 patients with histopathologically negative SNs expressed two or more mRNA markers. By multivariate analysis, patients at increased risk of metastases to the SN had thicker lesions ($p = 0.03$), were 60 years of age or younger ($p < 0.05$), and/or were MM-positive ($p < 0.001$). Patients with histopathologically melanoma-free SNs who were MM-positive, compared with those who were positive for one or fewer mRNA markers, were at increased risk of recurrence ($p = 0.02$). Patients who were MM-positive with histopathologically proven metastases in the SN were at greatest risk of disease relapse ($p = 0.01$). *Conclusion:* H & E staining and IHC underestimate the true incidence of melanoma metastases. MM expression in the SN more accurately reflects melanoma micrometastases and is also a more powerful predictor of disease relapse than are H & E staining and IHC alone.

Management of malignant melanoma of the head and neck using dynamic lymphoscintigraphy and gamma probe-guided sentinel lymph node biopsy.

Carlson GW, Murray DR, Greenlee R, Alazraki N, Fry-Spray C, Poole R, Blais M, Hestley A. Vansant J.

Emory University School of Medicine, Atlanta, GA, USA.

Archives of Otolaryngology – Head & Neck Surgery 126(3):433–7, 2000, March.

Background: The sentinel lymph node (SLN) biopsy is revolutionizing the surgical management of primary malignant melanoma. It allows accurate nodal staging, and targets patients who may benefit from regional lymphadenectomy and systemic therapy; however, its use in the management of head and neck melanoma has not been widely accepted. *Methods:* A retrospective review of patients treated for clinical stages I and II malignant melanoma of the head and neck with dynamic lymphoscintigraphy and gamma probe-guided SLN biopsy. *Results:* Fifty-eight patients (47 male and 11 female) were identified. Primary melanoma sites included the scalp (21), ear (8), face (13), neck (15), and eyelid (1). Primary tumor staging was T2 (11), T3 (24), and T4 (23). Dynamic lymphoscintigraphy visualized SLNs in 57 patients (98.3%). In 43 cases (75%) a single draining nodal basin was identified, and in 14 cases there were multiple draining nodal basins. Sentinel lymph nodes were successfully identified in 72 (96%) of 75 nodal basins. Positive SLNs were identified in 10 patients (17.5%). Sentinel lymph node positivity by tumor staging was T3, 16.7% and T4, 27.3%. Completion lymphadenectomy revealed residual disease in 3 patients (30%). Relapse occurred in 10 (21.3%) of the 47 patients with negative SLN biopsy results and 7 (70%) of those with positive results. *Conclusions:* Gamma probe-guided SLN localization in the head and neck region was successful in 96% of draining nodal basins. It can target regional lymphadenectomy in patients who may benefit from regional nodal dissection.

Judging the therapeutic value of lymph node dissections for melanoma.

Chan AD, Essner R, Wanek LA, Morton DL.

Roy E Coats Research Laboratories of the John Wayne Cancer Institute at Saint John's Health Center, Santa Monica, CA, USA.

Journal of the American College of Surgeons 191(1):16–22; discussion 22–3, 2000, July.

Background: The management of the regional lymph nodes remains controversial for early-stage melanoma and for those patients with lymph node metastases; American Joint Committee on Cancer stage III. This study examines the importance of quality of the surgical resection measured by the extent of lymph node dissection (quartile of the total number of lymph nodes removed) to determine if this factor is an important prognostic factor for survival. *Study design:* We reviewed our computer-assisted database of more than 8,700 melanoma patients prospectively collected from 1971 through the present to identify patients who underwent lymph node dissection for stage III melanoma. We included only patients who had their nodal dissections performed at our institute. Patients who underwent sentinel lymph node dissection were excluded. These patients were then analyzed as a group and by individual lymphatic basins: cervical, axillary, and inguinal basins. Univariate and multivariate analyses were used to examine the model that included tumor burden, thickness of the primary melanoma, gender, age, clinical status of the lymph nodes (palpable versus not palpable), and the primary site. The survival and recurrence rates were analyzed using the Cox proportional hazards model. *Results:* Five hundred forty-eight patients underwent regional lymph node dissections. Of these patients, 214 underwent axillary dissections, 181 inguinal dissections, and 153 cervical dissections. The extent of the nodal dissections was based on the quartile of nodes excised, ranging from 1 to 98 (mean $\pm$ SD = 25.8 $\pm$ 15.8). Patients were stratified by tumor burden and quartile of number of lymph nodes removed. The overall 5-year survival of patients with four or more lymph nodes having tumor and the highest quartile of lymph nodes removed was 44% and was 23% for the lowest quartile of total lymph nodes excised ($p = 0.05$). By univariate analysis, tumor burden ($p = 0.0001$), quartile of total lymph nodes removed ($p = 0.043$), and primary site ($p = 0.047$) were statistically significant for predicting overall survival. Gender, clinical status of the nodes, primary tumor thickness, age, and dissected basin were not significant ($p > 0.05$). By multivariate analysis only the tumor burden ($p = 0.0001$) and quartile of lymph nodes resected ($p = 0.044$) were statistically significant. *Conclusions:* The extent of lymph node dissection for melanoma when analyzed by quartiles is an independent factor in overall survival. This factor appears to be more important with increasing tumor burden in the lymphatic basin. The extent of lymph node dissection should be considered as a prognostic factor in the design of clinical trials that involve stage III melanoma.

Role for lymphatic mapping and sentinel lymph node biopsy in patients with thick ($\geqslant$ 4 mm) primary melanoma.

Gershenwald JE, Mansfield PF, Lee JE, Ross MI.

Department of Surgical Oncology, The University of Texas M.D. Anderson Cancer Center, Houston, TX, USA.

Annals of Surgical Oncology 7(2): 160–5, 2000, March.

Background: Historically, patients with thick ($\geqslant$ 4 mm) primary melanoma have not been considered candidates for elective lymph node dissection, because their risk for occult distant disease is significant. Sentinel lymph node (SLN) biopsy offers an alternative approach to assess disease in the regional nodal basin, but no studies have specifically addressed the role for this technique in patients with thick melanoma. Although adjuvant therapy benefits patients who develop nodal metastases, data that supports its routine use in all patients with thick melanoma is both limited and controversial. This study was performed to determine whether pathological status of the SLN is an important risk factor in this heterogeneous group and, thus, provides a rationale for SLN biopsy. *Methods:* The records of 131 patients with primary cutaneous melanoma whose primary tumors were at least 4 mm thick and who underwent lymphatic mapping and SLN biopsy were reviewed. Several known prognostic factors, i.e., tumor thickness, ulceration, Clark level, location, sex, as well as SLN pathological status were analyzed with respect to disease-free and overall survival. *Results:* Lymphatic mapping and SLN biopsy was successful in 126 (96%) of 131 patients who underwent the procedure. In 49 patients (39%), the SLN biopsy was positive by conventional histology, although it was negative in 77 patients (61%). The median follow-up was 3 years. Although presence of ulceration and SLN status were independent prognostic factors with respect to disease-free and overall survival, SLN status was the most powerful predictor of overall survival by univariate and multivariate analyses. *Conclusions:* Lymphatic mapping and SLN biopsy is a highly accurate method of staging lymph node basins at risk for regional metastases in patients with thick melanoma and identifies those patients who may benefit from earlier lymphadenectomy as well as patients with a more favorable prognosis. Pathological status of the SLN in these patients with clinically negative nodes is the most important prognostic factor for survival and is essential to establish stratification criteria for future adjuvant trials in this high-risk group.

Sentinel node biopsy for melanoma in the head and neck region.

Jansen L, Koops HS, Nieweg OE, Doting MH, Kapteijn BA, Balm AJ, Vermey A, Plukker JT, Hoefnagel CA, Piers DA, Kroon BB.

Department of Surgery, The Netherlands Cancer Institute/Antoni van Leeuwenhoek Hospital, Plesmanlaan 121, 1066 CX Amsterdam, The Netherlands.

Head & Neck 22(1):27–33, 2000, January.

Background: Lymphatic drainage in the head and neck region is known to be particularly complex. This study explores the value of sentinel node biopsy for melanoma in the head and neck region. *Methods:* Thirty consecutive patients with clinically localized cutaneous melanoma in the head and neck region were included. Sentinel node biopsy was performed with blue dye and a gamma probe after preoperative lymphoscintigraphy. Average follow-up was 23 months (range, 1–48). *Results:* In 27 of 30 patients, a sentinel node was identified (90%). Only 53% of sentinel nodes were both blue and radioactive. A sentinel node was tumor-positive in 8 patients. The sentinel node was false-negative in two cases. Sensitivity of the procedure was 80% (8 of 10). *Conclusions:* Sentinel node biopsy in the head and neck region is a technically demanding procedure. Although it may help determine whether a neck dissection is necessary in certain patients, further investigation is required before this technique can be recommended for the standard management of cutaneous head and neck melanoma.

Sentinel node biopsy before and after wide excision of the primary melanoma.

Karakousis CP, Grigoropoulos P.

State University of New York at Buffalo, Kaleida Health, Millard Fillmore Gates Hospital, NY, USA.

Annals of Surgical Oncology 6(8):785–9, 1999, December.

Background: Initially, the technique of sentinel node biopsy involved the use of blue dye alone and was later supplemented with the use of an intraoperative probe after radiocolloid injection near the melanoma site. Ideally, it should be done before wide excision. To our knowledge, there is no information in the literature regarding the applicability or reliability of this technique after wide excision. *Methods:* We conducted a retrospective review of 142 patients (1993–1999) with melanomas ≥ 1.0 mm or Clark's level $\geq$ IV. Of these, 116 patients had prior biopsy only, and 26 had wide excision. The mean melanoma thickness was 2.5 mm. The location of the primary lesion was in the upper extremity in 42 patients, the lower extremity in 33, the trunk in 49, and the head and neck area in 18. *Results:* The sentinel node was identified in 88 (93%) of 95 nodal basins using the blue dye alone and in 65 (98.5%) of 66 basins using dye plus probe. The sentinel node was positive in 35 (25%) of the 142 patients and 38 (24%) of the 161 nodal basins. In a mean follow-up of 30 months of 115 basins with negative sentinel nodes, 3 (3%) later developed a palpable positive node in the same basin. In the group of dye alone, the sentinel node was identified in 40 (100%) of 40 extremity primaries and in 48 (87%) of 55 trunk and head and neck primary lesions ($p = 0.02$). Nine (35%) of the 26 patients with previous wide excision (25 with primary closure or skin graft, 1 with flap rotation) and 10 (32%) of 31 of nodal basins had a positive node; in 8 of the 9 patients, the positive node was also the sentinel node. The only patient with a positive node incidentally removed along with a histologically negative sentinel node was the one with a previous wide excision and flap rotation. *Conclusions:* Previous wide excision of the melanoma does not appear to negate the reliability of sentinel node biopsy, provided that no flap rotation was used to cover the defect.

Surgical management of malignant melanoma using dynamic lymphoscintigraphy and gamma probe-guided sentinel lymph node biopsy: the Emory experience.

Murray DR, Carlson GW, Greenlee R, Alazraki N, Fry-Spray C, Hestley A, Poole R, Blais M, Timbert DS, Vansant J.

Department of Surgery, Emory University School of Medicine, Atlanta, GA, USA.

American Surgeon 66(8):763–7, 2000, August.

Sentinel lymph node (SLN) biopsy is revolutionizing the surgical management of primary malignant melanoma. It allows accurate nodal staging which targets patients who may benefit from regional lymphadenectomy and systemic therapy. This is a retrospective review of patients treated at Emory University for stage I and II malignant melanoma with gamma probe-guided SLN biopsy from 1/1/94 to 6/30/98. Three hundred sixty patients (males 228, females 132) were identified. Primary melanoma sites included: head and neck 58, trunk 148, and extremities 154 (upper 71, lower 83). Primary tumor staging was T1 9, T2 134, T3 153, and T4 64. SLNs were successfully identified in 99.7 percent of patients and 98.9 percent of nodal basins mapped. In 275 (76.6%) cases a single draining nodal basin was identified. In 84 (23.3%) cases there were multiple draining nodal basins. Positive SLNs were identified in 63 patients (17.5%). SLN positivity by tumor staging was T1 0 percent, T2 9.0 percent, T3 22.2 percent, and T4 26.6 percent. The overall recurrence rate was 11.9 percent. Recurrences by SLN status were SLN+, 27 percent and, SLN−, 8.8 percent. Regional recurrence occurred in 7 (2.4%) of the 297 with negative SLN biopsies and 7 (11.1%) of the 63 with positive SLN biopsies. Dynamic lymphoscintigraphy and gamma probe-guided SLN localization was successful in more than 98 percent of cases. Patients with negative SLN biopsies have a low risk of recurrence.

Significance of multiple nodal basin drainage in truncal melanoma patients undergoing sentinel lymph node biopsy.

Porter GA, Ross MI, Berman RS, Lee JE, Mansfield PF, Gershenwald JE.

Department of Surgical Oncology, The University of Texas M.D. Anderson Cancer Center, Houston, TX, USA.

Annals of Surgical Oncology 7(4):256–61, 2000, May.

Background: Although previous studies have demonstrated that truncal site is associated with an adverse prognosis, explanations for such risk are lacking. In addition, the number of nodal basins as well as the number of lymph nodes containing regional metastases are important prognostic factors in these patients. Because the lymphatic drainage pattern of truncal melanoma often includes more than one basin, we designed a study to evaluate (1) whether patients with multiple nodal basin drainage (MNBD) were at an increased risk of lymph node metastases identified by sentinel lymph node (SLN) biopsy, and (2) whether the histological status of an individual basin reliably predicted the status of the other draining basins in patients with MNBD. *Methods:* The records of 295 consecutive truncal melanoma patients who were managed primarily with intraoperative lymphatic mapping and SLN biopsy, between 1991 and 1997, were reviewed. All patients underwent preoperative lymphoscintigraphy, which established the number and location of draining nodal basins. Univariate and multivariate analyses of relevant clinicopathological factors were performed to assess which factors may predict the presence of a pathologically positive SLN. *Results:* At least one SLN was identified in 281 patients. MNBD was present in 86 (31%) patients, and a pathologically positive SLN was found in 56 (20%) patients. By multivariate analysis, the presence of MNBD (relative risk = 1.9; $p = 0.03$), tumor thickness ($p = 0.007$), and tumor ulceration (relative risk = 2.4; $p = 0.01$) were significant independent risk factors for the presence of at least one pathologically positive SLN. SLN pathology in one basin did not predict the histology of other basins in 19 (22%) of 86 patients with MNBD. *Conclusions:* MNBD is independently associated with an increased risk of nodal metastases in truncal melanoma patients. Because the histological status of an individual basin did not reliably predict the status of the other draining basins in patients with MNBD, it is important to adequately identify and completely assess all nodal basins at risk, as defined by lymphoscintigraphy, in truncal melanoma patients.

How many lymph nodes are enough during sentinel lymphadenectomy for primary melanoma?

Porter GA, Ross MI, Berman RS, Sumner WE, Lee JE, Mansfield PF, Gershenwald JE.

Department of Surgical Oncology, The University of Texas M.D. Anderson Cancer Center, Houston, TX, USA.

Surgery 128(2): 306–11, 2000, August.

Background: Sentinel lymph node (SLN) biopsy has been shown to reliably identify nodal metastases and the subsequent need for further surgical and adjuvant therapy in patients with cutaneous melanoma. Although SLN identification rates have improved with the addition of radioactive colloid to the blue dye technique, it remains unclear how many lymph nodes should be removed to accurately determine the histologic status of the nodal basin. The objective of this study was to determine the optimal extent of SLN biopsy in these patients. *Methods:* The records of 633 consecutive patients with melanoma (765 nodal basins) whose primary treatment included SLN biopsy with the use of a combination of blue dye and technetium Tc 99 labeled sulfur colloid were reviewed. SLN biopsy consisted of the removal of all of the blue-stained nodes and all nodes with radiotracer uptake activity of at least twice background. *Results:* SLN biopsy was successful in 765 of 772 basins (99%). A mean of 1.9 SLNs (median, 2 SLNs) per basin were excised. At least 3 SLNs were removed in 176 basins (23%). The overall histologic status of a basin was always established by the first or second SLN harvested (ie, in no patient was the third or subsequent SLN positive when 1 of the first 2 was not). Of the 124 basins containing lymphatic metastases, the SLN that contained the maximal radiotracer uptake (hottest) and/or stained blue was pathologically positive in 118 basins (95%). In only 6 of the 124 positive basins (5%) was the sole evidence of occult nodal metastases identified in an SLN that was neither blue-stained nor the

hottest. All but 1 of these SLNs had counts that were at least 66% of the hottest node in the basin. *Conclusions:* With a combined modality approach to SLN biopsy, removal of more than 2 SLNs did not provide information that upstaged any patient with primary melanoma. Removal of additional nonblue SLN(s) that contained radioactive counts of at least twice background but lower than two thirds of the SLNs with maximal radiotracer uptake affected patient management in less than 0.2% of all cases. These findings may be helpful in minimizing the extent of surgery and perhaps in reducing the costs and resource use associated with operating room time and pathologic examination.

Can elective lymph node dissection decrease the frequency and mortality rate of late melanoma recurrences?

Shen P, Guenther JM, Wanek LA, Morton DL.

Department of Surgical Oncology and the Roy E Coats Research Laboratories of the John Wayne Cancer Institute at Saint John's Health Center, Santa Monica, CA, USA.

Annals of Surgical Oncology 7(2):114–19, 2000, March.

Background: Although more than 90% of the morbidity and mortality from localized cutaneous melanoma occurs in the first decade after initial surgical treatment, melanoma can recur after a 10-year disease-free interval (DFI) with fatal consequences. We reviewed our melanoma data base of more than 8,500 prospectively acquired patients to identify clinicopathological factors that affect the type, rate of occurrence, and outcome of disease recurring 10 years or more after surgical treatment of primary cutaneous melanoma. *Methods:* From 1971 to 1997, 1907 melanoma patients treated at our cancer center reached or presented with a DFI of 10 years or more after surgical treatment of clinically localized melanoma. Of these, 217 (11%) patients had recurrences (mean DFI, 182 months). The sites of recurrence were local/in-transit in 26 (12%) patients, regional lymph nodes in 101 (47%) patients, and distant sites in 90 (41%) patients. *Results:* Univariate and multivariate analysis, using patient age and sex, type of initial treatment, and the site, Breslow thickness, and Clark level of the initial tumor, showed that the type of treatment for the primary tumor was a significant ($p = 0.0005$) prognostic factor in the development of late nodal recurrence. Of the 217 patients who had recurrences, 172 (79%) had undergone wide local excision for their primary melanoma, and 45 (21%) had undergone wide local excision plus elective lymph node dissection (ELND). The rates of nodal recurrence were 53% (92 of 172) and 20% (9 of 45), respectively, a significant ($p = 0.0001$) difference. When all patients with a DFI of 10 years or more were stratified by type of initial treatment, the ELND group demonstrated a significant improvement in disease-free survival and overall survival. *Conclusions:* The risk of late-recurring nodal disease increases and the chance of long-term survival decreases when wide local excision is performed without ELND. With the advent of sentinel lymphadenectomy, ELND can be selectively performed only for those nodal basins with occult tumor cells, thereby decreasing operative morbidity but allowing identification and early removal of nodal micrometastases.

Sentinel lymphadenectomy for staging patients with intermediate-level melanoma.

Smart KR, Cahoon BW, Dale PS.

Southeastern Surgical Oncology and the Division of Surgical Oncology, Mercer University School of Medicine, Macon, GA, USA.

American Surgeon 66(3):280–3, 2000, March.

Sentinel lymph node dissection (SLND) as originally described by D.L. Morton *et al.* (Surg Oncol Clin North Am 1992;1:247–59), is currently being used at most tertiary institutions for staging patients with intermediate-level melanomas. Identification and subsequent surgical resection of occult metastasis before the development of clinical disease may improve survival in these patients. This study is a retrospective review of patients with intermediate melanomas treated by the senior author (P.S.D.). Isosulfan blue dye and a radioactive technetium-labeled dye were used to identify the sentinel node. Sentinel nodes were evaluated by routine hematoxylin and eosin staining, immunohistochemical staining for S-100 and HMB-45, and later in the study with multipanel reverse transcriptase–polymerase chain reaction analysis. All patients were followed closely. Fifty-seven patients with primary melanoma were evaluated between December 1995 and June 1998. Thirty-two patients underwent SLND; two patients underwent SLND on two separate drainage basins, for a total of 34 procedures. The median age was 49 years (range, 19–77). There were 11 females and 21 males. The locations of the primary melanoma were: head and neck, seven; extremity, 8; and trunk, 18; 1 patient had a dual primary melanoma at presentation. Clark's levels of invasion among the patients were level III, 5; and level IV, 27; median Breslow thickness was 1.4 mm (range, 0.45–3.8 mm). A sentinel node was not identified in four procedures (11.1%). Twenty-two nodes (73%) were negative by all methods, and eight (27%) were positive by at least one method. All positive patients underwent complete lymphadenectomy, and routine hematoxylin and eosin stains identified no additional positive nodes. Median follow-up was 21 months (6–36 months). Two patients developed recurrent disease. The other 30 patients remain disease free at last follow-up. SLND is a low-morbidity technique that accurately stages patients with intermediate-level melanoma. Early intervention with complete therapeutic lymphadenectomy and possible interferon therapy may improve the survival of patients with stage III melanoma. A complete discussion of the technique for SLND and an update of this data is presented.

Popliteal lymph node metastasis from primary cutaneous melanoma.

Thompson JF, Hunt JA, Culjak G, Uren RF, Howman-Giles R, Harman CR.

Sydney Melanoma Unit, Royal Prince Alfred Hospital, Camperdown, Sydney, NSW, Australia.

European Journal of Surgical Oncology 26(2):172–6, 2000, March.

Aims: To document the incidence of popliteal lymph node involvement by metastatic melanoma and to consider the implications of this information for clinical management. *Methods:* From the computerized database of the Sydney Melanoma Unit, all patients with primary melanomas located at or distal to the knee were identified and their records were examined. Experience with those patients who developed popliteal node metastases was then reviewed. *Results:* Thirteen of 4262 patients (0.31%) with primary melanomas of the distal lower limb developed popliteal node metastases. Six of the 13 patients had previous, synchronous or subsequent groin node metastases. *Conclusions:* Popliteal lymph node involvement by metastatic melanoma is a rare event. The study results suggest only two indications for full popliteal node clearance – either a histologically positive sentinel node in the popliteal fossa or clinical evidence of metastatic disease in a popliteal node.

Sentinel lymph node biopsy for melanoma: experience with 234 consecutive procedures.

Wagner JD, Corbett L, Park HM, Davidson D, Coleman JJ, Havlik RJ, Hayes JT 2nd.

Department of Surgery, Indiana University School of Medicine at Indiana University Purdue University at Indianapolis, IA, USA. jdwagner@iupui.edu

Plastic & Reconstructive Surgery 105(6):1956–66, 2000, May.

Sentinel lymph node biopsy is increasingly used to identify occult metastases in regional lymph nodes of patients with melanoma. Selection of patients for sentinel lymph node biopsy and subsequent lymphadenectomy is an area of debate. The purpose of this study was to describe a large clinical series of these biopsies for cutaneous melanoma and to identify patients most likely to gain useful clinical information from sentinel lymph node biopsy. The Indiana University Melanoma Program computerized database was queried to identify all patients who underwent this procedure for clinically localized cutaneous melanoma. It was performed using preoperative technetium Tc 99 m lymphoscintigraphy and isosulfan blue dye. Pertinent demographic, surgical, and histopathologic data were recorded. Univariate and multivariate logistic regression and classification table analyses were performed to identify clinical variables associated with sentinel node and nonsentinel node positivity. In total, 234 biopsy procedures were performed to stage 291 nonpalpable regional lymph node basins. Mean Breslow's thickness was 2.30 mm (2.08 mm for negative sentinel lymph node biopsy, 3.18 mm for positive). The mean number of sentinel nodes removed was 2.17 nodes per basin (range, 1 to 8). Forty-seven of 234 melanomas (20.1 percent) and 50 of 291 basins (17.2 percent) had a positive biopsy. Positivity correlated with AJCC tumor stage: T1, 3.6 percent; T2, 8.1 percent; T3, 27.4 percent; T4, 44 percent. By univariate logistic regression, Breslow's thickness ($p = 0.003$, continuous variable), ulceration ($p = 0.003$), mitotic index $\geqslant 6$ mitoses per high power field ($p = 0.008$), and Clark's level ($p = 0.04$) were significantly associated with sentinel lymph node biopsy result. By multivariate analysis, only Breslow's thickness ($p = 0.02$), tumor ulceration ($p = 0.02$), and mitotic index ($p = 0.02$) were significant predictors of biopsy positivity.

Classification table analysis showed the Breslow cutpoint of 1.2 mm to be the most efficient cutpoint for sentinel lymph node biopsy result ($p = 0.0004$). Completion lymphadenectomy was performed in 46 sentinel node-positive patients; 12 (26.1 percent) had at least one additional positive non-sentinel node. Nonsentinel node positivity was marginally associated with the presence of multiple positive sentinel nodes ($p = 0.07$). At mean follow-up of 13.8 months, four of 241 sentinel node-negative basins demonstrated same-basin recurrence (1.7 percent). Sentinel lymph node biopsy is highly reliable in experienced hands but is a low-yield procedure in most thin melanomas. Patients with melanomas thicker than 1.2 mm or with ulcerated or high mitotic index lesions are most likely to have occult lymph node metastases by sentinel lymph node biopsy. Completion therapeutic lymphadenectomy is recommended after positive biopsy because it is difficult to predict the presence of positive nonsentinel nodes.

Predicting sentinel and residual lymph node basin disease after sentinel lymph node biopsy for melanoma.

Wagner JD, Gordon MS, Chuang TY, Coleman JJ 3rd, Hayes JT, Jung SH, Love C.

Department of Surgery/Plastic and Reconstructive Surgery, Indiana University School of Medicine, Indiana University-Purdue University at Indianapolis, Indianapolis, IA, USA.

Cancer 89(2): 453–62, 2000, July 15.

Background: The selection of patients for sentinel lymph node biopsy (SNB) and selective lymphadenectomy for histologically positive sentinel lymph nodes (SLND) are areas of debate. The authors of the current study attempted to identify predictors of metastases to the sentinel and residual nonsentinel lymph nodes in patients with melanoma. *Methods:* The Indiana University Interdisciplinary Melanoma Program computerized database was queried to identify all patients who underwent SNB for clinically localized cutaneous melanoma. Demographic, surgical, and histopathologic data were recorded. Univariate and multivariate logistic regression analyses were performed to identify associations with SNB and nonsentinel lymph node positivity. Classification tree and logistic procedures were performed to identify the ideal tumor thickness cutpoint at which to perform SNB. *Results:* Two hundred seventy-five SNB procedures were performed to stage 348 regional lymph node basins for occult metastases from melanoma. Of the 275 melanomas, 54 (19.6%) had a positive SNB, as did 58 of 348 basins (16.7%). Classification and logistic regression analysis identified a Breslow depth of 1.25 mm to be the most significant cutpoint for SNB positivity (odds ratio 8.8:1; $p = 0.0001$). By multivariate analyses, a Breslow thickness cutpoint $\geqslant 1.25$ mm ($p = 0.0002$), ulceration ($p = 0.005$), and high mitotic index (> 5 mitoses/high-power field; $p = 0.04$) were significant predictors of SNB results. SLND was performed in 53 SNB positive patients, 15 of whom (28.3%) had at least 1 additional positive lymph node. SLND positivity was noted across a wide range of primary tumor characteristics and was associated significantly with multiple positive SN, but not with any other variable. SNB result correlated significantly with disease free and overall survival. *Conclusions:* Patients with a Breslow tumor thickness $\geqslant 1.25$ mm, ulceration, and high mitotic index are most likely to have positive SNB results. SLND is recommended for all patients after positive SNB because it is difficult to identify patients with residual lymph node disease.

Lymphedema after sentinel lymph node biopsy for cutaneous melanoma: a report of 5 cases.

Wrone DA, Tanabe KK, Cosimi AB, Gadd MA, Souba WW, Sober AJ.

Massachusetts General Hospital Melanoma Center, Department of Dermatology, Massachusetts General Hospital, Boston, MD, USA.

Archives of Dermatology 136(4):511–14, 2000, April.

Background: Sentinel lymph node (SLN) biopsy has rapidly become the procedure of choice for assessing the lymph node status of patients with 1992 American Joint Committee on Cancer stages I and II melanoma. The procedure was designed to be less invasive and, therefore, less likely to cause complications than a complete lymph node dissection. To our knowledge, this is the first report in the literature documenting extremity lymphedema following SLN biopsy. *Observation*: We report 5 cases of lymphedema after SLN biopsy in patients being routinely followed up after melanoma surgery at the Massachusetts General Hospital Melanoma Center, Boston. Three cases were mild, and 2 were moderate. Potential contributing causes of lymphedema were present in 4 patients and included the transient formation of hematomas and seromas, obesity, the possibility of occult metastatic melanoma, and the proximal extremity location of the primary melanoma excision. Four of the patients underwent an SLN biopsy at our institution. We used the total number of SLN procedures ($n = 235$) that we have performed to calculate a 1.7% baseline incidence of lymphedema after SLN biopsy. *Conclusions*: Sentinel lymph node biopsy can be complicated by mild and moderate degrees of lymphedema, with an incidence of at least 1.7%. Some patients may have contributing causes for lymphedema other than the SLN biopsy, but many of these causes are difficult to modify or avoid.

18

Adjuvant therapy for melanoma

JEFFREY S WEBER, JULIE A WOLFE, AND VERNON K SONDAK

INTRODUCTION

Because of our limited success in treating metastatic melanoma, with no single agent having more than a 20% response rate, and the high failure rates associated with surgical therapy for locally and regionally advanced disease, the search for effective adjuvant therapy of melanoma has generated intense interest. Thus, few of the available cytotoxic chemotherapeutic agents have had more than limited efficacy against advanced disease, with response rates of no more than 15–20% for dacarbazine (DTIC), cisplatin, velban, taxol and temozolomide, indicating that single chemotherapy agents are unlikely to manifest activity as adjuvant therapy. That fact, combined with the assessment that melanoma is an immunogenic tumor susceptible to attack by the host's immune system, resulted in the testing of a remarkably broad spectrum of therapeutic agents – many of which have no applications in the treatment for other forms of cancer. The adjuvant therapy trials which were performed were often flawed and always greatly underpowered to detect a significant difference in survival between the arms. Not surprisingly, then, past reviews of the status of adjuvant therapy of melanoma have been little more than litanies of negative results. Occasionally, *post-hoc* (data-derived) subset analyses appeared promising in one or another trial, but the lack of a compelling rationale for the efficacy of the therapy in the particular subset analysed usually resulted in insufficient enthusiasm for further testing. The individual practitioner has had little motivation to treat melanoma patients with adjuvant therapy – despite the high risk of and lack of effective therapy for recurrent disease.

This situation changed after approval by the United States Food and Drug Administration (FDA) of interferon alfa-2b (IFN-α2b) for the post-surgical adjuvant therapy of high-risk melanoma in late 1995 and shortly thereafter by publication of the results of the clinical trial that resulted in this approval.[1] High-dose IFN-α2b became the standard of care and was utilized by many oncologists in the community. A major Intergroup adjuvant therapy trial in preparation was redesigned to incorporate high-dose IFN-α2b as the control arm. Yet the trial that showed benefit for IFN-α2b, the Eastern Cooperative Oncology Group (ECOG) Trial EST1684, suffered from many of the same ailments that plagued previous adjuvant therapy trials.[2,3] Unfortunately, the results of the confirmatory trial, E1690/SWOG 9111, have not reproduced the original positive results of the earlier trial, throwing the field back into confusion over the best alternatives for the adjuvant therapy of high-risk melanoma. That situation has fortunately been clarified by the recent data on the prematurely halted ECOG 1694/SWOG 9512 trial, which again suggested that relapse-free and overall survivals were improved with high-dose IFN-α2b.

Time and the maturation of several additional completed trials will further clarify the role of high-dose IFN-α2b adjuvant therapy, and of 20 years of work on allogeneic cellular vaccines as adjuvant therapy. However, the melanoma landscape has already been permanently changed, and adjuvant therapy research in this disease is in the process of a paradigm shift. The challenge now is to build on the successful model of large, randomized, well-powered phase III trials with appropriate control arms using new knowledge on antigen-specific immune responses to melanoma gained by basic immunologists over the last 5–10 years. Doing so in a rational manner, including adding more specific immune therapies to established IFN-α2b, will require improvements in several areas:

- increased understanding of the mechanisms of action of the available therapeutic agents (in particular allowing the rational design of combination therapies);
- better ability to prognosticate an individual's risk of recurrence (allowing the appropriate inclusion or exclusion of patients from protocol or non-protocol therapy); and
- a commitment to design and conduct clinical trials that possess sufficient statistical power to detect therapeutically meaningful differences.

The intent of this chapter is briefly but critically to analyse the many adjuvant therapy trials conducted to date – including those in progress and those closed to accrual but awaiting maturation of the results – and to describe briefly new and earlier phase trials of antigen-specific vaccines that may revolutionize the field. We hope to highlight the challenges for clinicians and clinical researchers alike as we take the adjuvant therapy of melanoma into the new millenium.

OVERVIEW OF METHODOLOGIC PROBLEMS IN MELANOMA ADJUVANT TRIALS

Virtually all of the adjuvant therapy trials reported to date have suffered from one or more basic methodologic problems that limit the degree of confidence which can be placed in their results.

Inadequate statistical power

Without an adequate sample size, a clinical trial will have very little power to detect a *clinically* significant difference as statistically significant. Most of the randomized, controlled trials of adjuvant therapy conducted in melanoma have had fewer than 250 patients per arm. For example, a 5% increase in 5-year survival for patients with melanoma metastatic to the regional lymph nodes (which would translate to at least 400–500 additional 5-year survivors in the USA annually) would require over 1250 patients per arm for a two-arm trial with 80% power to detect that difference. The largest randomized trials completed in melanoma to date have had 600–700 patients in total, and some of these have been multi-arm trials. Multi-arm trials with smaller patient groups will have lower statistical power than two-arm trials of the same total size, because of the need to account for multiple comparisons.

Improper or imbalanced control group

The results of a randomized, controlled trial are only as good as the control group utilized. Historical controls are clearly inappropriate in melanoma adjuvant trials and have led to recognizable and predictable errors.[4] Even consecutive series from a single institution or investigator are poor controls because the thoroughness with which patients are evaluated for metastatic disease has increased over the years (including the widespread use of sentinel node biopsies combined with immunohistochemical techniques to evaluate regional nodal metastases, magnetic resonance image (MRI) scanning to screen for central nervous system (CNS) metastases, and positron emission tomography (PET) scanning for the sensitive detection

of occult metastases), resulting in stage-migration and improved survival within stages in the absence of effective therapy. In randomized trials, the need for the use of a placebo has never fully been addressed.[5] Very few melanoma adjuvant trials have used a placebo control, which often presents a difficult decision for participating patients. Some studies have not used a no-treatment control of any kind, relying instead on allegedly inactive agents (such as the vaccinia viral oncolysate trial in which vaccinia virus alone was used as the control). When the study result is negative, the question of unrecognized activity of the control group arises and can obscure the results.[6] One of the biggest problems encountered in randomized, controlled trials of adjuvant therapy of melanoma to date, however, has been a known or potential imbalance of recognized prognostic factors between the treatment and control arms. For example, in the EST1684 trial of adjuvant high-dose IFN-α, there was a known imbalance between the treatment and control arms for the presence of ulceration in the primary tumor (favoring the control arm) for patients in the stratum with pT4N0M0 disease (thick primary, pathologically negative nodes). This limited the ability to generalize the positive results of this trial from node-positive patients to high-risk, node-negative patients. However, even more importantly, one of the primary prognostic factors for node-positive patients – the number of tumor-involved nodes – was not recognized at the time this study was designed.[1] Thus, it was unknown whether the treatment and control arms were balanced with respect to that crucial factor. The use of randomization does not guarantee that the two groups are equivalent in this regard; rather, it allows us to conclude that there is only a 5% or lesser chance that the two groups are sufficiently imbalanced to result in the erroneous conclusion that IFN-α2b is active when in fact it is not.

Heterogeneous risk groups

Compounding the problems inherent in trials with small sample sizes and potentially imbalanced risk factors is the inclusion of heterogeneous groups of at-risk patients in many of the adjuvant trials conducted to date. Current thinking, based in part on the existing TNM system for melanoma, would stratify patients into four risk categories as follows:

- low risk (stage I), primary tumor < 1.5 mm with negative nodes;
- intermediate risk (stage IIA), primary tumor 1.5–4.0 mm with negative nodes;
- high risk (stages IIB and III), primary tumor > 4.0 mm with negative nodes or any primary tumor with positive nodes, satellitosis, or in-transit metastases;
- very high-risk (stage IV), resected metastatic melanoma beyond the regional nodes.

Patients with non-cutaneous primaries, multiple (more than ten) positive nodes or gross extracapsular extension appear to be at higher risk than the average 'high-risk' patient, but precisely where they should fit into this classification scheme remains to be defined. The recently developed updated staging criteria now include such factors as ulceration of the primary lesion, which portends a worse prognosis for early-stage disease, and sentinel node positivity by immunohistochemical staining only, which suggests a better outcome for patients with stage III disease. The new staging criteria will completely change the accrual patterns to future adjuvant trials and render the use of historical controls impossible to interpret.

Lack of active agents

Perhaps nothing has posed a greater problem in devising melanoma clinical trials than the lack of effective agents. No available single agent has a greater than 20% objective response rate against measurable metastatic disease, and combination therapy has not yet been established to be superior to single agents. Dacarbazine and IFN-α are two of the active single agents in metastatic disease, and have been evaluated in several adjuvant therapy trials. Velban, cisplatin, taxol and temodol have 10–15% single-agent activity and are unlikely to be evaluated in randomized trials. Recently, several trials have been published suggesting that combination therapy, either with DTIC, cisplatin, bischloroethylnitrosourea (BCNU) and tamoxifen or DTIC plus IFN-α, has no survival advantage over DTIC alone.[7] Most of the other agents that have been investigated in the adjuvant setting have either no or minimal activity against metastatic disease. It has often been postulated – but never substantiated – that agents which lack activity against metastatic disease (particularly immunotherapeutic agents) could still prove efficacious in the adjuvant setting. Unfortunately, the mechanisms of action of these agents are poorly understood. When trials with these agents have yielded negative results, there has rarely been sufficient biologic information obtained to conclude whether the agent or agents actually achieved the desired surrogate or biologic effect. This has perpetuated the uncertainty regarding the adjuvant use of immunomodulatory agents, leaving few new leads upon which to build.

Variable or inadequate follow-up

Although patients with stage IV (disseminated) melanoma generally have a short median survival duration in the range of 7–9 months, patients with earlier-stage disease can have long disease-free intervals prior to relapse or recurrence. For this reason, an adequate length of patient follow-up to ensure that enough 'events' (relapse or death from disease) occur is critical in adjuvant therapy trials. There are instances of melanoma trials that were initially reported as positive, only to be reanalysed later and re-reported as negative.[8,9]

The methodologic problems described above are present to some extent in virtually every trial reported to date. They make comparisons of trials difficult, even when the trials are purporting to study similar interventions, and they preclude lending serious weight to the results of subset analyses. In the sections that follow, we provide an overview of the adjuvant trials conducted in melanoma to date, focusing on randomized, controlled trials that incorporate a no-treatment control arm, but also discussing new developments in antigen-specific therapy in detail. Generally, only the overall results of comparisons between the treatment arm and the control arm for disease-free survival and survival are presented. Results of multi-arm trials are considered separately for each treatment arm, recognizing that appropriate statistical adjustments for multiple comparisons may or, more likely, may not have been made. The reader is referred to the specified reference for more details about a particular trial.

NON-SPECIFIC IMMUNOSTIMULANTS

Bacille Calmette-Guérin

Morton demonstrated that intralesional injection of viable Bacille Calmette-Guérin (BCG) organisms could lead to the regression of intradermal metastases of melanoma, a local therapy that still has clinical use today.[10] Even more significantly, uninjected lesions occasionally regressed. This suggested that the human immune system could be primed to destroy distant melanoma and stimulated the conduct of clinical trials using BCG in the adjuvant setting. Although several non-randomized trials using historical controls and two small randomized trials of intralesional or intralymphatic BCG showed a statistically significant benefit in favor of BCG,[10,11] a number of other randomized trials failed to substantiate this benefit.[12–21] Virtually all of these trials were small and employed heterogeneous populations of patients at intermediate and high risk of recurrence. A small randomized trial employing the methanol-extracted residue of BCG was performed; no beneficial effect of treatment was found.[21]

Corynebacterium parvum

C. parvum is another micro-organism which non-specifically stimulates the human immune system, and has been used as an adjuvant in murine antitumor vaccination studies. It has an advantage compared with BCG in that viable organisms are not required for adjuvant efficacy. Based on data from murine studies, adjuvant treatment with *C. parvum* has been compared to untreated controls in two studies, neither of which demonstrated a significant overall benefit for the therapy.[22,23] *C. parvum* was also compared directly to BCG (without an untreated control group) in two adjuvant trials. Lipton found a statistically significant disease-free survival advantage for the subgroup of patients with positive nodes who were treated with *C. parvum*, but no such advantage for node-negative patients.[24] Balch conducted a slightly larger trial and found a non-significant increase in median survival in favor of the BCG-treated patients.[25] *C. parvum* has never found widespread adoption as a therapeutic agent in melanoma or any other malignancy.

Levamisole

Levamisole is an antihelminthic agent for which various immunomodulatory properties have been reported.[7] Four randomized, controlled trials of levamisole in melanoma have been conducted. In three of the four, no benefit for levamisole therapy was identified.[5,8,9] In one study, a significant increase in 5-year survival was seen in favor of levamisole. The significance of this difference disappeared, however, in multivariate analysis – raising the possibility of an imbalance of prognostic factors rather than a true treatment effect.[26]

Other non-specific immunostimulants

Transfer factor, an extract of disrupted leukocytes thought to transfer delayed-type hypersensitivity and act as a non-specific immunostimulant,[27] was tested in two small randomized, controlled trials in melanoma without evidence of efficacy.[28,29] Transfer factor has never found widespread adoption as a therapeutic agent in melanoma or any other malignancy. Isoprinosine, a mixture of inosine, adedoben, and dimepranol with putative immunostimulatory properties, has been tested in the adjuvant therapy of melanoma in several small randomized trials.[30,31] A suggestion of improved disease-free survival seen in one study was not confirmed in the other. A single small study of the thymic factor thymostimulin suggested a short-term advantage in disease-free and overall survival in favor of the treated group,[32] but two other studies did not.[33,34]

In conclusion, in the absence of a solid scientific rationale, the empiric use of non-specific immunostimulants would not seem to be worth pursuing in the adjuvant therapy of melanoma.

ACTIVE SPECIFIC IMMUNOTHERAPY

Unlike the non-specific immunostimulants described above, active specific immunotherapy is mediated by vaccine reagents which elicit a specific host immune response to known or unknown tumor-associated antigens. To date, only a limited number of melanoma-associated antigens have been defined, and peptide or whole-antigen vaccines have been developed for only a few of these, which are discussed below. Few vaccine trials have been conducted which included as part of the study appropriate immune monitoring to verify that the desired immunologic surrogate endpoint had been achieved. The lack of no-treatment control arms has also complicated the interpretation of several studies.

Autologous tumor vaccines

Because only a few melanoma-associated antigens have been defined, and because those few that are known may not be present or may not be sufficiently immunogenic in a given individual to mediate tumor regression (i.e., a 'tumor regression antigen'), a number of investigators have worked with autologous cellular tumor vaccines. This approach theoretically insures that all biologically relevant antigens are available for presentation to the immune system. Of course, this approach is limited to individuals with sufficient tumor to prepare a vaccine, is predicated on tumor regression antigens being present at a sufficiently high concentration on the tumor cell surface, with neither antigen down-modulation or active suppression being present, and presumes that antigens on tumor cells are capable of presentation to immune cells. This has restricted melanoma adjuvant trials to patients with bulky nodal or resectable distant metastatic disease. Such patients have a poor overall prognosis and are likely to have significant residual tumor burden and tumor-related immune suppression, making them less-than-ideal candidates for any immunotherapeutic approach. Even then, only enough tumor is usually obtained to provide for a limited number of vaccinations. Furthermore, the technical complexities inherent in harvesting tumor and preparing a vaccine have, to date, precluded multi-institutional trials to formally test the efficacy of autologous tumor vaccines. Two small randomized trials (15 and 31 patients respectively) comparing irradiated or neuraminadase-treated autologous tumor cells plus BCG to a control group found that the treatment group appeared to fare no better, or perhaps even worse, than the control group.[35–37] In addition, a somewhat larger randomized, controlled trial of adjuvant therapy with autologous tumor cells plus BCG in renal cell carcinoma failed to show any evidence of benefit for vaccine treatment.[38] Nonetheless, single-institution studies incorporating historical controls,[39] as well as the potential of genetically modifying tumor cells to render them more immunogenic,[40,41] continue to stimulate interest in this approach.

Allogeneic tumor cell vaccines

Allogeneic tumor cell vaccines, generally prepared from cultured cell lines or lysates, offer several important advantages over autologous vaccines: they are readily available, even for patients who lack sufficient tumor to produce an autologous tumor cell vaccine, and can be standardized, preserved, and distributed in a manner akin to that of any other pharmacologic or therapeutic agent, with specific potency tests and release criteria. This property allows for the use of multiple vaccinations over months or years and facilitates the performance of large-scale, multi-institutional, clinical trials. The majority of trials that have been completed to date, however, have been small, single-institution studies. None of these trials demonstrated an unequivocal benefit for immunotherapy with allogeneic tumor cells administered in conjunction with BCG when compared to an untreated[42] or a BCG-treated control group.[43] Considerable uncertainty remains as to the optimal immunologic adjuvant to use in conjunction with an allogeneic tumor cell vaccine, but there is reason to suspect that BCG may not be ideal.[44,45] Also controversial is the role of immunomodulators given concomitantly with vaccination, most notably cyclophosphamide. Two randomized studies have been conducted in which allogeneic melanoma vaccines were administered, without or with cyclophosphamide given for 3 days prior to vaccination. The results of these studies have been conflicting, with one suggesting no detectable difference[46] and one suggesting a decrease in suppressor cell activity and augmented antibody response.[47] The Southwest Oncology Group has recently closed a large (>600 patients) randomized trial comparing an allogeneic melanoma cell lysate (Melacine) co-administered with detoxified endotoxin/mycobacterial cell wall skeleton (DETOX), given without cyclophosphamide, to an untreated control group of patients with intermediate-thickness, node-negative melanoma (S9035).

C-VAX, a combination of allogeneic cell lines plus BCG, is currently being tested in a large, multi-institutional, randomized, double blind trial compared with BCG alone. Over 500 patients will be treated for 5 years, with overall survival as the key endpoint. In a recent single-arm trial,[48] C-VAX was administered to 77 patients with resected high-risk stage IV melanoma, and correlates of relapse-free and overall survival were assessed. It was found that there was a significant correlation between overall survival and development of IgM antibodies directed against TA-90, a recently characterized tumor-associated glycoprotein on melanomas. In this analysis, TA-90 IgM levels correlated more strongly with outcome than DTH to the vaccine components, suggesting that TA-90 antibodies may be a new prognostic marker for patients with resected high-risk melanoma.

Viral oncolysates

The allogeneic vaccine trials cited above incorporated an immunologic adjuvant to generate a sufficient local immune response so that priming of an immune response to tumor-associated antigens could occur. An alternative approach to allogeneic vaccination involves the use of a virus to lyse the tumor cells prior to inoculation. In theory, the admixture of viral and tumor proteins should provoke an intense non-specific immune response that would lead to recognition and rejection of tumor cells by the host. A pilot study of melanoma patients treated with Newcastle disease virus lysates of either autologous or allogeneic tumor cells for 5 years suggested an improved survival compared to historical controls.[49] This observation prompted two larger randomized trials using vaccinia viral lysates of allogeneic tumor. One trial incorporated a control arm in which patients were treated with vaccinia virus alone, without tumor cells.[6] The other trial used a no-treatment control arm.[50] Both studies demonstrated no evidence of benefit for the vaccinia oncolysate treatment. Although it is possible that a small immunomodulatory effect of vaccinia virus by itself could have obscured the beneficial effect of the viral oncolysate in one trial, the negative results of the other trial suggest that this is not the case. The results of these two randomized trials, in such marked contrast to the beneficial effect seemingly found in a non-randomized trial,[6,50] emphasize yet again the perils of relying on historical non-randomized control groups in evaluating melanoma therapy.[4]

DEFINED ANTIGEN VACCINES

Vaccination with autologous or allogeneic tumor cells represents an attempt to generate antitumor immunity by exposing the patient to a variety of tumor-associated antigens. In the last decade, a number of antigens present on melanoma cells that could potentially serve as targets for the human immune response have been identified and defined. Although all of these antigens may not be present on every tumor cell, as the number of defined antigens increases, the likelihood increases that at least one relevant antigenic target can be identified for every patient's melanoma. Still lacking, however, but in the process of development, are reliable and reproducible methods for immunizing humans against each of these defined antigens, and only one randomized, clinical trial utilizing a defined antigen vaccine has been completed to date.[51]

Gangliosides

Gangliosides are a group of related glycolipids present on melanoma cells and some non-neoplastic cells (particularly neural tissues and granulocytes). The various gangliosides differ in their expression on melanomas and normal tissues and in their intrinsic immunogenicity.[52–54] Ganglioside GD3, for example, is distributed widely on melanocytes, nevi, and practically all melanomas, as well as on some normal tissues, and naturally occurring anti-GD3 antibodies are rare. Administration of a monoclonal antibody to GD3 (in conjunction with macrophage-colony stimulating factor) resulted in objective regressions of melanoma metastases.[55] Ganglioside GM2 is expressed on a large percentage of melanoma tumors, is rarely detected on normal tissues, and about 5% of melanoma patients have naturally occurring anti-GM2 antibodies. Patients with anti-ganglioside antibodies (whether spontaneously occurring or secondary to therapy) appear to have a better prognosis than those without antibodies.[56,57] Livingston et al. conducted a small randomized trial comparing BCG to treatment with BCG plus purified GM2 ganglioside as adjuvant therapy for patients with node-positive melanoma. There was no overall significant difference between the two treatment arms.[56] Interpretation was hampered by the small size of the trial and the fact that there was an imbalance between the two arms with respect to the number of patients with pre-existing anti-GM2 antibodies. Since the completion of that study, the investigators have focused on ways to increase the humoral response to GM2 vaccination. By conjugating the GM2 to the xenogeneic protein keyhole limpet hemocyanin and replacing the BCG with the saponin-derived adjuvant QS-21, they were able to achieve high levels of IgG and IgM anti-GM2 antibodies in a very high percentage of patients.[51] Adjuvant therapy with GM2-KLH/QS-21 has been studied in two large cooperative group trials in the USA and abroad, and a recent Intergroup trial, in which patients received either 18 months of GM2-KLH/QS-21 or the EST 1684 high-dose IFN-α regimen for 1 year, has just ended accrual.

Another technique for stimulating an immune response to non-protein antigens such as gangliosides is by the administration of anti-idiotype antibodies. These 'anti-antibodies' are antibodies raised against anti-ganglioside antibodies so that the variable regions of the antibody are essentially mirror-images of the ganglioside itself, but composed of protein.[58] When an immune response occurs to this mirror-image protein, it is also cross-reactive against the original antigen.[59] To date, anti-idiotype antibodies have been produced against GD2 and GD3; these antibodies have undergone phase I and II testing and have been shown to be capable of generating high titers of anti-GD3 antibodies in patients with metastatic and resected melanoma. In a phase II trial of 47 patients with metastatic melanoma who received an anti-idiotype antibody with QS-21 adjuvant,[60] anti-anti-idiotype or Ab3 was documented in 40/47 patients. One complete responder and 18 stable patients were noted. The same investigators went on to immunize 44 patients without evidence of disease after resection, and 42 developed high-titer Ab3. The anti-idiotype antibodies have not yet been subjected to testing in randomized trials,[61,62] although this approach is planned for testing in a high-risk group of resected melanoma patients.

HLA-restricted melanoma-associated antigenic peptides

It is now recognized that T-cells recognize antigenic peptides in a human leukocyte antigen (HLA)-restricted manner, meaning that a given peptide must be presented to the T-cell in the antigen-binding groove of that particular HLA molecule in order to stimulate an immune response.[63,64] From a practical standpoint, this means that even if a tumor possesses a known tumor-regression antigen, the patient's HLA type will determine whether or not individual epitope peptides encoded by that antigen can be recognized. The search for tumor antigens recognized by human T-cells, and the definition of the restriction patterns of these antigens, have become a major focus of cancer research. At present, a number of HLA-restricted melanoma-associated antigenic peptides have been defined, and vaccines are being constructed and tested in appropriate patients (Table 18.1).[65] Initial experiments with the HLA-A1-restricted MAGE-3 peptide EVDPIGHLY given in aqueous solution at low (100–300 μg/injection) doses to 12 patients with metastatic melanoma indicated that six were able to complete three injections at monthly intervals, and three of the six had objective clinical responses.[66] Surprisingly, no evidence of boosted immunity was detected in the peripheral blood.

The MART-1 27–35 and 26–35, tyrosinase 1–9 and 368–376 as well as several gp100 peptides (280–288 and 457–467) have been tested alone and in combination in patients with metastatic or resected melanoma. Jaeger and colleagues immunized three metastatic melanoma patients intradermally with multiple peptides from MART-1, gp100, and tyrosinase in aqueous solution at 100 μg each weekly for four immunizations. When granulocyte-macrophage colony-stimulating factor (GM-CSF) was injected at 75 μg per dose subcutaneously as an adjuvant for 3 days prior to and 2 days after immunization with multiple antigen peptides, significant boosting of immune reactivity was seen compared to vaccination with peptides alone.[67] All three patients showed increased immune reactivity to tyrosinase peptide 1–9, and one had increased reactivity to MART-1 26–35. Objective clinical responses were seen in each patient, including two partial regressions in involved lymph nodal, cutaneous, and liver lesions, and one complete regression in a patient with subcutaneous disease.

Cebon and colleagues[68] immunized patients with metastatic melanoma using intradermally administered MART-1 26–35 peptide with interleukin-12 (IL-12) in increasing doses, given either subcutaneously or intravenously. The main toxicity of IL-12 by either route was flu-like symptoms. Of the first 15 patients, one complete response, one partial response, and one mixed response were noted. Immune assays for T-cell generation included delayed-type hypersensitivity (DTH), which was seen in patients with or without IL-12. Positive assays for

Table 18.1 *Defined HLA-restricted tumor-associated antigens in melanoma*

Antigen	HLA restriction pattern	Frequency in NAC population	Status of vaccine
gp100	HLA-A2	49.5	Currently in phase I testing
MART-1/MelanA	HLA-A2	49.5	Currently in phase I testing
TRP-1(gp75)	HLA-A31	25.7	Under development
Tyrosinase	HLA-A2	49.5	Currently in phase I testing
	HLA-B44	23.9	
	HLA-A24	15.3	
	HLA-DR4	31.3	
MAGE-1	HLA-A1	28.2	Currently in phase I testing
	HLA-Cw16		
MAGE-3	HLA-A1	28.2	Under development
	HLA-A2	49.5	
BAGE	HLA-Cw16		Not currently available
GAGE-1, GAGE-2	HLA-Cw16		Not currently available
N-acetylglucosaminyl-transferase-V	HLA-A2	49.5	Not currently available
p15	HLA-A24	15.3	Not currently available
β-catenin	HLA-A24	15.3	Not currently available
MUM-1	HLA-B44	23.9	Not currently available
CDK4	HLA-A2	49.5	Not currently available

NAC = North American Caucasian.

cytotoxic T-lymphocytes (CTL) were seen in patients with evidence of clinical benefit, but not in patients without regression.

A number of small pilot studies have been conducted in which patients with metastatic melanoma received multiple subcutaneous injections of a single peptide emulsified with IFN-α at 3-week intervals. MART-1 27–35, gp100 209–217, 154–162, and 280–288 have been used in these trials.[69,70] In one study, escalating doses of the gp100 209 (ITDQVPSFY), 280 (YLEPGPVTA), or 154 (KTWGQYWQV) peptides at doses from 1 mg to 10 mg were administered subcutaneously every 3 weeks with IFN-α.[71] Immune assays were performed using the above 'native' peptides for antigenic stimulation and substituted 209–2M (IMDQVPFSY) and 280–9V (YLEPG-PVTV) peptides. Strong evidence of boosted immune reactivity was seen in 90–100% of patients post-vaccination, as shown by an assay in which release of IFN-γ from peripheral blood mononuclear cells (PBMC) restimulated one to three times in the presence of IL-2 and peptide antigen was measured by enzyme-linked immunosorbent assay (ELISA). Seven of seven patients had boosted gp100 reactivity post-vaccine after only one restimulation with the 209–2M peptide, and 5/6 were boosted with one restimulation with the 280–9V peptide. Higher release of cytokine was seen after four immunizations than after two in most patients, and a greater level of reactivity was observed when substituted peptides were used in contrast to assays performed with 'native' peptides.

Boosted cytokine release was shown to correlate with cytolytic responses. When tumor cell lines expressing the correct major histocompatibility complex (MHC) restriction element and antigen were used as a stimulator in cytokine release assays, lower levels of cytokine were observed compared with T2 cells pulsed with the relevant peptide, suggesting that peptide density on the target was important for recognition by effector cells in PBMC. Objective partial and complete remissions were uncommon, with 1/20 patients having a complete regression. No clear correlation was observed between the level of immune response and the rare clinical responses, so no statement about clinical benefit could be made. In a second study of escalating doses of the MART-1 27–35 peptide administered subcutaneously every 3 weeks with incomplete Freund's adjuvant (IFA), 15/16 patients had evidence of boosting of immunity directed against the 'native' MART-1 27–35 peptide, with increased reactivity after four compared with fewer vaccinations.[72] No objective clinical responses were seen. At the university of Southern California/Norris Cancer Hospital, Los Angeles, California, we have treated 25 melanoma patients with high-risk resected stages III/IV disease with increasing doses of the MART-1 27–35 peptide emulsified with IFA every 3 weeks subcutaneously.[73] Ten of 22 patients had evidence of boosted immunity by cytokine release assays, and a correlation was observed between the absolute level of IFN-γ released after multiple re-stimulations of peptide-pulsed patient PBMC post-vaccination and time to relapse, with a p value of 0.003. The correlation of immune reactivity with time to relapse suggests that a positive response to peptide vaccination may incur clinical benefit.

The anchor amino acids that form hydrogen bonds between epitope peptides and class I MHC molecules can be modified to strengthen their binding, resulting in greater immunogenicity *in vitro* and *in vivo*. When such heteroclitic peptides derived from gp100 were used to restimulate PBMC from patients with metastatic melanoma immunized with a wild-type gp100 peptide, immune reactivity was detected with greater frequency and sensitivity.[72] Patients immunized with the heteroclitic gp100 peptide demonstrated a higher level of immune reactivity compared with the wild-type peptide. The MART-1 27–35 peptide has been shown to be 'naturally' processed and is immunodominant. However, the MART-1 26–35 peptide has been shown to be a better MHC binder and more immunogenic *in vitro*,[74] and was more effective at the detection and quantitation of MART-1-specific CTL in a flow cytometry assay when used for the generation of MHC/peptide tetramers.[75] Heteroclitic gp100 peptides combined with IFA have been used to immunize patients with metastatic melanoma, and more than 90% of the patients in one vaccine study had evidence of boosted immunity detected after one restimulation *in vitro*, suggesting that the substituted peptide was more immunogenic than 'natural' peptide *in vivo*.[76] When the same substituted gp100 peptide was injected, followed within several days by high-dose intravenous IL-2, surprisingly, no detectable augmented immune response was observed, but 13/31 patients had an antitumor response, including 12 partial responses and one complete response for an overall response rate of 42%, significantly greater than rates observed with IL-2 alone (15–20%).[76] The utility of a peptide vaccination added to high-dose IL-2 as an 'adjuvant' is currently being explored in two large multicenter, randomized trials. At our institution, the heteroclitic gp100 209–217 (210M) and tyrosinase 368–376 (370D) peptides emulsified in IFA with or without IL-12 as an adjuvant are being examined in a randomized, phase II trial in patients with high-risk resected stage III/IV melanoma, in which immune response is one endpoint and time to relapse is the clinical endpoint. Strong DTH skin-test responses to gp100 but not tyrosinase have been observed in 20/24 patients, and augmented immune responses to both gp100 and tyrosinase have been observed in 19/24 patients, suggesting that multiple melanoma peptides injected simultaneously with adjuvant result in boosted immunity to both antigens in virtually all patients with resected high-risk melanoma (JS Weber *et al.*, unpublished). Whether IL-12 administration results in augmented skin-test reactivity or increased antigen-specific immune responses measured by cytokine release or tetramer assays awaits a more detailed analysis.

MISCELLANEOUS AGENTS: HORMONES, COUMARIN, AND RETINOIDS

A small randomized, controlled trial using the progestational agent megestrol acetate (Megace) was conducted which demonstrated a trend for improved survival in favor of the treated group.[77] Although this difference failed to achieve statistical significance, it prompted a larger-scale evaluation by the North Central Cancer Treatment Group (NCCTG), whose results have not yet been published. On the theory that differentiation agents might be useful in the adjuvant setting, several studies have compared retinoic acid or 13-cis-retinoic acid to observation.[78,79] One additional trial compared BCG plus retinoic acid to BCG alone.[80] All of these studies failed to demonstrate a benefit for the adjuvant use of retinoids. A 27-patient study utilizing the anticoagulant coumarin (from which coumadin is derived) revealed an increased disease-free survival in the treated group.[81]

SINGLE-AGENT CYTOTOXIC CHEMOTHERAPY

Single agents with recognized but modest activity against advanced disease include dacarbazine (DTIC), the nitrosoureas (lomustine [BCNU], carmustine [CCNU] and semustine [methyl-CCNU]), the vinca alkaloids (vincristine, vinblastine, and vindesine), cisplatin, paclitaxel and bleomycin.[82] Single-agent therapy with dacarbazine results in objective responses in about 18–22% of patients with measurable metastatic disease. Response durations are generally short, and durable complete responses quite uncommon. Despite this modest activity, DTIC has been rather extensively evaluated in the adjuvant setting.[83] These trials have provided no evidence that DTIC has significant efficacy as a postsurgical adjuvant. One multi-arm trial incorporated single-agent methyl-CCNU in one treatment arm. There was a nonsignificant trend in favor of the chemotherapy arm,[84] but significant renal toxicity and the risk of treatment-induced myelodysplasia mitigated against further evaluation of this agent in the adjuvant setting.

MULTI-AGENT CYTOTOXIC CHEMOTHERAPY

Multi-agent chemotherapy has never been definitively documented to be superior to single-agent therapy when used for metastatic melanoma. A recent definitive phase III trial was performed under the auspices of the Eastern Cooperative Oncology Group (ECOG) to compare DTIC alone with the Dartmouth regimen of BCNU, CDDP, DTIC, and tamoxifen.[7] Two hundred and forty patients were randomized to the trial, in which median survival for DTIC was 6.3 months, compared with 7.7 months for the combination. There were no significant differences between the two groups in survival or response rate, suggesting that the Dartmouth regimen should no longer be used in the routine treatment of patients with metastatic melanoma. By default, DTIC remains the standard of care to which new experimental chemotherapies should be compared. Nonetheless, several adjuvant therapy trials have been conducted in which chemotherapy was combined with immunotherapy or in which multiple cytotoxic agents were employed.

Chemoimmunotherapy

Several small trials have explored postoperative adjuvant therapy with DTIC plus BCG, with or without a no-treatment arm.[85–88] DTIC plus BCG does not appear to have any efficacy in the adjuvant setting, which is hardly surprising in view of the lack of activity of the individual agents and the absence of any suggestion of synergy between them. DTIC with or without cyclophosphamide plus *C. parvum* also failed to prove superior to *C. parvum* alone,[89] or to a no-treatment control group.[90] BCG with or without *C. parvum* has been combined with DTIC-based multiagent chemotherapy in a few studies, all without a no-treatment control arm.[91–93] No suggestion of benefit for chemoimmunotherapy was seen in these studies. Finally, a small randomized trial of DTIC plus IFN revealed no evidence of benefit compared to a no-treatment control group.[94]

Multi-agent cytotoxic therapy

Multi-agent cytotoxic chemotherapy without immunotherapy has received relatively little attention in the postoperative adjuvant setting. Karakousis and Emrich found no benefit for the combination of DTIC and estramustine in a small, three-arm study comparing multi-agent chemotherapy or BCG to a no-treatment control group.[95] Four two-arm, randomized, controlled trials of multi-agent chemotherapy have been carried out. A trial using BCNU, dactinomycin, and vincristine,[96] and a small trial of DTIC, CCNU, and vincristine[97] both suggested a benefit for multi-agent chemotherapy, whereas other trials did not.[98] Interestingly, no adjuvant trials have been performed to date with cisplatin-containing combinations, although recent data discussed above in which a combination chemotherapy regimen failed to demonstrate a survival advantage over single-agent dacarbazine render any such adjuvant trials premature.

Preoperative (neoadjuvant) chemoimmunotherapy

Preoperative chemotherapy has become commonplace in the treatment of some tumor types, but has not found widespread application in melanoma. Nonetheless, patients with bulky nodal disease, resectable metastatic disease, and non-cutaneous primary melanomas (such as anorectal melanomas) would be logical candidates for a preoperative approach aimed at shrinking the tumor and assessing *in-vivo* chemosensitivity. A number of recent, non-randomized, phase II studies have revealed high response rates (40–65%) in patients with metastatic melanoma to chemoimmunotherapy regimens with cisplatin, velban, dacarbazine, IL-2, and IFN-α.[99,100] A similar regimen, including cisplatin, vinblastine, and DTIC administered concurrently with IL-2 and IFN-α,[101] has shown a 44% response rate used preoperatively, suggesting a possible role for this neoadjuvant approach. Patients who are candidates for this type of therapy, however, are also candidates for autologous tumor vaccines as well as postoperative IFN-α on cooperative group trials. Thus, the precise role of preoperative chemoimmunotherapy will need to be defined in a prospective, randomized study relative to these other approaches.

Intensive chemotherapy with autologous bone marrow support

A limited experience has been accumulated with autologous marrow support following intensive chemotherapy for metastatic melanoma. Although intensive chemotherapy for metastatic melanoma has not found widespread use, one small randomized trial was conducted in patients with multiple involved lymph nodes.[102] No advantage for the treatment group was found. Of interest was the high frequency of local/regional recurrence in this study, doubtless reflective of the high regional disease burden of eligible patients.

INTERFERONS AND OTHER CYTOKINES

Although their precise antitumor effects remain poorly understood, no agents have been more intensively studied in melanoma than the IFNs. This has resulted in multiple adjuvant trials involving these agents. Other cytokines, such as the ILS and tumor necrosis factor-α, have also undergone detailed evaluations, but as yet have received limited attention in the adjuvant setting.

Interferon gamma

The immunologic activities of IFN-γ have been extensively characterized – including studies in melanoma patients.[103–106] These studies provided a compelling rationale for the use of IFN-γ in the adjuvant treatment of melanoma.[107] A randomized trial of the Southwest Oncology Group, however, failed to indicate any benefit for adjuvant treatment with an immunologically active dose of IFN-γ in patients at intermediate and high risk of recurrence.[108] The results of this trial were disclosed early because of a suggestion that the treatment arm actually fared worse than the control arm,[109] prompting the National Cancer Institute of Canada to close its adjuvant therapy trial comparing levamisole and IFN-γ. A total of 89 patients were entered onto this study when it was closed; there was no apparent difference in disease-free or overall survival between the two groups.[110] The EORTC is currently conducting a multi-arm adjuvant trial in which one group receives IFN-γ; the results of these trials may address whether such treatment is indeed detrimental. Given the long list of favorable immunologic effects associated with IFN-γ, the lack of efficacy – and, indeed, the possibility of a detrimental effect – is difficult to explain, but should prompt a rethinking of the widely held tenet that immunologic agents which lack activity in metastatic disease are appropriate candidates for evaluation in the adjuvant setting.

Interferon alfa

Unlike IFN-γ, IFN-α does possess a reasonable degree of activity against metastatic melanoma,[111] in addition to a broad range of immunologic effects.[112] These properties have prompted several studies of IFN-α in the adjuvant setting (Table 18.2). These trials have employed varying doses, routes of administration, durations of therapy, and risk groups, making comparisons all but impossible. Nonetheless, on closer inspection some discernible patterns appear to be emerging.

One non-randomized trial evaluated a low-dose IFN-α regimen (2–3 million units (MU) subcutaneously twice or thrice weekly) administered for 20 months to patients at intermediate risk of recurrence. This study suggested an early increase in disease-free survival compared to historical controls, which disappeared once therapy was stopped.[113] Whether or not this represented a true biologic effect of IFN therapy is impossible to determine in a non-randomized trial, but this observation has nonetheless prompted concerns about the duration of IFN treatment in the adjuvant setting. The World Health Organization looked at a similar low-dose regimen (3 MU subcutaneously thrice weekly) administered for 3 years to patients with positive nodes in a randomized trial that has been completed but not yet subjected to a final analysis. Several interim analyses have been published or presented, initially with a suggestion of significant benefit,[114] and later without.[115] The mature results of this trial do not indicate a prolongation of survival for patients with stage III resected disease, nor do they shed light onto whether there is indeed a 'rebound' effect after IFN treatment is discontinued.

A different approach was taken by Creagan et al. and the North Central Cancer Treatment Group in a randomized trial of patients at intermediate and high risk of recurrence.[116] In this study, patients on the treatment arm received a 3-month course of high-dose (20 MU/m^2) IFN-α2a administered intramuscularly. Overall, there was no significant difference in outcome between the treatment and control arms. Patients in the high-risk group (involved nodes), however, had an increased disease-free survival (DFS) (40% versus 30% alive and well at 5 years), which reached statistical significance when adjusted for prognostic factors. Overall survival (OS) was also better in the node-positive patients who received IFN-α2a (47% versus 39% alive at 5 years), but not significantly so. No benefit was detected for the node-negative patients on this trial. The relatively small size of the study (262 patients overall, 160 node positive) severely limited the power to detect a significant treatment effect, and makes any conclusions about subset effects tenuous at best, but suggested that higher doses of IFN may be beneficial.

Like Creagan, Kirkwood et al. chose to employ a very high dose of IFN, this time IFN-α2b, but for a longer interval (1 year), in a randomized, controlled trial for ECOG.[1] Both node-positive and high-risk node-negative (T4N0M0) patients were included; the majority of patients had relapsed in the regional nodes after prior wide excision. The regimen involved an initial 'induction' phase of 20 MU/m^2 intravenously 5 days a week for 4 weeks, followed by a 'maintenance' phase of 10 MU/m^2 subcutaneously 3 days a week for 11 months. This regimen was deliberately chosen to be at or near the maximally tolerated dose and, indeed, was quite toxic. Treatment was reduced or discontinued in over half the patients, and there were two treatment-related deaths. The overall results, however, were positive: patients randomized to receive IFN-α2b had a significant 33% improvement in disease-free and a 27% improvement in overall survival compared to the control group. There was no evidence of an increased relapse rate after the IFN-α2b treatment ended; indeed, the results demonstrated a plateau of increased long-term survival. One observation was similar to the NCCTG trial: the beneficial effect was confined to node-positive patients. Indeed, in the small subset of node-negative patients (accounting for about 11% of the 280 total patients), the group randomized to receive IFN-α2b actually fared worse. The small size of this subset, and the presence of an imbalance between the treatment and control arms in the percentage of patients with ulcerated primaries, make it impossible to determine whether there is truly a difference in the response of node-positive and node-negative patients to IFN treatment. Despite the lack of a mature confirmatory trial, the FDA approved the use of adjuvant high-dose IFN-α2b for melanoma patients 'at high risk of recurrence' in December 1995. Doubtless, part of the rationale for approval on the basis of a single trial was the lack of efficacious adjuvant therapies for melanoma. It is also likely that the results of a quality-adjusted time without symptoms or toxicity (Q-TWiST) analysis, which confirmed the benefit of IFN-α2b therapy even after

Table 18.2 *Trials evaluating adjuvant therapy with interferon-α*

Author/institution	Reference	Treatment arms	Number per arm	Results/comments
Kokoschka/Vienna	113	IFN-α2b 2–3 MU sc 2–3$\times$/wk $\times$ 20 mos Concurrent controls	68	Nonrandomized
		Stage II & III	115	5-yr DFS, OS; NSD
Creagan/NCCTG	116	IFN-α2a 20 MU/m^2 im 3$\times$/wk $\times$ 12 wks vs Observation	131	5-yr DFS, OS; NSD
		Stage II & III	131	DFS for stage III patients significantly better with IFN
Kirkwood/ECOG	1	IFN-α2b 20 MU/m^2 iv 5$\times$/wk $\times$ 4 wk then 10 MU/m^2 sc 3$\times$/wk $\times$ 11 mos vs Observation	143	5-yr DFS: Significantly better with IFN (37% vs 26%)
		Stage IIB & III	137	5-yr OS: Significantly better with IFN (46% vs 37%)
Cascinelli/WHO	114	IFN-α2a 3 MU sc 3$\times$/wk $\times$ 3 yrs vs Observation	218	Final results pending
		Stage III	208	Most recent report 2-yr DFS, OS; NSD
Grob/French multicentre	120	IFN-α2a 3 MU sc 3$\times$/wk $\times$ 18 mos vs Observation	252	Final results pending
		Stage II	247	Preliminary report increased 2-yr DFS but not OS with IFN
Kirkwood/Intergroup	118	IFN-α2b 20 MU/m^2 iv 5$\times$/wk $\times$ 4 wk then 10 MU/m^2 sc 3$\times$/wk $\times$ 11 mos vs IFN-α2b 3 MU sc 3$\times$/wk $\times$ 2 yrs vs Observation Stage IIB & III	644 patients total	No differences in OS between the arms; HDI had a RFS advantage with $p < 0.05$ vs OBS
Eggermont/EORTC		IFN-α2b 1 MU sc OOD $\times$ 12 mos vs IFN-γ 0.2 mg sc 3$\times$/wk Stage IIB & III		Closed; results pending
Eggermont/EORTC		IFN-α2b 10 MU sc 5$\times$/wk $\times$ 4 wk then 10 MU sc 3$\times$/wk $\times$ 11 mos vs IFN-α2b 10 MU sc 5$\times$/wk $\times$ 4 wk then 5 MU sc 3$\times$/wk $\times$ 23 mos vs Observation Stage IIB & III		Open to patient accrual
Kirkwood/Intergroup		IFN-α2b 20 MU/m^2 iv 5$\times$/wk $\times$ 4 wk then 10 MU/m^2 sc 3$\times$/wk $\times$ 11 mos vs GM2/KLH plus QS-21 vaccine $\times$ 2 yrs Stage IIB & III		Preliminary report indicates increased DFS and OS with IFN; trial closed early by DSMB because of superior RFS with IFN compared to vaccine ($p < 0.001$)

NCCTG, North Central Cancer Treatment Group; ECOG, Eastern Cooperative Oncology Group; WHO, World Health Organization; EORTC, European Organization for the Research and Treatment of Cancer; NSD, no significant difference between treatment and control arms; DFS, disease-free survival; DSMB, Data Safety Monitoring Board; HDI, high-dose interferon; OS, Overall survival; RFS, relapse-free survival.

accounting for its significant toxicity,[117] also played a role in the FDA decision. This analysis was done retrospectively, without prospective collection of quality-of-life data from participants in the original ECOG trial, but still provides a basis for assuring patients that the significant toxicity of therapy appears justified.

One additional reservation must be stated regarding the ECOG trial: patients were not evaluated for a recognized prognostic factor, the number of positive lymph nodes. Thus, it is possible that there was an unrecognized imbalance between the treatment and control groups of node-positive patients that could have influenced the outcome.[2] A confirmatory study has been conducted as an ECOG-coordinated Intergroup trial, with accrual completed in June 1995. The preliminary results of the ECOG 1690/SWOG 9111/C9190 trial comparing observation, low-dose IFN-α and high-dose IFN-α for patients with resected lymph nodal melanoma were presented by Kirkwood at the American Society of Clinical Oncology (ASCO) in 1999 and recently published.[118] Six hundred and forty-two patients were accrued, and 163 had T4 lesions. No impact upon overall survival was seen for the high-dose or low-dose IFN regimens. Relapse-free survival (RFS), on the other hand, was prolonged for the patients on the high-dose regimen. Seven percent of the total group had sentinel lymph node biopsies. Interestingly, interstudy improvement for the control arm was seen, with a p value less than 0.001, suggesting that therapy in general, staging criteria, and supportive care had improved since the 1980s. Relapse-free survival time was clearly prolonged, as in the prior E1684 study, but the time from relapse to death in the control arm significantly increased, resulting in no survival difference. The explanation for this has been debated, with no clear-cut answer, but it was intriguing that patients who relapsed on the observation arm were more commonly treated with high-dose IFN or chemobiotherapy than patients on the treatment arms, which may account for the improvement on survival between the two studies. These data may suggest that IFN could be used up front as an adjuvant therapy or delayed until nodal relapse with equal utility. These data continued the controversy over the utility of IFN in the high-dose regimen, which has been shown to have significant toxicity. Recently, the third in a series of IFN adjuvant trials, ECOG 1694/SWOG 9512, completed accrual, in which 774 patients were allocated randomly to receive the EST 1684 1-year regimen of IFN or 96 weeks of a vaccine called GM-K, which generates anti-ganglioside antibodies (V Sondak, personal communication). The trial was stopped prematurely by the Data Safety Monitoring Board (DSMB) because relapse-free survival in the IFN arm was clearly superior to that in the vaccine arm ($p < 0.001$), meeting a milestone as determined in a planned interim analysis. Overall survival in eligible patients was also improved with short follow-up time, with $p = 0.04$. For the first time, benefit was seen in patients with node-negative stage IIB disease. These updated data again suggest that high-dose IFN is the standard of care in patients with resected stage III melanoma against which other regimens should be measured (see Editors' selected abstracts, Kirkwood, Ibrahim, Sosman, et al., page 482). An encouraging note stems from a recent multicenter pilot study through ECOG in which patients were randomly assigned to receive high-dose IFN for 1 year or IFN plus a GM2 vaccine.[119] The results of this trial indicated that no diminution in antibody responses to the vaccine was seen with concurrent high-dose IFN, suggesting that, as new vaccine strategies are developed, they may be added to the existing standard IFN-α regimen with a reasonable chance that the vaccine-induced immune response will not be diminished.

A subset of patients may benefit from briefer IFN regimens after resection of high-risk melanoma, but that group has not yet been defined. In a follow-up study for patients with node negative T3 lesions (E1697), patients will either be treated only with the 1-month dose intense intravenous portion of the E1690 study, or have observation only after a wide and deep excision. Most of these patients will have had a sentinel node biopsy, and this study marks the first time that an adjuvant study will enroll large numbers of sentinel node biopsy-negative individuals.

As indicated previously, neither the first two ECOG trial with IFN-α2b nor the NCCTG trial with IFN-α2a demonstrated a benefit for adjuvant IFN therapy in node-negative patients, although preliminary results from the recent 1694 trial were the first to suggest such benefit. A French multicenter trial has recently been completed using low-dose IFN-α2a (3 MU subcutaneously three times a week) in node-negative patients with melanomas > 1.5 mm in thickness. Preliminary results of this trial suggest a small but significant benefit for adjuvant IFN therapy in terms of disease-free but not overall survival.[120] The updated results of this trial have not suggested any survival advantage. Of future interest is an EORTC trial just underway which will compare two different intermediate-dose IFN-α2b regimens to a no-treatment control arm in patients with high-risk (stage IIB and III) melanoma.

Interleukin-2 and other cytokines

Besides IFN-α, IL-2 is the only other cytokine that has documented efficacy in advanced disease, an indication for which it was approved by the FDA. Unfortunately, significant toxicity has precluded evaluation of this agent in the adjuvant setting. The National Cancer Institute attempted to conduct an adjuvant trial of high-dose IL-2 in patients at extremely high risk of recurrence (≥ ten involved lymph nodes), but, even in this poor prognosis group, the severe toxicity of treatment led to premature closure of the study. There are currently insufficient data to justify the use of other cytokines in the systemic adjuvant therapy of melanoma patients.

REGIONAL ADJUVANT THERAPY

Not all adjuvant therapy need be administered systemically; regional treatments have also been extensively evaluated in melanoma. Elective lymph node dissection can be considered an 'adjuvant' to wide excision of the primary tumor; the results of clinical trials evaluating node dissections are discussed elsewhere in this book. The two other techniques for increasing regional control that have been evaluated in melanoma include external-beam radiation therapy and hyperthermic isolation limb perfusion.

External-beam radiation therapy

Radiation therapy has traditionally had a very limited role in the management of melanoma, primarily confined to the treatment of central nervous system metastases.[121] There is reason to suspect, however, that adjuvant treatment with radiation can decrease recurrence after lymph node dissection.[122] Surprisingly, only one small, randomized trial of adjuvant radiotherapy has been completed in cutaneous melanoma, and this yielded a negative result.[123] This study utilized conventional radiation fractions and a treatment break, both currently felt to be suboptimal for melanoma. A small, non-randomized phase II study of adjuvant radiation therapy delivered in large fractions to patients with lymph nodal melanoma in the neck suggested a very favorable survival and time to relapse compared with historical controls. Based on these promising phase II data, the Radiation Therapy Oncology Group initiated a randomized trial of postoperative irradiation using larger treatment fractions in patients undergoing neck dissections for melanoma. Accrual to this trial has been poor, however, and the approval of IFN-α as adjuvant therapy further jeopardized its success, resulting in the trial being modified to include IFN-α treatment for all randomized patients. It remains clear that patients with multiple lymph nodes involved with melanoma are at great risk of regional and distant recurrence. Such patients could potentially benefit from an integrated strategy involving both IFN and radiotherapy. Preliminary studies are necessary to define the optimal scheduling of these two modalities, but, if these can be conducted, a randomized trial comparing IFN alone to IFN plus radiation for melanoma patients with multiple involved nodes would seem to be worthwhile. Adjuvant radiation therapy is also being evaluated in the management of ocular melanoma, in a multicenter collaborative trial.[124]

Hyperthermic isolation limb perfusion

Extremity isolation limb perfusion is conducted as a surgical procedure under general anesthesia, by cannulating the main artery and vein to the arm or leg and diverting the blood flow in that extremity through a cardiac surgery bypass oxygenation apparatus. Tourniquets are applied to effectively isolate the entire limb from the systemic circulation, and antineoplastic agents are then introduced into the bypass circuit, perfusing the limb but not the systemic circulation. The temperature of the perfusate can be adjusted, and most perfusions are carried out at elevated temperatures (39–41.5 °C). The most commonly used drug for perfusion has been melphalan,[125] but cisplatin, dactinomycin, and, most recently, tumor necrosis factor-α with or without IFN-γ[126] have also been used. Although hyperthermic isolation limb perfusion with any of these agents induces a high rate of objective remissions in patients with measurable cutaneous ('in transit') metastases, response durations are typically short and these patients generally succumb to distant disease regardless of whether or not local control is achieved. Isolation limb perfusion has been evaluated in the adjuvant setting, with the goal of reducing in transit recurrences. Trial design has been hampered by the difficulty in defining a patient population at high enough risk of cutaneous recurrence who do not also have a prohibitively high risk of developing distant metastases. Several suggestive retrospective reviews led to two small, randomized trials, which showed evidence of an overall or disease-free survival benefit for adjuvant isolation limb perfusion with melphalan.[127,128] This prompted a large, international, Intergroup trial of adjuvant limb perfusion (over 700 patients). The final results as well as interim analysis revealed no evidence of a survival or disease-free survival benefit for melphalan perfusion.[129] Thus, once again, retrospective studies and small randomized trials suggested a benefit that was not confirmed in a well-designed, appropriately powered, randomized study. Given the technical complexity, risks, and lack of demonstrated benefit of this adjuvant therapy, its further routine use as adjuvant therapy for patients with resected in-transit limb melanoma should not be considered. Whether the availability of new perfusion therapies such as tumor necrosis factor-α will lead to a rethinking of this position remains to be seen. If so, any future adjuvant trials should probably be confined to patients with primary tumors at very high risk of local/regional recurrence (i.e., thick primaries with ulceration, satellitosis, or extensive angiolymphatic spread and/or patients with completely resected local or in-transit recurrences).

SUMMARY AND FUTURE CONSIDERATIONS

Who is an appropriate candidate for systemic adjuvant therapy?

Metastatic malignant melanoma remains a highly lethal disease; therefore, the prevention of its development is a clinical priority. Of the myriad of agents tested over the years, IFN-α2b was the only one to gain FDA approval on the basis of a survival advantage, albeit in a single, but well-designed, phase III, randomized trial. A confirmatory trial (ECOG 1690/SWOG9111) did not confirm this benefit, but a recently halted study suggests that it must be considered the standard of care for patients for whom adjuvant therapy is prescribed. But what should those patients do?

- *Resected stage III melanoma.* Otherwise healthy patients should be offered entry to randomized clinical trials comparing new approaches to adjuvant therapy with high-dose IFN-α2b. These patients should be given a clear understanding of the relapse-free and overall survival benefit and toxicity of therapy. A discussion of the results of the recent Q-TWiST analysis of the E1684 trial,[117] and the developments in the recent confirmatory three-arm trial,[118] as well as the prematurely halted ECOG 1694/SWOG 9512 trial is often a helpful exercise in allowing prospective patients to weigh the toxic costs of therapy against the possible gains in freedom from relapse and overall survival. Patients with multiple (≥ ten) involved lymph nodes, extracapsular invasion, or other risk factors for regional recurrence should also be considered for concomitant adjuvant external-beam radiation. Substantive questions remain about the use and proper scheduling of adjuvant radiation that are worthy of a large-scale clinical trial. If patients are to receive high-dose IFN-α, one possible practice is to initiate radiation therapy in these patients after the completion of the 1 month of intravenous IFN-α2b concomitant with the start of subcutaneous therapy. Patients with bulky nodal disease should be strongly considered for investigations of neoadjuvant chemoimmunotherapy or combination therapy with tumor vaccines.

- *Resected stage IV melanoma.* Resection of isolated melanoma metastases remains the best option for the curative treatment of metastatic melanoma in those few individuals amenable to this therapy. It should be offered to eligible patients whenever possible. Referral of these patients to treatment centers where aggressive surgery and investigational protocols are available is advocated. These patients should be strongly considered for investigations of adjuvant chemoimmunotherapy, allogeneic tumor vaccination, or phase II peptide or antigen-specific vaccine trials. Off protocol, adjuvant therapy with two to three cycles of chemoimmunotherapy or the use of high-dose IFN-α2b, if administered with careful, informed consent, is acceptable given the extremely high risk of relapse in this patient population.

- *Resected stage IIB melanoma.* Patients with thick (≥4.0 mm) primary tumors and clinically or pathologically negative lymph nodes ideally should be considered for participation in clinical trials assessing vaccines and other biologic therapies. This approach is justified by the high risk of recurrence combined with the equivocal benefit for IFN-α2b in this subgroup. Given the high risk of occult nodal involvement in these patients, lymphatic mapping and selective lymph node dissection should be employed when possible, and patients with pathologically positive nodes treated as outlined for stage III patients, although benefit for IFN-α seems possible but unclear in this subgroup.

- *Resected stage IIA melanoma.* Patients with intermediate-thickness primary tumors and clinically or pathologically negative lymph nodes are not candidates for adjuvant therapy with the 1-year regimen of high-dose IFN-α2b, but are at sufficient risk of relapse to justify participation in clinical trials incorporating a no-treatment control. Experimental approaches appropriate for this group include low-dose or brief high-dose IFN regimens, allogeneic vaccines, and defined antigens such as peptides or gangliosides. Given the moderate risk of occult nodal involvement in patients with intermediate-thickness primary melanomas, lymphatic mapping and selective lymph node dissection are reasonable for those patients who would be suitable candidates for adjuvant trials or off-protocol therapy if pathologically positive nodes are found. Although there is no rigorous evidence to date that earlier detection of nodal positivity by sentinel node mapping and subsequent initiation of IFN therapy alter the outcome, sentinel node mapping should generally be performed in patients with stage IIA disease. Expectant observation of clinically node-negative patients with the institution of adjuvant treatments including IFN only upon nodal relapse is also an acceptable, but less aggressive, strategy.

- *Resected stage I melanoma.* Patients with thin primary tumors and clinically negative lymph nodes are not candidates for adjuvant therapy, and if the primary tumor is less than 1 mm, have insufficient risk of occult nodal involvement to justify lymphatic mapping and selective lymph node dissection unless the lesion is ulcerated. Such patients are at high enough risk for the development of second primary melanomas (and non-melanoma skin cancers) to justify participation in experimental trials aimed at melanoma prevention – a fertile field of future research.

- *Resected non-cutaneous melanoma.* The use of adjuvant therapy in mucosal and choroidal melanomas must still be considered purely investigational, and should therefore ideally take place in the context of randomized, controlled phase III or pilot phase II trials. Because many patients with mucosal melanomas – and some patients with choroidal melanomas – are at very high risk of local/regional and distant recurrence, multicenter and cooperative group trials addressing multimodality therapy in these diseases should be developed. An increased understanding of the biologic and therapeutic differences (if any) between cutaneous and non-cutaneous melanomas would certainly facilitate the design and conduct of such trials.

REFERENCES

1. Kirkwood JM, Strawderman MH, Ernstoff MS, Smith TJ, Borden EC, Blum RH. Interferon alfa-2b adjuvant therapy of high-risk resected cutaneous melanoma: the Eastern Cooperative Oncology Group trial EST 1684. J Clin Oncol 1996; 14:7–17.

2. Balch CM, Buzaid AC. Finally, a successful adjuvant therapy for high-risk melanoma. J Clin Oncol 1996; 14:1–3.

3. Nathanson L. Interferon adjuvant therapy of melanoma. Cancer 1996; 78:944–7.

4. Balch CM. How patient referral bias can confuse interpretation of clinical results: elective lymph node dissections at the Sydney Melanoma Unit. J Am Coll Surg 1995; 180:490–2.

5. Spitler LE. A randomized trial of levamisole versus placebo as adjuvant therapy in malignant melanoma. J Clin Oncol 1991; 9:736–40.

6. Wallack MK, Sivanandham M, Balch CM, et al. A phase III randomized, double-blind, multiinstitutional trial of vaccinia melanoma oncolysate – active specific immunotherapy for patients with stage II melanoma. Cancer 1995; 75:34–42.

7. Saxman SB, Meyers ML, Chapman PB, et al. A phase III multicenter randomized trial of DTIC, cisplatin, BCNU and tamoxifen versus DTIC alone in patients with metastatic melanoma. Proc Am Soc Clin Oncol 1999; 536a:(Abstract 2068).

8. Stevenson HC, Green I, Hamilton JM, Calabro BA, Parkinson DR. Levamisole: known effects on the immune system, clinical results, and future applications to the treatment of cancer. J Clin Oncol 1991; 9:2052–66.

9. Loutfi A, Shakr A, Jerry M, Hanley J, Shibata HR. Double blind randomized prospective trial of levamisole/placebo in stage I cutaneous malignant melanoma. Clin Invest Med 1987; 10:325–8.

10. Morton DL. Immunological studies with human neoplasms. J Reticuloendothelial Soc 1971; 10:137–46.

11. Pinsky CM, Hirshaut Y, Oettgen HF. Treatment of malignant melanoma by intratumoral injections of BCG. Natl Cancer Inst Monogr 1973; 39:255.

12. Mastrangelo MJ, Sulit HL, Prehn LM. Intralesional BCG in the treatment of metastatic malignant melanoma. Cancer 1976; 37:684.

13. Morton DL, Eilber FR, Holmes EC, et al. BCG immunotherapy of malignant melanoma: summary of a seven year experience. Ann Surg 1974; 180:635–50.

14. Gutterman JU, Mcbride C, Freireich EJ, et al. Active immunotherapy with BCG for recurrent malignant melanoma. Lancet 1973; 1208–13.

15. Paterson AH, Wilans DJ, Jerry LM, et al. Adjuvant BCG immunotherapy for malignant melanoma. Can Med Assoc J 1984; 131:744.

16. Czarnetzki BM, Macher E, Suciu S, Thomas D, Steerenberg PA, Rumke P. Long-term adjuvant immunotherapy in stage I high risk malignant melanoma, comparing two BCG preparations versus non-treatment in a randomised multicentre study (EORTC Protocol 18781). Eur J Cancer 1993; 29A(9):1237–42.

17. Paterson AH, Willans DJ, Jerry LM, Hanson J, McPherson TA. Adjuvant BCG immunotherapy for malignant melanoma. Can Med Assoc J 1984; 131(7):744–8.

18. Silver HK, Ibrahim EM, Evers JA, Thomas JW, Murray RN, Spinelli JJ. Adjuvant BCG immunotherapy for stage I and II malignant melanoma. Can Med Assoc J 1983; 128(11):1291–5.

19. Byrne MJ, Van Hazel G, Reynolds PM, Lemish WM, Holman CD. Adjuvant immunotherapy with BCG in stage II malignant melanoma. J Surg Oncol 1983; 23(2):114–16.

20. Cochran AJ, Buyse ME, Lejeune FJ, Macher E, Revuz J, Rumke P. Adjuvant reactivity predicts survival in patients with 'high-risk' primary malignant melanoma treated with systemic BCG. EORTC Malignant Melanoma Cooperative Group Writing Committee. Int J Cancer 1981; 28(5):543–50.

21. O'Connor TP, Labandter HP, Hiles RW, Bodenham DC. A clinical trial of BCG immunotherapy as an adjunct to surgery in the treatment of primary malignant melanoma. Br J Plast Surg 1978; 31(4):317–22.

22. Christie GH, Bomford R. Mechanisms of macrophage activation by Corynebacterium parvum I. In vitro experiments. Cell Immunol 1975; 17:150–9.

23. Lipton A, Harvey HA, Lawrence B, et al. Corynebacterium parvum versus BCG adjuvant immunotherapy in human malignant melanoma. Cancer 1983; 51:57–66.

24. Lipton A, Harvey HA, Balch CM, et al. Corynebacterium parvum versus Bacille Calmette–Guerin adjuvant immunotherapy of stage II malignant melanoma. J Clin Oncol 1991; 9:1151–8.

25. Balch CM, Smalley RV, Bartolucci AA, et al. A randomized prospective clinical trial of adjuvant C. parvum immunotherapy in 260 patients with clinically localized melanoma (stage I): prognostic factors analysis and preliminary results of immunotherapy. Cancer 1982; 49:1079–86.

26. Lejeune FJ, Macher E, Kleeberg U, et al. An assessment of DTIC versus levamisole or placebo in the treatment of high risk stage I patients after surgical removal of a primary melanoma of the skin: a phase III adjuvant study. EORTC Protocol 18761. Eur J Cancer Clin Oncol 1988; 24:S81–90.

27. Lawrence HS. The transfer in humans of delayed skin sensitivity to streptococcal M substance and to tuberculin with disrupted leucocytes. J Clin Invest 1955; 34:219–30.

28. Bukowski RM, Deodhar S, Hewlett JS, Greenstreet R. Randomized controlled trial of transfer factor in stage II malignant melanoma. Cancer 1983; 51:269–72.

29. Miller LL, Spitler LE, Allen RE, Minor DR. A randomized, double-blind, placebo-controlled trial of transfer factor as adjuvant therapy for melanoma. Cancer 1988; 61:1543–9.

30. Martinez J, Miller L, Allen R, Spitler L. A randomized trial of isoprinosine as surgical adjuvant therapy of melanoma: final report. Proc Am Assoc Cancer Res 1990; 31:203.

31. Khayat D, Pompidou A, Soubrane C, et al. Results of two successive randomized prospective studies of nonspecific adjuvant immunotherapy of thin malignant melanoma. Fourth International Congress on Anti-cancer Chemotherapy, Paris, France, February 2–5, 1993, p. 118.

32. Azizi E, Brenner HJ, Shoham J. Postsurgical adjuvant treatment of malignant melanoma patients by the thymic factor thymostimulin. Arzneimittel Forschung 1984; 34:1043–6.

33. Bernengo MG, Doveil GC, Lisa F, Meregalli M, Novelli M, Zina G. The immunological profile of melanoma and the role of adjuvant thymostimulin immunotherapy in stage I patients. Thymic Factor Therapy: Serono Symp Publ 1984; 16:329–39.

34. Norris RW, Byrom NA, Nagvekar NM, Dean AJ, Mahaffey P, Hobbs JR. Thymostimulin plus surgery in the treatment of primary truncal malignant melanoma: preliminary results of a UK multi-centre clinical trial. Thymic Factor Therapy: Serono Symp Publ 1984; 16:341–8.

35. McIllmurray MB, Embleton MJ, Reeves WG, Langman MJS, Deane M. Controlled trial of active immunotherapy in management of stage IIB malignant melanoma. BMJ 1977; 1(6060):540–2.

36. McIllmurray MB, Reeves WG, Langman MJS, Deane M, Embleton MJ. Active immunotherapy in melanoma [letter]. BMJ 1978; 1(6112):579.

37. Aranha GV, McKhann CF, Grage TB, Gunnarsson A, Simmons RL. Adjuvant immunotherapy of malignant melanoma. Cancer 1979; 43:1297–303.

38. Galligioni E, Quaia M, Merlo A, et al. Adjuvant immunotherapy treatment of renal carcinoma patients with autologous tumor cells and Bacillus Calmette–Guérin. Five-year results of a prospective randomized study. Cancer 1996; 77:2560–6.

39. McCulloch PB, Dent PB, Blajchman M, Muirhead WM, Price RA. Recurrent malignant melanoma: effect of adjuvant immunotherapy on survival. Can Med Assoc J 1977; 117:33–6.

40. Dranoff G, Jaffee E, Lazenby A, et al. Vaccination with irradiated tumor cells engineered to secrete murine granulocyte–macrophage colony stimulating factor stimulates potent, specific, and long-lasting anti-tumor immunity. Proc Natl Acad Sci USA 1993; 90:3539–43.

41. Arca MJ, Krauss JC, Strome SE, Cameron MJ, Chang AE. Diverse manifestations of tumorigenicity and immunogenicity displayed by the poorly immunogenic B16-BL6 melanoma transduced with cytokine genes. Cancer Immunol Immunother 1996; 42:237–45.

42. Morton DL. Adjuvant immunotherapy of malignant melanoma: status of clinical trials at UCLA. Int J Immunother 1986; 2:31–6.

43. Hedley DW, McElwain TJ, Currie GA. Specific active immunotherapy does not prolong survival in surgically treated patients with stage IIB melanoma and may promote early recurrence. Br J Cancer 1978; 37:491–6.

44. Schultz N, Oratz R, Chen D, Zeleniuch-Jacquotte A, Abeles G, Bystryn JC. Effect of DETOX as an adjuvant for melanoma vaccine. Vaccine 1995; 13:503–8.

45. Helling F, Zhang A, Shang A, et al. GM2-KLH conjugate vaccine: increased immunogenicity in melanoma patients after administration with immunological adjuvant QS-21. Cancer Res 1995; 55:2783–8.

46. Oratz R, Dugan M, Roses DF, et al. Lack of effect of cyclophosphamide on the immunogenicity of a melanoma antigen vaccine. Cancer Res 1991; 51:3643–7.

47. Hoon DSB, Foshag LJ, Nizze AS, Bohman R, Morton DL. Suppressor cell activity in a randomized trial of patients receiving active specific immunotherapy with melanoma cell vaccine and low dosages of cyclophosphamide. Cancer Res 1990; 50:5358–64.

48. Hsueh EC, Gupta RK, Qi K, Morton DL. Correlation of specific immune responses with survival in melanoma patients with distant metastases receiving polyvalent melanoma cell vaccine. J Clin Oncol 1998; 16:2913–20.

49. Cassel WA, Murray DR, Phillips HS. A phase II study on the postsurgical management of stage II malignant melanoma with a Newcastle disease virus oncolysate. Cancer 1983; 52:856–60.

50. Hersey P, Coates P, McCarthy WH. Active immunotherapy following surgical removal of high risk melanoma: present status and future prospects. SBT93: Society for Biological Therapy, Proceedings of 8th Annual Scientific Meeting. Biological Therapy of Cancer–VIII. Nashville, TN, November 10–14, 1993, p. 24.

51. Livingston PO, Wong GYC, Adluri S, et al. Improved survival in stage III melanoma patients with GM2 antibodies: a randomized trial of adjuvant vaccination with GM2 ganglioside. J Clin Oncol 1994; 12:1036–44.

52. Hersey P. Ganglioside antigens in tissue sections of skin, naevi, and melanoma: implications for treatment of melanoma. Cancer Treat Res 1991; 54:137–51.

53. Hamilton WB, Helling F, Lloyd KO, Livingston PO. Ganglioside expression on human malignant melanoma assessed by quantitative immune thin-layer chromatography. Int J Cancer 1993; 53:566–73.

54. Tai T, Cahan LD, Tsuchida T, Saxton RE, Irie RF, Morton DL. Immunogenicity of melanoma-associated gangliosides in cancer patients. Int J Cancer 1985; 35:607–12.

55. Minasian LM, Yao TJ, Steffens TA, et al. A phase 1 study of anti-GD3 ganglioside monoclonal antibody R24 and recombinant human macrophage-colony stimulating factor in patients with metastatic melanoma. Cancer 1995; 75:2251–7.

56. Livingston PO, Ritter G, Srivastava P, et al. Characterization of IgG and IgM antibodies induced in melanoma patients by immunization with purified GM2 ganglioside. Cancer Res 1989; 49:7045–50.

57. Takahashi T, Chang C, Morton DL, Irie RF. IgM antibodies to ganglioside GM3 and GD3 induced by active immunization correlated with survival in melanoma patients. Proc Am Assoc Cancer Res 1995; 36:485.

58. Chatterjee MB, Foon KA, Köhler H. Idiotypic antibody immunotherapy of cancer. Cancer Immunol Immunother 1994; 38:75–82.

59. Mittelman A, Wang X, Matsumoto K, Ferrone S. Antiantiidiotypic response and clinical course of the disease in patients with malignant melanoma immunized with mouse antiidiotypic monoclonal antibody MK2-23. Hybridoma 1995; 14:175–81.

60. Foon KA, Lutzky J, Hutchins L, et al. Clinical and immune responses in melanoma patients immunized with an anti-idiotype (ID) antibody mimicking GD2. Proc Am Soc Clin Oncol 1999; 434a, Abstract 1672.

61. Saleh MN, Stapleton JD, Khazaeli MB, LoBuglio AF. Generation of a human anti-idiotypic antibody that mimics the GD2 antigen. J Immunol 1993; 151:3390–8.

62. McCaffery M, Yao TJ, Williams L, Livingston PO, Houghton AN, Chapman PB. Immunization of melanoma patients with BEC2 anti-idiotypic monoclonal antibody that mimics GD3 ganglioside: enhanced immunogenicity when combined with adjuvant. Clin Cancer Res 1996; 2:679–86.

63. Townsend ARM, Gotch RM, Davey J. Cytotoxic cells recognize fragments of the influenza nucleoprotein. Cell 1985; 42:457–67.

64. Townsend ARM, Rothbard J, Gotch FM, Bahadur G, Wraith P, McMichael AJ. The epitopes of influenza nucleoprotein recognized by cytotoxic T lymphocytes can be defined with short synthetic peptides. Cell 1986; 44:959–68.

65. Robbins PF, Kawakami Y. Human tumor antigens recognized by T cells. Curr Opin Immunol 1996; 8:628–36.

66. Marchand M, Weynants P, Rankin E, et al. Tumor regression responses in melanoma patients treated with a peptide encoded by MAGE-3. Int J Cancer 1995; 63:883–5.

67. Jaeger E, Ringhoffer M, Dienes H-P, et al. Granulocyte macrophage colony stimulating factor enhances immune responses to melanoma associated peptides in vivo. Int J Cancer 1996; 66:54–62.

68. Cebon JS, Jaeger E, Gibbs P, et al. Phase I studies of immunization with Melan-A and IL-12 in HLA-A2 positive patients with stage III and IV metastatic melanoma. Proc Am Soc Clin Oncol 1999; 18:434a, Abstract 1671.

69. Salgaller MM, Marincola FM, Cormier JN, et al. Immunization against epitopes in the human melanoma antigen gp100 following patient immunization with synthetic peptides. Cancer Res 1996; 56:4749–57.

70. Salgaller ML, Afshar A, Marincola FM, et al. Recognition of multiple epitopes of the human melanoma antigen gp100 by peripheral blood lymphocytes stimulated in vitro with synthetic peptides. Cancer Res 1995; 55:4972–7.

71. Cormier JN, Salgaller ML, Prevette T, et al. Enhancement of cellular immunity in melanoma patients immunized with a peptide from MART-1/Melan A. Cancer J Sci Am 1997; 3:37–44.

72. Parkhurst MR, Salgaller ML, Southwood S, et al. Improved induction of melanoma reactive CTL with peptides from melanoma antigen gp100 modified at HLA-A0201 binding residues. J Immunol 1996; 157:2536–48.

73. Wang F, Bade E, Kuniyoshi C, et al. Phase I trial of a MART-1 peptide vaccine with incomplete Freund's adjuvant for resected high-risk melanoma. Clin Cancer Res 1999; 5:2756–65.

74. Valmori D, Fonteneau JF, Lizana CM, et al. Enhanced generation of specific tumor-reactive CTL in vitro by selected Melan-A/MART-1 immunodominant peptide analogues. J Immunol 1998; 160:1750–8.

75. Romero P, Dunbar PR, Valmori D, et al. Ex vivo staining of metastatic lymph nodes by class I major histocompatibility complex tetramers reveals high numbers of antigen-experienced tumor specific cytolytic T lymphocytes. J Exp Med 1998; 188:1641–50.

76. Rosenberg SA, Yang JC, Schwartzentruber DJ, et al. Immunologic and therapeutic evaluation of a synthetic peptide vaccine for the treatment of patients with metastatic melanoma. Nat Med 1998; 4:321–7.

77. Creagan ET, Ingle JN, Schutt AJ, Schaid DJ. A prospective, randomized controlled trial of megestrol acetate among high-risk patients with resected malignant melanoma. Am J Clin Oncol 1989; 12:152–5.

78. Meyskens FL Jr, Liu PY, Tuthill RJ, et al. Randomized trial of vitamin A versus observation as adjuvant therapy in high risk primary malignant melanoma: a Southwest Oncology Group study. J Clin Oncol 1994; 12:2060–5.

79. Lotan R, Hendrix MJC, Lippman SM. Retinoids in the management of melanoma. In Marks R, ed. Retinoids in cutaneous malignancy. London, Blackwell Scientific, 1991, 133–56.

80. Meyskens FL Jr, Booth AE, Goff P, Moon TE. Randomized trial of BCG ± vitamin A for stages I

and II cutaneous malignant melanoma. In Salmon SE, ed. *Adjuvant therapy of cancer V*. New York, Grune & Stratton, 1987, 665–86.

81. Thornes RD, Daly L, Lynch G, *et al*. Treatment with coumarin to prevent or delay recurrence of malignant melanoma. J Cancer Res Clin Oncol 1994; 120:S32–4.

82. Houghton AN, Legha S, Bajorin DF. Chemotherapy for metastatic melanoma. In Balch CM, Houghton AN, Milton GW, Sober AJ, Soong S, eds. *Cutaneous melanoma*, 2nd edn. Philadelphia, J.B. Lippincott, 1992, 498–508.

83. Hill GJ II, Moss SE, Golomb FM, *et al*. DTIC and combination therapy for melanoma: III. DTIC (NSC 45388) Surgical Adjuvant Study COG Protocol 7040. Cancer 1981; 47:2556–62.

84. Quirt IC, DeBoer G, Kersey PA, *et al*. Randomized controlled trial of adjuvant chemoimmunotherapy with DTIC and BCG after complete excision of primary melanoma with a poor prognosis or melanoma metastases. Can Med Assoc J 1983; 128:929–33.

85. Wood WC, Cosimi AB, Carey RW, Kaufman SD. Randomized trial of adjuvant therapy for 'high-risk' primary malignant melanoma. Surgery 1978; 83:677–81.

86. Knost JA, Reynolds V, Greco FA, Oldham RK. Adjuvant chemoimmunotherapy stage I/II malignant melanoma. J Surg Oncol 1982; 19:165–70.

87. Sterchi JM, Wells HB, Case LD, *et al*. A randomized trial of adjuvant chemotherapy and immunotherapy in stage I and II cutaneous melanoma: an interim report. Cancer 1985; 55:707–12.

88. Castel T, Estapé J, Viñolas N, *et al*. Adjuvant treatment in stage I and II malignant melanoma: a randomized trial between chemoimmunotherapy and immunotherapy. Dermatologica 1991; 183:25–30.

89. Balch CM, Murray D, Presant C, Bartolucci AA. Ineffectiveness of adjuvant chemotherapy using DTIC and cyclophosphamide in patients with resectable metastatic melanoma. Surgery 1984; 95:454–9.

90. Karakousis CP, Didolkar MS, Lopez R, Baffi R, Moore R, Holyoke ED. Chemoimmunotherapy (DTIC and Corynebacterium parvum) as adjuvant treatment in malignant melanoma. Cancer Treat Rep 1979; 63:1739–43.

91. Banzet P, Jacquillat C, Civatte J, *et al*. Adjuvant chemotherapy in the management of primary malignant melanoma. Cancer 1978; 41:1240–8.

92. Quagliana J, Tranum B, Neidhardt J, Gagliano R. Adjuvant chemotherapy with BCNU, Hydrea and DTIC (BHD) with or without immunotherapy (BCG) in high risk melanoma patients: a SWOG study. Proc Am Assoc Cancer Res 1980; 21:399.

93. Misset JL, Delgado M, De Vassal F, *et al*. Immunotherapy or chemo-immunotherapy as adjuvant treatment for malignant melanoma: a G.I.F. trial. In Salmon SE, Jones SE, eds. *Adjuvant therapy of cancer III*. New York, Grune & Stratton, 1981, 225–35.

94. Kerin MJ, Gillen P, Monson JRT, Wilkie J, Keane FBV, Tanner WA. Results of a prospective randomized trial using DTIC and interferon as adjuvant therapy for stage I malignant melanoma. Eur J Surg Oncol 1995; 21:548–50.

95. Karakousis CP, Emrich LJ. Adjuvant treatment of malignant melanoma with DTIC + estracyt or BCG. J Surg Oncol 1987; 36:235–8.

96. Karakousis C, Blumenson L. Adjuvant chemotherapy with a nitrosourea-based protocol in advanced malignant melanoma. Eur J Cancer 1993; 29A:1831–5.

97. Hansson J, Ringborg U, Lagerlof B, Strander H. Adjuvant chemotherapy of malignant melanoma. A pilot study. Am J Clin Oncol 1985, 8:47–50.

98. Tranum BL, Dixon D, Quagliana J, *et al*. Lack of benefit of adjunctive chemotherapy in stage I malignant melanoma: a Southwest Oncology Group Study. Cancer Treat Rep 1987; 71:643–4.

99. Richards J, Mehta N, Ramming K, *et al*. Sequential chemoimmunotherapy in the treatment of metastatic melanoma. J Clin Oncol 1992; 10:1338–46.

100. Legha SW, Ring S, Eton O, *et al*. Development of a biochemotherapy regimen with concurrent administration of cisplatin, vinblastine, dacarbazine, interferon alfa and interleukin-2 for patients with metastatic melanoma. J Clin Oncol 1998; 16:1752–9.

101. Buzaid AC, Legha S, Bedikian A, *et al*. Neoadjuvant biochemotherapy in melanoma patients with local regional metastases (LRM). Proc Am Soc Clin Oncol 1996; 15:434.

102. Meisenberg BR, Ross M, Vredenburgh JJ, *et al*. Randomized trial of high-dose chemotherapy with autologous bone marrow support as adjuvant therapy for high-risk, multi-node-positive malignant melanoma. J Natl Cancer Inst 1993; 85:1080–5.

103. Herlyn M, Guerry D, Koprowski H. Recombinant alfa-interferon induces changes in expression and shedding of antigens associated with normal human melanocytes, nevus cells, and primary and metastatic melanoma cells. J Immunol 1985; 134:4226–30.

104. Kurzrock R, Rosenblum MG, Sherwin SA, *et al*. Pharmacokinetics, single-dose tolerance and biological activity of recombinant α-interferon in cancer patients. Cancer Res 1985; 45:2866–72.

105. Maluish AE, Urba WJ, Longo DL, *et al*. The determination of an immunologically active dose of

interferon-gamma in patients with melanoma. J Clin Oncol 1988; 6:434–45.

106. Schiller JH, Pugh M, Kirkwood JM, Karp D, Larson M, Borden E. Eastern Cooperative Group Trial of interferon gamma in metastatic melanoma: an innovative study design. Clin Cancer Res 1996; 2:29–36.

107. Jaffe HS, Herberman RB. Rationale for recombinant human interferon-gamma adjuvant immunotherapy for cancer. J Natl Cancer Inst 1988; 80:616–18.

108. Meyskens FL Jr, Kopecky K, Taylor CW, et al. Randomized trial of adjuvant human interferon gamma versus observation in high-risk cutaneous melanoma. J Natl Cancer Inst 1995; 87:1710–13.

109. Meyskens FL Jr, Kopecky K, Samson M, et al. Recombinant human interferon: adverse effects in high-risk stage I and II cutaneous malignant melanoma [Letter]. J Natl Cancer Inst 1990; 82:1071.

110. Osoba D, Zee B, Sadura A, Pater J, Quirt I. Measurement of quality of life in an adjuvant trial of gamma interferon versus levamisole in malignant melanoma. In Salmon SE, ed. Adjuvant therapy of cancer VII. Philadelphia, J.B. Lippincott, 1993, 412–20.

111. Parkinson DR, Houghton AN, Hersey P, Borden EC. Biologic therapy for melanoma. In Balch CM, Houghton AN, Milton GW, Sober AJ, Soong S, eds. Cutaneous melanoma, 2nd edn. Philadelphia, J.B. Lippincott, 1992, 522–34.

112. Pfeffer LM, Dinarello CA, Heberman RB, et al. Biologic properties of recombinant alpha-interferons: 40th anniversary of the discovery of interferons. Cancer Res 1998; 58(12):2489–99.

113. Kokoschka EM, Trautinger F, Knobler RM, Pohl-Markl H, Micksche M. Long-term adjuvant therapy of high-risk malignant melanoma with interferon α2b. J Invest Dermatol 1990; 95:S193–7.

114. Cascinelli N, Bufalino R, Morabito A, et al. Results of an adjuvant interferon study in the WHO melanoma programme. Lancet 1994; 343:913.

115. Caraceni A, Gangeri L, Martini C, et al. Neurotoxicity of interferon-alpha in melanoma therapy: results from a randomized, controlled trial. Cancer 1998; 83(3):482–9.

116. Creagan ET, Dalton RJ, Ahmann DL, et al. Randomized, surgical adjuvant clinical trial of recombinant interferon alfa-2a in selected patients with malignant melanoma. J Clin Oncol 1995; 13:2776–83.

117. Cole BF, Gelber RD, Kirkwood JM, Goldhirsch A, Barylak E, Borden E. Quality-of-life-adjusted survival analysis of interferon alfa-2b adjuvant treatment of high-risk resected cutaneous melanoma: an Eastern Cooperative Oncology Group study. J Clin Oncol 1996; 14:2666–73.

118. Kirkwood JM, Ibrahim JG, Sondak VK, et al. High- and low-dose interferon alfa-2b in high risk melanoma: first analysis of intergroup trial E1690/S9111/C9190. J Clin Oncol 2000; 18:2444–2458.

119. Kirkwood JM, Ibrahim J, Lawson JH, et al. High dose interferon alfa-2b does not diminish antibody response to GM2 vaccination in patients with resected melanoma: results of the multicenter Eastern Cooperative Oncology Group phase II trial E2696. J Clin Oncol 2001; 19(5):1430–6.

120. Grob JJ, Dreno B, Delaunay M, et al. Results of the French multicenter trial on adjuvant therapy with interferon alfa-2a in resected primary melanoma (>1.5 mm). Proc Am Soc Clin Oncol 1996; 15:437.

121. Schmidt-Ullrich RK, Johnson CR. Role of radiotherapy and hyperthermia in the management of malignant melanoma. Semin Surg Oncol 1996; 12:407–15.

122. Ang KK, Peters LJ, Weber RS, et al. Postoperative radiotherapy for cutaneous melanoma of the head and neck region. Int J Radiat Oncol Biol Phys 1994; 30:795–8.

123. Creagan ET, Cupps RE, Ivins JC, et al. Adjuvant radiation therapy in the treatment of regional nodal metastases from malignant melanoma: a randomized prospective study. Cancer 1978; 42:2206–10.

124. Kirkwood JM, Earle JD, Fine SL, Hawkins BS, Straatsma BR, Mowery RL. Five-year progress report: the Collaborative Ocular Melanoma Study. Proc Am Soc Clin Oncol 1992; 11:349.

125. Cumberlin R, De Moss E, Lassus M, Friedman M. Isolation perfusion for malignant melanoma of the extremity: a review. J Clin Oncol 1985; 3:1022–31.

126. Lienard D, Ewalenko P, Delmotte J-J, Renard N, Lejeune FJ. High-dose recombinant tumor necrosis factor alpha in combination with interferon gamma and melphalan in isolation perfusion of the limbs for melanoma and sarcoma. J Clin Oncol 1992; 10:52–60.

127. Ghussen F, Krüger I, Smalley RV, Groth W. Hyperthermic perfusion with chemotherapy for melanoma of the extremities. World J Surg 1989; 13:598–602.

128. Hafström L, Rudenstam C-M, Blomquist E, et al. Regional hyperthermic perfusion with melphalan after surgery for recurrent malignant melanoma of the extremities. J Clin Oncol 1991; 9:2091–4.

129. Lejeune FJ, Vaglini M, Schraffordt-Koops H, et al. A randomized trial on prophylactic isolation perfusion for Stage I high-risk (i.e., greater than 1.5-mm thickness) malignant melanoma of the limbs. An interim report. Special International Columbus Meeting on Surgical Oncology, Genoa, Italy, December 3–5, 1992, 75.

ANNOTATED BIBLIOGRAPHY

Balch CM. How patient referral bias can confuse interpretation of clinical results: elective lymph node dissections at the Sydney Melanoma Unit. J Am Coll Surg 1995; 180:490–2.

This article explores how retrospective reviews can yield misleading or erroneous results, in this case indicating a favorable impact of elective lymph node dissection when none, in fact, may have existed.

Creagan ET, Dalton RJ, Ahmann DL, et al. Randomized, surgical adjuvant clinical trial of recombinant interferon alfa-2a in selected patients with malignant melanoma. J Clin Oncol 1995; 13:2776–83.

This randomized trial evaluated adjuvant therapy with a 3-month course of high-dose intramuscular IFN-α2a compared to observation in 262 patients with stage II and III melanoma. Overall, there was no significant difference in disease-free or overall survival between the treatment and control arms. Node-positive patients had a statistically significant improvement in disease-free survival in a multivariate analysis.

Kirkwood JM, Strawderman MH, Ernstoff MS, Smith TJ, Borden EC, Blum RH. Interferon alfa-2b adjuvant therapy of high-risk resected cutaneous melanoma: the Eastern Cooperative Oncology Group trial EST 1684. J Clin Oncol 1996; 14:7–17.

This report documents the results of the first trial to show a benefit for adjuvant therapy (high-dose IFN-2b) on both relapse-free and overall survival in stage IIB and III melanoma.

Livingston PO, Wong GYC, Adluri S, et al. Improved survival in stage III melanoma patients with GM2 antibodies: a randomized trial of adjuvant vaccination with GM2 ganglioside. J Clin Oncol 1994; 12:1036–44.

This randomized trial evaluated 122 patients with resected stage III melanoma who were treated with either BCG alone or BCG plus the ganglioside GM2. Patients who had or developed anti-GM2 antibodies fared better than those without an antibody response. The study arms were imbalanced with respect to naturally occurring anti-GM2 antibodies, in favor of the control group. There was a trend toward improved disease-free and overall survival in the GM2/BCG arm among patients without pre-existing anti-GM2 antibodies.

Robbins PF, Kawakami Y. Human tumor antigens recognized by T cells. Curr Opin Immunol 1996; 8:628–36.

The authors review the HLA-restricted tumor antigens that have been described and the T cell epitopes which have been identified. Melanoma-associated antigens may be generated by several mechanisms, including transcription of normal, non-mutated genes, translation of alternative open reading frames, mutations of widely expressed genes, incomplete splicing, transcription from cryptic promoters, or post-translational modification. Many of these antigens are currently being evaluated in clinical trials as targets for adjuvant or combination therapy for melanoma patients.

Romero P, Dunbar PR, Valmori D, et al. Ex vivo staining of metastatic lymph nodes by class I major histocompatibility complex tetramers reveals high numbers of antigen-experienced tumor specific cytolytic T lymphocytes. J Exp Med 1998; 188:1641–50.

The first report of the presence of tumor-specific memory T cells in lymph nodes draining tumors in melanoma patients.

Commentary

CHRISTOS I STAVROPOULOS, MUTHUKUMARAN SIVANANDHAM, AND MARC K WALLACK

INTRODUCTION

The incidence of melanoma has increased from 5.7 in the 1970s to 13.3 per 100 000 in the 1990s in the USA, and it is expected to continue to rise.[1] It was estimated that nearly 42 500 new patients would present with melanoma in the year 2000 and about 40% of them were expected to have clinically positive metastases or clinically negative micrometastases.

Earlier diagnosis of primary malignant melanoma has resulted in an increased frequency of surgical cure. Metastatic melanoma, however, has long been considered an incurable disease, with a median survival of approximately 8 months.[2] Two recently completed, large overview studies of survival in American Joint Committee on Cancer (AJCC) stage IV melanoma included patients treated with both chemotherapy and biotherapy, and overall survival (OS) did not appear to be appreciably different from that of untreated patients.[3,4] These findings underscore the need for better adjuvant therapy to prevent recurrence and the development of systemic metastases, as well as more effective intervention to treat advanced disease. With regard to these efforts, Dr Weber and his colleagues provide a concise review of the current progress in adjuvant therapy for melanoma. In our commentary, we, too, focus primarily on recent data as they apply to the adjuvant setting, when possible, as well as highlighting some of the aforementioned studies.

In order to explore the adjuvant therapy for melanoma, it is important first to appreciate numerous recent developments. For example, in melanoma staging, there have been proposed changes, such as using simple integer break-point of tumor thickness, sentinel lymph node mapping and lymphadenectomy, prognostic/stratification criteria for patients with secondary melanoma based on sensitive markers such as lactate dehydrogenase (LDH) and reverse transcriptase–polymerase chain reaction (RT–PCR), and improved understanding of the underlying pathophysiology and natural history of melanoma.[5–12] It may now, in fact, be possible with the above approaches to better identify the population of melanoma patients that will benefit most from adjuvant therapy. These new advances have provided opportunities to stratify appropriately patients for future prospective, randomized clinical trials and therefore to render meaningful assessments of the relative impact of disease and treatment characteristics on long-term survival. Earlier phase I–III studies, including single-institution and retrospective reports, often studied a heterogeneous population (e.g., 'patients with melanoma'), as described by Weber *et al.* in this chapter, with varied prognoses and thus could not provide truly useful data.

Eton and associates at the University of Texas MD Anderson Cancer Center, using univariate and multivariate analyses of 318 stage IV patients, reported that normal serum levels of LDH and albumin, soft tissue and/or single visceral organ metastases (especially lung), female sex, and enrollment in the later part of this past decade were all independent positive predictors for survival.[11] Interestingly, the 11% of patients who lived longer than 2 years combined these favorable prognostic characteristics with a high frequency of surgical resection of residual or recurrent disease.[11] Furthermore, Borgstein *et al.* recently demonstrated that locoregional cutaneous recurrence appears to be highly predictable in the presence of histopathological signs of lymphatic invasion.[12] In a prospective study of 258 patients with clinical stage I melanoma who had undergone wide local excision (WLE) and sentinel lymph node (SLN) biopsy, 93% of patients with unequivocal signs of lymphatic invasion developed in-transit metastases, compared to 1.6% of those patients without evidence of lymphatic invasion ($p < 0.0001$).[12]

The presence of circulating melanoma cells in disease-free patients, detected with RT–PCR, has also been found to be an independent prognostic predictor of recurrence by several investigators.[13–16] Interestingly, Curry *et al.* recently hypothesized that therapy directed against MART-1 may reduce the establishment of disseminated metastases.[17] They analysed the prognostic significance of the patterns of expression of tyrosinase and MART-1 in 186 patients followed sequentially before and after the surgical removal of AJCC stage I, II, and III melanoma.[17]

Whereas patients with locoregional metastases had circulating melanoma cells that expressed tyrosinase and MART-1 at similar rates, patients with disseminated recurrence had a significantly lower incidence of MART-1-positive than of tyrosinase-positive circulating melanoma cells.[17]

There have also been many published series reporting the long-term survival after surgical excision for patients with metastatic melanoma to visceral sites, including the lung, gastrointestinal tract, brain, and adrenal gland.[7,18] Collectively, these studies suggest that, in the carefully selected patient who has isolated visceral metastatic melanoma, with no major coexistent morbidity, complete resection may be associated with a survival benefit. Although prospective randomized trials are lacking, the reported survival rates for patients chosen by an experienced surgical oncologist to undergo surgical excision of stage IV melanoma are better than any type of currently available systemic treatment.[2,19] The John Wayne Cancer Institute recently demonstrated, in a retrospective review of 83 melanoma patients with adrenal metastases, that surgical resection of all visible disease, including extra-adrenal disease, was associated with a median survival of 25.7 months, versus 9.2 months after palliative resection ($p = 0.02$).[18] The results of their ongoing adjuvant multicenter trial, in which patients are randomized to treatment with CancerVax (their polyvalent melanoma cell vaccine) or placebo after complete resection of distant melanoma metastases, stratified by site and number of resected lesions, are eagerly anticipated.[18]

Lastly, the Sunbelt Melanoma Trial integrates these advances in melanoma staging with interferon-alfa (IFN-α2b) adjuvant therapy and thus serves a prototype multicenter, prospective, randomized trial.[20] Eligibility includes all patients who are younger than 71 years old, with melanoma ≥1.0 mm Breslow thickness, without palpable lymph nodes and/or evidence of distant metastasis, and who otherwise do not have any contraindication to IFN-α2b therapy. Patients are initially subdivided into two protocols based on histologically and immunohistochemically determined SLN status. In one protocol, randomization is based on Breslow thickness stratification (1.0–2.0 mm, >2.0–4.0 mm, or >4.0 mm) and positive SLN status (e.g., positive SLN only or > one positive SLN/positive non-SLN/extracapsular extension). The other protocol considers only patients with negative SLN status. Using RT–PCR analysis to detect tyrosinase plus one of the markers MART-1, MAGE-3, or gp100, subsequent positive SLN patients, also stratified by tumor thickness, are then randomized to one of three treatment arms: observation, lymph node dissection, or lymph node dissection plus IFN-α2b. Patients confirmed negative SLN by RT–PCR are observed only. This study will determine if adjuvant IFN-α2b plus lymphadenectomy is superior to lymphadenectomy alone in terms of disease-free survival (DFS) and OS, as well as establish the value of RT–PCR as a molecular staging test. More importantly, the data will define precisely the subgroups of patients who benefit from the proposed adjuvant therapy. Given the improved surgical staging with SLN technology and better-defined pathologic[13–17] and clinical prognostic factors,[6–12,21] (neo)adjuvant therapy may indeed have an impact on survival in the appropriately selected patients with melanoma. Ongoing and future adjuvant trials will be able to select a homogeneous study population and thus render data that can be applied directly to a clinician's practice. These advances will offer a new look into surgical adjuvant therapy that can be truly an effective weapon against melanoma (i.e., chance for cure).

ADJUVANT THERAPY FOR MELANOMA

Several experimental treatments, including biotherapy, chemotherapy and radiotherapy, and their combinations, have been investigated in the adjuvant setting for patients who had undergone surgical resection of melanoma and are at high risk for recurrence. These therapies are elegantly reviewed individually by Weber and associates. Nevertheless, like most cancers, effective adjuvant therapy will probably entail a multidisciplinary strategy that may conceivably reduce recurrent and/or systemic disease to a resectable lesion(s), if not cure altogether. Here, we discuss the salient features of these adjuvant therapies, supplemented with recently available additional information.

Biotherapy

Numerous types of biotherapy have been studied for patients with melanoma in the surgical adjuvant setting. The list includes biological agents such as interferons, interleukins, colony-stimulating factors, viruses, bacteria, and melanoma antigens. They induce an anti-melanoma response either by direct cytotoxicity on melanoma cells or by eliciting specific or non-specific immunity to melanoma. Biotherapy is particularly interesting as an adjuvant therapy for melanoma because it has been shown to work best with minimal tumor burden and produces minimal toxicity. Moreover, the presence of melanoma-associated antigens such as glycolipid antigens (GD2, GD3, 9-0-acetyl GD3, GM2, and GM3), glycoprotein antigens (high molecular weight proteoglycan, melanoma transferrin, urinary tumor-associated antigen, and melanoma fetal-associated antigen), and peptide melanoma antigens (MAGE-1, MAGE-3, tyrosinase-1 and tryosinase-2, melanoma antigen reacting to T-cells-1 (MART-1)/melan-A, GP 100/pMel-17, NY-ESO-1, etc.) have displayed antibody and cytotoxic T-lymphocyte (CTL) responses. These antigenic characteristics of melanoma suggest clinical utility in immunomodulatory biotherapies and thus several such strategies have been developed for patients with melanoma.

Cytokine-based biotherapy

Interferons, interleukins, and colony-stimulating factors display immunomodulatory properties. IFN-α, IFN-γ, and interleukin-2 (IL-2) are the most studied cytokines in the experimental adjuvant therapy for patients with melanoma. The landmark Eastern Cooperative Oncology Group (ECOG) EST 1684 Trial showed that the use of high-dose IFN-α2b adjuvant therapy for 1 year produced a significantly prolonged DFS and OS in patients with stage IIB and III melanoma.[22] (An extended review of this therapy is presented by Weber et al.) Therefore, the US Food and Drug Administration (FDA) approved IFN-α2b for use in the adjuvant setting. Although subsequent trials (E1690 S9111/C9091) with high-dose IFN-α2b confirmed the significant improvement in DFS in stage IIB and III melanoma patients, they did not show significant improvement in OS.[23] Clinical trials with low-dose IFN-α2b for 2–3 years in the WHO trial[24] and high-dose IFN-α2a for 12 weeks in the North Central Cancer Treatment Group trial[25] also did not show a significant DFS and OS for melanoma patients at high risk for recurrence. Lastly, the Southwest Oncology Group studied low-dose IFN-γ adjuvant therapy for melanoma patients with stage II or III disease.[26] Patients were treated with 0.1 mg of IFN-γ subcutaneously three times weekly for 1 year. This therapy also did not produce an increase in OS or DFS.[26]

In several of the IFN therapy trials, high-dose IFN therapy alone produces some clinical efficacy, which suggests that IFNs act as a direct cytotoxic agent to melanoma rather than the induction of immunity. Because this effect has not yielded sound evidence with regard to prolonged survival, several investigators have also evaluated combination therapies of IFN-α2b with chemotherapy (discussed under the section 'Chemotherapy') in search of enhanced clinical efficacy. Although the toxicity of IFN-α2b adjuvant therapy is often a major problem, lack of other, less toxic alternatives have made it the standard of care at this time. Nonetheless, it is important to reiterate that the survival advantage with this therapy has not been clearly established. Consequently, experimental therapies with other cytokines, melanoma vaccine therapies, and/or their combinations are currently under investigation.

Unlike the IFNs, IL-2 does not show direct cytotoxicity against melanoma cells. Rather, IL-2 expands the tumor-specific CTL response and the non-specific killer lymphocytes. Because patients with advanced melanoma can prime their cellular antitumor response by virtue of the numerous melanoma antigens, high-dose IL-2 adjuvant therapy seems ideal for these patients. Clinical trial with high-dose IL-2 therapy showed both a disease-free interval (DFI) and OS advantage in patients with advanced-stage melanoma.[27] Therefore, the FDA approved the high-dose IL-2 therapy for these patients.[28] A recent review of eight clinical trials with 270 patients analysed high-dose bolus recombinant IL-2 therapy for patients with melanoma.[27] Patients were treated with either 600 000 or 720 000 IU kg^{-1} intravenously every 8 h for up to 14 doses. A second cycle of therapy was performed following 6–9 days of rest. The two cycles per course of IL-2 therapy were repeated every 6–12 weeks for up to five total cycles in responding patients. Sixteen percent of patients showed an objective response, 6% with a complete response, and 10% with a partial response. However, toxicity was severe, with a 2% mortality rate. The utility of IL-2 therapy in an adjuvant setting for melanoma patients at risk for recurrence has yet to be elucidated. However, low-dose IL-2 therapy in combination with either a melanoma vaccine or chemotherapy is another promising approach (both are discussed below).

Biotherapy with immunomodulating bacterial and viral agents

The immunopotentiating bacterial and viral agents *Bacillus Calmette–Guérin* (BCG)[29] and vaccinia vaccine virus[30] were two of the originally studied biologics as potential therapy for patients with melanoma. Morton *et al.*,[29] in 1970, used intralesional injections of BCG and showed regression of melanoma. Subsequently, several investigators confirmed the effectiveness of intratumoral BCG therapy. However, randomized, controlled trials using intralesional BCG for malignant melanoma failed to reproduce the earlier results. Although the use of BCG, *C. parvum*, and vaccinia virus therapy demonstrated encouraging results in preliminary clinical trials,[29–31] later trials failed to reproduce significant efficacy, as indicated by Weber *et al.*, and, thus, this form of non-specific immunotherapy for patients with melanoma was abandoned. Moreover, the identification of melanoma-associated antigens called for specific immunotherapy strategies rather than non-specific immunotherapy.

Biotherapy with melanoma vaccines

Specific immunotherapy in the form of melanoma vaccines was initiated over 25 years ago for patients with melanoma. A number of melanoma vaccines have been developed for study in the adjuvant setting. These vaccines are broadly grouped under the following categories: cell-lysate vaccines from allogeneic or autologous melanoma cells/tissues, whole-cell vaccines from autologous or allogeneic melanoma cells, anti-idiotypic antibodies to melanoma antigen epitopes, and purified or synthesized melanoma antigens. Weber and associates extensively review these. We focus on some of the more important trials in our discussion.

Morton *et al.* performed pioneering work in melanoma vaccine therapy.[32] They initially performed a clinical trial using allogeneic melanoma cells mixed with BCG. Only 35% of patients developed high levels of anti-melanoma antibodies, indicating the limitation of the use of this vaccine. Therefore, they constructed a new, polyvalent, allogeneic whole-cell vaccine using three melanoma cell lines that contain high concentrations of six representative melanoma antigens.[32] They conducted a clinical trial with this new vaccine using 24 million irradiated allogeneic melanoma cells mixed with BCG. This vaccine induced anti-melanoma humoral responses that correlated with increased survival. A phase II clinical trial was subsequently performed using this vaccine for patients with stage III and IV melanoma.[32] One hundred and thirty-six melanoma patients were immunized intradermally as follows: every 2 weeks for 4 weeks, then monthly for 1 year, every 3 months for the following year (four injections), and finally every 6 months thereafter. Only the first two vaccine injections contained irradiated melanoma cells mixed with BCG; subsequent injections contained only irradiated melanoma cells. Some patients also received biological response modifiers such as cimetidine, indomethacine, and cyclophosphamide. Minor toxicity such as local erythema, induration, and ulceration at the injection sites, as well as mild fever with occasional myalgias, arthralgias, and chills were also experienced. Patients were followed at 3-month intervals with preimmune and postimmune sera analyses for the presence of antibodies to melanoma antigens. Delayed-type hypersensitivity (DTH) responses against melanoma cells were also measured. Both stage III and IV patients receiving vaccine therapy survived significantly longer than those patients treated otherwise.[39] Those patients with a median survival of 30 months had a significantly higher IgM antibody response to melanoma antigens and a significantly higher DTH response (>10 mm) to melanoma cells. These interesting results led to a large phase III, multicenter, randomized clinical trial to elucidate the efficacy of this melanoma cell vaccine. Results of this trial are patiently awaited.

A non-randomized phase II adjuvant melanoma vaccine trial was performed by Mordoh *et al.*[33] for patients with stage III melanoma. This trial used 5 million irradiated allogeneic melanoma cells mixed with 5 million BCG organisms. Thirty patients were immunized intradermally as follows: one vaccine injection every 3 weeks (four injections), every 2 months for the rest of the first year, every 3 months in the second year, and then once every 6 months until the fifth year. Patients received cyclophosphamide 3 days before each vaccination. DTH and antibody responses were analysed. Twenty-four patients with the same stage of disease served as controls in this study. There was a significant DFI noted at 20 months, with 33.3% survival in the vaccine-treatment arm, compared to 4.1% survival in the control arm. Interestingly, a significant portion of patients who experienced the induction of an antibody response also demonstrated a positive DTH response. The true efficacy of this vaccine, nevertheless, needs to be confirmed in a randomized trial with a larger number of patients.

Berd *et al.*[34] used dinitrophenyl (DNP) as a hapten to modify autologous melanoma cells and used it as a vaccine for 62 patients with stage III melanoma and for 15 patients with stage IV melanoma. Each dose of the vaccine contained 5–25 million autologous tumor cells. All patients were initially sensitized with 1–5% dinitro-flurobenzine (DNFB) in acetone-corn oil on two consecutive days and received intravenous cyclophosphamide (300 mg/kg) 3 days before the DNFB to reduce suppressor T-cell activity. These patients were subjected to two different vaccine schedules. In the first schedule, the DNP-modified tumor cells were mixed with BCG and administered intradermally every 4 weeks for eight doses. Cyclophosphamide was given only for the first two doses. In the second schedule, 6 weekly vaccine injections were performed. Only the first three vaccines were modified with DNP. Patients were then followed every 2 months for 2 years and tested for DTH responses. With a median follow-up of 55 months, DFI of stage III patients treated with vaccine was 45% at 5 years and OS was 58% at that time point. In contrast, with a median follow-up of 73 months, the OS of stage IV patients >50 years of age and <50 years of age were 71% and 41%, respectively, at a 5-year time point. These survival rates were better than those of patients with no treatment. Additionally, there was significant survival in patients who showed a positive DTH response when compared to negative DTH responders: 71% versus 49% at 5 years. A phase III clinical trial with this vaccine is also in progress.

Our laboratory has investigated the use of vaccinia virus-modified melanoma cell lysate (VMO) for melanoma patients at high risk for recurrence. Based on significant clinical efficacy seen with VMO in a phase II trial, a phase III prospective, randomized, double-blind, multi-institutional trial was conducted to evaluate the efficacy of VMO vaccine in melanoma patients with high-risk stage III disease.[35] Patients were treated weekly for 13 weeks and then biweekly for 39 weeks or until recurrence. A total of 33 injections were administered to the patients unless any patient was withdrawn from the study. The toxicity of either VMO or vaccinia virus (V) was minimal. The final analysis, with a median follow-up of 46.3 months, showed that there was no significant difference in either DFI or OS with VMO compared to placebo V.[36] However, there was approximately a 10% difference in the OS with VMO at a 4-year time point in the first interim analysis (a median follow-up of 30.3 months),[35] which suggests that perhaps continuing the immunization beyond the 1-year therapy could have maintained the survival advantage with VMO. There was also a problem in the design of the trial. The control arm was not an observation control, but rather a vaccinia virus treatment arm that was also shown to produce anti-melanoma activity. Weber and colleagues highlighted these and other problems with clinical trial blueprints.

Another phase III randomized trial was performed with vaccinia melanoma cell-lysate (VMCL) vaccine to evaluate its efficacy in patients with stage III melanoma.[37]

Patient enrollment has been recently completed and an interim analysis of 648 patients in this trial showed survival advantage with VMCL (96 months) when compared to observation controls (80 months).[37]

Mitchell has also performed a phase III randomized clinical trial with a melanoma cell-lysate vaccine and the adjuvant DETOX as well as low-dose cyclophosphamide in patients with stage IV melanoma.[38] The vaccine treatment arm was compared to the control chemotherapy arm and there were no statistically significant differences in objective responses between them. The median survival of patients treated with this vaccine was 9.4, versus 12.1 months with chemotherapy alone. Interestingly, the toxicity of this vaccine therapy was far less than that observed with chemotherapy. This group has also performed a randomized clinical trial with a melanoma cell-lysate vaccine mixed with DETOX adjuvant for patients with stage II and stage III melanoma. The final analysis of data from this trial will be presented over the next few years.

McGee et al.[39] conducted a non-randomized clinical trial with a melanoma tissue lysate for 129 melanoma patients with stage I disease and 61 patients with stage II disease. Immunizations were given weekly for 8 weeks and then every 3 months for 24 months. The vaccine was administered in two portions, one intradermally and another subcutaneously. At 5 years' follow-up, patients with stage I melanoma did not show any significant survival when compared with their historical controls, which suggests that patients with stage I melanoma would not benefit with melanoma vaccine therapy. However, patients with stage II melanoma demonstrated a significantly increased survival rate when compared with historical controls (64% versus 40%, respectively).

Adjuvant therapy using purified melanoma antigens as vaccines has also been extensively studied. Livingston et al. studied GM2 therapy in a phase III randomized trial for patients with melanoma.[40] When compared with a control group receiving BCG alone, patients who induced antibodies to GM2 ($n = 56$) with the vaccine therapy showed a significant improvement in DFS. Currently, a modified GM2 vaccine (conjugated with the carrier keyhole lymphet hemocyanin and adjuvant QS21) has been studied in a large multi-institutional trial. This therapy is compared with a group receiving IFN-α2b alone. Interim results have not shown clinical efficacy with the GM2 vaccine. Anti-idiotypic antibodies to GD2, GD3, and high molecular weight proteoglycan antigens have also been tested as vaccines in the active specific immunotherapy of melanoma. Although preliminary trials have shown clinical responses with these therapies, randomized trials in the adjuvant setting have not been done.

Several new melanoma vaccine therapies based on the melanoma peptide antigens are currently under investigation as well. Weber et al. extensively covered these studies in their chapter. The preliminary clinical trials performed by Rosenberg *et al.*[41] with the gp100 melanoma peptide antigen and those performed by Cebon *et al.*[42] and Jaeger *et al.*[43] with MART-1 peptide antigen vaccination demonstrated promising clinical responses. It is also interesting to note that these vaccinations were supplemented with adjuvant cytokines such as granulocyte-macrophage colony-stimulating factor (GM-CSF), IL-2, and IL-12. These melanoma vaccines have a promising role in the active specific immunotherapy of melanoma. However, there is controversy concerning the use of a univalent immunodominant single-peptide melanoma vaccine therapy versus a polyvalent approach. Considering the immune escape mechanisms via melanoma antigen modulation on melanoma cells, a polyvalent vaccine strategy appears to be best suited for use in vaccine therapy.

Passive and adoptive immunotherapies

It is interesting to note in the above-mentioned GM2 vaccine trial that a group of patients who developed an anti-GM2 response experienced a DFS advantage.[40] This suggests that a passive immunotherapy with antibodies to melanoma antigens could benefit patients with melanoma. An earlier trial with a murine monoclonal antibody to GD3, however, produced only moderate responses.[44] In an another study, a human monoclonal antibody to melanoma-associated ganglioside GM2 (L55) was used to treat patients with melanoma. After completing two courses of this antibody therapy, complete tumor regression was noted in a patient with a right cheek lesion.[45] This study clearly suggests that patients with melanoma may benefit from passive antibody-based immunotherapy. Moreover, this antibody therapy should be tested for efficacy against those cutaneous melanoma lesions that are inoperable.

The clinical efficacy of adoptive immunotherapy using tumor-infiltrating lymphocytes for patients with melanoma has yet to be determined in randomized, control trials. Several phase I/II trials showed that patients with melanoma benefited by adoptive immunotherapy via enhanced tumor-specific CTL. Studies are now underway to produce melanoma-specific CTL responses by priming lymphocytes *in vitro* with melanoma antigen-pulsed dendritic cells, harnessing their potent capacity for antigen processing and presenting.[46] This therapy will play a critical role in future developments of adjuvant therapy for melanoma.

Chemotherapy

Systemic chemotherapy

There is considerable experience with single-agent chemotherapy in both therapeutic and adjuvant settings in metastatic melanoma, albeit disappointing, with most agents yielding responses of less than 10%.[2] The most commonly used agents include dacarbazine (DTIC),

carmustine, cisplatin, vincristine, vinblastine, and paclitaxel.[2,5] The highest reported objective response rates are seen with DTIC, carmustin, and cisplatin at approximately 20%; DTIC therapy is the US FDA-approved standard therapy for advanced melanoma.[2,5] A considerably smaller percentage of patients experience a complete response (5% of cases), but remissions are short lived (most last 3–6 months).[2,5] Accordingly, the 5-year survival rate of patients with advanced malignant melanoma who were treated with single-agent systemic chemotherapy is reportedly 2–6%, at best.[2,5,21,47,48]

Similarly, in the post-surgical adjuvant setting, single-agent chemotherapy (primarily DTIC or cisplatin) has not been shown to provide any significant clinical efficacy,[2] as Dr Weber and his colleagues alluded to earlier in their review. It is difficult to dispute data derived from large, randomized trials including observation-only control arms.[49,50] Patients at high risk of relapse following excision of their primary melanoma and/or nodal metastases did not experience a clear benefit with chemotherapy.[49,50] Currently, there is no defined role for adjuvant single-agent chemotherapy in patients with melanoma, although patients with advanced disease can be offered this modality as a palliative option.

New agents, however, might improve the ease of treatment delivery or the tolerability of treatment. Middleton *et al.*, for example, recently reported in a randomized phase III trial that temozolomide, a novel oral alkylating agent with a broad spectrum of antitumor activity and relatively mild toxicity, demonstrates efficacy equal to that of DTIC.[51] Although there was no significant difference between the two treatments with regards to OS, median DFS time and health-related quality of life were significantly increased in the temozolomide-treated group.[51] Moreover, there is increasing evidence that patients with intracranial metastases can benefit from the ability of temozolomide to penetrate the blood–brain barrier.[52–54]

Given the relatively dismal efficacy of single-agent chemotherapeutics, investigators have evaluated multi-agent chemotherapy combinations in patients with metastatic melanoma. Dr Weber and his colleagues appropriately noted that, historically, encouraging data have generally emerged from single-institution studies, but have simply not been reproduced in the more conclusive multicenter and cooperative group trials.

In single-institution phase II trials, many of these multi-agent regimens, often based on DTIC and/or cisplatin, collectively demonstrate a response rate in the range of 30–50%; <5% are remissions (<2% long term).[2,55–64] One of the more currently popular combinations is the 'Dartmouth' regimen, first reported by Del Prete and colleagues in 1984, consisting of DTIC, cisplatin, carmustine, and tamoxifen.[57] In multiple single-institution phase II trials, this regimen has demonstrated promising response rates of 40–50%.[56,57,62] Subsequent multi-institutional and cooperative group trials, however, could not confirm these observations.[65–68] Margolin and colleagues, for example, could only demonstrate a 15% objective response rate and a median survival of 9 months for 79 metastatic melanoma patients treated with the Dartmouth regimen.[66] Similarly, the ECOG could not demonstrate a survival advantage or significantly higher response rate with the Dartmouth regimen versus DTIC alone in their recently reported phase III randomized trial of 240 patients with advanced metastatic melanoma.[69] Furthermore, the Dartmouth regimen was significantly more toxic, with patients frequently experiencing bone marrow suppression, nausea, vomiting, and fatigue.[69]

The addition of tamoxifen to single-agent or multi-agent chemotherapy regimens has also been controversial. Tamoxifen was originally used in the Dartmouth regimen to modulate the sensitivity of tumor cells to cisplatin via calcium-channel inhibition.[2,57] In a small phase III cooperative group trial comparing DTIC alone versus DTIC plus tamoxifen, a significant improvement in response rate (28% versus 12%; $p = 0.03$) and survival (median, 48 weeks versus 29 weeks; $p = 0.02$) was noted in patients who received tamoxifen.[70] Nathan and colleagues also recently published data on a phase II trial showing an improved overall response rate (24%) with the addition of daily low-dose tamoxifen to outpatient paclitaxel 3-h infusions every 3 weeks in patients with metastatic melanoma.[71] Paclitaxel was historically associated with a 15% response rate and considerable toxicity as a 24-h infusion.[72] Lastly, the Hollings Cancer Center at the Medical University of South Carolina at Charleston has demonstrated favorable DFS and OS in 35 patients treated with cisplatin and tamoxifen following resection of all visible stage III and IV disease when compared to historical controls.[73]

Nevertheless, large multicenter, randomized phase III trials do not confirm these promising observations.[74–76] The National Cancer Institute of Canada Clinical Trials Group recently compared DTIC, carmustine, and cisplatin with or without high-dose tamoxifen in patients with metastatic melanoma.[74] The tamoxifen-treatment arm did not exhibit a significantly higher response rate, DFS, or OS.[74] The subsequent ECOG phase III trial (E-3690) compared the addition of tamoxifen to either DTIC alone or DTIC plus INF-α2b in 250 patients with metastatic melanoma and demonstrated nearly identical response rates and no difference in OS with the addition of tamoxifen.[75] A collaborative randomized phase III trial (North Central Cancer Treatment Group and Mayo Clinic) also reported that there was no meaningful clinical advantage in adding tamoxifen to the regimen of DTIC, carmustine, and cisplatin in the treatment of patients with advanced melanoma.[76]

In light of these findings, there is no convincing evidence to support the value of combination chemotherapy (with or without tamoxifen), relative to DTIC alone, in the 'routine' management of patients with recurrent and/or metastatic melanoma. It is feasible that this modality can serve a palliative role in the treatment of advanced melanoma. Further study is clearly indicated to better define the role of combination chemotherapy in the adjuvant setting as well.

Biochemotherapy

Both high-dose IFN-α2b and IL-2 have shown clinical utility in melanoma patients. The former demonstrated prevention of relapses and prolonged median survival when administered to patients at high risk for recurrence; the latter produced durable responses in a meaningful proportion of patients with distant metastases[77] (reviewed further in the appropriate sections of the chapter). Combinations of either of these two recombinant cytokines with other cytokines, each other, monoclonal antibodies, or various non-specific vaccines have yet to produce results superior to those of IL-2 alone.[78,79] In light of this, so-called biochemotherapy (or chemoimmunotherapy) – the combination of IL-2- and/or IFN-α2b-based immunotherapy with cytotoxic chemotherapy – has offered an encouraging therapeutic, possibly adjuvant, alternative for patients with melanoma. The rationale for this approach is based on preclinical models that have suggested additive or synergistic effects between the two groups of agents as well as proven individual activity in advanced melanoma and distinct toxicity profiles.[48,78]

Dr Weber and his colleagues summarized the brief clinical experience of biochemotherapy in the adjuvant setting of melanoma, with the expected conclusion that there is no clear role given the limited available studies and their contradictory findings. Indeed, data from phase III trials have not established clinical superiority of biochemotherapy regimens to either IL-2-based immunotherapy or cytotoxic chemotherapy alone.[75,79,80] Although we do not dispute these reputable data, we would like to offer the viewpoint that ongoing and future prospective, randomized adjuvant trials with biochemotherapy, including cisplatin-based regimens, are not premature, but, in fact, justified based on recently reported efficacy data and the unrealized potential of previously described molecular/surgical staging advances and clinical/pathologic stratification factors.

A review of the European Organization for Research and Treatment of Cancer (EORTC) database of 631 patients treated with high-dose IL-2-based regimens, 27 phase I and II protocols (conducted at 11 European institutions and at the University of Texas MD Anderson Cancer Center in Houston) demonstrated that the highest response rate (44.9%; $p < 0.001$) and median survival (11.4 months; $p = $ NS) were seen in the biochemotherapy treatment group.[81] Additionally, the 2-year survival rate was 23% and the 5-year survival rate was 13% among patients receiving IL-2 and IFN-α2b combinations.[81] Although not confirmed in prospectively randomized trials, these observations are in marked contrast to the reported 5-year survival rates of 2–6% achieved with chemotherapy alone.[2] To substantiate their initial data, this group has recently completed a prospective, randomized trial (EORTC 18951) to determine the contribution of high-dose IL-2 to long-term survival in patients treated with biochemotherapy.[82] The regimen consisted of a different cisplatin schedule, DTIC, and IFN-α2b with or without the addition of decrescendo high-dose IL-2. Interim analysis revealed that there were significantly more patients in the IL-2 treatment arm ($n = 10$) who were free of disease progression than in the non-IL-2 treatment arm ($n = 2$; $p = 0.026$) after a median follow-up of 1 year.[83] It will be important to see if this difference is maintained and if it translates into a significant survival advantage. Preliminary data from this trial have also demonstrated that patients in continuous complete remission ($n = 6$, thus far) have evidence of residual disease by RT–PCR-detected tyrosinase tumor antigens as well as synchronous melanoma-reactive T-cells using the enzyme-linked immunospot (ELISPOT) assay.[82] This group has also identified serum LDH, metastatic site (or number of involved organs), and performance status as useful stratification factors for future cytokine-based biochemotherapy randomized trials.[82]

In another comprehensive meta-analysis of 154 studies (>7000 patients with metastatic melanoma) comparing chemotherapy (DTIC-based or cisplatin-based regimens) with IL-2 alone, IL-2 plus IFN-α2b, and IL-2 plus IFN-α2b and chemotherapy, Allen et al. reported that the biochemotherapy treatment arm yielded the highest response rate (47%).[84] Likewise, the median response duration of 10 months in the biochemotherapy group was statistically superior to that achieved with either IL-2 alone (8 months) or chemotherapy alone (7 months).[84] Richards et al. were able to demonstrate efficacy with a combined regimen of IL-2 and IFN-α2b administered immediately after the first chemotherapy cycle and immediately before the second chemotherapy cycle of the Dartmouth regimen.[85] More than 10% of patients in their study (total $n = 84$), particularly patients with brain metastases, experienced a DFS beyond 4 years, suggesting a potential long-term benefit in some patients with advanced disease.[85] Interestingly, this regimen also produced a skin depigmentation which was associated with prolonged survival.[85] To alleviate the often severe toxicity commonly seen with cytokine-based biochemotherapy regimens, O'Day and colleagues recently evaluated the efficacy and toxicity profile of decrescendo dosing of IL-2, post-treatment granulocyte colony-stimulating factor (G-CSF), and low-dose tamoxifen in 45 patients with poor-prognosis metastatic melanoma.[86] Utilizing this different IL-2 dosing approach, toxicity, lengths of hospital stay, and readmission rates were significantly reduced. The overall response rate was 57%, the complete response rate was 23%, and the partial response rate was 34%. Interestingly, complete remissions were achieved in an additional 11% of patients by surgical resection of residual disease after this biochemotherapy regimen, suggesting a potential neoadjuvant role.

Legha and colleagues at the University of Texas MD Anderson Cancer Center have conducted a series of studies to establish the ideal combination and sequence of chemotherapy with biologic modifiers.[87] Generally, data from phase II trials have demonstrated that regimens in which chemotherapy was administered either prior to or concurrently with biotherapy appear to be the most effective.[87] For example, they recently utilized the concurrent administration of DTIC, cisplatin, vinblastine, intravenous IL-2, and subcutaneous IFN-α2b to treat 53 metastatic melanoma patients and achieved an overall response rate of 64%. Although 9% of patients have remained in remission for 50+ months, toxicity was usually severe and required hospitalization. A pilot study conducted at the Beth Israel Deaconess Medical Center by Atkins et al. modified this regimen (e.g., prophylactic antibiotics, frequent central line replacement, addition of G-CSF, decreased vinblastine dose) and achieved a significantly lower incidence of hematological toxicity, but not at the expense of effectiveness (response rate = 48%, complete response = 20%).[77] Based on this favorable outcome, ECOG has initiated a prospectively randomized phase III trial (E-3695) that will evaluate the modified biochemotherapy regimen described above versus the traditional regimen of cisplatin, vinblastine, and DTIC.[87] More importantly, patients will be stratified by extent of disease, prior use of IFN adjuvant therapy, and performance status – again, in the hope of identifying a homogeneous group of patients who are likely to benefit most.[48]

These data suggest that biochemotherapy, particularly with an IL-2-based regimen, may be superior to chemotherapy and/or biotherapy alone, albeit lacking confirmatory data from prospectively randomized trials. Notwithstanding, the available efficacy evidence outlined above, coupled with new developments in staging, natural history of advanced disease, prognostic/stratification factors, and the identification of more effective combinations and sequencing/dosing of biochemotherapy protocols, clearly validate ongoing and future adjuvant biochemotherapy trials.[88] The aforementioned Sunbelt Melanoma Trial, ECOG 3695, and EORTC 18951 represent a few of the many studies in progress that incorporate this current knowledge and will thus precisely delineate the role of biochemotherapy (and other systemic therapeutic/adjuvant modalities) in patients with melanoma.

Regional chemotherapy with isolated limb perfusion

Isolated limb perfusion (ILP), introduced by Creech and Krementz in 1958,[89] is a surgical procedure for the regional intravascular delivery of chemotherapeutics to an extremity with locally advanced melanoma. The basis of the therapy was maximum tumor kill but minimum systemic toxicity. Since Luck first reported efficacy with melphalan (*l*-phenylalanine mustard) in a murine pre-clinical model,[90] it has become the most widely used cyto-static agent for the treatment of extremity melanoma by ILP. ILP under mild hyperthermic conditions was first described by Stehlin in 1969 and is still practiced today.[91]

Multiple investigators have established the therapeu-tic efficacy of ILP for the treatment of locally recurrent extremity melanoma (i.e., satellites, in-transit metas-tases, positive nodes) and/or inoperable melanoma of the limbs.[92–98] Although the benefit of ILP on OS has not been clearly established, ILP as an adjunct to local surgery in recurrent melanoma has been demonstrated to result in lower locoregional recurrence rates.[99] Further-more, whether ILP can be used to eliminate micro-metastatic disease that is not removed by primary surgery (i.e., patients with high-risk primary extremity melanoma but no clinical evidence of metastatic disease) is also controversial.[100,101] In reporting their lifetime experience with ILP for more than 700 melanoma patients, Krementz *et al.* had nearly a 78.7% 20-year sur-vival rate (not actuarial and does include some patients with thin melanomas), nearly a 50% cure rate in those patients with satellitosis, and over a third of those indi-viduals with lymph node metastases were without relapse at 20 years.[102]

As is often the case, adjuvant ILP data have generally been derived from retrospective case-controlled studies in which patients treated with ILP were compared with historical controls treated by local wide excision (LWE) alone or from small single-institution reports in which a heterogeneous population of patients was used to estab-lish the benefit of ILP.[103] Ghussen *et al.* were the first to report data from a randomized phase III trial of adjuvant ILP.[104] A total of 107 patients were randomized into LWE only and ILP plus LWE arms, mostly including patients with stage II and III disease (satellitosis or in-transit metastases were excised prior to perfusion). The ILP treatment arm demonstrated a significant reduction in relapse rate (11% versus 48%); however, the survival data are controversial. Although 66% of the patients in the ILP treatment arm had stage II and III disease, remark-ably, 98% have survived beyond 5 years (only one death). Furthermore, the control group experienced an exceed-ingly high rate of early recurrences (39%). The small number of patients in this single-institution trial may have accounted for these biases.

The first large-scale, multicenter, prospectively ran-domized phase III trial evaluating the effect of ILP as an adjunct to surgery for high-risk melanoma in patients with no clinical evidence of metastases was recently reported by Schraffordt Koops and colleagues.[105] A total of 832 eligible patients over a 10-year period (1984–1994) were randomized to be treated by LWE only or ILP plus LWE, as part of the same operative procedure, using the

following stratification criteria: sex, anatomic site (upper versus lower limb), Breslow thickness (1.5–2.99 mm ver-sus 3.0–3.99 mm versus ≥4.0 mm), ulceration (present or absent), and previous biopsy (yes or no). The median follow-up duration was 6.4 years. The results demonstrate a transient benefit from ILP in terms of locoregional dis-ease control. For example, there was an increased disease-free interval in those ILP-treatment arm patients with lesions 1.5–2.99 mm and who did not undergo elective lymph node dissection (ELND). A similar reduction of in-transit metastases (6.6% versus 3.3%) and regional lymph node metastases (16.7% versus 12.6%) was found as well. Nevertheless, the data could not prove a clear benefit on OS. Given the potentially serious side-effects in the absence of an obvious survival advantage, the authors reasonably concluded that prophylactic ILP can-not be recommended as standard adjuvant therapy to LWE.[105] Lastly, others have evaluated adjuvant ILP as an alternative to delayed regional lymph node dissection and/or therapeutic ILP and all reported no impact on survival in patients treated by ELND or by delayed dis-section when clinically detectable node metastases.[103,106] Therefore, prophylactic ILP also does not appear to be an alternative to ELND, even for tumors of intermediate Breslow thickness.[103,106] Nonetheless, recent develop-ments may renew the controversy concerning ILP in the adjuvant setting for patients with melanoma. As dis-cussed above, Borgstein *et al.* have demonstrated the presence of lymphatic invasion as a significant predictor of locoregional cutaneous metastases and thus suggest that a possible subgroup of patients may indeed benefit from adjuvant ILP.[12] Furthermore, multiple reports of new combinations of tumor necrosis factor-α and/ or IFN-γ and/or melphalan have collectively yielded complete response rates of 78–90%, although a median survival duration of only 2 years.[103,107] These recent findings have led many in the surgical community who have experience with ILP to believe that it is the treat-ment of choice for the thick and/or primary lesion aris-ing on the extremity, although further study is necessary to verify this proposition.[108]

Radiation therapy

In their review, Dr Weber and his colleagues described the significant evolution of radiotherapy in the management of malignant melanoma. We would like to add to their comments with a brief historical perspective before turn-ing to recent data. Traditionally, malignant melanoma was regarded a radioresistant tumor,[109–111] although not without controversy from isolated studies having sug-gested otherwise.[112,113] It was not until the early 1970s that *in-vitro* studies demonstrated some potentially favor-able effects of radiation in this disease using large doses per fraction.[109,110] Multiple investigators subsequently reported high response rates in a variety of primary and metastatic melanomas using ≥ 4 Gy dosing in both elective and adjunctive regional RT settings.[114–119] Clearly, sufficient biologic and clinical evidence now exists to rebut the one-time belief that melanomas are uniformly radioresistant. This misconception has unfortunately limited the clinical experience at most cancer centers to patients with an overall poor prognosis (e.g., those with advanced, recurrent, and/or metastatic disease) and, consequently, data from prospective multicenter clinical trials.

Several newly reported retrospective studies demonstrate postoperative adjuvant radiation therapy was effective in reducing local recurrence in melanoma patients at high risk of locoregional failure.[120–124] Taken together, these studies produced 5-year OS rates ranging from 30% to 50% in those patients having received adjuvant radiation therapy for advanced lesions (AJCC/ International Union Against Cancer (UICC) stage IIB/III/IV). Although these findings compare favorably to published 'surgery-only' data,[2] randomized prospective trials are needed for validation. Moreover, there was considerable toxicity in the form of limb edema noted in most of these studies, despite hypofractionated dosing.

Seegenschmiedt and associates recently compiled their 20-year experience in using radiation therapy for patients with advanced melanoma.[120] One hundred and twenty-one patients out of the nearly 3000 consecutive patients in their melanoma registry received radiation therapy for palliation of UICC stage IIB/III/IV lesions; at 3 months follow-up, 64%, 44%, and 17% achieved a complete response, respectively. The complete responders survived longer than those patients without a complete response (median: 40 versus 10 months; $p < 0.01$), as expected. Furthermore, univariate analysis revealed that UICC stage ($p < 0.001$; also in multivariate analysis), head and neck primary lesions ($p < 0.05$), and total radiation dose > 40 Gy ($p < 0.05$) were significant prognostic factors for a complete response, whereas age, gender, and histology had no impact. The authors concluded that future prospective, randomized trials using palliative/adjuvant radiation therapy for advanced melanoma are justified based on their data demonstrating effective palliation as well as long-term local control.

While the results of randomized clinical trials are awaited, advances have been made in determining prognostic factors predictive of local recurrence – that is to say, selecting patients who may benefit from locoregional adjuvant radiation therapy.[12,125] To this end, a recent retrospective study from the Roswell Park Cancer Institute analysed patterns of failure in 338 positive lymph node melanoma patients who had undergone lymph node dissection (LND) of the involved nodal basin. On multivariate analysis, the following risk factors were significant of nodal basin recurrence following LND: cervical involvement, $>$ three positive nodes, clinically involved nodes, any node > 3 cm, or evidence of extracapsular extension. The authors concluded that adjuvant radiation therapy should be considered for those patients who met any of these criteria. Lastly, several new treatment methods have been evaluated to augment the response of malignant melanoma to radiation therapy. These include hyperthermia, boron neutron capture therapy, photodynamic therapy, radiosensitizers, and targeted radiolabeled antibodies and, for the most part, are still at the experimental level.[126]

SUMMARY

Despite several experimental adjuvant therapies, such as IFN-α2b therapy, chemotherapy with DTIC, combination chemotherapy, etc., having yielded moderate clinical benefit, toxicity continues to be problematic. Physicians and patients are therefore interested in therapies that are less toxic and more effective. The current treatment options are reviewed by Weber et al. and abstracted here. Patients with resected stage I melanoma disease are not candidates for IFN-α2b or chemotherapy. If patients have a genetic disposition to melanoma (i.e., familial melanoma), these patients are best suited for any type of vaccine therapy that can help prevent the development of a second primary. Patients with resected stage IIA (< 4 mm thickness) who have either clinically negative or pathologically negative nodal involvement are also not candidates for adjuvant therapy with IFN-α2b. Given the likelihood that this stage of disease may be a harbinger for nodal micrometastases, patients should be enrolled in one of the several clinical trials that are designed to study the diagnosis of micrometastases by RT–PCR-based molecular marker analysis aided by lymphatic mapping. Moreover, patients with genetic disposition to the development of melanoma should be enrolled in active specific immunotherapy trials.

The majority of patients with stage IIB melanoma (tumor thickness > 4 mm) are known to be at high risk for recurrence, particularly in the regional lymph node basin, even though they may be clinically free of disease. As Weber et al. suggest, these patients are ideal candidates for the lymphatic mapping and selective lymph node dissection followed by one of the many experimental biological therapies. Therapy for patients with stage III melanoma should be based on the number of involved nodes. High-dose IFN-α2b adjuvant therapy would be appropriate for these patients. However, toxicity and no improvement in the OS are still major concerns. There are several experimental vaccine and/or chemotherapy trials that are also suitable for patients with this stage of disease. Finally, patients with stage IV disease may receive palliative surgery, as indicated, and experimental adjuvant therapy via chemotherapy, radiotherapy, biological therapy, or variations in these modalities.

REFERENCES

1. American Cancer Society – facts and figures. Melanoma 1999; 10–11.
2. Balch CM, Reintgen D, Kirkwood JM, et al. Cutaneous melanoma. In DeVita VT, Hellman S, Rosenberg SA, eds. Cancer: principles and practice of oncology, 5th edn. Philadelphia, JB Lippincott Co, 1997, 1947–94.
3. Barth A, Wanek LA, Morton DL. Prognostic factors in 1521 melanoma patients with distant metastases. J Am Coll Surg 1995; 181:193–201.
4. Tomsu K, Van Eschen KB, Lee MA. Meta-analysis of median survival of patients with stage IV melanoma. Proc Am Soc Clin Oncol 1997; 16:1784.
5. Mastrangelo M, Bellet R, Kane M, et al. Chemotherapy of melanoma. In: Perry M, ed. The chemotherapy source book. Baltimore, Williams & Wilkins, 1992, 886–907.
6. Keilholz U, Eggermont AMM. The role of interleukin-2 in the management of stage IV melanoma: the EORTC Melanoma Cooperative Group Program. Cancer J Sci Am 2000; 6(Suppl. 1):S99–103.
7. Balch CM. Surgical treatment of advanced melanoma. In Balch CM, Houghton AN, Sober AJ, Soong SJ, eds. Cutaneous melanoma. Saint Louis, MI, QMP Publisher, 1998.
8. Garber C, Buttner P, Bertz J, et al. Primary cutaneous melanoma: identification of prognostic groups and estimation of individual prognosis for 5093 patients. Cancer 1995; 75:2484–91.
9. Schuchter L, Schulz DJ, Synnestvedt M, et al. A prognostic model for predicting 10-year survival in patients with primary melanoma. Ann Intern Med 1996; 125:369–75.
10. Huang X, Soong S, McCarthy WH, et al. Classification of localized melanoma by the exponential survival trees methods. Cancer 1997; 79:1122–8.
11. Eton O, Legha SS, Moon TE, et al. Prognostic factors for survival of patients treated systemically for disseminated melanoma. J Clin Oncol 1998; 16(3):1103–11.
12. Borgstein PJ, Meijer S, van Diest PJ. Are locoregional cutaneous metastases in melanoma predictable? Ann Surg Oncol 1999; 6(3):315–21.
13. Gershenwald JE, Colome MI, Lee JE, et al. Patterns of recurrence following a negative sentinel lymph node biopsy in 243 patients with stage I or II melanoma. J Clin Oncol 1998; 16(6):2253–60.
14. Curry BJ, Myers K, Hersey P. Polymerase chain reaction detection of melanoma cells in the circulation: relation to clinical stage, surgical treatment, and recurrence from melanoma. J Clin Oncol 1998; 16(5):1760–9.
15. Mellado B, Colomer D, Castel T, et al. Detection of circulating neoplastic cells by reverse-transcriptase polymerase chain reaction in malignant melanoma: association with clinical stage and prognosis. J Clin Oncol 1996; 14:2091–7.
16. Ghossein RA, Coit B, Brennan M, et al. Prognostic significance of peripheral blood and bone marrow tyrosinase messenger RNA in malignant melanoma. Clin Cancer Res 1998; 4:419–28.
17. Curry BJ, Myers K, Hersey P. MART-1 is expressed less frequently on circulating melanoma cells in patients who develop distant compared with locoregional metastases. J Clin Oncol 1999; 17(8):2562–71.
18. Haigh PI, Essner R, Wardlaw JC, et al. Long-term survival following complete resection of melanoma metastatic to the adrenal gland. Ann Surg Oncol 1999; 6:633–9.
19. Balch CM. Palliative surgery for stage IV melanoma: is it a primary treatment? Ann Surg Oncol 1999; 6(7):623–4.
20. McMasters KM, Sondak VK, Lotze MT, et al. Recent advances in melanoma staging and therapy. Ann Surg Oncol 1999; 6(5):467–75.
21. Ahmann DL, Creagan ET, Hahn RG, et al. Complete responses and long-term survivals after systemic chemotherapy for patients with advanced malignant melanoma. Cancer 1989; 63:224–7.
22. Kirkwood JM, Strawderman MH, Ernstoff MS, Smith TJ, Borden EC, Blum RH. Interferon alfa-2b adjuvant therapy of high-risk resected cutaneous melanoma: the Eastern Cooperative Oncology Group Trial EST 1684. J Clin Oncol 1996; 14(1):7–17.
23. Kirkwood JM, Ibrahim J, Sondak V, et al. Preliminary analysis of the E1690/S9111/C9190 Intergroup Postoperative Adjuvant Trial of high- and low-dose interferon alpha 2b in high-risk primary or lymph node metastatic melanoma. Proc Am Soc Clin Oncol 1999; (18):537a (Abstract 2072).
24. Grob JJ, Dreno B, Delauney M, et al. Randomized trial of interferon alpha 2a as adjuvant therapy in resected primary melanoma thicker than 1.5mm without clinically detectable nodal metastases. Lancet 1998; 351(9120):1905–10.
25. Creagan ET, Dalton RJ, Ahmann DL, et al. Randomized, surgical adjuvant clinical trial of recombinant interferon alfa-2a in selected patients with melanoma. J Clin Oncol 1995; 13:2776–83.
26. Meyskens FL, Kopecky K, Taylor CW, et al. Randomized trial of adjuvant human interferon gamma versus observation in high-risk cutaneous melanoma. J Natl Cancer Inst 1995; 87:1710–13.
27. Atkins MB. Interleukin-2 in metastatic melanoma: what is the current role. CA J Sci Am 2000; 6:S8–10.
28. Atkins MB, Lotze MT, Dutcher JP, et al. High-dose recombinant interleukin-2 therapy for patients with metastatic melanoma: analysis of 270 patients treated between 1985 and 1993. J Clin Oncol 1999; 17(7):2105.

29. Morton DL, Eilber FR, Holmes EC, *et al.* Immunological factors which influence response to immunotherapy in malignant melanoma. Surgery 1970; 68:158–64.

30. Hunter-Craig I, Westbury G. Use of vaccinia virus in the treatment of metastatic melanoma. BMJ 1970; 2:512–15.

31. Jones PC, Sze LL, Liu PY, *et al.* Prolonged survival for melanoma patients with elevated IgM antibody to oncofetal antigen. J Natl Cancer Inst 1981; 66:249–54.

32. Morton DL, Foshag LJ, Hoon DSB, *et al.* Prolongation of survival in metastatic melanoma after active specific immunotherapy with a new polyvalent melanoma vaccine. Ann Surg 1992; 216:463–82.

33. Mordoh J, Kairiyama C, Bover L, *et al.* Allogeneic cells vaccine increases disease-free survival in stage III melanoma patients. A non-randomized phase II study. Medicinia (Buenos Aires) 1997; 57:421–7.

34. Berd D, Maguire HC Jr, Schuchter LM, *et al.* Autologous hapten-modified melanoma vaccine as postsurgical adjuvant treatment after resection of nodal metastases. J Clin Oncol 1997; 15:2359–70.

35. Wallack MK, Sivanandham M, Balch C, *et al.* A phase III randomized, double-blind, multi-institutional trial of vaccinia melanoma oncolysate (VMO) active specific immunotherapy for patients with stage II (UICC) melanoma. Cancer 1995; 75:34–42.

36. Wallack MK, Sivanandham M, Balch CM, *et al.* Surgical adjuvant active specific immunotherapy for patients with stage III melanoma: the final analysis of data from a phase III, randomized, double-blind, multicenter vaccinia melanoma oncolysate trial. J Am Coll Surg 1998; 187:69–77.

37. Mastrangelo M. Conference report of the 3rd International Conference on Adjuvant Therapy of Melanoma. Melanoma Res 1999; 9:306–8.

38. Mitchell MS. Perspective on Allogeneic Melanoma Lysates in Active Specific Immunotherapy. Semin Oncol 1998; 25:623–5.

39. McGee JMC, Lytle GH, Malnar KF, *et al.* Melanoma tumor vaccine: five-year follow-up. J Surg Oncol 1991; 47:233–8.

40. Livingston PO, Wong GYC, Adluri S, *et al.* Improved survival in stage III melanoma patients with GM2 antibodies: a randomized trial of adjuvant vaccination with GM2 ganglioside. J Clin Oncol 1994; 12:1036–44.

41. Rosenberg SA, Yang JC, Schwartzentruber DJ, *et al.* Immunologic and therapeutic evaluation of a synthetic peptide vaccine for the treatment of patients with metastatic melanoma. Nat Med 1998; 4:321–7.

42. Cebon JS, Jaeger E, Gibbs P, *et al.* Phase I studies of immunization with Melan-A and IL-12 in HLA-A2 positive patients with stage III and IV metastatic melanoma. Proc Am Soc Clin Oncol 18:434a (Abstract 1671).

43. Jaeger E, Bernhard H, Romero P, *et al.* Generation of cytotoxic T-cell responses with synthetic melanoma-associated peptides in vivo: implications for tumor vaccines with melanoma-associated antigens. Int J Cancer 1996; 66(2):162–9.

44. Houghton AN, Mintzer D, Cordon-Caro C, *et al.* Mouse monoclonal IgG3 antibody detecting GD3 ganglioside. A phase I trial in patients with malignant melanoma. Proc Natl Acad Sci USA 1985; 82:1242–6.

45. Irie R, Matsuki T, Morton D. Human monoclonal antibody to ganglioside GM2 for melanoma treatment. Lancet 1989; 1:786–7.

46. Dunbar PR, Chen JL, Chao D, *et al.* Cutting edge: rapid cloning of tumor-specific CTL suitable for adoptive therapy of melanoma. J Immunol 1999; 162(12):6959–62.

47. Flaherty L, Unger J, Liu P, *et al.* Gender differences and predictors of survival in patients with metastatic melanoma of SWOG trials [abstract]. Proc Am Soc Clin Oncol 1996; 15:433a.

48. Flaherty LE. Rationale for Intergroup Trial E-3695 comparing concurrent biochemotherapy with cisplatin, vinblastine, and DTIC alone in patients with metastatic melanoma. Cancer J Sci Am 2000; 6(Suppl. 1):S15–20.

49. Veronesi U, Adamus J, Auebert C, *et al.* A randomized trial of adjuvant chemotherapy and immunotherapy in cutaneous melanoma. N Eng J Med 1982; 307:913–16.

50. Lejeune FJ, Macher E, Kleeberg U, *et al.* An assessment of DTIC versus levamisole or placebo in the treatment of high risk stage I patients after surgical removal of a primary melanoma of the skin: a phase III adjuvant study (EORTC 18761). Eur J Cancer 1988; 24(Suppl. 2):81–90.

51. Middleton MR, Grob JJ, Aaronson N, *et al.* Randomized phase III study of temozolomide versus dacarbazine in the treatment of patients with advanced metastatic malignant melanoma. J Clin Oncol 2000; 18:158–66.

52. Middleton M, Gore M, Tilgen W, *et al.* A randomized, phase III study of temozolomide (TMZ) versus dacarbazine (DTIC) in the treatment of patients with advanced, metastatic melanoma. Proc Natl Acad Sci USA 1999; 18:536a.

53. Summers Y, Calvert H, Lee SM, *et al.* Effect of temozolomide (TMZ) on central nervous system (CNS) relapse in patients with advanced melanoma (abstract). Proc Am Soc Clin Oncol 1999; 18:531a.

54. Gonzalez R, O'Day S, Gibbs P, *et al.* A preliminary analysis of a multicenter phase II study of biochemotherapy with temozolomide, cisplatin, interleukin-2, α-interferon, and granulocyte macrophage colony stimulating factor (GM-CSF)

for stage IV melanoma (abstract). Cancer Invest 2000; 18 (Suppl. 1):101–2a.

55. Legha SS, Ring S, Papadopoulos N, *et al*. A prospective evaluation of a triple-drug regimen containing cisplatin, vinblastine and dacarbazine (CVD) for metastatic melanoma. Cancer 1989; 64:2024–9.

56. McClay EF, Mastrangelo MJ, Bellet RE, *et al*. Combination chemotherapy and hormonal therapy in the treatment of malignant melanoma. Cancer Treat Rep 1987; 71:465–9.

57. Del Prete SA, Maurer LH, O'Donnell J, *et al*. Combination chemotherapy with cisplatin, carmustine, dacarbazine, and tamoxifen in metastatic melanoma. Cancer Treat Rep 1984; 68:1403–5.

58. Murren JR, DeRosa W, Durivage HJ, *et al*. High-dose cisplatin plus dacarbazine in the treatment of metastatic melanoma. Cancer 1991; 67:1514–17.

59. Fletcher WS, Green S, Fletcher JR, *et al*. Evaluation of cisplatinum and DTIC combination chemotherapy in disseminated melanoma. A Southwest Oncology Group Study. Am J Clin Oncol 1988; 11:589–93.

60. Seigler HF, Lucas VS Jr, Pickett NJ, *et al*. DTIC, CCNU, bleomycin and vincristine (BOLD) in metastatic melanoma. Cancer 1980; 46:2346–8.

61. York RM, Foltz AT. Bleomycin, vincristine, lomustine, and DTIC chemotherapy for metastatic melanoma. Cancer 1988; 61:2183–6.

62. McClay EF, Mastrangelo MJ, Berd D, *et al*. Effective combination chemo/hormonal therapy for malignant melanoma: experience with three consecutive trials. Int J Cancer 1992; 50:553–6.

63. Margolin KA, Liu P-Y, Flaherty LE, *et al*. Phase II study of carmustine, dacarbazine, cisplatin and tamoxifen in advanced melanoma: a Southwest Oncology Group study. J Clin Oncol 1998; 16:664–9.

64. Hill GJ, Krementz ET, Hill HZ, *et al*. DTIC and combination therapy for melanoma. Cancer 1984; 53:1299–305.

65. Flaherty LE, Liu PY, Mitchell MS, *et al*. The addition of tamoxifen to dacarbazine and cisplatin in metastatic malignant melanoma. A phase II trial of the Southwest Oncology Group (SWOG-8921). Am J Clin Oncol 1996; 19:108–13.

66. Margolin KA, Liu PY, Unger JM, *et al*. Phase II trial of biochemotherapy with interferon alpha, dacarbazine, cisplatin and tamoxifen in metastatic melanoma: a Southwest Oncology Group trial. J Cancer Res Clin Oncol 1999; 125(5):292–6.

67. Chemotherapy of disseminated melanoma with bleomycin, vincristine, CCNU, and DTIC (BOLD regimen). The Prudente Foundation Melanoma Study Group. Cancer 1989; 63:1676–80.

68. Fletcher WS, Daniels DS, Sondak VK, *et al*. Evaluation of cisplatin and DTIC in inoperable stage III and IV melanoma. A Southwest Oncology Group study. Am J Clin Oncol 1993; 16:359–62.

69. Chapman PB, Einhorn LH, Meyers ML, *et al*. Phase III multicenter randomized trial of the Dartmouth regimen versus dacarbazine in patients with metastatic melanoma. J Clin Oncol 1999; 17:2745–51.

70. Cocconi G, Bella M, Calabresi F, *et al*. Treatment of metastatic malignant melanoma with dacarbazine plus tamoxifen. N Engl J Med 1992; 327:516–23.

71. Nathan FE, Berd D, Sato T, *et al*. Paclitaxel and tamoxifen – an active regimen for patients with metastatic melanoma. Cancer 2000; 88:79–87.

72. Wiernik PH, Einzig AI. Taxol in malignant melanoma. Monogr Natl Cancer Inst 1993; 15:185–7.

73. McClay EF, McClay ME, Monroe L, *et al*. The effect of tamoxifen (TAM) and cisplatin (DDP) on the disease free survival (DFS) and overall survival (OS) in patients with surgically resected metastatic melanoma (abstract). Proc Am Soc Clin Oncol 1998; 17:522a.

74. Rusthoven JJ, Quirt IC, Iscoe NA, *et al*. Randomized, double-blind, placebo-controlled trial comparing the response rates of carmustine, dacarbazine, and cisplatin with and without tamoxifen in patients with metastatic melanoma. J Clin Oncol 1996; 14:2083–90.

75. Falkson CI, Ibrahim J, Kirkwood JM, *et al*. Phase III trial of dacarbazine versus dacarbazine with interferon alpha-2b versus dacarbazine with tamoxifen versus dacarbazine with interferon alpha-2b and tamoxifen in patients with metastatic malignant melanoma: an Eastern Cooperative Oncology Group study. J Clin Oncol 1998; 16(5):1743–51.

76. Creagan ET, Suman VJ, Dalton RJ, *et al*. Phase III clinical trial of the combination of cisplatin, dacarbazine, and carmustine with or without tamoxifen in patients with advanced malignant melanoma. J Clin Oncol 1999; 17:1884–900.

77. Atkins M, Shet A, Sosman J. Interleukin-2: clinical applications – melanoma. In DeVita VT, Hellman S, Rosenberg SA, eds. *Principles and practice of the biologic therapy of cancer*, 3rd edn. Philadelphia, Lippincott Williams & Wilkins, 2000, 50–73.

78. Atkins MB, Kunkel L, Sznol M, *et al*. High-dose recombinant interleukin-2 therapy in patients with metastatic melanoma: long-term survival update. Cancer J Sci Am 2000; 6(Suppl. 1):S11–14.

79. Keilholz U, Eggermont AMM. The role of interleukin-2 in the management of stage IV melanoma: the EORTC Melanoma Cooperative Group Program. Cancer J Sci Am 2000; 6(Suppl. 1):S99–103.

80. Rosenberg SA, Yang JC, Schwartzentruber DJ, *et al*. Prospective randomized trial of the treatment of patients with metastatic melanoma using chemotherapy with cisplatin, dacarbazine, and

tamoxifen alone or in combination with interleukin-2 and interferon-alfa-2b. J Clin Oncol 1999; 17:968–75.

81. Keilholz U, Goey SH, Punt CJ, et al. Interferon alfa-2b and interleukin-2 with or without cisplatin in metastatic melanoma: a randomized trial of the European Organization for Research and Treatment of Cancer Melanoma Cooperative Group. J Clin Oncol 1997; 15:2579–88.

82. Keilholz U, Conradt C, Legha SS, et al. Results of interleukin-2-based treatment in advanced melanoma: a case record-based analysis of 631 patients. J Clin Oncol 1998; 16(9):2921–9.

83. Keilholz U, Punt CJ, Gore M, et al. Dacarbazine, cisplatin and interferon alpha with or without interleukin-2 in advanced melanoma: interim analysis of EORTC Trial 18951 (abstract). Proc Am Soc Clin Oncol 1999; 18:530a.

84. Allen I, Kupelnick B, Kumashiro M. Efficacy of interleukin-2 in the treatment of metastatic melanoma – systemic review and meta-analysis. Cancer Ther 1998; 1:168–73.

85. Richards JM, Gale D, Mehta N, et al. Combination of chemotherapy with interleukin-2 and interferon alfa for the treatment of metastatic melanoma. J Clin Oncol 1999; 17(2):651–7.

86. O'Day SJ, Gammon G, Boasberg P, et al. Advantages of concurrent biochemotherapy modified by decrescendo interleukin-2, granulocyte colony-stimulating factor, and tamoxifen for patients with metastatic melanoma. J Clin Oncol 1999; 17(9):2752–61.

87. Legha SS, Ring S, Eton O, et al. Development and results of biochemotherapy in metastatic melanoma: the University of Texas M.D. Anderson Cancer Center experience. Cancer J Sci Am 1997; 15:2579–88.

88. McDermott DF, Mier JW, Lawrence DP, et al. A phase II pilot trial of concurrent biochemotherapy with cisplatin, vinblastine, dacarbazine (CVD), interleukin-2 (IL-2), and interferon alpha 2b (IFN) in patients with metastatic melanoma (abstract). Proc Am Soc Clin Oncol 1998; 17:507a.

89. Creech O Jr, Krementz ET, Ryan RF, et al. Chemotherapy of cancer: regional perfusion utilizing an extracorporeal circuit. Ann Surg 1958; 148:616–32.

90. Luck J. Action of P-di(2-chloroethyl)-amino-L-phenylalanine on Harding Passey mouse melanoma. Science 1956; 123:984–5.

91. Stehlin JS. Hyperthermic perfusion with chemotherapy for cancers of the extremities. Surg Gynecol Oncol 1969; 129:305–8.

92. Lejeune FJ, Deloof T, Ewalenko P, et al. Objective regression of unexcised melanoma in-transit metastases after hyperthermic isolation perfusion of the limbs with melphalan. Recent Results Cancer Res 1983; 86:268–76.

93. Storm FK, Morton DL. Value of therapeutic hyperthermic limb perfusion in advanced recurrent melanoma of the lower extremity. Am J Surg 1985; 150:32–5.

94. Santinami M, Belli F, Cascinelli N, et al. Seven years experience with hyperthermic perfusions in extracorporeal circulation for melanoma of the extremities. J Surg Oncol 1989; 42:201–8.

95. Di Filippo F, Calabro A, Giannarelli D, et al. Prognostic variables in recurrent limb melanoma treated with hyperthermic antiblastic perfusion. Cancer 1989; 63:2551–61.

96. Skene AI, Bulman AS, Williams TR, et al. Hyperthermic isolated perfusion with melphalan in the treatment of advanced malignant melanoma of the lower limb. Br J Surg 1990; 77:765–7.

97. Klaase JM, Kroon B, van Geel AN, et al. Prognostic factors for tumor response and limb recurrence-free interval in patients with advanced melanoma of the limbs treated with regional isolated perfusion with melphalan. Surgery 1994; 115:39–45.

98. Thompson JF, Hunt JA, Shannon KF, et al. Frequency and duration of remission after isolated limb perfusion for melanoma. Arch Surg 1997; 132:903–8.

99. Hafstrom L, Rudenstam C-M, Blomquist E, et al. Regional hyperthermic perfusion with melphalan after surgery for recurrent malignant melanoma of the extremities. J Clin Oncol 1991; 9:2091–4.

100. Franklin HR, Schraffordt Koops H, Oldhoff J, et al. To perfuse or not to perfuse? A retrospective comparative study to evaluate the effect of adjuvant isolated regional perfusion in patients with stage I extremity melanoma with a thickness of 1.5 mm or greater. J Clin Oncol 1988; 6:701–8.

101. Schraffordt Koops H, Kroon BBR, Oldhoff J, et al. Controversies concerning adjuvant regional isolated perfusion for stage I melanoma of the extremities. World J Surg 1992; 16:241–5.

102. Krementz ET, Ryan RF, Carter RD, et al. Hyperthermic regional perfusion for melanoma of the limbs. In Balch CM, Milton GW, eds. Cutaneous melanoma: clinical management and treatment results worldwide. Philadelphia, JB Lippincott, 1985, 171–95.

103. Fraker DL. Hyperthermic regional perfusion for melanoma and sarcoma of the limbs. Curr Probl Surg 1999; 36(11):845–908.

104. Ghussen F, Nagel K, Groth W, et al. A prospective randomized study of regional extremity perfusion in patients with malignant melanoma. Ann Surg 1984; 200:764–8.

105. Schraffordt Koops H, Vaglini M, Suciu S, et al. Prophylactic isolated limb perfusion for localized, high-risk limb melanoma: results of a multicenter randomized phase III trial. J Clin Oncol 1998; 16(9):2906–12.

106. Balch CM, Soong SJ, Bartolucci AA, et al. Efficacy of an elective regional lymph node dissection of

1 to 4 mm thick melanomas for patients 60 years of age and younger. Ann Surg 1996; 224:255–63.

107. Lienard D, Eggermont AM, Kroon BB, *et al.* Isolated limb perfusion in primary and recurrent melanoma: indications and results. Semin Surg Oncol 1998; 14:202–9.

108. Polk HC Jr. Surgical progress and understanding in the treatment of the melanoma epidemic. Am J Surg 1999; 178:443–8.

109. Barranco SC, Romsdahl M, Humphrey RM. The radiation response of human malignant melanoma cells grown in vitro. Cancer Res 1971; 31:830–3.

110. Dewey DL. The radiosensitivity of melanoma cells in culture. Br J Radiol 1971; 44:816–17.

111. Doss LL, Memula N. The radioresponsiveness of melanoma. Int J Radiat Oncol Biol Phys 1982; 8:1131–4.

112. Trott KR, von Lieven H, Kummermehr J, *et al.* The radiosensitivity of malignant melanomas, part I: Experimental studies. Int J Radiat Oncol Biol Phys 1981; 7:9–13.

113. Trott KR, von Lieven H, Kummermehr J, *et al.* The radiosensitivity of malignant melanomas, part II: Clinical studies. Int J Radiat Oncol Biol Phys 1981; 7:15–20.

114. Habermalz HJ, Fischer JJ. Radiation therapy of malignant melanoma: experience with high individual treatment doses. Cancer 1976; 38:2258–62.

115. Hornsey S. The relationship between total dose, number of fractions and fraction size in the response of malignant melanoma in patients. Br J Radiol 1978; 51:905–9.

116. Johanson CR, Harwood AR, Cummings BJ, *et al.* 0-7-21 Radiotherapy in nodular melanoma. *Cancer* 1983; 51:226–32.

117. Overgaard J, von der Maase H, Overgaard M, *et al.* A randomized study comparing two high-dose per fraction radiation schedules in recurrent or metastatic malignant melanoma. Int J Radiat Oncol Biol Phys 1985; 11:1837–9.

118. Ang KK, Byers RM, Peters LJ, *et al.* Regional radiotherapy as an alternative or adjuvant to nodal dissection for high risk cutaneous malignant melanoma of the head and neck – Preliminary results. Arch Otolaryngol Head Neck Surg 1990; 116(2):169–72.

119. Ang KK, Peters LJ, Weber RS, *et al.* Postoperative radiotherapy for cutaneous melanoma of the head and neck region. Int J Radiat Oncol Biol Phys 1994; 30:795–8.

120. Seegenschmiedt MH, Keilholz L, Altendorf-Hofmann A, *et al.* Palliative radiotherapy for recurrent and metastatic melanoma: prognostic factors for tumor response and long-term outcome: a 20-year experience. Int J Radiat Oncol Biol Phys 1999; 44(3):607–18.

121. Burmeister BH, Smithers BM, Poulsen M, *et al.* Radiation therapy for nodal disease in malignant melanoma. World J Surg 1995; 19:369–71.

122. Strom EA, Ross MI. Adjuvant radiation therapy after axillary lymphadenectomy for metastatic melanoma: toxicity and local control. Ann Surg Oncol 1995; 2(5):445–9.

123. Corry J, Smith JG, Bishop M, *et al.* Nodal radiation therapy for metastatic melanoma. Int J Radiat Oncol Biol Phys 1999; 44(5):1065–9.

124. Stevens G, Thompson JF, Firth I, *et al.* Locally advanced melanoma – results of postoperative hypofractionated radiation therapy. Cancer 2000; 88:88–94.

125. Lee RJ, Gibbs JF, Proulx GM, *et al.* Nodal basin recurrence following lymph node dissection for melanoma: implications for adjuvant radiotherapy. Int J Radiat Oncol Biol Phys 2000; 46(2):467–74.

126. Geara FB, Ang KK. Radiation therapy for malignant melanoma. Surg Clin North Am 1996; 76(6):1383–98.

Editors' selected abstracts

Intermediate dose recombinant interferon-alpha as second-line treatment for patients with recurrent cutaneous melanoma who were pretreated with low dose interferon.

Ascierto PA, Daponte A, Parasole R, Perrone F, Caraco C, Melucci M, Palmieri G, Napolitano M, Mozzillo N, Castello G.

Department of Clinical Immunology, National Cancer Institute, Naples, Italy.

Cancer 89(7):1490–4, 2000, October 1.

Background: Interferon (IFN) is widely considered the most effective agent in the adjuvant therapy of patients with cutaneous melanoma (CM). However, little is known about the effect of IFN on pretreated CM patients who experience disease recurrence. The authors conducted a Phase II study to determine whether intermediate doses of IFN could be beneficial for these patients. *Methods:* A series of 24 consecutive CM patients who had undergone surgery for local, in-transit, or lymph node disease recurrence during adjuvant therapy with low dose IFN (IFNalpha-2b, 3 million units [MU] per day, three times per week) were enrolled for second-line therapy with intermediate dose IFN (IFNalpha-2b, 10 MU per day) for one year. *Results:* IFN was discontinued in 7 patients (29.2%) because of toxicity. Several patients complained of impairment in their daily activities. Progression of disease was registered in 17 patients (70.8%), with a median disease free survival of 5.5 months (95% confidence interval, 3.4–14.2). The median follow-up for the

7 patients who did not experience disease recurrence was 15 months (range, 13–22 months). *Conclusions:* An increased dose of IFN as second-line adjuvant treatment was poorly tolerated and produced negative clinical outcomes in patients with CM. However, these patients probably were unresponsive to IFN regardless of the dosage level. In fact, the first adjuvant IFN treatment was ineffective in all patients. Thus, the key factor in the treatment of CM seems to be patient responsiveness to IFN rather than the total dosage achieved.

Adjuvant therapy of melanoma with interferon-alpha-2b is associated with mania and bipolar syndromes.

Greenberg DB, Jonasch E, Gadd MA, Ryan BF, Everett JR, Sober AJ, Mihm MA, Tanabe KK, Ott M, Haluska FG.

Massachusetts General Hospital, Boston, MD, USA.

Cancer 89(2):356–62, 2000, July 15.

Background: The use of a high dose regimen of interferon-alpha-2b (IFN) has recently been demonstrated to benefit patients with resected high risk melanoma. The incidence of melanoma is rising rapidly, and the use of this regimen is becoming increasingly common. IFN has been associated with numerous psychiatric side effects. *Methods:* The authors describe four melanoma patients treated with adjuvant IFN who developed a manic–depressive syndrome or mood instability with therapy, and they review the literature on mania and the mixed affective syndromes associated with IFN. *Results:* The authors suggest that IFN may induce a mixed affective instability, and that patients risk developing hypomania or mania as IFN doses fluctuate or as IFN-induced depression is treated with antidepressants alone. Mania is particularly associated with dose reductions or pauses in IFN treatment. The risk of mood fluctuation continues after treatment with IFN stops, and patients should be monitored for 6 months following completion of therapy. Gabapentin appeared effective as monotherapy for acute mania, as an antianxiety agent, as a hypnotic, and as a mood stabilizer in these individual cases. *Conclusions:* Mania and mood instability can occur in patients being treated with IFN therapy for melanoma. In this study, gabapentin was an effective mood-stabilizing agent for these patients.

Molecular markers in blood as surrogate prognostic indicators of melanoma recurrence.

Hoon DS, Bostick P, Kuo C, Okamoto T, Wang HJ, Elashoff R, Morton DL.

Department of Molecular Oncology, John Wayne Cancer Institute, Saint John's Health Center, Santa Monica, CA, USA.

Cancer Research 60(8):2253–7, 2000, April 15.

Improvement is needed in the ability to evaluate the prognosis of melanoma patients who are clinically disease-free but likely to develop recurrent metastatic disease. The detection of circulating melanoma cells in blood is a potential surrogate marker of subclinical residual disease. We assessed the prognostic clinical utility of a multimarker melanoma reverse transcriptase–PCR (RT–PCR) assay using blood of 46 patients who were clinically disease-free.

All patients were followed up for more than 4 years for disease recurrence. There was a significant correlation between number of RT–PCR markers present in blood and American Joint Committee on Cancer stage ($p = 0.009$). The number of RT–PCR markers detected in blood was an independent prediction factor of disease recurrence in a Cox proportional hazard model ($p = 0.02$). A risk factor model using American Joint Committee on Cancer stage and number of positive RT–PCR markers significantly predicted disease recurrence in 2, 3, and 4 years of follow-up. These studies demonstrate that molecular detection of circulating melanoma cells may be of significant prognostic value in determining early disease recurrence and may be useful for stratifying patients for adjuvant therapy.

Does endogenous immune response determine the outcome of surgical therapy for metastatic melanoma?

Hsueh EC, Gupta RK, Yee R, Leopoldo ZC, Qi K, Morton DL.

Roy E. Coats Research Laboratories, John Wayne Cancer Institute at Saint John's Health Center, Santa Monica, CA, USA.

Annals of Surgical Oncology 7(3):232–8, 2000, April.

Background: Although the presence of tumor cells in the blood of patients with metastatic melanoma suggests widely disseminated disease, many of these patients enjoy prolonged survival or cure after surgical resection. Our previous study of adjuvant vaccine therapy after complete resection of metastatic melanoma revealed a strong correlation between postoperative survival and elevated antibody titers to a 90-kDa tumor-associated antigen (TA90) expressed by melanoma cells of the vaccine. We hypothesized a similar correlation between postoperative survival and endogenous anti-TA90 antibody titers induced by the patient's melanoma in the absence of postoperative adjuvant immunotherapy. *Methods:* From 1970 to 1996, 64 patients underwent complete resection of distant melanoma metastases and did not receive postoperative adjuvant immunotherapy. Serum collected within 4 months after surgery was tested in a coded and blinded fashion for anti-TA90 IgG and IgM by enzyme-linked immunosorbent assay, and for total IgG and IgM (controls) by radial immunodiffusion. *Results:* Median follow-up for the study population was 19 months (range 3–147 months). There was no significant correlation between anti-TA90 IgG titer and total IgG level ($p = 0.4785$), or between anti-TA90 IgM and total IgM ($p = 0.0989$). Univariate analysis showed that postoperative anti-TA90 IgM titer as a continuous variable was significantly associated with overall survival (OS); i.e., the higher the anti-TA90 IgM titer, the longer the OS. Using an established cutoff titer of 800, median OS was 42 months for patients with high anti-TA90 IgM titers ($n = 28$) vs. 9 months for patients with low titers ($n = 36$) ($p = 0.0001$). There was no significant correlation between total IgG/IgM and survival ($p = 0.4107$ and 0.4044, respectively). Multivariate analysis identified anti-TA90 IgM as the most significant independent variable influencing OS after complete resection of distant melanoma metastases ($p = 0.0001$). *Conclusions:* We conclude that the endogenous immune response to metastatic melanoma determines the outcome after surgical therapy. Enhancement of this specific immune response may prolong the survival of patients with distant melanoma metastases.

High- and low-dose interferon alfa-2b in high-risk melanoma: first analysis of intergroup trial E1690/S9111/C9190.

Kirkwood JM, Ibrahim JG, Sondak VK, Richards J, Flaherty LE, Ernstoff MS, Smith TJ, Rao U, Steele M, Blum RH.

Department of Pathology, University of Pittsburgh Medical Center, PA, USA.

Journal of Clinical Oncology 18(12):2444–58, 2000, June.

Purpose: Pivotal trial E1684 of adjuvant high-dose interferon alfa-2b (IFNalpha2b) therapy in high-risk melanoma patients demonstrated a significant relapse-free and overall survival (RFS and OS) benefit compared with observation (Obs). *Patients and methods:* A prospective, randomized, three-arm, intergroup trial evaluated the efficacy of high-dose IFNalpha2b (HDI) for 1 year and low-dose IFNalpha2b (LDI) for 2 years versus Obs in high-risk (stage IIB and III) melanoma with RFS and OS end points. *Results:* A total of 642 patients were enrolled (608 patients eligible), of whom a majority (75%) had nodal metastasis (50% had nodal recurrence). Unlike E1684, E1690 allowed entry of patients with T4 (>4 mm) deep primary tumors, regardless of nodal dissection, and 25% of the patients entered onto this trial had deep primary tumors (compared with 11% in E1684). At 52 months' median follow-up, HDI demonstrated an RFS benefit exceeding that of LDI compared with Obs. The 5-year estimated RFS rates for the HDI, LDI, and Obs arms were 44%, 40%, and 35%, respectively. The hazards ratio for the intent-to-treat analysis of HDI versus Obs was 1.28 ($p^2 = 0.05$); for LDI versus Obs, it was 1.19 ($p^2 = 0.17$). By Cox analysis, the impact of HDI on RFS achieved significance ($p^2 = 0.03$). The RFS benefit was equivalent for node-negative and node-positive patients. Neither HDI nor LDI has demonstrated an OS benefit compared with Obs at this time. A major improvement in the median OS of patients in the E1690 Obs arm was noted in comparison with E1684 (6 years v 2.8 years). An analysis of salvage therapy for patients who relapsed on E1690 demonstrated that a significantly larger proportion of patients in the Obs arm received IFNalpha-containing salvage therapy compared with the HDI arm; this therapy was unavailable to patients during E1684, and patients with undissected regional nodes were not included in E1684. This study did not specify therapy at recurrence. Analysis of treatments received at recurrence demonstrated significantly more frequent use of IFNalpha2b at relapse from Obs than from HDI, which may have confounded interpretation of the survival benefit of assigned treatments in E1690. *Conclusion:* The results of the intergroup E1690 trial demonstrate an RFS benefit of IFNalpha2b that is dose-dependent and significant for HDI by Cox multivariable analysis.

High-dose interferon alfa-2b significantly prolongs relapse-free and overall survival compared with the GM2-KLH/QS-21 vaccine in patients with resected stage IIB-III melanoma: results of intergroup trial E1694/S9512/C509801.

Kirkwood JM, Ibrahim JG, Sosman JA, Sondak VK, Agarwala SS, Ernstoff MS, Rao U.

Division of Hematology–Oncology and Department of Pathology, Department of Medicine, University of Pittsburgh Cancer Institute Melanoma Center, University of Pittsburgh Medical Center, Pittsburgh, PA, USA.

Journal of Clinical Oncology 19(9):2370–80, 2001, May 1.

Purpose: Vaccine alternatives to high-dose interferon alfa-2b therapy (HDI), the current standard adjuvant therapy for high-risk melanoma, are of interest because of toxicity associated with HDI. The GM2 ganglioside is a well-defined melanoma antigen, and anti-GM2 antibodies have been associated with improved prognosis. We conducted a prospective, randomized, intergroup trial to evaluate the efficacy of HDI for 1 year versus vaccination with GM2 conjugated to keyhole limpet hemocyanin and administered with QS-21 (GMK) for 96 weeks (weekly $\times$ 4 then every 12 weeks $\times$ 8). *Patients and methods:* Eligible patients had resected stage IIB/III melanoma. Patients were stratified by sex and number of positive nodes. Primary end points were relapse-free survival (RFS) and overall survival (OS). *Results:* Eight hundred eighty patients were randomized (440 per treatment group); 774 patients were eligible for efficacy analysis. The trial was closed after interim analysis indicated inferiority of GMK compared with HDI. For eligible patients, HDI provided a statistically significant RFS benefit (hazard ratio [HR] = 1.47, $p = 0.0015$) and OS benefit (HR = 1.52, $p = 0.009$) for GMK versus HDI. Similar benefit was observed in the intent-to-treat analysis (RFS HR = 1.49; OS HR = 1.38). HDI was associated with a treatment benefit in all subsets of patients with zero to $\geq$ four positive nodes, but the greatest benefit was observed in the node-negative subset (RFS HR = 2.07; OS HR = 2.71 [eligible population]). Antibody responses to GM2 (i.e. titers $\geq 1 : 80$) at days 29, 85, 365, and 720 were associated with a trend toward improved RFS and OS ($p^2 = 0.068$ at day 29). *Conclusion:* This trial demonstrated a significant treatment benefit of HDI versus GMK in terms of RFS and OS in melanoma patients at high risk of recurrence.

The effect of tamoxifen and cisplatin on the disease-free and overall survival of patients with high risk malignant melanoma.

McClay EF, McClay ME, Monroe L, Baron PL, Cole DJ, O'Brien PH, Metcalf JS, Maize JC.

Department of Medicine, University of California, San Diego, La Jolla, CA, USA.

British Journal of Cancer 83(1):16–21, 2000, July.

The adjuvant treatment of high-risk malignant melanoma remains problematic. Previously we reported moderate success in the treatment of metastatic disease using tamoxifen, cisplatin, dacarbazine and carmustine. Based upon data that suggested tamoxifen and cisplatin were the active agents in this regimen, we initiated a phase II trial of this combination in the adjuvant setting. We treated 153 patients with 4 cycles of tamoxifen (160 mg/day, days 1–7) and cisplatin (100 mg/m^2, day 2) for 28-day intervals. Patients received an anti-nausea regimen of dexamethasone with ondansetron or granisetron. During the first 2 years of follow-up, patients were evaluated every 2 months with a history, physical exam, laboratory work and computed tomography scans of the chest, abdomen and pelvis every 4 months. Thereafter, patients were evaluated every 3 months and radiographic studies were performed if necessary. Currently, with a median follow-up of 36 months, the disease-free survival (DFS) is 68.4% and overall survival (OS) is 84.5%. Kaplan–Meier analysis predicts a 5-year DFS of 62% with an OS of 79%. Relapses after 20 months have been rare. No effect of gender or number of positive lymph nodes was noted, however, stage of disease prior to treatment was a factor. The major toxicity proved to be gastrointestinal in nature with nausea the most prevalent symptom. Minimal renal, haematologic and neurologic toxicity occurred. These preliminary results suggest that there is a positive impact of tamoxifen and cisplatin on both the DFS and OS of high-risk malignant melanoma patients. The 5-year projected DFS and OS compare favourably with those reported for the ECOG 1684 trial and warrant confirmation in a prospective randomized trial.

Adjuvant therapy of stage III and IV malignant melanoma using granulocyte–macrophage colony-stimulating factor.

Spitler LE, Grossbard ML, Ernstoff MS, Silver G, Jacobs M, Hayes FA, Soong SJ.

Northern California Melanoma Center, San Francisco, CA, USA.

Journal of Clinical Oncology 18(8):1614–21, 2000, April.

Purpose: To evaluate granulocyte–macrophage colony-stimulating factor (GM-CSF) as surgical adjuvant therapy in patients with malignant melanoma who are at high risk of recurrence. Patients and methods: Forty-eight assessable patients with stage III or IV melanoma were treated in a phase II trial with long-term, chronic, intermittent GM-CSF after surgical resection of disease. Patients with stage III disease were required to have more than four positive nodes or a more than 3-cm mass. All patients were rendered clinically disease-free by surgery before enrollment. The GM-CSF was administered subcutaneously in 28-day cycles, such that a dose of 125 μg/m^2 was delivered daily for 14 days followed by 14 days of rest. Treatment cycles continued for 1 year or until disease recurrence. Patients were evaluated for toxicity and disease-free and overall survival. Results: Overall and disease-free survival were significantly prolonged in patients who received GM-CSF compared with matched historical controls. The median survival duration was 37.5 months in the study patients versus 12.2 months in the matched controls ($p < 0.001$). GM-CSF was well tolerated; only one subject discontinued drug due to an adverse event (grade 2 injection site reaction). Conclusion: GM-CSF may provide an antitumor effect that prolongs survival and disease-free survival in patients with stage III and IV melanoma who are clinically disease-free. These results support institution of a prospective, randomized clinical trial to definitively determine the value of surgical adjuvant therapy with GM-CSF in such patients.

Locally advanced melanoma: results of postoperative hypofractionated radiation therapy.

Stevens G, Thompson JF, Firth I, O'Brien CJ, McCarthy WH, Quinn MJ.

Department of Radiation Oncology, Royal Prince Alfred Hospital, Sydney, Australia.

Cancer 88(1):88–94, 2000, January 1.

Background: High rates of locoregional recurrence have been reported from surgical series of locally advanced melanoma. In this study, the outcomes of patients treated with surgery and postoperative hypofractionated radiation therapy were reviewed to assess local recurrence and survival. Methods: From 1989 to 1998, 174 patients with International Union Against Cancer Stage I–III melanoma received postoperative radiation therapy, either as a component of their initial management or following surgery for recurrence. Radiation was delivered to the primary site in 35 cases and involved regional lymph nodes in 139. The indications for irradiation included microscopically positive surgical margins or other adverse pathologic features. All patients received a hypofractionated schedule of 30–36 grays (Gy) in 5–7 fractions over 2.5 weeks. Results: Recurrence within the radiation fields was identified in 20 patients (11%) at a median time of 6 months. There was no difference in recurrence rates for patients with microscopically positive margins compared with other indications for adjuvant treatment. The main complication of treatment was symptomatic arm lymphedema in 58% of patients following axillary dissection and postoperative irradiation. The median disease specific survival for the entire group was 25 months from radiation therapy, and the 5-year survival was 41%. The only factor that predicted significantly for decreased survival was infield recurrence (the median survival periods were 13 months and 35 months for those with and without infield recurrence, $p < 0.0001$). The median time to the development of distant metastasis was 19 months. Conclusions: Despite the high incidence of distant metastasis, locoregional control remains an important goal in the management of melanoma. Compared with published surgical data, postoperative adjuvant radiation therapy given according to a hypofractionated schedule was effective in reducing local recurrence in patients at high risk of locoregional failure.

19

Surgical management of cancer of the esophagus

CEDRIC G BREMNER

INTRODUCTION

Despite an increased resectability and decreased operative mortality rate, the overall international survival following surgery for esophageal cancer has not improved dramatically in the last 20 years. Earlam and Cunha-Melo published a critical review of the world results of the surgical treatment of esophageal cancer for the years 1953–1978,[1] and, in 1990, Müller et al. repeated the exercise for the previous 10 years.[2]

During this period, the resectability rate increased from 39% to 56% and hospital mortality decreased from 29% to 8%. However, the 5-year survival rate following surgery remained low at under 20%. Overall survival figures from the National Cancer Data Base[3] report a 3-year survival rate of 18% for patients with localized disease. Against this dismal background, however, are reports of significantly better results from units dedicated to esophageal surgery. Ellis reported an overall 5-year survival rate of 23% following esophagectomy,[4] updated recently to 24.7%.[5] The improvement in the mortality rate for esophagectomy has been reported only from centers dedicated to this type of surgery. The poor survival results of esophageal cancer have been ascribed to lack of a serosal barrier and a submucosal network of lymphatics that extends for the whole length of the esophagus. In an attempt to improve survival, surgical techniques have become more aggressive in some centers where en-bloc resections include radical lymphadenectomy. Others have attempted to treat micrometastases with chemotherapy and radiation therapy. The overall survival for en-bloc esophagectomy in selected patients is reported to be up to 60%.[6–9] Whereas overall reported results for the nation appear dismal, dedicated centers have shown a marked improvement in survival and a lower mortality rate. Müller's report included results from 21 units performing fewer than ten resections per year, with an overall operative mortality of 23%. This high mortality rate contrasts with the low mortality of 0–5% reported by 16 authors who performed more than ten procedures each year.

Despite these results, there is no consensus about the optimal method for treating cancer of the esophagus. Surgeons are divided about the best surgical approach, whether en-bloc resection is justified or not, and even whether a pyloroplasty should accompany resection or not. The role of adjuvant therapy likewise is in turmoil. Earlam's review[1] on the results of surgical treatment is still quoted by groups who advocate chemotherapy as an alternative to surgery, despite the fact that surgical results have improved. The responses to chemotherapy, even in early lesions, still do not match the more recent results of surgical therapy, and chemotherapy carries a mortality which equates to that of surgery.[10]

The purpose of this chapter is to highlight the controversial aspects of the surgical management of esophageal cancer and to make concluding remarks about the best management of this disease.

PATHOGENESIS

There is a distinct difference in the geographic pattern of esophageal cancer between Eastern and Western countries. Squamous cell cancer is still the commonest cancer worldwide, and high-risk areas include northeast Iran, the Transkei on the southeastern coast of South Africa, and the Linxian area in northern China. Squamous cell cancer affects more African–Americans than whites, while adenocarcinoma is more common in whites. In fact, the incidence of adenocarcinoma of the cardia has increased four-fold in the last decade.[11,12] White males who are smokers and who have Barrett's esophagus are particularly at risk. Barrett's esophagus is the result of gastro-esophageal reflux disease (GERD) and is an uncommon disease in the Far East and in black Africa, whereas it is extremely common in the Western world. Dietary factors may play a part. The addition of a high-fat diet to a rat model of Barrett's esophagus increased the prevalence of adenocarcinoma.[13] A high-fat diet and smoking appear to be related carcinogens or co-carcinogens in the development of adenocarcinoma of the cardia. Inactivation of the *p53* tumor suppressor gene appears to play a common role in the malignant degeneration associated with Barrett's epithelium.

There are also indicators as to the possible carcinogen sources for squamous cell cancer induction. Smoking may also play a role, and in some areas fungal contaminants of maize (*Fusarium*) may be important.[14] The high risk of developing esophageal cancer in certain areas and population groups raises the question of surveillance, and this is discussed below. N-nitroso compounds may be the carcinogens responsible for squamous esophageal cancer.[15]

SCREENING AND SURVEILLANCE FOR ESOPHAGEAL CANCER

Screening techniques for squamous cancer are used in some high-risk areas, and are mostly based on cytological examination of material obtained from brushing with an expandable brush delivered by swallowing either a capsule that dissolves or a balloon device. A balloon covered with fine mesh and pulled through the esophagus gives up to a 90% accuracy rate for the diagnosis of cancer,[16] and is the method commonly used in the Far East. Endoscopic brushing and suction abrasion tubes are alternative techniques. Cure rates for mucosal lesions treated surgically approximate 90%. When patients with severe dysplasia were followed, 8% progressed to cancer in 1–2 years, 21% in 2–5 years, 34% in 5–9 years, and 53% in 9–12 years.

In low-risk countries such as the USA, mass screening such as is practiced in China is not feasible. Jacob *et al.*[17] screened 255 asymptomatic high-risk USA veterans (>40 years of age; ethanol abuse > 20 years; cigarette smoking > 20 pack-years). Twenty-eight patients with squamous cell dysplasia were followed by balloon mesh cytology every 6 months for up to 36 months. Dysplasia persisted in two patients (7%), and progressed to cancer in a further two patients. This small return questions the usefulness of screening for squamous cancer in the USA.

Dye-spraying during endoscopy is a method which has been practiced for many years in Europe and Japan, but has not gained popularity in the USA. Endo *et al.*[18] used 2% toluidine blue or 0.5% methylene blue solution with 3% Lugol's solution. Unstained areas are specifically selected for biopsy. The 5-year survival rate following surgery for their group of 'early' cancer was 62%, but, when lymph node metastases were present, it was only 17%. Misumi *et al.*[19] from Japan used Lugol's iodine to demonstrate the absence of staining in malignant lesions, which was due to the absence of glycogen in those tissues. However, staining is not specific for cancer, and biopsies of these areas must be taken from confirmation of malignancy.

There are certain patients who are at a high risk for developing squamous or adenocarcinoma of the esophagus, and these include patients who have had a treated ENT cancer, caustic burns, achalasia with retention, and Barrett's esophagus. Patients who have a history of alcohol and tobacco abuse or who have had previous gastric surgery have a slightly increased risk for developing cancer, but do not merit surveillance. However, all patients who have Barrett's esophagus should have regular endoscopic and biopsy surveillance irrespective of the length of the columnar segment. Four quadrant biopsies taken at every 2 cm of the columnar length and from any area of mucosal abnormality should be made. The risk of esophageal adenocarcinoma is about 500 cancers per 100 000 patients with Barrett's esophagus per year.[20] High-grade dysplasia in a patient with Barrett's esophagus should be managed by esophagectomy for the following reasons:

1 it is difficult to ensure that there is no adenocarcinoma in a patient who presents with high grade dysplasia;[21–24]
2 there is a strong likelihood that if the patient with high-grade dysplasia does not have cancer, he or she will soon progress to cancer;[25–31]
3 detection of dysplasia or early esophageal adenocarcinoma on surveillance permits early referral` to surgery;
4 patients being operated on for high-grade dysplasia or esophageal cancer detected on surveillance have a better prognosis than patients who present for the first time with a cancer.[24]

In Peters' study, 17 patients with Barrett's esophagus were placed on a surveillance program.[24] Of nine patients who underwent esophagectomy for high-grade dysplasia, five had invasive cancer in the esophagectomy specimens. The survival of the patients diagnosed by surveillance biopsy was significantly better than that of a non-surveyed group.

Others have also reported on the advantages of surveillance in Barrett's esophagus. Lerut *et al.*[7] reported on a favorable staging with negative lymph nodes in 9 of 11 patients with adenocarcinoma diagnosed at screening. A European multicenter survey of 9743 patients with early esophageal cancer reported a 92.8% 5-year survival for intraepithelial tumors, 72.8% for intramucosal tumors, and 44% for submucosal tumors treated by esophagectomy.[32] Screening or follow-up examination detailed the early tumor in 28% of the cases.

Figure 19.1 summarizes the suggested surveillance program for Barrett's esophagus adapted from the recent International Society for Diseases of the Esophagus (ISDE)

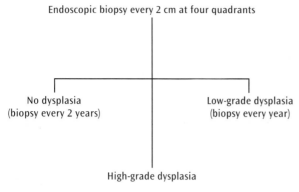

1. Review report to assure a good endoscopy was performed
2. Repeat biopsy if report uncertain
3. If endoscopy was adequate, obtain second pathology opinion
4. If high-grade dysplasia confirmed: esophageal resection

NB: vital staining and brush cytology are optional.

Figure 19.1 *Surveillance protocol for Barrett's columnar-lined esophagus (short and long segment).*

conference (unpublished) and the previous World Congress in Gastroenterology.[33]

PREOPERATIVE STAGING FOR CARCINOMA OF THE ESOPHAGUS

Excessive weight loss, supraclavicular nodes, and voice changes usually indicate advanced disease. Near to total esophageal obstruction usually indicates transmural spread. Akiyama's signs of axis deviation seen on barium studies indicate incurable and often irresectable cancer.[34] It has also been reported that the longer the lesion, the less likely is the potential for cure: a lesion of 9 cm long has no cure rate.[35] These advanced lesions are more the rule than the exception in Third World countries, and account largely for the poor prognosis quoted in reviews.

Inculet *et al.*[36] recommended computer tomography (CT) of the chest and upper abdomen, bone scans, and bronchoscopy for staging. They found CT scanning to be the best non-invasive test for detecting intra-abdominal and intrathoracic spread. CT scanning is able to measure the length of the lesion accurately, but is not the best method to evaluate tumor depth. Ultrasound has now gained the preference in many clinics to assess tumor depth. Botet *et al.*[37] from the Sloan-Kettering Cancer Center compared endoscopic ultrasound with dynamic CT scanning in 88 patients. Endoscopic ultrasound was more accurate in assessing regional lymph nodes (88%) than CT (73%). CT scanning, however, was more accurate in assessing metastases (90% versus 70%, respectively).

Table 19.1 *Cancer staging for esophageal cancer*

Primary tumor (T)

TX	Primary tumor cannot be assessed
T0	No evidence of primary tumor
Tis	Carcinoma-*in-situ*
T1	Tumor invades lamina propria or submucosa
T2	Tumor invades muscularis propria
T3	Tumor invades adventitia
T4	Tumor invades adjacent structures

Nodal involvement (N)

Regional lymph nodes are:
  Cervical esophagus – cervical nodes including
    the supraclavicular lymph nodes
  Intrathoracic esophagus – mediastinal and
    perigastric lymph nodes, excluding the celiac nodes
  Involvement of more distant nodes is considered
    distant metastasis

NX	Regional lymph nodes cannot be assessed
N0	No regional lymph node metastasis
N1	Regional lymph node metastasis

Distant metastasis (M)

MX	Presence of distant metastasis cannot be assessed
M0	No distant metastasis
M1	Distant metastasis

Stage grouping – clinical and pathologic staging

Stage 0	Tis	N0	M0
Stage I	T1	N0	M0
Stage IIA	T2	N0	M0
	T3	N0	M0
Stage IIB	T1	N1	M0
	T2	N1	M0
Stage III	T3	N1	M0
	T4	Any N	M0
Stage IV	Any T	Any N	M1

From American Joint Committee on Cancer. In Beahrs OH, Hensen DE, Hutter RVP, Kennedy BJ, eds. *Manual for staging cancer*, 4th edn. Philadelphia, JB Lippincott, 1992, 57–61.

Rice *et al.*[38] found endoscopic ultrasound to be 70% accurate (sensitivity, specificity, positive and negative predictive values). Magnetic resonance imaging (MRI) scanning has not improved on the accuracy of CT scanning. In fact, Lehr *et al.*[39] prospectively evaluated 60 patients who underwent surgery and concluded that the sensitivity of both CT and MRI was so low that the use of these techniques for staging was questionable.

STAGING FOR CANCER OF THE ESOPHAGUS

The American Joint Committee on Cancer (AJCC) Staging Systems for Esophageal Cancer are reproduced in Table 19.1. Clinical staging is inaccurate because of the difficulties in assessing lymph node involvement. The depth of penetration of the wall and nodal status are the

Table 19.2 *Staging protocol for carcinoma of the esophagus*

1. Physical examination
2. Chest x-ray
3. Barium swallow in all:
   localize the tumor
   assess degree of stenosis
   assess relation to adjacent organs
      (especially trachea)
4. Endoscopy and biopsy
   assess mobility, degree of differentiation,
      histological type
5. CT scan of chest and abdomen:
   local invasion?
   nodal status?
   distant metastasis?
6. Summarize result of staging: T1 T2 versus T3 T4
7. Bronchoscopy on T1 T2 lesions:
   ? carinal infiltration or indirect signs of compression
8. Bronchoscopy and biopsy on T3 T4 lesions
9. Laparoscopy optional
   There is no consensus as to value and 77% of
      surgeons do not use it
10. *Risk analysis*
    Mandatory in all patients prior to surgery
    Pulmonary and cardiac function are most relevant
    Hepatic and renal function should be evaluated

International Society for Diseases of the Esophagus, Consensus Meeting, Milan, 1995.

two most important prognostic features in esophageal cancer.[40]

A shortfall of the AJCC (1988) staging system for esophageal cancer is the limited stratification of patients into N0 and N1. There is good evidence that an intermediate nodal level offers good prognostic information.[41]

Table 19.2 summarizes a protocol for staging of esophageal cancer presented at the ISDE meeting in Milan in 1995 (unpublished).

SURGICAL TREATMENT OF ESOPHAGEAL CANCER

Surgical technique for high-grade dysplasia in Barrett's esophagus

Adenocarcinoma confined to the mucosa superficial to the lamina muscularis mucosa can be resected with a high probability of cure (92.8%).[7] The reason for this success is that there is no lymphatic node invasion in early lesions. There is, therefore, no reason to perform an en-bloc resection. A trans-hiatal resection with gastric pull-up is therefore the standard practice. Dr DeMeester at the University of Southern California has recently added a vagal sparing maneuver to the resection, and

replaced the esophagus with left colon. The function of the stomach is therefore maintained. To date, the results have been very encouraging, but have not yet been published.

The standard surgical treatment for esophageal cancer in most Western centers is esophagectomy without node dissection. There is considerable controversy about the benefits of 'en-bloc' excision, despite the improved results reported from several groups. The early metastasis to esophageal nodes and the widespread network of esophageal lymphatics are reasons to explain why removal without lymphadenectomy gives such poor results. Akiyama *et al.*[42,43] mapped out the lymphatic spread from operative specimens with lesions in the upper, mid and lower esophagus in great detail following en-bloc resection, and counted between 50 and 70 nodes per specimen. Between 5% and 9% of these nodes were positive for metastatic cancer. Importantly, distant lymph nodes were often involved in patients considered to be resectable for cure. Superior gastric nodes were involved in as many as 32% of patients with upper esophageal tumors, and cervico-thoracic node metastases were present in 42% of the patients with lower esophageal tumors. Cervical nodes were present in up to 20% of lower esophageal cancers. These data suggest that any surgery short of complete nodal resection from the celiac, mediastinal, and cervical lymphatic fields is unlikely to cure the majority of patients.

Palliative resection

The Ivor–Lewis procedure, popularized by Norman Tanner[44,45] in the UK and Sweet[46] in the USA, has been the standard technique used for two decades or more in the Western World. The stomach is mobilized via an abdominal incision, and the vascular supply from the right gastroepiploic vessels is preserved. A pyloroplasty or pyloromyotomy is optional. After closure of the abdomen, the esophagus is mobilized via a right thoracotomy, having repositioned the patient in the right lateral position. The esophagogastric anastomosis is made in the chest above the site of the azygos vein division (Figure 19.2). McKeown described an additional step to make the anastomosis in the neck region, so as to avoid the catastrophe of an intrathoracic leak at the anastomotic site.[47] Wong has reported on a low leakage rate (2.6%) from a high intrathoracic anastomosis using a stapling technique and 2.9% for hand-sewn anastomosis of tumors of the middle and distal esophagus.[48] Wong's expertise has developed during a vast experience of approximately 100 resections a year. He rarely found the cervical addition necessary because, in his experience, subepithelial spread was confined almost exclusively to the esophagus distal to the palpable tumor mass. Recurrence at the anastomosis was 8% if the proximal resection margin was 6–10 cm and was avoided completely only if the proximal length was > 10 cm. The 30-day

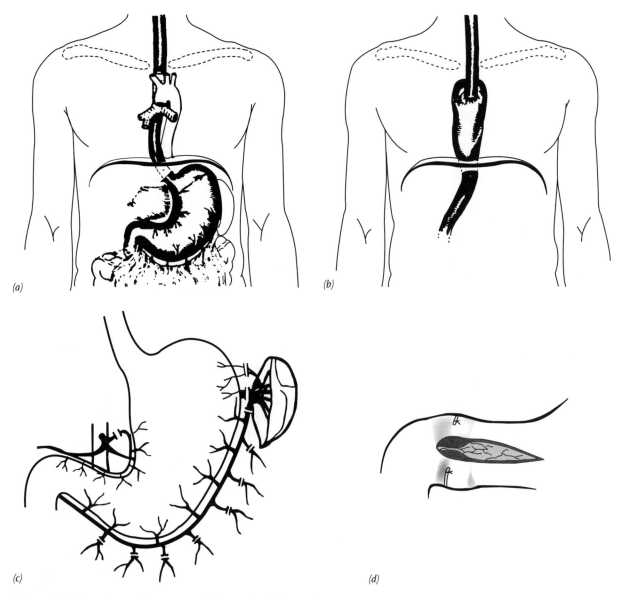

(a)

(b)

(c)

(d)

Figure 19.2 *The Ivor–Lewis (Tanner–Lewis) procedure for resection of esophageal cancer with gastric replacement. (From Bremner, 1989.[86])*

mortality in Wong's series was 6.9%, and the 3.5-year survival was 24.4% (41.3% for curative resections and 7.3% for palliative resections).

A left thoracotomy approach through the head of the non-resected eighth rib is used by Ellis and others.[5] The exposure to the upper abdomen is through a semilumar incision bordering the costal arch, avoiding transection of the arch. Margins of 5 cm or more on either side of the tumor are obtained and reconstitution is made by an end-to-side anastomosis. In the authors' experience, the palliation of the resection by this technique is considerably reduced by gastroesophageal reflux, and a higher anastomosis, preferably to the neck, is much preferred for this reason.

Ellis has reviewed the more recent results of the 'standard' approach from 14 reports published between 1990 and 1997.[5] He restricted the review to reports of 100 or

more cases. Resectability rates varied between 61.5% and 89.9% (median 75%), and mortality rates from 3.2% to 23% (median 7%). The 5-year survival rates ranged from 9% to 44.8% (median 21%). There was a median complication rate of 52%. Trans-hiatal esophagectomy has become more popular in the last 10 years because it avoids thoracotomy and achieves similar results to the open thoracotomy procedure (Figure 19.3).

Trans-hiatal versus transthoracic resection

Grey Turner introduced trans-hiatal esophagectomy in 1933, and Orringer popularized the procedure in the USA in the 1980s.[49] Up until this time, there had been no comparisons with the results of the standard Ivor–Lewis or McKeown transthoracic approaches. Orringer reported on his results of 100 patients with carcinoma of

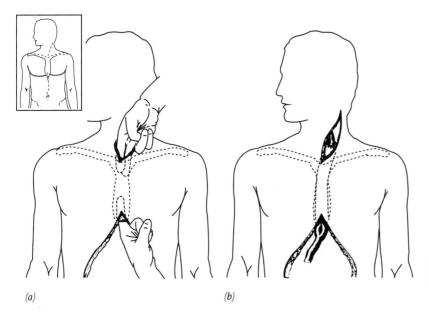

Figure 19.3 *Trans-hiatal esophagectomy. (From Bremner, 1989.[86])*

(a)   (b)

the esophagus (7 upper; 45 mid; 48 lower-third).[50] There was no operative mortality and a 6% hospital mortality rate. His 3-year survival for middle-third lesions was 17%, and 31% for distal third lesions. Orringer[51] recently reported on 1085 patients, and included the results of refinements he has made to the technique to improve the overall results. The hospital mortality rate was 4%, and blood loss averaged 689 mL. The anastomotic leak rate of 13% has been reduced to < 3% since the use of a side-to-side, stapled, cervical esophagogastric anastomosis. The need for an intensive care stay has also been eliminated, and the length of hospital stay reduced to 7 days. This again highlights the excellent results that can be obtained from a dedicated unit. Survival for this group was 23%. Survival for adenocarcinoma was better than that for squamous carcinoma. Stage 0 and I lesions had 5-year survival rates of 51% and 59%, respectively. Following Orringer's first report, the procedure has been used extensively throughout the world. Hankins *et al.*[52] reported on the results of 52 transthoracic and 26 trans-hiatal esophagectomies. The mortality rates (6% versus 8%), overall morbidity (75% versus 85%), and actuarial survival rates (10% at 5 years) were similar for both groups. Shahian,[53] Orringer,[49] and Fok[54] have compared their results of trans-hiatal and transthoracic esophagectomy. There was no difference in hospital mortality or survival between the two groups. In Orringer's large series of 583 patients, the mortality was 5% and he reported on good functional results in 70% of cases. Anastomotic stricture requiring repeated dilatation occurred in 12% of his cases. From a series of 295 esophagectomies (1981–94) Finley and Inculet[55] experienced a higher mortality (9%), a higher prevalence of delayed gastric emptying (11%), pneumonia (26%), reflux (20%), and dysphagia (53%) when esophagectomy was performed by a right thoracotomy and when compared

to the results of trans-hiatal esophagectomy. In Orringer's series, there were also two tears of the membranous trachea during resection of mid-esophageal lesions and one tracheal tear. In the series reported by Fok *et al.*[54] and Bonavina,[32] there was a survival advantage favoring the transthoracic over the trans-hiatal approach. Early lesions at these sites would be easily resectable by the trans-hiatal method. Large lesions, however, should have open thoracic procedures. Bolger *et al.* reported that chylothorax was commoner following trans-hiatal (10.5% of 95) than transthoracic (0.2% of 442) resection.[56] In summary, trans-hiatal esophagectomy is an acceptable approach for palliative resection of the esophagus and gives results which are comparable to those of the standard transthoracic approach. An anatomical understanding[57] and technical aids in performing this procedure as described by Orringer[51] are of infinite importance for furthering successful outcomes.

TRANS-HIATAL ESOPHAGECTOMY FOR MIDDLE AND UPPER-THIRD LESIONS

The location of tumors in close proximity to vital structures which could be disrupted during trans-hiatal esophagectomy (azygos vein, trachea, bronchus, recurrent laryngeal nerve) would deter many surgeons from practicing this procedure in these situations. Certainly, it would seem apparent that trans-hiatal esophagectomy for large lesions which have already spread through the wall at these sites would not be feasible. However, several authors have reported on the resection of lesions at these sites (Table 19.3). Early lesions at these sites would be easily resectable by the trans-hiatal method. Large lesions should have open thoracic procedures. Fixity of the tumor encountered during trans-hiatal esophagectomy

Table 19.3 *Site of lesions resected by trans-hiatal esophagectomy*

Author (Year)	Number in series	Site			Complication rate (%)	
		Upper	Mid	Lower	Mortality	Morbidity
Orringer (1984)[49]	100	7	45	48	6	2
Hankins *et al.* (1989)[52]	26	9	12	5	8	5

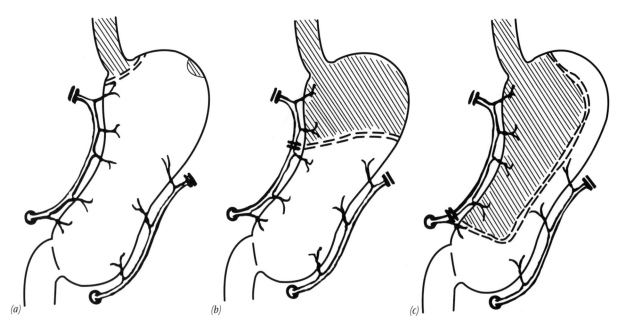

(a)   (b)   (c)

Figure 19.4 *Methods of preparing the stomach for esophageal replacement: (a) whole stomach, (b) distal two-thirds of the stomach, and (c) tabularized stomach. (After Bemelman et al., 1995.[59])*

should prompt immediate thoracotomy. A CT scan may be useful in assessing which patients have tumors confined to the esophageal wall and are suitable for blunt esophagectomy. For carcinomas of the thoracic inlet, the pharynx is not necessarily removed routinely. A mediastinotomy may be used in addition to a trans-hiatal dissection.[49,58]

EXTENT OF GASTRIC RESECTION DURING PALLIATIVE ESOPHAGOGASTRECTOMY

There are two reasons why the stomach should be tubularized by the removal of the lesser curve and esophagogastric junction. The first is to remove lesser curve nodes which may have metastatic deposits. If these are not removed, the involved nodes will be transposed to the chest and neck. The second reason is to improve gastric function. Bemelman *et al.* demonstrated that the type of gastric remnant used for reconstruction determines postoperative emptying.[59] Delayed gastric emptying was diagnosed when a patient was unable to resume a normal solid diet within 7 days of the 7-day postoperative esophagogram which was done routinely to exclude leaks. The tubularized stomach without pyloroplasty gave the best results, and

only one of 35 patients demonstrated a delay in emptying (Figure 19.4). The authors did not use gastric-emptying studies to validate their clinical assessment, but Bemelman had previously used a physical model to show that the smaller the internal volume of the gastric remnant, the lower the compliance of the gastric wall.[60] A small gastric tube leads to a rapid increase in intragastric pressure when the stomach is filled and facilitates gastric emptying.

IS A GASTRIC DRAINAGE PROCEDURE NECESSARY?

The argument for tubularizing the stomach as discussed previously is pertinent to the question as to whether or not a pyloroplasty or pyloromyotomy is necessary. Bemelman did not perform a pyloroplasty in 35 tubularized stomachs and had delay in emptying in one patient only.[59] The transposed stomach is vagotomized and has decreased motility. A need for a drainage procedure or not has been discussed by surgeons for 25 years. A prospective, randomized study of pyloroplasty versus no drainage in 200 patients from John Wong's practice concluded that pyloroplasty is recommended.[61] Thirteen patients who did not have a pyloroplasty in that series developed symptoms of gastric outlet obstruction, four developed pulmonary symptoms, and two had fatal aspiration. Mean daily gastric aspirates were 161 mL in the pyloroplasty group and 233 mL in the control group. Gastric emptying T 1/2 times were 6.6 minutes in the pyloroplasty group and 24.3 minutes in the control group. The gastric replacement technique used by Wong was of the Ivor–Lewis procedure without tubularizing the stomach. The answer to the question of whether or not pyloroplasty is necessary would appear to be related to the type of reconstruction used. If the stomach is not tubularized according to the method described by Bemelman et al.,[59] a pyloroplasty is essential; whereas, in the tubularized technique, it may be unnecessary. Balloon dilatation has been used to relieve gastric outflow obstruction when pyloroplasty was omitted in these techniques.[62] Duodenogastric reflux is another consideration and may take place irrespective of whether or not a pyloroplasty has been performed.[63] Further studies of duodenogastric reflux of the tubularized stomach would compliment Bemelman's gastric-emptying study.

STAPLED VERSUS HAND-SEWN ANASTOMOSIS

A prospective, non-randomized study by Fok et al. compared hand-sewn anastomosis in 33 patients using a continuous monofilament suture with 64 cases of stapled anastomosis (EEA; US Surgical Corporation) and 77 stapled anastomosis using an intraluminal stapler (ILS; Ethicon Ltd).[64] The anastomotic leakage rate was 3.4% with the hand-sewn technique and 3.5% with the stapled technique (4.7% for the EEA and 2.6% for the ILS). The incidence of stricture formation was 8.7% for the hand-sewn and either 20% for the EEA anastomosis or 10% for ILS anastomosis. The overall stricture rate was 14.7%. The 25-mm stapler had the highest stricture rate (28.6%), but the 29-mm and 33-mm staplers gave lower rates of 5.3% and 0%, respectively. Strictures were dilated in one or two sessions, with a satisfactory outcome in 75% of cases. An end-to-side anastomosis has been shown to minimize the leakage rate,[65] and this has been the author's preference for the last 25 years.

CURATIVE EN-BLOC ESOPHAGEAL RESECTION

The standard resection techniques practiced in the USA do not include lymph node en-bloc resection, and there is considerable controversy as to whether or not this procedure is acceptable. Akiyama et al.[42,43] have, for 15 years or more, stressed the importance of total esophagectomy and complete node dissection of the posterior mediastinum and upper abdomen for the cure of esophageal cancer (Table 19.4). Since then, there have been other reports from Europe and the USA confirming an increased survival rate. The operative mortality ranges between 1.4% and 10%. Table 19.5 summarizes the reported results of the standard resection. The results of en-bloc two-field and three-field resections reported from 1992 to 1999 are summarized in Table 19.6.

The purposes of lymphadenectomy are three-fold:

1 they are diagnostic to improve staging,
2 they are prophylactic against local recurrence,
3 to improve prognosis.

For correct pathologic staging, 15–20 nodes are needed and all efforts should be made to remove at least ten nodes from the chest. Not all lymphatic node resections are 'en bloc,' i.e., adding an envelope of tissues surrounding the esophagus and including nodes. The results of lymphatic dissection short of en bloc should not therefore be compared to the more major dissections described. To what extent lymphadenectomy prevents local recurrence remains conjectural. The reported results of en-bloc resections are difficult to compare with the results of standard procedures that do not resect lymph

Table 19.4 Percentage 5-year survival after esophagectomy with two-field and three-field node dissection

	Two field (n = 393)	Three field (n = 324)
Node negative	55	83.9
Node positive	27.9	43.1

From Akiyama H et al. (1994).[9]

Table 19.5 Survival after standard transthoracic (TT) or trans-hiatal (TH) resection

Author	n	Procedure	Operative mortality (%)	5-year survival (%)
Lieberman et al. (1995)[67]	258	TT	5.0	27.0
Horstman et al. (1995)[68]	87	TH	15.0	18.0
		TT	10.0	17.0
Ellis (1999)[5]	316	TT	3.3	24.7
	103	TH		
Altorki et al. (1997)[69]	50	TT		27.0
Orringer et al. (1999)[51]	800	TH	4.0	23.0

Table 19.6 *Survival after en-bloc esophagectomy*

Author	n	Procedure	Operative mortality (%)	5-year survival (%)
Akiyama et al. (1994)[9]	81	Three field	2.2	55
	111	Two field		38.3
Kato et al. (1993)[70]	43	Three field	2.3	73.2 (superficial cancer)
				68.6 (node positive)
				33.3 (cervical node positive)
Matsubara et al. (1994)[72]	171	Three field	5.3	54
Altorki et al. (1997)[69]	78	Two field	4.8	68 (node negative)
	33			34 (stage III)
Hagen et al. (1993)[71]	30	Two field		41
				75 (early)
				27 (advanced)
Nishimaki et al. (1998)[73]	190	Three field	1.6	41.5
Lerut et al. (1992)[7]				3–9.6 (30 overall)
	23			90 stage I
	46			56 stage II
	75			15.3 stage III
Nigro et al. (1999)[66]	44			26 overall
	7			85 (no nodes)
Torres et al. (1999)[74]	28			36
				44 (no nodes)

nodes because no trial has been done. Furthermore, there has been no uniformity of classification of tumor stage. However, from the reported results, it is obvious that survival is related to tumor depth and the extent of lymph node metastasis. Favorable results were reported from Skinner's series[40] when tumors did not completely penetrate the esophageal muscle layer. All had fewer than four positive regional nodes in the en-bloc-resected specimen. To quote Skinner, 'The principle should now be established that patients with metastases to one or a few lymph nodes can be cured by extensive surgery and that these lymph nodes need not be located only adjacent to the primary tumor.' More recently, Japanese surgeons have stressed the need to clear all three lymph node fields.

The survival rate after en-bloc esophagectomy for transmural tumors of the lower esophagus and gastroesophageal junction was 26% at 5 years in a series of 44 patients reported from the University of Southern California by Nigro et al.[66] The most important predictors of the likelihood of recurrent disease and 5-year survival were the presence and number of lymph node metastases and the ratio of involved to total removed nodes. Patients with more than four involved nodes or a node ratio (positive nodes to total number removed) greater than 0.1 had a high likelihood of recurrence and death. It is noteworthy that the median number of lymph nodes removed per patient after systematic mediastinal and abdominal lymphadenectomy was 51 (range 18–92). Seven patients had no lymph node metastases despite transmural tumor invasion, and had an 85% 5-year survival. This experience illustrates the important fact that tumors which have penetrated the wall to the serosa may

not have metastasized to lymph nodes, and also raises the question as to whether or not en-bloc esophagectomy was necessary in these cases. The fact that neither the CT scanning nor endoscopic ultrasonography can reliably detect metastatic nodes hampers the preoperative assessment as to whether or not metastatic nodes are present.

Altorki et al. reported on the survival data of 128 patients who underwent esophagectomy for cancer between 1988 and 1996.[69] Seventy-eight patients had an en-bloc resection and 50 had a standard resection. For node-negative disease, there was a 68% 5-year survival following radical resection and 27% following a standard resection. The mean number of resected nodes following en-bloc removal was 35.9 nodes per patient, and 19.5 nodes per patient after limited resection. The 5-year survival rate for stage III disease was 34% following the radical procedure and 11% following the standard resection.

A review of Table 19.6 shows that the results are varied and, without controlled trials, difficult to compare. However, the results of en-bloc resection appear to be improved when compared to the standard technique results as documented in Table 19.5. The morbidity from the en-bloc procedure is also high, especially for recurrent laryngeal nerve palsy.

EXTENT OF LYMPHADENECTOMY

Lymphadenectomy has usually been confined to abdominal and thoracic nodal clearance. The extent of the

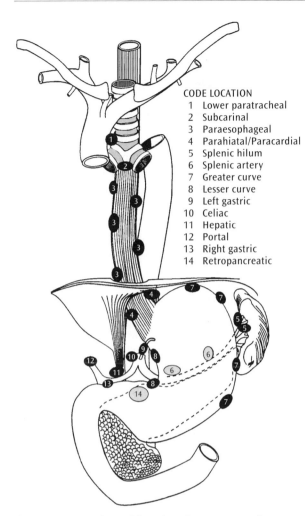

CODE	LOCATION
1	Lower paratracheal
2	Subcarinal
3	Paraesophageal
4	Parahiatal/Paracardial
5	Splenic hilum
6	Splenic artery
7	Greater curve
8	Lesser curve
9	Left gastric
10	Celiac
11	Hepatic
12	Portal
13	Right gastric
14	Retropancreatic

Figure 19.5 *Locations of lymph nodes. Frozen-section biopsies are performed at the beginning of the procedure to exclude disease at the margins of the resection (lymph node groups 12, 14, and 1). When these nodes are negative, en-bloc resection is performed with complete removal of lymph node groups 2 through 11 and 13. Included in the resection are a small number of tracheobronchial nodes (not shown), portal nodes, and retropancreatic nodes. (From Clark et al., 1994.[75])*

resection used by DeMeester is shown in Figures 19.5 and 19.6, and the reconstruction in Figure 19.7. He considers the en-bloc procedure to be appropriate only for lesions of the lower esophagus and cardia and does not advocate it for patients over the age of 75 years. Patients should ideally have a forced expiratory volume (FEV) of 2 L and a rest ejection fraction of over 40%. An algorithm for decisions in the management of patients with cancer of the esophagus and cardia is included in Figure 19.8. More recently, Japanese surgeons have stressed the need to clear the cervical nodes as well (three-field). Abdominal lymphadenectomy includes the celiac and splenic nodes in all cases. Thoracic lymphadenectomy includes three options:

1 standard lymphadenectomy which extends from the carina to diaphragm,

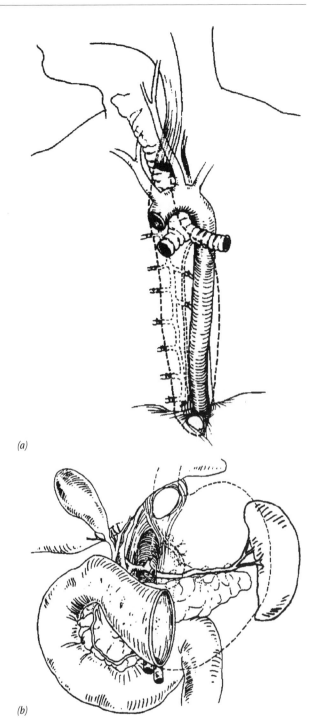

(a)

(b)

Figure 19.6 *(a) Outline of the boundaries for the thoracic portion of an en-bloc esophagogastrectomy. (b) Outline of the boundaries for the abdominal portion of an en-bloc esophagogastrectomy. (From DeMeester et al., 1988.[87])*

2 lymphadenectomy above the carina and including the right paratracheal nodes,
3 total lymphadenectomy including the left recurrent laryngeal nerve nodes.

All options are open, and there are differing opinions regarding the extent of nodal dissection. However, it is generally agreed that, for supracarinal tumors, a total

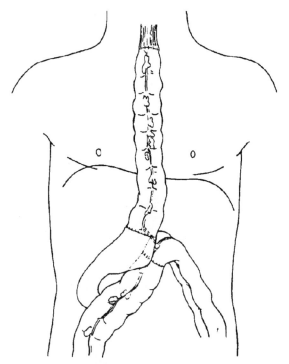

lymphadenectomy including removal of the cervical nodes should be performed.

LYMPH NODE METASTASES RELATED TO TUMOR DEPTH

Clark *et al.* reviewed the histopathology of specimens resected by en-bloc esophagectomy and found nodal metastases in two of six intramucosal lesions, six of nine intramural lesions, and 25 of 28 transmural lesions.[75] Akiyama found lymph nodes in 33 of 61 specimens (54%) which were confined to the submucosa, 23 of 33 (70%) which had invaded the muscularis propria, and in 81% of tumors which had reached the adventitia.[43] This high rate of metastasis in early lesions is disturbing and may explain the decreased survival of only 25% after esophagectomy without lymphadenectomy for tumors which have already reached the submucosal. A two-field, en-bloc resection for this lesion gave a 47.9% survival in Akiyama's two-field operation series and 82.5% in the three-field operation.[43]

TWO-FIELD OR THREE-FIELD EN-BLOC DISSECTION

Two-field en-bloc resection (abdominal and thoracic) is practiced by a few surgical teams in the West,[6,7,9,40] and

Figure 19.7 *Reconstruction of the gastrointestinal tract with left colon interposition after en-bloc resection. Distal anastomosis is made to the antral portion of the stomach, and proximal anastomosis to the esophagus in the neck. (Reprinted from Bremner and DeMeester, 1991,[88] as adapted from DeMeester et al., 1988.[87])*

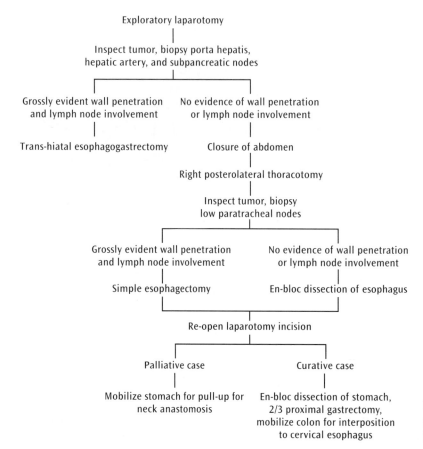

Figure 19.8 *Algorithm outlining surgical procedure and intraoperative decisions. (From Hagen et al., 1993.[89])*

three-field operations which include a cervical lymph node dissection have been reported to give improved results in Japanese studies.[43] The dissection removes nodes in close proximity to the recurrent laryngeal nerve, and the incidence of vocal cord paralysis was about 14%, as opposed to 2% following a two-field dissection. The recent report of Akiyama's formidable series[43] highlights his markedly improved results from three-field en-bloc resections. The three-field lymph node operation included abdominal, thoracic, and cervical dissections. The three-field, 5-year survival rate was 55%, and 38% for two-field dissections, with a hospital mortality rate of 5%. The results for node-negative and node-positive patients treated by two-field and three-field node dissections are listed in Table 19.6. Results such as these emanate from a dedicated unit in a large series (717) of curative resections. An important finding of these series was that 54% of lymph nodes were positive. This is important for those who plan to ablate early lesions using laser therapy. Matsubara *et al.* achieved similar good results with a three-field node dissection.[72] In 37% of cases, nodes were involved in the cervical mediastinal and gastric lymphatic fields. The results of en-bloc resection for nine centers are listed in Table 19.6. Lymph node involvement was noted in 44% of T1 tumors invading the lamina propria or submucosa and in 67% of T2 lesions and 84% of T3 and T4 lesions (see Table 19.1). The 5-year survival rate was 54% for tumors which had not metastasized to more than seven nodes, and 80% if no nodes were involved.

LEFT THORACOABDOMINAL APPROACH TO CARDIA LESIONS

This procedure is still practiced in several centers but has distinct disadvantages. The palliation may be substandard because of gastroesophageal reflux and reflux strictures at the esophagogastric anastomosis. Jackson *et al.* suggest that an increased survival is offered by total gastrectomy and Roux-en-Y reconstruction, which may be due to more extensive lymphadenectomy.[76] The average survival following a Roux-en-Y procedure was 12–20 months longer than when a partial gastric resection and esophagogastric anastomosis were made, depending on whether or not there was local spread.

EXTENT OF MARGINS FOR RESECTION

At least a 4 cm margin beyond the tumor is necessary, but 8 cm is preferable if possible. The tumor will be present in 4% of the resected margins that are 4 cm from the tumor and in none if the margin is 8 cm.[48]

PALLIATION FOR INOPERABLE ESOPHAGEAL CANCER

The best palliative procedure for inoperable esophageal cancer would:

1 require minimal hospital stay,
2 provide relief of dysphagia,
3 provide relief of pain,
4 have a low mortality and morbidity rate,
5 be inexpensive.

At best, these patients have only about 6 months to live and should be treated as expeditiously as possible. The therapeutic modalities available are laser ablation, bicap probe cautery, endoprosthesis, and brachytherapy. Laser therapy requires repeated procedures (four to five) and more days in the hospital than endoscopic intubation or brachytherapy, and both procedures achieve similar palliation from dysphagia. The results of treatment for lesions at the cardia were better with intubation than with laser therapy in Loizou's series.[77] Laser recanalization provided a better functional result for short lesions (lesions < 4 cm) and intubation for larger lesions in Alderson and Wright's series.[78] Kratz and associates compared the results of treatment with three different endoprosthetic tubes: Celestin, Proctor–Livingstone, and Atkinson.[79] Patients treated with Atkinson tubes experienced fewer complications and had a shorter hospital stay (4 days). The hospital death rate was 6% for the Atkinson tube, versus 42% for either the Celestin or Proctor–Livingstone tube. This high mortality with the Celestin and Proctor–Livingstone tubes was not experienced by other authors. Reilly and Fleischer compared the use and results of laser and the bicap tumor probe therapy.[80] An exophytic, non-circumferential tumor located in the distal or middle esophagus was treated preferably with the Yag laser. Long circumferential tumors which were predominantly submucosal were best treated with the bicap tumor probe because it offered quicker and safer palliation. Long strictures require more frequent treatment with the Yag laser than with bicap probes. Proximal or cervical lesions are also more easily treated with the bicap tumor probe. Both treatments have a similar benefit, and the bicap probe is considerably less expensive. The disadvantages of the bicap probe are that it cannot be used unless the lesion is circumferential and it is of no value if the lesion is tortuous.

BRACHYTHERAPY

This type of intervention is generally used as adjuvant therapy. It involves the endoscopic placement of a hollow sheath within the fluoroscopically marked borders of the tumor. The patient is then taken to a separate, shielded procedure room where the sheath is loaded with iridium or some other radioactive substance by a remote-control apparatus. This allows a large amount of radiation (approximately 1500 rad within 10–15 min) to be delivered directly to the 1 cm of tissue bordering the sheath. Obviously, it requires dilatation in order to place the catheter.

The literature on this technique quotes excellent palliation from dysphagia with virtually no need for recurrent therapy. It is a technically easy procedure which results in short admission times (80% of patients go home within 2 days).[81]

There are some significant hindrances to this becoming a widely used method of palliation, however. To set up a dedicated treatment room with the appropriate equipment is quite costly ($250K), and there are few centers presently actively involved in this type of treatment. Also significant is that it always requires the cooperation of two different services. Complications include transient post-procedure edema, dysphagia, and esophagitis.

THE ROLES OF RADIATION THERAPY AND CHEMOTHERAPY IN CANCER OF THE ESOPHAGUS

Radiation therapy alone for the treatment of carcinoma of the esophagus has given poor survival results, with a 3-year survival rate of only 6%.[82] The local lesion, however, is often well controlled and may even disappear after radiation therapy, but there is an inability to irradiate a field that will cover all the lymphatic regions of spread. Preoperative radiation has not improved the results, and postoperative radiotherapy has even shortened the survival rate.[83] Fok et al., reporting on an extensive experience in Hong Kong, experienced gastric ulceration in 17 of 24 patients, resulting in death from bleeding in five.[83] They conclude that postoperative radiotherapy should be limited to a specific group of patients with residual tumor in the mediastinum for which radiotherapy can significantly reduce the incidence of local recurrence obstructing the tracheal bronchial tree. Chemotherapy for esophageal cancer has also had disappointing results. Numerous agents have been used and, currently, cisplatin and 5-fluorouracil (5-FU), which are both radiosensitizers, are the favored drugs. Herskovic et al. reported on a trial of chemotherapy and radiotherapy compared with radiotherapy alone in a series of 121 patients.[10] The median survival was 8.9 months in the radiation-treated patients, compared with 12.5 months in the combined radiation and chemotherapy group, using cisplatin and 5-FU. The 24-month survival rates of 33% and 38% for the radiation and radiation–chemotherapy groups, respectively, are not as good as the survival rates for standard surgical resection and not as good as the 5-year survival rates for en-bloc

resection. Furthermore, severe and life-threatening side-effects occurred in 44% of patients with chemotherapy. Ten percent of the patients had T1 lesions and 82% had T2 lesions. It is disappointing that the early lesions did not respond better. Roth et al. randomly assigned patients with middle lower-third esophageal cancers to receive operation only or preoperative and postoperative therapy with cisplatin, vindesine, and bleomycin.[84] Patients who had experienced a weight loss of less than 10% of body weight responded to chemotherapy with a significantly prolonged survival (median >2 months) compared to non-responders. However, the numbers were small. Kelsen et al. recently published the first prospective trial comparing preoperative chemotherapy followed by surgery with surgery alone.[85] Preoperative chemotherapy with a combination of cisplatin and 5-FU did not improve overall survival in patients with squamous or adenocarcinoma of the esophagus.

The following guidelines related to adjuvant therapy have evolved from a consensus opinion held at the 1995 Milan meeting of the International Society of Diseases of the Esophagus:

1 *Radiotherapy.* Extensive randomized trials have not shown any overall improvement in the resection rate or survival following radiotherapy, and the use of radiotherapy alone should therefore be abandoned.

2 *Chemotherapy.* Extensive phase II and III trials have concluded that in 50% of patients there will be either a complete or partial response, but no improvement in overall survival.

3 *Chemotherapy and radiotherapy.* The combined use of chemotherapy and radiotherapy increases the mortality rate from 7% to 12%, but there is also an increase in response rate with no overall increase in survival. It is therefore advised that this therapy be used only in an investigational setting and not outside of trials. If the tumor is locally advanced, the mortality following combined therapy is also increased (9–16%) and survival may be increased.

CONCLUSIONS

Surgical resection still offers the best chance of cure for esophageal cancer, and the cure rate is related to the depth of invasion of the esophageal wall and to the presence and number of lymphatic nodal metastases. The mortality of esophageal resection is acceptably low only in units which perform the procedure frequently, and these patients should therefore only be treated by dedicated units. Although no control trials have been performed on the value of en-bloc resection, impressive results from several centers worldwide justify the procedure in dedicated units which have a low mortality rate. Tubularization of the gastric replacement appears to improve its function, with some possible vascular compromise. If en-bloc resection is not performed, the trans-hiatal approach has comparable results to transthoracic resection.

REFERENCES

1. Earlam R, Cunha-Melo JR. Oesophageal squamous cell carcinoma: a critical review of surgery. Br J Surg 1980; 67:381–90.

2. Müller JM, Erasmi H, Stelzner M, Zierer U, Pichlmaier H. Surgical therapy of oesophageal cancer. Br J Surg 1990; 77:845–57.

3. Menck HR, Garfinkel I, Dodd GD. Preliminary report of the National Cancer Data Base. Cancer 1991; 41:7.

4. Ellis FH Jr. Treatment of carcinoma of the esophagus or cardia. Mayo Clin Proc 1989; 64:945.

5. Ellis FH Jr. Standard resection for cancer of the esophagus and cardia. Surg Clin North Am 1999; 8(2):279–94.

6. DeMeester TR, Attwood SEA, Smyrk T, Therkildsen DH, Hinder RA. Surgical therapy in Barrett's esophagus. Ann Surg 1990; 212:528–41.

7. Lerut T, DeLeyn P, Coosemans W, Van Raemoonck D, Scheys I, Lesaffre E. Surgical strategies in esophageal carcinoma with emphasis on radical lymphadenectomy. Ann Surg 1992; 216:583–90.

8. Skinner DB. Cervical lymph node dissection for thoracic esophageal cancer. Ann Thorac Surg 1991; 51:884–5.

9. Akiyama H, Tsurumaru M, Udagawa H, Kajiyama Y. Radical lymph node dissection for cancer of the thoracic esophagus. Ann Surg 1994; 220:364–72.

10. Herskovic A, Martz MS, Al-Sarraf M, et al. Combined chemotherapy and radiotherapy compared with radiotherapy alone in patients with cancer of the esophagus. N Engl J Med 1992; 326:1629–30.

11. Hesketh PJ, Clapp RW, Doos WG, Spechler SJ. The increasing frequency of adenocarcinoma of the esophagus. Cancer 1989; 64:526–30.

12. Blot WJ, Devesa SS, Kneller RW, Fraumeni JF. Rising incidence of adenocarcinoma of the esophagus and gastric cardia. JAMA 1991; 265(10):1287–9.

13. Clark GWB, Smyrk TC, Mirvish SS, et al. Effect of gastroduodenal juice and dietary fat on the development of Barrett's esophagus and esophageal neoplasia. An experimental rat model. Ann Surg Oncol 1994; 1:252–61.

14. Yoshizawa LY, Katayama T. Comparative study on the natural occurrence of fusarium mycotoxins in corn and wheat from high and low risk areas for human esophageal cancer in China. Appl Environ Microbiol 1990; 56:3723–6.

15. Mirvish SS. Role of N-nitroso compounds (NOC) and N-nitrosation on the etiology of gastric, esophageal, nasopharyngeal and bladder cancer and contribution to cancer of known exposures to NOC. Cancer Lett 1995; 93: 17–48.

16. Lightdale CJ, Winawar SJ. Screening diagnosis and staging of esophageal cancer. Semin Oncol 1994; 11:101–12.

17. Jacob P, Kahrilas PJ, Desai T, et al. Natural history and significance of esophageal squamous cell dysplasia. Cancer 1990; 65:2731–9.

18. Endo M, Takeshita K, Yoshida M. How can we diagnose the early stage of esophageal cancer? Endoscopy 1986; 18 (Suppl. 3):11–18.

19. Misumi A, Harada K, Murakami A, et al. Early diagnosis of esophageal cancer; analysis of 11 cases of esophageal mucosal cancer. Ann Surg 1989; 210:732–9.

20. Spechler SS. Endoscopic surveillance for patients with Barrett esophagus: does the cancer risk justify the practice? Ann Intern Med 1987; 106:902–4.

21. Palley SL, Sampliner RE, Garewal HS. Management of high grade dysplasia in Barrett's esophagus. J Clin Gastroenterol 1989; 11:369–72.

22. Altorki NK, Sunagawa M, Little AG, Skinner DB. High grade dysplasia in the columnar lined esophagus. Ann J Surg 1991; 161:97–9.

23. Streitz JM Jr, Andrews CW Jr, Ellis FH Jr. Endoscopic surveillance of Barrett's esophagus: does it help? J Thorac Cardiovasc Surg 1993; 105:383–7.

24. Peters JH, Clark GWB, Ireland AP, Chandrosoma P, Smyrk TC, DeMeester TR. Outcome of adenocarcinoma arising in Barrett's esophagus in endoscopically surveyed and non-surveyed patients. J Thorac Cardiovasc Surg 1994; 108:813–22.

25. Spechler SS, Robbins AH, Rubins HB, et al. Adenocarcinoma and Barrett's esophagus: an overrated risk? Gastroenterology 1984; 87:927–33.

26. Sprung DJ, Ellis FH, Gibbs SP. Incidence of adenocarcinoma in Barrett's esophagus. Am J Gastroenterol 1984; 79:817A.

27. Cameron AJ, Ott BJ, Payne WS. The incidence of adenocarcinoma in columnar lined (Barrett's) esophagus. N Engl J Med 1985; 313:857–9.

28. Robertson CS, Mayberry JF, Nicholson DA, James PD, Atkinson M. Value of endoscopic surveillance in the detection of neoplastic change in Barrett's oesophagus. Br J Surg 1988; 75:760–3.

29. Van der Veen AH, Dees J, Blankenstein JD, Van Blankenstein M. Adenocarcinoma in Barrett's esophagus: an overrated risk. Gut 1989; 30:14–18.

30. Hameeteman W, Tytgat GN, Hovthoff HJ, Van den Tweel JG. Barrett's esophagus: development of dysplasia and adenocarcinoma. Gastroenterology 1989; 96:1249–56.

31. Iftikhar SY, James PD, Steele RJ, Hardcastle JD, Atkinson M. Length of Barrett's oesophagus: an important factor in the development of dysplasia and adenocarcinoma. Gut 1992; 33:1155–8.

32. Bonavina L. Early esophageal cancer: results of a European multicenter survey. Br J Surg 1995; 82:98–101.

33. Dent J, Bremner CG, Collen MJ, Hagitt RC, Spechler SG. Working party report to the World Congress of Gastroenterology, Sydney 1990. Barrett's esophagus. J Gastroenterol Hepatol 1991; 6:1–22.

34. Akiyama H, Kogure T, Itai Y. The esophageal axis and its relationship to resectability of carcinoma of the esophagus. Ann Surg 1972; 176:30–6.

35. DeMeester TR, Stein HJ. Surgical therapy for cancer of the esophagus and cardia. In Castell DO, ed. *The esophagus*. Boston, Little, Brown and Company, 1992, 299–341.

36. Inculet RI, Keller SM, Dwyer A, Roth JA. Noninvasive tests for the preoperative staging of carcinoma of the esophagus: a prospective study. Ann Thorac Surg 1985; 40:561–5.

37. Botet JF, Lightdale CJ, Zauber AG, Gerdes H, Brennan M, Urmacher C. Preoperative staging of esophageal cancer: comparison of endoscopic US and dynamic CT. Radiology 1991; 181:419–23.

38. Rice TW, Boyce GA, Sivak MV. Esophageal ultrasound and the preoperative staging of carcinoma of the esophagus. J Thorac Cardiovasc Surg 1991; 101:536–44.

39. Lehr L, Rupp M, Siewert JR. Assessment of resectability of esophageal cancer by computed tomography and magnetic resonance imaging. Surgery 1988; 103:344–50.

40. Skinner DB, Ferguson MK, Soriano A, Little A, Staszak VM. Selection of operation for esophageal cancer based on staging. Ann Surg 1986; 204:391–401.

41. Ellis FH, Watkins E Jr, Krasna MJ, Heatley GJ, Balogh K. Staging of carcinoma of the esophagus and cardia: a comparison of different staging criteria. J Surg Oncol 1993; 52:231–5.

42. Akiyama H, Tsurumaru M, Kawamura T, Ono Y. Principles of surgical treatment for carcinoma of the esophagus: analysis of lymph node involvement. Ann Surg 1981; 194:438–46.

43. Akiyama H, Tsurumaru M, Kajiyama Y. Radical lymph node dissection for cancer of the esophagus. Ann Surg 1994; 220:364–73.

44. Lewis I. The surgical treatment of carcinoma of the oesophagus with special reference to a new operation for growths of the middle third. Br J Surg 1946; 34:18–31.

45. Tanner NC. The present position of carcinoma of the oesophagus. Postgrad Med J 1947; 23:109–39.

46. Sweet RH. Surgical management of carcinoma of the mid-thoracic esophagus. Preliminary report. N Engl J Med 1945; 223:1.

47. McKeown KC. Total three-stage oesophagectomy for cancer of the oesophagus. Br J Surg 1976; 63:259–62.

48. Wong J. Esophageal resection for cancer: the rationale of current practice. Am J Surg 1987; 153:18–24.

49. Orringer MB. Transhiatal esophagectomy without thoracotomy for carcinoma of the thoracic esophagus. Ann Surg 1984; 200:282–8.

50. Orringer MB. Technical aids in performing transhiatal esophagectomy without thoracotomy. Ann Thorac Surg 1984; 38:128–32.

51. Orringer MB, Marshall B, Iannettoni MD. Transhiatal esophagectomy: clincal experience and refinements. Ann Surg 1999; 230(3):392–403.

52. Hankins JR, Attar S, Coughlin TR, et al. Carcinoma of the esophagus: a comparison of the results of transhiatal versus transthoracic resection. Ann Thorac Surg 1989; 47:700–5.

53. Shahian DM, Neptune WB, Ellis FH Jr, Watkins E. Transthoracic versus extra thoracic esophagectomy: mortality, morbidity, and long-term survival. Ann Thorac Surg 1986; 41:237–46.

54. Fok M, Siu KF, Wong J. A comparison of transhiatal and transthoracic resection for carcinoma of the thoracic esophagus. Am J Surg 1989; 158:414–19.

55. Finley RJ, Inculet RI. The results of esophagogastrectomy without thoracotomy for adenocarcinoma of the esophagogastric junction. Ann Surg 1989; 21:535–43.

56. Bolger C, Walsh TN, Tanner WA, Keeling P, Hennessy TPJ. Chylothorax after esophagectomy. Br J Surg 1991; 78:587–8.

57. Strano S, Bremner CG. Transhiatal blunt esophagectomy. Surg Gynecol Obstet 1988; 166:541–4.

58. Ong GB, Lam KH, Wong J. Resection for carcinoma of the superior mediastinal segment of the esophagus. World J Surg 1978; 2:497–504.

59. Bemelman WA, Taat CW, Slors JFM, Van Lanschot JJB. Delayed postoperative emptying after esophageal resection is dependent on the size of the gastric substitute. J Am Coll Surg 1995; 180:461–4.

60. Bemelman WA, Verburg J, Brummelkamp NH, Kloper PH. A physical model of the intrathoracic stomach. Am J Physiol 1988; 254:G168–75.

61. Fok M, Cheng SWK, Wong J. Pyloroplasty versus no drainage in gastric replacement of esophagus. Am J Surg 1991; 162:447–52.

62. Bemelman WA, Brummelkamp WH, Bartelsman JF. Endoscopic balloon dilatation of the pylorus after esophagogastrostomy without a drainage procedure. Surg Gynecol Obstet 1990; 170:424–6.

63. Mannell A, Hinder RA, San-Garde BA. The thoracic stomach: a study of gastric emptying, bile reflux and mucosal change. Br J Surg 1984; 71:438–41.

64. Fok M, Ahchong AK, Wong J. Comparison of a single layer continuous hand-sewn method and circular stapling in 580 oesophageal anastomosis. Br J Surg 1991; 78:342–5.

65. Chassin JL. Esophagogastrectomy: data favoring end-to-side anastomosis. Ann Surg 1978; 188:22–7.

66. Nigro JJ, DeMeester S, Hagen JA, et al. Node status in transmural esophageal adenocarcinoma and outcome

after enbloc esophagectomy. J Thorac Cardiovasc Surg 1999; 117:960–8.

67. Lieberman MD, Shriver CD, Bleckner S, et al. Carcinoma of the esophagus. Prognostic significance of histologic type. J Thorac Cardiovasc Surg 1995; 109:130–8.

68. Horstman O, Verreet PR, Becker H, Ohmann C, Roher HD. Transhiatal oesophagectomy compared with transthoracic resection and systemic lymphadenectomy for the treatment of oesophageal cancer. Eur J Surg 1995; 161:557–67.

69. Altorki N, Girardi L, Skinner D. En-bloc esophagectomy improves survival for stage III esophageal cancer. J Thorac Cardiovasc Surg 1997; 114:948–56.

70. Kato H, Tachimori Y, Mizobuchi S, Igaki H, Ochiai A. Cervical mediastinal and abdominal lymph node dissection (three-field dissection) for superficial carcinoma of the thoracic esophagus. Cancer 1993; 72:2879–82.

71. Hagen JA, Peters JH, DeMeester TR. Superiority of extended en-bloc esophagogastrectomy for carcinoma of the lower esophagus and cardia. J Thorac Cardivasc Surg 1993; 106:850–9.

72. Matsubara T, Ueda M, Yanagida O, Nakajima T, Nishi M. How extensive should lymph node dissection be for cancer of the thoracic esophagus? J Thorac Cardiovasc Surg 1994; 107:1073–8.

73. Nishimaki T, Suzuki T, Suzuki S, Kuwabara S, HataKeyama K. Outcomes of extended radical esophagectomy for thoracic esophageal cancer. J Am Coll Surg 1998; 186;306–12.

74. Torres AJ, Sanchez-Pernaute A, Hernando F, et al. Two-field radical lymphadenectomy in the treatment of esophageal carcinoma. Dis Esoph 1999; 12:137–43.

75. Clark GWB, Peters JH, Ireland AP, et al. Nodal metastasis and sites of recurrence after en bloc esophagectomy for adenocarcinoma. Ann Thorac Surg 1994; 58:646–54.

76. Jackson JW, Cooper DKC, Cuvendik L, Reece-Smith H. The surgical management of malignant tumors of the oesophagus and cardia: a review of the results in 292 patients treated over a 15 year period. Br J Surg 1979; 66:98–104.

77. Loizou LA, Rampton RCN, Atkinson M, Robertson C, Bown SG. A prospective assessment of quality of life after endoscopic intubation and laser therapy for malignant dysphagia. Cancer 1992; 70:386–91.

78. Alderson D, Wright PD. Laser recanalisation versus endoscopic intubation in the palliation of malignant dysphagia. Br J Surg 1990; 77:1151–3.

79. Kratz JM, Reed CE, Crawford FA, Stroud MR, Parker EF. A comparison of esophageal tubes: improved results with the Atkinson tube. J Thorac Cardiovasc Surg 1989; 97:19–23.

80. Reilly HF, Fleischer DE. Palliative treatment of esophageal carcinoma using laser and tumor probe

therapy. Gastroenterology Clin North Am 1991; 20:731–41.

81. Sawant D, Moghissi K. Management of unresectable oesophageal cancer: a review of 537 patients. Eur Cardiothorac Surg 1994; 8:113–17.

82. Diehl LF. Radiation and chemotherapy in the treatment of esophageal cancer. Gastroenterol Clin North Am 1991; 20:765–74.

83. Fok M, Sham JST, Choy D, Cheng S, Wong J. Postoperative radiotherapy for carcinoma of the esophagus: a prospective, randomized controlled trial. Surgery 1993; 113:138–47.

84. Roth J, Pass HI, Flanagan MM, Graeber GM, Roseberg JC, Steinberg S. Randomized clinical trial of preoperative and postoperative adjuvant chemotherapy with cisplatin, vindesine, and bleomycin for carcinoma of the esophagus. J Thorac Cardiovasc Surg 1988; 96:242–8.

85. Kelsen DP, Geinsberg R, Pajak TF, et al. Chemotherapy followed by surgery compared with surgery alone for localized esophageal cancer. N Engl J Med 1998; 339:1979–84.

86. Bremner CG. Carcinoma of the oesophagus. In Schwartz SI, Ellis H, eds. *Maingot's abdominal operations.* Connecticut, Appleton and Lange, 1989, 547–65.

87. DeMeester TR, Zaninotto G, Johanson K-E. Selective therapeutic approach to cancer of the lower esophagus and cardia. J Thorac Cardiovasc Surg 1988; 95:42–54.

88. Bremner RM, DeMeester TR. Surgical treatment of esophageal carcinoma. In Wong RKH, ed. *Gastroenterology clinics of North America,* Vol. 20, No. 4. Philadelphia, WB Saunders Co., 1991, 743–63.

89. Hagen JA, Peters JH, DeMeester TR. Superiority of extended en bloc esophagogastrectomy for carcinoma of the lower esophagus and cardia. J Thorac Cardiovasc Surg 1993; 106(5):850–9.

ANNOTATED BIBLIOGRAPHY

Akiyama H, Tsurmaru M, Udagawa H, Kajiyama Y. Radical lymph node dissection for cancer of the thoracic esophagus. Ann Surg 1994; 220(3):364–73.
Extended (three-field) radical lymph node dissection for esophageal squamous cancer can be accomplished with a low operative mortality and results in improved survival.

Bonavina L. Early esophageal cancer: results of a European multicenter survey. Br J Surg 1995; 82:98–101.
Patients with early tumors (pTis-T1 N0 M0) have a significantly improved survival and lower rate of local recurrence following transthoracic resection rather than trans-hiatal resection. Actuarial 5-year survival rates, excluding

operative deaths, were 93%, 73%, and 44% for intraepithelial, intramucosal, and submucosal tumors, respectively.

Ellis FH, Watkins E, Krasna MJ, Heatley GJ, Balogh K. Staging of carcinoma of the esophagus and cardia: a comparison of different staging criteria. J Surg Oncol 1993;52:231–5.

Change of the AJCC classification 1983 to 1988 for esophageal cancer did not improve prognostication for patients in the different staging levels. A flaw in the AJCC 1988 classification is the lack of an intermediate lymph node category, which gives better prognostic information.

Matsubara T, Ueda M, Yanagida O, Nakajima T, Nishi M. How extensive should lymph node dissection be for cancer of the thoracic esophagus? J Thorac Cardiovasc Surg 1994; 107(4):1073–8.

The commonest lymph node area for metastases from esophageal squamous cancer is the area around the recurrent laryngeal nerves. Patients with isolated metastases to this area have a significantly worse 5-year survival than patients with isolated metastases to the perigastric lymph nodes, who have a survival similar to that of node-negative patients.

20

Neoadjuvant therapy of esophageal carcinoma

BRIAN J KAPLAN AND MITCHELL C POSNER

INTRODUCTION

In 2001 it is estimated there will be 13 200 new cases of esophageal cancer and 12 500 deaths in the USA.[1] The incidence and mortality rates closely approximate one another, underscoring that esophageal cancer remains a highly lethal disease.[2] Unfortunately, the incidence of esophageal carcinoma is increasing in the USA[3] due to a sharp rise in adenocarcinoma of the esophagus.[4] Concomitant with the increased incidence of adenocarcinoma is an increase in lesions in the lower third of the esophagus.[5]

Patients with esophageal carcinoma treated with a single modality, i.e., chemotherapy (CT), radiotherapy (RT), or surgery alone, frequently fail at locoregional or distant sites. Surgery remains the mainstay of treatment. However, due to dismal 5-year survival rates following resection alone, efforts have focused on a multimodality therapeutic approach to esophageal cancer. Reports suggest that combination chemoradiotherapy (CRT) alone without resection yields survival equivalent to that reported in surgical series. However, local failure with chemoradiotherapy alone is substantial and therefore treatment with surgery and RT to control locoregional disease combined with CT directed at systemic disease is theoretically sound.

This chapter focuses on combined modality treatment of esophageal cancer and reviews the rationale for this approach, summarizes pertinent clinical trials, and discusses future directions.

PATIENT SELECTION

Almost all patients with esophageal carcinoma are potential candidates for multimodality therapy because they are at high risk for locoregional and systemic failure. Although patients who would benefit most from preoperative therapy remain to be defined, patients who are at low risk for distant and local recurrence could theoretically avoid potentially toxic additional therapy and be treated effectively with esophagectomy alone. Patients who meet these criteria might include those with high-grade dysplasia (carcinoma *in situ*) in Barrett's esophagus and patients with T1 or T2N0 disease. The selection of patients appropriate for neoadjuvant therapy as opposed to treating all patients is dependent on accurate and reproducible staging techniques. Unfortunately, computerized axial tomography (CAT) scan, the most widely utilized staging technique, is not sensitive enough in evaluating the depth of wall invasion by the primary tumor and/or lymph node status.

Endoscopic ultrasound (EUS), a combination high-frequency ultrasound probe and endoscope, is a more reliable tool to assess the depth of tumor and lymph node involvement. One large study to evaluate the role of EUS in esophageal cancer showed overall accuracies for predicting wall penetration and lymph node involvement of 92% and 78%, respectively.[6] Lightdale[7] found 86% accuracy in predicting cancer stage when EUS and CAT were used in a complementary fashion. EUS, however, is highly operator dependent and not routinely applied in most centers.

The advent of minimally invasive surgery has allowed for more accurate staging in a number of gastrointestinal neoplasms. Esophageal cancer is ideally suited for this approach because accurate preoperative staging is lacking and is critical to properly designed and interpreted clinical trials. Molloy *et al.*[8] evaluated laparoscopy in 244 patients with cancer of the gastric cardia and esophagus. Unresectable disease, defined in this study as hepatic metastasis, peritoneal disease, extensive lymph node involvement, or direct invasion of the colon or liver, was detected in 92 patients (38%). An additional 11 patients did not tolerate laparoscopy and, therefore, were not surgical candidates. Resection was successful in 72% of patients. In this study, 65 patients had definitive CAT scan evidence of metastatic disease. If these patients are eliminated from analysis, selective laparoscopy would detect an additional 38 patients (21%) who would not benefit from laparotomy. Krasna *et al.*[9,10] have applied both thoracoscopy and laparoscopy, either used separately or in tandem, in staging esophageal cancer. In a pilot study,[10] 45 patients were staged with thoracoscopy, and both thoracoscopy and laparoscopy were used in 19 patients. Thoracoscopic staging detected positive regional lymph nodes with 93% accuracy and laparoscopy with 94% accuracy. Laparoscopy detected positive celiac nodes in 5/18 patients (28%) that were not detected on preoperative CAT scan. Although laparoscopy can detect metastatic disease, it is less sensitive in assessing the depth of wall invasion and nodal status.

By combining laparoscopy with laparoscopic ultrasound in the evaluation of these patients, a more comprehensive staging can theoretically be accomplished. Finch et al.[11] evaluated 26 patients with potentially resectable gastric or esophageal cancer using CAT scan, laparoscopy, and laparoscopic ultrasound. The sensitivity and specificity of predicting resectability were 100% and 91%, with laparoscopic ultrasound 100% and 73%, and 75% and 60% for CAT scan, respectively. Metastases were detected with an 82% sensitivity with laparoscopic ultrasound and with 55% sensitivity with CAT scan. Using laparoscopic ultrasound, no patient was overstaged. For T stage, laparoscopic ultrasound was 92% accurate, laparoscopy 42% accurate, and CAT scan 60% accurate. Lymph node metastases were detected with an accuracy rate of 89% for laparoscopic ultrasound, 44% for laparoscopy, and 62% for CAT scan. These results are comparable to N staging using EUS.[7] Minimally invasive techniques show promise in the evaluation of patients with esophageal cancer and can potentially select those subgroups that might benefit from preoperative therapy. Multi-institutional studies are needed to further delineate the role and feasibility of these techniques.

As discussed later in this chapter, neoadjuvant CRT is being used with increased frequency. The use of CAT scan and EUS to assess response to this treatment may provide useful information. Unfortunately, preliminary data call into question their use for this purpose. In one study,[12] post-treatment CT scans were reviewed retrospectively in 50 patients who underwent preoperative CRT and compared to pathologic tumor response. Post-treatment CAT scans accurately staged T classification in 42% of patients, overstaged 36% of patients, and understaged 20%. CAT scan had a sensitivity and specificity of 65% and 33%, respectively. The authors concluded that CAT scan is inadequate in assessing pathologic response and T stage after preoperative CRT. EUS does not appear to have any advantage over CAT scan in this role. EUS was evaluated retrospectively in 59 patients after CRT.[13] The accuracy in predicting T stage was 37%. In another study,[14] 87 patients with squamous cell carcinoma (SCC) were evaluated. EUS was 47.9% accurate in predicting T stage and 71.3% accurate for nodal disease. It appears that radiation-induced fibrosis and edema make staging in this situation inaccurate.

It is evident that selecting patients for clinical trials based on routine preoperative staging techniques is not straightforward. Wide application of the above-mentioned novel modalities may improve the accuracy of staging. At the present time, however, the vast majority of patients are candidates for investigational therapy once a diagnosis of esophageal cancer is confirmed.

NEOADJUVANT THERAPY

Neoadjuvant (preoperative or induction) therapy for esophageal cancer has been delivered in four ways:

1 by preoperative RT,
2 by preoperative CT,
3 by combined preoperative CRT,
4 by CRT as primary therapy.

The advantages and disadvantages of each approach based on data from clinical trials is discussed below.

Preoperative radiotherapy

Radiotherapy given preoperatively has several theoretical advantages, including increased resectability rates by reducing tumor volume, decreased tumor seeding at time of surgery, and improved tolerance. Preoperative radiation allows for the greatest number of well-oxygenated tumor cells, theoretically making radiation more effective. The potential disadvantages of preoperative RT include overtreating patients based on clinical staging, and increased postoperative morbidity, especially if the anastomosis is in the radiated field. In addition, by delivering RT alone, only locoregional disease is addressed.

There have been four randomized studies comparing preoperative RT and surgery to surgery alone (Table 20.1). The doses delivered in these trials (20–40 Gy) are considered inadequate by today's standards. In addition, the time interval between the completion of RT and surgery was short – 8 days to 2–4 weeks. More patients would theoretically benefit if this interval was increased to allow the full effects of RT to take place, although this would have to be weighed against increased fibrosis leading to a more technically difficult resection.

Launois et al.[15] randomized 109 patients with SCC of the esophagus to receive either surgery alone or RT consisting of 40 Gy in 8–12 fractions followed by surgery in less than 8 days. There was no difference in resectability rate, operative mortality, and actuarial 5-year survival. Local failure rate, a key determinant of the efficacy of RT, was not mentioned in this study. Arnott et al. randomized patients with either SCC or adenocarcinoma to receive either low-dose RT, consisting of a total of 2000 Gy in 10-Gy fractions over 2 weeks, followed by surgery, or surgery alone.[16] Again, no difference was noted in resectability rates, operative mortality, and 5-year actuarial

Table 20.1 *Prospective, randomized, preoperative RT trials*

Author	Number of patients	Dose (Gy)/ number of fractions	Resectable (%) RT/surgery	Local failure (%) RT/surgery	Operative mortality (%) RT/surgery	5-year survival RT/surgery
Lanouis	109	40/10	76/70	NA/NA	23/23	9.5/11.5
Arnott	176	20/10	74/72	NA/NA	15/13	9/17
Mei	206	40/20	93/85	13/12	5/6	35/30
Gignoux	208	33/10	47/58	46/67	24/18	10/9

RT, radiotherapy; NA, not available.

Table 20.2 *Prospective, randomized, preoperative CT trials*

Author	Number of patients	Agents	Resectable (%) CT/surgery	Complete response (%)	Operative mortality (%) CT/surgery	Survival (3 year) CT/surgery
Roth	36	CP/V/BL	35/30	6	12/0	25/5
Schlag	69	CP/5-FU	71/77	NA	21/12	NA
Nygaard	91	CP/BL	58/69	NA	15/13	3/9
Kelsen	440	CP/5-FU	76/89	NA	6/6	20/25

CT, chemotherapy; NA, not available; CP, cisplatin; V, vindesine; BL, bleomycin; 5-FU, 5-fluorouracil.

survival. Gignoux *et al.* reported on 208 patients with SCC in a European Organization for the Research and Treatment of Cancer (EORTC) trial.[17] Patients were randomized to receive either 33 Gy in ten fractions followed by surgery within 8 days or surgery alone. Local recurrence was less in the RT group (46% versus 67%, $p < 0.05$). Other parameters, including resectability rate, operative mortality and 5-year survival were no different between the two groups. Mei *et al.* randomized 206 patients to a surgery-only group and a preoperative RT group.[18] RT consisted of 40 Gy and surgery was performed after a 2–4-week period. There was no difference between the two groups in resection rate or operative mortality. Five-year survival was slightly improved in the preoperative RT group (35%) compared to the surgery-alone group (30%) ($p > 0.05$).

It is clear, based on these randomized studies, that preoperative RT does not improve overall survival, although it may decrease local recurrence. Once again, these studies have two major drawbacks:

1 the dose of RT is low compared to today's CRT trials,
2 there was a short time interval between completion of RT and surgery.

Preoperative RT alone should not be recommended for most patients with esophageal cancer. Patients with advanced disease not amenable to surgery may benefit from RT for palliation.

Preoperative chemotherapy

The use of neoadjuvant CT aimed at the prevention and treatment of systemic disease is attractive, because the majority of patients have occult disseminated disease at the time of presentation.[19,20] In addition, patients who present with tumors apparently limited to the submucosa (T1) have a 30% incidence of lymph node involvement.[20] Preoperative CT shares some of the benefits associated with induction RT, including the theoretical advantage of allowing tumor shrinkage, facilitating resection and decreasing local recurrence. Patients who exhibit a good response to preoperative CT may benefit from adjuvant postoperative CT. The potential disadvantage of preoperative CT is that chemoresistant tumor cells may develop. Single chemotherapeutic agents used in the neoadjuvant setting have included, 5-flourouracil (5-FU), etoposide, cisplatin (CP), mitomycin-c, bleomycin, and vindesine. The response rates for single-agent CT are between 15% and 28%.[21] If combination CP-based CT is used, as in all phase II and III trials addressing this issue, locoregional response rates increase from 45% to 75%.[21] Early trials were phase II, single-arm studies of patients with SCC treated with CP-based combination CT. Although an increased percentage of patients in these phase II trials was reported to have prolonged survival compared to historical controls (especially those who had an objective response), these studies were not designed to answer a survival question. In order to address that issue, phase III trials were conducted comparing surgery alone to preoperative CT and surgery (Table 20.2).

Roth *et al.* randomized 36 patients with SCC to receive surgery alone (19 patients) or induction CT plus surgery followed by postoperative CT (17 patients).[21] CT consisted of CP, vindesine, and bleomycin. The postoperative complication rate was 47% in the surgery arm and 29% in the CT plus surgery arm (not statistically significant). There were two deaths in the CT arm, both occurring postoperatively, and none in the surgery arm. In the CT group, 35% were resected with free margins and 21% in the surgery-only group. Median follow-up was 30 months and there were no differences in median survival or actuarial 5-year survival between the two groups. One patient had a pathologic complete response and seven partial responses (>50% reduction in two perpendicular diameters as measured by serial radiographic exams) were noted. Actuarial survivals at 3 years (25% in the CT group and 5% in the surgery-alone group) were not statistically different. Patients with either a complete or partial response had significantly prolonged survival compared to non-responders (20 versus 6 months, respectively). The authors concluded that preoperative CT was well tolerated, was not associated with increased morbidity or mortality, and is beneficial in responders.

Based on positive results from a phase II study[22] using a similar regimen to that above, Schlag initiated a phase III trial.[23] Seventy-seven patients with SCC of the esophagus were eligible, 46 of whom agreed to be randomized, 24 to surgery alone and 22 to preoperative CT. Of the non-randomized patients, 13 received CT and 18 received surgery alone. CT consisted of 5-FU (1000 mg/m^2 per day by 24-h continuous infusion for 5 days) and CP (20 mg/m^2 on days 1–5). Patients were re-evaluated after one cycle of CT and, if no change or tumor progression was noted, underwent immediate surgery while responders received two more cycles of CT. Toxicity was significant, with two treatment-related deaths secondary to myelotoxicity and early termination of CT in one patient secondary to nephrotoxicity. The response to CT was based on clinical criteria. Complete and major (decrease in tumor size by 50% judged by esophagogram or endoscopy) response was observed in 2 (6%) and 11 (32%) patients, respectively, with 9 (26%) patients demonstrating progressive disease. Patients who underwent CT had no improvement in resectability, but did have an increase in postoperative complications (sepsis, respiratory disorders) and operative mortality (19% versus 10%). Responders to CT had a higher survival rate than non-responders ($p = 0.02$). There was no difference in overall survival, with a median survival of 10 months in both groups. The authors concluded that there is no survival benefit to preoperative CT, although it was associated with significant treatment-related morbidity and mortality.

A Scandinavian phase III trial had four treatment arms:[24] RT followed by surgery (48 patients), CRT followed by surgery (47 patients), surgery only (41 patients), and CT followed by surgery (50 patients). CT consisted of two cycles of bleomycin and CP. Resectability rates, morbidity, and operative mortality rates were not significantly different between the groups. The authors pooled survival data from patients who received RT as part of their treatment (alone or combined with CT) and compared them to data from patients in the other arms treated with either surgery alone or CT. The 3-year actuarial survival was greater in the two groups receiving RT compared to the others ($p < 0.05$).

A recent multi-institutional, randomized, prospective trial compared CT followed by surgery to surgery alone.[25] Patients with both adenocarcinoma and SCC were included. Patients randomized to the preoperative CT arm received three cycles of CP and 5-FU, followed by surgery 2–4 weeks later. Two additional cycles of CT were given to patients after surgery if they did not progress. The survival rates in all registered patients (median possible duration of participation 55.4 months) were not significantly different. CT was well tolerated and did not increase the morbidity or mortality of surgery. Patterns of failure were not different in the two arms.

The only trial to compare preoperative CT to preoperative RT was conducted at the Memorial Sloan–Kettering Cancer Center.[26] CT consisted of CP, vindesine, and bleomycin for two cycles. RT was administered to a total dose of 55 Gy. In this trial, utilizing a crossover design, patients who received CT preoperatively received RT postoperatively and vice versa if their tumors were unresectable or T3 lesions. There was no difference in resectability, operability, or operative mortality. Actuarial 5-year survival was 20% in both groups.

Although these clinical trials are limited by small sample size and other design flaws, the available results suggest that preoperative CT does not improve resectability, disease-free survival, or overall survival compared to surgery alone. Unless large, randomized studies show a benefit to induction CT, it has a limited role in the treatment of patients with esophageal cancer.

Preoperative chemoradiotherapy

The failure of single-modality induction therapy has led to the investigation of combination treatment in an attempt to address both systemic disease and locoregional disease. Radiation, used preoperatively, allows tumor shrinkage and, theoretically, enhances resectability. In addition, tumor seeding is reduced. The addition of CT to RT allows treatment of occult micrometastic disease and may also lead to further tumor downstaging. Furthermore, certain chemotherapeutic agents are radiosensitizers.[27] The combination of RT and CT has additive effects and has the potential to improve the therapeutic index. Finally, patients treated preoperatively who have responded to CT may be more appropriately treated with postoperative adjuvant therapy.

There are also a number of theoretical disadvantages of neoadjuvant therapy. Chemoresistance may develop, limiting the effectiveness of treatment. Preoperative treatment may also increase surgical morbidity, including anastomotic dehiscence and wound complications.

Table 20.3 *Phase II preoperative CRT trials*

Author	Number of patients	RT dose (cGy)	Agents	Resectable (%)	Complete response (%)	Operative mortality (%)	5-year survival
Franklin	30	3000	5-FU/MTC	76	20	13	30[a]
Leichman	21	3000	5-FU/CP	71	24	27	NA
Wolfe	165	4500	CP/VP16 (SCC) CP/5-FU (adeno)	NA	40 SCC 20 adeno	5	25[b]
Hoff	68	3000	CP/VP 16/5-FU/LV	91	21	2	51[c]
Stahl	72	4000	CP/VP 16/5-FU/LV	61	22	15	33[a]
Seydel	41	3000	5-FU/CP	66	20	4	8[a]
Poplin	106	3000	5-FU/CP	49	17	11	16[a]
Forastiere	43	3750–4500	5-FU/CP/VB	84	24	2	34[b]
Bates	35	4500	5-FU/CP	100	51	9	43[c]

[a]Three-year survival.
[b]Five-year survival.
[c]Two-year survival.
CRT, chemoradiotherapy; NA, not available; CP, cisplatin; BL, bleomycin; 5-FU, 5-fluorouracil; MTC, mitomycin C; VN, vincristine; VB, vinblastine; VP16, etoposide; LV, leucovorin; SCC, squamous cell carcinoma; adeno, adenocarcinoma.

In addition, induction CRT precludes accurate, adequate surgical staging and, therefore, patients who may not benefit from CRT (i.e., those with early-stage disease) are treated and exposed to the potential toxicity associated with aggressive therapy.

Non-randomized trials

In the early 1980s, a number of single-institution phase II trials were initiated using combination CRT in the preoperative setting (Table 20.3). One of the earliest studies addressing neoadjuvant CRT for esophageal cancer[28] was based on earlier work done by Nigro *et al.*[29] using CRT in SCC of the anus. In this study, 30 patients with SCC with localized disease were treated with curative intent, and an additional 25 patients with locally advanced or disseminated disease were treated with palliative intent. The regimen consisted of mitomycin C (10 mg/m^2 bolus on day 1) and 5-FU (1000 mg/m^2 on days 1–4 and 29–32 by continuous infusion). Radiation was given on days 1–21, to a total dose of 3000 cGy. Surgery was performed a minimum of 4 weeks following the completion of RT. Patients with histological evidence of residual tumor following surgery were treated with an additional 2000 cGy and a single course of CT. In the group undergoing CRT for curative intent, 23/30 (77%) underwent attempted resection. At the time of exploration, five had metastatic disease. In the remaining 18, six had no evidence or tumor, three had intramural disease, and nine had transmural disease. The median survival for those resected was 18 months. Local recurrence occurred in only two patients. The morbidity was low, with 13% of patients having postoperative pneumonia. Operative mortality was 13%, with two deaths related to complications of pneumonia.

In a follow-up study, the group from Wayne State University, Detroit, MI, treated 21 patients with SCC.[30] RT was given to a total dose of 3000 cGy, in 15 fractions over 3 weeks. CT consisted of 5-FU (100 mg/m^2 continuous infusion on days 1–4 and 29–32) and CP (100 mg/m^2 intravenous bolus on days 1 and 29). At exploration, 15 patients underwent curative resection with clear margins. Two patients refused surgery and four were unresectable. The operative mortality was substantial (27%), with all deaths due to respiratory failure. Five patients had no evidence of tumor in the resected specimen. The median survival was 18 months overall and 24 months in the group with no residual cancer in the resected esophagus, with no local recurrences noted in the latter group. All patients in both trials[28,30] who had microscopic disease in the resected specimen developed local recurrences.

A large, retrospective, single-institution trial of induction CRT[31] evaluated 229 patients, with 165 ultimately undergoing esophagectomy (93 with adenocarcinoma and 72 with SCC). The chemotherapeutic regimens for the two histologies were different, based on the investigators' belief that 5-FU was more effective for adenocarcinoma. Patients with adenocarcinoma received CP (20 mg/m^2 per day for 5 days) and 5-FU (1000 mg/m^2 per day for 5 days). Patients with SCC received CP (20 mg/m^2) and etoposide (60 mg/m^2) for 5 days. RT was delivered for 5 weeks for a total dose of 45 Gy. The surgical approach included both transthoracic and trans-hiatal esophagectomy. The overall 5-year survival for both histologic groups was 25%. If there was no evidence of tumor in the resected specimen, the 5-year survival was 60% for adenocarcinoma and 40% for SCC. In a group of patients treated with CRT without resection, 18% of SCC patients survived 5 years, whereas no patients with adenocarcinoma survived 3 years. In addition, no patient with SCC treated off protocol with surgery alone survived 3 years.

Based on the above-mentioned phase II single-institution trials, two multi-institutional phase II trials were initiated, one from the Radiation Therapy Oncology Group (RTOG) and one from the Southwestern Oncology Group (SWOG). The RTOG trial evaluated 41 patients with SCC.[32] Radiation was administered to a total of 3000 cGy over 3 weeks. CT consisted of 5-FU (1000 mg/m^2 continuous infusion for 96 h) and CP (100 mg/m^2 intravenous bolus on the first day of radiation). On days 29–32, CT was repeated. Patients with no evidence of metastatic disease were explored. If at final pathology the specimen contained residual cancer, an additional 2000 cGy was given. Of the patients entered in the study, 66% were resected (27/41). In the group not resected, there were two treatment-related deaths, four refused surgery, one was unresectable, three had progression of disease, and four were unfit for surgery. In the resected group, 30% had no evidence of tumor in the resected specimen. The mean survival of all patients in the trial was 13 months, and 3-year survival was 8%. All patients with no residual tumor in the resected specimen were alive at 3 years. The operative mortality rate was 4%. The authors concluded that patients who have no residual tumor in the resected specimen benefit most from neoadjuvant CRT, and raised the issue of whether surgery is unnecessary in complete responders.

In a phase II trial from SWOG, 106 patients received the same regimen as above.[33] Four patients did not complete CT, leaving 102 eligible patients. Eleven patients refused surgery, 14 had progressive disease, and six were not operative candidates. Seventy-one underwent surgery, 16 of whom had unresectable disease, and 13 had incomplete resections. Complete resection was possible in 24 patients and 18 patients had no evidence of residual disease on pathological exam (17%). Severe toxicity included leukopenia (eight patients), esophagitis (one patient), stomatitis (seven patients), nausea/vomiting (eight patients), and thrombocytopenia (one patient). Life-threatening toxicity included nausea/vomiting in two patients, leukopenia in two patients, and thrombocytopenia in one patient. The overall resectability rate was 49% (55/113) and operative mortality was 11%. Median survival was 12 months overall. In the group that underwent surgery, the median survival was 14 months and 32 months in those who had complete pathologic response. These two multi-institutional trials suggest that induction CRT may benefit patients with esophageal cancer, especially complete responders.

A study from the University of Michigan group reported on a more intense CRT regimen in the treatment of patients with either adenocarcinoma or SCC.[34] Forty-three patients were treated with CP, vinblastine, and 5-FU continuous infusion combined with radiation over a 21-day period. Radiation was delivered in 250-cGy

fractions to a total dose of 3750 cGy in the first 20 patients, and in subsequent patients the dose of radiation was increased to 4500 cGy. Twenty-two patients had SCC and 23 patients had adenocarcinoma. Trans-hiatal esophagectomy was performed on day 42. There were two deaths in the preoperative period secondary to sepsis. Of the remaining 41 patients, 36 were resected for cure. On examination of the resected specimen, 10/41 (24%) had no evidence of residual tumor. In a final analysis from this trial,[35] the 5-year survival rate was 34% at 78.7 months' median follow-up. The median survival of all patients was 29 months. Median survival for patients with adenocarcinoma was 32 months, and 23 months for patients with SCC. In patients who had a complete pathologic response, median survival was 70 months and 5-year survival was 60%, whereas patients who had residual disease in the resected specimen had a median survival of 26 months and 32% were alive at 5 years. The authors state that surgery is an important component of multimodality therapy because almost one-third of patients who had evidence of residual disease in the specimen were alive at 5 years, with no local recurrences. The authors compared their series to historical surgical series and concluded that CRT led to a doubling of survival rates.

A study from Bates et al.[36] tried to address the issue of whether surgery is essential after neoadjuvant CRT and tried to identify a group of patients in whom surgery could be omitted based on preoperative esophagogastroduodenoscopy (EGD). Thirty-five patients with localized disease, defined as esophageal cancer with or without periesophageal adenopathy, were evaluated. The majority of patients (80%) in this study had SCC. CT consisted of 5-FU (1000 mg/m^2 per day on days 1–4 and 29–32) and CP (100 mg/m^2 on day 1). Radiation was given to a total dose of 45 Gy in 25 fractions. The toxicity of CT was minimal and there were no treatment-related deaths. Ninety-seven percent of patients completed the full neoadjuvant CRT regimen. Approximately 2–8 weeks after completing CRT, patients underwent an Ivor–Lewis esophagectomy. The median survival and disease-free survival rates for the 35 patients who received trimodality therapy were 25.8 months and 32.8 months, respectively. Eighteen patients had a pathologic complete response (51%). The median survival and 3-year survival rate for those achieving a complete response were 36.8 months and 61%, respectively, whereas patients who had residual tumor in the surgical specimen had median survival and a 3-year survival rate of 12.9 months and 25%, respectively. There were three perioperative deaths (8.6%), all occurring early in the series. Twenty-two patients underwent EGD prior to resection, and 17 (77%) had no evidence of tumor on biopsy. On final pathologic evaluation, seven (41%) patients with a presumptive complete response as determined by EGD had residual tumor in the resected specimen. The authors concluded that patients should not be excluded from resection based on EGD. In addition, 25% of patients who had residual tumor in the surgical specimen survived 3 years, suggesting that esophagectomy was beneficial.

A study from Kane et al. also addressed the issues of whether esophagectomy is a necessary component of multimodality treatment and whether preoperative CRT was associated with increased perioperative morbidity and mortality.[37] CT consisted of 5-FU (300 mg/m^2 continuous infusion), CP (20 mg/m^2), and interferon (IFN; 3 million units). Forty-four patients were enrolled in the trial, 16 were treated on a 28-day cycle (RT to a total dose of 4000 cGy) and the other 28 patients on a 21-day cycle (RT to a total dose of 4600 cGy). Thirty-seven patients underwent curative esophagectomy. These patients were compared to a cohort who underwent esophagectomy only during this same time period and served as controls. Adenocarcinoma comprised the predominant histology in both groups. There were no statistical differences in the two groups with regard to age, sex, race, histological features, or type of resection. All patients in the CRT group were clinically staged and all were stage II (66%) or stage III (34%). In the control group, all patients were staged post-resection and the majority were either stage II (36%) or stage III (53%). Analysis of intraoperative factors revealed that mean operating time and estimated blood loss were significantly less in the CRT group. There was no statistically significant difference in postoperative parameters, including hospital stay, days in the intensive care unit, or days on mechanical ventilation. Patients in the CRT group required fewer blood transfusions ($p < 0.05$). There was no significant difference between the CRT group and control group regarding 30-day hospital mortality (5.4% and 3.3%, respectively) and morbidity.

Eighty percent of the entire group had a 'major pathological response,' consisting of 24% with a complete response and 56% with a partial response (microscopic residual disease in the resected specimen). Eighteen patients are alive with no evidence of disease at 30-month median follow-up. Of those alive and disease free, 50% were complete responders, whereas the other half had residual disease in the resected esophagus, suggesting that esophagectomy is a critical component of treatment.

The above phase II studies and others[38] laid the framework for further investigation into the use of induction CRT. These studies had many flaws. The chemotherapuetic agents used varied, sample size was small, and RT regimens were not consistent. The early studies included patients with SCC exclusively, whereas more recent studies predominantly enrolled patients with adenocarcinoma. The biology of these two histologies is probably discordant and, therefore, it is inappropriate to combine these two entities in a single trial and difficult to interpret the results that are generated. Moreover, as with all phase II studies, bias may be introduced when attempting to make conclusions regarding efficacy.

Phase III trials

The first randomized study to examine CRT followed by surgery compared to surgery alone in SCC of the esophagus was from France.[39] After initial evaluation, 86 patients fulfilled the inclusion criteria and were randomized. Forty-one patients were treated with neoadjuvant CRT consisting of CP (100 mg/m^2 intravenous bolus on days 1 and 21) and 5-FU (600 mg/m^2 continuous infusion on days 2–5 and days 22–25). Sequential external-beam radiation was delivered in ten fractions to a total dose of 20 Gy on days 8–19. The two groups were matched for age, sex, tumor location, size, and grade. The operative mortality (8.5% for the CRT group and 7% for the surgery groups) and morbidity (average postoperative stay 27 days) were the same for each group. The 3-year actuarial survival was 19.2% for the CRT group and 13.8% for the surgery group (not statistically different). The complete pathologic response rate was 10%, which is lower than in the previously mentioned studies.

Two prospective, randomized trials evaluating neoadjuvant CRT have recently been published. Walsh et al. conducted a phase III trial randomizing 113 patients with adenocarcinoma of the esophagus to either preoperative CRT plus surgery or surgery alone.[40] CRT consisted of two cycles of 5-FU (15 mg/kg for 5 days) and CP (75 mg/m^2 on day 7 in weeks 1 and 6). Radiotherapy was given in 15 fractions to a total dose of 40 Gy over a 3-week period. Surgery was performed 8 weeks after starting therapy. A major drawback of the study is that there was a total of 11 'protocol violations,' ten in the neoadjuvant CRT group. All of these patients were eliminated from the analysis and, therefore, conclusions were not based on intent-to-treat analysis. The 90-day in-hospital mortality was 6% (five deaths in the neoadjuvant CRT group and two deaths in the surgery only arm). In the CRT group, 23/58 (40%) of patients had involved lymph nodes or metastatic disease at the time of surgery, compared to 45/55 (82%) patients in the surgery-only arm ($p < 0.001$), indicating either downstaging as a result of treatment or pretreatment stratification inequalities between groups. A complete pathologic response was demonstrated in 13 (23%) patients, 11 of whom were alive at 2–43 month follow-up. Three-year survival was 32% for patients assigned to multimodality therapy, compared with 6% for those assigned to surgery. The median survival was 32 months in the CRT group and 11 months in the surgery-only group ($p = 0.01$). There are a number of criticisms of this study. The 'protocol violations' are mainly related to treatment toxicity or progression of disease and should be included in an intent-to-treat analysis. In addition, preoperative staging was suboptimal by today's standard. CAT scans were only performed if patients had equivocal findings on chest radiographs or liver sonograms, and EUS was not performed. There is no assurance that the groups were matched for stage based on just physical examination and endoscopy.

Table 20.4 *Phase II preoperative CRT trials*

Author	Number of patients (CRT/surgery)	RT dose (cGy)	Agents	Resectable (%) (CRT/surgery)	Complete response (%) (CRT)	Operative mortality (%) (CRT/surgery)	3-year survival (%) (CRT/surgery)
LePrise	86 (41/45)	2000	5-FU/CP	85/84	10	8.5/7	19/14
Bosset	282 (143/139)	1850	CP	81/68	26	17/5	36/34
Walsh	113 (58/55)	4000	CP/5-FU	NA	25	9/4	32/6[a]

[a]$p < 0.05$.
CRT, chemoradiotherapy; RT, radiotheraphy; NA, not available; CP, cisplatin; 5-FU, 5-fluorouracil.

Bossett *et al.* reported a phase III study examining neoadjuvant CRT in patients with SCC.[41] Patients who were randomized to receive CRT were given single CP (80 mg/m^2) 0–2 days before each course of radiotherapy. Radiotherapy consisted of two 1-week courses, separated by 2 weeks, to a total of 37 Gy (18.5 Gy each course) divided into 3. 7-Gy fractions. There were 139 patients in the surgery-alone group and 143 patients in the CRT group. Ultimately, 275 patients came to resection; five were eliminated from the CRT group (three had disease progression, one refused treatment, and there was one preoperative death) and two from the surgery-only group (disease progression). The postoperative mortality in the CRT group (17%) was significantly increased when compared to the surgery-alone arm (5%) ($p = 0.012$). The pathologic tumor stage and nodal status after preoperative treatment were significantly lower in the CRT group compared to the surgery-alone group which, as mentioned above, can be attributed to either downstaging as a result of treatment or stratification flaws based on preoperative staging. The overall median survival was the same for both groups at a median follow-up of 55.2 months. There was a difference between the deaths that were attributable to cancer in the two groups: 87 of 101 (86.1%) cancer deaths in the surgery-alone group and 69 of 102 (67.6%) cancer deaths in the CRT group ($p = 0.002$).

The data presented in the above studies do not support the use of preoperative CRT outside investigational trials (Table 20.4). These studies have varying histologies, small patient numbers, different chemotherapeutic and radiotherapy regimens, multiple study design flaws, and are single institutional. A large, multi-institutional, prospective, randomized study with uniform CRT regimens and surgical approaches will help clarify this issue.

Combined chemoradiotherapy without surgery in the treatment of esophageal carcinoma

Although surgery is the preferred treatment for patients with resectable esophageal carcinoma, CRT as primary treatment is the subject of a number of trials. The potential advantages of this therapy include:

1 avoiding operative intervention and its attendant morbidity and mortality,
2 salvage esophagectomy is feasible if patients develop local recurrences or persistent disease. In a number of the above-mentioned studies, patients who had no evidence of tumor in the resected specimen fared best, raising the question of whether resection provides any additional benefit. CRT used as primary therapy has disadvantages of suboptimal relief of dysphagia, high local recurrence rates or residual disease and can be associated with significant toxicity.

Phase II trials

The Wayne State University group initiated a trial of the use of combined CRT without surgical intervention.[42] The premise of the study was that in an earlier trial from this same group,[30] the only patients who benefited from surgery were those who had no evidence of tumor in the resected specimen. Twenty patients with biopsy-proven SCC of the esophagus were enrolled. The CT consisted of 5-FU (1000 mg/m^2 on days 1–4 and 29–32), CP (100 mg/m^2 on days 1 and 29), mitomycin C (10 mg/m^2 administered on day 57) and bleomycin (20 mg/m^2 intravenous infusion on days 57–60 and 78–81). RT consisted of 200-cGy fractions, 5 days a week for the first 3 weeks to a total of 3000 cGy. Two radiation boosts were given on days 99–103 and 106–110, each of 200-cGy fractions. The total radiation dose was 5000 cGy. The major toxicity from this protocol was pulmonary; 50% of patients developed radiographic evidence of pneumonitis and dyspnea was noted in 16 patients. The median overall survival was 22 months. In the group of patients who were clinically free of tumor, the median survival was 35 months. Eighty percent of the patients survived 1 year from entry into the trial. This study laid the groundwork for future trials investigating the role of combined multi-modality therapy without surgery in selected patients and reserving surgery for salvage therapy.

A subsequent trial from the Wayne State group[43] focused on intensifying CRT in an effort to improve local control and improve survival, with surgery reserved for

Table 20.5 *Phase III CRT as primary therapy trials*

Author	Number of patients	RT dose (cGy)	Agents	Complete response (%)	Median survival (months)
Herskovic	61	5000	5-FU/CP	NA	12.5[a]
	60	6400	–		8.9[a]
Araujo	28	5000	5-FU/MTC	75	8
	31	5000	–	58	8

[a]$p < 0.05$.

CRT, chemoradiotherapy; RT, radiotherapy; NA, not available; CP, cisplatin; 5-FU, 5-fluorouracil; MTC, mitomycin C.

patients with residual disease after treatment. Twenty-six patients with both SCC and adenocarcinoma were entered in the study. CT consisted of 5-FU ($300 \, mg/m^2$ continuous infusion) for 5 weeks concurrent with RT. CP ($25 \, mg/m^2$ per day) was administered on days 1–3, and 21–23. Radiation consisted of 4000–5000 cGy for 5–6 weeks. Two more monthly cycles consisting of 5-FU ($300 \, mg/m^2$) for 21 days and CP ($75 \, mg/m^2$) on days 43 and 71 were administered. Patients were then restaged with CT of the abdomen and chest and endoscopy following CRT. After these evaluations, if there was no evidence of disease, patients were deemed to have a complete response and were treated with three additional cycles of CT. The remaining patients with residual disease were treated with esophagectomy if they were resectable and had no distant disease. At restaging, 17/26 (65%) of patients had a clinical complete response. Three patients underwent esophagectomy, one recurred and two died in the perioperative period. The median survival was 37 months in the complete-response group and 9 months in patients who did not have a complete response. The survival for the entire group was 24 months. There was major toxicity in this trial, with 19 patients requiring hospitalization for esophagitis, infection, or catheter-related thrombosis. In addition, 15 patients required dose reduction or delay in CRT.

Another phase II study of CRT as primary treatment for esophageal carcinoma involved 90 patients.[44] Fifty-seven patients with both stage I and II SCC and adenocarcinoma of the esophagus were treated definitively with 5-FU ($1000 \, mg/m^2$ continuous infusion for 4 days on days 2 and 29), and mitomycin C ($10 \, mg/m^2$ intravenous bolus on day 2). Radiotherapy in this group consisted of 6000 cGy in 6 weeks, administered concomitantly with the above-mentioned CT. Thirty-three patients with stage III/IV esophageal cancer were treated with palliative intent with the same CT regimen and a lower radiation dose of 5000 cGy. The median follow-up was 45 months. The median survival for the definitively treated group was 18 months, compared to 8 months for the palliative group. The patterns of failure of the definitively treated group were local recurrence in 48% and distant failure in 72%. Both therapies were well

tolerated, with only 3.3% of the entire group requiring hospitalization.

Phase III trials (Table 20.5)

The first phase III trial addressing CRT alone was reported in 1992.[45] One hundred and twenty-one patients were randomized to either CRT alone or RT alone. In the combined modality arm, CT consisted of 5-FU ($1000 \, mg/m^2$ for 4 days in weeks 1, 5, 8, and 11) and CP ($75 \, mg/m^2$ on the first day of each cycle). Radiation was administered to a total dose of 5000 cGy in the CRT group and to a total dose of 6400 cGy in the RT-alone group. Patients with both SCC and adenocarcinoma were included, with 84% of the combined therapy group and 92% of the radiation group having SCC. The 2-year survival rate was 10% in the radiation-only group and 38% in the CRT group, with a median survival time of 8.9 months in the RT group and 12.5 months in the combined therapy group ($p < 0.001$). The recurrence rate, both local and distant, was lower in the CRT group, but local recurrence was still considerable (40%) and only 58% had improvement of dysphagia. There was one death in the CRT group secondary to renal and bone marrow failure. Life-threatening side effects were noted in 20% of the combined therapy group and in 3% of the radiation arm. The authors concluded that CRT provides better control of both local disease and distant metastasis and improves survival when compared to RT alone. As the median survival of patients in the CRT arm was similar to that reported in surgical series with resection alone, the authors raised the question of whether surgery is a necessary component of multimodality therapy.

Randomization in the above trial closed when a highly significant survival advantage for the combined CRT arm was noted, but the trial was kept open to accrue more patients into the CRT arm. At 5-year follow-up, 27% of the combined therapy group were alive, compared to none in the RT group ($p < 0.0001$). The 2-year local recurrence rate was 59% in the RT-only arm and 45% in the combined CRT arm. The rate of distant metastasis at 2 years was 37% in the RT-only arm and 21% in the combined therapy arm.

A South American study examined the role of CRT as primary treatment.[46] Fifty-nine patients with stage II SCC were randomized to receive RT alone (50 Gy) or CRT alone (mitomycin C 10 mg/m^2 bleomycin 15 units weekly for 5 weeks, and 5-FU 1000 mg/m^2/24 h continuous infusion for 72 h). Twenty-eight patients received CRT alone and 31 RT alone. Complete response and overall survival were seen in 58% of the RT group and in 75% of the CRT group and overall 6% and 16%, respectively ($p = 0.16$).

Primary CRT is well tolerated in patients with esophageal cancer. Survival data indicate that there it is more efficacious than RT alone (Table 20.5). A randomized, prospective trial comparing primary CRT to preoperative CRT and surgery is a reasonable study and the only way to address the issue of the efficacy of resection in the management of esophageal cancer.

CONCLUSIONS

The management of esophageal cancer has evolved from single to multimodality treatment. Patients can now be staged more accurately with the advent of the CAT scan, EUS, laparoscopy, and thoracoscopy. However, these staging modalities have their shortcomings. Accurate staging is paramount to selecting patients who might benefit from preoperative therapy. The morbidity and mortality associated with surgery have decreased due to improvement of the techniques and of perioperative care.

The utility of upfront CRT is not clear. A large, multi-center, prospective, randomized study will substantiate its role in patients with esophageal cancer. The use of CRT is clearly superior to that of RT alone. Obligate esophagectomy could be omitted in certain subgroups if complete tumor sterilization could be confirmed without examining the resected specimen. This may well be one of the most crucial areas of future investigation. At the present time, esophagectomy remains the mainstay of treatment, and the role of preoperative CRT and CRT alone is yet to be defined. The treatment of esophageal cancer remains a challenge.

REFERENCES

1. American Cancer Society. *Cancer facts and figures – 1997.* Atlanta, GA, American Cancer Society, 1997.
2. Parker SL, Tong T, Bolden S, Wingo PA. Cancer statistics. CA 1996; 46:5.
3. Blot WJ, Devessa SS, Kellner RW, Fraumeni JF Jr. Rising incidence of adenocarcinoma of the esophagus and gastric cardia. JAMA 1991; 265:1287–9.
4. Mayer RJ. Overview: the changing nature of esophageal cancer. Chest 1993; 103:404s.
5. Daley JM, Karnell LH, Menck HR. National Cancer Data Base report on esophageal carcinoma. Cancer 1996; 78:1820–8.
6. Botet JF, Lightdale CH, Zauber PG, *et al.* Preoperative staging of esophageal carcinoma: comparison of results with endoscopic sonography + dynamic CT. Radiology 1991; 181:419–25.
7. Lightdale CH. Staging of esophageal cancer I: Endoscopic ultrasonography. Semin Oncol 1994; 21:438–46.
8. Molloy RG, McCourtney JS, Anderson JR. Laparoscopy in the management of patients with cancer of the gastric cardia and esophagus. Br J Surg 1995; 82:352–4.
9. Krasna MJ, Flower JL, Attar S, *et al.* Combined thoracoscopic/laparoscopic staging of esophageal cancer. J Thorac Cardiovasc Surg 1996; 111: 806–7.
10. Krasna MJ. The role of thoracoscopic lymph node staging in esophageal cancer. Int Surg 1997; 82:7–11.
11. Finch MD, John TG, Garden OJ, *et al.* Laparoscopic ultrasonography for staging gastroesophageal cancer. Surgery 1996; 121:10–17.
12. Jones DR, Parker LA, Detterbeck FC, Egan TM. Inadequacy of computed tomography in assessing patients with esophageal carcinoma after induction chemoradiotherapy. Cancer 1999; 85:1026–32.
13. Zuccaro GJR, Rice TW, Goldblum J, *et al.* Endoscopic ultrasound cannot determine suitability for esophagectomy after aggressive chemoradiotherapy for esophageal cancer. Am J Gastroenterol 1997; 94:906–12.
14. Lasterza E, deManzoni G, Guglielmi A, *et al.* Endoscopic ultrasonography in the staging of esophageal carcinoma after preoperative radiotherapy and chemotherapy. Ann Thorac Surg 67:1466–9.
15. Launois B, Delarue D, Campion JP, Kerbaol M. Preoperative radiotherapy for carcinoma of the esophagus. Surg Gynecol Obstet 1981; 153:690.
16. Arnott SJ, Duncan W, Kerr GR, *et al.* Low dose preoperative radiotherapy for carcinoma of the oesophagus: results of a randomized clinical trial. Radiother Oncol 1992; 24:108.
17. Gignoux M, Roussel A, Paillot B, *et al.* The value of a preoperative radiotherapy in esophageal cancer: results of a study of the EORTC. World J Surg 1987; 11:426.
18. Mei W, Xian-Zhi G, Weibo Y, *et al.* Randomized clinical trial on the combination of preoperative irradiation and surgery in the treatment of esophageal carcinoma: a report of 206 patients. Int J Radiat Oncol Biol Phys 1989; 16;325.

19. Anderson I, Ladd T. Autopsy findings in squamous cell carcinoma of the esophagus. Cancer 1981; 50:1587–90.

20. Mannard AM, Chasle J, Marnay J, et al. Autopsy findings in 111 cases of esophageal cancer. Cancer 1981; 48:329–35.

21. Roth JA, Pass HI, Flanagan MM, et al. Randomized clinical trial of preoperative and postoperative adjuvant chemotherapy with cisplatin, vindesine, and bleomycin for carcinoma of the esophagus. J Thorac Cardiovasc Surg 1988; 96:242–8.

22. Schlag P. Results of surgery in multimodality therapy of esophageal cancer. Onkologie 1991; 14:13–20.

23. Schlag PM. Randomized trial of preoperative chemotherapy for squamous cell cancer of the esophagus. Arch Surg 1992; 127:1446–50.

24. Nygaard K, Hagen S, Hansen HS, et al. Pre-operative radiotherapy prolongs survival in operable esophageal carcinoma: a randomized multicenter study of pre-operative radiotherapy and chemotherapy. The second Scandinavian trial in esophageal cancer. World J Surg 1992; 16:1104–10.

25. Kelsen DP, Ginsberg R, Pajak TF, et al. Chemotherapy followed by surgery compared with surgery alone for localized esophageal cancer. N Engl J Med 1998; 339:1979–84.

26. Kelsen DP, Minsky BD, Smith M, et al. Preoperative therapy for esophageal cancer randomized comparison of chemotherapy vs. radiation therapy. J Clin Oncol 1990; 8:1352–61.

27. Vokes EE, Weichselbaum RR. Concomitant chemoradiotherapy: rationale and clinical experience in patients with solid tumors. J Clin Oncol 1990; 8:911–34.

28. Franklin R, Steiger Z, Vaishampayan G, et al. Combined modality therapy for esophageal squamous cell carcinoma. Cancer 1983; 51:1062–71.

29. Nigro ND, Vaitkevicius VK, Considene B Jr. Combined therapy for cancer of the anal canal preliminary report. Dis Colon Rectum 1974; 17:354.

30. Leichman L, Steiger Z, Seydel HG. Preoperative chemotherapy and radiation therapy for patients with cancer of the esophagus: a potentially curative approach. J Clin Oncol 1984, 2:75.

31. Wolfe WG, Vaughn AL, Seigler HF, et al. Survival of patients with carcinoma of the esophagus treated with combined modality therapy. J Thoracic Cardiovasc Surg 1993; 105:749.

32. Seydel HG, Leichman L, Byhardt R, et al. Preoperative radiation and chemotherapy for localized squamous cell carcinoma of the esophagus: a RTOG study. Int J Radiat Oncol Biol Phys 1988; 14:33.

33. Poplin E, Fleming T, Leichman L, et al. Combined therapies for squamous-cell carcinoma of the esophagus, a Southwest Oncology Group Study 9 SWOG-8037. J Clin Oncol 1987; 5:622–8.

34. Forastiere AA, Orringer MB, Perez-Tamayo C, et al. Concurrent chemotherapy and radiation therapy followed by transhiatal esophagectomy for local regional cancer of the esophagus. J Clin Oncol 1990; 8(1):119–27.

35. Forastiere AA, Orringer MB, Perez-Tamayo C, et al. Preoperative chemotherapy and radiation therapy followed by transhiatal esophagectomy for carcinoma of the esophagus: final report. J Clin Oncol 1993; 11:118–23.

36. Bates BA, Detterbeck FC, Bernard SA, et al. Concurrent radiation therapy and chemotherapy followed by esophagectomy for localized esophageal carcinoma. J Clin Oncol 1996; 14:156.

37. Kane JM, Shears LL, Riberio U, et al. Is esophagectomy following upfront chemoradiotherapy safe and necessary? Arch Surg 1997; 132:481.

38. Hoff SJ, Stewart JR, Sawyers JL, et al. Preliminary results with neoadjuvant therapy and resection for esophageal carcinoma. Ann Thorac Surg 1993; 56:282–7.

39. Le Prise E, Etienne PL, Meunier B, et al. A randomized study of chemotherapy, radiation therapy and surgery versus surgery for localized squamous cell carcinoma of the esophagus. Cancer 1994; 73:1779.

40. Walsh TN, Noonan N, Hollywood D, et al. A comparison of multimodal therapy and surgery for esophageal adenocarcinoma. N Engl J Med 1996; 355:462.

41. Bossett JF, Gingoux M, Triboulet JP, et al. Chemoradiotherapy followed by surgery compared with surgery alone in squamous-cell cancer of the esophagus. N Engl J Med 1997; 337:161.

42. Leichman L, Herskovic A, Leichman CG, et al. Nonoperative therapy for squamous cell cancer of the esophagus. J Clin Oncol 1987; 5:365.

43. Poplin EA, Khanuja PS, Kraut MJ, et al. Chemoradiotherapy of esophageal carcinoma. Cancer 1994; 74:1217.

44. Coia LR, Engstrom PF, Paul AR, et al. Long term results of infusional 5-FU, mitomycin-C and radiation as primary management of esophageal carcinoma. Int J Radiat Oncol 1990; 20:29.

45. Herskovic A, Martz K, Al-Saraf M, et al. Combined chemotherapy and radiotherapy compared with radiotherapy alone in patients with cancer of the esophagus. N Engl J Med 1992; 326:1593.

46. Araujo CM, Souhami L, Gil RA, et al. A randomized trial comparing radiation therapy versus concomitant radiation therapy and chemotherapy in carcinoma of the thoracic esophagus. Cancer 1991; 67:2258–61.

Commentary 1 (on Chapters 19 and 20)

CLARK B FULLER AND ROBERT J McKENNA JR

Chapters 19 and 20 are very good updates that summarize the current state of the art for surgical treatment and the multimodality treatment of esophageal cancer. Over recent years, the risk of operative treatment for esophageal cancer has substantially decreased. The use of currently available surgical treatment has been optimized and has acceptable morbidity and mortality.[1] The increase in resectability rates and the decrease in operative mortality, while commendable, are not reflected in improved survival and thus highlight the need for a more complete understanding and less dogmatic approach to esophageal cancer.

The most telling statement from these chapters is that it is estimated that there will be 13 200 new cases of esophageal cancer this year and 12 500 deaths due to esophageal cancer. In recent years, the surgical technique for esophageal disease has improved and multimodality treatment has started to show some efficacy.[2] Despite these improvements, the prognosis for esophageal cancer is still dismal. Why is this? What can be done? What is the impact of treatment on the quality of life?

SURGICAL TREATMENT

The vast majority of esophageal resections are performed as either an Ivor–Lewis procedure or a transhiatal esophagectomy. As the authors note, the results are remarkably similar. While an Ivor–Lewis esophagogastrectomy allows the surgeon to perform a much more complete regional resection of the esophagus and the surrounding lymphatic tissue, the survival is essentially the same as that following the trans-hiatal esophagectomy. Therefore, the reality of esophageal surgery is that surgeons should perform the procedure that they can perform with the least morbidity and mortality. At first glance, the two-field or three-field resection seems to offer better survival than the other procedures. However, selection bias is probably the reason for this apparent difference. A randomized, prospective trial would be needed to determine if the more radical procedures really do provide better survival. All of the procedures described are acceptable treatments for esophageal cancer, and none of the procedures offers a clearly superior survival for patients.

The authors provide the reader with a detailed description and excellent discussion of the information that is available regarding the technical details of the procedures. Experts in the field of esophageal surgery, however, do have widely disparate technical approaches

for the operations. The authors advocate the gastric tube for esophageal replacement, while Orringer uses the stomach,[3] with resection of only a minimal amount of cardia. There is currently renewed interest in a minimally invasive approach to esophagectomy.[4] Early results show that the procedure requires a long operative time, but perhaps a shorter length of stay in hospital. More follow-up is needed to determine if this is a reasonable approach to esophageal surgery. Again, this shows that surgeons should monitor their results and perform the procedure that provides the best functional result with the lowest morbidity and mortality.

QUALITY OF LIFE

The cure rate for surgical treatment of esophageal cancer is very low and the life expectancy is short. The incidence of anastomotic leak is 10–15%, and at least 35% of patients require esophageal dilatation. At least one major complication occurred in 46% of patients following esophagectomy. The incidence of significant toxicity following induction therapy is as follows: death (14.7%), pneumonitis (14.7%), and severe mucositis (38%). Because the incidence and types of treatment complications are significant, quality-of-life assessment is an important part of the evaluation of the treatment for esophageal cancer.

Esophagectomy has a significant negative impact on self-assessed quality of life.[5] A recent prospective, longitudinal study examined the quality of life in patients with esophageal carcinoma after palliative and potentially curative resections of esophageal cancer. Most aspects of quality of life, except dysphagia, were worse initially after the operation. Six weeks after resection, patients reported worse function, symptoms, and quality-of-life scores compared to preoperative levels for the 9 months prior to resection. All aspects of quality of life, except the relief of dysphagia, deteriorated until death for the patients who died within 2 years after the operation. For patients who survived at least 2 years, the quality-of-life scores returned to preoperative levels in 6–9 months. In both groups, dysphagia improved after surgery and the improvement was maintained until death. Palliation is, therefore, marginal for patients who are not cured by esophagectomy.

The American College of Surgeons Patient Care Evaluation Study showed the current state of care for esophageal cancer in the USA. The operative mortality was an impressive 3.6%, but complications occurred in

Table 1 *Incidence and survival of esophageal cancer by stage*

Pathologic stage	I	II	III	IV
Patients with that stage (%)	13.6	25.7	26.5	31.7
Survival at 1 year (%)	70	57.4	41.2	17.8

46% of patients. Only early-stage cancer is cured by today's best treatment, and only a small percentage of patients have early-stage cancer (Table 1). The use of multimodality treatment was common and did not appear to increase the postoperative morbidity, but it has not increased the survival.[2] This means that identification of these patients is important for treatment planning. Perhaps esophagectomy should be reserved for patients who have true early-stage cancer.[6]

Table 1 shows the incidences of esophageal cancer by stage and the survival at 1 year for each stage.

FUTURE DIRECTIONS

Pathogenesis

Whereas much is known about the risk factors associated with squamous cell cancer, it is the apparent sequence of gastroesophageal reflux, mucosal injury, epithelial transformation from squamous to columnar-lined esophagus (CLE), accumulation of genetic mutations, and the development of frank adenocarcinoma that has generated the greatest interest. CLE, also referred to as Barrett's esophagus, is found in approximately 10% of patients with gastroesophageal reflux. Ninety percent of esophageal adenocarcinomas originate from CLE. Furthermore, clinical studies and evidence from animal models implicate alkaline reflux, duodenal–gastric–esophageal reflux, and antisecretory medications as mediators of mucosal injury and subsequent dysplastic changes. At a molecular level, these risk factors initiate and sustain mutations of the *p53* tumor suppressor gene, which allows clonal populations of high-risk proliferating cells to exist. Cytochrome p450 and gluthathione-S-transferase (GST) are both found in CLE and can activate chemical carcinogens or detoxify carcinogenic metabolites, respectively, and thus play a role in the metaplasia–dysplasia–carcinoma sequence. The prevalence of other mutations that might contribute to malignant transformation is under study. It is hoped that this will lead to the identification of people at high risk for esophageal cancer and the early detection of the disease.

Surveillance

The increasing incidence of esophageal cancer and its apparent relationship to CLE as a precursor lesion highlight the need for appropriate management of patients with Barrett's esophagus. Once CLE has elements of severe dysplasia, invasive carcinoma may coexist in 30–40% of patients and elective trans-hiatal esophagectomy should be considered. This relationship creates a need for either routine endoscopic surveillance and biopsy in patients with CLE or antireflux surgery coupled with maximal acid suppression. The latter option has not produced results that unequivocally show metaplastic regression and improved outcome. A recent report indicated that routine screening and surveillance biopsies in patients with CLE and esophagectomy in those with severe dysplasia are associated with improved survival. Furthermore, surveillance is required following antireflux procedures because the metaplastic changes may still progress to become increasingly dysplastic, even cancerous. A potential alternative is eradication of the dysplasia or CLE with laser therapy, ultrasound ablation, or photodynamic therapy (PDT). PDT utilizes an intravenously administered photosensitizer which is selectively taken up by dysplastic or malignant cells and produces tissue necrosis via a light-activated generation of singlet oxygen. Photosensitivity, esophageal stricture formation, search for the ideal photosensitizer, and long-term follow-up limit the use of PDT, but early results are encouraging.

Staging

There is considerable room for improvement in the clinical staging of esophageal cancer. A better system will provide more accurate grouping of patients for comparison, prognosis, triage, and therapy modulation. Currently, there is a disparity between clinical and pathologic staging in two-thirds of cases. The TNM system was revised in 1997 to separate distant metastases into cervical lymph node involvement with upper esophageal tumors and celiac nodes with lower tumors from tumors with more distant metastases. Although this division of distant metastases is statistically significant, it lacks clinical relevance.

The present staging modalities of computerized tomography (CT) scan, endoscopic ultrasound, and positron emission tomography (PET) scan all have limitations with regard to sensitivity, specificity, and accuracy. A new concept is surgical staging that employs thoracoscopy and laparoscopy to sample lymph node stations and periesophageal tissue much like mediastinoscopy in lung cancer. Prospective trials evaluating PET scan and surgical staging are presently underway (ACOSOG Z0050 and CALBG 9380, respectively). Currently, minimally invasive staging has little clinical relevance because the survival rates are so low. For the treatment of lung cancer, the preoperative identification of stage III disease is important because neoadjuvant treatment has been proven to increase survival. That is not true for esophageal cancer. As more effective treatment becomes available, this will probably be more important.

Finally, the use of molecular markers to stage esophageal cancer, to detect micrometastases, and to predict chemosensitivity may further refine the staging system. Such a system could exclude some patients from surgical treatment or match the disease with different surgical procedures.

THE NEED FOR BETTER TREATMENT

Unfortunately, 75% of patients have nodal metastases at the time of diagnosis, 30% of patients present with disseminated disease, and over 90% of esophageal cancer patients die of their disease. The morbidity and mortality of currently available treatment have been minimized, and the survival from these treatments has been maximized. Unfortunately, that has not been enough. Survival is still dismal. The biggest impact on the survival for patients with esophageal cancer will come from the development of more effective non-surgical treatment for the disease.

REFERENCES

1. Ellis FH, Williamson WA, Heatley GJ. Cancer of the esophagus and cardia: does age influence treatment selection and surgical outcomes. J Am Coll Surg 1998; 187:345–51.
2. Alexander EP, Lipman T, Harmon J, Wadleigh R. Aggressive multimodality therapy for stage III esophageal cancer: a phase I/II study. Ann Thorac Surg 2000; 69:363–8.
3. Orringer MB, Marshall B, Iannettoni MD. Eliminating the cervical esophagogastric anastomotic leak with a side-to-side stapled anastomosis. J Thorac Cardiovasc Surg 2000; 119:277–88.
4. Nguyen NT, Schauer P, Luketich JD. Minimally invasive esophagectomy for Barrett's esophagus with high-grade dysplasia. Surgery 2000; 127(3):284–90.
5. Blazeby JM, Farndon JR, Donovan J, Alderson D. A prospective longitudinal study examining the quality of life of patients with esophageal carcinoma. Cancer 2000; 88:1781–7.
6. Maier A, Tomaselli F, Gebhard F, Rehak P, Smolle J, Smolle-Juttner FM. Palliation of advanced esophageal carcinoma by photodynamic therapy and irradiation. Ann Thorac Surg 2000; 69:1006–90.

Commentary 2 (on Chapter 20)

TOM R DeMEESTER

The proposal to use adjuvant chemotherapy in the treatment of esophageal cancer was made when it became evident that most patients develop postoperative systemic metastasis without local recurrence. This observation led to the hypothesis that undetected systemic micrometastases were present at the time of diagnosis and, if effective systemic therapy were added to local regional therapy, survival should improve.

Recently, this hypothesis has been supported by the observation of epithelial tumor cells in the bone marrow in 37% of patients with esophageal cancer who were resected for cure. These patients had a greater prevalence of relapse at 9 months after surgery compared to those patients without such cells.[1] Such studies emphasize that hematogenous dissemination of viable malignant cells occurs early in the disease and that systemic chemotherapy may be helpful if the cells are sensitive to the agent. On the other hand, systemic chemotherapy may be a hindrance, because of its immunosuppressive properties, if the cells are resistant. Unfortunately, current technology is not able to test tumor cell sensitivity to chemotherapeutic drugs. Therefore, the choice of drugs rests solely on their clinical effectiveness against grossly similar tumors.

The decision to encourage preoperative rather than postoperative chemotherapy was based on the perceived ineffectiveness of chemotherapeutic agents when used after surgery and on animal studies suggesting that agents given before surgery were more effective. The claim that patients who received chemotherapy before resection were less likely to develop resistance to the drugs was, in reality, only opinion and unsupported by data. Similarly, the claim that drug delivery is enhanced because blood flow is more robust before the patients undergo surgical dissection is also flawed in that, if enough blood reaches the operative site to heal the wound or anastomosis, then the flow should be sufficient to deliver chemotherapeutic drugs. An agreed-upon benefit that can be attributed to preoperative chemotherapy in esophageal carcinoma is its ability, if effective, to facilitate surgical resection, particularly squamous cell tumors above the level of the carina. Reducing the size of the tumor may provide a safer margin between the tumor and the trachea or larynx and allow an anastomosis to a

Table 1 *Esophageal carcinoma: randomized preoperative chemotherapy versus surgery alone*

Authors	Year	n = C/S	Cell type	Regimen	CR (%)	Survival: C versus S
Roth et al.[2]	1988	19/20	Squamous	P,V,B	6	NS
Nygaard et al.[3]	1992	50/41	Squamous	P, B	–	NS
Schlag[4]	1992	21/24	Squamous	P, 5-FU	5	NS

P, cisplatin; V, vindesine; B, bleomycin; 5-FU, 5-fluorouracil; C, preoperative chemotherapy; S, surgery only; CR, complete response to chemotherapy; NS, not significant.

tumor-free cervical esophagus just below the cricopharyngeus. An involved margin at this level usually requires a laryngectomy to prevent subsequent local recurrence.

DOES PREOPERATIVE CHEMOTHERAPY IMPROVE SURVIVAL?

Three randomized, prospective studies with squamous cell carcinoma have shown no survival benefit with preoperative chemotherapy, i.e., neoadjuvant therapy, over surgery alone (Table 1).[2–4] Similar studies for adenocarcinoma have not been done. For squamous cell tumors, a complete response to chemotherapy occurred only in 6% of patients. Some proponents of neoadjuvant therapy have emphasized the benefits by focusing only on patients who responded to treatment, leaving nonresponders out of the equation. This is inappropriate in that the success of surgery could be similarly inflated by focusing only on those in whom all tumor could be completely removed and comparing their survival to those in whom tumor was left behind, i.e., R_0 and R_1 versus R_2 resections. Survival for the former group is statistically better.[5] Other proponents have pointed to the increase in the 'disease-free' interval of patients who received neoadjuvant therapy as a justification for its use. This cannot be assumed to be irrefutable in that the intensity and frequency of the hunt for recurrent disease can vary depending on the investigator prejudices, and patients who have an increased disease-free interval may develop metastasis in organs that are less likely to be scrutinized. Further, an increase in the disease-free interval without an increase in survival requires that the interval between recurrent disease and death is accelerated. This suggests that a more aggressive clone of tumor cells was selected out by the chemotherapy or the therapy has crippled the patient's ability to mount an immunological response to the tumor. The observation that many patients who have histochemical evidence of bone marrow metastasis from solid organ tumor have become long-term survivors suggests that such an immunological response could occur and may be an important factor in survival after surgical resection.

With the exception of the potential to improve the resectability of tumors located above the carina, the benefits cited by those in favor of preoperative chemotherapy are questionable. A review of the literature would suggest that investigators have allowed their quest for prolonged survival to assume secondary importance as they have become more intrigued with the opportunity neoadjuvant therapy provides for an *in-vivo* assessment of the tumoricidal effectiveness of a drug or combination of drugs. Studies on survival take up to 5 years to complete, whereas studies on tumor chemosensitivity can be completed within 3 months and can be objectively studied by evaluating the resected specimens. In summary, preoperative chemotherapy alone can potentially downstage the tumor, particularly squamous cell carcinoma. It may also delay the appearance of metastases. However, there is no evidence that it can prolong the survival of patients with resectable carcinoma of the esophagus. Most failures are due to distant metastatic disease underscoring the need for improved systemic therapy. Further, postoperative septic and respiratory complications are more common in patients receiving chemotherapy.

DOES PREOPERATIVE CHEMORADIOTHERAPY IMPROVE SURVIVAL?

Preoperative chemoradiotherapy using the drug combinations of platinum with 5-fluorouracil (5-FU) has been reported by several investigators to be beneficial in both adenocarcinoma and squamous cell esophageal carcinoma, but, particularly for squamous cells, by increasing the number of complete pathological responses of the primary tumor prior to resection. There have been only five randomized, prospective studies utilizing this strategy, three with squamous cell carcinoma, one with both squamous cell carcinoma and adenocarcinoma, and one with only adenocarcinoma (Table 2).[3,6–9] All but one have shown no survival benefit with preoperative chemoradiotherapy over surgery alone. Most authors report substantial morbidity and mortality associated with the treatment. Despite this, many have been encouraged by the observation that some patients, who have had a complete response, have remained free of recurrence at 3 years.

Table 2 *Esophageal carcinoma: randomized preoperative chemoradiotherapy versus surgery alone*

Authors	Year	n = C/S	Cell type	Regimen	Survival: C versus S
Nygaard et al.[3]	1992	47/41	Squamous	P, B, 35 Gy	NS
Le Prise et al.[6]	1994	41/45	Squamous	P, 5-FU, 20 Gy	NS
Apinop et al.[7]	1994	35/34	Squamous	P, 5-FU, 40 Gy	NS
Urba et al.[8]	1995	50/50	Squamous + adenocarcinoma	P, 5-FU, V, 45 Gy	NS
Walsh et al.[9]	1996	48/54	Adenocarcinoma	P, 5-FU, 40 Gy	$p = 0.01$

P, cisplatin; 5-FU, 5-fluorouracil; B, bleomycin; V, vinblastine; C, preoperative chemotherapy; S, surgery only; NS, not significant.

Table 3 *Results of neoadjuvant therapy in adenocarcinoma of the esophagus*

Institution	Year	Number of patients	Regimen	CR (%)	Survival (%)
M.D. Anderson	1990	35	P, E, 5-FU	3	42 at 3 y
SLMC	1992	18	P, 5-FU, RT	17	40 at 3 y
Vanderbilt	1993	39	P, E, 5-FU, RT	19	47 at 4 y
Michigan	1993	21	P, VBL, 5-FU, RT	24	34 at 5 y
MGH	1994	16	P, 5-FU	0	42 at 4 y
MGH	1994	22	EAP	5	58 at 2 y

A, adriamycin (doxorubicin); CR, pathologic complete response; E, etoposide; 5-FU, 5-fluorouracil; VBL, vinblastine; P, cisplatin; RT, radiation therapy; SLMC, St Louis University Medical Center; MGH, Massachusetts General Hospital. From Wright et al.[11]

The study reported by Walsh[9] and associates represents the one positive outcome and deserves special comment. Several concerns have arisen about this trial:

1 Before the results are accepted as gospel, it must be kept in mind that three other studies have not shown any benefit to this approach and that the report of this study is only an interim analysis at 3 years. Things could change with further follow-up. If one more death occurs in the multimodal group, the p-value would go from 0.01 to 0.03 and, with two deaths, to >0.05.[10]

2 The number of early-stage tumors was low in the surgery group and therefore there was a worse survival than is generally reported following resection. In contrast, nothing is known about the initial stage of the multimodal therapy group. The number in each arm is small and there could be a stage bias.

3 There is no clear account of the kind of surgical resection performed, i.e., R_0, R_1, or R_2.

4 Withdrawals from the protocol may have resulted in a selection that favored the outcome of multimodal therapy in that ten patients were withdrawn from that arm compared to only one from the surgical arm. Five of the ten withdrawals from the multimodal therapy arm completed a full course of chemotherapy.

5 Fifty-one patients (45%) of the original 113 were excluded from randomization, which questions whether the studied population is an accurate representation of the disease as seen in the clinics.

Consequently, caution must be exercised in emphasizing the effects of chemotherapy with a multimodal approach in that the addition of preoperative radiation therapy to chemotherapy elevates the complete response rate and inflates the benefit of chemotherapy. With chemoradiation, the complete response rates for adenocarcinoma range from 17% to 24%. When radiation was removed, the complete response fell to 0–5%, which suggests that the effects of chemotherapy are negligible (Table 3).[11] If radiotherapy is the factor responsible for improved response rate, surgery alone could do the job as well, as numerous studies in the past have shown that the combination of surgery and radiation does not provide any beneficial survival advantage.

THE ULTIMATE QUESTION REGARDING CHEMOTHERAPY

Most medical and radiation oncologists, dismayed by the high local recurrence and distant failure rates after trans-hiatal or standard transthoracic esophagectomy, have called into question the relevance of surgery in the treatment of esophageal cancer. In their minds, it has become a medical disease, despite sound evidence to the contrary. Surgeons who perform a more extended en-bloc resection and lymphadenectomy for cure of appropriately staged disease have shown

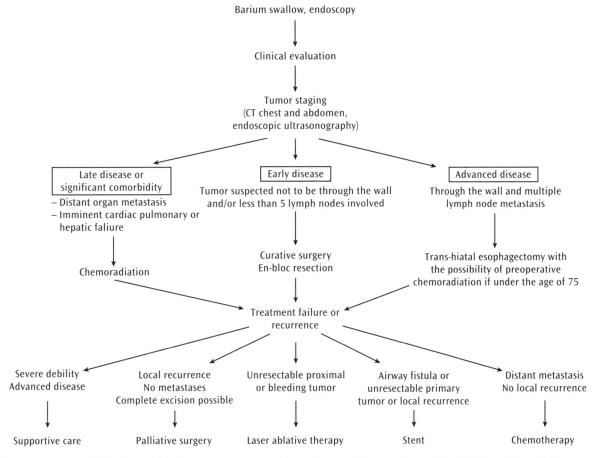

Figure 1 *Suggested global algorithm for the management of carcinoma of the esophagus. (Modified from the guidelines prepared by DeMeester et al., 1994.[14])*

gratifyingly low local recurrence rates in long-term survivors.[12]

The ultimate question is: should patients with carcinoma of the esophagus go through two to three cycles of chemotherapy on the 5% chance that they may get a complete response in the primary tumor and with little evidence that a lesser response will control systemic disease? Prudence would encourage going directly to surgery and avoiding the morbidity associated with preoperative chemotherapy, particularly chemoradiation therapy. Some studies have shown that the rates of infection, anastomotic breakdown, incidence of adult respiratory distress syndrome, and long-term use of a respirator were greater in patients receiving adjuvant therapy compared to those with surgery alone.[4]

Most treatment failures in patients with adjuvant therapy are due to distant disease. This underscores the need to understand that systemic therapy requires further improvement before it can be unconditionally recommended to patients. Rather than calling into question the relevance of surgery, oncologists need to answer the question: is chemotherapy with the newer agents, given at the time of systemic recurrence, after resection, effective in prolonging survival?'[13] Perhaps the newer agents

are more effective at this stage if patients have not received chemotherapy before.

SUMMARY

In summary, current data would support using chemoradiotherapy preoperatively to reduce tumor size in a young person with squamous cell carcinoma above the carina, and using chemotherapy as salvage therapy for patients who have not had previous chemotherapy and develop recurrent systemic disease after surgical resection. A global management algorithm that incorporates this use of chemoradiotherapy is shown in Figure 1.

REFERENCES

1. Thorban S, Rodeu JO, Nekarda H, Funk A, Pantel K, Siewert R. Disseminated epithelial tumor cells in bone marrow of patients with esophageal cancer: detection

and prognostic significance. World J Surg 1996; 20:567–73.

2. Roth JA, Pass HI, Flanagan MM, *et al.* Randomized clinical trial of preoperative and postoperative adjuvant chemotherapy with cisplatin, vindesine, and bleomycin for carcinoma of the esophagus. J Thorac Cardiovasc Surg 1988; 96:242–8.

3. Nygaard K, Hagen S, Hansen HS, *et al.* Pre-operative radiotherapy prolongs survival in operable esophageal carcinoma: a randomized multicenter study of pre-operative radiotherapy and chemotherapy. World J Surg 1992; 16:1104–10.

4. Schlag PM, for the Chirurgische Arbeitsgemeinschaft fuer Onkologie der Deutschen Gesellschaft fuer Chirurgie Study Group. Randomized trial of preoperative chemotherapy for squamous cell cancer of the esophagus. Arch Surg 1992; 127:1446–50.

5. Hermanek P. pTNM and residual tumor classification: problems of assessment and prognostic significance. World J Surg 1995; 19:184–90.

6. Le Prise E, Etienne P, Meunier B, *et al.* A randomized study of chemotherapy radiation therapy, and surgery versus surgery for localized squamous cell carcinoma of the esophagus. Cancer 1994; 73:1779–84.

7. Apinop C, Puttisak P, Preecha N. A prospective study of combined therapy in esophageal cancer. Hepato-Gastroenterol 1994; 41:391–3.

8. Urba S, Orringer M, Turrisi A, *et al.* A randomized trial comparing transhiatal esophagectomy to

preoperative concurrent chemoradiation followed by esophagectomy in locoregional esophageal carcinoma. Proceedings of the American Society of Clinical Oncology's annual meeting in Los Angeles, California, May 20–23, 1995; 14:199(A).

9. Walsh TN, Noonan N, Hollywood D, *et al.* A comparison of multimodal therapy and surgery for esophageal adenocarcinoma. N Engl J Med 1996; 335:462–7.

10. Badwe RA, Vaidya JS, Bhansali M. Multimodal therapy for esophageal adenocarcinoma. N Engl J Med 1996; 336:374–6.

11. Wright CD, Mathisen DJ, Wain JC, *et al.* Evolution of treatment strategies for adenocarcinoma of the esophagus and gastroesophageal junction. Ann Thorac Surg 1994; 58:1574–9.

12. Clark GWB, Peters JH, Ireland AP, *et al.* Nodal metastasis and sites of recurrence after en bloc esophagectomy for adenocarcinoma. Ann Thorac Surg 1994; 58(3):646–54.

13. Raoul JL, LePrise E, Meunier B, *et al.* Combined radiochemotherapy for postoperative recurrence of esophageal cancer. Gut 1995; 37:174–6.

14. DeMeester TR, Kimmey MB, Kozarek RA, Levin B, Spechler S, Tytgat GNJ. In Ninety-fifth annual American Gastroenterological Association's Clinical Practice Section Symposium on Esophageal Cancer, May 15–18, 1994, New Orleans, LA.

Editors' selected abstracts (for Chapters 19 and 20)

Bone marrow-disseminated tumor cells in patients with carcinoma of the esophagus or cardia.

Bonavina L, Soligo D, Quirici N, Bossolasco P, Cesana B, Deliliers GL, Peracchia A.

Department of General and Oncologic Surgery, University of Milan, Bone Marrow Transplantation Unit, Fondazione Matarelli, and Epidemiology Unit, Ospedale Maggiore di Milano, Milano, Italy.

Surgery 129(1):15–22, 2001, January.

Background: The long-term prognosis after surgical therapy for esophageal carcinoma depends on tumor stage and completeness of resection. Similarly to other epithelial tumors, the presence of micro deposits of neoplastic cells in the bone marrow may indicate residual disease and the potential for recurrence. This study assesses the prevalence of bone marrow-disseminated tumor cells in patients undergoing surgical resection for esophageal carcinoma. In addition, we investigated the agreement between immuno-histochemical and molecular techniques for the detection of micrometastases in a subgroup of patients. *Methods:* Between January 1998 and November 1999, forty-eight patients with adenocarcinoma of the esophagogastric junction ($n = 29$) or squamous cell carcinoma of the thoracic esophagus ($n = 19$) and no evidence of overt metastatic disease entered the study. An immunohisto-chemical assay (capable of detecting 1 carcinoma cell in 7×10^5 bone marrow cells) was used to test bone marrow obtained by flushing a resected rib or by needle aspiration either of the iliac crest or of a rib. A polymerase chain reaction (PCR) molecular technique was also used to identify bone marrow and peripheral blood epithelial cells. *Results:* Cytokeratin-positive cells were found in 79.1% of the bone marrow samples obtained from the rib, and in only 8% of the needle aspirates either from the iliac crest or from a contiguous rib. This difference is probably explained by the improved removal of metastatic cells with the flushing of the rib. Comparable results were obtained at a qualitative level by the PCR technique on bone marrow. In addition, PCR-positive results were found in 3 of 18 peripheral blood samples. There was no association with tumor type, neo-adjuvant therapy, or lymph node status. Patients with a pT3 or pT4 tumor showed, at a borderline statistical level, a higher proportion of cytokeratin-positive cells in the flushed rib. *Conclusions:* Bone marrow-disseminated tumor cells are present in the resected rib of a high proportion of patients undergoing esophagectomy for carcinoma, and immunohistochemistry seems to be the method of choice for their quantitative assessment. However, the prognostic and therapeutic implications of this finding need further investigation.

Transhiatal versus transthoracic esophagectomy: complication and survival rates.

Boyle MJ, Franceschi D, Livingstone AS.

Department of Surgery, Sylvester Comprehensive Cancer Center, University of Miami Hospitals and Clinics/Jackson Memorial Hospital, Miami, FL, USA.

American Surgeon 65(12):1137–41, 1999, December.

The classic approach for esophagectomy is via a combined thoracic and abdominal approach. Concerns persist regarding the adequacy of this approach as a cancer operation. A study was carried out to compare these approaches, with particular reference to complication rates and long-term survival. The charts of all adult patients undergoing esophagectomy for carcinoma at the University of Miami/Jackson Memorial Hospital between July 1991 and June 1996 were reviewed. Patients who had transabdominal resections alone or colon interpositions were excluded. Of 65 esophageal resections, 38 (58%) were performed transhiatally (THE) and 27 (42%) were performed via the transthoracic (TTE) route. Treatment groups were matched for age and site, stage, and histology of tumor. Similarly, the treatment groups were homogeneous with respect to distribution of neoadjuvant chemotherapy/radiation. The number of patients experiencing any postoperative complication was similar in both treatment groups, occurring in 22 THE (58%) and 17 TTE (63%) patients ($p > 0.05$). Anastomotic leak occurred in five THE patients (13%) and one TTE patient (4%) ($p > 0.05$). The single TTE patient with a leak died within 3 months without leaving the hospital. All five THE patients who developed a leak left the hospital. Although there was a tendency toward a higher percentage of patients in the TTE group to suffer respiratory failure and sepsis and a higher percentage of THE patients to experience anastomotic leak, these did not reach statistical significance. Again, although perioperative mortality tended to be higher in the TTE group, this did not reach statistical significance. Four and 5-year survival rates were similar in both groups. Whereas a 4-year cumulative survival difference of 42% for THE patients and 31% in TTE patients extended at 58 months to 28% and 8%, respectively, these did not reach statistical significance. Similarly, analysis by stage and preoperative treatment type ($\pm$ neoadjuvant chemotherapy/radiation) failed to demonstrate any survival difference between the two groups. These findings demonstrate that there is little difference in operative morbidity and mortality between THE and TTE routes. Anastomotic leaks that occur after cervical anastomosis tend to run a more benign course. Survival data do not support routine TTE as a superior oncological operation, despite the theoretical benefit of better lymphatic clearance. We continue to advocate THE because it allows a cervical anastomosis without thoracotomy and we feel it is better tolerated by patients.

Methylene blue-directed biopsies improve detection of intestinal metaplasia and dysplasia in Barrett's esophagus.

Canto MI, Setrakian S, Willis J, Chak A, Petras R, Powe NR, Sivak MV Jr.

Division of Gastroenterology and Institute of Pathology, University Hospitals of Cleveland–Case Western Reserve University, Department of Anatomic Pathology, The Cleveland Clinic Foundation, and Louis Stokes Cleveland VAMC, OH, USA.

Gastrointestinal Endoscopy 51(5):560–8, 2000, May.

Background: Endoscopically applied methylene blue selectively stains specialized columnar epithelium in Barrett's esophagus. *Methods:* The diagnostic yield and cost of cancer surveillance in patients with Barrett's esophagus using methylene blue-directed biopsies (MBDB) were compared with surveillance using a 'jumbo' random biopsy technique in a prospective, sequential, controlled trial. Esophagogastroduodenoscopy was performed with either MBDB or random biopsy in a randomized sequence. The proportions of various types of epithelia in each biopsy were estimated and dysplasia was graded in a blinded fashion. *Results:* Forty-three patients with short- ($n = 8$), limited- ($n = 10$), and long-segment ($n = 25$) Barrett's esophagus were studied. Using MBDB technique, the average number of biopsies obtained per patient was significantly lower and the proportion of specialized columnar epithelium in each specimen was significantly higher compared with random biopsy. Dysplasia or cancer was diagnosed in significantly more MBDB specimens (12% vs. 6%, $p = 0.004$). Despite fewer biopsies per patient using MBDB, dysplasia or cancer was diagnosed in significantly more patients (44% vs. 28%, $p = 0.03$) than by random biopsy technique. MBDB cost less and detected more cancers than random biopsy. *Conclusions:* MBDB is a more accurate and cost-effective technique than random biopsy for diagnosing specialized columnar epithelium and dysplasia/cancer, particularly in long-segment Barrett's esophagus.

Resectable esophageal carcinoma: local control with neoadjuvant chemotherapy and radiation therapy.

Chidel MA, Rice TW, Adelstein DJ, Kupelian PA, Suh JH, Becker M.

Department of Radiation Oncology, Cleveland Clinic Foundation, OH, USA.

Radiology 213(1):67–72, 1999, October.

Purpose: To evaluate the usefulness of neoadjuvant chemotherapy and radiation therapy before esophagectomy for invasive cancer of the esophagus or gastroesophageal junction (GEJ). *Materials and methods:* The authors conducted a retrospective analysis of 154 patients who underwent esophagectomy for invasive cancer between September 1, 1991, and December 31, 1995. The end points evaluated were overall, disease-free, local–regional relapse-free, and systemic relapse-free survival. *Results:* Seventy of the 154 patients received neoadjuvant combined-modality therapy (CMT) consisting of concurrent cisplatin and fluorouracil administration and accelerated, hyperfractionated radiation therapy. The remaining 84 patients underwent immediate esophagectomy. With a median follow-up of 34.7 months, the 3-year overall, disease-free, and distant metastatic relapse-free survival rates were 38.0%, 41.9%, and 56.0%, respectively. Although neoadjuvant therapy did not appear to prevent distant metastases, there was a dramatic effect on local control. After CMT, the 5-year local control rate was 90% compared to 64% after surgery ($p < 0.001$). Tumors in the GEJ recurred more frequently ($p = 0.01$); however, multivariate analysis showed CMT was the only independent predictor of local control. Postoperative mortality was 15.7% after CMT versus 5.9% without CMT ($p = 0.05$). *Conclusion:* Local control of esophageal cancer is excellent following neoadjuvant chemotherapy and radiation therapy. However, the effects of CMT on overall and disease-free survival are less clear due to significant differences between the treatment groups.

Esophageal cancer: results of an American College of Surgeons Patient Care Evaluation Study.

Daly JM, Fry WA, Little AG, Winchester DP, McKee RF, Stewart AK, Fremgen AM.

Department of Surgery, New York Presbyterian Hospital–Weill Medical College of Cornell University, NY, USA.

Journal of the American College of Surgeons 190(5):562–72, 2000, May.

Background: The last two decades have seen changes in the prevalence, histologic type, and management algorithms for patients with esophageal cancer. The purpose of this study was to evaluate the presentation, stage distribution, and treatment of patients with esophageal cancer using the National Cancer Database of the American College of Surgeons. *Study design:* Consecutively accessed patients ($n = 5044$) with esophageal cancer from 828 hospitals during 1994 were evaluated in 1997 for case mix, diagnostic tests, and treatment modalities. *Results:* The mean age of patients was 67.3 years with a male to female ratio of 3:1; non-Hispanic Caucasians made up most patients. Only 16.6% reported no tobacco use. Dysphagia (74%), weight loss (57.3%), gastrointestinal reflux (20.5%), odynophagia (16.6%), and dyspnea (12.1%) were the most common symptoms. Approximately 50% of patients had the tumor in the lower third of the esophagus. Of all patients, 51.6% had squamous cell histology and 41.9% had adenocarcinoma. Barrett's esophagus occurred in 777 patients, or 39% of those with adenocarcinoma. Of those patients that underwent surgery initially, pathology revealed stage I (13.3%), II (34.7%), III (35.7%), and IV (12.3%) disease. For patients with various stages of squamous cell cancer, radiation therapy plus chemotherapy were the most common treatment modalities (39.5%) compared with surgery plus adjuvant therapy (13.2%). For patients with adenocarcinoma, surgery plus adjuvant therapy were the most common treatment methods. Disease-specific overall survival at 1 year was 43%, ranging from 70% to 18% from stages I to IV. *Conclusions:* Cancer of the esophagus shows an increasing occurrence of adenocarcinoma in the lower third of the esophagus and is frequently associated with Barrett's esophagus. Choice of treatment was influenced by tumor histology and tumor site. Multimodality (neoadjuvant) therapy was the most common treatment method for patients with esophageal adenocarcinoma. The use of multimodality treatment did not appear to increase postoperative morbidity.

The pattern of metastastatic lymph node dissemination from adenocarcinoma of the esophagogastric junction.

Dresner SM, Lamb PJ, Bennett MK, Hayes N, Griffin SM.

Northern Esophago-Gastric Cancer Unit, Royal Victoria Infirmary, Newcastle upon Tyne, UK.

Surgery 129(1):103–9, 2001, January.

Background: The incidence of adenocarcinoma of the esophagogastric junction is rapidly increasing, and the extent of lymphadenectomy for such tumors remains controversial. The aim of this study was to identify the pattern of dissemination by examination of all lymph nodes retrieved from resected tumors of the esophagogastric junction. *Methods:* The endoscopic and pathologic reports of patients who underwent R0 resection for adenocarcinoma of the esophagogastric junction between January 1996 and November 1999 were examined. Patients with type 1 tumors (distal esophagus) underwent subtotal esophagectomy with 2-field lymphadenectomy. Patients with type 2 (gastric cardia) tumors underwent transhiatal D2 total gastro-esophagectomy. Lymph node groups were dissected from the main specimens and examined separately. *Results:* One hundred and four type 1 and 48 type 2 tumors were studied. Median nodal recovery was 23 lymph nodes (type 1, 22 lymph nodes; type 2, 23 lymph nodes). Seventy-eight percent of the type 1 tumors with nodal metastases had dissemination in both the abdomen and mediastinum. The common abdominal sites were the paracardiac and the left gastric stations. Within the mediastinum, paraesophageal, paraaortic and tracheobronchial metastases were more often encountered. Type 2 tumors had positive lymph nodes most frequently in the left and right paracardiac, lesser curve (N1 group), and left gastric (N2 group) territories. Nodal status correlated with increasing depth of tumor invasion ($p = 0.002$). *Conclusions:* The pattern of nodal dissemination for cardia tumors concurs with that described by other studies. The current definition of nodal fields in the abdomen and mediastinum for esophageal tumors relates to experience with squamous carcinomas. Our results demonstrate a different pattern of dissemination for junctional esophageal adenocarcinomas. The nodal stations to be resected in radical lymphadenectomies for such tumors should be redefined.

Phase II evaluation of preoperative chemoradiation and postoperative adjuvant chemotherapy for squamous cell and adenocarcinoma of the esophagus.

Heath EI, Burtness BA, Heitmiller RF, Salem R, Kleinberg L, Knisely JP, Yang SC, Talamini MA, Kaufman HS, Canto MI, Topazian M, Wu TT, Olukayode K, Forastiere AA.

Departments of Oncology, Surgery, Medicine, and Pathology, Johns Hopkins University School of Medicine, Baltimore, MD, USA.

Journal of Clinical Oncology 18(4):868–76, 2000, February.

Purpose: This phase II trial evaluated continuous-infusion cisplatin and fluorouracil (5-FU) with radiotherapy followed by esophagectomy. The objectives of this trial were to determine the complete pathologic response rate, survival rate, toxicity, pattern of failure, and feasibility of administering adjuvant chemotherapy in patients with resectable cancer of the esophagus treated with preoperative chemoradiation. *Patients and methods:* Patients were staged using computed tomography, endoscopic ultrasound, and laparoscopy. The preoperative treatment plan consisted of continuous intravenous infusion of cisplatin and 5-FU and a total dose of 44 Gy of radiation. Esophagogastrectomy was planned for approximately 4 weeks after the completion of chemoradiotherapy. Paclitaxel and cisplatin were administered as postoperative adjuvant therapy. *Results:* Forty-two patients were enrolled onto the trial. Of the 39 patients who proceeded to surgery, 29 responded to preoperative treatment: 11 achieved pathologic complete response (CR) and 18 achieved a lower posttreatment stage. Five patients had no change in stage, whereas eight had progressive disease (four with distant metastases and four with increases in the T and N stages). At a median follow-up of 30.2 months, the median survival time has not been reached and the 2-year survival rate is 62%. The median survival of pathologic complete responders has not been reached, whereas the 2-year survival rate of this group is 91% compared with 51% in patients with complete tumor resection with residual tumor ($p = 0.03$). *Conclusion:* An excellent survival rate, comparable to that of our prior preoperative trial, was achieved with lower doses of preoperative cisplatin and 5-FU concurrent with radiotherapy.

The role of laparoscopy in preoperative staging of esophageal cancer.

Heath EI, Kaufman HS, Talamini MA, Wu TT, Wheeler J, Heitmiller RF, Kleinberg L, Yang SC, Olukayode K, Forastiere AA.

Department of Medical Oncology, Johns Hopkins Oncology Center, Baltimore, MD, USA.

Surgical Endoscopy 14(5):495–9, 2000, May.

Background: Diagnostic laparoscopy has been used to determine resectability and to prevent unnecessary laparotomy in patients with advanced esophageal cancer. The objective of this prospective study was to evaluate the role of laparoscopy in conjunction with computed tomography (CT) scan in staging patients with esophageal cancer. *Methods:* From March 1995 to October 1998, 59 patients with biopsy-proven esophageal cancer underwent diagnostic laparoscopy with concurrent vascular access device and feeding jejunostomy tube placement. *Results:* Laparoscopy changed the treatment plan in 10 of 59 patients (17%). Of the patients with normal-appearing regional or celiac nodes, 78% were confirmed by biopsy to be tumor free, whereas 76% of patients with abnormal-appearing nodes were confirmed by biopsy to have node-positive disease. *Conclusions:* Diagnostic laparoscopy is useful for detecting and confirming nodal involvement and distant metastatic disease that potentially would alter treatment and prognosis in patients with esophageal cancer.

The recurrence pattern of esophageal carcinoma after transhiatal resection.

Hulscher JB, van Sandick JW, Tijssen JG, Obertop H, van Lanschot JJ.

Department of Surgery, Academic Medical Center/University of Amsterdam, The Netherlands.

Journal of the American College of Surgeons 191(2):143–8, 2000, August.

Background: There is much controversy about the optimal resection for carcinoma of the esophagus. Little is known about the pattern of recurrence after transhiatal resection for esophageal carcinoma. *Study design:* We retrospectively reviewed the charts of 149 patients who underwent transhiatal esophagectomy for carcinoma of the mid or distal esophagus or gastroesophageal junction between June 1993 and June 1997. Recurrence was classified as locoregional or distant recurrence. Nine patients with macroscopically evident tumor left after resection and three patients (2.0%) who died in the hospital were excluded from the analysis. This left 137 patients; 105 men and 32 women with a median age 65 years (range 37 to 84 years). *Results:* There were 95 adenocarcinomas (69.3%) and 42 squamous cell carcinomas (30.7%). Overall the median followup was 24.0 months (range 1.4 to 69.2 months). For patients alive at the end of followup without recurrence, the median followup was 36.5 months (range 23.6 to 69.2 months). Seven patients died of other causes. The median interval between operation and recurrence was 11 months (range 1.4 to 62.5 months) for patients who had recurrence, with no significant difference in interval between locoregional and systemic recurrence. Seventy-two of the 137 patients (52.6%) developed recurrent disease. Thirty-two patients (23.4%) developed locoregional recurrence only, 21 patients (15.3%) developed systemic recurrence only, and 19 patients (13.9%) had a combination of both. In only 8.0% of all patients was there recurrence in the cervical lymph nodes. The most frequent sites of distant recurrence were liver (37.5%), bone (25.0%), and lung (17.5%). Recurrence was related to postoperative lymph node status ($p < 0.001$) and the radicality of the operation ($p < 0.001$) in multivariate analysis. Recurrence was not associated with localization or histologic type of the tumor. *Conclusions:* Recurrence after transhiatal resection is an early event. Almost 40% of patients developed locoregional recurrent disease. For this patient group a more extended procedure may be of benefit, especially in the patients (23.4%) with locoregional recurrence in whom this is the only site of recurrent disease. But the potential benefit of a more extended procedure has to be balanced against a possible increase in perioperative morbidity and mortality.

Factors affecting morbidity, mortality, and survival in patients undergoing Ivor Lewis esophagogastrectomy.

Karl RC, Schreiber R, Boulware D, Baker S, Coppola D.

Departments of Surgery, Biostatistics, and Pathology, University of South Florida, Tampa, FL, USA.

Annals of Surgery 231(5):635–43, 2000, May.

Objectives: To examine the safety of transthoracic esophagogastrectomy (TTE) in a multidisciplinary cancer center and to determine which clinical parameters influenced survival and the rates of death and complications. *Summary background data:* Although the incidence of cancer at the gastroesophageal junction has been rising rapidly in the United States, controversy still exists about the safety of surgical procedures designed to remove the distal esophagus and proximal stomach. Alternatives to TTE have been proposed because of the reportedly high rates of death and complications associated with the procedure. *Methods:* Data from 143 patients treated by TTE by one author (1989–1999) were entered into a computerized database. Preoperative clinical parameters were tested for effect on death, complications, and survival. *Results:* The patient population consisted of 127 men and 16 women. One hundred twenty-one patients had a history of tobacco abuse, and 118 reported the regular ingestion of alcohol. One hundred fifteen patients had adenocarcinoma, 16 had squamous cell cancer, 6 had another form of esophageal tumor, and 6 had high-grade dysplasia associated with Barrett epithelia. Fifty-six patients had adenocarcinomas arising in Barrett epithelium. Twenty-eight patients were treated with neoadjuvant chemoradiation before surgery. Three patients died within 30 days of surgery (mortality rate 2.1%). Five patients (3.5%) had a documented anastomotic leak; three died. Overall, 42 patients had complications (29%). Twenty-six had pulmonary complications (19%). The mean length of stay in the intensive care unit was 3.35 days; the mean hospital length of stay was 13.54 days. The overall 3-year survival rate was 29.6%. *Conclusions:* A high ASA score and the development of complications predicted an increased length of stay. The presence of diabetes predicted the development of complication and an increased length of stay. None of the other parameters tested predicted perioperative death or complications. Only disease stage, diabetes, and blood transfusion affected overall survival. From these results with a large series of patients with gastroesophageal junction cancers, TTE can be performed with a low death rate (2.1%), a low leak rate (3.5%), and an acceptable complication rate (29%).

Minimally invasive esophagectomy.

Luketich JD, Schauer PR, Christie NA, Weigel TL, Raja S, Fernando HC, Keenan RJ, Nguyen NT.

Section of Thoracic Surgery, University of Pittsburgh Medical Center Health System, PA, USA.

Annals of Thoracic Surgery 70(3):906–11, 2000, September.

Background: Open esophagectomy can be associated with significant morbidity and delay return to routine activities. Minimally invasive surgery may lower the morbidity of esophagectomy but only a few small series have been published. *Methods:* From August 1996 to September 1999, 77 patients underwent minimally invasive esophagectomy. Initially, esophagectomy was approached totally laparoscopically or with mini-thoracotomy; thoracoscopy subsequently replaced thoracotomy. *Results:* Indications included esophageal carcinoma (*n* = 54), Barrett's high-grade dysplasia or carcinoma in situ (*n* = 17), and benign miscellaneous (*n* = 6). There were 50 men and 27 women with an average age of 66 years (range 30 to 94 years). Median operative time was 7.5 hours (4.5 hours with >20

case experience). Median intensive care unit stay was 1 day (range 0 to 60 days); median length of stay was 7 days (range 4 to 73 days) with no operative or hospital mortalities. There were four nonemergent conversions to open esophagectomy; major and minor complication rates were 27% and 55%, respectively. *Conclusions:* Minimally invasive esophagectomy is technically feasible and safe in our center, which has extensive minimally invasive and open esophageal experience. Open surgery should remain the standard until future studies conclusively demonstrate advantages of minimally invasive approaches.

Adenocarcinoma of the esophagogastric junction: results of surgical therapy based on anatomical/topographic classification in 1,002 consecutive patients.

Rudiger Siewert J, Feith M, Werner M, Stein HJ.

Chirurgische Klinik und Poliklinik and Institut fur Pathologie und Pathologische Anatomie, Klinikum rechts der Isar, Technische Universitat Munchen, Munich, Germany.

Annals of Surgery 232(3):353–61, 2000, September.

Objective: To assess the outcome of surgical therapy based on a topographic/anatomical classification of adenocarcinoma of the esophagogastric junction. *Summary background data:* Because of its borderline location between the stomach and esophagus, the choice of surgical strategy for patients with adenocarcinoma of the esophagogastric junction is controversial. *Methods:* In a large single-center series of 1,002 consecutive patients with adenocarcinoma of the esophagogastric junction, the choice of surgical approach was based on the location of the tumor center or tumor mass. Treatment of choice was esophagectomy for type I tumors (adenocarcinoma of the distal esophagus) and extended gastrectomy for type II tumors (true carcinoma of the cardia) and type III tumors (subcardial gastric cancer infiltrating the distal esophagus). Demographic data, morphologic and histopathologic tumor characteristics, and long-term survival rates were compared among the three tumor types, focusing on the pattern of lymphatic spread, the outcome of surgery, and prognostic factors in patients with type II tumors. *Results:* There were marked differences in sex distribution, associated intestinal metaplasia in the esophagus, tumor grading, tumor growth pattern, and stage distribution between the three tumor types. The postoperative death rate was higher after esophagectomy than extended total gastrectomy. On multivariate analysis, a complete tumor resection (R0 resection) and the lymph node status (pN0) were the dominating independent prognostic factors for the entire patient population and in the three tumor types, irrespective of the surgical approach. In patients with type II tumors, the pattern of lymphatic spread was primarily directed toward the paracardial, lesser curvature, and left gastric artery nodes; esophagectomy offered no survival benefit over extended gastrectomy in these patients. *Conclusion:* The classification of adenocarcinomas of the esophagogastric junction into type I, II, and III tumors shows marked differences between the tumor types and provides a useful tool for selecting the surgical approach. For patients with type II tumors, esophagectomy offers no advantage over extended gastrectomy if a complete tumor resection can be achieved.

Adenocarcinoma of the esophagus with and without Barrett mucosa.

Sabel MS, Pastore K, Toon H, Smith JL.

Roswell Park Cancer Institute, Buffalo, NY, USA.

Archives of Surgery 135(7):831–5, 2000, July.

Hypothesis: Previous studies have demonstrated an improved prognosis in patients with Barrett adenocarcinoma as compared with esophageal adenocarcinoma without Barrett. It has been suggested that an earlier presentation due to gastroesophageal reflux disease (GERD) may lead to detection of adenocarcinoma at an earlier stage. *Design:* The records of 178 patients with esophageal adenocarcinoma presenting to Roswell Park Cancer Institute (Buffalo, NY) between 1991 and 1996 were reviewed. *Main outcome measures:* The clinical presentation, work-up, therapy, and outcome were compared between patients with Barrett esophagus ($n = 66$) and those without endoscopic or pathologic evidence of Barrett esophagus ($n = 112$). *Results:* There were several favorable prognostic signs in the Barrett group, including smaller tumors, lower grade, and earlier stage. More patients in the Barrett group had surgically resectable tumors, resulting in an improved overall survival. However, there were no differences in the type or duration of symptoms. Overall, very few patients presented because of GERD, and only slightly more in the Barrett group (14% vs 4%). While survival greatly improved in patients diagnosed with Barrett due to GERD, this did not account for the difference in prognosis. *Conclusions:* Improved prognosis and survival for the Barrett group is not due to earlier presentation due to symptoms of GERD. It is more likely that all esophageal adenocarcinoma arises from Barrett esophagus, and that it is obscured by larger tumors. Reviews limited to resected patients greatly overestimate the number of adenocarcinoma cases diagnosed due to GERD. Increased efforts to identify high-risk patients and initiate screening are necessary to diagnose adenocarcinoma at an earlier stage.

Effect of operative volume on morbidity, mortality, and hospital use after esophagectomy for cancer.

Swisher SG, Deford L, Merriman KW, Walsh GL, Smythe R, Vaporicyan A, Ajani JA, Brown T, Komaki R, Roth JA, Putnam JB.

Departments of Thoracic and Cardiovascular Surgery, Medical Informatics, Gastrointestinal Oncology, and Radiation Oncology, The University of Texas M.D. Anderson Cancer Center, Houston, TX, USA.

Journal of Thoracic and Cardiovascular Surgery 119(6):1126–32, 2000, June.

Objective: We sought to evaluate the effect of operative volume, hospital size, and cancer specialization on morbidity, mortality, and hospital use after esophagectomy for cancer. *Methods:* Data derived from the Health Care Utilization Project was used to evaluate all Medicare-reimbursed esophagectomies for treatment of cancer from 1994 to 1996 in 13 national cancer institutions and 88 community hospitals. The complications of care, length of stay, hospital charges, and mortality were assessed according to hospital size ($\geqslant 600$ beds vs < 600 beds), cancer specialization (national cancer institution vs community hospital), and operative volume (esophageal [$\geqslant 5$ Medicare esophagectomies per year vs < 5 Medicare esophagectomies per year] and nonesophageal operations [$\geqslant 3333$ cases per year vs < 3333 cases per year]). *Results:* Mortality was lower in national cancer institution hospitals (4.2% [confidence interval, 2.0%–6.4%] vs 13.3% [confidence interval, 4.2%–26.2%], $p = 0.05$) and in hospitals performing a large number of esophagectomies (3.0% [confidence interval, 0.09%–5.1%] vs 12.2% [confidence interval, 4.5%–19.8%], $p < 0.05$). Multivariate analysis revealed that the independent risk factor for operative mortality was the volume of esophagectomies performed (odds ratio, 3.97; $p = 0.03$) and not the number of nonesophageal operations, hospital size, or cancer specialization. Hospitals performing a large number of esophagectomies also showed a tendency toward decreased complications (55% vs 68%, $p = 0.06$), decreased length of stay (14.7 days vs 17.7 days, $p = 0.006$), and decreased charges ($39,867 vs $62,094, $p < 0.005$). *Conclusions:* These results demonstrate improved outcomes and decreased hospital use in hospitals that perform a large number of esophagectomies and support the concept of tertiary referral centers for such complex oncologic procedures as esophagectomies.

Epithelial cells in bone marrow of oesophageal cancer patients: a significant prognostic factor in multivariate analysis.

Thorban S, Rosenberg R, Busch R, Roder RJ.

Department of Surgery, Technische Universitat Munchen, Germany.

British Journal of Cancer 83(1):35–9, 2000, July.

The detection of epithelial cells in bone marrow, blood or lymph nodes indicates a disseminatory potential of solid tumours. 225 patients with squamous cell carcinoma of the oesophagus were prospectively studied. Prior to any therapy, cytokeratin-positive (CK) cells in bone marrow were immunocytochemically detected in 75 patients with the monoclonal anti-epithelial-cell antibody A45-B/B3 and correlated with established histopathologic and patient-specific prognosis factors. The prognosis factors were assessed by multivariate analysis. Twenty-nine of 75 (38.7%) patients with oesophageal cancer showed CK-positive cells in bone marrow. The analyses of the mean and median overall survival time showed a significant difference between patients with and without epithelial cells in bone marrow ($p < 0.001$). Multivariate analysis in the total patient population and in patients with curative resection of the primary tumour confirmed the curative resection rate and the bone marrow status as the strongest independent prognostic factors, besides the T-category. The detection of epithelial cells in bone marrow of oesophageal cancer patients is a substantial prognostic factor proved by multivariate analysis and is helpful for exact preoperative staging, as well as monitoring of neoadjuvant therapy.

Randomized trial of preoperative chemoradiation versus surgery alone in patients with locoregional esophageal carcinoma.

Urba SG, Orringer MB, Turrisi A, Iannettoni M, Forastiere A, Strawderman M.

University of Michigan Medical Center, Ann Arbor, MI, USA.

Journal of Clinical Oncology 19:305–13, 2001.

Purpose: A pilot study of 43 patients with potentially resectable esophageal carcinoma treated with an intensive regimen of preoperative chemoradiation with cisplatin, fluorouracil, and vinblastine before surgery showed a median survival of 29 months in comparison with the 12-month median survival of 100 historical controls treated with surgery alone at the same institution. We designed a randomized trial to compare survival for patients treated with this preoperative chemoradiation regimen versus surgery alone. *Materials and methods:* One hundred patients with esophageal carcinoma were randomized to receive either surgery alone (arm I) or preoperative chemoradiation (arm II) with cisplatin 20 mg/m^2/d on days 1 through 5 and 17 through 21, fluorouracil 300 mg/m^2/d on days 1 through 21, and vinblastine 1 mg/m^2/d on days 1 through 4 and 17 through 20. Radiotherapy consisted of 1.5-Gy fractions twice daily, Monday through Friday over 21 days, to a total dose of 45 Gy. Transhiatal esophagectomy with a cervical esophagogastric anastomosis was performed on approximately day 42. *Results:* At median follow-up of 8.2 years, there is no significant difference in survival between the treatment arms. Median survival is 17.6 months in arm I and 16.9 months in arm II. Survival at 3 years was 16% in arm I and 30% in arm II ($p = 0.15$). This study was statistically powered to detect a relatively large increase in median survival from 1 year to 2.2 years, with at least 80% power. *Conclusion:* This randomized trial of preoperative chemoradiation versus surgery alone for patients with potentially resectable esophageal carcinoma did not demonstrate a statistically significant survival difference.

21

Surgical management of gastric cancer

WALTER LAWRENCE Jr

INTRODUCTION

For 2001, gastric cancer is estimated to be the cause of only 2.3% of all cancer deaths in the USA and it will rank eighth in mortality, in terms of anatomic site of cancer origin.[1] This represents a striking decline in both incidence and mortality from 1930, when gastric cancer was the number one cause of cancer mortality and represented 38% of all cancer deaths in the USA.[2-4] This decline, occurring mainly between 1930 and 1985, is shown graphically in Figure 21.1, where it is contrasted with mortality data for cancers of the colon and rectum. Because this unique decrease in mortality occurred specifically in the USA, not in most other countries[5-6] and not in association with significant alterations in treatment methods, it is presumed that some exogenous factor (or factors) affecting incidence was responsible. Possible explanations include various dietary alterations, particularly changes in methods of food preservation (with more emphasis on frozen foods over the last several

decades), and possibly an increase in the intake of vitamin C by our population.[7-9] Another potential causative factor for gastric cancer that has received considerable attention in the last few years is chronic *Helicobacter pylori* infection.[10-16] A relationship of the possible antibiotic control of *H. pylori* to the decreasing incidence of peptic ulcers now appears likely, and a similar mechanism may well be operative for the decrease in incidence of some forms of gastric cancer. Clarification of factors affecting carcinogenesis will be of great importance to the development of prevention strategies in those countries where gastric cancer is still a relatively common, often fatal, disease.[17]

Many think the decrease in the frequency of gastric cancer in the USA makes this disorder a less important challenge to surgical oncologists here. It should be pointed out, however, that this decrease in gastric cancer incidence actually 'plateaued' somewhat after 1985. Gastric cancer incidence continued to decrease slightly after 1985, but the disease has not disappeared! Evidence

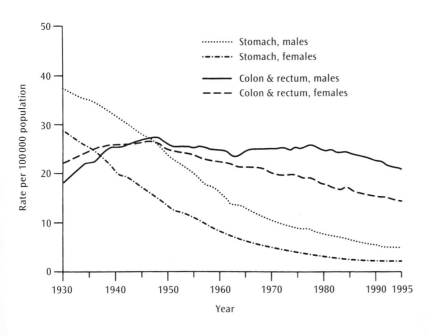

Figure 21.1 *Trend in mortality of gastric cancer in the USA contrasted with that for colon cancer. (Modified from* Cancer facts and figures – 2000.[1])

for this fact comes from the patterns-of-care study of gastric cancer conducted by the American College of Surgeons and reported by Wanebo and coworkers,[4] as well as from the reported data from the National Cancer Data Base (NCDB) studies comparing the years 1985 and 1986 with 1991.[2,18] Operations for gastric cancer are less frequent, but radical gastrectomy is still an operative strategy that requires expertise, and it must be included in the armamentarium of the surgical oncologist.

Another trend in gastric cancer presentation over the last few decades is a shift in the anatomic location of the primary lesions. A number of authors have pointed out that there has been a distinct change from the predominantly distal gastric cancers in earlier years to a greater frequency of lesions in the proximal stomach.[3,19,20] Of some concern is the fact that proximal gastric cancers have a worse prognosis when compared to distal lesions, and the operative approach to the cancer certainly is more complex and more morbid for proximal lesions, due to the need for an esophageal anastomosis. The cause of this shift in anatomic location of gastric cancer is unclear. However, recent observations on *H. pylori* may provide a partial explanation because this chronic infection is associated with atrophic gastritis, the precancerous change most often associated with the 'intestinal type' that is characteristic of distal gastric cancer.[14,15] The reduction in infection by this organism (due to the widespread use of antibiotics?) may have led to a decrease in distal gastric cancer. Also, the proximal trend in anatomic site may be related, in some way, to the marked increase in incidence of adenocarcinoma of the distal esophagus that has been observed over recent years.[21]

New diagnostic, staging, and therapeutic techniques available to us have changed the patterns of care of many diseases for which operation has been a mainstay of treatment. Radiologic imaging, endoscopic advances, ultrasound, interventional radiologic approaches, and laparoscopy are outstanding examples. How this has affected our management of gastric cancer or will do in the future deserves discussion in this chapter.

Yet another trend worth noting is the apparent relative increase in the incidence of primary gastric lymphoma.[22,23] At one time, this was a rare type of gastric cancer, but now the diagnosis is more frequently made, often prior to operation. It is important for the surgical oncologist to be fully acquainted with the potential for non-operative therapy for primary gastric lymphoma to be able to participate on the management team for this disorder as new concepts of treatment evolve.

DIAGNOSIS OF GASTRIC CANCER

The lesson learned first with cancer of the cervix, and then with cancers of the breast and prostate, is that a diagnosis of cancer at an early stage of disease leads to a better outcome than when diagnosis is made at more advanced stages. The ultimate approach, other than primary prevention, is the screening of asymptomatic, 'high-risk' individuals, as this 'secondary' prevention has detected (and allowed the effective treatment of) not only early stage cancers, but precancerous lesions as well. In some Japanese centers, the validity of this concept of screening for gastric cancer has been demonstrated by the early detection of cancers that are confined to the mucosa, or 'early gastric cancer.'[24,25] These early gastric cancers detected by screening have had a higher cure rate, as one might expect, and the relatively rare early gastric cancers that have been diagnosed in the USA have a comparable prognosis.[26,27] In Japan, such diagnoses have led to less aggressive treatment strategies in selected cases.[28] The problem for us, of course, is that the yield from any attempt at gastric cancer screening in the USA would be far too low to ever approach cost-effectiveness, except for a very few 'high-risk' populations (e.g., patients with pernicious anemia and, possibly, patients who have previously undergone partial gastrectomy for benign disease).[29,30] Despite the lack of feasibility of gastric cancer screening programs in the USA, the increasing use of upper gastrointestinal endoscopy over the last several decades has allowed more precise, and possibly earlier, diagnosis of gastric lesions. Previously, we relied primarily on radiologic procedures for diagnosis and these were not as sensitive as endoscopy. Double contrast radiologic study has increased accuracy, but biopsy capability with endoscopy adds the advantage of precision regarding both the diagnosis of cancer and determination of the specific variety.

Continued efforts to make a specific diagnosis for patients older than 40 who have persistent, vague upper gastrointestinal symptoms are essential if we are to make diagnoses of gastric cancer at a curable stage. The recent popular, but unfortunate, trend toward prolonged therapeutic trials of symptom-relieving medications before conducting detailed diagnostic procedures is to be discouraged, despite the cost savings that have been attributed to this approach.

STAGING OF GASTRIC CANCER

A few words on the staging of gastric cancer are appropriate, as staging concepts are relevant to the recent discussions of alterations in our operations, particularly the concepts expressed by Japanese investigators relating to early gastric cancer and to extended lymph node dissections. *Clinical* staging of the gastric cancer patient has been based on the extent of disease as shown by physical examination and by diagnostic radiologic or endoscopic studies. The prognosis of carcinoma may be affected by other parameters such as carcinoembryonic antigen (CEA) or other tumor markers,[31] histologic grading, *p53* expression,[32] cell proliferation kinetic indicators, and tumor DNA ploidy pattern,[33–35] but none of these parameters is incorporated in the TNM staging system now in use. The prognostically valuable part of the TNM staging system of the American Joint Committee on Cancer (AJCC) has depended almost entirely on information obtained from a pathologic specimen.[36] Pathologic staging, as opposed to the clinico-diagnostic stage, appears to be the most prognostically useful staging process, other than the clinical determination of 'inoperability.' However, computed tomography (CT) and the relatively new procedures of endoscopic ultrasound (EUS) and laparoscopy may improve our ability to stage patients *prior* to open surgical intervention.

A preoperative staging procedure available only over the past 20 years is CT.[37] Most surgeons have argued that the algorithm for deciding on operative treatment is not altered by preoperative CT findings, just as has been argued for patients with colon cancer, because an operation is still indicated for palliation, if not for cure. The major additional findings with CT are those of unsuspected liver metastases and extragastric metastatic disease. However, CT does allow somewhat more accurate T-staging,[38] and allows some estimation of regional lymph node spread,[39] as well as detecting distant metastasis not appreciated on physical examination. This additional information is often useful, as it may lead to the clinical decision not to operate or to employ preoperative non-operative therapy. In the latter case, these staging findings are useful later for assessing treatment response.

EUS allows the endoscopist to visualize all layers of the gastric wall and to identify the full extent of the primary neoplasm in terms of its depth of invasion (T1, T2, T3, T4), and this leads to further refinement of pretreatment T-evaluation.[40–45] Assessment of lymph node status by EUS is less precise than T-evaluation, and often adds little to the information already obtained by CT, but it is useful in some instances for identifying obvious regional lymph node involvement. Regional lymph nodes can be needle-biopsied under ultrasound guidance during the procedure.[46] The role of EUS for the staging of gastric cancer is not quite as clear as it is in the staging of esophageal and rectal cancers, where it clearly affects surgical decision making. However, it may prove to have a similar role for gastric cancer in the future. Also, the added information regarding stage obtained from laparoscopy would clearly justify its use.[47–49]

Concepts of pathologic staging are important to the surgical oncologist when it comes to assessing the role of various aspects of the operation for gastric cancer, particularly the lymph node dissection. The extent of the primary tumor (T), lymph node spread (N), and the most recent AJCC pathologic stage groupings are shown in Table 21.1.[36] Both histopathologic type and grade of gastric cancer have an impact on prognosis, but these features are not now elements of the standard, agreed-upon staging systems of the AJCC or the International Union

Against Cancer (UICC). It is apparent from the NCDB,[2,18] and other similar clinical data sources, that the stage grouping employed in the AJCC system does have a significant impact on prognosis, as would be expected, because the system was constructed on the basis of clinical outcomes. This staging system has been, and will continue to be, useful for making various non-randomized comparisons of differing treatment strategies until convincing randomized treatment data are available.

OPERATIVE TREATMENT OF GASTRIC CANCER

Before there were any non-operative therapies available for cancer, Dr Theodor Billroth performed the first resection of gastric cancer with survival of the patient in 1881 (Figure 21.2). Operative resection remains the mainstay of therapy, despite the continued frequency of treatment failure with gastric cancer. Possibly the only major recent therapeutic advance in the surgical area has been an increase in the safety of major operations of all types. The decrease in the incidence of gastric cancer, and in the number of operations required for peptic ulcer disease, has led younger surgeons to have considerably less

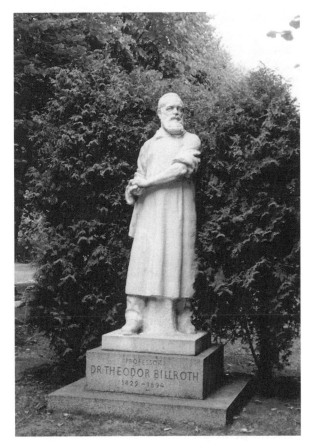

Figure 21.2 *Statue of Billroth in front of the hospital where he performed the first successful gastrectomy for cancer in 1881, in Vienna, Austria.*

Table 21.1 *TNM staging for stomach cancer*

Classification	Definition		
Primary tumor (T)			
TX	Primary tumor cannot be assessed		
T0	No evidence of primary tumor		
Tis	Carcinoma *in situ*; intraepithelial tumor without invasion of lamina propia		
T1	Tumor invades lamina propria or submucosa		
T2	Tumor invades the muscularis propria or the subserosa		
T3	Tumor penetrates the serosa (visceral peritoneum) without invasion of adjacent structures		
T4	Tumor invades adjacent structures		
Regional lymph nodes (N)			
NX	Regional lymph node(s) cannot be assessed		
N0	No regional lymph node metastasis		
N1	Metastasis in 1–6 regional nodes		
N2	Metastasis in 7–15 regional nodes		
N3	Metastasis in more than 15 regional lymph nodes		
Distant metastasis (M)			
MX	Presence of distant metastasis cannot be assessed		
M0	No distant metastasis		
M1	Distant metastasis		
AJCC/UICC stage grouping			
Stage 0	Tis	N0	M0
Stage IA	T1	N0	M0
Stage IB	T1	N1	M0
	T2	N0	M0
Stage II	T1	N2	M0
	T2	N1	M0
	T3	N0	M0
Stage IIIA	T2	N2	M0
	T3	N1	M0
	T4	N0	M0
Stage IIIB	T3	N2	M0
Stage IV	T4	N1	M0
	T1	N3	M0
	T2	N3	M0
	T3	N3	M0
	T4	N2	M0
	T4	N3	M0
	Any T	Any N	M1

From American Joint Committee on Cancer.[36]

familiarity with gastric resection, a justification for reviewing here some of the technical features of the operative approach to gastric cancer. These include general principles of resection, decisions regarding the extent of the resection itself, the appropriate extent of the lymph node dissection accompanying this resection, the method and importance of the post-resection reconstruction employed, and the potential role of laparoscopy in the overall management of gastric neoplasms.

General principles

Gastrectomy was one of the most commonly performed operations in the USA when it was utilized to treat many peptic ulcer patients. Now that peptic ulcer disease has decreased in incidence and lesser procedures, such as parietal cell vagotomy, are employed, gastric resection has become an infrequent operation. Another fact worth emphasizing is that resection of the stomach for cancer is a completely different operation from the one usually employed for peptic ulcer disease. Not only is it necessary to be certain there are broad gross margins around the cancer in the stomach (and in the esophagus for proximal gastric lesions), but the removal of potentially involved regional lymph nodes is generally considered an important part of the procedure. There is no way that supplemental non-operative treatment can make up for narrow or questionable margins around the primary lesion (as there is when we use adjuvant radiation for the treatment of narrow margins at operation for breast cancer or soft tissue sarcoma). Although the presence of lymph node spread worsens the prognosis, some gastric cancer patients with lymph node metastases appear to be cured as a result of regional lymphadenectomy. This supports the inclusion of regional lymph nodes in the resection, but, at present, there is uncertainty concerning the optimal extent of lymphadenectomy.

In line with the above, *wide* resection of the primary lesion in the stomach and en-bloc excision of actual or potential lymphatic extensions of the neoplasm are indicated if a regionally localized process is found at the time of abdominal exploration. The detailed operative techniques for this so-called 'radical' subtotal or total gastrectomy are presented with illustrations elsewhere, and the reader is referred to those books for details of both the resections and the reconstructions employed.[50–51]

Partial versus total gastric resection

The optimal extent of gastric resection for cancer was first seriously questioned in the 1940s by Lahey and Marshall,[52] and McNeer et al.,[53] who proposed the concept of removal of the entire organ for cancer, rather than removing only that portion of the stomach actually involved by the process. The concept was based on a study of the sites of 'failure' after subtotal gastrectomy.[54] It was hoped that total gastrectomy would improve the rather poor end results of the time. Part of the rationale for this proposal was that total gastrectomy allowed a more thorough lymph node dissection, as will be discussed subsequently, but the major reason advanced was the concept that the entire organ was 'at risk,' just as is the case with the breast that harbors a breast cancer. No randomized trial data were brought to bear on this idea of routinely removing the entire organ of origin of the cancer, but subsequent, non-randomized comparison data on post-resection outcomes failed to support routine total gastrectomy for all patients as superior to 'custommade' resections based on the observed local extent of the neoplasm.[55] These same data impacted on the approach in the USA to surgical decisions regarding the extent of lymph node dissection, as discussed below. Although there are no data in the USA that demonstrate routine total gastrectomy has a survival advantage,[56] many of us feel that total gastrectomy is superior to partial proximal gastrectomy for *proximal* gastric lesions, for reasons unrelated to either the extent of lymph node dissection or the expected cure rate. These reasons include avoiding the reflux esophagitis that is often associated with minimal proximal gastric resection, and the avoidance of an inadequate distal gastric reservoir when the proximal resection is more extensive. With this exception, the extent of operation on the stomach recommended by

most surgeons varies with the anatomy of the specific lesion and is determined by both the location in the stomach and the local extent of the neoplasm.

Inclusion of adjacent organs

As with other primary cancers in the abdomen, more advanced gastric cancers often become adherent to, or locally invade, adjacent anatomical structures. This extension adversely impacts on prognosis, to some extent, but this finding is not nearly as concerning as the presence of lymphatic spread or peritoneal spread if a complete resection of the involved adjacent structures is feasible. One of the more common sites for this local adherence problem is the region of the transverse mesocolon and the middle colic vessels. If there is no distant spread of the cancer in the abdomen, the mesocolon and middle colic vessels can be resected with the stomach, leaving the adherent tissue attached to the gastric specimen. Adequate collateral blood supply in the transverse mesocolon will usually allow sacrifice of the proximal middle colic vessels, without resection of the transverse colon, but the colon should be resected also if there is any question about the adequacy of its blood supply. The posterior portion of the stomach, particularly the proximal stomach, is not infrequently adherent to the body or tail of the pancreas, and this is an indication for an en-bloc resection of the body and tail of the pancreas along with the spleen. Occasionally, the left lateral segment of the liver is adherent to a proximal gastric cancer, and this lateral segment can be resected 'in continuity' with the gastrectomy, also. Although all of these extensions of gastrectomy are reasonably well tolerated by the patient, and accepted by most surgeons, it is more difficult to say whether resection of the head of the pancreas and duodenum with distal subtotal or total gastrectomy is justified when there is local extension of the gastric cancer to this portion of the pancreas. Pancreatoduodenectomy is a major and morbid extension of subtotal or total gastrectomy for cancer, but it should be remembered that the 'standard' Whipple operation for primary cancer of the pancreas also removes the distal stomach and produces an anatomic defect not too dissimilar to that which would be required for resection of a distal gastric cancer invading the head of the pancreas. The difference, of course, is that a primary gastric cancer with operative findings requiring inclusion of the pancreatic head might well involve other adjacent tissues that would not be thoroughly resected by this type of operation. This is undoubtedly the reason so few resections of this type are carried out. Three such extended operations performed by the author in the past resulted in local recurrence within 12 months in two instances, but long-term survival without recurrence occurred with the other patient. Consideration of resection of adjacent adherent organs, rather than limiting the operation to palliative removal of the gastric lesion only, is supported by the fact that our results from using non-operative therapies for residual gastric cancer are so disappointing.

An interest in including splenectomy with gastric resection for cancer was prompted years ago by the observation that splenic hilar lymph nodes often contained metastatic deposits.[57] The concept that survival might be enhanced by removing all potentially involved lymph nodes was applied to this specific location long before the more recent proposals for a more systematic and thorough attack on multiple lymph node groups in the upper abdomen. However, older data on patterns of lymphatic spread demonstrated clearly that there was a flaw in the idea of an isolated removal of the spleen in addition to a conventional lymphatic dissection for gastric cancer. The detailed lymphatic studies we carried out on specimens removed by 'extended total gastrectomy' (total gastrectomy with distal pancreatectomy and splenectomy), reported in 1953, never demonstrated involved lymph nodes in the splenic hilum *unless* one or more nodes in the chain of pancreato-lienal lymph nodes were involved as well (Figure 21.3).[53,58] This finding demonstrated that the route of lymphatic spread was from the peripancreatic area to the splenic hilum portion of this lymphatic chain. It showed also that there was a fallacy in isolated splenic resection along with gastrectomy, unless the nodes along the body and tail of the pancreas were removed as well. Subsequent clinical studies have failed to support the addition of simple splenectomy to gastric resection, except in those instances in which direct invasion or adherence to the spleen was observed.[59,60] An increase in morbidity and mortality has also been described for this extension of the operation.[61]

Extent of lymph node dissection for 'curative' gastrectomy for gastric cancer

It has been known for some time that the overall end results after operations for gastric cancer in Japan are superior to the results that have been obtained in most of the USA and Europe.[62] A number of non-randomized comparisons of operative results from Japan support the concept that these improved results in Japan *might* be due to the use of more extensive regional lymph node dissections by Japanese surgeons than by most surgeons elsewhere in the world.[63–68] This concern regarding the extent of lymphadenectomy for gastric cancer remained unresolved until recently due to the limited data that were available from randomized clinical trials.

Lymphatic spread has long been recognized as a major prognostic determinant for gastric cancer, and it is not surprising that this difference noted between the end results in Japan and those in the USA and Europe was attributed to the more extensive lymph node dissections often conducted by Japanese surgeons. Other factors confuse the situation, however. The possibility that underlying

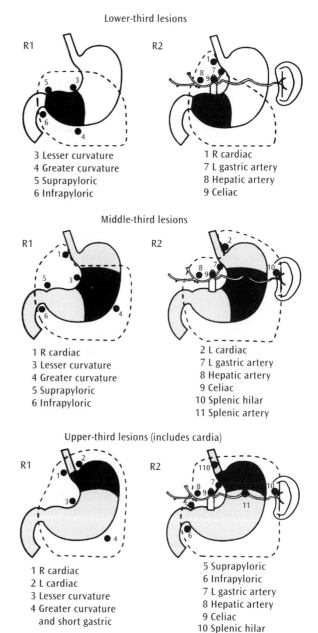

Figure 21.3 *The scope of gastric lymphadenectomy based on the location of the primary cancer. (Reprinted with permission of the American Medical Association, from Smith et al., 1991.[131])*

racial or ethnic differences in these various populations might herald a different biology of these tumors in Japanese and Caucasian patients has been suggested (and rejected),[69] but a major factor considered has been stage differences between these different populations at the time of operation.[70] The proportion of cancers that are 'early gastric cancers,' which result in a much better survival rate, has progressively increased in Japan since the mid-1950s. On this basis, it has been suggested that the difference in postoperative outcome observed between Japanese series and other series results entirely from differences in the stage of disease (or stage 'migration') rather than the extent of lymphadenectomy employed.[62] Others refute this explanation. Another possible explanation is a pathologic one. Major differences in diagnostic criteria for gastric carcinoma between Japanese and Western pathologists have been shown in a recent study.[71] This may well contribute to the higher incidence and the better prognosis after treatment for gastric carcinoma in Japan overall, and also help to explain the geographic differences in survival noted. Nevertheless, the questions regarding the reasons for differences in treatment results and the optimal extent of lymphadenectomy still remain unanswered.

Japanese surgeons continue to be meticulous in their description of multiple anatomic groups of regional lymph nodes that may become involved with metastatic disease. They have developed a uniform classification of gastric resection in terms of the extent of stomach removal and the extent of lymph node dissection using a rather complex staging classification of lymph nodes (N1–N4).[62] The Japanese terminology for differing levels of lymph node dissection is relevant to this discussion of the potential value of more extensive dissections (Figure 21.3). It is as follows:

1 R1 resection includes en-bloc dissection of N1 nodes as defined in an earlier TNM classification (where N related to distance from the primary lesion rather than the number of involved nodes, as defined in the 1997 version).[36]

2 R2 resection includes N1 and N2 lymph nodes using the earlier classification for N. If distal subtotal gastrectomy is employed, the spleen and distal pancreas are *not* removed. With total gastrectomy, splenectomy is performed and distal pancreatectomy is included if the serosa, the greater curvature or the posterior wall of the stomach is involved.

3 R3 resection means complete resection of N1, N2, and N3 lymph nodes in the earlier TNM classification. N3 lymph nodes were generally considered distant metastases in the AJCC classification. Now that the AJCC N classification is strictly related to the actual number of involved nodes, this classification of the extent of lymphadenectomy is not well described in terms of current TNM categories.

In addition to multiple reports from the Far East supporting the value of extended lymphadenectomy, successful efforts to emulate these improved results have been reported from the West by Siewert *et al.*[72,73] (Germany), Jatzko *et al.*[74] (Austria), and by Volpe *et al.*[75,76] (USA). These reports of non-randomized comparisons of the outcomes following extended lymph node dissection with earlier surgical results using more limited lymph node dissection have further increased the suspicion around the world that extended

lymphadenectomy is 'better.' However, recent retrospective evaluation from the USA using the American College of Surgeons database failed to show survival benefit from the N2 dissection.[77]

While many surgeons in both the Eastern and Western worlds stress the need for the more extensive dissections, most surgeons in Western countries remain skeptical of the advantage of these possibly morbid extensions. Before addressing the recent randomized trials that relate to this question, it is probably worthwhile to review earlier information that led to a general bias toward a more conservative lymphadenectomy in the USA than employed in Japan. After personal armchair enthusiasm in earlier years for the potential benefit of an extensive lymphadenectomy by means of a routine 'extended total gastrectomy,'[53] this author retrospectively compared the overall results of gastric resection for cancer during two different time intervals at a major cancer center.[55] The first time period (1945–1950) was an era when the resection policy was 'conservative,' what in Japan is now called an R1 type of dissection. The second time period was 1950–1955, a period in which more than half of the gastric cancer patients at this same cancer center were treated by an 'extended total gastrectomy.'[78] This extended procedure included routine resection of the body and tail of the pancreas and spleen, in order to remove the secondary orbit of lymph nodes, the so-called pancreatolienal nodes (Figure 21.4). This was an operation similar to the so-called R2 resection.[53] Assessment in 1960 of the survival of *all* patients for these two time periods failed to show any differences in overall survival, nor was there a difference in survival for all patients undergoing

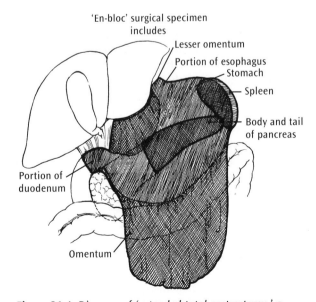

Figure 21.4 *Diagram of 'extended total gastrectomy,' a total gastrectomy combined with distal pancreatectomy and splenectomy. This procedure was intended to accomplish more extensive lymph node dissection. (From Lawrence, 1990.[50])*

'curative' resection during these two time periods.[55] This lack of survival benefit in the later interval, when the policy for curative resection stressed more extensive lymphadenectomy, led to a significant revision of this author's thoughts at that time. Gilbertson's retrospective analysis of 1983 cases of gastric cancer at the University of Minnesota operated between 1936 and 1963 echoed these findings.[79] During an earlier interval (1936–1958), when conservative resection was the order of the day, the operative mortality was lower and the overall survival slightly higher than in the later period (1958–1963), when there was widespread use of extensive lymph node dissections. This finding was similar to our own. My personal conclusion on the basis of all these data was that routine extension of elective lymphadenectomy to include the pancreato-lienal nodes was probably not justified. The intriguing observations from Japan of better survival after extended lymphadenectomy clearly lead to the need for data from randomized trials to answer this question.

The key question is whether R2 dissection adds significant survival benefit to that achieved by R1 dissection. We often develop enthusiasm for a new treatment approach, based on non-randomized retrospective comparisons, only to be disappointed when a subsequent randomized clinical trial fails to support our initial concepts based on 'historic controls.' Randomized clinical trials have been conducted to answer this question regarding the optimal extent of lymphadenectomy. The first completed trial, a small trial from South Africa reported by Dent et al.,[80] failed to show a survival benefit from R2 dissection when these patients were compared with a group undergoing R1 dissection. A more recent trial reported from Hong Kong compared R1 subtotal gastrectomy with R3 total gastrectomy for *antral* cancers.[81] This study failed to show survival benefit after extensive lymphadenectomy, and the morbidity was significantly greater in the R3 group. A much larger trial reported recently from the Netherlands – a prospective, randomized comparison of R1 with R2 dissections – evaluated adherence in this trial to the specific surgical– pathologic guidelines.[82] Although the morbidity with more extensive dissection in this study was increased,[83] some considered it 'acceptable.'[84] The overall design and size of the Dutch trial, including significant efforts to standardize the operations, gave hope of obtaining a convincing answer to the question posed. This study was completed and a recent report has demonstrated that, despite improved survival data in both groups, D2 survival was no better than after D1 dissection.[85] This randomized trial of 711 patients appears to settle the question for Western patients.

It should be stressed that there are no *randomized* trial data thus far that support the contention that more extensive (R2 or R3) lymphatic dissection is justified for Western patients, but, alternatively, there may not be adequate evidence to discount completely the possible value of more extensive dissections in Japanese patients. However, any benefit in this latter population must be small, if present. The accepted policy of only performing a 'standard' regional dissection of perigastric lymph nodes (R1 in Japanese terms) is probably appropriate *at this time* for resectable gastric cancer in the USA, rather than routinely conducting these more extensive lymph node dissections that clearly appear to be associated with an increase in morbidity.

Reconstruction after gastrectomy for gastric cancer

After distal partial gastrectomy for gastric cancer, it is generally recommended that continuity be restored by gastrojejunostomy rather than gastroduodenostomy because this approach avoids the problem of possible gastric outlet obstruction if locally recurrent carcinoma develops. Autopsy studies in the distant past pointed out the high frequency of recurrent disease in the 'bed of the stomach' in and around the pancreas in those patients demonstrating treatment failure.[54] This pattern of recurrent disease would tend to cause gastric outlet obstruction more often if gastroduodenostomy has been established rather than anterior gastrojejunostomy. There is no physiologic advantage to gastroduodenostomy as there is no evidence that the absorption of nutrients or the symptoms following this operation are any different.

After total gastrectomy, the most troublesome part of the reconstruction is the esophageal anastomosis. This needs to be performed as precisely as possible to avoid subsequent leakage, because this is the major cause of morbidity and mortality after total gastrectomy. The esophageal anastomosis can be performed equally well by direct suture anastomosis or by stapling instruments. Despite a focus on other aspects of the reconstruction after total gastrectomy in earlier years, it is now clear that the most important feature of the reconstruction after resection of the cardia or the entire stomach is a precise esophageal anastomosis (Figure 21.5)!

The specific details of reconstruction after total gastrectomy for cancer have received considerable attention over the years. Methods employed have ranged from simple to complex techniques, but all methods have been difficult to assess due to great individual patient variability in response to food intake after these major alterations in upper gastrointestinal anatomy. Until recently, most surgeons developed a preference for one method of reconstruction or another, often based on assumptions regarding the relative importance of a pouch of some kind and the importance of 'routing' of foodstuffs.

Reconstruction after total gastrectomy initially employed a simple approach involving correction of the operative defect by either esophagojejunostomy or esophagoduodenostomy, the former being the most

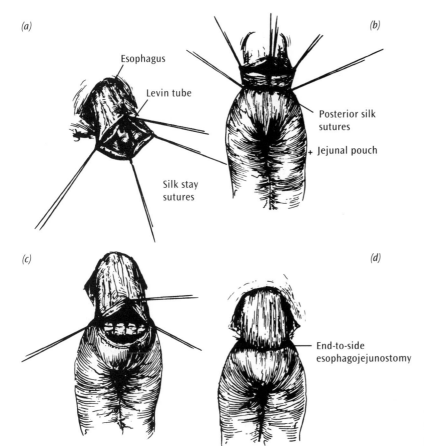

(a)

Esophagus

Levin tube

Silk stay
sutures

(b)

Posterior silk
sutures

Jejunal pouch

(c)

(d)

End-to-side
esophagojejunostomy

Figure 21.5 *Esophageal anastomosis after total gastrectomy utilizing suture technique. (From Lawrence, 1990.[50])*

commonly employed due to the greater ease of approximating the esophagus and the jejunum. Malnutrition after initial recovery from the operative procedure was a frequent accompaniment of total gastrectomy when such simple reconstructive procedures were employed. Because postgastrectomy malnutrition and reduced 'quality of life,' as manifested by decreased food capacity, postprandial unpleasant symptoms, and problems in body weight maintenance seemed to be related in some way to both the absence of the stomach and a potentially faulty reconstruction, new and more complex ideas for reconstruction were developed (Figures 21.6 and 21.7). The goal of all these efforts was to increase total nutritional intake by both increasing capacity and decreasing postprandial symptoms, thereby leading to better weight maintenance overall.

The broad questions that have developed regarding the actual technique of reconstruction are:

1 Is an intestinal reservoir substitute for the missing stomach useful in achieving increased total food intake?
2 Is 'duodenal passage' of foodstuff preferable to bypass of the duodenum by a Roux-en-Y anastomosis?
3 Do any of these reconstruction procedures actually delay the transit of foodstuff in such a way that they thereby reduce so-called dumping symptoms?

Until recently, most surgeons presumed they knew the correct answers to these questions and based their choice of reconstructive approach on these assumptions. They might favor a jejunal reservoir, or they might reject this approach as a non-beneficial addition. They might route the foodstuff through the duodenum, often with a jejunal reservoir segment, or, alternatively, use a Roux-en-Y reconstruction in which the duodenum is bypassed. Also, the transit in the small bowel may be modified by the Roux-en-Y anastomosis itself. The marked variability in the nutritional response of individual patients and the relatively small series of total gastrectomy patients that were studied objectively made definitive answers to the above questions difficult to obtain. In the last few years, however, prospective, randomized trials have addressed these specific questions and it would appear that the preferred method of reconstruction after total gastrectomy can now be defined on a more scientific basis.

Is a reservoir a significant addition to reconstruction after total gastrectomy? The first clinical trial that objectively addressed this question was a 1987 randomized study by Troidl *et al.*[86] comparing simple esophagojejunostomy with enteroenterostomy between two jejunal loops, to a double lumen jejunal pouch proximal to a Roux-en-Y anastomosis. Evaluation of postprandial symptoms and evaluation of weight maintenance following gastrectomy

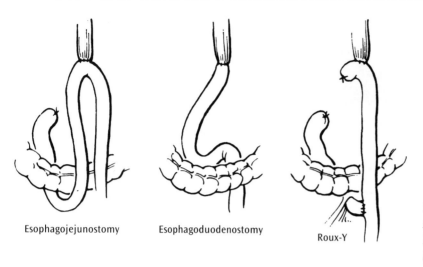

Esophagojejunostomy   Esophagoduodenostomy   Roux-Y

Figure 21.6 *Diagrams demonstrating simple means of reconstructing the intestinal tract after total gastrectomy. (From Lawrence, 1962.[92])*

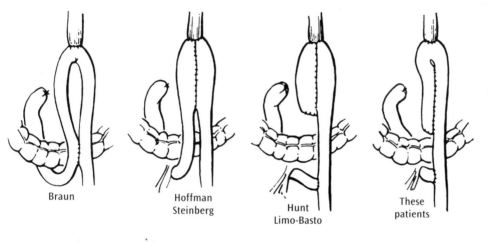

Braun   Hoffman Steinberg   Hunt Limo-Basto   These patients

Figure 21.7 *Diagrams of simple methods for construction of a jejunal reservoir after total gastrectomy. The diagram on the right demonstrates the operation preferred by the author, an operation preserving blood supply to the jejunum at the site of esophageal anastomosis. (From Lawrence, 1962.[92])*

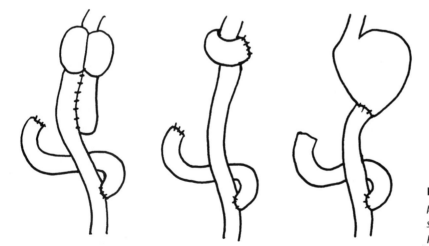

Figure 21.8 *Three groups of postgastrectomy reconstructions studied by Buhl et al.[87] (Each has Roux-en-Y anastomosis.)*

both showed benefit in favor of the pouch and Roux-en-Y anastomosis. Whether or not this observed benefit can be attributed totally to the jejunal reservoir might be considered presumptuous, because the Roux-en-Y anastomosis could delay intestinal transit significantly and, thus, be the major explanation for the superiority of results in the pouch group. A subsequent non-randomized study of 104 subjects by Buhl *et al.*[87] specifically assessed the role of the jejunal pouch. (Figure 21.8) All patients in this study had a Roux-en-Y anastomosis (and bypass of the duodenum), and the group with a double lumen jejunal pouch clearly did better nutritionally than the group without a pouch. The creation of a pouch from the jejunum gave nutritional results that were quite similar to those obtained with another group of concurrent patients who had only distal *partial* gastrectomy. These data gave further support to the benefit of a jejunal pouch as part of the reconstruction.

Is 'duodenal passage' important? A study by Nakane *et al.*[88] addressed the possible increased or decreased benefit of reconstruction by Roux-en-Y anastomosis by randomizing jejunal pouch reconstructions by this route versus the same pouch using 'duodenal passage' instead. A third experimental group had a Roux-en-Y anastomosis without a jejunal pouch and served as an additional control. In this study, the patients with the pouch and the Roux-en-Y anastomosis achieved greater food intake and greater weight recovery than the other experimental groups, thereby appearing to confirm the superiority of the pouch and Roux-en-Y combination over other methods of reconstruction. A study by Fuchs *et al.*[89] did not fully support those findings, however.

Is there a reason why reconstruction after total gastrectomy by jejunal pouch with Roux-en-Y anastomosis should give better simulation of normal gastric function than other reconstructive methods? A possible explanation of long standing has been that the jejunal pouch can function effectively as a reservoir if there is a pseudopyloric function introduced by using the Roux-en-Y anastomosis. Initial evidence for this anastomosis functioning in this fashion came from postsurgical radiologic studies described in the 1950s by Dr Limo-Basto of Portugal.[90] Whether the delay in transit following barium-impregnated meals he demonstrated was due to transection of the circular muscle of the jejunum or to partial obstruction at the Roux-en-Y anastomotic site was unclear. However, a significant reduction in motility has been demonstrated in the human jejunum after a double lumen jejunal pouch has been created, when compared to the motility of a simple efferent jejunal limb.[91] It would appear from this study that the rate of transit in the region of the jejunal pouch may be slowed enough to contribute to the desired storage function without completely relying on the concept of a pseudopylorus advanced by Limo-Basto, but both mechanisms may be operative in slowing transit.

From the data summarized above, it appears that a jejunal pouch reservoir with distal Roux-en-Y anastomosis after total gastrectomy is superior to reconstruction without a pouch (Figure 21.9). This approach is probably superior to using the same type of pouch via the duodenal route (rather than Roux-en-Y anastomosis), but clinical trial data results are somewhat conflicting on this point. Last, but not least, the type of reconstruction supported by these clinical trial data is easily and rapidly constructed by either suture or stapling techniques. After years of preferring this approach of jejunal pouch with Roux-en-Y anastomosis on clinical grounds only,[92] there are now clinical trial data to support this approach.

If proximal *partial* gastrectomy is chosen for a specific case, a precise anastomosis between the transected esophagus and the anterior wall of the gastric remnant is carried out. Some form of pyloroplasty (or pyloromyotomy) is advisable under these circumstances, because the resection includes truncal vagotomy and carries the potential for partial obstruction at the pylorus. As noted earlier, the author does not favor proximal partial gastrectomy because of the possibility of either acid reflux problems in the esophagus or inadequate gastric reservoir when the resection is more extensive.

Palliative resections

A significant number of patients who are explored with the hope of resection have unfavorable operative findings, such as serosal implants, liver or ovarian metastases, or metastases in lymph nodes outside the limits of a radical en-bloc resection. This was the case in almost two-thirds of patients in a large prechemotherapy series who were operated on with the hope that a curative gastric resection was possible.[93] The addition of CT scanning in more recent years has allowed the identification of many of these patients with incurable disease prior to operation, but some patients still have not had adverse findings of incurability detected until the time of celiotomy. This has been the justification for the recommendation by some that laparoscopy should precede operative exploration in patients with gastric cancer,[48] but most surgeons advocate some form of resection, whether or not signs of incurability exist. The benefit of palliative resection over simple gastrojejunostomy, gastrostomy, or jejunostomy has been appreciated for a long time. Resection, when feasible, achieves a higher rate of symptomatic relief, and longer survival.[93,94]

In earlier years, palliative distal gastrectomy became well accepted, but total gastrectomy for palliation was rarely employed due to the expectation of much higher morbidity and mortality than exists now. Indications for total gastrectomy, as a palliative procedure, included distal outlet obstruction or a patient in whom the only anatomic reason for incurability was distant lymphatic spread. Palliative gastrectomy (partial or total) under this latter circumstance has yielded significantly longer survival intervals than with patients undergoing palliative resection for liver or peritoneal metastases.[93] With the passage of time, and improved postoperative management, there has been a marked decrease in morbidity and mortality following total gastrectomy. There is now general agreement, as noted above, that total gastrectomy is sometimes a worthwhile palliative procedure, even in the presence of advanced disease.[95] However, not all patients with signs of incurability are suitable for total gastrectomy, particularly those whose projected survival times are quite short.

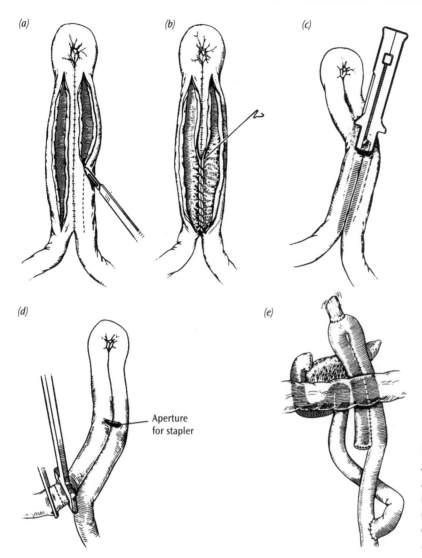

Figure 21.9 *Reconstruction after total gastrectomy with double lumen jejunal pouch and Roux-en-Y anastomosis. (a) and (b), hand-sewn technique; (c) and (d), stapled technique; (e), completed reconstruction. (From Lawrence, 1993.[51])*

Role of laparoscopy

With the advent of laparoscopic techniques in surgery, and the extension of this technology to virtually all surgical specialties, we must evaluate this approach for patients with neoplasms of the stomach. Laparoscopy can be considered both as an approach for pretreatment evaluation[47–49,96] (for staging) and as a means of definitive operative resection.[97–99] Let us address the latter first, as the role determined to be optimal for laparoscopy in gastric resection would impact considerably on our pre-resection strategy.

The use of laparoscopy for gastric resection is a feasible approach, as has been demonstrated by a number of surgeons familiar with these techniques.[97–100] The inability to remove the operative specimen of the stomach adequately without an incision makes it necessary to perform the operation as a 'laparoscopic-assisted resection,' rather than making it a pure laparoscopic endeavor. The difficulty in assessing the extent of tumor without palpation, the greater complexity of the lymphatic dissection and reconstruction required for gastric cancer, the multiple variations in the resection that may be required for gastric cancer, and the infrequent use of this procedure lead this author to predict that it will not soon become 'standard practice' for the curative treatment of gastric cancer. The potential advantages of a laparoscopically assisted gastrectomy seem relatively small when compared with the potential obstacles to the adequate technical performance of this operation. On the other hand, some palliative operations may soon be best accomplished laparoscopically.

As noted above, the optimal palliative procedure for gastric cancer, when feasible, is resection rather than either a bypass or an external stoma.[93] The latter procedures are more feasible than resection for the laparoscopic surgeon, however, and this author is concerned that increasing use of the laparoscope in surgical practice may tend to reduce the proportion of patients with incurable disease who receive a palliative gastrectomy, in favor of the more convenient bypass procedure. On the other hand, a non-resectional laparoscopic procedure for a patient with a predictably short survival may facilitate palliation by allowing a quicker recovery from the operation itself. Time will tell where laparoscopic gastric resection fits into our armamentarium for gastric cancer, but the infrequency of gastric resection overall makes it seem likely that the open approach will prevail for now.

What is the potential role for the pre-resection evaluation or staging of gastric cancer patients by laparoscopy? Even if the surgeon prefers open operation for radical 'curative' gastrectomy, abdominal exploration by laparoscopy may be useful, just as has been proposed for the pre-resection staging evaluation of other abdominal cancers, particularly cancer of the pancreas. The finding of unexpected signs of incurability (e.g., peritoneal 'implants' or small surface liver metastases not detected on preoperative imaging tests) on staging laparoscopy will make this approach advisable *if*:

1 these clinical findings occur frequently enough to make this approach worthwhile;
2 subsequent operative treatment is achieved without an open operation; or
3 a positive finding will lead to a non-operative treatment strategy.[101–104]

It might well be possible to estimate, on preoperative evaluation of the patient, whether palliative resection by laparoscopy would be a feasible approach for that individual patient if signs of incurability were detected on laparoscopy or other work-up. For example, a cancer in the distal stomach might be quite amenable to a laparoscopic palliative resection if there were new, unexpected findings of spread on laparoscopic 'exploration,' while a patient with a lesion in a location that would require total gastrectomy might be more expeditiously managed by an open operative technique from the start. Laparoscopic exploration appears to be advantageous for some patients, and not others, and this determination can be made on the basis of both the location and the extent of disease noted at the time of the initial diagnosis. My personal conclusion is that laparoscopy should be used 'selectively' for patients with gastric cancer, but, presently, it is not a necessary part of the treatment plan.

NON-OPERATIVE TREATMENT OF GASTRIC CANCER

Radiotherapy

Postoperative radiotherapy after resection for adenocarcinoma of the stomach has not been utilized routinely after either curative or palliative gastrectomy. This results from the difficulty of employing a large enough field to encompass the entire volume for potential residual disease. More recently, there has been some interest in the combined use of external-beam radiation and chemotherapy as an adjuvant following curative resection for adenocarcinoma of the stomach when there is extension of the lesion through all walls of the stomach or into regional lymph nodes. The potential value of this combined adjuvant approach and the possible value of intraoperative radiation at the time of resection are being explored in clinical trials.[105,106] These randomized trials have been prompted by preliminary studies suggesting possible benefit from both of these approaches, but the actual role of radiation in the 'curative' treatment of gastric cancer is not clearly established. However, radiation has proven to be useful for palliation by relieving localized areas of obstruction, particularly in the region of the cardia or local recurrence at the site of an esophageal anastomosis.

Chemotherapy

We continue to have a great interest in the possible benefit of adjuvant chemotherapy for patients with gastric cancer due to a high failure rate following resection. Although striking benefits from chemotherapy have not been seen yet for adenocarcinoma of the stomach, clinical trials continue in the hope that some progress will be made.

Many chemotherapeutic agents have been utilized as single agents for the palliation of advanced gastric cancer, but the results generally have been disappointing. 5-Fluorouracil (5-FU) has been used for many years, with some responses, but no significant increase in survival time.[107] This is undoubtedly the reason why this agent and other single agents have shown no survival benefit when used as adjuvant therapy *after* 'curative' gastric resection. Multiple trials of postoperative combination chemotherapy have also been disappointing, with no improvement in overall survival. These combinations have included 5-FU plus methyl-CCNU, 5-FU plus adriamycin plus mitomycin C (FAM), and mitomycin C plus 5-FU plus cytosine arabinoside. The benefit noted from combining radiation with chemotherapy in the treatment of rectal cancer has led to interest in a trial utilizing a combination of 5-FU and radiation following 'curative' gastric resection. Another ongoing trial utilizing a similar approach tests 5-FU plus leucovorin plus radiation in patients with resected gastric cancer.

Some surgeons have proposed or conducted encouraging phase II trials of chemotherapy *prior* to gastric resection for high-grade carcinomas,[102,104,108–110] but there are no phase III trials demonstrating a survival advantage for this approach, as with most other primary sites of cancer for which 'neoadjuvant' chemotherapy has been employed. The trials of adjuvant treatment before or after operation that are now ongoing require our continued attention, but adjuvant chemotherapy, preoperatively or postoperatively, cannot be recommended as a routine plan at present. A phase II study from Italy has shown that the chemotherapeutic combination of cisplatin, epirubicin, and leucovorin preceding 5-FU has about three times the response rate of the standard drug combinations that have been utilized in earlier adjuvant chemotherapy trials.[111] If confirmed, this is another chemotherapy combination that must be considered for a future adjuvant clinical trial in patients undergoing 'curative' resection of gastric cancer.

The intraperitoneal administration of adjuvant chemotherapy has been described by several groups. One report showed improved survival when compared to a historic control group,[104] one randomized trial showed no survival benefit on early analysis, but subset analysis of stage III suggested benefit,[112] and one randomized trial showed increased complications and no survival benefit.[113]

Another type of adjuvant therapy that is showing promise, and has some support in randomized clinical trials, is the use of combined adjuvant immunotherapy and chemotherapy. This approach has been explored in Japan,[114] and Dr J.P. Kim from Korea reported a larger phase III randomized trial of this approach in 1992.[115] In a three-armed study comparing postoperative combined immunotherapy and chemotherapy, postoperative adjuvant chemotherapy only, and no adjuvant therapy, the 5-year survival rates were significantly improved in the group receiving immunochemotherapy when compared with the survival of each of the other groups. A randomized phase III adjuvant trial of FAM chemotherapy with or without the biologic response modifier OK-432 suggested, but did not prove, survival benefit.[116] These interesting data should encourage additional adjuvant clinical trials to attempt confirmation of these findings.

SPECIAL MANAGEMENT PROBLEMS

Peptic ulcer versus cancer

Ulcero-cancer of the stomach appears to be a discrete gross pathologic type of gastric cancer with some favorable clinical features (higher resectability and cure rates) than some of the other gross forms, particularly the infiltrative type. For this reason, it is particularly important to differentiate this favorable malignant lesion from benign gastric ulcer as early as possible in the clinical course. When radiologic diagnosis prevailed, and endoscopy was less frequently employed, surgical resection was usually recommended for gastric ulcer due to the difficult problem of differentiating benign from malignant lesions. Flexible endoscopy has led to much greater precision in diagnosis because the gross visual examination, and the ability to biopsy, have added a great deal to our diagnostic accuracy. If both the endoscopic appearance *and* the biopsy findings strongly support the diagnosis of a benign gastric ulcer, a therapeutic trial rather than resection certainly seems justified, as the

diagnostic accuracy with these criteria exceeds 95%. However, follow-up radiologic and/or gastroscopic examination should show definite evidence of healing within 3–4 weeks. Eventually, complete healing is required or some form of operation will be indicated. Not only is the possibility of neoplasm an indication for a surgical approach under these circumstances, but some aspects of benign gastric ulcer (particularly significant bleeding episodes) are often indications for surgical intervention as well.

Another peptic ulcer 'problem' that has cancer implications is the patient presenting with a perforated gastric ulcer. Perforation of a gastric cancer as its first clinical presentation is quite rare, but it has always been taught that the diagnosis of cancer should be a consideration with acute gastric perforations. It is considered appropriate to carry out local excision of a perforated gastric ulcer at the time of emergency laparotomy for this condition so that histologic evaluation of the ulcer can be accomplished. If a frozen-section diagnosis of cancer is unexpectedly made with a distal perforation, an emergency distal gastrectomy is probably the most appropriate approach if there has not been major peritoneal contamination and/or a long time interval since the perforation occurred.[117] If resection of a perforated cancer would require an esophageal anastomosis, or if there is considerable peritoneal soilage, closure of the biopsy defect may be the most suitable emergency procedure. Resection under these difficult circumstances might be more wisely deferred until such time as the patient has fully recovered from the initial emergency operative procedure. Unfortunately, the prognosis of perforated gastric cancer is poor, just as with free peritoneal perforation of colon cancer.

Gastric polyps

A 'polyp' of the stomach may be an adenomatous polyp, a cancer of the stomach in the gross configuration of a 'polyp,' an inflammatory polyp, or a benign or malignant neoplasm of epithelial or mesodermal origin. The relative rarity of gastric polyps tends to eliminate consideration of the adenomatous polyp as a significant precancerous lesion in the epidemiologic sense, but the management of benign adenomatous lesions of the stomach is still confused by differing concepts of their neoplastic potential.

There are two features suggesting some relationship between adenomatous polyps and cancer of the stomach. The first is the fact that there is a high incidence of simultaneous adenomatous polyps in patients with established gastric cancer (as high as 25%), and the second is that there is a high incidence of achlorhydria and atrophic gastritis in patients with adenomatous polyps just as there is with gastric cancer. Earlier studies of adenomatous polyps showed 10–15% of these lesions had on their surface what was considered 'carcinoma *in situ*,' but there was little evidence that many of these microscopic lesions proceeded to clinical cancer.[118] Polypoid lesions in the stomach larger than 2 cm in diameter do appear to have a higher risk of associated cancer than the smaller lesions that are often incidental findings at the time of gastroscopy.

Although gastric polyps are not a frequent clinical problem, the following is a reasonable clinical strategy for dealing with these potentially neoplastic lesions. When single or multiple polypoid lesions cause symptoms, such as bleeding or obstruction, surgical intervention is certainly indicated. The solitary polyp or multiple lesions of limited extent can often be treated by a limited resection. If there are no symptoms, the biopsy is benign, and the polypoid lesion is definitely less than 2 cm in diameter, it can be safely observed by serial gastroscopic examinations if it cannot be conveniently excised endoscopically. However, if a single lesion is larger than 2 cm in diameter, surgical excision is indicated for complete pathologic study of the entire lesion in question. If there is diffuse polyposis, rather than a single lesion, partial gastrectomy may be required to eliminate the abnormality, but there is no evidence at present for a causative relationship between this lesion and cancer that is comparable to the relationship between familial polyposis and colon cancer. The 'bottom line' is that small, unimpressive polypoid lesions of the stomach can be observed endoscopically, but larger lesions, or multiple lesions, probably deserve operative removal.

GASTRIC LYMPHOMA

In the past, primary extranodal lymphoma in the stomach represented a small proportion of gastric cancers (less than 3%) and the diagnosis was usually made on an operative specimen after resection of the involved stomach had been accomplished. The decision process then addressed the need for added non-surgical therapies. A side issue at the time was a group of gastric lesions that confused pathologists and clinicians somewhat, the so-called 'pseudo-lymphomas.'[119] There are three major developments that have altered this clinical schema somewhat:

1 There has been an increased incidence of primary gastric lymphoma in our population (now approximately 10% of gastric cancers), a development that has taken place while adenocarcinoma has been decreasing in incidence.[22,23]

2 Non-operative programs for primary lymphoma of the stomach, particularly chemotherapy regimens, have become much more effective in terms of curative potential.[120]

3 Recent pathologic assessment of these lesions has identified mucosa-associated lymphoid tissue (MALT) lymphomas,[121] a concept that includes, among other

superficial lesions, those that we previously termed 'pseudo-lymphoma'; this has clarified the selection for patients who might be treated without anticancer therapy, and has eliminated the entity term pseudo-lymphoma.

In addition to standard hematologic studies, CT examination of the chest and abdomen/pelvis and bone marrow aspiration or biopsy are indicated if non-Hodgkin's lymphoma is found on endoscopic biopsy. However, it may be wise to precede this with EUS[122] examination because a superficial lesion limited to the mucosa on this examination would be considered a MALT lymphoma. This process may respond completely to antibiotic therapy directed at *H. pylori* (e.g., metronidizole, clarythrocin, and omeprazole) and require no anticancer therapy.[123,124] If antibiotics prove ineffective, radiation to the local lesion may be the optimal therapeutic approach.[125] Deeper wall extension noted on EUS should prompt the staging studies listed above (CT) before deciding on treatment. EUS has an accuracy of 90% in the evaluation of gastric lesions, and CT is considered quite accurate for staging extragastric disease. As the diagnosis is often made endoscopically, some degree of pretreatment staging can and should be accomplished.

Although, in the past, discussions on non-operative therapies occurred *after* resection was completed, now the treatment strategy and the order of therapies can receive multidisciplinary discussion at the outset. This has changed our thinking about primary gastric lymphoma.[120,126–129] Those lymphomas demonstrated as having a MALT component have a considerably better prognosis than deeper lesions, and it appears that neither resection nor radiation offers any additional survival advantage when compared with chemotherapy alone in stage I and II gastric lymphomas. Earlier concerns that a primary chemotherapy program for deeper lymphomas might lead to significant danger of gastric perforation, as occurs on occasion with primary chemotherapy of small-bowel lymphomas, have not been realized. Upper gastrointestinal bleeding may be a reasonable indication for preforming primary resection *before* chemotherapy in this group of patients, however. For those gastric lymphomas that invade the entire gastric wall, primary resection with an R1 regional node dissection is probably still an appropriate approach, but ultimate prognosis is clearly enhanced in this group of patients by the use of adjuvant postoperative chemotherapy programs. The principal adjuvant treatment of earlier years, postoperative radiation therapy, appears to be playing a much smaller overall role in the management of this form of cancer. All of the above observations and considerations regarding primary gastric lymphoma emphasize the importance of multidisciplinary discussions between pathologist and clinicians from the various oncology specialties. The surgical oncologist must be aware of all new developments so that surgery will maintain the appropriate role in the overall management of this disorder.

MANAGEMENT OF OTHER TUMORS OF THE STOMACH

Other than primary lymphoma, the most common cancer of mesodermal origin in the stomach was known as leiomyosarcoma. It is noteworthy that what were termed benign leiomyomas were much more frequent than their malignant counterpart. While some leiomyosarcomas were clearly infiltrative lesions on gross examination, and clearly cancers, other low-grade sarcomas were only differentiated from benign leiomyomas by the frequency of mitotic figures on histologic section. This problem in differentiating these lesions led in recent years to the classification of the entire group as 'gut stromal tumors.'[130] Less common types of sarcoma that arise in the stomach are classified histogenetically as liposarcoma, fibrosarcoma, carcinosarcoma, and malignant tumors of vascular origin. All of these mesodermal lesions are quite uncommon, and together represent less than 3% of all gastric cancers. Appropriate treatment for all is gastric resection, as for a primary adenocarcinoma of the stomach, and, whereas the removal of the immediately adjacent regional lymph nodes seems appropriate, metastatic spread to these nodes is unlikely. There is no established role for adjuvant radiation or chemotherapy with any of these lesions, if they are completely resected, and the palliative role of non-operative therapies is uncertain.

Other rare types of malignant gastric tumor are carcinoids, plasmacytomas, and metastatic cancers. Carcinoids are generally small, firm, yellow, well-circumscribed submucosal lesions, as they are in other locations, but some present as rather large lesions (>2 cm) that look quite similar to primary adenocarcinomas. Carcinoid tumors may spread to regional lymph nodes, so a gastric resection similar to that employed for adenocarcinoma is appropriate. Surgical oncologists should be aware of these lesions, as well as the plasmacytomas and the rare metastatic lesions in the stomach, because the management strategy may be modified by the specific diagnosis in each instance.

SUMMARY

Gastric cancer continues to be a significant cause of cancer mortality in some parts of the world, but its incidence progressively decreased in the USA in the years 1930 to 1985, when it seemed to have 'plateaued.' There has been a relative increase in proximal gastric cancers, compared to the antral location, and there appears to be a real increase in the incidence of primary gastric lymphoma. The cause of these observed trends is

unknown. Changes in diet and food preservation, and changes in the frequency of *H. pylori* infection, may be important.

Where earlier stage lesions appear to be more frequent (as in Japan), the prognosis of gastric cancer is better. The diagnosis of gastric cancer at as early a stage as possible appears important. However, screening populations for asymptomatic, favorable prognosis mucosal lesions is not feasible in most part of the world. Because staging does impact on both the prognosis and treatment strategy for carcinoma, improvements in the accuracy of pretreatment staging are important. The contribution of CT to this staging process has not been great and the role of EUS continues to be evaluated. Both staging techniques have proven useful in treatment planning for gastric lymphoma.

Surgical resection has remained the mainstay of treatment for gastric cancer, with the extent of resection determined by the need to obtain wide gross margins around the primary gastric tumor. Resection of adherent anatomic structures is also indicated, but the added value of extended lymphadenectomy over adequate regional lymphadenectomy is unclear at this time. A more extended lymphatic dissection is proposed by both Japanese surgeons and some Western surgeons, who do seem to obtain better overall results than most surgeons in the USA and Europe. However, both retrospective comparisons and the results of early randomized clinical trials outside Japan have failed to support the concept of extended lymphadenectomy. Also, some differences in diagnostic criteria between Japanese and Western pathologists confuse some of the reported clinical data.

The role of laparoscopy in the management of gastric cancer remains unclear, and the role of adjuvant therapies after gastric resection for adenocarcinoma is not clearly established. Early data suggest some benefit from adjuvant chemotherapy programs that combine chemotherapy and immunotherapy, and there is interest in the potential value of preoperative chemotherapy, but these approaches require further study. However, it is clear that chemotherapy plays an important role in the management of gastric lymphoma. The entire spectrum of gastric cancer requires the continued participation of the general surgeon, or surgical oncologist, because surgery remains the critical primary intervention.

REFERENCES

1. *Cancer facts and figures* – 2000. Atlanta, GA, American Cancer Society, Inc.
2. Lawrence W Jr, Menck HR, Steele GD Jr, Winchester DP. The National Cancer Data Base Report on Gastric Cancer. Cancer 1995; 75:1734–44.
3. Zheng T, Mayne ST, Holford TR, *et al.* The time trend in age period cohorts effects on incidence of

adenocarcinoma in the stomach in Connecticut from 1959–1989. Cancer 1993; 72:330–40.

4. Wanebo HJ, Kennedy BJ, Chmiel J, *et al.* Cancer of the stomach (a patient care study by the American College of Surgeons). Ann Surg 1993; 218:583–92.

5. Correa PA. A human model of gastric carcinogenesis. Cancer Res 1988; 48:3554–60.

6. Parkin DM, Laara E, Muir CS. Estimates of the worldwide frequency of sixteen major cancers in 1980. Int J Can 1988; 41:184–97.

7. Chyou PH, Nomura AM, Hankin JH, Stemmermann GM. A case-cohort study of diet and cancer. Cancer Res 1990; 50:7501–4.

8. Risch HA, Jain M, Choi NW, *et al.* Dietary factors and the incidence of cancer of the stomach. Am J Epidemiol 1985; 12:947–59.

9. You WC, Blot WJ, Chang Y-S, *et al.* Allium vegetables and reduced risk of stomach cancer. J Natl Cancer Inst 1989; 81:162–4.

10. Parsonnet J, Vandersteen D, Goats J, *et al.* *Helicobacter pylori* infection in intestinal and diffuse-type gastric adenocarcinomas. J Natl Cancer Inst 1991; 83:640–3.

11. Talley NJ, Zinsmeister AW, DiMagno EP, *et al.* Gastric adenocarcinoma and *Helicobacter pylori* infection. J Natl Cancer Inst 1991; 83:1734–8.

12. Tatsuta M, Iishi H, Okuda S, *et al.* The association of *Helicobacter pylori* with differentiated type early gastric cancer. Cancer 1993; 72:1841–5.

13. Kuipers EJ, Uyterlinde AM, Pena AS, *et al.* Long-term sequelae of *Helicobacter pylori* gastritis. Lancet 1995; 345:1525–8.

14. Endo S, Ohkusa T, Saito Y, *et al.* Detection of *Helicobacter pylori* infection in early stage gastric cancer (a comparison between intestinal and diffuse type gastric adenocarcinomas). Cancer 1995; 75:2203–8.

15. Shibata T, Imoto I, Ohuchi Y, *et al. Helicobacter pylori* infection in patients with gastric carcinoma in biopsy, and surgical resection specimens. Cancer 1996; 77:1044–9.

16. Zhang H-M, Wakisaka N, Maeda O, Yamamoto T. Vitamin C inhibits the growth of a bacterial risk factor for gastric carcinoma: *Helicobacter pylori.* Cancer 1997; 80:1897–903.

17. Correa P. Human gastric carcinogenesis: a multistep and multifactorial process – first ACS Award Lecture on Cancer Epidemiology and Prevention. Cancer Res 1992; 52:6735–40.

18. Hundahl S, Menck HR, Mansour EG, Winchester DP. The National Cancer Data Base Report on Gastric Carcinoma. Cancer 1997; 80:2333–41.

19. Meyers WC, Damiano RJ, Postlethwait RW, Rotolo FS. Adenocarcinoma of the stomach: changes in patterns over the last four decades. Ann Surg 1987; 205:1–8.

20. Salvon-Harman JC, Cady B, Nikulasson S, *et al.* Shifting proportions of gastric adenocarcinomas. Arch Surg 1994; 129:381–9.

21. Devesa SS, Blot WJ, Fraumeni JF Jr. Changing patterns in the incidence of esophageal and gastric carcinoma in the United States. Cancer 1998; 83:2049–53.

22. Hayes J, Dunn E. Has the incidence of primary gastric lymphoma increased? Cancer 1989; 63:2073–6.

23. Severson RK, Davis S. Increasing incidence of primary gastric lymphoma. Cancer 1990;66:1283–7.

24. Yamazaki H, Oshima A, Murakami R, *et al.* A long term follow-up study of patients with gastric cancer detected by mass screening. Cancer 1989; 63:613–17.

25. Hisamichi S, Tsubono Y, Fukad A. Screening for gastric cancer: appraisal of the Japanese experience. Gastrointest Cancer 1995; 1:87–93.

26. Bringaze WL, Chappius CW, Cohn I Jr, Correa P. Early gastric cancer (21 year experience). Ann Surg 1986; 204:103–7.

27. Moreaux J, Bougaran J. Early gastric cancer (25 year experience). Ann Surg 1994; 217:347–55.

28. Nakamura K, Morisaki T, Sugitani A, *et al.* An early gastric carcinoma treatment strategy based on analysis of lymph node metastasis. Cancer 1999; 85:1500–5.

29. Greene FL. Management of gastric remnant carcinoma based on the results of a fifteen year endoscopic screening program. Ann Surg 1996; 223:701–8.

30. Fisher SG, Davï F, Nelson R, *et al.* A cohort study of stomach cancer risk in man after gastric surgery for benign disease. J Natl Cancer Inst 1993; 85:1303–10.

31. Nakane Y, Okamura S, Akehira K, *et al.* Correlation of preoperative carcinoembryonic antigen levels and prognosis of gastric cancer patients. Cancer 1994; 73:2703–8.

32. Poremba C, Yandell DW, Huang Q, *et al.* Frequency and spectrum of p53 mutations in gastric cancer. Virchows Arch 1995; 426:447–55.

33. Rugge M, Sonego F, Panozzo M, *et al.* Pathology and ploidy in the prognosis of gastric cancer with no extra-nodal metastasis. Cancer 1994; 73:1127–33.

34. Ohyama S, Yonemura Y, Miyazaki I. Prognostic value of S-phase fraction and DNA ploidy studied with in vivo administration of bromodeoxyuridine on human gastric cancers. Cancer 1990; 65:116–21.

35. Kimura H, Yonemura Y. Flow cytometric analysis of nuclear DNA content in advanced gastric cancer and its relationship with prognosis. Cancer 1991; 67:2588–93.

36. Fleming ID, Cooper JS, Henson DE, *et al.* (eds.) *AJCC cancer staging manual*, 5th edn. Philadelphia, Lippincott-Raven, 1997.

37. Sussman SK, Halvorsen RA, Illescas FF, *et al.* Gastric adenocarcinoma: CT vs surgical staging. Radiology 1988; 167:335–40.

38. Minami M, Kawauclii N, Itai Y, *et al*. Gastric tumors: radiologic–pathologic correlation and accuracy of T staging with dynamic CT. Radiology 1992; 185:173–8.

39. Fukuya T, Hiroshi H, Hayashi T, *et al*. Lymph node metastases: efficacy of detection with helical CT in patients with gastric cancer. Radiology 1995; 197:705–11.

40. Smith JW, Brennan MF, Botet JF, *et al*. Preoperative endoscopic ultrasound can predict the risk of recurrence after operation for gastric carcinoma. J Clin Oncol 1993; 11:2380–5.

41. Dittler HJ, Siewert JR. Role of endoscopic ultrasonography in gastric carcinoma. Endoscopy 1993; 25:162–6.

42. Colin Jones DG, Rösch T, Dittler L. Staging of gastric cancer by endoscopy. Endoscopy 1993; 25:34–8.

43. Greenberg J, Durkin M, VanDrunen M, Ranha GV. Computed tomography or endoscopic ultrasonography in preoperative staging of gastric and esophageal tumors. Surgery 1994; 116:696–702.

44. Botet JF, Lightdale CJ, Zauber AG. Preoperative staging of gastric cancer: comparison of endoscopic U.S. and dynamic CT. Radiology 1991; 181:426–32.

45. Ajani JA, Mansfield PF, Ota DM. Potentially resectable gastric carcinoma: current approaches to staging and preoperative therapy. World J Surg 1995; 19:216–20.

46. Wiersema MJ, Cochman ML, Cramer HM, *et al*. Endosonography-guided real-time fine-needle aspiration biopsy. Gastrointest Endosc 1994; 40:700–7.

47. Watt I, Stewart I, Anderson D, *et al*. Laparoscopy, ultrasound, and computed tomography and cancer of the esophagus and gastric cardia: a prospective comparison for detecting intra-abdominal metastases. Br J Surg 1989; 76:1036–9.

48. Lowy AM, Mansfield PF, Leach SD, Ajani J. Laparoscopic staging for gastric cancer. Surgery 1996; 119:611–14.

49. Sendler A, Dittler HJ, Feussner H, *et al*. Preop staging of gastric cancer as precondition for multimodal treatment. World J Surg 1995; 19:501–8.

50. Lawrence W Jr. Radical gastrectomy. In Nora P, ed. *Operative surgery: principles and techniques*, 3rd edn. Philadelphia, WB Saunders, 1990, 544–61.

51. Lawrence W Jr. Total gastrectomy. In Daly J, Cady B, eds. *Atlas of surgical oncology*. Mosby, 1993, 241–61.

52. Lahey FH, Marshall SF. Should total gastrectomy be employed in early carcinoma of the stomach? Experience with 139 total gastrectomies. Ann Surg 1950; 132:540–65.

53. McNeer G, Sunderland DA, McInnis G, *et al*. A more thorough operation for gastric cancer (anatomic basis and description of technique). Cancer 1951; 4:957–67.

54. McNeer G, Vandenberg H Jr, Donn FY, Bowden L. Critical evaluation of subtotal gastrectomy for the cure of cancer of the stomach. Ann Surg 1951; 134:2–7.

55. Lawrence W Jr, McNeer GP. An analysis of the role of radical surgery for gastric cancer. Surg Gynecol Obstet 1960; 111:691–6.

56. Harrison LE, Karpeh MD, Brennan MF. Total gastrectomy is not necessary for proximal gastric cancer. Surgery 1998; 123:127–30.

57. Fly OA, Dockerty MB, Waugh JM. Metastases to the regional nodes of the splenic hilus from carcinoma of the stomach. Surg Gynecol Obstet 1956; 102:279–86.

58. Sunderland DA, McNeer G, Ortega LG, Pierce LS. The lymphatic spread of gastric cancer. Cancer 1953; 6:987–96.

59. Marehara Y, Moriguchi S, Yoshida M, *et al*. Splenectomy does not correlate with the length of survival in patients undergoing curative total gastrectomy for gastric carcinoma. Cancer 1991; 67:3006–9.

60. Brady MS, Rogatko A, Dente L, Shiu MH. Effect of splenectomy on morbidity and survival following curative gastrectomy for carcinoma. Arch Surg 1991; 126:359–64.

61. Otsuji E, Yamguchi Y, Sawaik K, *et al*. End results of simultaneous splenectomy in patients undergoing total gastrectomy for gastric carcinoma. Surgery 1996; 120:40–4.

62. Noguchi Y, Imada T, Matsumoto A, *et al*. Radical surgery for gastric cancer (a review of the Japanese experience). Cancer 1989; 64:2053–62.

63. Maruyama K, Gunven P, Okabayashi K, *et al*. Lymph node metastases of gastric cancer (general pattern in 1931 patients). Ann Surg 1989; 210:596–602.

64. Kaibara M, Sumi K, Yonekawa M, *et al*. Does extensive dissection of the lymph nodes improve the results of surgical treatment of gastric cancer? Am J Surg 1990; 159:218–21.

65. Adachi Y, Kamakura T, Mori M, *et al*. Role of lymph node dissection and splenectomy for node-positive gastric carcinoma. Surgery 1994; 116:837–41.

66. Baba H, Maehara Y, Takeuchi H, *et al*. Effect of lymph node dissection on the prognosis in patients with node-negative early gastric cancer. Surgery 1994; 117:165–9.

67. Baba H, Maehara Y, Inutsuka S, *et al*. Effectiveness of extended lymphadenectomy in non-curative gastrectomy. Am J Surg 1995; 169:261–4.

68. Maehara Y, Tomoda M, Tomisaki S, *et al*. Surgical treatment and outcome for node negative gastric cancer. Surgery 1997; 121:633–9.

69. Hundahl SA, Stemmermann GN, Oishi A. Racial factors cannot explain superior Japanese outcomes in stomach cancer. Arch Surg 1996; 131:170–5.

70. Bollschweiler E, Boettcher K, Hoelscher AH, *et al*. Is the prognosis for Japanese and German patients with gastric cancer really different? Cancer 1993; 71:2918–25.

71. Schlemper RJ, Itabasi M, Kato Y, *et al.* Differences in diagnostic criteria for gastric carcinoma between Japanese and Western pathologists. Lancet 1997; 349:1725–9.

72. Siewert JR, Böttcher K, Stein J, Roder JD (and the German Gastric Cancer Group). Relevant prognostic factors in gastric cancer (ten year results of the Gastric Cancer Study); Ann Surg 1998; 228:449–61.

73. Siewert JR, Kestlemeier R, Busch R, *et al.* Benefits of D2 lymph node dissection for patients with gastric cancer and PN0 and PNI metastases. Br J Surg 1996; 83:1144–7.

74. Jatzko GR, Lisborg PH, Denk H, *et al.* A ten year experience with Japanese-type radical lymph node dissection for gastric cancer outside of Japan. Cancer 1995; 76:1302–12.

75. Volpe CM, Koo J, Miloro SM. The effect of the extended lymphadenectomy on survival in patients with gastric adenocarcinoma. J Am Coll Surg 1995; 181:56–64.

76. Volpe CM, Driscoll DL, Mallio SM, Douglass HO Jr. Survival benefit of D2 resection for proximal gastric cancer. J Surg Onc 1997; 64:231–6.

77. Wanebo HJ, Kennedy BJ, Winchester DP, *et al.* Gastric carcinoma: does lymph node dissection alter survival? J Am Coll Surg 1996; 183:616–24.

78. McNeer G, Lawrence W Jr, Ortega LG, Sunderland DA. Early results of extended total gastrectomy for cancer. Cancer 1956; 9:1153–9.

79. Gilbertson VA. Results of treatment of gastric cancer (an appraisal of efforts from more extensive surgery and a report of 1,983 cases). Cancer 1969; 23:1305–8.

80. Dent DM, Maddes MV, Price SK. Randomized comparison of R1 and R2 gastrectomy for gastric carcinoma. Br J Surg 1988; 75:110–12.

81. Robertson CS, Chung SCS, Woods SDS, *et al.* A prospective randomized trial comparing R-1 sub-total gastrectomy with R-3 total gastrectomy for antral cancer. Ann Surg 1994; 220:176–82.

82. Bunt AMG, Hermans J, Boon MC, *et al.* Evaluation of the extent of lymphadenectomy in a randomized trial of Western vs Japanese type surgery in gastric cancer. J Clin Oncol 1994; 12:4117–22.

83. Bonenkamp JJ, Songun I, Hermans J, *et al.* Randomized comparisons of morbidity after D1 and D2 dissection for gastric cancer in 996 Dutch patients. Lancet 1995; 345:745–8.

84. Adachi Y, Mimori K, Mori M, *et al.* Morbidity after D2 and D3 gastrectomy for node-positive gastric carcinoma. J Am Coll Surg 1997; 184:240–4.

85. Bonenkamp JJ, Hermans J, Sasako M, Van de Velde CJH (for the Dutch Gastric Cancer Group). Extended lymph node dissection for gastric cancer. N Engl J Med 1999; 340:908–14.

86. Troidl H, Kusche J, Vestweber K-H, *et al.* Pouch versus esophagojejunostomy after total gastrectomy: a randomized clinical trial. World J Surg 1987; 11:699–712.

87. Buhl K, Lehnert T, Schlag P, Herfarth C. Reconstruction after gastrectomy and quality of life. World J Surg 1995; 19:558–64.

88. Nakane Y, Okumura S, Akehira K, *et al.* Jejunal pouch reconstruction after total gastrectomy for cancer: a randomized controlled trial. Ann Surg 1995; 222:27–35.

89. Fuchs KH, Theide A, Engemann R, *et al.* Reconstruction of the food passage after total gastrectomy: randomized trial. World J Surg 1995; 19:698–706.

90. Limo-Basto E. Problemas da technica da gastrectomia total. Arqh Patol 1956; 28:206–35.

91. Thomas H, Heimbucher J, Fuchs KH, *et al.* The mode of roux en y reconstruction affects motility in the efferent limb. Arch Surg 1996; 131:63–6.

92. Lawrence W Jr. Reservoir construction after total gastrectomy: an instructive case. Ann Surg 1962; 155:191–8.

93. Lawrence W Jr, McNeer G. The effectiveness of surgery for palliation of incurable gastric cancer. Cancer 1958; 11:28–32.

94. Haugstvedt T, Viste A, Eide GE, *et al.* The survival benefit of resection in patients with advanced stomach cancer: the Norwegian multi-center experience. World J Surg 1989; 13:617–22.

95. Monson JRT, Donohue JH, McIlraith DC, *et al.* Total gastrectomy for advanced cancer – a worthwhile palliative procedure. Cancer 1991; 68:1863–8.

96. Forse RA, Babineau T, Bleday R, Steele G Jr. Laparoscopy/thoracoscopy for staging (1. Staging endoscopy in surgical oncology). Semin Surg Oncol 1993; 9:51–5.

97. Goh P, Kum CK. Laparoscopic Billroth II gastrectomy: a review. Surg Oncol 1993; 10(Suppl.):13–18.

98. Ballesta-Lopez C, Bastida-Villa X, Catarchi M, *et al.* Laparascopic Billroth II subtotal gastrectomy with gastric stump suspension for gastric malignancies. Am J Surg 1996; 171:289–92.

99. Mayers TM, Orebaugh MG. Totally laparoscopic Billroth I gastrectomy. J Am Coll Surg 1998; 186:100–3.

100. Zhang D, Shimoyama S, Kaminishi M. Feasibility of pylorus-preserving gastrectomy with a wider scope of lymphadenectomy. Arch Surg 1998; 133:993–7.

101. Ajani JA, Mayer RJ, Ota DM, *et al.* Preoperative and postoperative combination chemotherapy for potential resectable gastric carcinoma. J Natl Cancer Inst 1993; 85:1839–44.

102. Yonemura Y, Sawa T, Kinoshita K, *et al.* Neoadjuvant chemotherapy for high grade advanced cancer. World J Surg 1993; 17:256–62.

103. Fink U, Stein HJ, Schuhmacher C, Wilke HJ. Neoadjuvant chemotherapy for gastric cancer: update. World J Surg 1995; 19:509–16.

104. Crookes P, Leichman CG, Leichman L, *et al*. Systemic chemotherapy for gastric carcinoma followed by postoperative intraperitoneal therapy. Cancer 1997; 79:1767–75.

105. Gunderson LL, Nagorney DM, Martenson JA, *et al*. External beam plus intra-operative irradiation for gastro intestinal cancers. World J Surg 1995; 19:191–7.

106. Sindelar WF, Kinsella TJ, Tepper JE. Randomized trial of intra-operative radiotherapy in carcinoma of the stomach. Am J Surg 1993; 165:178–87.

107. MacDonald JS, Schnall SF. Adjuvant treatment of gastric cancer. World J Surg 1995; 19:221–5.

108. Kelson D, Karpeh M, Schwartz G, *et al*. Neoadjuvant therapy of high risk cancer. J Clin Oncol 1996; 14:1818–28.

109. Lowy AM, Mansfield PF, Leach SD, *et al*. Response to neoadjuvant chemotherapy best predicts survival after curative resection of gastric cancer. Am J Surg 1999; 229:303–8.

110. Becker K, Fumagalli U, Mueller JD, *et al*. Neoadjuvant chemotherapy for patients with locally advanced gastric carcinoma. Cancer 1999; 85:1484–9.

111. Cocconi G, Bella M, Zironi S. Fluorouracil, doxorubin, mitomycin combination versus PELF chemotherapy in advanced cancer: a prospective randomized trial of the Italian Oncology Group for Clinical Research. J Clin Oncol 1994; 12:2687–93.

112. Yu W, Whang I, Suh I, *et al*. Prospective randomized trial of early post-operative intraperitoneal chemotherapy as an adjuvant to resectable gastric cancer. Ann Surg 1998; 228:347–54.

113. Rosen HR, Jatzko G, Repse S, *et al*. Adjuvant intraperitoneal chemotherapy with carbon-absorbed mitomycin in patients with gastric cancer. J Clin Oncol 1998; 16:2733–8.

114. Kyoto Research Group for Digestive Organ Surgery. A comprehensive multi-institutional study on postoperative adjuvant immunotherapy with oral Streptococcal preparation OK-432 for patients after gastric cancer surgery. Ann Surg 1992; 216:44–54.

115. Kim JP, Kwon OJ, Oh ST, Yang HK. Results of surgery on 6589 gastric cancer patients and immunochemosurgery as the best treatment of advanced gastric cancer. Ann Surg 1992; 216:269–79.

116. Kim Si-Y, Park HC, Yoon C, *et al*. OK-432 and 5-fluorouracil, doxorubicin, and mitomycin C (FAM-P) versus FAM chemotherapy in patients with curatively resected gastric cancer. Cancer 1998; 83:2054–9.

117. Gertsch P, Yip SKH, Chow LWC, Lauder IJ. Free perforation of gastric cancer (results of surgical treatment). Arch Surg 1995; 130:177–81.

118. Berg JW. Histological aspects of the relation between gastric adenomatous polyps and gastric cancer. Cancer 1958; 11:1149–55.

119. Orr RK, Lininger JR, Lawrence W Jr. Gastric pseudo lymphoma (a challenging clinical problem). Ann Surg 1984; 200:185–94.

120. Maor MH, Velasquez WS, Fuller LM, Silvermintz KB. Stomach conservation in stages Ie and IIe gastric non-Hodgkin's lymphoma. J Clin Oncol 1990; 8:266–71.

121. Hoshida Y, Kuskabe H, Furukawa H, *et al*. Reassessment of gastric lymphoma in light of the concept of mucosa-associated lymphoid tissue lymphoma. Cancer 1997; 80:1151–9.

122. Shuder G, Hildebrandt U, Kreissler-Haag B, *et al*. Role of endosonography in the surgical management of non-Hodgkin's lymphoma of the stomach. Endoscopy 1993; 25:509–12.

123. Bayerdorffer E, Neubauer A, Rudolph B, *et al*. Regression of primary gastric lymphoma of mucosa-associated lymphoid tissue after cure of *Helicobacter pylori* infection. Lancet 1995; 345:1591–4.

124. Neubauer A, Thiede C, Morgner A. Cure of *Helicobacter pylori* infection and duration of remission of low grade gastric MALT lymphoma. J Natl Cancer Inst 1997; 89:1350–5.

125. Fung CY, Grossbard ML, Linggood RM, *et al*. Mucosa-associated lymphoid tissue lymphoma of the stomach (long term outcome after local treatment). Cancer 1999; 85:9–17.

126. Shiu MH, Karas M, Nisce L, *et al*. Management of primary gastric lymphoma. Ann Surg 1982; 195:196–202.

127. Shiu MH, Nisce LZ, Pinna A, *et al*. Recent results of multi-modal surgery of gastric lymphoma. Cancer 1986; 58:1389–99.

128. Rosen CB, Van Heerden JA, Martin JK, *et al*. Is aggressive surgical approach to the patient with gastric lymphoma warranted? Ann Surg 1987; 205:634–9.

129. Gobbi PG, Dionigi P, Barbieri F, *et al*. The role of surgery in the multi-modal treatment of primary gastric non-Hodgkin's lymphoma. Cancer 1990; 65:2528–36.

130. Ludwig DJ, Traverse W. Gut stromal tumors and their clinical behavior. Am J Surg 1997; 173:390–4.

131. Smith JW, Shiu MH, Kelsey L, Brennan MF. Morbidity of radical lymphadenectomy in the curative resection of gastric carcinoma. Arch Surg 1991; 126:1469–73.

ANNOTATED BIBLIOGRAPHY

Adachi Y, Kamakura T, Mori M, *et al*. Role of lymph node dissection and splenectomy in node positive gastric carcinoma. Surgery 1994; 116:837–41.

This is a careful study of the survival of gastric cancer patients subjected to R1, R2, or R3 dissections. A group of

240 patients were treated by one or other of these lymph node dissection plans and all patients received postoperative chemotherapy. The selection of the type of lymph node dissection for each patient was not determined by randomized clinical trial, but the various clinical pathologic data for patients in each of the three groups show a rather homogeneous distribution of patients in terms of these factors. The survival rate was not significantly different among R1, R2, and R3 dissections, the 10-year survival rates being 57%, 50%, and 40%, respectively. There were no survival differences between R2 and R3 dissections, even when the patients were stratified by the level of lymph node metastases observed in the pathologic specimens. The study also failed to demonstrate any survival differences between those patients who had routine splenectomy and those who did not. Although subsequent randomized clinical trials seem to settle this question about the extent of lymph node dissection for gastric cancer effectively, these observations demonstrate long-term efficacy of the most extended dissection (R3) with routine splenectomy to be limited.

Bonenkamp JJ, Hermans J, Sasako M, Van de Velde CJH (for the Dutch Gastric Cancer Group). Extended lymph node dissection for gastric cancer. N Engl J Med 1999; 340:908–14.

This is the report of the randomized clinical trial that we were all waiting for to settle the question regarding value (or lack of value) from extended lymph node dissection for gastric cancer. Retrospective data from Japan, and some Western countries, demonstrated increased survival after extended lymphadenectomy, whereas some other reviews and *small* randomized trials of either a limited (D1) lymph node dissection or an extended (D2) lymph node dissection showed increased morbidity with D2 dissection and no increase in 5-year survival over that achieved with D1 dissection. This carefully controlled trial involving 711 patients appears to settle this question, at least for Western patients. Despite improved survival overall, D2 patient survival was no better than D1 patient survival.

Correa P. Human gastric carcinogenesis: a multistep and multifactorial process. Cancer Res 1992; 52:6735–40.

This pathologist has made human gastric carcinogenesis his life's work. He links epidemiologic, pathologic, and clinical observations in a description of factors causing this disease. The interrelationship between inflammation and atrophy of the gastric mucous membrane, subsequent metaplasia, digestive enzymes, mucins, antigens, carcinogens, and bacterial infection of the stomach are all clearly discussed from the standpoint of both carcinogenesis and the potential for prevention interventions.

Hallissey MT, Dunn JA, Ward LC, Allum WH. The Second British Stomach Cancer Group Trial of adjuvant radiotherapy or chemotherapy in resectable gastric cancer: five year follow up. Lancet 1994; 343:1309–12.

This is a prospective, randomized, controlled trial of adjuvant radiotherapy or cytotoxic chemotherapy with mitomycin, doxorubicin, and fluorouracil after gastrectomy for adenocarcinoma. Four hundred and thirty-six patients were entered; 145 were allocated to surgery alone, 153 to receive adjuvant radiotherapy, and 138 to adjuvant combination chemotherapy. The overall 2-year and 5-year survivals were 33% and 17%. No survival advantage was shown for those patients receiving either type of adjuvant therapy compared with those patients undergoing surgery alone. The authors stress that surgery remains the standard treatment for this condition and the use of adjuvant treatments should continue to be restricted to controlled clinical trials.

Kim JP, Kwon OJ, Oh ST, Yang HK. Results of surgery on 6589 gastric cancer patients and immunochemosurgery as the best treatment of advanced gastric cancer. Ann Surg 1992; 216:269–79.

The total series from 1970 to 1990 from Seoul National University Hospital included 6589 gastric cancer operations! To evaluate 'immunochemosurgery,' two randomized trials were initiated in 1976 and 1981, the first comparing potential benefits of 5-fluorouracil, mitomycin C, cytosine arabinoside and OK 432 with surgery alone. This showed significant benefit in favor of combined therapy (44.6% versus 23.4% 5-year survival). The second trial had a chemotherapy arm (mitomycin C and 5-fluorouracil), a surgery-only arm and a combined treatment arm (5-fluorouracil, mitomycin C and OK 432). The 5-year survival rate for combined immunochemosurgery (45.3%) was significantly better than adjuvant chemotherapy (29.8%) or surgery only (24.4%). The authors urge further randomized clinical trials to confirm the benefit demonstrated in this study.

Noguchi Y, Imada T, Matsumoto A, Coit DG, Brennan MF. Radical surgery for gastric cancer (a review of the Japanese experience). Cancer 1989; 64:2053–62.

This article, by authors from both Yokahoma and New York, reviews the experience of gastric cancer in Japan as the results appear to be superior to those obtained in the USA and Europe. It appears that the survival differences noted are due mainly to a stage 'shift' resulting from a much higher frequency of mucosal or early gastric cancer in Japan and meticulous histopathologic evaluation of surgical specimens leading to more accurate staging. Extended operations to include directly adjacent organs do not seem to improve survival rates for gastric cancer, but these authors express the view that a meaningful clinical trial would be useful to clarify the question regarding the value (or lack thereof) of extended lymph node dissection. We have the results of such trials and these early results do not encourage extended lymphadenectomy.[85]

Sawyers JL. Gastric carcinoma. Curr Prob Surg 1995; 32:101–88.

This is a thorough review of all aspects of gastric cancer by an outstanding and experienced surgeon. The history of gastric surgery is delightfully presented and all the current controversies regarding cause, diagnosis, and treatment are outlined in greater detail than is possible in this volume.

The reader wishing more detailed information will find this monograph and appended bibliography extremely useful.

Schlemper RJ, Itabasi M, Kato Y, *et al*. Differences in diagnostic criteria for gastric carcinoma between Japanese and Western pathologists. Lancet 1997; 349:1725–9.
This fascinating 'clinical' trial shows a marked discrepancy in diagnostic criteria of Eastern (Japan) and Western

(US) pathologists. Many precancerous lesions diagnosed by Western pathologists became early cancers when reviewed by Japanese pathologists. Although this does not explain the discrepancy in end results noted between the Japanese and Western worlds, it does suggest a reason for the marked differences in stages of disease.

Commentary

BRUCE E STABILE

GASTRIC CANCER: CURRENT SURGICAL MANAGEMENT ISSUES

For more than a century, surgeons have been frustrated by their inability to effect cure of gastric cancer. As the safety of gastric resection improved, the radicality of the operation expanded, but without significant gains in long-term survival. Moreover, the benefits of postoperative adjuvant radiotherapy and chemotherapy were found to be minimal. These factors quite naturally led to a nihilistic view of the disease; indeed, the role of surgery has long been considered palliative in the vast majority of cases. Consequently, in the USA and Europe, most surgeons have adopted a somewhat conservative operative approach that does not adhere to the principles of surgical resection for cancer. In reality, poor outcomes have largely been related to late diagnosis and inaccurate tumor staging rather than to any fundamental inadequacy of operative intervention. The large Japanese experience with gastric cancer has, at least, given reason for cautious optimism regarding the efficacy of aggressive lymph node dissection as a component of gastric resection. These data combined with recent advances in the understanding of the etiology, early diagnosis, accurate staging, and delivery of effective adjuvant therapies have renewed and enlivened the debate surrounding the role of surgery for gastric cancer. Although the findings of a few recent, randomized trials have not supported a role for more radical operation, the controversy is far from settled. Additionally, other important issues remain unresolved that will long require the energies of surgeons interested in improving the lot of patients afflicted with gastric cancer.

EPIDEMIOLOGY AND PATHOGENESIS

Humans are the only known host for *Helicobacter pylori* and it appears that the infection is transmitted by the fecal–oral and oral–oral routes. Notably, the beginning of the decline in the incidence of gastric cancer in the USA

antedated the introduction of antibiotics by a number of years. Improvements in public sanitation, personal hygiene, and living conditions during the early part of the twentieth century were probably important in reducing infection rates, particularly among children. This hypothesis is supported by US data showing pediatric infection rates of only 2–3% in middle-class suburbs versus 60–70% in inner-city neighborhoods.[1] Infection at an early age is associated with the development of pangastritis, progressive mucosal atrophy, and an increased risk of subsequent gastric cancer. The cytotoxin-associated gene A (*cagA*) that is found in particular strains of *H. pylori* has recently been shown to be associated with a relative risk of 2.94 for developing gastric adenocarcinoma.[2] The rapid and routine acquisition of *H. pylori* infection in childhood probably explains the higher rates of gastric cancer in underdeveloped as compared to developed countries. The recent leveling off of the prevalence of gastric cancer in the USA may, in part, be due to the recent immigration of populations from underdeveloped countries where the infection is epidemic. Mucosa-associated lymphoid tissue (MALT) lymphoma of the stomach has an even higher association with *H. pylori* infection than does gastric adenocarcinoma, although the presence of the *cagA* gene appears not to be a factor in MALT lymphoma.[3] Whereas both intestinal and diffuse histologic varieties of adenocarcinoma are associated with *H. pylori* infection, other environmental and host factors are clearly also operative in gastric carcinogenesis.[2–5] Diets high in salt, fat, nitrites, and polycylic hydrocarbons have all been implicated.[6] Cigarette smoking and exposure to aflatoxin are also associated with increased risks. Pernicious anemia, an autoimmune disease leading to chronic atrophic gastritis, is a well-established example of a predisposing host factor for gastric carcinoma.[7]

Although there has been substantial elucidation of the risk factors for gastric cancer, it is clear that our understanding remains very incomplete. This is illustrated by the unexplained recent increase in proximal gastric cancer in white males in the USA.[8,9] Some of these tumors probably arise in severely dysplastic Barrett's epithelium in the distal esophagus of individuals with chronic gastroesophageal reflux disease (GERD).[10] Others probably derive from the mucosa of the gastric cardia itself. In any event, proximal gastric adenocarcinomas do not appear to be closely related to *H. pylori* infection, and speculation as to their origin abounds.[11]

DIAGNOSIS

Unless gastric cancer is discovered at an early stage, the prognosis is extremely poor, regardless of therapy. Unlike in Japan, aggressive screening for the disease is not cost-effective and therefore is not practiced in the USA. Nonetheless, it is incumbent upon all physicians who treat abdominal conditions to maintain a low threshold for ordering upper gastrointestinal endoscopy in high-risk patients. Such patients include not only those with pernicious anemia and prior partial gastric resection, but also symptomatic patients having a prior history of benign gastric ulcer and immigrants from areas where *H. pylori* infection in childhood is common (especially Eastern Asia, Central and South America, and Eastern Europe).[12,13] The age of the patient at the time of immigration and the length of time since immigration are largely irrelevant; it is the duration of infection that is important to the process of carcinogenesis. Very noteworthy is the fact that the disease appears to be afflicting large numbers of patients at an earlier age. In some recent reports, up to 15% of patients have been 40 years of age or younger.[14]

It is not uncommon for patients with symptomatic gastric cancer to escape diagnosis for many months despite having access to medical care. The delay can usually be attributed to a failure by the primary care provider to appreciate the more subtle secondary symptoms and signs of cancer such as anorexia, early satiety, weight loss, fatigue, and anemia that uncommonly accompany benign conditions such as peptic ulcer and GERD. Dyspeptic pain unresponsive to standard antisecretory therapy should also suggest the possibility of cancer and should prompt early upper gastrointestinal endoscopy and biopsy of any gastric lesion encountered. Failure to endoscope the patient with atypical pain or some additional worrisome symptom or sign is the single most redressable cause for the delayed diagnosis of gastric cancer. Such delay can have a profoundly deleterious effect on the progression and curability of the disease. Fortunately, it is within the easy means of the healthcare profession to remedy this situation with simple education and clinical training.

STAGING

Recent technologic developments have greatly increased the accuracy of preoperative gastric tumor staging. This in turn has allowed refinement of treatment algorithms designed to enhance cure rates and minimize unnecessary operations. Computed tomography (CT) and magnetic resonance imaging (MRI) scans have been most useful in the discovery of distant metastases to liver, lungs, and ovaries. They have been much less accurate in defining peritoneal and lymph node metastases, and particularly poor in assessing the depth of penetration of the primary tumor.[15] It is in these more difficult areas that the newer modalities of endoscopic ultrasonography (EUS) and laparoscopy have had an impact.

Comparison studies for both tumor (T) and lymph node (N) staging have demonstrated a clear superiority of EUS over CT. The accuracy of CT for T staging has been only 20–30%, whereas that for EUS has been 80–90%.[15,16] For N staging, the figures have been 30–40% and 70–80% for CT and EUS, respectively. The high degree of concordance between preoperative EUS and the pathologic stage of gastric cancer has allowed accurate prediction of the risk of recurrence after operation.[17] EUS has also been found to be useful in the detection of small-volume malignant ascites and occult left lobe hepatic metastases not appreciated by CT. EUS-guided fine-needle aspiration (FNA) has been successfully employed to obtain cytologic confirmation of malignant cells in lymph nodes, liver, and ascitic fluid, thus avoiding laparotomy in selected patients with incurable disease.[18]

There is currently no indirect imaging modality capable of detecting non-bulky metastatic peritoneal tumor implants, the discovery of which has usually been made at the time of exploratory laparotomy for an attempt at curative resection. Laparoscopy prior to the laparotomy permits minimally invasive visualization and biopsy of metastatic deposits for frozen-section histologic examination as well as aspiration of occult ascites or peritoneal lavage for immediate cytologic evaluation.[19] Small liver metastases (< 1 cm) and distant lymph node (N3) tumor spread can also be detected by laparoscopy and are aided by the use of laparoscopic ultrasonography (LUS).[19,20] Available data suggest that laparoscopic staging alters the clinical stage as determined by conventional means in more than one-third of cases.[20] The combined modalities of EUS and laparoscopy with LUS and FNA are presently being introduced at many centers as components of the preoperative staging sequence, with the goal of reserving aggressive 'curative' resection for patients without advanced disease and 'palliative' gastrectomy for incurable patients in need of symptomatic relief. The clinical efficacy and cost-effectiveness of these newer staging approaches remain to be established.

GASTRECTOMY FOR CURE

American and European surgeons traditionally have not embraced the concept of an aggressive or radical operative approach to gastric cancer. There have been several cogent reasons for this:

1 the usually advanced stage of the disease;
2 the lack of scientifically valid data to support any putative benefit;
3 the concern over the associated additional morbidity and mortality;
4 lack of familiarity with the required operative technique.

Most of these deterrents remain despite the extensive Japanese literature supporting aggressive resection.[11] With the decline in training experience with gastrectomy for any and all causes and the continued absence of randomized trial results supporting radical operation, there appears to be little compelling reason for Western surgeons to change their approach. However, some mitigating considerations do pertain. There is, for instance, little question that earlier diagnosis and more accurate preoperative staging will permit better patient selection for curative operative strategies. Non-existent or inappropriate patient stratification has been a major problem in several of the randomized prospective trials that have failed to show efficacy of extensive (D2 or D3) lymph node dissection.[21,22] Inclusion of stage IV (T4, N2, M0) patients beyond any reasonable possibility of surgical cure clearly dilutes the statistical probability of demonstrating superiority of radical operation.[22,23] Small sample sizes or patient subsets have also made the likelihood of type 2 statistical errors highly probable in most studies.[21–24] In the large Dutch trial, the 10% operative mortality, 43% complication rate, and 18% reoperation rate for D2 resection patients also raise the issue of the readiness of participating surgeons to safely perform the more radical operation.[23] That trial also included all stages of disease except distant metastasis (M1). Thus, inaccurate preoperative staging together with poor study design and inadequate patient stratification probably precluded all of the randomized trials conducted to date from proving efficacy of aggressive surgery for gastric cancer.

In the absence of acceptable data from randomized trials, Western surgeons are left with only retrospective and non-randomized prospective data on which to base their operative choice. Particularly pertinent is the large prospective multicenter German trial that showed statistically significant increased 5-year survival rates for stages II and IIIA patients treated with curative intent by radical (D2) gastrectomy and lymph node dissection versus standard (D1) gastrectomy.[25] Importantly, there was no increased mortality or morbidity with radical operation. The importance of patient stratification was well illustrated by the lack of benefit of D2 operation for patients with stages I, IIIB, and IV disease. Retrospective analysis of D1 versus D2 resection in stage-stratified patients further supports the safety and efficacy of the latter operation.[26–28]

While a reasonable argument can be made for aggressive D2 lymphadenectomy with gastrectomy for gastric cancer, the routine inclusion of distal pancreatectomy and splenectomy is not justifiable. Available data have shown no survival benefit with pancreaticosplenectomy when performed to ensure complete lymphadenectomy of the splenic artery and hilar node groups.[29] Furthermore, the extended operation has been accompanied by increased rates of mortality, anastomotic dehiscence, pancreatic fistulization, and other serious complications.[29,30] These poor results do not, however, diminish the potential efficacy of lymphadenectomy along the splenic artery without pancreaticosplenectomy. This dissection can be safely performed in most patients and may be appropriate for clinical stage II and IIIA cancers of the proximal and mid-stomach.[29] Certainly, pancreaticosplenectomy is appropriate for potentially curable T4 tumors directly invading these organs. For distal gastric tumors involving the head of the pancreas, a somewhat more conservative approach would seem appropriate. Because of the added morbidity and mortality associated with pancreaticoduodenectomy (Whipple operation), it should be reserved only for the occasional patient operatively staged to have a T4, N0, M0 distal gastric adenocarcinoma. En-bloc resection of a portion of the transverse colon or mesocolon is entirely justified for otherwise potentially curable T4 tumors.[31] A complete preoperative bowel preparation should be prescribed for patients with distal gastric tumors in any proximity to the colon.

The adequacy of the extent of gastric resection is undeniably a critical determinant of long-term survival. A microscopic positive resection margin confers the highest relative risk of death from the disease.[26] The emerging consensus opinion is that total gastrectomy need not be performed except to ensure an adequate proximal margin. Nevertheless, the safety of total gastrectomy is currently as great as for subtotal gastrectomy and the operation should be used without hesitation in order to render the patient tumor free.[32,33]

In general, the biology and stage of the tumor are the most important prognostic factors in gastric cancer. The surgeon's ability to affect the course of the disease is inherently somewhat limited. Optimal surgical care is required to maximize the relatively small therapeutic opportunity. Adequate margins of resection, aggressive regional lymphadenectomy, minimal blood loss, and a secure restorative anastomosis are the critical elements under the surgeon's control that must be achieved if the patient's best interests are to be served.

RECONSTRUCTION AFTER GASTRECTOMY

Distal gastrectomy for antral carcinoma offers the option of Billroth I gastroduodenostomy or Billroth II gastrojejunostomy for reconnection of the digestive tract. Conventional wisdom has dictated that the latter procedure is superior because it provides a greater distal margin of resection, removes a greater number of juxtapyloric lymph nodes, and reduces the likelihood of anastomatic obstruction due to local recurrence of tumor. Unfortunately, there have been few reliable data to support these assumptions. A recent randomized, prospective trial comparing the two anastomatic techniques in patients with antral cancers has somewhat clarified the issue. Specifically, there were no significant differences in perioperative morbidity or mortality, resection margins, numbers of lymph nodes removed, anastomatic strictures, digestive complaints, or long-term survival.[34] There were, however, more anastomatic fistulas and a trend toward more local tumor recurrences at the hepatic pedicle after the Billroth I operation. It would appear that a Billroth I anastomosis is an acceptable reconstruction for early-stage antral cancers without nodal involvement that allow distal gastrectomy with wide margins and a low probability of local recurrence. However, in the absence of any demonstrated disadvantage of the Billroth II gastrojejunostomy, it continues to be preferred in the vast majority of cases because of its demonstrated safety and ease of construction.

Controversy still abounds regarding the efficacy of jejunal pouch reconstruction after total gastrectomy. The complexity of the physiologic consequences of both simple Roux-en-Y and a myriad of jejunal pouch configurations has made analysis of the issue laborious and difficult. The findings of retrospective studies have failed to allow a consensus opinion and most surgeons have continued to use the Roux-en-Y anastomosis because of its simplicity.[35] The few published prospective, randomized trials have similarly lacked concordance.[36,37] Detailed analysis of the long-term nutritional consequences of the randomized procedures has not demonstrated any advantage of jejunal pouch reconstruction.[37] Dietary support is probably a more important determinant of nutritional status than is the use of a pouch reservoir after total gastrectomy.[37,38]

ROLE OF LAPAROSCOPY

Laparoscopy is rapidly gaining acceptance as a legitimate staging procedure that is complementary to CT and EUS.[19,20] It is, however, superfluous and contraindicated in patients with incurable but clearly resectable gastric cancers who require palliative gastrectomy for bleeding, obstruction, or severe pain. On the other hand, laparoscopy to rule out occult distant metastases prior to embarking on laparotomy and planned curative gastrectomy in minimally symptomatic patients with small primary tumors seems logical and appropriate. Thus, proper patient selection based on clinical status and preoperative assessment with CT and EUS is needed for the cost-effective utilization of staging laparoscopy in gastric cancer.

The role of therapeutic laparoscopic surgery has largely been limited to bypass procedures and occasional palliative resections performed by skilled practitioners.[39,40]

Palliative resection is often a formidable open operation, particularly for very proximal or very distal bulky tumors. It is not reasonable to expect that such resections will be routinely, safely, or expeditiously performed using laparoscopic techniques. However, simple proximal bypass of unresectable distal obstructing gastric cancers with laparoscopic stapled side-to-side gastrojejunostomy is very feasible and may soon become the preferred approach. An additional application of therapeutic laparoscopic surgery appears to be endoscopically facilitated wedge excision of small-diameter stromal cancers and early gastric adenocarcinomas not requiring lymph node dissection.[41,42] Obviously, highly accurate preoperative EUS staging of T and N status is a mandatory prerequisite to such an approach.

ADJUVANT THERAPIES

The results of postoperative adjuvant radiotherapy and chemotherapy for gastric cancer have been poor, even when used in combination.[43,44] Although there has been some support for intraoperative radiotherapy, its ability to impart a significant survival advantage remains unproven.[45] The most promising role for radiotherapy and chemotherapy appears to be as a combined neoadjuvant treatment program designed to downstage the disease and render it more curable by surgical resection. A recent Irish randomized trial compared preoperative fluorouracil, cisplatin, and radiation followed by surgery to surgery alone for adenocarcinomas of the gastric cardia and distal esophagus associated with Barrett's epithelium.[46] The combined multimodal therapy group evidenced dramatic downstaging on histologic examination of surgical specimens and statistically significant improvements in 3-year survival (37% versus 7%). These results appear to have been directly related to the 25% complete tumor response verified histologically in the group that received the neoadjuvant chemoradiation therapy. While certainly promising, the efficacy of combination neoadjuvant chemoradiation therapy awaits further evaluation in patients with gastric cancers in locations other than the cardia.

It appears that major future advances in the treatment of gastric cancer may lie in the emerging field of immunotherapy. The encouraging preliminary results reported from Korea and Japan with combination chemotherapy plus the immunomodulator OK-432 deserve the attention of Western investigators.[47,48] It must be remembered, however, that the effectiveness of this and all other adjuvant regimens is predicated on the principle that a 'curative' surgical resection of the primary tumor and all macroscopic regional metastatic deposits can and will be effected. Until genetic therapies and new preventative strategies are developed and implemented, it will remain the responsibility of the surgeon to provide the primary and most effective treatment modality available for gastric cancer.

SPECIAL MANAGEMENT PROBLEMS

Gastric ulceration

The problem of differentiation between benign and malignant gastric ulcer has been largely solved by the use of flexible fiberoptic upper gastrointestinal endoscopy as the diagnostic procedure of choice for non-trivial dyspeptic pain complaints. Because the cost of this procedure has become competitive with that of upper gastrointestinal contrast radiography, the latter has fallen out of favor due to its lack of specificity. Because all gastric ulcers should be biopsied to rule out cancer, initial radiographic studies are superfluous in most cases. Endoscopy with biopsy and brush cytology accurately diagnoses gastric cancer in more than 95% of patients.[49,50] It should be appreciated, however, that small ulcerated cancers can evidence mucosal healing in response to medical therapy. Follow-up endoscopic evaluation is thus mandatory for all gastric ulcers.

That ulcerated cancers of the stomach have a more favorable prognosis is probably related more to their association with pain symptoms and earlier diagnosis than to any inherent differences in biologic behavior. The current state of knowledge suggests that the tumor stage (T, N, M) and the histologic type (intestinal or diffuse) are important determinants of clinical outcome.[51–53] Gross morphology of the tumor is much less important, although it is somewhat related to both its histology and T stage. This is exemplified by superficial spreading or early gastric cancers which are T1 tumors usually of intestinal histologic type.[54–56]

Gastric polyps

There is little question but that adenomatous gastric polyps greater than 2 cm in diameter are premalignant lesions and should be excised.[57] Some three-quarters of adenomatous polyps fall into this larger size range, in which the prevalence of malignancy has been reported to be as high as 27%.[58] When few in number, large adenomatous polyps can usually be managed by endoscopic excision. Laparoscopic wedge resection aided by intraoperative endoscopic localization has proven useful for large sessile lesions.[42] Multiple large adenomatous polyps should prompt partial or even total gastrectomy. This is particularly mandated by the presence of severe dysplasia on biopsy.

Early gastric cancer

By definition, early gastric cancers are confined to the mucosa or submucosa and therefore are T1 lesions.[56] They are usually of intestinal-type histology, may be multiple, are most commonly found in the antrum, and are common in Japan but rather rare in Western countries.[11,56,59] Because the tumors have relatively limited lymphatic access (submucosal tumors only), the incidence of lymph node metastasis is only about 10%.[56] These early cancers are quite curable, with 5-year survival rates exceeding 80% that approximate the survival of age-matched controls.

The treatment of early gastric cancer is excision and this has traditionally been accomplished by distal gastrectomy.[11,55,56] For tumors confined to the mucosa, a D1 lymphadenectomy encompassing only the perigastric nodes is sufficient. In Japan, EUS-guided endoscopic mucosal excisions, laser ablations, and intralesional chemical injections have been used in high-risk patients.[60–63] Such lesions are also amenable to endoscopically assisted laparoscopic wedge resection. Tumors invading the submucosa should be treated by D2 radical gastrectomy with regional lymphadenectomy in order to encompass any micrometastases to N2 as well as N1 level nodal basins.[11,56,64]

SUMMARY

Gastric cancer remains a vexing problem for surgeons and oncologists. The recently defined etiologic role of *H. pylori* in the disease has stimulated renewed interest in both therapeutic and preventative strategies. This comes at an appropriate time when the prevalence of the disease may actually again be on the rise in the USA due to recent immigration patterns and other unknown factors. Fiberoptic endoscopy has afforded a greater opportunity than ever before for early diagnosis, and early diagnosis is the key to improving the traditionally dismal outcome associated with gastric cancer. EUS is redefining preoperative tumor staging and will allow the development of new and more exacting treatment algorithms encompassing neoadjuvant multimodal therapies, minimally invasive tumor resections, aggressive radical gastrectomy and regional lymphadenectomy, and non-operative palliations tailored to address individual patient needs. In the near future, immunomodulating agents can be expected to play an important role as well. Ultimately, genetic therapies and innovative prevention programs will probably have a profound impact on the mortality and morbidity caused by gastric cancer. Until then, it is incumbent upon surgeons to remain informed and committed to the prudent application of new concepts and technical advances relevant to this challenging disease.

REFERENCES

1. Malaty HM, Evans DG, Evans DG Jr, Graham DY. *Helicobacter pylori* infection in Hispanics: comparison with blacks and whites of similar age and socioeconomic class. Gastroenterology 1992; 103:813–16.

2. Rugge M, Busatto G, Yih-Homg S, *et al*. Patients younger than 40 years with gastric carcinoma. *Helicobacter pylori* genotype and associated gastritis phenotype. Cancer 1999; 85:2506–11.

3. Go MF, Vakil N. *Helicobacter pylori* infection. Clin Perspect Gastroenterol. 1999; 2:141–53.

4. Sakagami T, Dixon M, O'Rourke J, *et al*. Atrophic gastric changes in both *Helicobacter felis* and *Helicobacter pylori* infected mice are host dependent and separate from antral gastritis. Gut 1996; 39:639–48.

5. Parsonnet J, Friedman G, Vandersteen DP, *et al*. *Helicobacter pylori* and the risk of gastric carcinoma. N Engl J Med 1991; 325:1127–31.

6. Boeing H. Epidemiological research in stomach cancer: progress over the last ten years. J Cancer Res Clin Oncol 1991; 117:133–43.

7. Correa P. Chronic gastritis: a clinico-pathological classification. Am J Gastroenterol 1988; 83:504–9.

8. Blot WJ, Devesa SS, Kneller RW, Fraumeni JF Jr. Rising incidence of adenocarcinoma of the esophagus and gastric cardia. JAMA 1991; 265:1287–9.

9. Pera M, Cameron AJ, Trastek VF, *et al*. Increasing incidence of adenocarcinoma of the esophagus and esophagogastric junction. Gastroenterology 1993; 104:510–13.

10. Lagergren J, Bergstrom R, Lindgren A, Nyren O. Symptomatic gastroesophageal reflux as a risk factor for esophageal adenocarcinoma. N Engl J Med 1999; 340:825–31.

11. Sawyers JL. Gastric carcinoma. Curr Prob Surg 1995; 32:101–88.

12. Hansson L-E, Myren O, Hsing AW, *et al*. The risk of stomach cancer in patients with gastric or duodenal ulcer disease. N Engl J Med 1996; 335:242–9.

13. Bonacini M, Valenzuela JE. Changes in the relative frequency of gastric adenocarcinoma in southern California. West J Med 1991; 154:172–4.

14. Theuer CP, de Virgilio C, Keese G, *et al*. Gastric adenocarcinoma in patients 40 years of age or younger. Am J Surg 1996; 172:473–7.

15. Pollack BJ, Chak A, Slvak MF Jr. Endoscopic ultrasonography. Semin Oncol 1996; 23:336–46.

16. Caletti G, Ferrari A, Brocchi E, Barbara L. The accuracy of endoscopic ultrasonography in the diagnosis and staging of gastric cancer and lymphoma. Surgery 1993; 113:14–27.

17. Smith JW, Brennan MF, Botet JF, *et al*. Preoperative endoscopic ultrasonography can predict the risk of recurrence after operation for gastric carcinoma. J Clin Oncol 1993; 11:2380–5.

18. Chang KJ, Katz KD, Darbin TE, *et al*. Endoscopic ultrasound-guided fine-needle aspiration. Gastrointest Endosc 1994; 40:694–9.

19. Stell DA, Carter CR, Stewart I, Anderson JR. Prospective comparison of laparoscopy, ultrasonography and computed tomography in the staging of gastric cancer. Br J Surg 1996; 83:1260–2.

20. Conlon KC, Karpeh MS Jr. Laparoscopy and laparoscopic ultrasound in the staging of gastric cancer. Semin Oncol 1996; 23:347–51.

21. Dent DM, Madden MV, Price SK. Randomized comparison of R_1 and R_2 gastrectomy for gastric carcinoma. Br J Surg 1988; 75:110–12.

22. Robertson CS, Chung SCS, Woods SDS, *et al*. A prospective randomized trial comparing R_1 subtotal gastrectomy with R_3 total gastrectomy for antral cancer. Ann Surg 1994; 220:176–83.

23. Bonenkamp JJ, Songun I, Hermans J, *et al*. Randomized comparison of morbidity after D1 and D2 dissection for gastric cancer in 996 Dutch patients. Lancet 1995; 345:745–8.

24. Bonenkamp JJ, Hermans J, Sasako M, *et al*. Extended lymph-node dissection for gastric cancer. N Engl J Med 1999; 340:908–14.

25. Siewert JR, Bottcher K, Roder JD, *et al*. Prognostic relevance of systemic lymph node dissection in gastric carcinoma. Br J Surg 1993; 80:1015–18.

26. Shiu MH, Moore E, Sanders M, *et al*. Influence of the extent of resection on survival after curative treatment of gastric carcinoma. Arch Surg 1987; 122:1347–51.

27. Pacelli F, Doglietto GB, Bellantone R, *et al*. Extensive versus limited lymph node dissection for gastric cancer: a comparative study of 320 patients. Br J Surg 1993; 80:1153–6.

28. Smith JW, Brennan MF. Surgical treatment of gastric cancer. Surg Clin North Am 1992; 72:381–99.

29. Kodera Y, Yamamura Y, Shimizu Y, *et al*. Lack of benefit of combined pancreaticosplenectomy in D2 resection for proximal-third gastric carcinoma. World J Surg 1997; 21:622–8.

30. Cuschieri A, Fayers P, Fielding J, *et al*. Postoperative morbidity and mortality after D1 and D2 resections for gastric cancer: preliminary results of the MRC randomised controlled surgical trial. Lancet 1996; 347:995–9.

31. Korenaga D, Okamura T, Baba H, *et al*. Results of resection of gastric cancer extending to adjacent organs. Br J Surg 1988; 75:12–15.

32. Bozzetti F, Marubini E, Bonfanti G, *et al*. Total versus subtotal gastrectomy. Surgical morbidity and mortality rates in a multicenter Italian randomized trial. Ann Surg 1997; 226:613–20.

33. Gouzi JL, Huguier M, Fagniez PL, *et al*. Total versus subtotal gastrectomy for adenocarcinoma of the gastric antrum. A French prospective controlled study. Ann Surg 1989; 209:162–6.

34. Chareton B, Landen S, Manganas D, *et al*. Prospective randomized trial comparing Billroth I and Billroth II procedures for carcinoma of the gastric antrum. J Am Coll Surg 1996; 183:190–4.

35. Heberer G, Teichmann RK, Kramling H-J, Gunther B. Results of gastric resection for carcinoma of the stomach: the European experience. World J Surg 1988; 12:374–81.

36. Troidl H, Kusche J, Vestweber K-H, *et al*. Pouch versus esophagojejunostomy after total gastrectomy: a randomized clinical trial. World J Surg 1987; 11:699–712.

37. Bozzetti F, Bonfanti G, Castellani R, *et al*. Comparing reconstruction with Roux-en-Y to a pouch following total gastrectomy. J Am Coll Surg 1996; 183:243–8.

38. Braga M, Zuliani W, Foppa L, *et al*. Food intake and nutritional status after total gastrectomy: results of a nutritional follow-up. Br J Surg 1988; 75:477–80.

39. Ballesta-Lopez C, Bastida-Villa X, Catarchi M, *et al*. Laparoscopic Billroth II subtotal gastrectomy with gastric stump suspension for gastric malignancies. Am J Surg 1996; 171:289–92.

40. Mayers TM, Orebaugh MG. Totally laparoscopic Billroth I gastrectomy. J Am Coll Surg 1998; 186:100–3.

41. Di Lorenzo N, Sica GS, Gaspari AL. Laparoscopic resection of gastric leiomyoblastoma. Surg Endosc 1996; 10:662–5.

42. Leong HT, Siu WT, Li MK. Gasless laparoscopic excision of bleeding gastric polyps. J Laparoscopic Surg 1996; 6:189–91.

43. Kelson DP. Adjuvant and neoadjuvant therapy for gastric cancer. Semin Oncol 1996; 23:379–89.

44. Karpeh MS, Kelson DP. Combined modality therapy of gastric cancer. Surg Oncol Clin North Am 1997; 6:741–7.

45. Abe M, Shibamoto Y, Takahasi M, *et al*. Intraoperative radiotherapy in carcinoma of the stomach and pancreas. World J Surg 1987; 11:459–64.

46. Walsh TN, Noonan N, Hollywood D, *et al*. A comparison of multinodal therapy and surgery for esophageal adenocarcinoma. N Engl J Med 1996; 335:462–7.

47. Kim JP, Kwon OJ, Oh SUT, *et al*. Results of surgery on 6,598 gastric cancer patients and immunochemosurgery as the best treatment of advanced gastric cancer. Ann Surg 1992; 216:269–79.

48. Kim JP, Park HC, Yoon C, *et al*. OK-432 and 5-fluorouracil, doxorubicin and mitomycin C (FAM-P) versus FAM chemotherapy in patients with curatively resected gastric cancer. Cancer 1998; 83:2054–9.

49. Graham D, Schwartz J, Cain G, *et al*. Prospective evaluation of biopsy number in the diagnosis of esophageal and gastric carcinoma. Gastroenterology 1982; 82:228–31.

50. Gupta JP, Jain AK, Agrawal BK, *et al*. Gastroscopic cytology and biopsies in diagnosis of gastric malignancies. J Surg Oncol 1983; 22:62–4.

51. Maruyama K. Progress in gastric surgery in Japan and its limits of radicality. World J Surg 1987; 11:418–25.

52. Lauren P. The two histological main types of gastric carcinoma: diffuse and so-called intestinal type carcinoma. Acta Pathol Microbiol Scand 1965; 64:31–49.

53. Ming SC. Gastric carcinoma: a pathological classification. Cancer 1977; 39:2475–85.

54. Green P, O'Tolle K, Weinberg L, *et al*. Early gastric cancer. Gastroenterology 1981; 81:247–56.

55. Kodama VI, Inokuchi K, Soejima K, *et al*. Growth patterns and prognosis in early gastric carcinoma. Cancer 1981; 51:320–6.

56. Farley DR, Donohue JH. Early gastric cancer. Surg Clin North Am 1992; 72:401–21.

57. Laxen F, Sipponen P, Ikamaki T, *et al*. Gastric polyps: their morphologic and endoscopic characteristics and relation to gastric carcinoma. Acta Pathol Microbiol Immunol Scand 1982; 90:221–8.

58. Ming SC, Goldman H. Gastric polyps: a histogenetic classification and its relation to carcinoma. Cancer 1965; 18:721–6.

59. Tsukuma M, Mishima T, Oshima A. Prospective study of 'early' gastric cancer. Int J Cancer 1983; 31:471–6.

60. Akahoshi K, Chijiiwa Y, Tanaka Y, *et al*. Endosonography probe-guided endoscopic mucosal resection of gastric neoplasms. Gastrointest Endosc 1995; 42:248–52.

61. Sakita T. Early cancer of the stomach treated successfully with an endoscopic neodymium-YAG laser. Am J Gastroenterol 1981; 76:441–5.

62. Hirao M, Masuda K, Asanuma T, *et al*. Endoscopic resection of early gastric cancer and other tumors with local injection of hypertonic saline–epinephrine. Gastrointest Endosc 1988; 34:264–9.

63. Maehara Y, Okuyama T, Oshiro T, *et al*. Early carcinoma of the stomach. Surg Gynecol Obstet 1993; 177:593–7.

64. Whiting JL, Fielding JWL. Radical surgery for early gastric cancer. Eur J Surg Oncol 1998; 24:263–6.

Editors' selected abstracts

Laparoscopy-assisted Billroth I gastrectomy compared with conventional open gastrectomy.

Adachi Y, Shiraishi N, Shiromizu A, Bandoh T, Aramaki M, Kitano S.

First Department of Surgery, Oita Medical University, Japan.

Archives of Surgery 135(7):806–10, 2000, July.

Background: Although several studies compare surgical results of laparoscopic and open colonic resections, there is no study of laparoscopic gastrectomy compared with open gastrectomy. *Hypothesis:* When compared with conventional open gastrectomy, laparoscopy-assisted Billroth I gastrectomy is less invasive in patients with early-stage gastric cancer. *Design:* Retrospective review of operative data, blood analyses, and postoperative clinical course after Billroth I gastrectomy. *Setting:* University hospital in Japan. *Patients:* The study included 102 patients who were treated with Billroth I gastrectomy for early-stage gastric cancer from January 1993 to July 1999: 49 with laparoscopy-assisted gastrectomy and 53 with conventional open gastrectomy. *Main outcome measures:* Demographic features examined were operation time; blood loss; blood cell counts of leukocytes, granulocytes, and lymphocytes; serum levels of C-reactive protein, interleukin 6, total protein, and albumin; body temperature; weight loss; analgesic requirements; time to first flatus; time to liquid diet; length of postoperative hospital stay; complications; proximal margin of the resected stomach; and number of harvested lymph nodes. *Results:* Significant differences ($p < 0.05$) were present between laparoscopy-assisted and conventional open gastrectomy when the following features were compared: blood loss (158 vs 302 mL), leukocyte count on day 1 (9.42 vs 11.14 × 10^9/L) and day 3 (6.99 vs 8.22 × 10^9/L), granulocyte count on day 1 (7.28 vs 8.90 × 10^9/L), C-reactive protein level on day 7 (2.91 vs 5.19 mg/dL), interleukin 6 level on day 3 (4.2 vs 26.0 U/mL), serum albumin level on day 7 (35.6 vs 33.9 g/L), number of times analgesics given (3.3 vs 6.2), time to first flatus (3.9 vs 4.5 days), time to liquid diet (5.0 vs 5.7 days), postoperative hospital stay (17.6 vs 22.5 days), and weight loss on day 14 (5.5% vs 7.1%). There was no significant difference between laparoscopy-assisted and conventional open gastrectomy with regard to operation time (246 vs 228 minutes), proximal margin (6.2 vs 6.0 cm), number of harvested lymph nodes (18.4 vs 22.1), and complication rate (8% vs 21%). *Conclusions:* Laparoscopy-assisted Billroth I gastrectomy, when compared with conventional open gastrectomy, has several advantages, including less surgical trauma, less impaired nutrition, less pain, rapid return of gastrointestinal function, and shorter hospital stay, with no decrease in operative curability. When performed by a skilled surgeon, laparoscopy-assisted Billroth I gastrectomy is a safe and useful technique for patients with early-stage gastric cancer.

Extended lymph-node dissection for gastric cancer. Dutch Gastric Cancer Group.

Bonenkamp JJ, Hermans J, Sasako M, van de Velde CJ.

Department of Surgery, Leiden University Medical Center, The Netherlands.

New England Journal of Medicine 340(12):908–14, 1999, March 25.

Background: Curative resection is the treatment of choice for gastric cancer, but it is unclear whether this operation should include an extended (D2) lymph-node dissection, as recommended by the Japanese medical community, or a limited (D1) dissection. We conducted a randomized trial in 80 Dutch hospitals in which we compared D1 with D2 lymph-node dissection for gastric cancer in terms of morbidity, postoperative mortality, long-term survival, and cumulative risk of relapse after surgery. *Methods:* Between August 1989 and July 1993, a total of 996 patients entered the study. Of these patients, 711 (380 in the D1 group and 331 in the D2 group) underwent the randomly assigned treatment with curative intent, and 285 received palliative treatment. The procedures for quality control included instruction and supervision in the operating room and monitoring of the pathological results. *Results:* Patients in the D2 group had a significantly higher rate of complications than did those in the D1 group (43 percent vs. 25 percent, $p < 0.001$), more postoperative deaths (10 percent vs. 4 percent, $p = 0.004$), and longer hospital stays (median, 16 vs. 14 days; $p < 0.001$). Five-year survival rates were similar in the two groups: 45 percent for the D1 group and 47 percent for the D2 group (95 percent confidence interval for the difference, −9.6 percent to +5.6 percent). The patients who had R0 resections (i.e., who had no microscopical evidence of remaining disease), excluding those who died postoperatively, had cumulative risks of relapse at five years of 43 percent with D1 dissection and 37 percent with D2 dissection (95 percent confidence interval for the difference, −2.4 percent to +14.4 percent). *Conclusions:* Our results in Dutch patients do not support the routine use of D2 lymph-node dissection in patients with gastric cancer.

Gastroesophageal reflux disease, use of H2 receptor antagonists, and risk of esophageal and gastric cancer.

Farrow DC, Vaughan TL, Sweeney C, Gammon MD, Chow WH, Risch HA, Stanford JL, Hansten PD, Mayne ST, Schoenberg JB, Rotterdam H, Ahsan H, West AB, Dubrow R, Fraumeni JF Jr, Blot WJ.

Fred Hutchinson Cancer Research Center, and University of Washington, School of Public Health & Community Medicine, Department of Epidemiology, Seattle, USA.

Cancer Causes Control 11(3):231–8, 2000, March.

Objective: The incidence of esophageal adenocarcinoma has risen rapidly in the past two decades, for unknown reasons. The goal of this analysis was to determine whether gastroesophageal reflux disease (GERD) or the medications used to treat it are associated with an increased risk of esophageal or gastric cancer, using data from a large population-based case-control study. *Methods:* Cases were aged 30–79 years, newly diagnosed with esophageal adenocarcinoma ($n = 293$), esophageal squamous cell carcinoma ($n = 221$), gastric cardia adenocarcinoma ($n = 261$), or non-cardia gastric adenocarcinoma ($n = 368$) in three areas with population-based tumor registries. Controls ($n = 695$) were chosen by random digit dialing and from Health Care Financing Administration rosters. Data were collected using an in-person structured interview. *Results:* History of gastric ulcer was associated with an increased risk of non-cardia gastric adenocarcinoma (OR 2.1, 95% CI 1.4–3.2). Risk of esophageal adenocarcinoma increased with frequency of GERD symptoms; the odds ratio in those reporting daily symptoms was 5.5 (95% CI 3.2–9.3). Ever having used H2 blockers was unassociated with esophageal adenocarcinoma risk (OR 0.9, 95% CI 0.5–1.5). The odds ratio was 1.3 (95% CI 0.6–2.8) in long-term (4 or more years) users, but increased to 2.1 (95% CI 0.8–5.6) when use in the 5 years prior to the interview was disregarded. Risk was also modestly increased among users of antacids. Neither GERD symptoms nor use of H2 blockers or antacids was associated with risk of the other three tumor types. *Conclusions:* Individuals with long-standing GERD are at increased risk of esophageal adenocarcinoma, whether or not the symptoms are treated with H2 blockers or antacids.

The National Cancer Data Base Report on poor survival of U.S. gastric carcinoma patients treated with gastrectomy: Fifth Edition American Joint Committee on Cancer staging, proximal disease, and the 'different disease' hypothesis.

Hundahl SA, Phillips JL, Menck HR.

Department of Surgery, The Queen's Medical Center, Honolulu, Hawaii, USA.

Cancer 88(4):921–32, 2000, February 15.

Background: A high proportion of U.S. patients with gastric carcinoma do not receive surgical treatment. To sharpen staging criteria and facilitate comparisons with surgical series, an analysis of patients whose treatment included gastrectomy was undertaken. In addition, to evaluate the 'different disease' hypothesis as an explanation for superior Japanese results, outcomes for Japanese Americans were examined. *Methods:* Data were obtained from National Cancer Data Base (NCDB) reports of 50,169 gastric carcinoma cases diagnosed during the years 1985–1996 and treated with gastrectomy. In addition to demographic and treatment information, 5-year and 10-year relative survival rates are presented, with stage defined according to fifth edition American Joint Committee on Cancer (AJCC) staging procedures. *Results:* Stage-stratified 5-year and 10-year relative survival rates were as follows: Stage IA, 78%/65%; Stage IB, 58%/42%; Stage II, 34%/26%; Stage IIIA, 20%/14%; Stage IIIB, 8%/3%; and Stage IV, 7%/5%. Stage-stratified survival for Japanese Americans was higher. Males had a poorer prognosis than females, and the male-to-female ratio for Japanese Americans was lower. Proximal tumors were associated with a worse prognosis than distal tumors; the proportion of Japanese Americans with proximal disease was less than in the overall patient group. Japanese Americans underwent resection of adjacent organs less frequently. In this series, adjuvant therapy did not substantially affect survival. Overall, 20% were 10-year survivors; of these, 67% were lymph node negative and 98% had ≤8 involved lymph nodes. Five-year stage-stratified survival increased for cases with ≥15 lymph nodes analyzed. Stage migration was evident in cases with ≤15 nodes examined. *Conclusions:* The current AJCC/International Union Against Cancer TNM staging system fails to accommodate the effect of proximal location on prognosis. Largely because Japanese Americans present with fewer proximal tumors, have a lower male-to-female ratio, and undergo adjacent organ resection less frequently, stage-stratified survival for Japanese Americans appears to be superior. In the U.S., surgical undertreatment of patients with this disease appears to be a problem.

Effect of microscopic resection line disease on gastric cancer survival.

Kim SH, Karpeh MS, Klimstra DS, Leung D, Brennan MF.

Department of Surgery, Memorial Sloan-Kettering Cancer Center, New York, NY, USA.

Journal of Gastrointestinal Surgery 3(1):24–33, 1999, January–February.

To study the effect of residual microscopic resection line disease in gastric cancer, we compared 47 patients with positive margins to 572 patients who underwent R0 resections using a multivariate analysis of factors affecting outcome. Although the presence of positive margins was a significant and independent predictor of outcome for the entire group (*n* = 619), this factor lost significance in patients who had undergone D2 or D3 lymph node dissections (*n* = 466). Subset analysis within the D2/D3 group determined that this finding was limited mainly to those patients with >5 positive nodes (*n* = 189). The survival of patients who had nodes (*n* = 277) was significantly worsened by a microscopically involved margin. Supporting this observation, intraoperative reexcision of microscopic disease based on frozen section analysis resulted in a significant improvement in overall survival in patients with nodes but not in those with >5 positive nodes. We conclude that the significance of a positive microscopic margin in gastric cancer is dependent on the extent of disease. This factor is not predictive of outcome in patients who have undergone complete gross resection and have pathologically proved advanced nodal disease. Thus the goal in these cases should be an R0 resection when feasible but with the realization that the presence of ≥5 positive nodes (N2 disease according to the 1997 American Joint Committee on Cancer criteria) will mainly determine outcome and not microscopic residual cancer at the margin.

Is gastric carcinoma different between Japan and the United States?

Noguchi Y, Yoshikawa T, Tsuburaya A, Motohashi H, Karpeh MS, Brennan MF.

First Department of Surgery, Yokohama City University School of Medicine, Yokohama, Japan.

Cancer 89(11):2237–46, 2000, December 1.

Background: Analyses of surgical results for gastric carcinoma often lead to the conclusion that gastric carcinoma occurring in Japan is different from that diagnosed in the U.S. *Methods:* To elucidate factors that might explain the differences in surgical results between the two countries, the authors compared data from a cancer center and a university hospital in Japan and a specialist cancer hospital in the U.S. (Memorial Sloan-Kettering Cancer Center [MSKCC]). *Results:* The mean age and body mass index were significantly greater in patients in the U.S. The N category appeared to be determined less accurately at MSKCC compared with the Japanese centers. The occurrence of early gastric carcinoma was not confined to Japanese patients because 20% of U.S. patients who underwent surgery were determined to have early stage disease. However, mucosal (in situ) carcinoma was detected rarely, and the proportion of advanced stage disease was greater in the U.S. Lesions in the upper gastric body, including the gastroesophageal junction, occurred in >50% of cases at MSKCC but in only 20% of cases at the Japanese centers (*p* < 0.001). D2 lymph node dissection was possible with low morbidity and minimum mortality (31% and 3%, respectively, at MSKCC). The 5-year survival rates, stratified by tumor location and T category, revealed more similar results between Japan and the U.S. than had been reported previously. The marked difference between Japanese and American institutions only was observed for T1 and T2 tumors occurring in the lower gastric body and for T3 tumors occurring in the middle and upper third of the stomach. *Conclusions:* Based on the findings of the current study, it would appear that the more favorable outcome noted for gastric carcinoma patients in Japan primarily is explained by the differences in tumor location, a greater frequency of early stage disease, and more accurate staging compared with gastric carcinoma patients in the U.S. Results of gastric carcinoma treatment comparable to those obtained in Japan can be obtained in Western centers.

Early and late recurrence after gastrectomy for gastric carcinoma. Univariate and multivariate analyses.

Shiraishi N, Inomata M, Osawa N, Yasuda K, Adachi Y, Kitano S.

Department of Surgery I, Oita Medical University, Oita, Japan.

Cancer 89(2):255–61, 2000, July 15.

Background: To the authors' knowledge, there are few studies regarding the predictors of early and late recurrence after gastrectomy for gastric carcinoma, and it is unknown whether prognostic factors can be applied to the timing of recurrence. The current study analyzed patients who died of recurrent gastric carcinoma and clarified histopathologic indicators associated with early and late recurrence. *Methods:* The study included 138 patients who died of recurrent gastric carcinoma after gastrectomy that was performed in the Department of Surgery I, Oita Medical University, between 1982–1995. Clinicopathologic findings were compared between 104 patients who died within 2 years after gastrectomy (early recurrence group) and 34 patients who died >2 years after gastrectomy (late recurrence group). Multivariate analysis was performed to determine the independent factors correlated with the timing of recurrence. *Results:* When compared with the late recurrence group, the early recurrence group was characterized by a tumor size ≥ 5 cm (92% in the early recurrence group vs. 74% in the late recurrence group), positive lymphatic invasion (64% vs. 38%), extended lymph node metastasis (73% vs. 35%), Stage III or IV disease (87% vs. 62%), and limited lymph node dissection (32% vs. 3%). The mean survival time was influenced by the lymphatic invasion ($p < 0.01$), vascular invasion ($p < 0.05$), level of lymph node metastasis ($p < 0.01$), stage of disease ($p < 0.01$), and extent of lymph node dissection ($p < 0.01$). On multivariate analysis, survival time was found to be associated independently with the stage of disease (Stage I, II vs. Stage III, IV) or the level of lymph node metastasis (N0, N1 vs. N2, N3). *Conclusions:* The stage of disease and level of lymph node metastasis were found to be the most significant factors independently associated with the survival time after

gastrectomy for gastric carcinoma. Patients with more advanced stage of disease (Stage III, IV) or those with extended lymph node metastasis (N2, N3) frequently died of recurrence within 2 years after gastrectomy.

Outcome of patients with proximal gastric cancer depends on extent of resection and number of resected lymph nodes.

Volpe CM, Driscoll DL, Douglass HO Jr.

Division of Surgical Oncology, Roswell Park Cancer Institute, State University of New York at Buffalo, NY, USA. cmvol@aol.com

Annals of Surgical Oncology 7(2):139–44, 2000, March.

Background: Studies have shown that the survival of patients with gastric adenocarcinoma is related to the number of regional lymph nodes with metastases. The probability of identifying node-positive cancers increases with the number of lymph nodes resected and examined. It has been recommended that at least 15 lymph nodes be removed and examined for adequate staging. Prospective randomized studies have shown the lymph node yield is much greater with the D2 resection than the D1. This study evaluated the relative contribution of both the number of resected lymph nodes and the extent of gastric resection (D1/D2) on the outcome of patients with proximal gastric cancer. *Methods:* The medical records of 114 patients with adenocarcinoma of the proximal stomach, who underwent a curative gastric resection, were reviewed. Patients were stratified into four groups, i.e., two groups, D1/D1.5 and D2/D2.5, based on the extent of resection, and two groups based on the number of lymph nodes removed, fewer than 15 lymph nodes and 15 or more lymph nodes. Survival was determined by the method of Kaplan–Meier and differences compared by the log-rank test. Multivariate analysis was performed by using the Cox model. *Results:* The number of resected lymph nodes had no effect on the survival of the group as a whole. A significant improvement in survival was noted for patients with a D2 or greater resection. The median survival of patients with 15 or more lymph nodes resected improved from 25 months to 42 months when treated with an extended resection, (D2 or D2.5). Resection of 15 or more lymph nodes alone, or combined with an extended resection, resulted in a statistically significant improvement in survival for patients in American Joint Committee on Cancer Staging (AJCC) stage II. *Conclusions:* Both resection of 15 or more lymph nodes and extended lymphadenectomy contributed to the survival advantage observed in patients with AJCC stage II gastric cancer. The D2 gastric resection prolonged the median survival time and improved the 5-year survival rate for patients with 15 or more resected lymph nodes.

22

Surgical management of cancer of the pancreas

KAREN E TODD AND HOWARD A REBER

INTRODUCTION

Pancreatic cancer causes approximately 27 000 deaths per year in the USA.[1] It is the fourth leading cause of cancer death in men and the fifth leading cause in women.[2] The 1-year survival rate after diagnosis is less than 20%, and the overall 5-year survival is 3%.[3] Ninety percent of the exocrine tumors of the pancreas are ductal adenocarcinomas,[4] and approximately three-quarters of these arise in the head of the pancreas. These tumors are usually diagnosed at an earlier stage than cancers in the body or tail of the gland because they cause jaundice when they obstruct the intrapancreatic portion of the common bile duct.[5] Pancreatic cancer is an aggressive lesion. Fewer than 10% of patients have tumor confined to the pancreas at the time of diagnosis; over 40% have locally advanced disease, and more than half have distant spread.[6,7]

In 1935, Whipple performed a two-stage resection for a carcinoma of the ampulla of Vater, and by 1942 he had perfected a one-stage operation similar to that performed today. In the hands of experienced pancreatic surgeons around the world, the operative mortality rate of this operation is now about 2–3%.

The purpose of this chapter is to discuss the preoperative diagnosis and staging, surgical options, postoperative care, and survival of patients with pancreatic cancer.

INITIAL EVALUATION

The main goals in the initial evaluation and management of a patient with pancreatic cancer are to establish the diagnosis *with a high degree of certainty*, to identify those patients who would benefit from laparotomy, and to optimize their condition for operation.[8]

DIAGNOSIS AND STAGING

Approximately 75% of patients have tumors of the pancreatic head, while the remainder develop their disease in the body and tail of the gland.[9] This is important because lesions of the head, close to the bile duct, may produce obstructive jaundice when they are still small and curable. Biliary obstruction, in the absence of other symptoms, is associated with a better prognosis. Persistent back pain is associated with a worse prognosis. Painless jaundice, anorexia, and weight loss are only the presenting symptoms in 7% of patients; the majority present with significant pain. Body and tail tumors almost always produce symptoms late and are usually quite advanced at the time of diagnosis. Very few are resectable and the outlook is even poorer than with head lesions.[10] Physical examination and laboratory tests are consistent with the diagnosis of obstructive jaundice.[11] The total bilirubin level tends to be greater with malignant obstruction than with obstruction from benign causes (15 versus 5 mg/dL). Serum amylase elevation is seen in only 5% of patients with pancreatic cancer.[12–18]

The most important factor determining outcome is whether the tumor is resectable. In general, larger tumors are less likely to be resectable. Thus, efforts have been focused toward early diagnosis when the tumor is still small. This has been difficult because pancreatic cancer remains asymptomatic or produces only vague symptoms at an early stage. One center compared the interval between the first symptoms and diagnosis in patients treated from 1973 to 1980 with those treated from 1981 to 1988.[7] From 1981 to 1988, the diagnosis was made within 1 month of the onset of symptoms, 2 months sooner than in the earlier time period. This was probably related to the use of newer diagnostic tests such as computerized tomography (CT) scans and endoscopic retrograde cholangiopancreatography (ERCP). Nevertheless, the cure rate was not improved.

To improve survival, diagnosis probably has to be made years before the patient is symptomatic. Screening tests for pancreatic cancer are being investigated.[19] The results of CA 19-9, a monoclonal antibody to the Lewis blood group antigen, have been the most encouraging.[20] However, the test is more likely to be positive when the tumor is large, so it is not likely to be able to diagnose early lesions. The test has a sensitivity of about 80%, and a specificity of about 90%. Gastric and colorectal cancers may be associated with an elevated CA 19-9 as well. CA 19-9 may have some utility in following patients after resection to determine response to adjuvant therapy and to detect evidence of recurrence.[21]

Some recent studies show that ductal pancreatic adenocarcinomas are associated with a high rate of genetic alterations. These include the presence of k-ras oncogenes in as many as 85% of cases, and *p53* mutations in at least half.[22,23] It is still uncertain at what stage in the development of the cancer these changes occur, but the genetic abnormalities have been detected in cancers that are still small and asymptomatic. This is an exciting area of research, and probably represents the most productive line of activity for efforts aimed at the early diagnosis of this disease.

Certain patients who are at higher risk for pancreatic cancer should be aggressively worked up. Examples are individuals who have a heavy cigarette-smoking history, an unexplained recent weight loss of greater than 10% of body weight, unexplained upper abdominal or lumbar back pain, new-onset dyspepsia, recent onset of diabetes mellitus or glucose intolerance, 'idiopathic' or chronic pancreatitis, or those with unexplained steatorrhea.[24]

DIAGNOSTIC TECHNIQUES

Recent advances in diagnostic techniques have improved our ability to detect pancreatic cancer, to stage the tumor, and to obtain tissue for diagnosis. In all patients in whom pancreatic cancer is suspected, an abdominal CT scan and ERCP are the two most valuable studies for diagnosis. If both the ERCP and CT scan are normal, the diagnosis of ductal adenocarcinoma of the pancreas is extremely unlikely. A number of other diagnostic tests are also available, and the important ones are examined below with respect to the risk, cost, and impact of the information acquired on patient management.

Non-invasive techniques

Ultrasound

Ultrasound (US) is a relatively inexpensive test with a sensitivity of 70% and a specificity of over 90% for the diagnosis of pancreatic cancer.[25] However, in 20% of patients the examination is unreliable due to body habitus or overlying bowel gas. US has its greatest value in the discrimination between intrahepatic and extrahepatic biliary obstruction. Extrahepatic obstruction from a periampullary malignancy would be expected to show dilated intrahepatic and extrahepatic biliary radicles. It can also identify gallstones that may be the cause of obstruction. Although US provides some information about the relationship of the tumor to surrounding structures, CT is much better in this regard.

Computerized tomography

CT has a sensitivity of at least 80% and a specificity of 95% for the diagnosis of pancreatic cancer.[26] These data were derived from experience with conventional imaging techniques; the newer helical (spiral) CT equipment provides images of even greater quality and precision. Lesions of 2 cm or greater should be detectable. CT is more reliable than US because it visualizes the entire pancreas and the presence of bowel gas does not interfere. It also provides information about the level of biliary obstruction, when it is present. CT also gives information about tumor resectability, such as the presence of liver metastases and the involvement of major blood vessels such as the superior mesenteric and portal veins, the superior mesenteric artery, and the celiac artery and its branches. Enlarged lymph nodes can be seen, but it is important to point out that inflammatory nodes cannot be distinguished from neoplastic ones.[26,27] Thus, the presence of large nodes should not be the reason that a CT scan is interpreted as showing an 'unresectable' tumor. CT scanning has a false-positive rate of less than 10%, which is usually attributed to focal pancreatitis, or variations in normal pancreatic anatomy.

In our experience, the ability of CT to predict 'resectability' is about 75%.[24] Errors are usually due to small liver or peritoneal metastases that were undetected. The ability of a CT scan to predict that a tumor will be 'unresectable' has been reported to be as high as 95%. Our own experience suggests that the accuracy of such a prediction is related to the expertise of the radiologist, the nature of the CT finding on which the prediction is based, and the experience and philosophy of the surgeon. Thus, if the apparent presence of liver metastases is the basis for the prediction of unresectability, the level of reliability is high. If the radiologist finds evidence for tumor invasion of the superior mesenteric vein, with less than circumferential narrowing of the vessel, the implications of such a finding are less clear. For example, we will often resect such a tumor including a segment of the vein in an effort to palliate a patient who seems to be a reasonable candidate. The pathologist eventually may determine that the adherence to the vein was only inflammatory, or that tumor had extended only to the adventitia of the vessel. Whereas we do not believe that many such patients are cured by the resection, some may be, and some are undoubtedly palliated. In any case, the tumors clearly were 'resectable.' A more accurate term to use in these efforts to stage a tumor preoperatively might be 'resectable for cure.'

Angiography

In a study by Freeny et al., angiography did not add any significant information with respect to staging.[28] This has been our experience as well, especially with the superb vascular imaging now possible with the spiral CT technique.

Magnetic resonance imaging

MRI is reported to provide slightly better pancreatic tissue contrast than CT, but spatial resolution is inferior.[29] It was hoped that MRI would be superior to CT in outlining the blood vessels, but such an advantage has not been demonstrated.

Invasive techniques

Endoscopic retrograde cholangiopancreatography

ERCP has a sensitivity of 95% and a specificity of 85%, in the diagnosis of pancreatic cancer.[30] The procedure can be performed successfully in more than 90% of patients and it detects some tumors not seen on CT. The classic finding that suggests pancreatic cancer is obstruction of both the bile and pancreatic ducts in the head of the pancreas, the so-called 'double-duct sign.' At the time of ERCP, brushings for cytology may be obtained from the pancreatic duct, which has a sensitivity of about 60% in proving the diagnosis of malignancy.[31] Some have argued that ERCP should be done routinely in these patients because it may be possible to determine the origin of the tumor (e.g., ampulla of Vater instead of the pancreas). Although this may be true in some cases, it usually does not affect subsequent management, because the operation that is required is the same for all of the periampullary malignancies.[31] ERCP can also be used for stent placement, which has an important role in the palliation of patients who do not require surgery. Stents should not be used routinely for preoperative decompression, however.

Despite its value, there is some evidence that ERCP tends to be an overused study. If a patient has a history typical for pancreatic cancer (e.g., pain, jaundice, weight loss) with a mass in the head of the pancreas evident on CT scan, then an ERCP is unnecessary for the diagnosis and generally adds nothing to the work-up that is of value to either the patient or the surgeon.

Endoscopic ultrasound

Endoscopic ultrasound (EUS) may be able to detect small lesions not seen with other studies, but the experience with this new technology is still being accumulated.[32] It also may prove useful to assess vascular involvement by the tumor, and provide information about resectability. A recent prospective study by Rosch et al. compared EUS with transabdominal ultrasound (TRUS), CT, and angiography in 60 patients with pancreatic or ampullary cancer. In the 40 patients who underwent surgery, EUS was superior to abdominal ultrasound and CT in determining tumor size and extent, and lymph node metastases. The involvement of the portal venous system was correctly assessed in 95% of patients.[33] On the other hand, abdominal ultrasound is known to be inferior to standard CT; the study did not employ spiral CT scanning, which is the current state-of-the-art, and most experienced pancreatic surgeons do not use angiography as part of the work-up at all.

Percutaneous trans-hepatic cholangiography

Percutaneous trans-hepatic cholangiography (PTC) also provides information about biliary ductal anatomy in patients with bile duct obstruction. However, ERCP is probably safer, and it is preferred in those with periampullary tumors. PTC is the procedure of choice in most patients with proximal bile duct tumors (e.g., Klatskin tumor), however. It opacifies the intrahepatic ducts, and precisely defines the level of the tumor and its degree of involvement of the hepatic ducts and their branches. This is important to the surgeon in making decisions about resectability.

Fine-needle aspiration

Preoperative fine-needle aspiration (FNA) for cytology can be obtained percutaneously using a fine-gauge needle under CT or US guidance. The characteristic signs of malignancy are single or irregularly arranged clusters of cells exhibiting pleomorphism, large vesicular nuclei, and prominent nucleoli.[34] The sensitivity is 85% and the specificity is almost 100%.[34] Complications include hemorrhage, pancreatitis, pancreatic fistula, and seeding of the needle tract with cancer cells, all of which are uncommon.[34] We do not believe that this study should be done routinely in the work-up of these patients. It is uncomfortable for the patient, it is associated with considerable cost, and, in patients who are operative candidates, it does not change management. We use the study in situations in which the cytologic diagnosis of malignancy will have a clear impact on subsequent management. For example, in a patient with a tumor in the body of the pancreas who has no symptoms for which surgical palliation is required, FNA could confirm the diagnosis, and chemotherapy and/or radiation could be given. In a patient with obstructive jaundice and a mass in the head of the pancreas, who may not be a candidate for resection because of coexisting medical problems, FNA would be useful to confirm the diagnosis. Then a stent could be placed for palliation, and surgery simply to obtain tissue for diagnosis would have been avoided. *It is important to stress that a negative FNA never rules out the possibility of malignancy.*

The argument that preoperative knowledge of the diagnosis of cancer simplifies or speeds up the operation may be valid if the surgeon is inexperienced. However, most pancreatic surgeons do not require histologic proof of malignancy before proceeding with resection. We decide to resect on the basis of the patient's history and the gross findings at operation. Of course, this issue is always discussed preoperatively with the patient. With this approach, experienced surgeons err less than 10% of the time (i.e., a resection is performed for what turns out to be benign disease). This is acceptable because the mortality rate of resection is quite low, and the majority of patients who undergo resection for benign disease have chronic pancreatitis, for which resection is also appropriate.

Laparoscopy

Laparoscopy has been used to stage patients with pancreatic cancer, but its place in the management of patients with periampullary malignant disease continues to evolve. Some surgeons have favored its use in the majority of cases, as a routine part of the work-up before laparotomy. In some instances, laparoscopy was done as a separate procedure in the outpatient setting, and the findings guided the subsequent work-up. More often, it was performed immediately before laparotomy under the same anesthetic; if evidence of unresectability was found, the operation was concluded. There is some evidence that it was a cost-effective approach and that it spared many patients the discomfort of an unnecessary laparotomy.[35] Warshaw *et al.*'s experience is quoted widely.[36] They found that 40% of patients without apparent extrapancreatic involvement on conventional CT, and thus judged to have resectable lesions, had hepatic or peritoneal metastases at laparoscopy. However, the data that supported that philosophy were published between 1986 and 1990, and helical CT scans were not used in these cases. We have not used laparoscopy in patients who appear to have resectable lesions on *helical* CT, and who are good candidates for resection. It should be pointed out that even helical CT scans do not show the very small hepatic or peritoneal metastases (2–3 mm) that may be present. But the newer technique shows vascular involvement much more reliably than the conventional scans did, and we have found that most patients who have these small metastases also have been considered unresectable because of vascular involvement. As stated previously, resection was possible in 75% of our patients who were judged to have 'resectable' cancers of the head of the pancreas after CT scan. Of the remaining 25% of the total who did not have resectable cancers, small liver or peritoneal metastases, which might have been seen laparoscopically, were the reason in only half. Thus, if all of our patients had undergone laparoscopy as a routine, at best, only 12.5% might have been spared subsequent laparotomy. This seems to us to be too low a yield to justify the additional operative time and expense of the procedure. The remaining patients who were falsely designated as resectable on the basis of helical CT evaluation had locally extensive tumor which was assessed as unresectable only after mobilization of the pancreas from the superior mesenteric and portal veins at laparotomy. This would not have been safe to do laparoscopically.

Although laparoscopy still has certain limitations as a staging tool, progress is being made in this area.[37,38] Advanced laparoscopic techniques and improved instrumentation (e.g., laparoscopic US) may allow the surgeon to perform a more complete and accurate assessment of resectability. Laparoscopy also may have a useful therapeutic role. Rhodes *et al.*[39] reported 15 patients who were treated palliatively with cholecystojejunostomy (7), gastroenterostomy (5), or both procedures (3). The average hospital stay was 4 days and the patients appeared to recover more rapidly. Thus, the role of laparoscopy may again increase.

We do use laparoscopy, *selectively*, in certain circumstances. Examples include some patients with pancreatic cancer and CT evidence of liver or other metastases, body or tail cancers, and some patients with ascites who probably have peritoneal metastases.

An algorithm for the evaluation of a patient with suspected cancer of the pancreas is presented in Figure 22.1. Under ideal circumstances, this should be done with the cooperation of the surgeon who will perform the operation and at an institution with experience in the care of

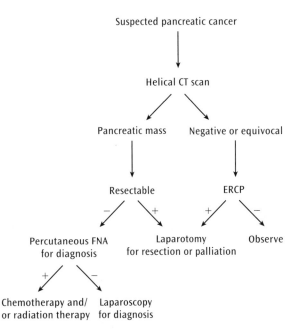

Figure 22.1 *An algorithm for the work-up and treatment of suspected pancreatic cancer. CT, computerized tomography; ERCP, endoscopic retrograde cholangiopancreatography; FNA, fine-needle aspiration.*

patients with these tumors. Helical CT scan may be the only test required. If it shows a mass in the head of the pancreas without evidence of metastatic disease, laparotomy may be undertaken without further studies. If the CT suggests hepatic, peritoneal, or distant metastases, percutaneous FNA may be appropriate if a positive biopsy would obviate the need for surgery. If the mass involves the body and tail of the gland, there is usually evidence of metastatic disease or advanced local spread. Because these patients seldom benefit from palliative operations, percutaneous FNA is often indicated to provide a tissue diagnosis before starting chemotherapy and/or radiation therapy. Occasionally, these tumors appear resectable, or the biopsy is negative or equivocal; then laparoscopy for further assessment may be reasonable. The patient should undergo laparotomy under the same anesthetic if the lesion appears resectable.

If the CT is normal or the findings are equivocal in a patient with suspected pancreatic cancer, ERCP is indicated. If both the CT and ERCP are normal, pancreatic cancer is extremely unlikely.

PREOPERATIVE MANAGEMENT

As in all patients about to undergo major surgery, it is important to optimize cardiac, pulmonary, and renal function preoperatively. This can usually be done in the outpatient setting. Although these patients have often lost weight, delay of the operation in order to restore nutrition with parenteral alimentation is rarely indicated. When it is, a biliary stent should be placed endoscopically if the patient is jaundiced.

Because jaundice is associated with defects in hepatic, renal, and immune function, some have suggested that postoperative morbidity in these patients might be improved by drainage of the biliary tract before surgery.[40] Several studies have failed to show such a benefit.[41-43] Pitt et al.[41] were unable to identify any difference in outcome, and hospital stay was longer for the drainage group than for the non-drainage group. McPherson and colleagues[42] reported a higher mortality in the drainage group, primarily as a result of septic complications related to the percutaneous catheter.

OPERATIVE MANAGEMENT

Historical perspective

Halsted reported the first ampullary resection for tumor in 1899,[44] and he successfully reimplanted the biliary and pancreatic ducts directly into the duodenum. This was done to avoid the technical challenge of reconstruction when the duodenum was also removed. In 1935, Whipple et al.[45] described a two-stage pancreaticoduodenectomy for a tumor of the ampullary region. At the

first operation, biliary decompression was achieved by draining the gallbladder into the stomach, and a gastrojejunostomy was also performed. After several weeks, a limited resection of the duodenum and pancreas was carried out, without any pancreatic anastomosis. In 1937, Brunschwig[46] reported an extension of this procedure that included resection of most of the head of the pancreas and duodenum. He performed an anastomosis between the cut end of the pancreas and jejunum. In 1945, Whipple[47] revised his original operation, incorporating Brunschwig's modifications. The technique used today is quite similar. It involves a partial gastrectomy (antrectomy), cholecystectomy, and removal of the distal common bile duct, head of the pancreas, duodenum, proximal jejunum, and regional lymph nodes. Reconstruction requires a pancreaticojejunostomy, hepaticojejunostomy, and a gastrojejunostomy.

Determination of resectability

Tumor size

Apart from the usual pessimism associated with the diagnosis of pancreatic cancer, many physicians are particularly discouraged if the tumor is large, and may even fail to refer the patient to a surgeon. It is true that small pancreatic tumors (<2 cm diameter) are more likely to be resectable than larger ones. Nevertheless, the majority of pancreatic cancers located in the head of the gland are larger than that by the time the diagnosis is made and an operation is performed. At the University of Erlangen in Germany, of all resections of tumors in the head of the gland, 15% were 1–2 cm in diameter, 33.4% were 2–3 cm, 23.3% were 3–4 cm, and 27.8% were >4 cm. At UCLA Medical Center over the period 1989–1994, 26% of the resections were for tumors 1–2 cm in diameter, 17% were 2–3 cm, 22% were 3–4 cm, 26% were 4–5 cm, and 9% were >5 cm in diameter.[48] Thus, it should be apparent that no patient should be denied the chance for a resection because of a tumor that is considered 'too large'. It is true that larger tumors as a group are less likely to be resectable than small ones, and that the average length of survival after resection is shorter in patients who had larger tumors. A recent retrospective study showed that primary tumor size was the strongest determinant of prognosis in patients with resectable cancers.[49] The 5-year survival for patients with tumors <2.5 cm was 33%; it was 12% for patients with larger tumors. No patient with a tumor larger than 5 cm survived for more than 5 years. The reasons for this are uncertain, but it is not because large tumors are more malignant. In fact, even small tumors have usually metastasized to lymph nodes (86%) by the time they are diagnosed, and are likely to exhibit other characteristics associated with a poor prognosis, e.g., pancreatic capsular invasion (50%), perineural invasion (60%), and microvascular invasion (75%). The likelihood of these findings is no greater with the larger lesions. Larger tumors may be less amenable to resection because they often invade adjacent major vessels or other nearby structures. In addition, as small tumors grow to become large ones, distant sites of metastatic disease also enlarge and are more likely to be clinically apparent, which precludes resection.

Vascular invasion

In the absence of distant metastases (e.g., peritoneum, serosal surfaces of other organs, lymph nodes outside the usual limits of the resection, liver), resectability depends on whether the tumor has invaded major vascular structures. We usually will not resect if the tumor has invaded the superior mesenteric or portal vein, and will never resect if the superior mesenteric artery or the hepatic artery is involved. There are two circumstances in which we will remove tumors with venous invasion, excising the involved segment of the vein with the specimen. Occasionally, when the preoperative discussion has convinced us of the patient's desire for an aggressive approach to the problem, we will undertake the resection with prior knowledge that the vein is involved. In other cases, lateral or posterior involvement of the vein only becomes apparent after the neck of the pancreas has been transected as part of the Whipple. The segment of vein is removed either as a sleeve resection or as a lateral segment from the side of the vessel, provided that this does not narrow the vein significantly. Sleeve resections are usually repaired by an end-to-end anastomosis; a graft is rarely needed. There is evidence that venous resections under those conditions are associated with a survival similar to that seen in patients who undergo resection when the vessels are not involved. Nevertheless, we view this as a palliative resection, and recommend adjuvant treatment later.

Pancreaticoduodenectomy

Modifications of the operation

The Whipple procedure with preservation of the stomach and pylorus (*pylorus-preserving Whipple*) was described by Watson in 1944.[50] In 1978, Traverso and Longmire reported their experience with a similar operation to treat chronic pancreatitis.[51] Because of concern that the standard Whipple resection was associated with excessive morbidity (excessive weight loss, diarrhea, dumping), many surgeons have adopted this pylorus-preserving modification in patients with pancreatic cancer as well. Here, the stomach and pylorus are preserved, which maintains gastric reservoir function, and postoperative gastric emptying is closer to normal. It is widely believed that the modified procedure minimizes the nutritional disturbances, and that it can be done more quickly and easily. It has generally been accepted that this does not compromise the chance for cure of the cancer.

We have recently completed the only randomized, prospective study of the standard Whipple and the pylorus-preserving variant. There were no differences in any of the postoperative complications, nutritional parameters, the frequency or type of gastrointestinal symptoms, weight loss, or in the ease or time required to perform the two operations. The 22 patients in the study were all operated upon by one surgeon, and were evaluated 9–12 months after the operation. Thus, the procedures appear to be equivalent. We did not compare the operations with regard to their efficacy as treatment for the underlying cancer, however. We now perform the two operations interchangeably, and usually select the pylorus-preserving modification in patients with smaller, less extensive tumors.

In 1973, Fortner[52] reported a '*regional pancreatectomy*' which included resection of portions of the portal vein and hepatic or superior mesenteric arteries in some cases. Morbidity and operative mortality rates were high, and there was no evidence that outcome was improved by this technique.

More recently, Japanese surgeons reviewed material from autopsy data that showed metastatic involvement of para-aortic lymph nodes at some distance from the primary tumor in the head of the pancreas. These nodes were not included in the standard Whipple resection.[53] Autopsies performed in patients who died after the standard Whipple procedure from recurrent disease indicated that the tumor had recurred locally or in these regional nodes.[54] Thus, it seemed logical to perform a more radical operation which removed these lymph nodes and adjacent soft tissues. An early study from Japan reported a 38% 3-year survival in patients who underwent such a wider resection, compared to a 13% 3-year survival in patients who had the standard Whipple resection.[55] These data were supported by other groups.[56] Takahashi *et al.* reported on results from this so-called *extended Whipple resection* combined with portal vein resection. They reported an increase in resectability rate when the portal vein was resected, and felt that the procedure was well tolerated and safe to perform.[57]

The operation involves pancreaticoduodenectomy, and sometimes total pancreatectomy, along with extensive retroperitoneal lymph node and soft-tissue resection as well as superior mesenteric and portal vein and occasionally superior mesenteric artery resection. The lymphadenectomy consists of a wide retroperitoneal dissection of the lymph nodes from the celiac axis to the iliac bifurcation, and laterally to the kidneys. The nodes removed include the pyloric, superior and inferior pancreatic head, common bile duct, anterior pancreaticoduodenal, and superior mesenteric lymph nodes as well as a para-aortic and celiac lymphadenectomy and neurectomy performed *en bloc*. The superior mesenteric, portal and splenic veins, hepatic and mesenteric arteries, and celiac axis are skeletonized. This extensive dissection adds 60–90 minutes to the operation.[58]

Reber *et al.* examined data from 651 Japanese pancreatic cancer patients who underwent the extended resection. Survival rates 5 years postoperatively ranged from 0% to 30%, with a mean survival of 13%. This was similar to the 9% survival rate of 1700 patients who had the standard Whipple resection in the USA.[58] Reber *et al.* stressed that a variety of issues prevented a meaningful evaluation of these results. Some of the patients had also received adjuvant therapy. A different staging system was used in many of the Japanese series, compared to those in use in Western countries, including the USA. Thus, differences in survival could be due to differences in disease stage rather than treatment.[58]

Yeo and Cameron also compared the standard versus the extended Whipple.[59] They reported a recent retrospective study by Satake *et al.*[60] comparing standard and radical resection of the pancreas in 185 patients with tumors less than 2 cm in size. There was no difference in 5-year survival (27%) between the two groups. A study from Memorial Sloan-Kettering Cancer Center showed that the difference in survival between the standard and radical resection groups in that institution was not statistically significant.[61]

Although a prospective, randomized study would be necessary to determine whether the extended resection is superior to the standard Whipple operation, so far this has not been done. Most surgeons in the USA do not perform this operation.

Priestly *et al.*[62] described *total pancreatectomy* for an islet cell tumor in 1944 and this technique was subsequently used for adenocarcinoma to try to improve the results of the Whipple procedure. It was thought that the cancer was multicentric in up to 35% of cases, and that total pancreatectomy might improve cure rates. Later experience suggested that the tumor was usually unifocal, and the operation, which did not improve outcome, has largely been abandoned.

Technical aspects of reconstruction

The pancreatic anastomosis

A variety of techniques have been used for the pancreaticojejunostomy, including end-to-end and end-to-side reconstructions, and one-layer or two-layer anastomoses, with or without a pancreatic duct stent. Each has its own proponents, suggesting that each is satisfactory in the hands of experienced surgeons. We have had experience with a number of different types, and have come to favor a two-layer, end-of-pancreas to side-of-jejunum anastomosis, without a stent. The duct is incorporated into the anastomosis by passing several sutures of the inner layer through the duct lumen. We use interrupted 3–0 silk sutures for the outer layer; a continuous 3–0 polyglycolic acid absorbable suture is used for the inner layer. Anastomosis to the side of the jejunum allows the creation of an opening that fits the pancreatic remnant

perfectly every time. Our pancreatic fistula rate with this approach is about 8%; it should be less than 10%.

Although some have claimed that a pancreaticogastrostomy is a safer technique than attaching the pancreas to the jejunum, we have had little experience with it. A recent prospective trial at Johns Hopkins which compared the two procedures found no advantage when the stomach was used.

The pancreatic anastomosis is drained with a closed suction drain (e.g., number 10 Jackson Pratt or equivalent), which is removed after the patient is eating, just before discharge from the hospital. Somatostatin, to decrease pancreatic secretions and minimize the incidence of a pancreatic fistula, is only used in patients who had a soft, friable pancreas at the time of the operation. When it is used, it is discontinued 24 h before pulling the pancreatic drain. If a fistula develops, as evidenced by the discharge of fluid with a high amylase concentration, the drain is not removed, and somatostatin is continued or started. Today, the morbidity of a pancreatic fistula is quite low. Virtually all pancreatic fistulae close by themselves, and the patient may be discharged from the hospital with the drain in place. When the drainage stops, the drain is pulled in the office.

The biliary anastomosis

We attach the end of the bile duct to the side of the jejunum, with a single layer of interrupted 4–0 polyglycolic acid absorbable sutures. A T-tube stent is used only if the bile duct is less than 1 cm in diameter, which is increasingly common today because many patients have had their jaundice relieved preoperatively with an endoscopically placed stent. This anastomosis is also drained to the outside, and the drain is removed after the patient is eating. The T-tube is clamped prior to discharge, and is removed about 3–4 weeks postoperatively at the first office visit. No cholangiograms are obtained in the usual uncomplicated case.

The gastric anastomosis

In the standard Whipple resection in which an antrectomy has been performed, the reconstruction is a retrocolic Hoffmeister-type reconstruction, with either an isoperistaltic or antiperistaltic gastrojejunostomy. If a pylorus-preserving Whipple has been done, the duodenojejunostomy is also done in a retrocolic fashion. The anastomoses are hand sewn in two layers.

POSTOPERATIVE MANAGEMENT

Patients rarely require admission to an intensive care unit, and are typically managed on the gastrointestinal surgical floor quite safely. The nasogastric tube is removed on the morning of the first postoperative day, after either the standard Whipple operation or its pylorus-preserving modification. Oral fluids are begun after peristaltic activity returns, usually on the fourth or fifth postoperative day. Over the next 3 days, intake is advanced to a regular diet, served in five to six divided portions. Patients are usually discharged on the ninth or tenth postoperative day.

If the patient is unable to tolerate oral intake, and vomiting suggests impaired gastric emptying, we re-insert a nasogastric tube, and usually obtain an abdominal CT scan. This occasionally reveals a fluid collection near the stomach, which may represent an undrained pancreatic fistula or other process. Percutaneous drainage and culture of the fluid should be done. Although delayed gastric emptying occurs from other unknown causes, it is important not to overlook such a treatable condition. Gastric function usually returns when the fluid collection is treated appropriately, or after a period of nasogastric suction if no other abnormalities are found.

PALLIATIVE WHIPPLE RESECTION

Because the Whipple resection is now done around the world with operative mortality rates less than 5%, pancreatic surgeons have discussed the possibility that it might be done for palliation. Indeed, there is anecdotal evidence that patients may live longer and enjoy a better quality of life if the tumor is removed than if it is not. Several recent reports which support the performance of the Whipple for palliation were not appropriately designed to answer the question, however.[63] All of the patients who underwent resection appeared to have lesions resectable for cure, according to the authors' usual criteria. The designation of one of the groups as the 'palliative Whipple' group was made retrospectively, when the pathology report showed that tumor extended to the resection margin. However, the issue at hand is whether a resection should be done in a patient whose disease is obviously incurable, e.g., one in whom liver metastases are evident at the time of exploration. That question has not been answered. We have not performed resections in patients with hepatic, peritoneal, or other distant metastases. We have done knowingly non-curative resections in selected patients with locally extensive disease (vascular or adjacent soft-tissue involvement), with the hope that they would provide palliation. Our anecdotal experience is encouraging.

OUTCOME

A review of UCLA patients treated between 1981 and 1988[7] showed mean survival rates of:

1. 22.1 ± 3.3 months for patients undergoing resections;
2. 7.1 ± 0.8 months after palliative bypass;
3. 4.8 ± 0.6 months with no intervention.

A recent review showed that the 5-year survival for pancreatic cancer after resection was 9%.[64]

Various prognostic indicators for survival after resection for pancreatic cancer have been evaluated. Geer and Brennan reviewed 799 patients admitted with a diagnosis of pancreatic cancer at the Memorial Sloan-Kettering Cancer Center. Their results showed that lymph node involvement, poor histologic tumor differentiation, and tumors greater than 2.5 cm in size were associated with a significantly reduced survival.[61]

Cameron *et al.*, at the Johns Hopkins Hospital, analysed 89 patients with carcinoma of the head of the pancreas who underwent pancreaticoduodenectomy. The strongest predictive factor for survival was negative lymph node status: a median survival of 55.8 months was seen in node-negative patients versus 11 months for node-positive patients. Patients receiving three or more units of blood also had a significantly decreased survival compared with patients receiving two units of blood or less (10.2 months versus 24.7 months).[65] A group at the Mayo Clinic also examined prognostic factors after pancreaticoduodenectomy. Malignant infiltration of the pancreatic capsule, proximity of tumor to lymphatic and blood vessels, round cell infiltrate at the tumor margin, and epithelial atypia in the uninvolved pancreatic ducts were all significantly associated with a poor prognosis.[66]

Bottger *et al.* reviewed the course of 41 patients after resection of pancreatic cancer and found, in a multivariate analysis, that DNA content was the strongest indicator of prognosis.[67] A group at Johns Hopkins found a significant difference in survival between diploid and aneuploid tumors (25 months versus 10.5 months). They also found that ploidy and proliferative index were independent prognostic factors.[68]

There is increasing evidence that the best outcomes in patients with pancreatic cancer are achieved at major centers with the most experience (>20 Whipple resections a year), and at the lowest cost.[69] This appears to be related not only to surgical expertise, but also to the expertise of the staff of numerous other ancillary services (e.g., nursing, radiology, gastrointestinal endoscopy), who all gain experience in the management of large numbers of these challenging patients.

REFERENCES

1. Gold EB. Epidemiology of and risk factors for pancreatic cancer. Surg Clin North Am 1995; 75:819–43.
2. Silverberg E, Boring CC, Squires TS. Cancer statistics, 1990. Cancer 1990; 40:9–26.
3. National Cancer Institute. *Annual cancer statistics review 1973–1988.* NIH Publication No. 91-2789. Bethesda, MD, Department of Health and Human Services, 1991.

4. Cubilla AL, Fitzgerald P. Pathology of cancer of the exocrine pancreas. In Howard JM, Jordan GL, Reber HA, eds. *Surgical diseases of the pancreas.* Philadelphia, Lea and Febiger, 1987, 627–40.

5. Lillemoe KD. Current management of pancreatic carcinoma. Ann Surg 1995; 221:133–48.

6. Fontham E, Correa P, Cohn I Jr. Epidemiology of cancer of the pancreas. In Howard JM, Jordan GL, Reber HA, eds. *Surgical diseases of the pancreas.* Philadelphia, Lea and Febiger, 1987, 613–26.

7. Singh SM, Longmire WP Jr, Reber HA. Surgical palliation for pancreatic cancer. The UCLA experience. Ann Surg 1990; 212:132–9.

8. Braasch JW. Pancreaticoduodenal resection. Curr Probl Surg 1988; 25(5):321–63.

9. Cubilla AL, Fitzgerald PJ. Pancreas cancer. I. Duct adenocarcinoma. Pathol Ann 1978; 1:241.

10. Way LW. Diagnosis of pancreatic and other periampullary cancers. In Howard JM, Jordan GL, Reber HA, eds. *Surgical diseases of the pancreas.* Philadelphia, Lea and Febiger, 1987, 641–53.

11. Bowden L, Pack GT. Cancer of the head of the pancreas. A collective review of the experience of the gastric service of the Memorial Cancer Center, 1926–1958. GEN 1969; 23:339–67.

12. Moosa AR, Levin B. The diagnosis of 'early' pancreatic cancer. The University of Chicago experience. Cancer 1981; 47(Suppl.):1688–97.

13. Ariyama J, Shirakabe H, Ikenobe H, Kurosawa A, Owman T. The diagnosis of the small resectable pancreatic carcinoma. Clin Radiol 1977; 28:437–44.

14. Takagi K, Takahashi T, Hori M, *et al.* Small carcinoma of head of the pancreas discovered by the clue of transitory elevation of urinary amylase level. Stomach and Intestine 1980; 15:637–40 (summary in English).

15. Suzuki T, Uchida K, Tobe T. Six cases of small pancreatic cancer. Stomach and Intestine 1980; 15:641–5 (summary in English).

16. Abe M, Hara Y, Kiyonari H, *et al.* Early diagnosis of cancer of body of the pancreas. Jpn J Gastroenterol 1981; 78:1676 (Japanese).

17. Ozaki H, Ohkura H, Nakamura K, Yoshimori M, Oka Y, Kishi K. Small carcinoma of the head of the pancreas: report of a case. Stomach and Intestine 1980; 647–51 (summary in English).

18. Ozaki H. Improvement of pancreatic cancer treatment: from the Japanese experience in the 1980s. Int J Pancreatol 1992; 1:5–9.

19. Podolsky DK. Serologic markers in the diagnosis and management of pancreatic carcinoma. World J Surg 1984; 8:822–30.

20. Malesci A, Tommasini MA, Bonato C. Determination of CA 19-9 antigen in serum and pancreatic juice for differential diagnosis of pancreatic adenocarcinoma from chronic pancreatitis. Gastroenterology 1987; 92:60–7.

21. Howard JM. Carcinoma of the exocrine pancreas: current progress. Int J Pancreatol 1992; 12:1–3.

22. Poston GJ, Gillespie J, Guillou PJ. Biology of pancreatic cancer. Gut 1991; 32:800–12.

23. Tada M, Omata M, Ohto M. Clinical application of gene mutations for diagnosis of pancreatic adenocarcinoma. Gastroenterology 1991; 100:233–8.

24. Moosa AR, Gamagami RA. Diagnosis and staging of pancreatic neoplasms. Surg Clin North Am 1995; 75:871–90.

25. Lawson TL. Sensitivity of pancreatic ultrasonography in the detection of pancreatic disease. Radiology 1978; 128:733–6.

26. Freeny PC, Marks WM, Ryan JA. Pancreatic ductal adenocarcinoma: diagnosis and staging with dynamic CT. Radiology 1988; 166:125–33.

27. Ward EM, Stephens DH, Sheedy PR II. Computed tomographic characteristics of pancreatic cancer: an analysis of 100 cases. Radiographics 1983; 3:547–65.

28. Freeny PC, Traverso LW, Ryan JA. Diagnosis and staging of pancreatic adenocarcinoma with dynamic computed tomography. Am J Surg 1993; 165:600–6.

29. Sindelar WF, Kinsells TJ, Mayer RJ. Cancer of the pancreas. In DeVita VT Jr, Hellman S, Rosenberg SA, eds. *Cancer: principles and practice of oncology.* Philadelphia, J.B. Lippincott Co, 1985, 691–735.

30. Frick MP. Accuracy of endoscopic retrograde cholangiopancreatography (ERCP) in differentiating benign and malignant pancreatic disease. Gastrointest Radiol 1982; 7:241.

31. Yang R, Leichman L, Ralls PW, Cohen H, Karanjia ND, Reber HA. Carcinoma of the exocrine pancreas. In Valenzulea JE, Reber HA, Ribet A, eds. *Medical and surgical diseases of the pancreas.* New York, Igaku-Shoin, 1991, 155–78.

32. Tio TL, Tytgat GNJ. Endoscopic ultrasonography in staging local resectability of pancreatic and periampullary malignancy. Scand J Gastroenterol 1986; 21:135–42.

33. Rosch T, Braig C, Gain T, *et al.* Staging of pancreatic and ampullary carcinoma by endoscopic ultrasonography: comparison with conventional sonography, computed tomography, and angiography. Gastroenterology 1992; 102:188–99.

34. Dickey JE, Haaga JR, Stellato TA. Evaluation of computed tomography-guided percutaneous biopsy of the pancreas. Surg Gynecol Obstet 1986; 163:497–503.

35. Conlon KC, Dougherty E, Klimstra D, Coit DG, Turnbull ADM, Brennan MF. The value of minimal access surgery in the staging of patients with potentially resectable perpancreatic malignancy. Ann Surg 1996; 223:134–40.

36. Warshaw AL, Tepper JE, Shipley WU. Laparoscopy in the staging and planning of therapy for pancreatic cancer. Am J Surg 1986; 151:76–80.

37. Cuesta MA, Meijer S, Borgstein PJ, Mulder LS, Sikkenk AC. Laparoscopic ultrasonography for

hepatobiliary and pancreatic malignancy. Br J Surg 1993; 80:1571–4.

38. John TG, Greig JD, Carter DC, Garden OJ. Carcinoma of the pancreatic head and periampullary region: tumor staging with laparoscopy and laparoscopic ultrasonography. Ann Surg 1995; 221:156–64.

39. Rhodes M, Nathanson L, Fielding G. Laparoscopic biliary and gastric bypass: a useful adjunct in the treatment of carcinoma of the pancreas. Gut 1995; 36:778–80.

40. Nakayama T, Ikeda A, Okuda K. Percutaneous transhepatic drainage of the biliary tract. Gastroenterology 1978; 74:554–9.

41. Pitt HA, Gomes AS, Lois JF. Does preoperative percutaneous biliary drainage reduce operative risk or increase hospital cost? Ann Surg 1985; 201:545–53.

42. McPherson GAD, Benjamin IS, Hodgson HJF. Preoperative percutaneous transhepatic biliary drainage: the results of a controlled trial. Br J Surg 1984; 71:371–5.

43. Hatfield ARW, Terblanche J, Fataar S. Preoperative external biliary drainage in obstructive jaundice. Lancet 1982; 2:896–9.

44. Halsted WS. Contributions to the surgery of the bile passages, especially the common bile duct. Boston Med Surg J 1899; 141:645–54.

45. Whipple AO, Parsons WB, Mullins CR. Treatment of carcinoma of ampulla of Vater. Ann Surg 1935; 102:763–79.

46. Brunschwig A. Resection of the head of the pancreas and duodenum for carcinoma – pancreaticoduodenectomy. Surg Gynecol Obstet 1937; 65: 681–4.

47. Whipple AO. Pancreaticoduodenectomy for islet carcinoma: five-year follow-up. Ann Surg 1945; 121:847–52.

48. Reber HA. Small pancreatic tumors: is size any indication of cure? J HPB Surg 1995; 2:384–6.

49. Fortner JG, Klimstra DS, Senie RT, Maclean BJ. Tumor size is the primary prognosticator for pancreatic cancer after regional pancreatectomy. Ann Surg 1996; 223(2):147–53.

50. Watson K. Carcinoma of ampulla of Vater: successful radical resection. Br J Surg 1944; 31:368–73.

51. Traverso LW, Longmire WP Jr. Preservation of the pylorus in pancreaticoduodenectomy. Surg Gynecol Obstet 1978; 146:959–62.

52. Fortner JG. Regional resection of cancer of the pancreas: a new surgical approach. Surgery 1973; 73:307–20.

53. Nagai H, Kuroda A, Morioka Y. Lymphatic and local spread of T1 and T2 pancreatic cancer: a study of autopsy material. Ann Surg 1985; 204:65–71.

54. Griffin JF, Smalley Sr, Jewell W. Patterns of failure after curative resection of pancreatic carcinoma. Cancer 1990; 66:56–61.

55. Ishikawa O, Ohhigashi H, Sasaki Y, et al. Practical usefulness of lymphatic and connective tissue clearance for the carcinoma of the pancreas head. Ann Surg 1988; 208:215–20.

56. Tsuchiya R, Tsunoda T, Yamaguchi T. Operations of choice for resectable carcinoma of the head of the pancreas. Int J Pancreatol 1990; 6:295–306.

57. Takahashi S, Ogata Y, Tsuzuki T. Combined resection of the pancreas and portal vein for pancreatic cancer. Br J Surg 1994; 81:1190–3.

58. Reber HA, Ashley SW, McFadden D. Curative treatment for pancreatic neoplasms. Surg Clin North Am 1995; 75:905–12.

59. Yeo CJ, Cameron JL. Arguments against radical (extended) resection for adenocarcinoma of the pancreas. Adv Surg 1994; 27:273–84.

60. Satake K, Nishiwaki H, Yokomatsu H, et al. Surgical curability and prognosis for standard versus extended resections for T1 carcinoma of the pancreas. Surg Gynecol Obstet 1992; 175:259–65.

61. Geer RJ, Brennan MF. Prognostic indicators for survival after resection of pancreatic adenocarcinoma. Am J Surg 1993; 165:68–73.

62. Priestly JT, Comfort MW, Radcliffe J Jr. Total pancreatectomy for hyperinsulinism due to an islet cell adenoma. Survival and cure at 16 months after operation. Presentation of metabolic studies. Ann Surg 1944; 119:211–15.

63. Lillemoe KD, Cameron JL, Yeo CJ, et al. Pancreaticoduodenectomy: does it have a role in the palliation of pancreatic cancer? Ann Surg 1996; 223(6):718–28.

64. Livingston EH, Welton ML, Reber HA. Surgical treatment of pancreatic cancer. The United States experience. Int J Pancreatol 1991; 9:153–7.

65. Cameron JL, Crist DW, Sitzmann JV, et al. Factors influencing survival after pancreaticoduodenectomy for pancreatic cancer. Am J Surg 1991; 161:120–5.

66. Mannell A, van Heerden JA, Weiland LH, Ilstrup DM. Factors influencing survival after resection of ductal adenocarcinoma of the pancreas. Ann Surg 1986; 203:403–7.

67. Bottger TC, Storkel S, Wellek S, Stockle M, Junginger T. Factors influencing survival after resection of pancreatic cancer: a DNA analysis and histomorphologic study. Cancer 1994; 73:63–73.

68. Allison DC, Bose KK, Hruban RH, et al. Pancreatic cancer cell DNA content correlates with long-term survival after pancreaticoduodenectomy. Ann Surg 1991; 214:648–56.

69. Gordon TA, Burleyson GP, Tielsch JM, Cameron JL. The effects of regionalization on cost and outcome for one general high-risk surgical procedure. Ann Surg 1995; 221:43–9.

Commentary

THEODORE X O'CONNELL

Drs Todd and Reber have presented a very excellent and complete review of all aspects of pancreatic carcinoma, based not only on an extensive literature review but also on their own very impressive personal experience. This commentary is basically planned to emphasize some of their points by comparison and/or contrast and at times playing the devil's advocate to stimulate additional thinking, perhaps in a new or different direction.

The major problem of pancreatic carcinoma is its basic biologic behavior. Paper after paper over many decades has shown that survival has not improved significantly. The majority of patients with pancreatic cancer are not resectable and, even in those that are resectable, only 10–20% enjoy a 5-year survival. There is no substantial proof in any scientific report that earlier diagnosis, any type of screening, or more aggressive operations have produced any significant benefit to these patients.

PREOPERATIVE DIAGNOSIS AND MANAGEMENT

Again, Drs Todd and Reber have presented an extensive analysis of multiple tests used in the diagnosis and staging of pancreatic carcinoma, emphasizing the significant problem of the high number of false positives and false negatives. However, I wish to present a very practical approach to the work-up of these patients and not to reiterate all the possible tests that could be used.

The vast majority of the patients with surgically treatable disease have carcinoma in the head of the pancreas. Therefore, most patients present with jaundice. In general, in patients with jaundice, cancer should be the initial diagnosis until proven otherwise, especially if they have no other reasons to have jaundice such as evidence of hepatitis, stones in the common duct, recent biliary operations with the possibility of iatrogenic stricture or other diseases associated with bile duct strictures such as inflammatory bowel disease, etc. The purpose of the preoperative work-up is not so much to prove the diagnosis, which is already a given, with multiple different tests all of which have a significant false-negative rate, but to determine which patients are unresectable due to liver metastases, extensive lymph node metastases, peritoneal carcinomatosis, and vascular invasion. By preoperative staging, patients who are clearly not resectable or curable by surgical means can avoid an unnecessary exploration. The practical approach to patients with jaundice who have a high suspicion of carcinoma usually consists of only two tests:

1 *CA19-9*. CA19-9 should not be used as a screening test in asymptomatic individuals due to the fact that a significantly sized lesion needs to be present for the test to be positive. In addition, there are false positives with other tumors producing elevations such as upper gastrointestinal cancers, colon cancers, etc. Also, there are no studies to prove that CA19-9 is a worthwhile screening test that improves patient outcome. However, in patients with jaundice, an elevated CA19-9 is very helpful. Obviously, if the patient is jaundiced and has a significantly elevated CA19-9, then the assumption is that the patient has a malignancy as the cause, be it pancreatic, ampullary, or bile duct carcinoma. On the other hand, a negative test, especially a false-negative test, is of no help; however, the test is easy to perform, inexpensive, and non-invasive and can be helpful in planning treatment and in early discussions with the patient.

2 *Helical (spiral) computerized tomography.* It should be emphasized that helical computerized tomography (CT) is not used so much to make a definitive diagnosis of pancreatic cancer, but rather to determine resectability. The problem with using the CT to make a definitive diagnosis is the high rate of false negatives (approximately 20%). Often, the reason for the false negative is a relatively small cancer in the head of the pancreas that cannot be adequately imaged on the CT scan. However, these small lesions are often the earliest and the most resectable and therefore, simply because the CT scan does not show a definite pancreatic mass does not mean that the patients do not have cancer, especially a resectable cancer. The presence of a mass in the head of the pancreas may be helpful but is not 100% diagnostic because false positives can be produced by pancreatic head pancreatitis, enlarged lymph nodes, other neoplasms, etc. Usually, the CT scan will show intrahepatic and extrahepatic biliary duct dilatation that extends down to the pancreatic level. If it does, then one can assume that this is due either to pancreatic cancer or a periampullary lesion and proceed accordingly. Obviously, if there is no extrahepatic biliary dilatation or when the dilatation extends only partially down the duct, other diagnoses should be suspected and substantiated with either endoscopic retrograde cholangiopancreaticography (ERCP) or percutaneous trans-hepatic cholangiography (PTC). Therefore, the CT scan is not used to make the diagnosis of pancreatic cancer but to establish evidence of unresectable disease.

Although no test is perfect in the investigation of unresectability, helical CT scans have a low incidence of false positives that would preclude the patient from potentially curable operation. The small incidence of false negatives (approximately a third) can be accepted because the majority of patients who are found at operation to have additional disease not appreciated on CT scan can still have a palliative bypass and benefit from the operation. Again, perhaps in the future even better studies can be developed to determine resectability; however, helical CTs seem to be the best test at the present time.

The only two tests that I would do on a regular basis would be CA19-9 and helical CT scans, although other tests such as laparoscopy can be done on an individual basis for patients in whom there is a high suspicion of unresectable disease, but which has not been proven on the helical CT. This is especially true if one suspects carcinomatosis due to the presence of ascites or omental or mesenteric thickening on CT.

I agree wholeheartedly that ERCP should not be done routinely. The reasons for this include:

1 The real purpose of preoperative testing is to determine resectability and this is not possible with an ERCP.
2 There are potential complications of ERCP, including cholangitis, perforations, etc.
3 The operation for ampullary, distal bile duct, or pancreatic cancers is exactly the same, that is, a pancreatico-duodenectomy.

Knowledge of a specific diagnosis preoperatively usually will not change the operative plans. Also, when an ERCP is done, a stent may be placed. This is done to help prevent cholangitis, which is caused by the introduction of bacteria into the obstructed duct during ERCP. The preoperative placement of stents has not proven to be of significant benefit and may make the subsequent surgery more difficult by decreasing the diameter of the bile duct and causing periductal inflammation. Numerous reports have also shown a higher rate of postoperative sepsis when a preoperative ERCP stent is used.

ERCP stenting however does have a place in two circumstances:

1 when the patient is obviously not resectable, as determined by the CT scan or physical findings, a stent can produce palliation without the need for operation,
2 if the patient is currently not an operative candidate due to evidence of severe malnutrition, stenting may help decompress the liver and return the patient to operative status by improving the nutritional environment.

At the present time, endoscopic ultrasound has not significantly added to the findings of high-quality helical CT scans.

Fine-needle aspiration (FNA) of the pancreatic mass again should not be routinely employed. There is a 15–20% false-negative rate associated with this because of the sampling error primarily caused by pancreatitis surrounding the pancreatic cancer. Also, the results do not generally change management. If the FNA is positive

and the patient is otherwise resectable, you proceed to operation. If the test is negative, we still must assume that this is a cancer that has been missed because of the false negatives and still proceed with operation. The only time that FNA probably should be considered is when there is a mass in the body or tail of the pancreas that is not clearly an adenocarcinoma. A FNA may prove a diagnosis of something that may be surgically treatable, such as a non-functioning islet cell cancer.

OPERATIVE MANAGEMENT

After a helical CT scan that does not show evidence of unresectable disease, an operation is undertaken. The experienced surgeon then has to make the intraoperative decision that the patient has a resectable periampullary or pancreatic cancer (with or without a positive biopsy) and then proceed with a pancreaticoduodenectomy (Whipple). In a small percentage of cases, even with an experienced surgeon, a Whipple will be done for benign disease, i.e., pancreatitis of the head. This is acceptable treatment for this diagnosis and avoids not treating a small resectable pancreatic cancer.

Although it has been said that the size of the cancer is not a contraindication to surgical resection, it does have an impact on the surgical decision making and on outcome. A large tumor means that it has been present for a long time or is a very aggressively growing lesion. Although large size is not an absolute contraindication to resection, it is quite clear that patients with larger lesions have decreased survival rate, an increased rate of unresectability due to vascular invasion, and more difficult surgery with increased intraoperative and postoperative complications.

Modifications of Whipple procedure

1 *Pyloric sparing.* I think either a pyloric sparing or standard Whipple can be used, depending on the surgeon's choice and the individual anatomical variation seen at the time of operation. There has been little evidence to show that there is any difference in survival or long-term nutritional effects between the two procedures.
2 *Extended Whipple.* This includes any combination of resection of the superior mesenteric vein and/or superior mesenteric artery, total pancreatectomy and/or extensive lymph node resections outside the peripancreatic area. In general, I think these procedures are example of the surgeons 'hope springs eternal'. There is absolutely no evidence that any of these procedures increases survival significantly and certainly may increase the complication rate. As far as resecting vessels, there have been multiple studies to show that there is no real survival benefit to this. The reason for

this is that the patients generally fail with distant disease, that is, either liver or peritoneal metastases, and therefore removing the vessels does not have any impact on the occurrence of the metastases. Also, those patients who have vessel involvement have a poorer prognosis and a greater chance of having distant micrometastases than patients whose vessels are clear.

Drs Todd and Reber mentioned that at times they will do a vessel resection; however, I question the benefit of this. One of the rationales is 'the patient wants it'. I do not think this is a good argument. Patients may want a lot of things that the evidence clearly shows are of no benefit to them. Rather than just doing an operation that is not going to benefit the patient, patients should be counseled that this type of extensive operation will clearly not benefit them and may actually shorten both the quantity and quality of their lives. The other reason to do a partial resection of the vein is more understandable. This is the case when the surgeon initially finds that the anterior surface of the vein is free, but then, when the pancreas is split, discovers that the lateral or posterior surface of the vein is involved. This is particularly true when the cancer arises in the uncinate process. Unfortunately, at that point, the surgeon has nothing else to do but to proceed with the Whipple by taking a portion of the vein. Certainly, if the surgeon knew this was the case before hand, the Whipple would not have even been started.

Not surprisingly, extensive node dissections have not proven to be of any benefit. The lymph node positivity, especially of lymph nodes distant from the pancreas, is an indicator of systemic disease but not a determinate. The majority of patients do not fail locally in lymph nodes but distantly in the liver and/or peritoneum. If the lymph nodes in the retroperitoneal, celiac, or para-aortic area are negative, then obviously the patient cannot benefit from having them removed. If they are positive, this is an indicator of distant disease and the patient is not benefited by their removal.

Pancreatic anastomosis

The method of pancreatic anastomosis has always been controversial, because one of the major complications of pancreaticoduodenectomy is pancreatic fluid leak and subsequent pancreatic fistula. Obviously, the pancreatic anastomosis can be handled in multiple fashions, including end-to-end or end-to-side anastomosis or simply closing the end of the pancreas with a thoracic anastomosis (TA) stapler or, especially in a diabetic patient, a total pancreatectomy. Again, the technique used must be individualized based on the training of the surgeon and any patient specifics, including consistence of the gland

and size of the pancreatic duct. My method is quite similar to that of Drs Todd and Reber. However, I generally telescope the end of the pancreas into the end of the jejunal limb using a two-layer anastomosis with a running 3-0 polypropylene suture externally and a running 3-0 polyglactin suture internally. Using this method, we have had a very small percentage of leaks, well under 10%. All of the anastomoses are drained by a closed suction drainage and, if there is a small leak, it is controlled by this drain. If there is no distal obstruction, this small fistula will close when the drainage tube is removed. The biliary jejunal anastomosis is usually done with a single layer of 4-0 running polyglactic suture. A T-tube is generally placed with a limb across the anastomosis to help decompress the jejunum leading to the pancreatic anastomosis.

I agree that there is no need to place most patients in the intensive care unit after the operation unless there are intraoperative complications or there is some significant comorbid disease. Patients are generally eating by the fifth postoperative day and are usually discharged by the seventh to tenth day postoperatively. At times, there is initial intolerance of feeding, especially when the pyloric-sparing Whipple is performed. However, I do not routinely get a CT scan as suggested, because I feel it is generally not positive or helpful. The problem seems to be due to anastomotic edema and/or gastric atony. This problem can usually be easily treated with motility agents and a little patience.

PALLIATIVE TREATMENT

It must be realized that most of our efforts in treating patients with pancreatic cancer at this time are, in reality, palliative. The majority of Whipples that we do, even though we think that they are curative, actually turn out to be palliative because there is distant microscopic disease of which we are not aware. This is the reason that even extensive surgeries still show a 5-year survival rate that does not exceed 20%. Therefore, at least 80% of pancreaticoduodenectomies for pancreatic cancer are palliative. However, I do not recommend an obviously purposeful palliative Whipple when patients have obvious distant disease in the liver, peritoneal metastasis, distant lymph nodes, etc. This is exposing patients to excessive morbidity to produce palliative results, which can easily be obtained by simple bypass procedures. Although some published series indicate that patients treated with palliative Whipples live longer than those not having Whipples, it must be emphasized that these are not randomized, prospective studies and probably those patients having a Whipple are younger, have comparatively less distant disease, and have lesions that the surgeon can more easily resect. Therefore, I think this is a problem with 'an apples and oranges' comparison between patients, with palliative Whipples being compared to those patients with either bypass or no treatment at all. There is no justification for a knowingly palliative Whipple simply because current results show decreased morbidity and mortality rates from the operation itself, unless there is a proven increase in survival. Just because you can do an operation with fewer side-effects, if it does not produce the desired results, there is no reason to do it.

FUTURE TREATMENT

Although there is not much mention of adjuvant therapies in the chapter, this is obviously where a lot of the emphasis needs to be placed. There is some evidence that there is a minor impact of chemoradiation after Whipple; however, this result is not marked and most of the patients fail outside of the radiated area. Over the past years, doing extensive preoperative work-up, especially with helical CT, has decreased the amount of unnecessary operations. This has increased the rate of resection per operation and saved many patients from needless operations. This is certainly a significant move forward to be as selective as we can in the care of our patients. Also, I think more experience and better preoperative staging have perhaps decreased the absolute number of Whipples done, and have also increased slightly the percentage of the patients who have 5-year survivals after Whipples. However, it may not have increased the absolute number of patients surviving 5 years. In the years ahead, I think we should continue to try to devise new methods such as positron emission tomography (PET) scan, molecular markers, etc. to select even better those patients who have truly local disease and can benefit from pancreaticoduodenectomy.

The review states that centers that do more Whipples per year have a better outcome at a lower cost, but this is not entirely true. This is a generalization and generalizations are generally not entirely accurate. Even in the quoted articles, there are institutions that do few Whipples per year that have results identical to those of the major specialized institutions. Also, multiple other articles have presented excellent results with a smaller number of patients. This all needs to be individualized by specific outcome results, not just on the number of Whipples done per year. Obviously, if the results are poor with high morbidity and mortality, then those institutions should not be doing Whipples, no matter how many they do per year.

I think all of us, as surgeons, need to come to the understanding of the biology of pancreatic cancer. We have to understand that by the time patients are seen, the vast majority already have distant disease and cannot benefit from a pancreaticoduodenectomy and even bigger and supposedly better operations, including extensive lymph node resections, vascular resections, etc. We must respond to the biology of this disease and understand that this is a systemic disease when first seen and that effective adjuvant therapy needs to be developed to significantly change the survival outcomes in patients with pancreatic carcinoma.

Editors' selected abstracts

Radical resection of periampullary tumors in the elderly: evaluation of long-term results.

Bathe OF, Levi D, Caldera H, Franceschi D, Raez L, Patel A, Raub WA Jr, Benedetto P, Reddy R, Huston D, Sleeman D, Livingstone AS, Levi JU.

Department of Surgery, Division of Surgical Oncology, Sylvester Comprehensive Cancer Center, University of Miami, FL, USA.

World Journal of Surgery 24(3):353–8, 2000, March.

Increasingly, patients of advanced age are coming for evaluation of periampullary tumors. Although several studies have demonstrated the safety of resecting periampullary tumors in older patients, few long-term survival data have been reported. Between 1983 and 1992 various periampullary masses were resected in 70 patients over age 65 (range 65–87 years). Total pancreatectomy was performed in 11 patients, and 59 patients underwent pancreaticoduodenectomy. The mean duration of hospitalization was 17 ± 15 days. Major complications occurred in 27 patients (39%), and operative mortality rate was 8.5%. Overall median survival was 24 months; and 5-year survival was 25%. Perioperative outcome was compared in patients aged 65 to 74 years and in patients ≥ 75 years old. The older age group required longer periods in the surgical intensive care unit postoperatively, but the long-term survival was similar in the two age groups. Radical resection with the intent to cure periampullary tumors is safe in selected patients of advanced age, and long-term survival is in the range of expected survival for younger patients with the same tumors.

Pancreatic carcinoma deemed unresectable at exploration may be resected for cure: an institutional experience.

Chao C, Hoffman JP, Ross EA, Torosian MH, Eisenberg BL.

Department of Surgery, Fox Chase Cancer Center, Philadelphia, PA, USA.

American Surgeon 66(4):378–85, 2000, April.

Only a minority of patients with a diagnosis of pancreatic adenocarcinoma (PA) have disease amenable to curative resection. Between April 1987 and March 1999, 40 patients with pancreatic adenocarcinoma deemed unresectable at exploration at other institutions were considered for neoadjuvant treatments and then re-evaluated for possible re-exploration. We retrospectively compared the clinical outcomes, including overall survival (OS), among three groups: Group A, 22 previously unresectable patients who were subsequently successfully resected, 20 after induction therapy; Group B, 31 patients who received preoperative chemoradiotherapy before their only operation; and Group C, 33 patients who were primarily resected, 27 of whom were then treated with adjuvant therapy. Of those resectable from Group A, 5 required portal venorrhaphy and 3 had hepatic artery reconstruction. Eighteen of the 40 patients were unresectable because of progression of disease with a mean OS of 8 months; 12 were assessed at second laparotomy; 6 were excluded from second operation on the basis of preoperative imaging studies. Kaplan–Meier curves showed no differences in OS among the three groups: OS in Group A was 34 months; Group B, 21; and Group C, 13 ($p = 0.15$). Margin status was comparable in all three groups ($p = 0.52$). As expected, nodal positivity was greatest in Group C ($p = 0.001$). There were no operative mortalities in Group A, and the morbidity rate was comparable with that of Groups B and C. Upon re-evaluation, many tumors (54%) previously deemed 'unresectable' were surgically extirpated for cure with a median survival comparable with that of patients who did not undergo previous exploration.

Quality of life and outcomes after pancreaticoduodenectomy.

Huang JJ, Yeo CJ, Sohn TA, Lillemoe KD, Sauter PK, Coleman J, Hruban RH, Cameron JL.

Departments of Surgery, Oncology, and Pathology, The Johns Hopkins Medical Institutions, Baltimore, MD, USA.

Annals of Surgery 231(6):890–8, 2000, June.

Objective: To assess the quality of life (QOL) and functional outcome of patients after pancreaticoduodenectomy. *Summary background data:* Pancreaticoduodenectomy is gaining acceptance and is being performed in increasing numbers for various malignant and benign diseases of the pancreas and periampullary region. There is a general impression that pancreaticoduodenectomy can severely impair QOL and alter normal activities. Only a few small studies have evaluated QOL after pancreaticoduodenectomy. *Methods:* A standard QOL questionnaire was sent to 323 patients surviving pancreaticoduodenectomy who had undergone surgery at The Johns Hopkins Hospital between 1981 and 1997. Thirty items on a visual analog scale were categorized into three domains: physical (15 items), psychological (10 items), and social (5 items). Scores are reported as a percentile, with 100% being the highest possible score. The same QOL questionnaire was also sent to laparoscopic cholecystectomy patients and healthy controls. A separate component of the questionnaire asked about functional outcomes and disabilities. *Results:* Overall QOL scores for the 192 responding pancreaticoduodenectomy patients in the three domains (physical, psychological, social) were 78%, 79%, and 81%, respectively. These QOL scores were comparable to those of the 37 laparoscopic cholecystectomy patients and the 31 healthy controls. The pancreaticoduodenectomy patients were subgrouped into chronic pancreatitis, other benign disease, pancreatic adenocarcinoma, and other cancers. Patients who underwent resection for chronic pancreatitis and pancreatic adenocarcinoma had significantly lower QOL scores in the physical and psychological domains compared with the laparoscopic cholecystectomy patients and the healthy controls. Common problems after pancreaticoduodenectomy were weight loss, abdominal pain, fatigue, foul stools, and diabetes. *Conclusions:* This is the largest single-institution experience assessing QOL after pancreaticoduodenectomy. These data demonstrate that as a group, patients who survive pancreaticoduodenectomy have near-normal QOL scores. Many patients report weight loss and symptoms consistent with pancreatic exocrine and endocrine insufficiency. Most patients have QOL scores comparable to those of control patients and can function independently in daily activities.

Impact of laparoscopic staging in the treatment of pancreatic cancer.

Jimenez RE, Warshaw AL, Rattner DW, Willett CG, McGrath D, Fernandez-del Castillo C.

Department of Surgery, Massachusetts General Hospital and Harvard Medical School, Boston, MA, USA.

Archives of Surgery 135(4):409–14, 2000, April.

Hypothesis: Staging laparoscopy in patients with pancreatic cancer identifies unsuspected metastases, allows treatment selection, and helps predict survival. *Design:* Inception cohort. *Setting:* Tertiary referral center. *Patients:* A total of 125 consecutive patients with radiographic stage II to III pancreatic ductal adenocarcinoma who underwent staging laparoscopy with peritoneal cytologic examination between July 1994 and November 1998. Seventy-eight proximal tumors and 47 distal tumors were localized. *Interventions:* Based on the findings of spiral computed tomography (CT) and laparoscopy, patients were stratified into 3 groups. Group 1 patients had unsuspected metastases found at laparoscopy and were palliated without further operation. Group 2 patients had no demonstrable metastases, but CT indicated unresectability due to vessel invasion. This group underwent external beam radiation with fluorouracil chemotherapy followed in selected cases by intraoperative radiation. Patients in group 3 had no metastases or definitive vessel invasion and were resection candidates. *Main outcome measure:* Survival. *Results:* Staging laparoscopy revealed unsuspected metastases in 39 patients (31.2%), with 9 having positive cytologic test results as the only evidence of metastatic disease (group 1). Fifty-five patients (44.0%) had localized but unresectable carcinoma (group 2), of whom 2 (3.6%) did not tolerate treatment, 20 (36.4%) developed metastatic disease during treatment, and 21 (38.2%) received intraoperative radiation. Of 31 patients with potentially resectable tumors (group 3), resection for cure was performed in 23 (resectability rate, 74.2%). Median survival was 7.5 months for patients with metastatic disease, 10.5 months for those receiving chemoradiation, and 14.5 months for those who underwent tumor resection ($p = 0.01$ for group 2 vs. group 1; $p < 0.001$ for group 3 vs. group 1). *Conclusions:* Staging laparoscopy, combined with spiral CT, allowed stratification of patients into 3 treatment groups that correlated with treatment opportunity and subsequent survival. Among the 125 patients, laparoscopy obviated 39 unnecessary operations and irradiation in patients with metastatic disease not detectable by CT. Laparoscopic staging can help focus aggressive treatment on patients with pancreatic cancer who might benefit.

Results of total pancreatectomy for adenocarcinoma of the pancreas.

Karpoff HM, Klimstra DS, Brennan MF, Conlon KC.

Department of Surgery, Memorial Sloan-Kettering Cancer Center, New York, NY, USA.

Archives of Surgery 136(1):44–7, 2001, January.

Hypothesis: Total pancreatectomy for infiltrating ductal adenocarcinoma is not superior to pancreaticoduodenectomy or distal pancreatectomy. *Design:* A retrospective analysis of a prospective database of patients. *Setting:* Memorial Sloan-Kettering Cancer Center, New York, NY. *Patients:* All patients ($n = 488$) undergoing pancreatic resection. *Main outcome measures:* Duration of operation, estimated blood loss, complications, length of stay, number of positive lymph nodes, presence of a positive margin, and survival times were analyzed. *Results:* Thirty-five patients were identified who underwent total pancreatectomy, 28 of whom had adenocarcinoma. Median length of stay was 32 days; 19 (54%) developed postoperative complications, of which 63% were infectious. Thirty-day mortality was 3% (1 patient). Median survival was 9.3 months (range, 0.6–172 months). There was no significant difference between patients with and without adenocarcinoma in terms of duration of operation, estimated blood loss, complications, length of stay, or number of readmissions. In patients with adenocarcinoma, margin or nodal status were not significant survival variables. Patients undergoing total pancreatectomy for adenocarcinoma had a significantly worse overall survival than those undergoing total pancreatectomy for other reasons ($p < 0.001$), or compared with a contemporaneous cohort with adenocarcinoma undergoing pancreaticoduodenectomy ($n = 409$) and distal pancreatectomy ($n = 51$) (7.9 vs. 17.2 months; $p < 0.002$). *Conclusions:* Total pancreatectomy can be performed safely with low mortality; survival is predicted by the underlying pathologic findings: patients undergoing total pancreatectomy for adenocarcinoma have a uniformly poor outcome. Those undergoing total pancreatectomy for benign disease or nonadenocarcinoma variants can have long-term survival. In patients who require total pancreatectomy for ductal adenocarcinoma, the survival is so poor as to bring into question the value of the operation.

Is CT angiography sufficient for prediction of resectability of periampullary neoplasms?

Saldinger PF, Reilly M, Reynolds K, Raptopoulos V, Chuttani R, Steer ML, Matthews JB.

Department of Medicine, Beth Israel Deaconess Medical Center, Harvard Medical School, Boston, MA, USA.

Journal of Gastrointestinal Surgery 4(3):233–7, 2000, May–June.

The optimal preoperative evaluation of periampullary neoplasms remains controversial. The aim of this study was to analyze the accuracy of helical computed tomography (CT) and CT angiography with three-dimensional reconstruction in predicting resectability. Between March 1996 and May 1999, a total of 100 patients with periampullary neoplasms were prospectively staged by helical CT and CT angiography with three-dimensional reconstruction. Vascular involvement was graded from 0 to 4, with grade 0 representing no vascular involvement and grade 4 total encasement of either the superior mesenteric vein or artery. Patients with grade 4 lesions were considered unresectable. Sixty-eight patients underwent surgical exploration with intent to perform a pancreaticoduodenectomy. Forty-four lesions were grade 0, five were grade 1, eight were grade 2, and 11 were grade 3. Resectability for grades 0 to 3 was 96%, 100%, 50%, and 9%, respectively, for an overall resectability rate of 76%. Resectability in patients with vascular encroachment (grade 2) is usually determined by the extent of local disease rather than the presence of extrapancreatic disease. Resection is rarely possible in patients with evidence of vascular encasement (grade 3). Additional imaging modalities such as diagnostic laparoscopy are superfluous in patients with no evidence of local vascular involvement on CT angiography (grades 0 and 1) because of the high resectability rate and infrequency of unsuspected distant metastatic deposits.

The impact of laparoscopy and laparoscopic ultrasonography on the management of pancreatic cancer.

Schachter PP, Avni Y, Shimonov M, Gvirtz G, Rosen A, Czerniak A.

Departments of Surgery, Gastroenterolgy, and Radiology, E. Wolfson Medical Center, Sackler School of Medicine, Tel Aviv University, Tel Aviv, Israel.

Archives of Surgery 135(11):1303–7, 2000, November.

Hypothesis: Laparoscopy and laparoscopic ultrasonographic (LAPUS) examinations combined with a biopsy of the pancreatic lesion contribute significantly in the determination of resectability of pancreatic cancer. *Design:* A prospective evaluation of the impact of laparoscopy and LAPUS on surgical decision making in patients with pancreatic cancer. *Setting:* A general community hospital; the department of surgery serves as referral for pancreatic surgery. *Patients:* During a 36-month period, 94 patients with pancreatic lesions were prospectively examined. Twenty-seven patients were found to have advanced disease. The remaining 67 patients were examined by laparoscopy and LAPUS to determine the resectability of the pancreatic tumor. *Results:* Laparoscopy and LAPUS contributed new, additional data in 40 patients (60%). Advanced disease was found in 30 patients, precluding curative resection. The study indicated potentially resectable tumors in 37 patients (55%), including 3 defined by conventional imaging studies as probably unresectable, and these patients were operated on with the intention of curative resection. Thirty-three patients underwent resection, and 4 (6%) were found to have nonresectable disease and form the false-positive group of the study. A summary of the results shows that the study resulted in a change of the decision regarding surgical intervention in 24 patients (36%) and avoided unnecessary laparotomies in 21 (31%). The study had a sensitivity of 100%, a specificity of 88%, and a false-positive rate of 6%. The positive predictive value of the study is 89%, and the negative predictive value is 100%. *Conclusions:* Although rather invasive, procedures that require general anesthesia and hospitalization, laparoscopy and LAPUS significantly contribute to the staging of patients with potentially resectable pancreatic cancer, avoiding unnecessary explorative laparotomies. These procedures should be performed in all patients with potentially resectable pancreatic cancer before explorative laparotomy.

The increasing problem of unusual pancreatic tumors.

Sheehan M, Latona C, Aranha G, Pickleman J.

Department of Surgery, Loyola University Medical Center, Maywood, IL, USA.

Archives of Surgery 135(6):644–8, 2000, June.

Hypothesis: Patients presenting with a pancreatic mass often have a curable lesion rather than the more common adenocarcinoma. Greater awareness of this among nonsurgeons is necessary. *Design:* Retrospective case series. *Setting:* Tertiary care referral hospital. *Patients:* All patients who presented with a pancreatic mass during the 8 years from 1990 to 1998 were studied. Patients with a history of chronic pancreatitis, a functioning pancreatic neuroendocrine tumor, or pancreatic adenocarcinoma were excluded. Forty patients were identified, demographic and clinical characteristics recorded, and long-term follow-up obtained. *Interventions:* Therapy included either a Whipple procedure or distal pancreatectomy. Two patients underwent a biliary bypass. *Main outcome measures:* Tumor histology, morbidity, and survival. *Results:* Three hundred thirty-six patients with a pancreatic mass were treated during this 8-year period. Two hundred ninety-six of these had pancreatic adenocarcinoma. Forty (11.9%) of the 336 patients had other types of pancreatic tumors. Two-thirds of these patients were female, with an average age of 57 years. Seventy-five percent of these tumors were either malignant or potentially malignant. In several instances, cystic tumors were diagnosed as inflammatory pseudocysts and managed accordingly. Fourteen (35%) of 40 patients had no symptoms and their tumor was found on a computed tomographic scan performed for another indication. Percutaneous biopsy was performed in 9 patients, of whom 5 were assigned an incorrect diagnosis. There were no operative deaths, although the postoperative complication rate was 23%. *Conclusions:* In this series, nearly 12% of patients presenting with a pancreatic mass did not have pancreatic adenocarcinoma, but rather more favorable lesions amenable to operation. Preoperative biopsy should not be carried out. Curative procedures can be safely performed in centers seeing a large number of patients with pancreatic tumors, and the long-term results of extirpation are excellent.

Resected adenocarcinoma of the pancreas – 616 patients: results, outcomes, and prognostic indicators.

Sohn TA, Yeo CJ, Cameron JL, Koniaris L, Kausbal S, Abrams RA, Sauter PK, Coleman J, Hruban RH, Lillemoe KD.

Departments of Surgery, Pathology and Oncology, The Johns Hopkins Medical Institutions, Baltimore, MD, USA.

Journal of Gastrointestinal Surgery 4:567–79, 2000.

This large-volume, single-institution review examines factors influencing long-term survival after resection in patients with adenocarcinoma of the head, neck, uncinate process, body, or tail of the pancreas. Between January 1984 and July 1999 inclusive, 616 patients with adenocarcinoma of the pancreas underwent surgical resection. A retrospective analysis of a prospectively collected database was performed. Both univariate and multivariate models were used to determine the factors influencing survival. Of the 616 patients, 526 (85%) underwent pancreaticoduodenectomy for adenocarcinoma of the head, neck, or uncinate process of the pancreas, 52 (9%) underwent distal pancreatectomy for adenocarcinoma of the body or tail, and 38 (6%) underwent total pancreatectomy for adenocarcinoma extensively involving the gland. The mean age of the patients was 64.3 years, with 54% being male and 91% being white. The overall perioperative mortality rate was 2.3%, whereas the incidence of postoperative complications was 30%. The median postoperative length of stay was 11 days. The mean tumor diameter was 3.2 cm, with 72% of patients having positive lymph nodes, 30% having positive resection margins, and 36% having poorly differentiated tumors. Patients undergoing distal pancreatectomy for left-sided lesions had larger tumors (4.7 vs. 3.1 cm, $p < 0.0001$), but fewer node-positive resections (59% vs. 73%, $p = 0.03$) and fewer poorly differentiated tumors (29% vs. 36%, $p < 0.001$), as compared to those undergoing pancreaticoduodenectomy for right-sided lesions. The overall survival of the entire cohort was 63% at 1 year and 17% at 5 years, with a median survival of 17 months. For right-sided lesions the 1- and 5-year survival rates were 64% and 17%, respectively, compared to 50% and 15% for left-sided lesions. Factors shown to have favorable independent prognostic significance by multivariate analysis were negative resection margins (hazard ratio [HR] = 0.64, confidence interval [CI = 0.50 to 0.82, $p = 0.0004$), tumor diameter less than 3 cm (HR = 0.72, CI = 0.57 to 0.90, $p = 0.004$), estimated blood loss less than 750 mL (HR = 0.75, CI = 0.58 to 0.96, $p = 0.02$), well/moderate tumor differentiation (HR = 0.71, CI = 0.56 to 0.90, $p = 0.005$), and postoperative chemoradiation (HR = 0.50, CI = 0.39 to 0.64, $p < 0.0001$). Tumor location in head, neck, or uncinate process approached significance in the final multivariate model (HR = 0.60, CI = 0.35 to 1.0, $p = 0.06$). Pancreatic resection remains the only hope for long-term survival in patients with adenocarcinoma of the pancreas. Completeness of resection and tumor characteristics including tumor size and degree of differentiation are important independent prognostic indicators. Adjuvant chemoradiation is a strong predictor of outcome and likely decreases the independent significance of tumor location and nodal status.

Does prophylactic octreotide decrease the rates of pancreatic fistula and other complications after pancreaticoduodenectomy? Results of a prospective randomized placebo-controlled trial.

Yeo CJ, Cameron JL, Lillemoe KD, Sauter PK, Coleman J, Sohn TA, Campbell KA, Choti MA.

Department of Surgery, Johns Hopkins Hospital,
Baltimore, MD, USA.

Annals of Surgery 232(3):419–29, 2000, September.

Objective: To evaluate the endpoints of complications (specifically pancreatic fistula and total complications) and death in patients undergoing pancreaticoduodenectomy. *Summary background data:* Four randomized, placebo-controlled, multicenter trials from Europe have evaluated prophylactic octreotide (the long-acting synthetic analog of native somatostatin) in patients undergoing pancreatic resection. Each trial reported significant decreases in overall complication rates, and two of the four reported significantly lowered rates of pancreatic fistula in patients receiving prophylactic octreotide. However, none of these four trials studied only pancreaticoduodenal resections, and all trials had high pancreatic fistula rates (> 19%) in the placebo group. A fifth randomized trial from the United States evaluated the use of prophylactic octreotide in patients undergoing pancreaticoduodenectomy and found no benefit to the use of octreotide. Prophylactic use of octreotide adds more than $75 to the daily hospital charge in the United States. In calendar year 1996, 288 patients received octreotide on the surgical service at the authors' institution, for total billed charges of $74,652. *Methods:* Between February 1998 and February 2000, 383 patients were recruited into this study on the basis of preoperative anticipation of pancreaticoduodenal resection. Patients who gave consent were randomized to saline control versus octreotide 250 microg subcutaneously every 8 hours for 7 days, to start 1 to 2 hours before surgery. The primary postoperative endpoints were pancreatic fistula, total complications, death, and length of hospital stay. *Results:* Two hundred eleven patients underwent pancreaticoduodenectomy with pancreatic-enteric anastomosis, received appropriate saline/octreotide doses, and were available for endpoint analysis. The two groups were comparable with respect to demographics (54% male, median age 66 years), type of pancreaticoduodenal resection (60% pylorus-preserving), type of pancreatic-enteric anastomosis (87% end-to-side pancreaticojejunostomy), and pathologic diagnosis. The pancreatic fistula rates were 9% in the control group and 11% in the octreotide group. The overall complication rates were 34% in the control group and 40% in the octreotide group; the in-hospital death rates were 0% versus 1%, respectively. The median postoperative length of hospital stay was 9 days in both groups. *Conclusions:* These data demonstrate that the prophylactic use of perioperative octreotide does not reduce the incidence of pancreatic fistula or total complications after pancreaticoduodenectomy. Prophylactic octreotide use in this setting should be eliminated, at a considerable cost savings.

23

Principles of adjuvant and neoadjuvant therapy: applications in gastric and pancreatic cancer

SYMA IQBAL AND HEINZ-JOSEF LENZ

Neoadjuvant therapy, defined as chemotherapy or radiation therapy administered prior to, rather than after, a definitive surgical procedure, has a variety of theoretical advantages and disadvantages.

WHAT ARE THE POTENTIAL ADVANTAGES OF NEOADJUVANT THERAPY?

The intact vasculature of the tumor that exists prior to surgery results in well-oxygenated tumor cells that may be more susceptible to the effects of radiation. In addition, drugs may better perfuse the tumor prior to disruption of the blood supply that occurs during extirpation. Effective neoadjuvant therapy may downstage a tumor so that subsequent surgery is technically simpler; or it may render a tumor initially deemed unresectable resectable; or may allow a surgical procedure that is less morbid, such as a segmental mastectomy instead of a modified radical mastectomy, or a primary colorectal anastomsis instead of a colostomy.[1-3] Other tumors for which neoadjuvant chemotherapy has been incorporated into clinical use to reduce the extent of surgical resection include bladder carcinoma, laryngeal cancer, osteogenic sarcoma, and soft-tissue sarcomas.[1]

The use of neoadjuvant therapy in the management of gastric and pancreatic cancer is of considerable interest because of the dismal outcome associated with potentially curative surgical resection and the ineffectiveness of postoperative (adjuvant) therapy with drugs or radiation.

In gastric and pancreatic cancer, local recurrence, peritoneal seeding, and liver metastases are the most common patterns of treatment failure. Supporters of neoadjuvant therapy argue that with preoperative therapy there may be a reduction in the number of viable cells being shed into the circulation at the time of surgery, and such therapy may render more patients resectable.[2] The high

frequency of very narrow or positive margins of excision after resection of pancreatic and gastric cancers supports the concern that surgery alone may be inadequate for local control. Preoperative radiation may destroy the spread of cancer within the connective tissues such as perineural spaces and lymphatic vessels at a microscopic level. It may also decrease the ability of tumor cells to implant upon the surgical incisions at the time of operation.[4] By offering preoperative therapy, sterilization of cancer cells at the boundaries of resection may be achieved prior to manipulation, thereby reducing the incidence of positive margins. Peritoneal tumor cell implantation caused by the manipulation at surgery may also be prevented by preoperative chemoradiation. Preoperative therapies allow earlier exposure of micrometastases to a therapeutic agent. The potential for peritoneal seeding is a major argument in favor of preoperative therapy in patients with gastric and pancreatic cancer.[5]

An objective response to preoperative chemotherapy provides important *in-vivo* evidence that a patient may benefit from continued therapy with the same drug regimen. On the other hand, a poor response may identify a patient for whom another drug regimen or an alternative method of treatment should be used. Histologic examination of residual tumor following a partial response to preoperative chemotherapy may yield valuable information concerning the specific characteristics of the non-responsive tumor cells. Progression of disease in the face of neoadjuvant therapy may identify patients who should not be subjected to laparotomy, thereby sparing such patients the risk of operative morbidity and mortality.

A frequent problem in postoperative adjuvant therapy studies is that therapy may be delayed if a patient has a prolonged postoperative course with complications. By delivering all components of the multimodality treatment initially, postoperative recovery will not have an effect on the delivery of complete therapy. There is increased patient tolerance to preoperative therapy, as the patient will not yet have undergone the stress of surgery, thereby allowing the full dose of radiation and/or chemotherapy to be delivered. Technically, giving radiation therapy initially with no recent operation and no fixed small bowel in the radiation therapy port should improve patient tolerance and the ability to deliver the planned radiation dose.[4]

WHAT ARE THE DISADVANTAGES OF NEOADJUVANT THERAPY?

Resectability

The disadvantages of neoadjuvant chemotherapy include delaying definitive surgery, thereby risking progression of the tumor during neoadjuvant therapy and the patient becoming unresectable. However, this may be a potential advantage (as discussed earlier) as patients who have aggressive tumors that seem curable with a surgical resection can avoid the potential morbidity by declaring progressive disease within the time interval of neoadjuvant therapy.

True staging

In evaluating patients after preoperative chemotherapy and resection, the true pathologic stage of the cancer may be obscured as a result of the preoperative treatment altering tumor margins and converting histologically positive nodes to negative. The true stage is often important in determining the necessity for further therapy and in assessing the prognosis. Another potential disadvantage related to such tumor 'downstaging' is that a dramatic clinical response may result in the performance of a more conservative procedure than may be appropriate for curative resection.[5]

Imaging studies and other modalities used for preoperative evaluation are imperfect and may lead to inaccurate clinical conclusions regarding the origin and true pathologic stage of a given tumor, thereby leading to inappropriate neoadjuvant therapy. For example, in one study, 17 of 42 patients who had resections for probable pancreatic carcinoma in fact had periampullary adenocarcinoma of non-pancreatic origin. In this setting, the value of adjuvant chemoradiation is unproven and would have been inappropriate.[6]

Toxicity

The performance status of patients can significantly decrease during chemoradiation. For example, using the performance status scale developed by the Eastern Cooperative Oncology Group (ECOG), Jessup *et al.*[7] reported that, among patients with pancreatic cancer, preoperative therapy was associated with a deterioration in performance status, with the ECOG score rising to 2.2 from 1.2 initially. The main limiting toxicity of chemotherapy and radiation in this setting is often gastrointestinal toxicity, and some patients during the time of chemotherapy and radiation will even require parenteral nutrition for nutritional support. By performing surgery first, patients could potentially receive feeding tubes and enteral feeding during therapy, avoiding a loss of performance status.

Tumor complications

In patients with gastric or pancreatic cancers, symptoms of tumor burden or location, such as obstruction, may develop which require an intervention, such as stenting or drainage. Surgery initially could avoid the possibility of requiring such invasive procedures, which have inherent risks.

Refusal of curative surgery

Lastly, preoperative therapy that produces an excellent response may mislead patients to inappropriately decline operative intervention. With available neoadjuvant regimens, the standard of care with these gastrointestinal tumors calls for surgical resection.

GASTRIC CANCER

Complete resection of all gross disease with negative margins on pathologic review remains the only potentially curative therapy for gastric cancer.[8] In patients with gastric cancer, only those in a small subgroup, ranging from approximately 30% to 50% of patients, have a potentially resectable cancer.[8] Even after complete removal of tumor, recurrence is common, with local–regional and distant failure. Patients at especially high risk for tumor recurrence after resection are those with TNM classification T3 or T4 tumors, and any N lymph node metastasis. Most patients diagnosed and resected in the USA are at high risk. In contrast, in Japan, approximately 30–40% of patients are staged with a T1 or T2 lesion and, therefore, are low risk, whereas only 5–10% of patients in the USA present with early disease. Five-year survival rates with surgery alone, for patients with early-stage disease, have been reported to be as high as 80–90% worldwide.[9,10] Gastric cancers with deeper invasion (T3, T4) or nodal involvement (N1, N2) are associated with decreased survival, depending on the degree of invasion. Patients with N1 or N2 staging have a 5-year survival of 10–20%, whereas Japanese authors report survival rates of 25–60%.[9]

Adjuvant therapy is chemotherapy or radiation therapy, or a combination of both that is administered to patients after they have undergone a potentially curative resection of tumor to reduce the risk of tumor recurrence, locally and systemically. In these patients, the margins of resection must be histologically negative, and there must be no evidence of distant metastasis. There have been several studies addressing the use of adjuvant therapy in gastric carcinoma because of the high rate of recurrence following a potentially curative resection. These trials have failed to show a definite survival benefit. However, there has been a trend toward improved survival, but it is unknown which patients will benefit from adjuvant therapy. It is hoped that analysis of the trial undertaken by the Southwestern Oncology Group (SWOG 9008) will clarify the role of adjuvant therapy in gastric cancer. In this trial, patients were randomized to receive adjuvant chemoradiation therapy with 5-fluorouracil (5-FU) and radiation or no adjuvant therapy. Preliminary data show a survival advantage in the adjuvant chemoradiation arm.

A meta-analysis of adjuvant chemotherapy in gastric cancer showed a trend toward increased survival, which, however, did not reach statistical significance.[11] No difference in survival was found when patients with locally advanced but resected gastric cancer received either radiation or chemotherapy.[12]

Efforts to combine chemotherapy and radiation led to two phase III adjuvant studies. In the first, Dent et al. treated 142 patients randomly assigned postoperatively to either no additional therapy or to 2000 cGy plus 5-FU. No difference in overall survival was shown between the two groups.[13] In a second study, Moertel et al. looked at combined chemoradiotherapy. Sixty-two patients with curative resections with negative margins were randomized to no therapy versus combined chemoradiotherapy. Patients receiving adjuvant therapy had a significantly longer disease-free survival and overall survival.[14] Because of conflicting data, the question still remains open as to whether chemoradiation should be used in the adjuvant setting. Some of the criticism of the postoperative therapy studies involved the significant delay in starting treatment of up to 4–10 weeks, whereas Japanese studies do not have such a delay, and the outcome of Japanese studies shows a survival advantage with adjuvant treatment.[15]

Resectable gastric carcinoma

Because of high failure rates despite curative resections with negative margins of excision and adjuvant chemotherapy, Ajani et al. designed a trial in which patients with apparently resectable gastric cancer received both preoperative (neoadjuvant) and postoperative (adjuvant) chemotherapy consisting of etoposide, 5-FU, and cisplatin (EFP).[5] All 25 patients entered into the study underwent surgery. Six of the 25 patients (24%) had a complete clinical response (CCR). There were no complete pathologic responses, but three patients (12%) had only microscopic cancer in the resected specimens. Seven of the 25 patients (28%) had incomplete resections

because of metastatic disease. Median overall survival was reported as 15 months. Peritoneal carcinomatosis was the most common site of failure.

In a subsequent trial, Ajani and associates studied patients with potentially resectable tumors who had responded to preoperative chemotherapy.[3] The drug regimen provided etoposide, doxorubicin, and cisplastin (EAP). The 48 patients in this study received three cycles of chemotherapy before resection, and those who responded received two cycles of chemotherapy postoperatively. Six of the 48 patients (13%) had CCR, and 41 of 48 (85%) underwent surgery; 37 of the 41 (90%) had curative resections, representing 77% of the 48 patients entered into the study. The median survival of patients was 15.5 months, similar to that of the first report. However, this study was complicated by a substantial degree of toxicity: 19 patients (40%) were hospitalized for grade 3 and 4 hematologic and non-hematologic toxicity including nausea, vomiting, and diarrhea. Despite systemic chemotherapy preoperatively and postoperatively, the rate of local–regional failure remained significant. Potentially resectable patients who underwent curative surgery still had relatively poor survival rates.

Crookes et al., in 1997, evaluated gastric cancer amenable to curative resection to determine the feasibility and response to preoperative systemic chemotherapy followed by postoperative intraperitoneal chemotherapy to target better control of peritoneal recurrence.[16] Fifty-nine patients with resectable gastric cancer received two cycles of 5-FU, leucovorin, and cisplatin. Those with complete resection, including negative microscopic margins, received two cycles of intraperitoneal floxuridine (FUDR) and cisplatin. Fifty-six of the 59 (95%) had laparotomy for resection, 40/56 (71%) had gastric resection performed for cure, and 15/56 (27%) had palliative surgery. Thirty-one of the 40 (78%) patients resected for cure completed postoperative intraperitoneal chemotherapy. Nine of the 40 (23%) patients resected for cure had recurrent disease. Median follow-up at the time of publication for all 59 patients was 45 months. Calculated median survival was reported as greater than 4 years. These follow-up data support decreased recurrence and increased survival with preoperative systemic chemotherapy and postoperative intraperitoneal therapy compared with historical controls.[16]

In another study using postoperative intraperitoneal chemotherapy, Kelsen et al. reported on patients with gastric cancer who received neoadjuvant chemotherapy with 5-FU, adriamycin, and methotrexate (FAMTX), and postoperative intravenous 5-FU and intraperitoneal cisplatin–fluorouracil. Thirty-four of the 56 patients (61%) had curative resections; 75% of patients received postoperative intraperitoneal therapy. For the 61% of patients with potentially curative resections, median survival was 31 months. Intra-abdominal failure pattern improved with this combined systemic and intraperitoneal therapy. Whereas assessing objective regression to preoperative treatment is difficult, the number of patients found to have pT1 and pT2 disease was unexpectedly high, suggesting downstaging by preoperative therapy.[17]

To date, there has been no published study randomizing patients to either surgery alone or preoperative and postoperative therapy including intraperitoneal chemotherapy.

Unresectable gastric carcinoma

For patients who have tumors that are determined to be initially unresectable, chemotherapy has been offered with the goal of downstaging, to allow the possibility of subsequent resection.

In a study by Wilke et al.[18] 34 patients with locally advanced, unresectable gastric cancer determined at laparotomy received EAP. Second-look surgery with removal of residual tumor was performed in cases of complete or partial remissions (CR/PR) after the chemotherapy. Successful resection was followed by two cycles of EAP for consolidation therapy. Twenty-three of 33 (70%) evaluable patients had a CR or PR after EAP, including a 21% rate (7 of 33 patients) of clinical CR. Two patients had a minor remission (MR) or no change, and seven had progressive disease. Nineteen of the 23 responders and one patient with MR underwent second-look surgery. Five clinical CRs were pathologically confirmed; ten patients with clinical partial responses were rendered free of disease after resection. Twenty patients were disease free after EAP, surgery, and consolidation therapy. After a median follow-up of 20 months for disease-free patients, the relapse rate was 60% (12 of 20). The median survival for all patients was 18 months and for disease-free patients 24 months.

In another study by Verschueren et al.,[19] 17 patients who were inoperable at the time of laparotomy were given four courses of methotrexate and 5-FU. Seven patients became resectable after chemotherapy. Median survival was 14 months. These studies indicate that preoperative chemotherapy may allow some tumors to become resectable; however, if overall survival is improved, it has not yet been demonstrated.

Locally advanced gastric cancer

Another group of patients is those who are considered 'locally advanced.' The definition of locally advanced varies. It may refer to localized disease that the surgeon believes cannot be resected with negative margins, or it can refer to high-risk disease that may be resectable but at increased risk for recurrence, for example T3 or T4 tumors or tumors with nodal involvement. In many studies of 'locally advanced disease,' the authors do not define their criteria.

Ducreux et al., in 1993, conducted a phase II study evaluating long-term survival in locally advanced diseases, including cases of linitis plastica.[20] Of 30 patients who were entered into study, 15 patients had enlarged lymph nodes on computerized tomography (CT) scan and 15 patients had linitis. Patients received two to three cycles of 5-FU and cisplatin. There were 28 evaluable patients, among whom there was one CR and 14 PRs. Among the 28 patients who underwent surgery, complete resection was possible in 23 (82%). Median survival was 16 months.

There are few trials comparing surgery alone for locally advanced disease versus surgery after neoadjuvant therapy. Kang et al., in 1996, reported on 51 patients with locally advanced gastric cancer who received two to three cycles of EFP followed by surgery or underwent surgery alone.[21] Twenty-four patients were treated preoperatively. More patients were able to undergo curative resection in the treated group compared with the surgery-alone group (75% versus 56%, $p = 0.014$), thereby implying downstaging occurred to a significant degree. No survival data were reported.

Schwartz et al. conducted a phase 2 trial in an attempt to improve the rate of curative resections, disease-free survival, and overall survival in high-risk patients with T3–4, N any, M0.[22] Twenty-nine patients received three cycles of FAMTX preoperatively and three cycles of postoperative intraperitoneal therapy with 5-FU and cisplatin. Sixteen of 23 patients (70%) were resectable, 13 of the 23 (57%) had negative margins, and four patients had progressive disease on FAMTX. Six patients were still receiving therapy at the time of publication. Pathologic downstaging occurred in 6 of the 18 (33%) patients evaluated by endoscopic ultrasound. No survival data were reported.

In a study by Fink and associates,[23] the effect of preoperative outpatient chemotherapy with EAP was evaluated prospectively in 30 patients who had been shown by preoperative staging (including endosonography and surgical laparoscopy) to have gastric carcinoma stages IIIA, IIIB, or IV. Hematological side-effects were common and necessitated hospitalization in 13 of 30 patients. Complete clinical response to neoadjuvant therapy was observed in 8 of 27 (30%) evaluable patients. Resection was performed in 27 of 30 patients, with complete macroscopic and microscopic tumor removal in 24. There were no deaths and no major morbidity following operation. On multivariate analysis, complete clinical response ($p < 0.01$) and complete tumor resection ($p < 0.01$) were the major independent predictors of long-term survival after neoadjuvant chemotherapy. Actuarial survival after complete tumor removal appeared superior with neoadjuvant therapy compared with results in a control population matched for age, sex, and tumor stage who had primary resection ($p = 0.07$). Recurrence occurred in 17 of 23 evaluable patients who had complete tumor removal, with relapse in the tumor bed or area of lymphatic drainage in 11. The authors concluded that their data showed that neoadjuvant therapy in patients with locally advanced gastric carcinoma is feasible and appears to increase the rate of complete tumor removal, but that more powerful and less toxic regimens would be required to improve the response rate and to delay or avoid recurrence after neoadjuvant chemotherapy.

In summary, gastric cancer trials have suggested a trend toward increased survival benefit with neoadjuvant systemic chemotherapy delivered alone or in combination with intraperitoneal therapy. Downstaging was consistently demonstrated, and this might have contributed to increased resection rates without, however, demonstrating a survival benefit. There are no randomized trials evaluating neoadjuvant therapy versus adjuvant therapy versus surgery alone. There is evidence that a few percent of patients who achieve a complete pathological response may benefit from neoadjuvant chemotherapy/radiation. Delineating molecular predictors of response to therapy may allow the selection of patients who will be long-term survivors.

PANCREATIC CANCER

The standard surgical treatment for cancer involving the head of the pancreas remains the pancreaticoduodenectomy, a procedure first described by Whipple et al. in 1934. Initially, high operative morbidity and mortality rates led to modifications of the operation. Current perioperative mortality rates are about 2%. However, 'curative' radical resection can be performed in only 5–25% of patients at presentation, and only 5–25% of these patients who undergo resection will be alive after 5 years.[7] Pancreatic cancer is generally resistant to chemotherapeutic agents, and very few agents have demonstrated significant activity. In fact, data reveal that the use of multiple agents does not have superiority over the use of gemcitabine alone, or gemcitabine-containing regimens. A definitive role for radiation therapy alone or in combination with chemotherapy has not been fully established.

Burris et al.[24] evaluated the comparative effectiveness of gemcitabine on various clinical symptoms and survival in 126 patients with advanced symptomatic pancreas cancer. Patients were randomized to receive either a gemcitabine-based or 5-FU-based regimen. The primary efficacy measure was clinical benefit response, which was a composite of measurements of pain (analgesic consumption and pain intensity), Karnofsky performance status, and weight. Clinical benefit required a sustained improvement of a minimum duration of 4 weeks in at least one parameter without worsening in any others. Other measures of efficacy included response rate, time to progressive disease, and survival. Clinical benefit response was experienced by 23.8% of gemcitabine-treated patients compared with 4.8% of 5-FU-treated patients ($p = 0.0022$). The median survival durations were 5.65 and 4.41 months for gemcitabine-treated and 5-FU-treated patients, respectively ($p = 0.0025$). The survival rate at 12 months was 18% for gemcitabine patients and 2% for 5-FU patients. Treatment was well

tolerated. The authors concluded that gemcitabine was more effective than 5-FU in the alleviation of some disease-related symptoms in patients with advanced, symptomatic pancreas cancer. Gemcitabine also conferred a modest survival advantage over treatment with 5-FU.

Ishikawa et al. studied the effects of preoperative irradiation (50 Gy) in 18 patients with carcinoma of the head of the pancreas. Sixteen patients (89%) underwent resection of the tumor. In 13 of the 16 cases, the population of 'severely degenerative' cancer cells represented more than one-third of all the malignant cells and were likely to be located at the periphery of the tumor. The authors considered this histologic pattern a favorable indication of operative curability.[25] In a subsequent study, Ishikawa and associates retrospectively analysed the outcome in 54 patients with pancreatic head cancer deemed to be resectable by preoperative diagnostic techniques. Twenty-three patients had received preoperative irradiation (50 Gy) and 31 had not. Pancreatic resection with intent to cure was possible in 17 patients (74%) who received neoadjuvant radiation, and 19 (61%) of the non-irradiated group, but the difference was not statistically significant.[26] One-year survival in the irradiated group was 75%, compared with 43% in the non-irradiated group; however, 3-year and 5-year survival rates were the same in both groups, 28% versus 32%, and 22% versus 26%, respectively. The irradiated group had a significantly lower incidence of regional recurrence within 1.5 postoperative years compared with the non-irradiated group, whereas deaths due to hepatic metastasis were markedly higher, indicating that control of both local tumor recurrence and distant disease is imperative.

There is some evidence that multimodality therapy can prolong survival when compared with surgery alone. In 1978, the Gastrointestinal Tumor Study Group (GITSG) carried out a multi-institutional trial of radiation therapy alone and in combination with 5-FU for locally unresectable pancreatic carcinoma. One hundred and six patients were randomized to one of three radiation treatment programs initiated 3–6 weeks after surgery: radiation therapy alone to 6000 rad; 6000 rad plus 5-FU; or 4000 rad plus 5-FU. Patient survival was the primary study parameter. Both 4000 rad plus 5-FU and 6000 rad plus 5-FU were associated with a significantly longer patient survival than radiation to 6000 rad alone. Median survival rates were 36 weeks, 40 weeks, and 20 weeks, respectively. The survival difference between 4000 rad plus 5-FU and 6000 rad plus 5-FU was not statistically significant.[27]

Trials in patients who have had complete resection include the GITSG 1987 phase III evaluation of postoperative adjuvant chemoradiation.[28] Although this trial was closed early due to poor patient accrual, the data did demonstrate a statistically significant doubling in median survival and a slight improvement in 5-year survival in patients who received adjuvant chemoradiation compared to postoperative observation only. Reported median survival was 21 months compared with 11 months in the observation group, a difference that was statistically significant. The 5-year survival was 19% versus 5%. The rationale for the addition of chemotherapy to radiation therapy was radiosensitization by 5-FU. From data thus far accrued, there is no evidence that adjuvant chemotherapy alone has improved either local control or survival. A role for adjuvant chemotherapy plus radiation therapy for patients who undergo pancreaticoduodenctomy for adenocarcinoma of the pancreas is based on the GITSG study. It is theorized that the survival advantage observed in patients who received adjuvant radiotherapy in addition to chemotherapy was caused by a decrease in local–regional tumor recurrence. This hypothesis is supported by the high incidence of local recurrence observed in patients treated with pancreaticoduodenectomy alone and by the limited activity of systemic 5-FU in patients with metastatic disease.

In many of the adjuvant trials, patients initially enrolled failed to complete the protocol because of a prolonged postoperative course or refusal of further therapy. Consequently, there has been recent interest in providing therapy *preoperatively*, especially in view of some evidence from adjuvant studies that chemotherapy and radiation therapy may favorably affect survival.

Locally advanced and resectable pancreatic cancer

Hoffman and associates at the Fox Chase Cancer Center have published a series of reports detailing the results of ongoing prospective trials of preoperative chemoradiation for patients with localized adenocarcinoma of the pancreas.[4,29–32] The neoadjuvant regimen consisted of preoperative 5-FU and mitomycin C given with external-beam radiation therapy. Initially, patients were eligible for entry if there was no evidence of metastatic disease. Subsequently, eligibility was modified to allow the entry only of patients considered by the surgical consultant to have potentially resectable lesions. In their 1993 report,[4] the authors concluded that resectability was probably enhanced and nodal metastases and resection margins were downstaged by the preoperative program. In subsequent studies from the Fox Chase Cancer Center,[29,30] the authors reported that patients who recovered from a curative resection had a median survival from the time of tissue diagnosis of 45 months, with a median disease-free survival of 27 months. The authors concluded that the preoperative 5-FU–mitomycin–radiation regimen enhanced tumor-free resection margins and offered the possibility of prolonged survival to patients with truly localized pancreatic tumor. In contrast, the data demonstrated that the chemoradiation regimen did not cure or even render resectable most tumors that were more than 4 cm in diameter, that obstructed the portal or superior mesenteric veins, or that encased the superior mesenteric artery.

In 1991, the Eastern Cooperative Oncology Group initiated a prospective, multi-institutional trial of the same neoadjuvant regimen that had undergone pilot trials at the Fox Chase Cancer Center.[31] Fifty-three patients with localized adenocarcinoma of the pancreas were assessable for analysis. Forty-one of the treated patients proceeded to surgery, among whom only 24 were suitable for resection. Median survival for the entire group and for the 24 patients with resection was 9.7 and 15.7 months, respectively. The disappointing survival rate was deemed to reflect the advanced state of most resected cancers (positive peritoneal cytology in three patients; margins within 2 mm in 13; involved lymph nodes in four; and need for superior mesenteric vein resection in four patients).

Neoadjuvant versus adjuvant therapy

No prospective trials have been done comparing postoperative and preoperative chemoradiation. Available data do not consistently demonstrate any significant differences in the two approaches.

In a report from Pendurthi et al.,[32] two groups of patients with adenocarcinoma of the pancreas treated with either preoperative chemoradiation (preop CTRT) or postoperative chemoradiation (postop CTRT) were retrospectively analysed for various treatment-related parameters. A total of 70 patients with pancreatic adenocarcinoma was enrolled into preop CTRT protocols at the Fox Chase Cancer Center. Twenty-five patients with adenocarcinoma of the head of the pancreas underwent pancreaticoduodenectomy with curative intent. After the closure of the preop CTRT protocols, 23 pancreatic resections were performed without preop CTRT. After surgery, these patients were advised to undergo CTRT. These two cohorts of patients are compared for various relevant parameters. Treatment breaks resulting in greater than 1 week delay in the radiotherapy occurred in 2 (8%) of 25 patients in the preop CTRT group (myelotoxicity in one case and biliary sepsis in one case), whereas no treatment breaks greater than 1 week occurred in those receiving postop CTRT. Eleven patients in preop CTRT had grade 3 or 4 toxicity, whereas none was noted in those with postop CTRT. There was one postoperative death in the preop CTRT group and none in the postop CTRT group. Mean time to the start of CTRT was 45 days (range, 20–66 days) after pancreaticoduodenectomy. Five of 23 patients (22%) in the postop CTRT group did not receive treatment for various reasons. Average estimated operative blood loss, length of operation, and length of postoperative stay were similar in the two groups. Pathological findings in the resected specimens showed significantly fewer involved nodes in the preop CTRT group (28% versus 87%; $p = 0.0006$), whereas similar numbers of nodes per patient were counted in each group (14 versus 22, $p = 0.11$). More negative resection margins were observed in the preop CTRT group (28% versus 56%; $p =$ not significant). A significantly greater amount of fibrosis replacing the tumor was observed in the preop CTRT group (70% versus 40%; $p = 0.0001$). There were no significant survival differences observed (median 20 months versus 25 months; $p = 0.48$) in follow-up that ranged from 4 to 76 months (median 44 months for surviving patients) for the preop group and 4 to 40 months (median 16 months for surviving patients) for those with postop CTRT. Local failure either alone or as a component of distant failure occurred in 16% (4 of 25 patients) with preop CTRT and 17% (3 of 18 patients) with postop CTRT. Analysis of differences between those treated with preoperative and postoperative CTRT demonstrates similarity in toxicity and effects. However, 22% of patients intended for postoperative therapy did not receive treatment.

Spitz et al. also studied preoperative and postoperative chemoradiation strategies in patients treated with pancreaticoduodenectomy.[33] One hundred and forty-two patients with localized adenocarcinoma of the pancreatic head deemed resectable were treated using either preoperative or postoperative chemoradiation. Preoperative therapy consisted of radiation at a dose of 50.4 Gy (standard fractionation) or 30 Gy (rapid fractionation), combined with continuous infusion 5-FU. The postoperative therapy offered was 50.4 Gy with standard fractionation combined with continuous infusion 5-FU. No patient who received preoperative chemoradiation experienced a delay in surgery because of chemoradiation toxicity, but 6 of 25 (24%) eligible patients did not receive postoperative therapy because of delayed recovery. No significant difference in toxicities from therapy was observed between groups. At a median follow-up of 19 months, no significant differences in survival were observed between treatment groups. Median survival was 19 months for those who received preoperative therapy and 17 months for patients who received postoperative adjuvant therapy. Patients who did not undergo pancreaticoduodenectomy had a median survival of 7.2 months. No patient who received preoperative chemoradiation and pancreaticoduodenectomy experienced local recurrence, yet survival was limited because of the development of liver metastases. There was a trend to a decreased rate of microscopic retroperitoneal margin positivity in the preoperative group.

Evans et al. presented the M.D. Anderson Cancer Center experience with neoadjuvant multimodality therapy and compared the results with postoperative adjuvant therapy alone after resection.[34,35] Patients received preoperative 5-FU and radiation. Thereafter, in their two reports, 60–80% of patients underwent successful pancreatic resection. Histologic evidence of chemoradiation-induced tumor-cell injury was present in every resected specimen, but without a complete pathologic response. Median survival was 18 months for the resected patients and 6.7 months for the non-resected patients. The first site of tumor recurrence was liver or lung in 15 (83%) patients, again demonstrating improved local–regional disease control for resected patients, but with poor survival rates due to a high incidence of distant failure. There was no improvement in survival compared to historical control patients undergoing resection and postoperative chemoradiation.

Locally advanced pancreatic cancer

The role of neoadjuvant chemotherapy for locally advanced disease was addressed by Weese et al.[36] Sixteen patients with locally advanced disease received combination treatment with infusional 5-FU and mitomycin C and radiation therapy (5040 cGy in 28 fractions). Ten patients were resected, and the resection margins were tumor free. Median survival of the six patients who did not have a resection was 7 months; median survival of those who underwent resection had not been reached by the time of publication. In another study, neoadjuvant chemoradiation led to significant worsening of the overall performance status that apparently limited the possibility of a planned resection.[37]

Unresectable pancreatic cancer

Jessup et al.[7] undertook a study to determine whether continuous infusion of fluorouracil combined with external-beam radiation therapy could improve the resectability and survival of patients with pancreatic carcinoma initially considered unresectable. Sixteen patients with unresectable disease confined to the pancreas and celiac nodes were treated, and their outcome was compared with that of 24 patients with potentially resectable disease who were treated concurrently. The neoadjuvant therapy was completed with acceptably few toxic effects but with only a minor decrease in tumor size. Two patients underwent resection and remained free of disease 20 and 22.5 months later. However, the median survival of the entire neoadjuvant group was 8 months. All 24 patients with potentially resectable carcinoma underwent surgical exploration. Fifteen of the 24 (63%) patients underwent resection and survived a median of 12.5 months. The authors concluded that the neoadjuvant chemoradiation may have improved outcome and resectability for two (13%) of 16 patients with an initially unresectable lesion, but more effective therapy would have to be developed to improve outcome.

DISCUSSION AND CONCLUSIONS

Frequently, patients are found to have an unresectable carcinoma at the time of an anticipated curative operation because of suboptimal clinical staging. Commonly employed preoperative screening tests, including CT or magnetic resonance imaging (MRI), do not accurately stage the depth of tumor invasion (T stage) or identify regional nodal involvement (N stage), and thus do not identify the high-risk patient before surgical exploration. However, endoscopic ultrasonography (EUS) has been shown to be highly accurate in assessing the T stage and shows promise for improving the staging of nodal disease. EUS may be useful in separating *preoperatively* high-risk versus low-risk patients. More recently, laparoscopy with laparoscopic ultrasound appears to be an additional useful technique to identify high-risk patients, who nevertheless may be potentially curable. Exact determination of the tumor stage before treatment is essential to assess the clinical and histopathological response to neoadjuvant therapy and to document a benefit to this approach.

In view of the studies of pancreatic cancer reviewed here (Table 23.1), it must be concluded either that there is no difference in efficacy between preoperative and postoperative chemoradiotherapy, or that a difference may be obscured by selection factors. For gastric cancer, there is evidence that neoadjuvant chemotherapy in combination with postoperative intraperitoneal therapy may result in improved survival by better local–regional control (Table 23.2). The key limiting factor in the overall efficacy of current adjuvant or neoadjuvant regimens for gastric and pancreas cancer is the frequency of systemic failures despite improved local–regional control.[38,39] This problem can only be addressed with more efficient anticancer drugs.

Only patients in whom negative margins of excision can be achieved after pancreatic and gastric resections have a survival benefit from surgical extirpation of the primary tumor. The median survival of patients who undergo surgery and are found to have a positive margin is no different from that of patients with locally advanced disease treated with palliative chemoradiation without surgical resection.

In the future, it would be of great value to be able to identify patients who are most likely to respond to neoadjuvant therapies. Preliminary data suggest that it may even now be possible to predict response to chemotherapy with 5-FU and cisplatin. For example, two molecular markers, thymidylate synthase (TS) and *ERCC-1*, have been identified which appear to predict

Table 23.1 *Neoadjuvant therapy for pancreatic carcinoma*

Authors	Patients	Chemotherapy	Patients resected for cure (%)	Survival (months)
Hoffman et al. (1993)[4]	Stage I–III Some unresectable 39 patients	5-FU Mitomycin 50.4 Gy XRT	44	19
Hoffman et al. (1995)[29]	Unresectable 34 patients	5-FU Mitomycin 50.4 Gy XRT	44	45
Hoffman et al. (1995)[30]	Localized 63 patients	5-FU Mitomycin 50.4 Gy XRT	40 Before 1990, 24 After 1990, 47	22
Hoffman et al. (1998)[31]	Localized 64 patients	5-FU Mitomycin 50.4 Gy XRT	45	Resected: 15.7 Overall: 9.7
Pendurthi et al. (1998)[32]	Preop vs postop chemo Localized 70 patients	5-FU Mitomycin 50.4 Gy		Preop: 20 Postop: 25
Spitz et al. (1997)[33]	Localized and resectable 142 patients	5-FU/30 Gy hyperfract. or 50.4 Gy XRT		Preop: 19 Postop: 17
Evans et al. (1992)[34]	Localized 28 patients	5-FU 50.4 Gy XRT	61	Resected: 18 Nonresected: 6.7
Weese et al. (1990)[36]	Localized 16 patients	5-FU Mitomycin 50.4 Gy XRT	67	Resected: not reported Unresected: 7
Jessup et al. (1993)[37]	Unresectable but localized 23 patients	5-FU 45–50.4 Gy XRT	3 of 23 total resectable	Overall survival: 9
Jessup et al. (1993)[7]	Unresectable 16 patients	5-FU	2 of 16	Overall survival: 8

chemo, chemotherapy; 5-FU, 5-fluorouracil; XRT, radiation therapy.

Table 23.2 *Neoadjuvant therapy for gastric carcinoma*

Authors	Patients	Chemotherapy	Patients resected for cure (%)	Survival (months)
Verschueren *et al.* (1993)[19]	Unresectable 17 patients	MTX/5-FU	40	14
Ducreux *et al.* (1993)[20]	Locally advanced, 28 patients	5-FU/CDDP	77	16
Wilke *et al.* (1989)[18]	Locally advanced, unresectable, 34 patients	EAP	70	18
Fink *et al.* (1995)[23]	Stage IIIa, IIIb, IV, 30 patients	EAP	80	17
Kang *et al.* (1996)[21]	Locally advanced, 51 patients	EFP	63	N/A
Schwartz *et al.* (1993)[22]	High risk, 29 patients	FAMTX preop 5-FU/CDDP IP with 5-FU IV postop	56	N/A
Kelsen (1996)[8]	High risk, 60 patients	FAMTX preop 5-FU/CDDP IP with 5-FU IV postop	61	15.3
Ajani *et al.* (1991)[5]	Resectable 25 patients	EFP	72	15
Ajani *et al.* (1993)[3]	Resectable 48 patients	EAP	77	15.5
Crookes *et al.* (1997)[16]	Resectable 59 patients	Preop 5-FU/LV/CDDP Postop IP 5-FUDR/CDDP	71	>4 years

CDDP, cisplatin; EAP, etoposide, doxorubicin, cisplatin; EFP, etoposide, 5-FU, cisplatin; FAMTX, 5-FU, doxorubicin, methotrexate; FU, fluorouracil; FUDR, floxuridine; IP, intraperitoneal; IV, intravenous; LV, leucovorin.

response and survival in patients with localized gastric cancer who have been treated with neoadjuvant therapy.

Lenz and associates,[40,41] at the University of Southern California, have demonstrated an inverse relationship between the amount of TS within a primary adenocarcinoma of the stomach and the response and survival of patients receiving 5-FU-based therapy. Before systemic chemotherapy with protracted infusion 5-FU and a single dose of cisplatin, the genetic expression of TS (TS mRNA level) was determined. Sixty-five patients with primary gastric cancer had a median TS mRNA level of 4.6×10^3. Thirty-five percent of patients had measurable responses in their primary tumors. The difference in mean gastric cancer TS mRNA levels in responding and resistant patients was statistically significant ($p < 0.001$). The median survival time was 43+ months for treated patients with TS mRNA levels less than the median, and 6 months for those with TS mRNA levels greater than the median ($p = 0.003$).

ERCC-1 is the excision repair cross-complementing gene that functions to prevent mutations and other injuries to DNA, specifically those induced by cisplatin. Cisplatin cytotoxicity is associated with the induction of DNA intrastrand and interstrand cross-links. Studies from the University of Southern California indicate that relatively high levels of intratumoral *ERCC-1* increased the resistance of gastric cancer to cisplatin therapy, whereas lower levels were associated with sensitivity to the drug.[40,42] Thus, among a cohort of patients with gastric cancer receiving 5-FU and cisplatin, those with values below the median *ERCC-1* expression had a

significantly higher rate of tumor response than those with gene expression above the median (79% versus 29%, $p = 0.001$). Corresponding improvement in survival was also observed (> 24 months with low expression versus 5.4 months with high gene expression, $p = 0.034$). Patients with low levels of both TS and *ERCC-1* had significantly greater responses. Patients with high levels of both markers should be treated with non-TS and *ERCC-1*-affected agents, such as taxanes, gemcitabine, and CPT-11.

In the future, specific molecular markers may be identified which will allow tailoring of therapy to the individual patient. A high frequency of *ras* and *p53* mutations and expression of various growth factor receptors (such as epidermal growth factor (EGF), fibroblast growth factors (FGF), or insulin-like growth factors (IGF)) have been identified in pancreatic and gastric cancers. *Ras* mutations occur in approximately 70–90% of pancreatic tumors. *p53* is a protein that controls DNA integrity and repair. *Ras* and *p53* mutations are associated with poor differentiation and shortened survival in patients with certain tumors. The various growth factor receptors (such as EGF receptor (EGFR), Her2/Neu receptors, or FGF receptors) or growth factors (such as transforming growth factor-alpha, TGF-α, or FGF) may be involved in autocrine or paracrine growth of neoplastic pancreatic cells. This increased knowledge about the biology of pancreatic cancer has led to preclinical evaluation of novel approaches attempting specifically to target these detrimental features of pancreatic tumors. These novel approaches include gene therapy, vaccines, farnesyl transferase inhibitors to target mutated *ras* function, tyrosine kinase inhibitors to block the function of growth factor receptors, antibodies or fusion toxins aimed at EGF receptor or cell surface antigens, and antisense oligonucleotides targeted to genes important for the proliferation or survival of pancreatic cancer.[43] Additional experimental approaches include the use of anti-angiogenesis agents and agents interfering with signal transduction proteins.

REFERENCES

1. Chu E, DeVita VT Jr. Principles of cancer management: chemotherapy. In DeVita VT Jr, Hellman S, Rosenberg SA, eds. *Cancer: principles and practice of oncology*, 6th edn. Philadelphia, Lippincott–Williams and Wilkins, 2001, 289–306.

2. Hoffman JP, O'Dwyer P, Agarwal P, *et al*. Preoperative chemoradiotherapy for localized pancreatic carcinoma. Cancer 1996; (Suppl.) 78(3):592–7.

3. Ajani J, Mayer R, Ota D, *et al*. Preoperative and postoperative combination chemotherapy for potentially resectable gastric carcinoma. J Natl Cancer Inst 1993; 85(22):1839–44.

4. Hoffman JP, Weese JL, Solin LJ, *et al*. A single institutional experience with preoperative chemoradiotherapy for stage I–III pancreatic adenocarcinoma. Am Surg 1993; 59:772–81.

5. Ajani J, Ota D, Jessup JM, *et al*. Resectable gastric carcinoma: an evaluation of preoperative and postoperative chemotherapy. Cancer 1991; 68:1501–6.

6. Hoffman JP, Cooper HS, Young NA, *et al*. Preoperative chemotherapy or chemoradiotherapy for the treatment of adenocarcinoma of the pancreas and ampulla of Vater. J Hepatobiliary Pancreat Surg 1998; 5:251–4.

7. Jessup JM, Steele G, Mayer RJ, *et al*. Neoadjuvant therapy for unresectable pancreatic adenocarcinoma. Arch Surg 1993; 128:559–64.

8. Kelsen DP. Adjuvant and neoadjuvant therapy for gastric cancer. Semin Oncol 1996; 23(3):379–89.

9. Noguchi Y, Imada T, Matsumot A, *et al*. Radical surgery for gastric cancer, a review of the Japanese experience. Cancer 1989; 64:2053–62.

10. Cady B, Rossi RL, Silverman ML, *et al*. Gastric adenocarcinoma: a disease in transition. Arch Surg 1989; 124:303.

11. Hermens J, Beonenkamp JJ, Boon MC, *et al*. Adjuvant therapy after curative resection for gastric cancer: meta-analysis of randomized trials. J Clin Oncol 1993; 11:1441.

12. Hallissey MT, Dunn JA, Ward LC, *et al*. The second British Stomach Cancer Group trial of adjuvant radiotherapy or chemotherapy in resectable gastric cancer: five-year follow up. Lancet 1994; 343:1309–12.

13. Dent D, Werner I, Novis B, *et al*. A prospective randomized trial of combined oncological therapy for gastric carcinoma. Cancer 1979; 44:385–91.

14. Moertel CG, Childs DS, O'Fallon JR, *et al*. Combined 5 fluorouracil and radiation therapy as a surgical adjuvant for poor prognosis gastric carcinoma. J Clin Oncol 1984; 2:1249–54.

15. Lise M, Nitti D, Marchet A, *et al*. Adjuvant therapy for gastric cancer: a review. Anti-Cancer Drugs 1991; 2(5):433–45.

16. Crookes P, Leichman CG, Leichman L, *et al*. Systemic chemotherapy for gastric carcinoma followed by postoperative intraperitoneal therapy: a final report. Cancer 1997; 79:1767–75.

17. Kelsen D, Karpeh M, Schwartz G, *et al*. Neoadjuvant therapy of high risk gastric cancer: a phase II trial of preoperative FAMTX and postoperative intraperitoneal fluorouracil-cisplatin plus intravenous fluorouracil. J Clin Oncol 1996; 14(6):1818–28.

18. Wilke H, Preusser P, Fink U, *et al*. Preoperative chemotherapy in locally advanced and nonresectable gastric cancer: a phase II study with etoposide, doxorubicin, and cisplatin. J Clin Oncol 1989; 7(9):1318–26.

19. Verschueren RJC, Willemse PHB, Sleijfer DT, *et al*. Combined chemotherapeutic–surgical approach of locally advanced gastric cancer. Proc ASCO 1993; 12:355.

20. Ducreux M, Rougier P, Lasser P, *et al*. Neoadjuvant chemotherapy in locally advanced gastric carcinoma: does it increase long-term survival? Proc ASCO 1993; 12:670.

21. Kang YK, Choi DW, Im Y, *et al*. A phase III randomized comparison of neoadjuvant chemotherapy followed by surgery versus surgery for locally advanced stomach cancer. Proc ASCO 1996; 15:503.

22. Schwartz G, Kelsen D, Christman K, *et al*. A phase II study of neoadjuvant FAMTX (5-FU/adriamycin/ methotrexate) and postoperative intraperitoneal 5-FU and cisplatin in high risk patients with gastric cancer. Proc ASCO 1993; 12:572.

23. Fink U, Schuhmacher C, Stein HJ, *et al*. Preoperative chemotherapy for stage III–IV gastric carcinoma: feasibility, response and outcome after complete resection. Br J Surg 1995; 82:1248–52.

24. Burris HA, Moore MJ, Andersen J, *et al*. Improvements in survival and clinical benefit with gemcitabine as first-line therapy for patients with advanced pancreas cancer: a randomized trial. J Clin Oncol 1997; 15(6):2403–13.

25. Ishikawa O, Oshigasi H, Teshima T, *et al*. Clinical and histopathological appraisal of preoperative

irradiation for adenocarcinoma of the pancreaticoduodenal region. J Surg Oncol 1989; 40:143–51.

26. Ishikawa O, Oshigasi H, Imaoka S, *et al.* Is the long-term survival rate improved by preoperative irradiation prior to Whipple's procedure for adenocarcinoma of the pancreatic head. Arch Surg 1994; 129:1075–80.

27. Gastrointestinal Tumor Study Group. A multi-institutional comparative trial of radiation therapy alone and in combination with 5-fluorouracil for locally unresectable pancreatic carcinoma. Ann Surg 1978; 189(2):205–8.

28. Gastrointestinal Tumor Study Group. Further evidence of effective adjuvant combined radiation and chemotherapy following curative resection of pancreatic cancer. Cancer 1987; 59:2006–10.

29. Hoffman JP, Weese JL, Solin LJ, *et al.* A pilot study of preoperative chemoradiation for patients with localized adenocarcinoma of the pancreas. Am J Surg 1995; 169:71–8.

30. Hoffman JP, Weese JL, Ahmad N, *et al.* Preoperative chemoradiation and radiation therapy for patients with pancreatic carcinoma without demonstrable metastatic disease: the Fox Chase Cancer Center Experience. Semin Surg Oncol 1995; 11:141–8.

31. Hoffman JP, Lipsitz S, Pisansky T, *et al.* Phase II trial of preoperative radiation therapy and chemotherapy for patients with localized resectable adenocarcinoma of the pancreas: an Eastern Cooperative Oncology Group study. J Clin Oncol 1998; 16(1):317–23.

32. Pendurthi TK, Hoffman JP, Ross E, *et al.* Preoperative versus postoperative chemoradiation for patients with resected pancreatic adenocarcinoma. Am Surg 1998; 64:686–92.

33. Spitz FR, Abbruzzese JL, Lee JE, *et al.* Preoperative and postoperative chemoradiation strategies in patients treated with pancreaticoduodenectomy for adenocarcinoma of the pancreas. J Clin Oncol 1997; 15(3):928–37.

34. Evans DB, Rich TA, Byrd DR, *et al.* Preoperative chemoradiation and pancreaticoduodenectomy for adenocarcinoma of the pancreas. Arch Surg 1992; 127:1335–9.

35. Evans J, Abbruzzese J, Lee K, *et al.* Preoperative chemoradiation and pancreaticoduodenectomy for adenocarcinoma of the pancreas. Proc ASCO 1993; 12:692.

36. Weese JL, Nussbaum ML, Paul AR, *et al.* Increased resectability of locally advanced pancreatic and periampullary carcinoma with neoadjuvant chemoradiotherapy. Int J Pancreatol 1990; 7:177–85.

37. Jessup JM, Colacchio T, Valone F, *et al.* Phase I/II neoadjuvant trial for locally advanced pancreas adenocarcinoma. Proc ASCO 1993; 12:595.

38. Ajani JA, Ota D, Jackson D. Current strategies in the management of locoregional and metastatic gastric carcinoma. Cancer 1991; (Suppl.) 67:260–5.

39. Kelsen D. The use of chemotherapy in the treatment of advanced gastric and pancreas cancer. Semin Oncol 1994; 21(4):58–66.

40. Lenz HJ, Leichman CG, Leichman L, *et al.* Molecular markers as indicators of response and outcome in primary gastric cancer. Proc Gastric Cancer Res 1997; 22:1295–1300.

41. Lenz HJ, Leichman CG, Danenberg KD, *et al.* Thymidylate synthase mRNA level in adenocarcinoma of the stomach: a predictor for primary tumor response and overall survival. J Clin Oncol 1996; 14:176–82.

42. Metzger R, Danenbergb K, Danenberg P, *et al.* Excision repair cross complementing (ERCC)-1 gene in primary gastric cancer: a determinant of response to cisplatin-based chemotherapy. Proc ASCO 1996; 15:A505.

43. Clark JW, Glicksman A, Wanebo HJ, *et al.* Adjuvant and systemic therapy for pancreatic cancer. Semin Surg Oncol 1995; 11:149–53.

FURTHER READING

Evans DB, Byrd DR, Mansfield PF. Preoperative chemoradiotherapy for adenocarcinoma of the pancreas. Am J Clin Oncol 1991; 14(4):359–64.

Evans TRJ, Lofts FJ, Mansi JL, *et al.* A phase II study of continuous-infusion 5-fluorouracil with cisplatin and epirubicin in inoperable pancreatic cancer. Br J Cancer 1996; 73:1260–4.

Prott FJ, Schonekaes K, Preusser P, *et al.* Combined modality treatment with accelerated radiotherapy and chemotherapy in patients with locally advanced inoperable carcinoma of the pancreas: results of a feasibility study. Br J Cancer 1997; 75(4):597–601.

Robertson JM, Shewach DS, Lawrence TS. Preclinical studies of chemotherapy and radiation therapy for pancreatic carcinoma. Cancer 1996; Suppl. 78(3):674–8.

Rothenberg ML, Moore MJ, Cripps MC, *et al.* A phase II trial of gemcitabine in patients with 5-FU refractory pancreas cancer. Ann Oncol 1996; 7:347–53.

Tepper J, Nardi, G, Suit H. Carcinoma of the pancreas: review of MGH experience from 1963 to 1973: analysis of surgical failure and implications for radiation therapy. Cancer 1976; 37:1518–24.

Commentary

WILLIAM H ISACOFF

Adjuvant therapy may be defined as the use of one or more therapeutic interventions following surgical resection of a malignant neoplasm with curative intent. It is recommended to patients who are judged to have a high probability of relapse due to occult residual disease when all known and clinically obvious disease has been removed. Aggressive prophylactic treatment is therefore justified for these patients in an attempt to significantly prolong the disease-free period or, in some, with the hope that it will result in a cure. To recommend treatment in the 'adjuvant' context is to place that particular individual at some immediate risk of toxic side-effects and adverse reactions as well as enduring social and economic sacrifice from treatment with a view toward long-term gains in overall survival. Therapy which is being prescribed in the adjuvant setting should have proven efficacy in the management of patients with advanced disease. Additionally, the specific treatment being recommended should have been tested in phase III adjuvant trials to prove that it prolongs survival when compared to a surgery-only treated group.

Drs Iqbal and Lenz present an accurate review and analysis of current adjuvant therapeutic approaches for patients with gastric and pancreatic cancer. The chapter summarizes useful information which is important to clinical oncologists who manage patients with gastric and pancreatic cancer.

GASTRIC CANCER

Gastric cancer is a common disease, with a 5-year survival rate usually of less than 20%. Worldwide, it remains one of the leading causes of cancer-related deaths. In early stages, surgery is the treatment of choice. Several studies have investigated the possible role of chemotherapy after curative resection to see if survival may be improved when compared to surgery alone. The utility of adjuvant chemotherapy in gastric cancer remains unproven and controversial.

Adjuvant chemotherapy

Two comprehensive review papers on the use of adjuvant chemotherapy for gastric cancer have recently been reported.[1,2] In an analysis of 12 selected trials of adjuvant combination chemotherapy for resected gastric cancer, Yao et al. found that only three regimens demonstrated a survival benefit, which could not be substantiated in subsequent randomized trials. They concluded that the design of clinical trials needed to be improved, with better preoperative staging, standardized surgical techniques, inclusion of adequate numbers of patients, and the continued use of a surgery-alone control group. At present, based on the available data, the routine use of postoperative chemotherapy should be discouraged.

Cirera et al. recently reported the results of a randomized trial of adjuvant mitomycin C plus tegafur in patients with resected gastric cancer.[3] One hundred and fifty-six patients were randomized to receive surgery with or without mitomycin C and 3 months of tegafur. The median survival for the treated group was 74 months, compared to 29 months for the control group. The treated group had a 5-year survival of 56%, compared to 36% in the control group. These results should be interpreted with some degree of caution. The number of patients with T1 or T2 tumors was less than 10%. Therefore, 90% of patients had poor-prognosis disease. Survival of IIIb and IV disease is extremely poor, with only 10–15% alive at 5 years. The control group had a 36% 5-year survival. In another recent, well-designed, randomized trial by Nakajima et al., 579 patients were randomized between surgery or surgery plus mitomycin, 5-fluorouracil (5-FU), and oral uracil and tegafur following surgery.[4] There was no survival benefit.

Mari et al. performed a meta-analysis of published randomized trials to evaluate the efficacy of adjuvant chemotherapy after curative resection for gastric cancer.[5] In their analysis, chemotherapy produced a small survival benefit, but they warned that the data should be interpreted with caution, stating that meta-analysis based on summary data derived from the literature may be influenced by a series bias. They concluded that, although promising results have been seen in smaller trials, the use of systemic adjuvant chemotherapy has not been substantiated by larger prospective, randomized trials, and that this approach is still considered as investigational.

Adjuvant chemoradiation therapy

Data from a number of phase II single-institution trials on the use of postoperative adjuvant irradiation plus chemotherapy show that treatment is well tolerated, decreases the incidence of local failure, and may improve median and overall survival. At the annual meeting of the American Society of Clinical Oncology, May 2000, Macdonald et al. presented the results of a large intergroup trial in which more than 600 high-risk patients with completely resected gastric cancer were randomized to a surgery-alone control group versus postoperative irradiation plus chemotherapy.[6] The treatment consisted of one cycle of 5-FU ($425 \, mg/m^2$) plus leucovorin (LV) ($20 \, mg/m^2$) in a daily $\times$ 5 regimen, followed by 4500 cGy given with 5-FU/LV ($400 \, mg/m^2$ and $20 \, mg/m^2$) on days 1 through 4, and on the last 3 days of radiation. One month after completion of radiation, two cycles of daily 5-FU/LV were given at monthly intervals. With 4 years of median follow-up, 3-year disease-free survival is 49% for the treatment group and 32% for the control group. The 3-year overall survival is 52% for the treatment group and 41% for the control group ($p = 0.03$). The median survival was 27 months for the control arm, compared to 25 months for the treatment arm. It was concluded that postoperative chemoirradiation should now be considered a standard of care for high-risk, resected, locally advanced adenocarcinoma of the stomach and gastroesophageal junction.

PANCREATIC CANCER

Curative pancreaticoduodenectomy is feasible in only 10–15% of patients with pancreatic adenocarcinoma. Patients with surgically resected disease survive between 11 and 18 months, with less than 20% surviving 5 years.

Adjuvant therapy: prospective, randomized trials

In 1974, the Gastrointestinal Tumor Study Group (GITSG) organized the first prospectively randomized trial to evaluate the effects of postoperative adjuvant chemoradiation in patients with pancreatic cancer who have undergone curative resection.[7] This trial attempted to recruit patients with histologically negative margins who could be entered into study between 4 and 10 weeks postoperatively. Only 49 patients were randomized over an 8-year interval, with five patients withdrawing from the study without being treated. The radiation was given as two courses of 2000 Gy each, with a planned two-week rest. 5-FU chemotherapy was given on the first 3 days of each half of the radiotherapy at a dose of $500 \, \text{mg/m}^2$ as an intravenous bolus injection. Following radiotherapy, the 5-FU was continued weekly at $500 \, \text{mg/m}^2$ for 2 years. Patients treated with chemoradiotherapy had an improved survival compared to patients treated with surgery only. The median survivals were 20 months and 11 months, respectively. The study was terminated prematurely because of poor accrual and the observation that there was a significant difference in survival between the treated and control groups. In order to confirm the benefit of the treatment in the randomized study, the GITSG elected to reopen the treatment arm of the study to enroll a new cohort of patients, all of whom would receive radiation and 5-FU after curative resection.[8] An additional 30 patients were accrued and the study was closed. In the confirmatory trial, patients had a median survival of 18 months. By 1990, there were 10-year follow-up data from the randomized trial, and 5-year follow-up data from the confirmatory trial.[9] None of the patients in the control group was alive, whereas 19% of the patients in the treatment group were still alive.

In another prospectively randomized trial utilizing chemoradiation, the European Organization for Research and Treatment of Cancer (EORTC) assigned patients after curative resection to observation or adjuvant treatment which consisted of radiotherapy 40 Gy given as a split course and 5-FU $500 \, \text{mg/m}^2$ daily × 3 during each course of radiation, the same as the GITSG trial but without maintenance 5-FU chemotherapy.[10] A total of 119 patients with pancreatic cancer was accrued onto the trial, 58 of whom received treatment. The preliminary analysis of the data shows no difference in survival. The median survivals for the treated and the control groups are 15.7 and 12.9 months, respectively.

Two additional prospectively randomized trials are currently ongoing. The European Study Group for Pancreatic Cancer (ESPAC) is currently conducting an adjuvant pancreatic study designed to answer two questions:

- Is there a role for chemoradiation?
- Is there a role for chemotherapy?

Thus far, 530 patients with pancreatic ductal adenocarcinoma have been randomized. Preliminary results show no evidence of benefit for chemoradiation treatment. There is some evidence of a survival benefit for patients having chemotherapy. Patients are no longer being accrued to radiotherapy. The trial continues to randomize patients between chemotherapy with 5-FU/LV and surgery.[11]

The Radiation Therapy Oncology Group (RTOG) in July 1998 activated a phase III trial of adjuvant chemotherapy for patients with resected pancreatic cancer. Their objective is to determine whether 5-FU base chemoradiation preceded and followed by gemcitabine improves overall survival; local, regional, and distant disease control; and disease-free survival when compared to 5-FU base chemoradiation preceded and followed by 5-FU.

Adjuvant therapy: single institutional trials

Since the early 1980s, there have been a large number of single-institution, non-randomized trials utilizing non-split-course higher dose radiotherapy in combination with more aggressive chemotherapeutic regimens.[12–14] What have we learned? Prior to the use of adjunctive therapy, sites of local–regional failure were responsible for a substantial number of relapses, which could be significantly reduced with chemoradiotherapy. Reducing the rate of local–regional failure has resulted in only a modest improvement in survival.

Sites of distant metastases involving the liver, peritoneum, and extra-abdominal location are of equal, if not greater, importance than locally recurrent disease.[15–18] If adjuvant therapy is to have any meaningful impact on influencing the survival of patients with pancreatic cancer, it must not only address and eliminate disease at the resected site locally, but eradicate distant micrometastases as well.

The foregoing data allow one to reasonably conclude that, for the majority of patients with resectable gastric or pancreatic cancer, adjuvant therapies have in general been minimally effective in influencing outcome. Even the most recent work of Macdonald and colleagues, although encouraging, has been the only large trial to date showing benefit for those patients in the postoperative-treated group. The systemic therapy used in this trial was 5-FU and LV. If designed today, systemic therapy chosen for patients with gastric cancer would be potentially more active, yielding even better results.

Simply stated, the systemic approaches currently employed in gastric and pancreatic cancer are not effective in eradicating microscopic disease and do not prevent recurrent disease outside the field of surgery and radiation. Are there techniques and innovative approaches that are available today to change these dismal results? Dr Lenz suggests in his discussion that we should be more selective in how we choose therapy for patients undergoing adjuvant treatment. He sites a number of studies undertaken by himself and his colleagues at the University of Southern California demonstrating the predictive value of measuring the genetic expression of thymidylate synthase (TS) and the excision repair cross-complementing gene (ERCC-1) in tumor samples from patients with gastric cancer. Indeed, patients with low levels of gene expression do have significantly improved responses and prolonged survival.

This concept of genetic pharmacology has been used to predict the utility of chemotherapeutic intervention in patients with adenocarcinoma of the stomach, colon, and esophagus. Since the early 1990s, most gastrointestinal oncologists have been aware of the predictive value in measuring TS in RNA expression. It affords us the opportunity to more rationally select patients who will have a higher probability of responding to 5-FU. These predictive tests do not improve therapy, but will allow for the intelligent selection of patients who are likely to benefit from treatment. Unfortunately, these tests are not currently used in clinical practice. Not one cooperative group in a multi-institutional setting has prospectively utilized the measurement of TS mRNA in tumor tissue in the decision making of whether or not 5-FU should be included as part of the treatment regimen. If one knows that a patient's tumor overexpresses TS mRNA and therefore has less than a 10% chance of responding to 5-FU, why expose that patient to the risk, toxicity, and expense of ineffective treatment? Additionally, if there are possibly other more effective treatment possibilities, why waste the time? Dr Lenz certainly raises an important issue concerning how we can improve outcome through better drug selection. As yet, this extremely useful technology has not found its way to the clinic.

CAN WE IMPROVE UPON THE WAY WE DOSE AND SCHEDULE CHEMOTHERAPY?

Lastly, I would like to address the issue of how we can improve the therapeutic benefit of the marginally effective drugs being used to treat patients with gastric and pancreatic cancer. Two recently published editorials by Kamen et al.[19] and by Fidler and Ellis[20] raise the possibility that the chemotherapeutic approach for most malignant diseases should be reassessed. It is suggested that prolonged administration of low-dose chemotherapy may, in fact, be more effective than high-dose pulse therapy. We are reminded that for the past two decades many clinical trials have focused on achieving higher doses of chemotherapy. The concept of dose intensity may have erroneously evolved in such a way as to embrace the concept that 'more is better.' This evolution has culminated in the use of high-dose chemotherapy and the use of autologous blood progenitor stem cell support. After 20 years of hype and enthusiasm, surrounded by controversy, high-dose chemotherapy for patients with breast cancer has not been found to be better than standard, conventional-dose chemotherapy. Several randomized trials of both advanced breast carcinoma and the adjuvant setting so far have shown no advantage for high-dose chemotherapy with hematopoietic stem cell support when compared to standard-dose chemotherapy.[21]

Kamen et al.[19] point out that the idea of a log dose survival curve, developed by Skipper, was a consequence of in-vitro models to study the biology of chemotherapy on cell kill. In those in-vitro experimental models, the dose–response effect is only valid for log-phase, non-mitogenic cells when non-cell-cycle-specific agents are used. Skipper et al. state that the model would not apply for antimetabolites, and would have only limited application in vivo.[22] Yet the oncology community has for three decades applied this model to the clinic and has embraced the 'more is better' approach. Drug regimens have been designed to kill as many tumor cells as possible by using the 'maximum tolerated doses' (MTDs) of cytotoxic agents. When drugs are utilized at their MTDs, dose-limiting toxicities such as myelosuppression, neurotoxicity, and gastrointestinal side-effects put restrictions on their continued use. These constraints have resulted in the episodic use of chemotherapy at the MTDs of the drugs, followed by rest periods to allow healthy, normal tissues to recover from the toxic side-effects. The time required for the recovery of normal tissue also permits malignant cells to recover. Thus, scheduling becomes an important element in the design of chemotherapeutic protocols. Aside from dose (concentration), the other critical variable in the success of drug therapy is schedule (time). How much drug can be given over what period of time? Is it better to give high doses of treatment over short periods of time (pulse therapy) with harsh side-effects, or will less toxic doses (low dose) given repetitively over longer time intervals be better?

At the heart of this debate is the question of whether low-dose prolonged or continuous therapy may have other potential advantages. Two recent papers by Klement et al.[23] and Browder et al.[24] reveal the anti-angiogenic capability of commonly used chemotherapeutic drugs by simply developing alternative dosing schedules. More than 30 years ago, Folkman proposed the concept of developing anti-angiogenic drugs to treat cancer.[25] Angiogenesis is the process of new blood vessel formation. It is an essential capability of cancer, and a compelling body of evidence argues that tumor growth depends on it. In both studies cited above, cyclophosphamide and vinblastine, when used in a conventional MTD regimen, showed only a modest delay in tumor growth. In contrast, when cyclophosphamide and vinblastine were given at lower doses regularly, tumor growth was significantly impaired. In both studies, when chemotherapy was given as a low dose continuously and combined with experimental angiogenic inhibitors, the majority of drug-resistant carcinomas were eradicated. Each investigator has demonstrated the value of combining low-dose continuous chemotherapy with experimental angiogenesis inhibitors. Using an angiogenesis bioassay in normal mice, Browder et al. confirmed that 'metronomic' dosing of cyclophosphamide was anti-angiogenic. Kamen et al. have proposed a 'new' old concept for the design of chemotherapeutic regimens, namely, *high-time chemotherapy*.[19] High-time therapy would seek the longest time for drug exposure at a given concentration based on patient tolerance. The focus of drug administration would not be how much, but rather how long without interruption. Are there data to substantiate this approach? Etoposide, for example, given as an oral daily dose for 21 days is less toxic and more effective than a similar dose administered as a 24-h infusion.[26]

Recently, Luykx-de Bakker et al. performed a study in patients with locally advanced breast cancer in which six cycles of moderately high-dose doxorubicin, cyclophosphamide, and granulocyte–macrophage colony-stimulating factor were given to 42 patients prior to local therapy.[27] The response rate was 98%. Essential to the success of this approach was the fact that the primary tumor and draining axillary lymph nodes remained *in situ* for a prolonged period of time. In theory, the primary tumor may keep micrometastases dormant by producing anti-angiogenic peptides. Based on these findings, a large international group study is underway comparing preoperative and postoperative therapy to prolonged neoadjuvant treatment.

Gracchetti et al. combined 5-FU, LV, and oxaliplatin administered as a chronomodulated schedule to patients with colorectal cancer with liver metastases.[28] The chronomodulated schedule was used to take advantage of the improved tolerability associated with this mode of administration. In previous trials, chemotherapy with this mode of administration was significantly less toxic

with increased efficacy. In this current report, 151 patients were treated. The response rate was 59%, with a median overall survival of 24 months. Surgery with curative intent was undertaken in 77 patients, with complete resection of all liver metastases achieved in 58 patients. The median survival of the 77 operated patients was 48 months and the 5-year survival rate 50%. The median duration of chemotherapy prior to surgical resection was 5.5 months. This is another example of what one may consider prolonged continuous therapy that is minimally toxic, given for prolonged periods of time to achieve higher than expected response rates and survival.

Attempts to improve the therapeutic effects of 5-FU have included changing its route of administration to protracted infusion, combining it with biochemical modulators, and adding other chemotherapeutic agents. Isacoff et al. treated 41 patients with advanced colon cancer with continuous-infusion 5-FU, intravenous bolus LV, oral daily Persantine, and intravenous bolus mitomycin C. Twenty-five patients responded to therapy.[29] There were ten complete responses. The treatment regimen was safe, with a low toxicity profile. Currently, patients are receiving the same four-drug combination with the 5-FU, LV, and mitomycin being dose adjusted to patient tolerance, so as to allow for at least four consecutive weeks of uninterrupted therapy followed by a 1-week or 2-week rest. Encouraged by these results, we have used the same four drugs to treat 70 patients with locally advanced, unresected pancreatic cancer.[30] Thirty-eight percent of patients achieved response to therapy. Of the responding patients, nine were downstaged to justify a second-look operation, seven of whom underwent curative pancreaticoduodenectomies. The median survival of the entire group is 15.5 months, with a 1-year survival of 70%. The median survival of all responding patients is 24 months. Of those patients who were downstaged and underwent surgical resection, the median survival was 30 months.

Browder has also observed that the low-dose, continuous exposure of 5-FU has anti-angiogenic activity.[24] It is therefore critical to realize that another important potential chemotherapeutic target may be the tumor vasculature. Scheduling as well as dose may be essential in the chemotherapeutic effects on this target. Browder et al. point out that other drugs have antiendothelial effects which have been demonstrated *in vitro*.[24] These effects have been observed for cyclophosphamide, 5-FU, mitomycin C, vincristine, vinblastine, doxorubicin, etoposide, the toxanes, topotecan, and camptosar.

CONCLUSION

As mentioned previously, a large number of factors make it difficult to interpret data from adjuvant trials in gastric and pancreatic cancer. Newer prospective trials must be designed with the intent to accrue adequate numbers of patients to treatment and control arms in order to permit sufficient statistical power to detect meaningful differences in treatment outcome. In addition, techniques for improved preoperative staging should be implemented. Surgical techniques should be standardized. Molecular markers that predict response to chemotherapy and correlate with prognosis should be used more frequently in clinical practice. Newer drug strategies need to be developed that would be less toxic and more effective.

REFERENCES

1. Yao JC, Shimada K, Ajani JA. Adjuvant therapy for gastric carcinoma: closing out the century. Oncology 1999; 13:1485–94.

2. Gunderson LL, Donohue JH, Burch PA. Stomach cancer. In Abeloff MD, Armitage JO, Lichter AS, Niederhuber JE, eds. *Clinical oncology*. Philadelphia, Churchill Livingstone, 2000, 1545–85.

3. Cirera L, Balil A, Batiste-Alentorne, *et al.* Randomized clinical trial of adjuvant mitomycin plus Tegafur in patients with resected Stage III gastric cancer. J Clin Oncol 1999; 17(12):3810–15.

4. Nakajima T, Nashimoto A, Kitamura M, *et al.* Adjuvant mitomycin and fluorouracil followed by oral uracil plus Tegafur in serosa-negative gastric cancer: a randomized trial. Lancet 1999; 354:273–7.

5. Mari E, Floriani I, Tinazzi A, *et al.* Efficacy of adjuvant chemotherapy after curative resection for gastric cancer: a meta-analysis of published randomized trials: a study of the GISCAD. Ann Oncol 2000; 11:837–44.

6. Macdonald JS, Smaller S, Benedetti J, *et al.* Postoperative combined radiation and chemotherapy improves disease-free survival (DFS) and overall survival (OS) in resected adenocarcinoma of the stomach and GE junction: results of Intergroup Study INT-0116 (SWOG 9008). Proc Am Soc Clin Oncol 2000; 19(1a), Abstract.

7. Kalaser MH, Ellenberg SS. Pancreatic cancer: adjuvant combined radiation and chemotherapy following curative resection. Arch Surg 1985; 120:899–903.

8. Gastrointestinal Tumor Study Group. Further evidence of effective adjuvant combined radiation and chemotherapy following curative resection of pancreatic cancer. Cancer 1987; 59:2006–10.

9. Douglass HO Jr. Adjuvant therapy for pancreatic cancer. World J Surg 1995; 19:270–9.

10. Klinkelbijl JH, Jeekel J, Sahmoud T. Adjuvant radiotherapy and 5-fluorouracil after curative resection of cancer of the pancreas and periampullary region: Phase III trial of the EORTC Gastrointestinal Tract Cancer Cooperative Group. Ann Surg 1999; 230:776–84.

11. Neoptolemos JP, Dunn JA, Moffitt JA, *et al.* ESPAC-1 interim results: a European randomized study to assess the roles of adjuvant chemotherapy (5FU + folinic acid) and adjuvant chemoradiation (40 Gy + 5FU) in resectable pancreatic cancer. Proc Am Soc Clin Oncol 2000; 19:238a, Abstract.

12. Whittington R, Bryer MP, Haller DG, *et al.* Adjuvant therapy of resected adenocarcinoma of the pancreas. Int J Radiat Oncol Biol Phys 1991; 21:1137–43.

13. Foo ML, Gunderson LL, Hagornee DM, *et al.* Patterns of failure in grossly resected pancreatic ductal adenocarcinoma treated with irradiation + 5 fluorouracil. Int J Radiat Oncol Biol Phys 1993; 26:483–9.

14. Yeo CJ, Abrams RA, Grochow LB, *et al.* Pancreaticoduodenectomy for pancreatic adeno-carcinoma: postoperative adjuvant chemoradiation improves survival. A prospective single-institution experience. Ann Surg 1997; 225:621–6.

15. Griffin JF, Smalley SR, Jewell W, *et al.* Patterns of failure after curative resection of pancreatic cancer. Cancer 1990; 66:56–61.

16. Westerdahl J, Anden-Sandberg A, Ihse I. Recurrence of exocrine pancreatic cancer – local or hepatic? Hepato-Gastroenterol 1993; 40:384–7.

17. Amikura K, Kobari M, Matsuno S. Time of occurrence of liver metastasis in carcinoma of the pancreas. Int J Pancreatol 1995; 17:139–46.

18. Pister WT, Abbruggese JL, Ajani JA, *et al.* Rapid-fraction preoperative chemoradiation, pancreaticoduodenectomy, and intraoperative radiation therapy for resectable pancreatic adenocarcinoma. J Clin Oncol 1998; 16:3843–50.

19. Kamen BA, Rubin E, Asner J, Glatstein E. High-time chemotherapy or high-time for low dose. J Clin Oncol 2000; 18:2935–7.

20. Fidler I, Ellis LM. Chemotherapeutic drugs – more really is not better. Nat Med 2000; 6:500–2.

21. Coleman RE. High dose chemotherapy: rationale and results in breast carcinoma. Cancer 2000; 88(Suppl.):3059–64.

22. Skipper HE, Schabal FM, Mellet LB. Implications of biochemical cytokinetic, pharmacologic and toxicologic relationships in the design of optimal therapeutic schedules. Cancer Chemother Rep 1970; 54:431–50.

23. Klement G, Barachal S, Rak J, *et al.* Continuous low-dose therapy with vinblastine and VEGF receptor-2 antibody induces sustained tumor regression without overt toxicity. J Clin Invest, 2000; 105:R15–24.

24. Browder T, Butterfield C, Kraling B, *et al.* Antiangiogeneic scheduling of chemotherapy improves efficacy against experimental drug resistant cancer. Cancer Res 2000; 60:1878–87.

25. Folkman J. Tumor angiogenesis: therapeutic implication. N Engl J Med 1971; 285:1182–6.

26. Hainsworth JD, Greco FA. Etoposide: twenty years later. Ann Oncol 1995; 6:325–41.

27. Luykx-de Bakker SA, Verheul HMN, deGraijl TD, Pinedo HM. Prolonged neoadjuvant treatment in locally advanced tumours: a novel concept based on biological considerations. Ann Oncol 1999; 10:155–60.

28. Gracchetti S, Itzhaki M, Gruia G, *et al.* Long term survival of patients with unresectable colorectal cancer liver metastases following infusional chemotherapy with 5-fluorouracil, oxaliplatin, leucovorin, and surgery. Ann Oncol 1999; 10:663–70.

29. Isacoff WH, Eilber FR, Kuchenbecker SL, *et al.* Continuous infusion 5-fluorouracil given with calcium leucovorin, dipyridamole, and mitomycin-c in patients with advanced colorectal carcinoma: a Phase II trial. J Infusional Chemother 1994; 4:107–11.

30. Todd KE, Gloor B, Lane JS, *et al.* Resection of locally advanced pancreatic cancer after downstaging with continuous infusion 5-fluorouracil, mitomycin-c, leucovorin, and dipyridamole. J Gastrointest Surg 1998; 2:159–66.

Editors' selected abstracts

Results of irradiation or chemoirradiation for primary unresectable, locally recurrent, or grossly incomplete resection of gastric adenocarcinoma.

Henning GT, Schild SE, Stafford SL, Donohue JH, Burch PA, Haddock MG, Gunderson LL.

Division of Radiation Oncology, Mayo Clinic and Mayo Foundation, Rochester, MN, USA.

International Journal of Radiation Oncology, Biology, Physics 46(1):109–18, 2000, January 1.

Objective: To evaluate the results of irradiation chemotherapy for patients with unresectable gastric carcinoma. *Materials and methods:* The records of 60 patients with a gastric or gastroesophageal junction adenocarcinoma and a locally advanced unresectable primary ($n = 28$), a local or regional recurrence ($n = 21$), or gross residual disease following incomplete resection ($n = 11$) were retrospectively reviewed. Patients were treated with external beam irradiation (EBRT) alone or external beam plus intraoperative irradiation (IOERT), and 55 of the 60 (92%) patients received 5-FU based chemotherapy. *Results:* The median survival for the entire cohort was 11.6 months. There was no significant difference in median survival between each of the three treatment groups. In examining the extent of disease there was a significant difference in survival based on the number of sites involved. Nine patients with disease limited to a single non-nodal site appeared to represent a favorable subgroup compared to the rest of the patients (median survival of 21.8 months vs. 10.2 months, $p = 0.03$). In the patients with recurrent disease, the number of sites involved ($p = 0.05$), and total dose adding external beam dose to IOERT dose (> 54 Gy vs. $\leqslant 54$ Gy, $p = 0.06$) were of borderline significance in regard to survival. *Conclusions:* In patients with either primary unresectable, locally or regionally recurrent, or incompletely resected gastric carcinoma, the overall survival is similar, and related to the extent of disease based on the number of regional sites involved. The patients with a single non-nodal site of disease represent a favorable subgroup and patients with recurrent disease may benefit from total irradiation doses > 54 Gy.

Results of irradiation or chemoirradiation following resection of gastric adenocarcinoma.

Henning GT, Schild SE, Stafford SL, Donohue JH, Burch PA, Haddock MG, Trastek VF, Gunderson LL.

Division of Radiation Oncology, Mayo Clinic and Mayo Foundation, Rochester, MN, USA.

International Journal of Radiation Oncology, Biology, Physics 46(3):589–98, 2000, February 1.

Purpose: To evaluate the results of postoperative irradiation ± chemotherapy for carcinoma of the stomach and gastroesophageal junction. *Methods and materials:* The records of 63 patients who underwent resection for stomach cancer were retrospectively reviewed. Twenty-five patients had complete resection with no residual disease but with high-risk factors for relapse. Twenty-eight had microscopic residual and 10 had gross residual disease. Doses of irradiation ranged from 39.6 to 59.4 Gy with a median dose of 50.4 Gy in 1.8 Gy fractions. Fifty-three of the 63 (84%) patients received 5-fluorouracil (5-FU)-based chemotherapy. *Results:* The median duration of survival was 19.3 months for patients with no residual disease, 16.7 months for those with microscopic residual disease, and 9.2 months for those with gross residual disease ($p = 0.01$). The amount of residual disease also significantly impacted locoregional control ($p = 0.04$). Patients with linitis plastica did significantly worse in terms of survival, locoregional control, and distant control than those without linitis plastica. The use of 4 or more irradiation fields was associated with a significant decrease in the rate of Grade 4 or 5 toxicity when compared to the patients treated with 2 fields ($p = 0.05$). *Conclusions:* There was a significant association between survival and extent of residual disease after resection as well as the presence of linitis plastica. Distant failures are common and effective systemic therapy will be necessary to improve outcome. The toxicity of combined modality treatment appears to be reduced by using greater than 2 irradiation fields.

Novel allogeneic granulocyte–macrophage colony-stimulating factor-secreting tumor vaccine for pancreatic cancer: a phase I trial of safety and immune activation.

Jaffee EM, Hruban RH, Biedrzycki B, Laheru D, Schepers K, Sauter PR, Goemann M, Coleman J, Grochow L, Donehower RC, Lillemoe KD, O'Reilly S, Abrams RA, Pardoll DM, Cameron JL, Yeo CJ.

Departments of Oncology, Surgery, and Pathology, The Johns Hopkins Medical Institutions, Baltimore, MD, USA.

Journal of Clinical Oncology 19(1):145–56, 2001, January 1.

Purpose: Allogeneic granulocyte–macrophage colony-stimulating factor (GM-CSF)-secreting tumor vaccines can cure established tumors in the mouse, but their efficacy against human tumors is uncertain. We have developed a novel GM-CSF-secreting pancreatic tumor vaccine. To determine its safety and ability to induce antitumor immune responses, we conducted a phase I trial in patients with surgically resected adenocarcinoma of the pancreas. *Patients and methods:* Fourteen patients with stage 1, 2, or 3 pancreatic adenocarcinoma were enrolled. Eight weeks after pancreaticoduodenectomy, three patients received 1×10^7 vaccine cells, three patients received 5×10^7 vaccine cells, three patients received 10×10^7 vaccine cells, and five patients received 50×10^7 vaccine cells. Twelve of 14 patients then went on to receive a 6-month course of adjuvant radiation and chemotherapy. One month after completing adjuvant treatment, six patients still in remission received up to three additional monthly vaccinations with the same vaccine dose that they had received originally. *Results:* No dose-limiting toxicities were encountered. Vaccination induced increased delayed-type hypersensitivity (DTH) responses to autologous tumor cells in three patients who had received $\geqslant 10 \times 10^7$ vaccine cells. These three patients also seemed to have had an increased disease-free survival time, remaining disease-free at least 25 months after diagnosis. *Conclusion:* Allogeneic GM-CSF-secreting tumor vaccines are safe in patients with pancreatic adenocarcinoma. This vaccine approach seems to induce dose-dependent systemic antitumor immunity as measured by increased postvaccination DTH responses against autologous tumors. Further clinical evaluation of this approach in patients with pancreatic cancer is warranted.

Outcome of pancreaticoduodenectomy and impact of adjuvant therapy for ampullary carcinomas.

Lee JH, Whittington R, Williams NN, Berry MF, Vaughn DJ, Haller DG, Rosato EE.

Department of Radiation Oncology, University of Pennsylvania School of Medicine, Philadelphia, PA, USA.

International Journal of Radiation Oncology, Biology, Physics 47(4):945–53, 2000, July 1.

Purpose: To determine the clinical outcomes and potential impact of adjuvant chemoradiation in patients undergoing surgical resection of ampullary carcinoma. *Patients and methods:* Between 1988 and 1997, 39 patients underwent pancreaticoduodenectomy for ampullary adenocarcinomas. Clinical and pathologic factors, adjuvant therapy records, and disease status were obtained from chart review. Thirteen (33%) patients received adjuvant chemoradiation. Radiation therapy was delivered to the surgical bed and regional nodes to a median dose of 4,860 cGy with concurrent bolus or continuous infusion of 5-fluorouracil. Outcomes measures included locoregional control, disease-free survival, and overall survival. Univariate analysis was used to assess the impact of various patient- and tumor-related factors and the use of adjuvant therapy. Twenty (51%) patients with tumor invasion into the pancreas (T3) or node-positive disease were classified in a 'high-risk' subgroup. *Results:* After a median follow-up of 45 months for survivors, overall 3-year survival was 55%. Survival was significantly worse for patients with positive nodes (23% vs. 73%, $p < 0.001$) and high-risk status (30% vs. 80%, $p = 0.002$). Disease-free survival was 54% at 3 years. There were 3

postoperative deaths, and these patients (all high risk) are excluded from further analysis on adjuvant therapy. In univariate analysis, the use of adjuvant chemoradiation had no clear impact on local–regional control or overall survival. However, by controlling for risk status in multivariate analysis, the use of adjuvant therapy reached statistical significance for overall survival ($p = 0.03$). Among the high-risk patients, 7 (77%) of 9 patients receiving adjuvant therapy remained disease-free during follow-up compared with only 1 (14%) of 7 patients not receiving adjuvant therapy ($p = 0.012$). *Conclusion:* Despite the relatively favorable prognosis of ampullary carcinomas compared with other pancreaticobiliary tumors, patients with nodal metastases or T3 disease are at high risk for disease relapse. The use of adjuvant chemoradiation may improve long-term disease control in these patients.

Adjuvant chemoradiotherapy for 'unfavorable' carcinoma of the ampulla of Vater: preliminary report.

Mehta VK, Fisher GA, Ford JM, Poen JC, Vierra MA, Oberhelman HA, Bastidas AJ.

Department of Radiation Oncology, Stanford University Medical Center, Stanford, CA, USA.

Archives of Surgery 136(1):65–9, 2001, January.

Hypotheses: Adjuvant chemoradiotherapy decreases the risk of local recurrence in patients with adenocarcinoma of the ampulla of Vater and high-risk features. Adjuvant chemoradiotherapy for this population can be administered safely and without much morbidity. *Design:* Controlled, prospective, single-arm study. *Setting:* Tertiary care referral hospital. *Patients:* From June 1995 to March 1999, 12 patients (7 men and 5 women; median age, 66 years; age range, 38–78 years) with 'unfavorable' ampullary carcinoma were treated with adjuvant chemoradiotherapy. All patients underwent pancreaticoduodenectomy, and all pathologic findings were confirmed at Stanford University Medical Center, Stanford, Calif. Unfavorable features were defined as involved lymph nodes ($n = 10$), involved surgical margins ($n = 1$), poorly differentiated histological features ($n = 3$), tumor size greater than 2 cm ($n = 6$), or the presence of neurovascular invasion ($n = 4$). *Interventions:* Four to 6 weeks after undergoing pylorus-preserving pancreaticoduodenectomy with regional lymphadenectomy, patients began adjuvant chemoradiotherapy consisting of concurrent radiotherapy (45 Gy) and fluorouracil by protracted venous infusion (225–250 mg/m^2 per day, 7 days per week) for 5 weeks. *Main outcome measures:* Local recurrence, distant recurrence, overall survival rate, and treatment-related toxic effects. *Results:* All patients completed the prescribed treatment course. Toxic effects were assessed twice a week during treatment and graded according to the National Cancer Institute Common Toxicity Criteria Scale. One patient required a treatment interruption of 1 week for grade III nausea/vomiting. No grade IV or V toxic effects were observed. At median follow-up of 24 months (range, 13–50 months), 8 of 12 patients were alive and disease free. One patient was alive but had disease recurrence. Three patients died of this disease (liver metastases). Actuarial overall survival at 2 years was 89%, and median survival was 34 months. One surviving patient developed a local recurrence and a lung lesion. Actuarial overall survival and median survival were better than in a parallel cohort with resected high-risk pancreatic cancer ($n = 26$) treated with the same adjuvant chemoradiotherapy regimen (median survival, 34 vs 14 months; $p < 0.004$). *Conclusions:* Adjuvant chemoradiotherapy for carcinoma of the ampulla of Vater is well tolerated and might improve control of this disease in patients with unfavorable features.

Interferon-based adjuvant chemoradiation therapy improves survival after pancreaticoduodenectomy for pancreatic adenocarcinoma.

Nukui Y, Picozzi VJ, Traverso LW.

Department of General Surgery, Virginia Mason Medical Center, Seattle, Washington, USA.

American Journal of Surgery 179(5):367–71, 2000, May.

Background: Based on a 2-year survival of 43%, the Gastrointestinal Tumor Study Group (GITSG) recommended adjuvant 5-FU-based chemoradiation for resected patients with adenocarcinoma of the pancreatic head. Here we report improved survival over the GITSG protocol with a novel adjuvant chemoradiotherapy based on interferon-alpha (IFNalpha). *Methods:* From July 1993 to September 1998, 33 patients with adenocarcinoma of the pancreatic head underwent pancreaticoduodenectomy (PD) and subsequently went on to adjuvant therapy (GITSG-type, $n = 16$) or IFNalpha-based ($n = 17$) typically given between 6 and 8 weeks after surgery. The latter protocol consisted of external-beam irradiation at a dose of 4,500 to 5,400 cGy (25 fractions per 5 weeks) and simultaneous three-drug chemotherapy consisting of (1) continuous infusion 5-FU (200 mg/m^2 per day); (2) weekly intravenous bolus cisplatin (30 mg/m^2 per day); and (3) IFNalpha (3 million units subcutaneously every other day) during the 5 weeks of radiation. This was then followed by two 6-week courses of continuous infusion 5-FU (200 mg/m^2 per day, given weeks 9 to 14 and 17 to 22). Risk factors for recurrence and survival were compared for the two groups. *Results:* A more advanced tumor stage was observed in the IFNalpha-treated patients (positive nodes and American Joint Committee on Cancer [AJCC] stage III = 76%) than the GITSG group (positive nodes and stage III = 44%, $p = 0.052$). The 2-year overall survival was superior in the IFNalpha cohort (84%) versus the GITSG group (54%). With a mean follow-up of 26 months in both cohorts, actuarial survival curves significantly favored the IFNalpha group ($p = 0.04$). *Conclusions:* With a limited number of patients, this phase II type trial suggests better survival in the interferon group as compared with the GITSG group even though the interferon group was associated with a more extensive tumor stage. The 2-year survival rate in the interferon group is the best published to date for resected pancreatic cancer. The interferon/cisplatin/5-FU-based adjuvant chemoradiation protocol appears to be a promising treatment for patients who have undergone PD for adenocarcinoma of the pancreatic head.

Preoperative chemoradiation for patients with pancreatic cancer: toxicity of endobiliary stents.

Pisters PW, Hudec WA, Lee JE, Raijman I, Lahoti S, Janjan NA, Rich TA, Crane CH, Lenzi R, Wolff RA, Abbruzzese JL, Evans DB.

Pancreatic Tumor Study Group, The University of Texas M.D. Anderson Cancer Center, Houston, TX, USA.

Journal of Clinical Oncology 18(4):860–7, 2000, February.

Purpose: A recent multicenter study of preoperative chemoradiation and pancreaticoduodenectomy for localized pancreatic adenocarcinoma suggested that biliary stent-related complications are frequent and severe and may prevent the delivery of all components of multimodality therapy in many patients. The present study was designed to evaluate the rates of hepatic toxicity and biliary stent-related complications and to evaluate the impact of this morbidity on the delivery of preoperative chemoradiation for pancreatic cancer at a tertiary care cancer center. *Patients and methods:* Preoperative chemoradiation was used in 154 patients with resectable pancreatic adenocarcinoma (142 patients, 92%) or other periampullary tumors (12 patients, 8%). Patients were treated with preoperative fluorouracil (115 patients), paclitaxel (37 patients), or gemcitabine (two patients) plus concurrent rapid-fractionation (30 Gy; 123 patients) or standard-fractionation (50.4 Gy; 31 patients) radiation therapy. The incidences of hepatic toxicity and biliary stent-related complications were evaluated during chemoradiation and the immediate 3- to 4-week postchemoradiation preoperative period. *Results:* Nonoperative biliary decompression was performed in 101 (66%) of 154 patients (endobiliary stent placement in 77 patients and percutaneous transhepatic catheter placement in 24 patients). Stent-related complications (occlusion or migration) occurred in 15 patients. Inpatient hospitalization for antibiotics and stent exchange was necessary in seven of 15 patients (median hospital stay, 3 days). No patient experienced uncontrolled biliary sepsis, hepatic abscess, or stent-related death. *Conclusion:* Preoperative chemoradiation for pancreatic cancer is associated with low rates of hepatic toxicity and biliary stent-related complications. The need for biliary decompression is not a clinically significant concern in the delivery of preoperative therapy to patients with localized pancreatic cancer.

The feasibility of dose escalation using concurrent radiation and 5-fluorouracil therapy following pancreaticoduodenectomy for pancreatic carcinoma.

Regine WF, John WJ, McGrath P, Strodel WE, Mohiuddin M.

Department of Radiation Medicine, University of Kentucky, Lexington, KY, USA.

Journal of Hepatobiliary Pancreatic Surgery 7(1):53–7, 2000.

We evaluated the feasibility of dose escalation using external beam radiation therapy (RT) and 5-fluorouracil (5-FU) following pancreaticoduodenectomy for pancreatic carcinoma. Fourteen patients who underwent pancreaticoduodenectomy for stage I–III adenocarcinoma of the pancreas received postoperative high-dose chemoradiation. RT was given at 1.8-Gy daily fractions to total doses of 54 Gy for patients with negative surgical margins ($n = 12$), and 64.8 Gy for those with gross residual disease ($n = 2$). Concurrent 5-FU was given as a continuous infusion (CI) at 225 mg/m^2 per day ($n = 9$) beginning on day 1 and continuing until the completion of RT, or by bolus injection at 500 mg/m^2 per day ($n = 5$) during weeks 1 and 4 of RT. Follow-up ranged from 32 to 36 months (median, 35 months). All patients were able to complete the planned high-dose postoperative chemoradiation and none required a treatment break. No grade 4 acute toxicity was observed. Grade 3 acute toxicity was limited to 2 patients. Two patients developed grade 3 ($n = 1$) or 4 ($n = 1$) subacute toxicity, all gastrointestinal-related. There have been no fatal toxicities and no grade 3 or 4 late toxicity has been observed. The 3-year survival is 21%. Dose escalation of postoperative 5-FU chemoradiation following pancreatico-duodenectomy for pancreatic carcinoma is well tolerated. Further dose-intensification of postoperative adjuvant therapy in these patients appears feasible and is being evaluated in a recently activated national trial.

Palliative superselective intra-arterial chemotherapy for advanced nonresectable gastric cancer.

Shchepotin IB, Chorny V, Hanfelt J, Evans SR.

Department of Surgery, George Washington University, Washington, DC, USA.

Journal of Gastrointestinal Surgery 3(4):426–31, 1999, July–August.

From November 1988 to May 1996, a prospective randomized study was undertaken to assess the efficacy of superselective intra-arterial chemotherapy for surgically proved unresectable gastric carcinoma. Each patient had undergone endoscopy as well as abdominal and pelvic CT scanning for staging. Patients with evidence of liver metastasis, peritoneal carcinomatosis, enlarged retroperitoneal lymph nodes, or locally advanced disease beyond curative resection were excluded from the study. A total of 386 patients with potentially curable disease were randomized to one of three treatment groups: (1) control; (2) systemic intravenous chemotherapy; or (3) superselective intra-arterial chemotherapy. On completion of preoperative chemotherapy, all patients underwent operative exploration with curative intent. A total of 74 consecutive patients were found to be unresectable, as evidenced by the presence of liver metastasis, peritoneal carcinomatosis, enlarged retroperitoneal lymph nodes, or locally extensive disease not detected by preoperative CT scanning. The median survival time in the control group and after intravenous chemotherapy was only 91 and 96 days, respectively, as compared to 401 days in the patients receiving intra-arterial chemotherapy. The results confirmed that superselective intra-arterial chemotherapy conferred a highly significant survival advantage compared to control or systemic intravenous chemotherapy adjusted for all patient characteristics ($p < 0.0001$).

Survival advantage of combined chemoradiotherapy compared with resection as the initial treatment of patients with regional pancreatic carcinoma. An outcomes trial.

Snady H, Bruckner H, Cooperman A, Paradiso J, Kiefer L.

Department of Medicine, Mt Sinai Medical Center, New York, NY, USA.

Cancer 89(2):314–27, 2000, July 15.

Background: Resection of pancreatic carcinoma is resource-intensive with a limited impact on survival. Chemotherapy and/or radiotherapy (RT) have been shown to be effective palliation. To examine whether preoperative chemoradiotherapy as the initial treatment improves survival for patients with a regional pancreatic adenocarcinoma with a minimal chance of being resected successfully, an outcomes trial was conducted. *Methods:* Patients with radiologically regional tumors were staged by laparotomy and/or computed tomography followed by endoscopic ultrasonography, angiography, and/or laparoscopy. Those with locally invasive, unresectable, regional pancreatic adenocarcinoma initially were treated with simultaneous split-course RT plus 5-fluorouracil, streptozotocin, and cisplatin (RT-FSP) followed by selective surgery (Group 1). Patients determined to have a resectable tumor initially underwent resection without preoperative chemoradiotherapy, with or without postoperative chemoradiotherapy (Group 2). *Results:* Over 8 years 159 patients presenting with nonmetastatic pancreatic adenocarcinoma were administered RT-FSP or underwent surgery for resection. Group 1, comprised of 68 patients initially treated with RT-FSP, had a 0% mortality rate within 30 days of entry. In 20 of 30 patients undergoing surgery after RT-FSP, tumors were downstaged and resected. Group 2, comprised of 91 patients who initially underwent successful resection, had a 5% mortality rate within 30 days of entry. Postoperatively, 63 of these patients received chemotherapy with or without RT. The median survival for Group 1 was 23.6 months compared with 14.0 months for Group 2 ($p = 0.006$) despite more advanced disease cases in Group 1. Survival favored RT-FSP regardless of whether lymph nodes were malignant. The dominant prognostic factor of earlier stage pancreatic carcinoma having an expected survival advantage was reversed by the initial nonoperative treatment. *Conclusions:* Based on a reversal of the expected trend that patients with earlier stage resectable carcinoma (T1,2, N0,1, M0) who undergo removal of their tumors survive longer than patients with more advanced regional disease (T3, N0,1, M0), survival was found to improve significantly for patients reliably staged as having locally invasive, unresectable, nonmetastatic pancreatic adenocarcinoma when initially treated with RT-FSP.

Preoperative chemotherapy, radiotherapy, and surgical resection of locally advanced pancreatic cancer.

Wanebo HJ, Glicksman AS, Vezeridis MP, Clark J, Tibbetts L, Koness RJ, Levy A.

Department of Surgery, Boston University School of Medicine and Roger Williams Medical Center, Providence, RI, USA.

Archives of Surgery 135(1):81–7, 2000, January.

Hypothesis: Neoadjuvant therapy has the potential to induce regression of high-risk, locally advanced cancers and render them resectable. Preoperative chemoradiotherapy is proposed as a testable treatment concept for locally advanced pancreatic cancer. *Design:* Fourteen patients (8 men, 6 women) with locally advanced pancreatic cancer were surgically explored to exclude distant spread of disease, to perform bypass of biliary and/or gastric obstruction, and to provide a jejunostomy feeding tube for long-term nutritional support. A course of chemotherapy with fluorouracil and cisplatin plus radiotherapy was then initiated. Reexploration and resection were planned subsequent to neoadjuvant therapy. *Main outcome measures:* Tumor regression and survival. *Interventions:* Surgically staged patients with locally advanced pancreatic cancer were treated by preoperative chemotherapy with bolus fluorouracil, 400 mg/m^2, on days 1 through 3 and 28 through 30 accompanied by a 3-day infusion of cisplatin, 25 mg/m^2, on days 1 through 3 and 28 through 30 and concurrent radiotherapy, 45 Gy. Enteral nutritional support was maintained via jejunostomy tube. *Results:* Of 14 patients who enrolled in the protocol and were initially surgically explored, 3 refused the second operation and 11 were reexplored; 2 showed progressive disease and were unresectable and 9 (81%) had definitive resection. Surgical pathologic stages of the resected patients were: Ib (2 patients), II (2 patients), and III (5 patients). Pancreatic resection included standard Whipple resection in 1 patient, resection of body and neck in 1 patient, and extended resection in 6 patients (portal vein resection in 6, arterial resection in 4). One patient who was considered too frail for resection had core biopsies of the pancreatic head, node dissection, and an interstitial implant of the tumorous head. Pathologic response: 2 patients had apparent complete pathologic response; 1 patient had no residual cancer in the pancreatectomy specimen, the other patient who had an iridium 192 interstitial implant had normal core biopsies of the pancreatic head. Five patients had minimal residual cancer in the resected pancreas or microscopic foci only with extensive fibrosis, and 2 patients had fully viable residual cancer. Lymph node downstaging occurred in 2 of 4 patients who had positive peripancreatic nodes at the initial surgical staging. There was 1 postoperative death at 10 days. Sepsis, prolonged ileus, and failure to thrive were major complications. In the definitive surgery group the median survival was 19 months after beginning chemoradiotherapy and 16 months after definitive surgery. The absolute 5-year survival was 11% of 9 patients, 1 is surviving 96 months (with no evidence of disease) after chemoradiotherapy and extended pancreatic resection including resection of the superior mesenteric artery and the portal vein for stage III cancer. In the nonresected group the mean survival was 9 months (survival range, 7–12 months) after initiation of chemoradiotherapy. *Conclusion:* A pilot study of preoperative chemoradiotherapy with infusional cisplatin and radiation induced a high rate of clinical pathologic response in patients with locally advanced pancreatic cancer and merits further study in these high-risk patients.

24

Sphincter-preserving surgery in the management of rectal cancer

MARVIN L CORMAN AND JOSEPHINE TSAI

FACTORS INFLUENCING THE CHOICE OF OPERATION

To save or not to save the sphincter is a perennial question. Is there a level below which an anastomosis should not be attempted? When is an abdominoperineal resection inappropriate or an anterior resection the operation of choice? Unfortunately, there are no consistent answers to these questions. Some would advise with the simple adage: if you can feel the lesion, you should not perform a sphincter-saving operation – the rule of the index finger. But this is much too simplistic an approach and may prejudice the surgeon to embark upon the inappropriate operation.

Conversely, too often, surgeons, in a zealous effort to avoid a colostomy and to re-establish intestinal continuity, compromise on the margins of resection. The consequences are often tragic: recurrent disease, anastomotic obstruction, unremitting pelvic pain, and the requirement for subsequent surgery, including a colostomy. Obviously, an abdominoperineal resection is no panacea, but it is an operation that can be accomplished with relative safety and is at least as effective as any other modality of treatment for curing carcinoma of the rectum.

The alternatives to abdominoperineal resection are numerous and are discussed individually. However, if another resective procedure is contemplated, it should rarely be other than an anterior resection. If one embarks upon what may be called an esoteric sphincter-saving operation (e.g., abdomino-anal pull-through, abdominosacral resection, electrocoagulation, transanal excision, transcoccygeal excision), one must be able to justify it as the optimal treatment of the patient under the circumstances.

In recent years, many surgeons have utilized a more scientific approach to determining the proper surgical alternative. Factors that are helpful in determining the choice of operation for cancer in the rectum are summarized here:

- level
- macroscopic appearance (ulcerated, polypoid)
- extent of circumferential involvement
- fixity
- degree of differentiation (histologic appearance)
- tumor cell DNA content
- endorectal ultrasound determination
- magnetic resonance imaging (MRI) assessment
- body habitus
- gender
- age
- metastatic disease
- other systemic disease
- other conditions that might contraindicate colostomy (e.g., blindness, severe arthritis, mental incapacity).

The American Society of Colon and Rectal Surgeons has established practice parameters for the preoperative evaluation and treatment of rectal cancer.[1]

Level of the lesion

The distance of the lower edge of the tumor from the anal verge is probably the single most important variable that aids the surgeon in the choice of operation. This distance should be carefully measured using the rigid proctosigmoidoscope, and the result recorded. The flexible sigmoidoscope is not as accurate for this determination. When measuring, care must be taken to spread the buttocks so that the instrument can be seen emerging from the anus, not from the buttock fat.

The preconceived notion that a tumor that is 7 cm from the anal verge requires abdominoperineal resection but the one at 8 cm can be treated by anterior resection is erroneous. Other factors may prove the opposite to be true in both cases (e.g., fixity, size, degree of differentiation, pelvic anatomy, etc.). Generally, if the lower edge of the tumor does not impinge upon the puborectalis muscle and is at least 2 cm above the anorectal ring, a sphincter-preserving procedure is possible.

Macroscopic appearance

Generally, the distal margin of resection should be approximately 4 cm below the tumor, but for infiltrative carcinomas one may not be safe from the risk of anastomotic recurrence with a margin of <7 cm. The length of distal intramural spread of tumor in resected specimens is extremely variable. Three-quarters of the rectal tumors in one study were demonstrated to have no intramural spread.[2] A small, exophytic, well-differentiated lesion may be adequately removed with a 1-cm cuff of normal distal bowel. Ascertaining the appearance of the lesion, whether ulcerated, scirrhous (infiltrative), or polypoid, is very helpful in aiding the surgeon in the choice of operation.

Extent of circumferential involvement

Usually, more highly aggressive tumors tend to involve a greater circumference of the bowel wall when they present. Under these circumstances, a greater margin of resection is required. An anterior resection may be a poor choice, even though resection and anastomosis can be technically effected.

Fixity

Fixity of the tumor in the pelvis implies a poor prognosis. There is a greater likelihood of residual tumor following resection, and anastomotic recurrence is a frequent sequela. An abdominoperineal resection, although no guarantee of obviating the problem of recurrent disease, would probably offer better palliation, because the need for subsequent reoperation would be less likely. The presence of a fixed tumor might also encourage the surgeon to consider preoperative radiotherapy.

Histologic appearance

A biopsy is, of course, mandatory and is done routinely, usually at the time of initial discovery of the lesion. Ideally, the material obtained should be from the edge of the lesion, because much useful information can be obtained. For example, an expanding margin implies that the area of invasion is pushing or reasonably well circumscribed, whereas an infiltrating margin suggests diffuse or widespread penetration of normal tissue. It is important to be aware of the specific histologic appearance

of a malignant tumor. Is it poorly differentiated, moderately well differentiated, or well differentiated? Generally, tumors regarded as poorly differentiated have highly irregular glands or no glandular differentiation.[3] The more anaplastic, the more aggressive is the lesion; and the more aggressive, the greater is the resection margin that would be required. The chance of local recurrence is much higher with a poorly differentiated cancer than with one that is well differentiated. It is axiomatic that one must choose the most favorable cancers for performing less than a radical resection (see later). Therefore, one cannot overestimate the importance of degree of differentiation (Broder's classification), depth of penetration, and the presence or absence of venous or perineural invasion (PNI) in making the appropriate choice. Shirouzu and colleagues evaluated whether PNI is an independent prognostic factor in individuals who underwent curative surgery.[4] There was a significant difference in local recurrence rates between those individuals with stage III lesions who were found to have PNI and those without PNI. Also, the investigators found that patients with PNI and stage III lesions had a significantly lower survival rate.

Saclarides and colleagues attempted to determine which features were predictors of nodal metastases.[5] They utilized nine histologic and morphologic features of 62 radically excised rectal cancers to determine which were associated with nodal disease. Statistically significant variables were worsening differentiation, increasing depth of penetration, microtubular configuration of >20%, the presence of venous invasion or PNI, and, of course, lymphatic invasion. Exophytic tumor morphology, mitotic count, and tumor size were not significant predictors.[5] In an analysis of all the variables or combination of factors, Broder's classification was the strongest predictor of nodal disease.

Tumor cell DNA content

As with other solid cancers, malignant tumors of the bowel may demonstrate abnormalities in their chromosomal composition.[6] Reports of DNA measurements in human cancers suggest that flow cytometry assays of DNA ploidy have prognostic value.[6–10] Even with small rectal cancers, it appears that DNA content seems to provide useful prognostic information.[11] Thus, this may affect the choice of operation. A DNA histogram of normal colonic epithelium reveals that >90% of the cells have a single diploid peak. Carcinomas that are near-diploid have a better prognosis than those that are aneuploid. Aggressive tumor behavior appears to correlate especially closely with aneuploidy in locally treated rectal cancers.[7] Although, as of this writing, the available data have not been subjected to long-term follow-up evaluation, analysis of DNA distribution may ultimately prove to be more accurate a predictor of extent of involvement and, therefore, prognosis, than is degree of differentiation.

Computed tomography

Since its introduction, computed tomography (CT) had been thought to be a reasonably effective means for determining the depth of invasion of rectal cancer preoperatively.[12–16] Unfortunately, this has not proved to be the case. One thing is certain, however; CT is of great value in identifying metastatic disease, especially in the liver and elsewhere within the abdomen.

Magnetic resonance imaging

Magnetic resonance imaging (MRI) has also been used for preoperative assessment, but it has not been of particular advantage when compared with CT.[17,18] McNicholas and colleagues evaluated MRI in 20 consecutive patients with rectal cancer who were to undergo curative surgery.[19] MRI staging concurred with histologic staging in 18 of 20 patients if Dukes' classification was used, but in only 14 if the Astler–Coller model was employed. The technique was effective in all but one patient with microscopic muscle wall invasion. The overall accuracy was 95%. Thaler and colleagues compared the utility of endoluminal ultrasound (see below) with MRI in the preoperative staging of rectal cancer.[20] There was no statistically significant difference between the two methods in identifying T-staging. Nodal staging was correct in 80% by ultrasound but only in 60% by MRI. A comprehensive preoperative staging, i.e., nodal and tumor extent, was correctly made in 68% utilizing endoluminal ultrasound, but in only 48% utilizing MRI. However, these differences were not statistically significant.

Magnetic resonance imaging with endorectal coil

A recent improvement in MRI technique is the use of surface MRI coils to allow a higher definition of image to be obtained with a smaller field of view.[21] In this way, a more local, accurate staging might be possible. Like endoluminal ultrasound, the technology is now available for the office evaluation of patients (Medrad, Inc., Pittsburgh, PA). Initial reports indicated that this modality was promising for local staging of rectal cancer,[22] but later observations suggest that the use of a pelvic phased-array coil does not improve the staging accuracy of MRI to a clinically useful level.[21]

Endorectal or transrectal ultrasound examination

Endorectal ultrasound (Brüel & Kjaer Instruments, Inc., North Billerica, MA) has developed into an extremely useful tool for the preoperative assessment of patients with rectal cancer.[23–31] After a small enema is administered, the probe is introduced into the rectum beyond the tumor. A balloon is filled with approximately 50 mL of water, and an acoustic contact is produced between the rotating part of the transducer and the rectal wall.[32] During withdrawal, the monitor is observed and the findings recorded. Each of the layers of the rectum can be sonographically visualized, with a tumor usually appearing as a hypoechoic disruption of the rectal wall. The procedure may also reveal if underlying lymph nodes are affected. Most studies indicate a sensitivity and a specificity for bowel wall involvement of >90%.[33–35] An additional benefit has been recognized in that detection of invasive carcinoma within an otherwise villous lesion can be achieved with this technique.[36,37] In the experience of Hildebrandt and colleagues, lymph node metastases can be predicted with an accuracy of 72% and inflammatory lymph nodes with a specificity of 83%.[38] Most investigators, however, have expressed concern about the lack of specificity in distinguishing benign from malignant nodes.[39,40] Accurate preoperative staging with endorectal ultrasound implies the patients may be selected for a less than radical operation[41] (Figure 24.1). However, a number of investigators have commented that tumors of the lower rectum are incorrectly staged much more frequently than those of the middle and upper rectum.[42]

There is uniformity of agreement that optimal results can only be obtained if there is consistency in technique and in interpretation. Certainly, accuracy improves considerably with increased experience.[43] It is, therefore, preferable for the surgeon to be the individual responsible for performing and evaluating the study. As one gains experience with this instrument, patients with limited rectal wall involvement may be offered a less than radical surgical alternative to the treatment of their condition. In addition, the technique offers the opportunity for clear visualization of the full thickness of an anastomotic area in those patients who have undergone restoration of rectal continuity, especially with respect to the possibility of early detection of recurrent cancer, and for the effect of preoperative radiotherapy.[44–48] Further information can be obtained by means of ultrasonographically guided biopsies.[49]

A number of studies have been published comparing transrectal ultrasound (TRUS) examination, MRI, and CT. Roubein and colleagues showed that CT agreed with histopathology in 33% of cases, whereas TRUS agreed in 78%.[40] Some opine that TRUS is not sufficiently reliable for the evaluation of neoplasms because of interobserver differences.[50] However, this is a minority viewpoint. Goldman and colleagues found that TRUS had an accuracy of 81%, a sensitivity of 90%, and a specificity of 67%, whereas the corresponding figures for CT were 52%, 67%, and 27%.[51] Milsom and colleagues found that endoluminal ultrasound accurately predicted wall and

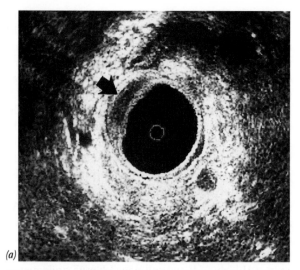

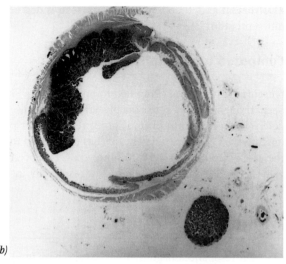

(a)   (b)

Figure 24.1 *Endorectal ultrasound. (a) Sonogram of a rectal cancer confined to wall of the bowel. The black cavity is the water-filled balloon, with the white circle in the center corresponding to the transducer. A hyperechoic lymph node can be seen at the lower right. (b) Corresponding photomicrograph of the excised specimen confirms the depth of invasion by tumor. The lymph node at the lower right was free of tumor.*

lymph node status with 95% confidence intervals of 0.88 to 0.99 and 0.87 to 0.99, respectively, in 81 patients.[52] Others confirm the increased reliability of TRUS when compared with CT and MRI in the preoperative assessment,[17,53,54] but when recurrent disease is being sought, MRI and CT are at least as accurate as TRUS, if not more so.[55,56] It has also been shown that preoperative radiation therapy makes TRUS and CT less effective for staging, but the absence of lymph nodes before and after radiation can be considered reliable.[57–60]

A new modality has been recently introduced, that of three-dimensional endoluminal ultrasound.[61,62] Although it has many of the limitations associated with conventional TRUS, it seems to provide significantly greater information for spatial relationships. This is particularly useful if one is to consider biopsy of extrarectal lymph nodes, for example.[63] Whether this modality will ultimately result in improved staging of rectal cancer awaits further investigations.

Other factors

The preceding factors concern the tumor, itself. The following variables that may influence the choice of operation are related to the patient.

Body habitus

A rectal resection carried out on an asthenic patient usually permits a technically lower anastomosis than does an operation for the same level of lesion in an obese individual. In preoperative evaluation and counseling, therefore, the factor of body habitus may lead the surgeon to present an optimistic or pessimistic view of the likelihood of re-establishing intestinal continuity.

Gender

As anastomotic procedure is more likely to be possible in women than in men. A broad pelvis, furthermore, usually permits a wider resection, whereas a narrow pelvis tends to impede dissection, potentially limiting the adequacy of tumor margins and the use of conventional anastomotic techniques. This is especially true when one performs a low anterior resection.

Age

A resection involving an anastomosis is a higher-risk procedure than an abdominoperineal resection; morbidity is greater, and operative mortality is higher. Furthermore, the possible need for a second operation (e.g., closure of a colostomy) increases the risk still further. Although resection is not absolutely contraindicated in elderly patients, these individuals may be less suitable for staged operations.

Other conditions

Avoiding a colostomy in a patient who cannot cope with an appliance or a stoma is an unusual, albeit legitimate, reason for choosing an alternative procedure. The quality of life may be poor, indeed, if a patient must be relegated to a nursing home or terminal-care facility because he or she cannot manage a stoma at home. This can happen if the individual is blind, has severe impairment in the use of hands (e.g., arthritis), or cannot be taught. Obviously, alternatives exist to support the patient, such as care by a family member, a visiting nurse, or a home helper. Of course, there may be no choice except to create a stoma to cure the disease or to effectively palliate the condition.

Comment

In the choice of operation, the surgeon must consider all of the above factors and make a recommendation based upon what is the appropriate procedure for each individual. A tumor may require treatment for one patient that is quite different from that required for the same lesion in the same location in another.

Each operation for carcinoma of the rectum, excluding abdominoperineal resection, is discussed in the following pages on its own merits.

LOW ANTERIOR RESECTION

The first resection of the sigmoid colon was performed in 1833 by Reybard of Lyons,[64] but for the next 100 years practically all operative approaches to the treatment of carcinoma either involved extirpation of the rectum or another sphincter-saving procedure, such as the various modifications of the pull-through operation. It was not until the 1940s, and even the 1950s in some centers, that conventional anastomotic techniques were felt safe enough to be employed for most cases of carcinoma of the rectum when intestinal continuity might be re-established. Generally, it was the work of Dixon and of Wangensteen that contributed much to the ultimate success of this operation.[65–67]

Indications

The most important factor that determines the likelihood of performing an anastomosis is the level of the lesion. Although favorable factors such as good differentiation, diploid histogram, limited bowel wall penetration with endorectal ultrasound, small size, and polypoid configuration may safely reduce the distal margin of resection to 1 cm or 2 cm, in my opinion it is the rare patient who should be considered for a low anterior resection when the tumor is < 7 cm from the anal verge. When compared with other resective sphincter-saving operations, the low anterior resection is the one that is preferred. To embark upon an esoteric approach, one must believe rather strongly that an abdominoperineal resection is inappropriate and a low anterior resection with conventional sutured or stapled anastomosis is technically impossible to accomplish.

Technique

There is often confusion about what constitutes a low anterior resection. This operation requires complete mobilization of the rectum from the hollow of the sacrum and division of the lateral ligaments with the middle hemorrhoidal arteries. Anastomosis is effected in the extraperitoneal rectum, that is, distal to the visceral peritoneum. Unless these criteria are met, the procedure is not, by definition, a low anterior resection.

The patient may be positioned in the perineolithotomy (Lloyd–Davies) position or supine on the operating table. When the surgeon feels confident that an anterior abdominal approach will permit anastomosis by a conventional suture method, the supine position is preferred. However, if there is some doubt whether an anastomosis can be effected readily from above or if a transanal stapling technique is contemplated, the perineolithotomy position should be adopted. One of the concerns of placing the patient in the perineolithotomy position is its association with the development of a compartment syndrome. This occurs when an elevated pressure in an osteo-fascial compartment compromises local perfusion.[68] This can result in neurovascular damage and permanent disability. A number of authors emphasize the importance of prevention and early diagnosis.[68–70] The use of intermittent sequential compression of the lower limbs is strongly encouraged to prevent venous stasis.[70]

By using the perineolithotomy position, alternative anastomotic techniques can be employed, if necessary, or an abdominoperineal resection can be synchronously performed should an anastomotic procedure be considered unwise or technically impossible to accomplish. I do not believe that irrigating the rectum prior to resection is important; this is not, in itself, an indication for using this position in my opinion. However, I recognize that well-respected authorities believe that irrigation limits the likelihood of suture-line recurrence.

An exploratory laparotomy is performed and a determination made of the possibility and advisability of performing a resection; this is based on the presence or absence of metastatic disease and the fixity of the tumor in the pelvis. It may not be possible, however, to determine resectability until the rectum has been fully mobilized.

On occasion, the surgeon may elect to perform a resection on a patient who has previously undergone a polypectomy and in whom an invasive carcinoma was found. At laparotomy, it is sometimes impossible to identify the site of the lesion; this may then necessitate a blind resection. To avoid this potential dilemma, the area that has been excised can be infiltrated with India ink a day or more prior to the operation. This produces a black pigment in the lymphatics and permits ready identification of the tumor area from within the pelvis.

Arthur H. Keeney has said, 'Pray before surgery, but remember that God will not alter a faulty incision.' The location of the incision is extremely important, not only for the obvious reason of access to the abdomen, but also to avoid interference with the subsequent placement of the stoma. A midline hypogastric incision is advised, extending through the umbilicus if necessary. After the insertion of a self-retaining (Balfour, Bookwalter, etc.) retractor, the abdomen is explored for evidence of metastatic disease, the presence of synchronous colon lesions, or other pathology. The small intestine is packed into the upper abdomen using three moist pads. Rarely should it be necessary to exteriorize the bowel. By keeping the viscera warm and moist and within the abdomen, there is less likelihood of postoperative ileus, and a nasogastric tube may be avoided. This can be more easily accomplished if the incision can be kept below the umbilicus.

Mobilization of the sigmoid colon and rectum commences along the left colic gutter, lysing the developmental adhesions. Mobilization of the splenic flexure is not routinely performed. The peritoneum on the left lateral aspect is incised, and the left ureter is identified and retracted laterally. Injury to the ureter most commonly occurs during this phase of the procedure, at the level of the iliac artery; it should always be visualized and protected. Incision of the peritoneum is continued anteriorly to the base of the bladder.

The left hand is then passed beneath the inferior mesenteric vessels, and a peritoneal incision is performed in a similar fashion on the right side. The mesenteric vascular pedicle is ligated between clamps; one should always check to be certain that the left ureter has not been incorporated. It is less important to visualize the right ureter because it should not be involved in this aspect of the dissection. Exceptions to this dictum include a congenital anomaly or a history of prior surgery that might have caused medial deviation of this structure. Injury to the right ureter is usually caused at the time of pelvic floor reconstruction by mobilization and suture of the peritoneum on that side.

Ligation of the inferior mesenteric artery at its origin is unnecessary because, in my experience and that of others, nodal involvement at that level is found only in patients with incurable cancer, and survival rates are not improved.[71] In a study of >4000 patients who underwent surgery for rectal carcinoma at St Mark's Hospital, Harrow, England, no improved survival was seen when the inferior mesenteric artery was ligated above the origin of the left colic artery.[72] Ligation distal to the first branch of the inferior mesenteric artery ensures a viable blood supply to the bowel. Pelvic peritoneal incisions are then joined across the base of the bladder (or at the vaginal apex in women).

I am also not an advocate of so-called en-bloc pelvic lymphadenectomy, although I recognize that some institutions, through their retrospective studies, believe that survival rates are increased.[73] Others have demonstrated that patients with Dukes' A tumors do not benefit from lateral lymph node dissection and that local recurrence rates in those with Dukes' B and C lesions are not significantly decreased.[74]

Attention is then turned to the retrorectal space. Often, surgeons commence blunt dissection at the level of the sacral promontory, but when doing so the plane may be improperly entered, and the presacral vessels can

be torn. This can result in rather profuse bleeding. Hemorrhage, in fact, is often due to bleeding from basivertebral veins through the sacral foramina and not from injury to the presacral venous plexus.[75] When such vessels are encountered, an attempt at ligation may be unsuccessful, especially if the bleeding emanates directly from bone. Rather than attempt to electrocoagulate and accept additional blood loss, direct pressure with a large pad for a few minutes is suggested. Failure to achieve hemostasis may necessitate the use of packing,[76,77] or even the application of a hemorrhage occluder pin (thumbtack) placed into the sacrum.[78] I believe that the risk of bleeding can be minimized if the dissection is performed, as much as possible, under direct visualization and by sharp dissection. Gentle anterior traction is placed on the rectosigmoid and the scissors inserted anterior to the sacral promontory. The presacral space is relatively avascular and usually readily entered. The loose areolar tissue is identified and incised. The presacral nerves can usually be seen quite clearly and can, therefore, be displaced out of harm's way.

Once the presacral space has been opened as far as convenient by retraction and under direct visualization, the right hand can be inserted and the dissection carried out bluntly. It is often helpful to drape a gauze sponge over the fingers to facilitate this maneuver. But it is still preferable to perform as much of the dissection under direct visualization, cutting with the scissors as distally as possible. The rectum is freed to the tip of the coccyx in a plane anterior to the sacral fascia, avoiding injury to the presacral veins.

Attention is then turned to the anterior part of the dissection. The posterior wall of the bladder and seminal vesicles (or uterus and posterior vaginal wall in women) are ideally demonstrated visually. This is accomplished by using a 7-inch St Mark's pattern retractor with turned-back lip (Thackray, Inc., Woburn, MA) and by a combination of sharp and blunt dissection. Denonvilliers' fascia must be incised in order to separate the rectum completely from the prostate and the seminal vesicles. By means of retraction of the bladder and prostatic area and countertraction on the rectum, the dissection is carried distally until the inferior margin of the prostate and the urethra with its contained catheter can be palpated. In women, the posterior vaginal wall is swept anteriorly to the point where it is to be incised or removed. Dissection is facilitated by placing the left hand as distally as possible and compressing the anterior rectal wall.

Attention is then turned to the lateral ligaments and to the middle hemorrhoidal vessels. The space distal to the lateral ligaments is entered using long scissors, and the scissors are spread in the anterior–posterior plane. The index finger of the left hand is then passed beneath the ligament and the adjacent vessels on the right side. There is often a firm fascial band that must be traversed bluntly. The ligament is then straddled with the index and long fingers of the left hand and retracted medially. A single crushing clamp is used, and the lateral ligament and the middle hemorrhoidal vessel transected medial to the clamp. Back-bleeding from the artery rarely occurs, but can easily and safely be controlled by rotating the rectum and directly visualizing the bleeding point. When the lateral ligament has been divided, the rectum on that side is readily mobilized.

The left lateral ligament is divided in a similar way, but the maneuver is slightly more difficult to perform. The left index and long fingers again straddle the structures, but the rectum is pushed toward the right side, and the clamp is applied adjacent to the dorsum of the hand. Upon completion of this step, the rectum is completely isolated anteriorly, laterally, and posteriorly. A few fibrous strands may require division, but no important vascular structures need to be controlled in order to complete the pelvic dissection.

Having been satisfied that an anastomosis can be performed, the surgeon's next task is to divide the mesorectum. Right-angle clamps are placed posteriorly and the mesentery divided above the clamps. Tension on the proximal bowel permits separation of the mesentery from the posterior rectal wall. With a very low anastomosis, there is usually little or no mesentery to divide.

Total mesorectal excision

Although tumor at the margin of resection and a second primary lesion are potential sources of recurrent disease, these are in all probability quite uncommon causes of recurrence. It is generally believed that the overwhelming majority of suture-line recurrences are due to residual tumor left in the pelvis (the so-called tangential or lateral margin) that subsequently grows into the lumen through the anastomosis.

A number of reports have emphasized the importance of mesorectal spread of the tumor in determining risk of recurrence and survival.[79–81] From Heald's group in Basingstoke, England, emphasis has been placed on removing the tongue of mesorectum, total mesorectal excision (TME), to reduce the incidence of recurrence.[81,82] They report no local recurrences with a resection margin of > 1 cm and only a 3.6% incidence of recurrence if the margin is less. In theory, failure to excise the mesorectum completely has the potential to leave gross or microscopic residual disease; this may predispose to local failure.[83] In Norway and Sweden, rectal cancer surgery has essentially been removed from general surgical training programs, and surgery is now essentially exclusively performed by TME surgeons.[84] Heald and colleagues go so far as to state that TME appears to be an oncologically superior operation to abdominoperineal excision.[85] The primary basis for this statement is that, in their opinion and experience, three-quarters of patients with cancer of the lower one-third of the rectum can be offered sphincter-sparing surgery. Heald further suggests that optimal TME surgery

can be widely implemented with the expectation that outcome improvement could be four times as great as that achievable by adjuvant therapy.[84,86]

One of the concerns that has been expressed concerns the increased morbidity associated with removing the mesentery to the rectum distal to the anastomosis. Devascularization may be a consequence, with an increased incidence of anastomotic leak. Hainsworth and colleagues suggest that the operation is not appropriate for the treatment of tumors in the upper third of the rectum for that reason.[87] Arbman and colleagues compared the results of resection by means of TME with those from an earlier period of cases performed without that operation.[88] Actuarial analysis demonstrated a significant reduction in local recurrence rate as well as an increase in survival with the latter technique. The problem with the study, however, is that the second group of patients underwent surgery by a limited number of surgeons familiar with TME. Others express enthusiasm for the technique, commenting also that the procedure is compatible with autonomic nerve preservation as well as sphincter preservation.[89,90]

The problem with accepting without question these remarkable results is that, when an abdominoperineal resection is performed (removing all of the mesorectum), the risk of recurrence in the pelvis is significantly higher than that which is reported by Heald and colleagues as well as other investigators. For me, this is a conundrum which defies explanation. The fact is, local recurrence has been demonstrated to be closely related to tumor at the lateral rectal margins.[91–93] In the experience of Ng and colleagues, 53% of patients with lateral resection margin involvement developed recurrent tumor.[92] In the experience of Adam and associates, tumor involvement of the circumferential margin was seen in 25% of 144 specimens for which the surgeon thought the resection was potentially curative.[91] Seventy-eight percent developed local recurrence under these circumstances. As with abdominoperineal resection, TME adds nothing to the conventional operation when a surgeon is confronted with lateral tumor spread.

Opinion

It is difficult for me to understand what the excitement is about when reading reports of the use of TME. The operation, as described by Heald, is essentially the same as the procedure that most surgeons experienced in removing the rectum for cancer have employed for many years. The only difference, perhaps, is the removal of the tongue of mesorectum distal to the site of a low rectal tumor. At least, that is what I read in the literature. For me, however, there is no such tongue when a low rectal cancer is resected. The mesorectum does not exist at this level. Furthermore, I do not understand why this operation is such a success in individuals with circumferential tumor involvement or where the tumor spreads laterally. The only conclusion that I can reach is that surgeons who have reported such a remarkably successful experience with the application of this technique are doing something which I truly do not understand or are selecting their patients on the basis of those most amenable to this modification. Finally, as expressed by others, I am most concerned about devascularizing the rectum for any extensive distance below my anastomosis.

Lymphadenectomy

A number of surgeons continue to recommend systemic lymphadenectomy with lateral node dissection in order to minimize the likelihood of recurrence. Moriya and colleagues reported a 5-year survival rate of 69% in their patients who did not undergo extended resection, as compared with a rate of 76% for those who did.[94] With respect to inguinal node metastases from rectal adenocarcinoma, an unusual manifestation indeed, Graham and Hohn found no 5-year survivors irrespective of the method of management.[95] They still recommend therapeutic node dissection for purposes of local control and possible cure.

Conventional suturing

A crushing clamp is applied, usually 5 cm below the distal margin of the tumor; an angled or curved clamp placed in the anteroposterior plane is preferred. Only one is used.

Anchoring sutures are placed, and the bowel is divided distal to the clamp. Long Allis clamps may be used to identify the cut edge of the rectum. With the proximal bowel divided and the specimen removed, an open end-to-end anastomosis is performed. Interrupted No. 3-0 or No. 4-0 long-term, absorbable sutures are recommended, but the type of suture material is of less importance than is the meticulous approach to the technique employed. Simple, interrupted sutures are placed as a single layer, taking deeper bites in the muscularis and minimal mucosa (the rectum has no serosa at this level). With a low anastomosis it is easier to place all of the sutures into the posterior row initially, before tying. It is usually more convenient to place the initial suture through the sigmoid on the ventral aspect of the mesenteric side and then through the right anterolateral part of the rectum. The knots are then secured and the anterior row completed. The last suture is usually a horizontal mattress suture in order to invert the mucosa. A single layer is considered adequate, although the surgeon may prefer to pull the anterior peritoneum over the anastomosis with Lembert sutures. A continuous suture technique, such as has been described, is also perfectly satisfactory. Deen advises the use of a Foley catheter to prevent bowel contamination and to facilitate placement of the sutures.[96] The floor of the pelvis is not reconstituted, but is vigorously irrigated with saline.

A useful step in the procedure is to place or secure omentum around the anastomosis.[97–100] This can be accomplished by freeing it from the transverse colon, with care to avoid injury to the blood supply. The appropriately tailored omentum is then brought down the lateral gutter into the pelvis, and an anchoring suture is placed below and posterior to the anastomosis to secure it.

Use of drains

The routine use of drains for pelvic anastomoses is not advised. In a number of studies, the presence of a drain did not influence the postoperative morbidity or mortality. Furthermore, if the anastomosis leaked, the presence of a drain did not prevent the need for reoperation, nor does pus or feces emerge from the drain in those individuals in whom a leak occurs.[101–103]

Stapled anastomosis

In 1978, the United States Surgical Corporation introduced a circular stapling device (similar to the Russian stapler, PKS) which was uniquely advantageous for effecting low colorectal anastomoses. The end-to-end anastomosis (EEA [reusable] and CEEA [disposable]) staplers and the intraluminal stapler create an inverted, circular anastomosis with two staggered rows of staples, and remove tissue doughnuts (rings) of bowel from each end to create an adequate lumen. Cartridges are available in several diameters: 25, 28, and 31 mm with the CEEA, and 21, 25, 29, and 33 mm with the ILS.

Double-stapling technique

The rectal stump is closed by means of a linear stapler and an end-to-end anastomosis is performed using the so-called double-stapling technique.[104–107] It offers a relatively safe method of performing a low colorectal anastomosis, which might not otherwise be technically possible.

In this approach, the distal rectum is closed with a linear stapling instrument. Eisenstat and colleagues suggest, however, that linear closure may be effected more easily by means of the GIA90 in certain individuals whose body habitus precludes the application of the technique.[108] Ganchrow and Facelle suggest application of the Roticulator so that further excision of the distal rectal stump can be achieved if the surgeon feels that the margin is inadequate.[109] As implied from the above, I find it sufficiently difficult to apply one Roticulator. My preference is to use the 30-mm instrument for low-rectal double-stapled anastomoses. At this level, the rectal diameter is usually relatively narrow, and there is minimal or no mesorectum to deal with. This permits the lowest application that I can achieve with the stapling device.

After dilatation of the anus has been performed, the well-lubricated circular stapling device is inserted into the rectum with the trocar tip. Alternatively, the center rod can be advanced with the EEA or ILS instrument and an incision made directly over the rod. The center rod is passed through the closed rectum adjacent to or through the staple line, so that, when the anastomosis is complete, the linear row of staples will be partially excised. Theoretically, if there is intact bowel wall between the circular and linear rows of staples, the tissue might become ischemic, and necrosis could result. This is of less concern, however, if the operation is performed at a later date, such as when a Hartmann pouch is reconnected to the colon. The stab wound in the rectum may be reinforced with a suture around the center rod if the surgeon is concerned about the possibility of an incomplete 'doughnut.' This may not be technically possible to accomplish, however. A singular advantage of the detachable anvil and shaft is the ability of the surgeon to facilitate securing of the proximal purse string. A simple alternative for placing this purse string is to ligate the bowel around the center rod. Debridement of the mesentery can then be undertaken expeditiously. The extension is then reattached to the instrument shaft, and the knob is turned in a clockwise fashion until the marking site appears on the handle, indicating adequate approximation of the two ends closed. The stapler is closed and fired. The anastomosis is secure because of the fact that tissue and staple lines are held firmly in place prior to the staple-cutting stage.[110] The intersecting staple is usually transferred to the removed doughnut; the knife will bend the intersecting staple rather than cut it.[110]

The anastamosis may be inspected by placing saline solution in the pelvis and looking for bubbles when air is insufflated into the rectum and with the proximal bowel occluded with fingers or a non-crushing clamp (Figure 24.2).

Comment

There is little doubt that the various stapling techniques can permit a secure anastomosis. The savings in time, albeit minimal, as well as the reduced risk of injury from needles in this AIDS-conscious environment will inevitably lead to almost complete replacement of conventional suturing for the great majority of surgeons. Fazio has outlined the important principles for minimizing complications related to the use of staplers.[111] It is worth restating them here:

- Use the largest caliber instrument that the anastomosis will accommodate.
- Place the purse strings so that excessive bulk of tissue does not appear around the shaft.
- Ensure that the purse string can be snugged up close to the shaft.
- Reinforce the purse string if concerned about the possibility of a gap.
- Use the detachable anvil-shaft, especially if faced with a 'formidable' pelvis.
- Repair any identified defect.
- Failure to effect a satisfactory repair mandates a diverting colostomy.[111]

Concomitant colostomy

The decision about whether to perform a protective colostomy at the time of low anterior resection is often not a matter of objective analysis but one of emotion. Karanjia and colleagues believe that diversion of the fecal stream should be routinely applied for any individual who undergoes an anastomosis <6 cm from the anal verge.[112] Others suggest that selective defunctioning of low colorectal anastomoses can produce low rates of anastomotic breakdown while limiting the morbidity associated with a temporary stoma.[113]

Probably the most common reason for subsequent anastomotic complications is tension on the suture line.

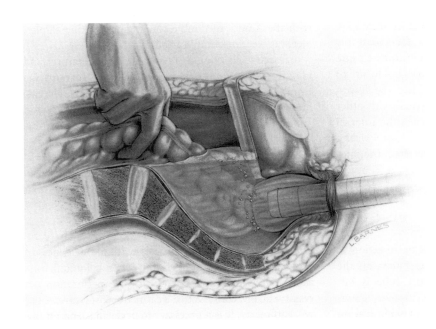

Figure 24.2 *Method of testing for the integrity of low rectal anastomosis. Inspection can be achieved by means of the rigid sigmoidoscope. By the insufflation of air with saline in the pelvis, bubbles may be seen. The leak site can then be identified and possibly repaired.*

This may compromise healing, not only because of distraction of the anastomosis itself, but also because of vascular insufficiency. Although mobilizing the splenic flexure is rarely necessary in the performance of a low anterior resection, every effort must be made to free the proximal bowel so that there is no tension. Placing the omentum around the anastomosis also helps to minimize the risk of leak.

If the above precautions are taken, a transverse colostomy is usually unnecessary. Pelvic sepsis, blood loss, other systemic disease, and poor nutritional status, however, are relative indications for protecting the anastomosis. However, if the patient is felt to have a limited survival, an abdominoperineal resection or a Hartmann resection is preferred. By creating a sigmoid colostomy rather than the more difficult-to-manage transverse colostomy, better palliation can be achieved in this situation.

The routine use of proximal colostomy with low anterior resection has been shown through reports to reduce mortality but not the morbidity of anastomotic septic and fistula complications.[114,115]

There has been some evidence to suggest that fecal diversion is accompanied by depression of collagen turnover in the wall of the excluded colon.[116] It is, therefore, possible that the presence of a colostomy proximal to an anastomosis may actually contribute to or cause breakdown. However, in controlled animal studies with and without a proximal colostomy, Senagore and colleagues demonstrated no significant difference in anastomotic blood flow, inflammatory scores, incidence of leak or stenosis, or bursting pressure.[117] They concluded that neither the presence of a proximal colostomy nor the choice of technique contributed any adverse effects to anastomotic healing. There is no question, however, that prolonged defunctioning of the rectum does result in mucosal hypoplasia and a transient, reversible, diversion colitis.[118]

Overall morbidity rates in our experience were 21% for colostomy construction and 49% for colostomy closure.[119] Although the morbidity of colostomy closure is decreasing, it is still an important concern. Closure of the colostomy without resection produces the lowest incidence of complications when compared with other types of closure. If a colostomy is created, the interval between creation and closure should be at least 6 weeks. The longer the subsequent closure is deferred, the safer the procedure will be.

Postoperative care

Postoperative care following low anterior resection is essentially the same as that for any operation on the colon. Prophylactic use of a nasogastric tube is not advised. An indwelling urinary catheter, however, is suggested for about 6 or 7 days. The amount of manipulation necessary to excise the rectum and effect a low anastomosis is equivalent to that required for an abdominoperineal resection. A progressive diet is instituted after the patient has passed flatus, or sooner, at the surgeon's personal preference. Discharge follows toleration of the diet, and after bowel and bladder functions are relatively normal. This usually requires approximately 7 days, but with economic concerns the overriding issue, this is not always possible.

Complications

Intraoperative complications

The most significant intraoperative complication is ureteral injury, which is usually recognized and repaired during the operation. Other intraoperative complications include bladder, urethral and seminal vesicle injuries. Specific intraoperative difficulties related to the use of the stapler include serosal tears, incomplete 'doughnuts,' instrument failure, and difficulty extracting.[120,121]

Postoperative complications

Anastomotic bleeding

Hemorrhage from the anastomosis is seen in approximately 1% of patients.[122] This may be due to inadequate hemostasis at the suture line itself, or to rupture of a hematoma in the pelvis through the posterior wall of the anastomosis. The former situation usually presents within the first 48 h, whereas the latter may not become apparent for 7 days or more. The problem may be managed expectantly, although one must be concerned about an anastomotic dehiscence. Endoscopic electrocoagulation may be used effectively in the early postoperative period to control anastomotic bleeding.[123] Hemorrhage was thought to be a problem with the single row of staples associated with the early Russian instrument, but, with the American double row of interlocking staples, bleeding is a rare complication.[124]

Cirocco and Golub reviewed the literature and identified 17 patients with postoperative hemorrhage from a combined total of 775 (2.2%) after stapled colorectal anastomoses that required blood transfusion and/or emergency surgery.[123] Non-operative therapy was successful in 82%. The frequency of this complication is probably more common than is evident from the literature, but the fact that the vast majority spontaneously cease and do not go on to anastomotic leak implies that this is a relatively minor concern.

Obstruction at the anastomosis

Obstruction at the anastomosis without evidence of sepsis is not commonly seen, but when colonic ileus is associated with an intact ileocecal valve, perforation can result. Usually, conservative treatment (nasogastric tube) will suffice; rarely is it necessary to perform a laparotomy.

Digital rectal examination may be helpful, but the use of a rectal tube is relatively contraindicated because of the danger of perforating the anastomosis. If unrelieved, this may be one of the few indications for cecostomy.

Sepsis and anastomotic leak

Anastomotic sepsis and fecal fistula are among the more serious concerns in the postoperative period and are the primary causes of operative mortality. A number of factors have been associated with these complications, including disease of the bowel itself (inflammation), inadequate blood supply, tension on the suture line, inaccurate suture placement, trauma, and failure to obtain a watertight seal.[115,125,126] In one report, blood transfusion, itself, was determined to be an independent risk factor for postoperative infectious complications.[127] Our results in a study of 152 patients indicate that diseases that affect local blood flow and response to infection (anemia, atherosclerotic disease, and diabetes) are important risk factors.[122] Others have demonstrated that factors predictive of anastomotic leaks include chronic obstructive pulmonary disease, peritonitis, bowel obstruction, malnutrition, use of corticosteroids, and perioperative blood transfusion.[128]

When a leak occurs, it is usually located on the posterior aspect of the anastomosis. Foster and colleagues demonstrated a midline paucity of vessels both anteriorly and posteriorly by means of angiography of cadaver specimens.[129] They suggest that one of the reasons why wrapping the omentum is protective is that neovascularization may be stimulated.

Management of the anastomotic leak

The presence of fever, leukocytosis, and peritoneal signs should cause the surgeon to consider performing abdominal drainage and proximal diversion.[130] A contrast study with Gastrografin (the use of barium is contraindicated) may demonstrate a leak into the abdomen or into the presacral (retrorectal) space. At the time of reoperation, care should be taken to make certain that drainage of the affected area is adequate, but the anastomosis itself should be left alone. Unless it is completely or almost completely disrupted, it is assumed that eventual healing will take place. An attempt at suture repair is usually an exercise in futility, but even if 'successful,' a proximal colostomy or ileostomy should always be performed.

Occasionally, a patient will have an anastomotic leak but fail to develop abdominal signs and symptoms suggestive of this complication. It is usually evident, however, that one is not having an uneventful postoperative course. Fever and leukocytosis should certainly arouse suspicion. Diarrhea, rectal pain, tenesmus, low back pain, and sciatic symptoms may be due to an abscess in the presacral space, a consequence of an anastomotic leak. Rectal examination may demonstrate a mass, and cautious proctoscopy may confirm the breakdown or the presence of purulent material. CT will usually demonstrate the abscess; the procedure can also be used to guide the placement of a transgluteal or transabdominal catheter in the hope that laparotomy and colostomy can be avoided. In my experience, however, this technique is of particular benefit only for those individuals who present at least 2 weeks after the operation. Inevitably, a diversionary procedure will be necessary if the patient develops an abscess during the postoperative period.

Colostomy closure

The question of when to close the colostomy often arises, especially if there remains evidence of a small leak. My own philosophy is to close the colostomy if the tract as demonstrated on the water-soluble enema is relatively short and at least 2 months have elapsed since the original procedure. One cannot argue with the concept of delaying closure for another 4–6 weeks and repeating the study. However, it is inappropriate to compel the patient to tolerate a difficult stoma for a longer time; the leak may never completely heal, and the colostomy should, therefore, be removed. If the tract is long or if it communicates with the abdomen, and if such a radiologic appearance fails to improve, reresection is advised.

Anastomotic leak – results of studies

The complication rate of anastomotic leak following anterior resection has, in the past, been variously reported to be from 15% to 77%.[114,115,122,125,126,131–135] More recently, however, studies seem to indicate a trend to lower rates (<10%).[136–141] This may be due to the more frequent use of the transanal circular stapling device, in addition to the implementation of intraoperative air testing and direct visualization by means of the sigmoidoscope. This was clearly demonstrated in the prospective trial performed by Beard and colleagues from the Leicester Royal Infirmary, England.[142] There were three clinical leaks (4%) in the 'test group,' and 10 were noted (14%) in the 'no-test' group. These differences, both for clinical and for radiologic leaks, were statistically significant. For anastomoses below the peritoneal reflection, protection is afforded, as mentioned earlier, if the floor of the pelvis is left open and omental wrapping is employed.

The presence of drains is associated with an increased incidence of anastomotic complications, although when one analyses published data it is possible that only less secure anastomoses are drained. However, there is certainly support for the concept that drains adversely affect anastomotic healing.[143,144]

The incidence of anastomotic breakdown following stapled anastomoses has been reported by Heald and Leicester.[124] They noted 13 clinical leaks in 100 stapled anastomoses. They attributed their high breakdown rate primarily to the low level of the anastomosis (all occurred below 7 cm). They caution that blood supply is more adequate if the left colon is fully mobilized and used for the anastomosis rather than the sigmoid colon (conserving the inferior mesenteric artery). In an experience from the same unit with leakage from stapled low anastomoses after TME, major anastomotic leaks associated with peritonitis or a pelvic collection were identified in 11.0% of patients.[145] An additional 6.4% were found to have minor, asymptomatic leaks that were detected by radiologic study.

The group from the Mayo Clinic, Rochester, MN, reported a controlled randomized trial. In a controlled trial of 118 patients reported by McGinn and colleagues, the incidence of clinical leaks with sutured anastomoses was 3% (radiologic 7%), whereas the rate with the stapled technique was 12% (radiologic 24%).[146] Other randomized trials comparing the two techniques have failed to demonstrate any statistically significant difference in leakage rate.[147–149]

The group from the Cleveland Clinic, Cleveland, OH, reported the results of 125 intestinal anastomoses using the Proximate ILS circular stapler.[150] Radiologic evaluation of 79 patients with Gastrografin demonstrated a leak in three (3.8%). There was only one clinically apparent leak in the series. A more recent report from the same institution comprised more than 1000 patients who underwent stapled anastomoses.[151] Clinically apparent anastomotic leaks developed in 2.9%, with inapparent anastomotic dehiscence occurring in 7.7%. However, the incidence of anastomotic leaks above the level of 7 cm from the anal verge was only 1%. The authors further concluded that diabetes mellitus, the use of pelvic drains, and the duration of surgery were significantly related to the occurrence of anastomotic leaks.

Pelvic abscess

In the absence of an anastomotic leak, if the pelvic floor has not been reconstituted, a pelvic abscess should be a rare complication. Additional treatment may be unnecessary if the abscess spontaneously drains through the anastomosis or through the vagina. If surgical drainage is required, it is usually accomplished from below. CT-guided drainage is another possible option. If signs of peritonitis are present, laparotomy is required for drainage, and a concomitant colostomy should also be performed.

Fecal fistula

Fecal fistula may develop early in the postoperative period as a consequence of an anastomotic leak (see earlier discussion). Usually, this complication requires abdominal drainage and a diversionary procedure. However, if the fistula arises at a later time, perhaps following drainage of an abdominal abscess, and connects with the abdominal wall, it can usually be treated expectantly if there is absence of sepsis and the patient

continues to have bowel movements. Without distal obstruction or persistent tumor, the fistula will usually close within a matter of a few weeks. If drainage is considerable, a colostomy appliance may be used.

Late complications

Stricture

Benign stricture following anterior resection is usually a consequence of an anastomotic breakdown with subsequent fibrosis (Figure 24.3). If there is dehiscence of > 50% of the circumference, healing will usually result in stricture formation. Stricture has been shown to develop more frequently following a diversionary colostomy, even in the absence of a leak, if a stapled anastomosis has been performed.[152] Apparently a stapled anastomosis may 'need' the effect of dilatation by the passage of stool; conventional suture technique appears to be associated with stenosis less commonly if a diversionary operation is undertaken. In a survey of members of the American Society of Colon and Rectal Surgeons, preoperative risk factors for the development of this complication were obesity and abscess.[153] Anastomotic leak, incomplete tissue 'doughnut,' postoperative radiation, and pelvic infection were also felt to be contributing factors.

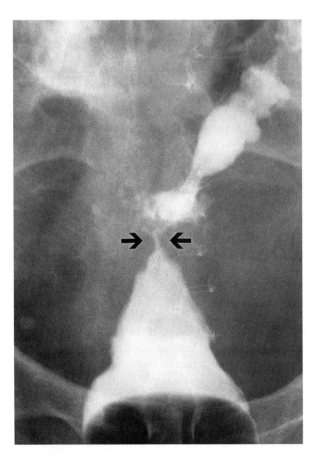

Figure 24.3 *Barium enema reveals rectal stricture following anastomotic leak. This was benign.*

Management

Non-surgical treatment of an anastomotic stricture consists of the use of stool softeners, enemas, or suppositories. Dilatation can be performed manually if it is within reach of the finger. For higher strictures (i.e., at a level of 8–12 cm) a double-ended Hegar's dilator (17–18 mm) or a flexible bougie may be used. Another alternative is to pass a narrow (1.1 cm) sigmoidoscope with its obturator through the stricture, gradually dilating the opening with the serial passage of instruments of increasing diameter. For higher level strictures, Hood and Lewis recommend a curved metal dilator, modeled after the Lister urethral dilator, because the curvature of the sacrum and the angulation of the bowel may make passage impossible.[154] The application of the technique of endoscopic balloon dilatation, with or without the use of a guide wire, has also been reported.[155–160] Most patients require two to four dilatations, repeated at 3-month intervals.[161] There is a risk, of course, of perforating the bowel, a particular concern if the stricture is above the level of the peritoneal reflection. One must weigh the morbidity of the procedure itself against the alternative of a major abdominal operation.

If a symptomatic stricture persists, transanal lysis with a sharp knife or electrocautery in the posterior midline may ameliorate the condition. The use of the optical urethrotome knife has also been described,[162] as well as a device called a 'staple cutter' (a variation of a bone cutter).[163] Following the procedure, frequent office visits with dilatation as necessary are recommended for a number of weeks. Alternatively, if possible, a proctoplasty is preferred, closing the proctotomy in a transverse fashion. Analogous to the Heinecke–Mikulicz pyloroplasty as applied to the rectum, it is hoped that the diameter can be maintained without recurrent stenosis. The application of the technique used for endoscopic papillotomy has also been suggested for the treatment of stricture,[164] as has Eder Puestow dilatation over a guide wire, the technique employed for the management of esophageal strictures.[165] Another option is the use of a endo-stapler.[166] The Wallstent prosthesis has also been advocated for relieving obstruction, not only for malignant tumors, but also for benign stricture.[167]

If all such treatments are of no avail, reresection may be indicated. An alternative to a standard resection is to pass the circular stapling instrument transanally without the anvil, with the center rod traversing the stricture. An enterotomy is created proximal to the strictured anastomosis, and the rod is visualized. The anvil is replaced and the instrument closed and fired. A single tissue 'doughnut' is created, which is the actual stricture. The enterotomy is then closed. Ovnat and colleagues describe the same method, using multiple applications of the circular stapler to create a larger lumen.[168]

One must always keep in mind that the cause of the stricture may be recurrent tumor. Evaluation by means of CT scan may be helpful, but biopsy or cytologic study is mandatory for establishing the diagnosis.[169] Obviously, the use of dilatation as a palliative tool has some merit,[170,171] but most successful reports employ cutting and ablating tools, such as the laser and electrocoagulator, for malignant disease.

Virtually all of the reports concerning the management of rectal strictures are essentially individual case studies. The long-term effectiveness of the various modalities has not been subjected to critical analysis. One exception is the publication of Johansson of a prospective study of 18 patients with rectal stricture.[172] Through the use of endoscopic balloon dilation, two-thirds had complete relief of their obstructive symptoms. Two of the patients considered the results to be poor, and four were not subjected to follow-up evaluation. One perforation developed as a consequence of the procedure.

Incontinence and irregular bowel function

Low anterior resection, irrespective of anastomotic technique, may be associated with control problems and other bowel management difficulties.[173,174] One concern about the stapling technique is the fact that sphincter disruption can occur from dilatation associated with the passage of the instrument. Direct injury to the sphincter during transanal instrumentation has been demonstrated by a number of techniques, including endorectal ultrasound.[175,176] Long-term functional outcome may also be impaired as a consequence of anastomotic leakage.[177]

Studies by Pedersen and colleagues of anorectal function following low anterior resection revealed that most patients demonstrate an abnormal rectoanal inhibitory reflex.[178] Rectal compliance was also lower 3 months after operation, but had returned to normal in every individual by 12 months. Nakahara and colleagues found that all of their patients who underwent low anterior resection with anastomosis by the circular stapling device suffered from frequent bowel actions and soiling.[179] These symptoms improved to a virtually normal state by 6 months, as did rectal sensation and reservoir capacity. However, abnormal rectoanal inhibitory reflex, anal canal resting pressure, and maximum squeeze pressure persisted. O'Riordain and colleagues found that, in the majority of patients who underwent low anterior resection, the rectoanal inhibitory reflex is abolished and remains absent throughout the first year.[180] However, in their experience, this reflex had recovered by the end of the second postoperative year in all patients. Lewis and associates opine that continence after anterior resection is related to the sampling response that the anal sphincter develops to activity within the neorectum.[181,182] The length of the residual rectum is felt to be of critical importance in maintaining effective function.

Inflammatory reaction, narrowing at the anastomosis, sensory impairment, and bowel denervation may all contribute to impairment of control and irregular bowel habits. However, as long as the anal canal and sphincter muscles have been preserved and there is no anatomic abnormality, the symptoms usually resolve in a matter of a few months. 'Slowing' medications should rarely be used because of the risk of precipitating a fecal impaction. Most patients are able to regulate themselves by paying slightly more attention to their diet than has been their custom. Eventually, in most instances, all such restrictions become unnecessary.

Recurrence and survival results following anterior resection

We have reported our experience with anterior resection in 152 patients.[122] The mean age for both men and women was 62 years. There were two in-hospital deaths, a mortality rate of 1.3%. There was no statistically significant difference in survival rates between abdominoperineal resection and anterior resection in those with Dukes' A and Dukes' B lesions. However, patients with Dukes' C tumors who underwent abdominoperineal resection had a significantly poorer survival rate than those who had a lesion sufficiently proximal to permit an anterior resection.

The most difficult problem following anterior resection is the management of locally recurrent disease. There is a dramatic decrease in the frequency of recurrence when the lesion is >13 cm from the anal verge.[183] Furthermore, it has been shown that most recurrences involve tumors that initially penetrated the rectal wall and extended into the surrounding tissue.[184] In our experience, 88% of recurrent malignant lesions in so-called curative cases followed resections for this type of tumor.[183]

In order to minimize the risk of recurrence and the necessity of performing additional surgery, it may be possible to identify preoperatively the individual at a high risk.

In summary, the incidence of anastomotic recurrence in our experience is as follows:

- increases with more distal lesions
- increases with resection margins of <6 cm
- is higher with ulcerating tumors
- is low with exophytic lesions
- is prohibitively high with poorly differentiated growths
- is low with well-differentiated tumors
- is low when the tumor does not penetrate the bowel
- is high with Dukes' B and C lesions
- is high in the presence of metastatic disease.

Therefore, in selecting patients for sphincter-saving procedures, the preoperative assessment is most important. If the tumor is low-lying (<8 cm from the anal verge), but especially if it is poorly differentiated, fixed, infiltrative or ulcerating, then a sphincter-saving operation may be relatively contraindicated. However, controversy concerning the ideal distal margin for anterior resection is unresolved. Vernava and colleagues prospectively studied 243 patients, and found that there was no significant difference in local or distant recurrence or survival when each centimeter interval was studied down to 1 cm.[185] However, those with a distal margin of <0.8 cm had a statistically significantly increased incidence of anastomotic recurrence when compared with those of a greater distal margin. The concept of a 5-cm rule would, therefore, be antiquated.

Recurrence has been attributed to unresected tumor (in the pelvis or the bowel wall itself),[186–198] to a zone of potentially malignant mucosa,[193] to a new primary tumor,[193,199,200] to spillage of viable malignant cells,[193,201–208] and to implantation by suture material.[209] It has also been demonstrated that recurrence rates are higher for the same stage of lesion in men when compared with women.[210] This is presumably because the pelvic anatomy is such that the operation can be undertaken with a greater distal and lateral margin in women than can be accomplished in most men.

A number of measures have been propounded which have been reported to reduce recurrence rates,[206,211–217] but in these non-randomized studies one wonders if the alleged improved results are a consequence of patient selection or due to attention to other details, such as a wide resection. I do not believe the type of suture material is important. I do not utilize the no-touch technique, and I do not perform rectal irrigation with cytotoxic agents.

Results with stapled anastomoses

Because it is possible for surgeons to effect re-establishment of intestinal continuity for relatively low-lying lesions, concern has been expressed about the risk of tumor recurrence following stapled anastomosis. There has been a case report of tumor implantation in the anal canal, possibly as a consequence of trauma from the insertion of the circular stapler.[218] Malignant cells have also been demonstrated in up to 90% of tissue doughnuts.[219] However, the real question is whether surgeons are compromising on the adequacy of the distal margin, and the corollary question is: is it truly important? A few studies suggest that there may be a higher rate of recurrence with the circular stapling device, but most investigators believe that this may be attributable to factors other than the length of the distal margin of resection (e.g., anatomic considerations, anastomotic leak).[146,220–222] Most reports reveal no increase in local recurrence when the stapler is used, and some believe the incidence is actually reduced (when compared with the suture technique), because one may possibly obtain a greater distal margin.[223–226] Akyol and colleagues suggest that the use of stapling instruments could be associated with a reduction in the incidence of local recurrence and cancer-specific mortality by as much as 50%.[227] Others have shown that tumor recurrence and cancer-specific mortality were higher in sutured patients and in those who sustained anastomotic leaks.[228] A number of studies have demonstrated that there is no statistically significant correlation between the incidence of recurrence and the length of distal margin when one controls for the other variables, unless the margin is minimal (<2 cm).[229–235] In a pathologic study of 42 colorectal cancers reported by Hughes and colleagues, only two demonstrated intramural spread, the maximum length being 2 cm.[232] Others have observed that all potentially curable carcinomas would have been adequately resected with a distal margin of only 1.5 cm.[234] In general, local recurrence rates following low anterior resection are essentially the same as the rates for abdominoperineal resection when comparing the same degree of differentiation and stage of tumor.[236,237]

Management of recurrence following anterior resection

When anastomotic recurrence develops, it usually presents within 2 years following resection. The patient may be without symptoms, but a suspicious area is identified either by palpation (digital examination) or by proctosigmoidoscopy as part of the cancer follow-up. Many patients who present with recurrent cancer in the pelvis do not have disseminated disease, and under these circumstances the carcinoembryonic antigen (CEA) level is often not elevated. When symptoms develop, they may include bleeding, change in the caliber of the stool, and pelvic, abdominal, or sacral pain. Biopsy or scrapings for cytologic examination will usually confirm the diagnosis, but barium enema examination and CT scan may also be helpful. Positron emission tomography (PET) has been used to follow-up individuals with colorectal malignancy to differentiate between recurrent tumor and scar. The method employs the injection of fluorine-18-labeled deoxyglucose (FDG) to assess tumor metabolism. In the experience of Strauss and colleagues, non-malignant lesions had a low FDG accumulation as compared with the high levels seen with recurrent cancer.[238,239] Based on subsequent histologic confirmation, the test was 100% accurate in their hands. The only hope for cure is reresection; this usually involves an abdominoperineal resection. Prior to undertaking reoperation, however, it is imperative to determine whether the patient has evidence of disseminated disease. Because of the possibility of retroperitoneal extension of the tumor and the likelihood of urinary tract involvement, a CT scan or intravenous pyelogram is mandatory.

Results of reoperation

Studies of abdominoperineal resection following anastomotic recurrence have limited numbers of patients and are difficult to interpret.[240] Overall cure rates are certainly <25% in those considered resectable for cure. Wanebo and colleagues reported limited success with a combined abdominosacrectomy, with more than one-half of the patients requiring a bladder resection.[241] The operative mortality was 12%.

It is my feeling that cure is rarely achieved, except in those situations in which a second primary lesion is found rather than recurrent disease, or when the pathologist reports that the recurrence is confined to, but does not breach, the bowel wall. This may be the rare circumstance when mucosal seeding produces the recurrence rather than inward growth of residual pelvic disease.

Ricardo *et al.* cite the first report of the use of brachytherapy for locally recurrent rectal cancer. For 28 patients, mean follow-up and local control were, respectively, 26 months and 37% for gross residual disease and 34 months and 66% for microscopic residual disease.[242]

OTHER ANASTOMOTIC TECHNIQUES

Transanal or coloanal anastomosis

An alternative technique for re-establishing intestinal continuity is the transanal or coloanal anastomosis, described initially by Parks in 1972.[243] A hand-sewn technique is usually employed, using a round-bodied modification of a Turner-Warwick urethroplasty needle, or a long-term absorbable suture on a 5/8 circle needle (Figure 24.4). Using a Parks self-retaining, three-bladed anal retractor, paired Gelpi retractors placed at right-angles to each other, a Lone Star Retractor, or a Bookwalter rectal kit (Codman, Randolph, MA), a transanal anastomosis can be effected. This is the technique employed for re-establishing continuity after colectomy, proctectomy, and ileal pouch for inflammatory bowel disease. The sutures incorporate the full thickness of the colon with the anal canal and the underlying internal sphincter. An alternative approach is to use a double-stapling technique.

Results

Enker and colleagues reported their experience with 41 individuals treated by this anastomotic technique.[244] The mean distance of the tumor from the anal verge was 6.7 cm. At the time of their publication, the median follow-up period was only 31 months, with 73% free of disease. The authors recommend that every patient should undergo a temporary diverting colostomy and that the left colon be completely mobilized to avoid tension on the anastomosis. A more recent report from the same institution (Memorial Sloan-Kettering Cancer Center) involved 134 patients.[245] Actuarially corrected 5-year survival for all patients was 73%. Mesenteric implants, positive microscopic resection margin, T3 tumor, PNI, blood vessel invasion, and high tumor grade

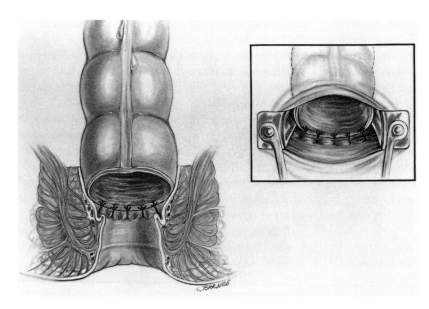

Figure 24.4 *A Parks retractor facilitates the insertion of sutures for coloanal anastomosis.*

were associated with increased risk for pelvic recurrence. Enker *et al.* and others report at least a satisfactory experience, both in terms of bowel function and of recurrent disease.[244,246–251] In the experience of the Memorial Sloan-Kettering Cancer Center, the median stool frequency was two per day, with 22% of patients reporting four or more stools in 24 h.[252] Stool frequency tended to decrease with time, with the use of postoperative adjuvant radiotherapy influencing the frequency and difficulty of evacuation. Poor sphincter function is significantly more common in women than in men.[253] All agree that the surgical morbidity is significantly higher than that of low anterior resection.

Transanal or coloanal anastomosis with colonic reservoir

A J-shaped colonic reservoir has been employed to supplement the coloanal anastomotic option described above in an effort to improve bowel function,[254–256] a virtually non-existing problem if you consult the references in the prior section. The technique is essentially the same as that for a J-shaped ileal reservoir except that the colon is used. Banerjee and colleagues developed a model for ideal pouch size.[257] According to the authors, ideal pouch dimensions are 6–7 cm of undistended bowel circumference, with limb lengths of 8–10 cm. All investigators emphasize the importance of mobilizing the splenic flexure and preserving the first branch of the inferior mesenteric artery.

Results

Drake and colleagues reported the Mayo Clinic experience with 29 individuals suffering from either benign or malignant disease.[258] Anastomotic stricture was found in 28%, and a 3.4% leak rate was noted. Fourteen percent could not have their colostomy or ileostomy closed. In a

later report incorporating the experience from both the Mayo and Cleveland clinics, involving 117 patients, most of whom had undergone a straight coloanal anastomosis, satisfactory fecal continence was achieved in 78%.[259] No J-pouch patient had frequent incontinence. Five-year survival was 69%, but 62% had complications (anastomotic leak 18%). Some institutions have found that stool frequencies are fewer with this method, especially during the first year,[260–266] than with patients reconstructed without a reservoir, but others note that approximately 25% of individuals must evacuate with a small enema.[255,256,267] Conversely, Nicholls and colleagues compared the St Mark's Hospital experience with the colonic reservoir and straight coloanal anastomoses.[268] They found no significant difference in balloon expulsion testing, defecation proctography, or methyl cellulose evacuation in the two groups. Frequencies of defecation and daytime soiling were inversely correlated with the maximal tolerable volume.[269] Hallböök and colleagues performed a randomized comparison of straight and J-pouch anastomoses in 100 consecutive patients with rectal cancer in whom a sphincter-saving procedure was considered appropriate.[270] The incidence of symptomatic anastomotic leakage was lower in the pouch group (2% versus 15%). At 1 year, the pouch patients had significantly fewer bowel movements in 24 h and fewer nocturnal evacuations, less urgency and incontinence.[270] Those familiar with the technique report no increase in morbidity or mortality attributable to the reservoir itself.

Comment

This procedure may be usefully applied in the uncommon situation in which intestinal continuity cannot be re-established by another method, especially as one always strives to avoid a colostomy for benign conditions. However, as of this writing, I have found few cancer patients to be candidates for its implementation. Body habitus, at least in my experience, is rarely the reason for my inability or unwillingness to perform a low anterior resection.

ACKNOWLEDGEMENT

Portions of this chapter have been taken from Corman ML, *Colon and Rectal Surgery*, 4th edition, Philadelphia, Lipincott Williams & Wilkins, 1998, 738–826.

REFERENCES

1. Task Force. American Society of Colon and Rectal Surgeons. Practice parameters for the treatment of rectal carcinoma. Dis Colon Rectum 1993; 36:989.
2. Williams NS, Dixon MF, Johnston D. Reappraisal of the 5 centimetre rule of distal excision for carcinoma of the rectum: a study of distal intramural spread and of patients' survival. Br J Surg 1983; 70:150.
3. Jass JR, Love SB, Northover JMA. A new prognostic classification of rectal cancer. Lancet 1987; 1:1303.
4. Shirouzu K, Isomoto H, Kakegawa T. Prognostic evaluation of perineural invasion in rectal cancer. Am J Surg 1993; 165:233.
5. Saclarides TJ, Bhattacharyya AK, Britton-Kuzel C, *et al.* Predicting lymph node metastases in rectal cancer. Dis Colon Rectum 1994; 37:52.
6. Tribukait B, Hammarberg C, Rubio C. Ploidy and proliferation patterns in colorectal adenocarcinomas relating to Dukes' classification and to histopathological differentiation. Acta Pathol Microbiol Immunol Scand (A) 1983; 91:89.
7. Chang K-J, Enker WE, Melamed M. Influence of tumor cell DNA ploidy on the natural history of rectal cancer. Am J Surg 1987; 153:184.
8. Jones DJ, Moore M, Schofield PF. Prognostic significance of DNA ploidy in colorectal cancer: a prospective flow cytometric study. Br J Surg 1988; 75:28.
9. Melamed MR, Enker WE, Banner P, *et al.* Flow cytometry of colorectal carcinoma with three-year follow-up. Dis Colon Rectum 1986; 29:184.
10. Wolley RC, Schreiber K, Koss LG, *et al.* DNA distribution in human colon carcinomas and its relationship to clinical behavior. J Natl Cancer Inst 1982; 69:15.
11. Heimann TM, Miller F, Martinelli G, *et al.* Significance of DNA content abnormalities in small rectal cancers. Am J Surg 1990; 159:199.
12. Cance WG, Cohen AM, Enker WE, Sigurdson ER. Predictive value of a negative computed tomographic scan in 100 patients with rectal carcinoma. Dis Colon Rectum 1991; 34:748.
13. Clark J, Bankoff M, Carter B, Smith TJ. The use of computerized tomography scan in the staging and follow-up study of carcinoma of the rectum. Surg Gynecol Obstet 1984; 159:335.
14. Koehler PR, Feldberg MAM, van Waes PFGM. Preoperative staging of rectal cancer with computerized tomography. Cancer 1984; 54:512.
15. Shank B, Dershaw DD, Caravelli J, *et al.* A prospective study of the accuracy of preoperative computed tomographic staging of patients with biopsy-proven rectal carcinoma. Dis Colon Rectum 1990; 33:285.
16. van Waes PFGM, Koehler PR, Feldberg MAM. Management of rectal carcinoma: impact of computed tomography. Am J Roentgenol 1983; 140:1137.
17. Guinet C, Buy J-N, Ghossain MA, *et al.* Comparison of magnetic resonance imaging and computed tomography in the preoperative staging of rectal cancer. Arch Surg 1990; 125:385.
18. Hodgman CG, MacCarty RL, Wolff BG, *et al.* Preoperative staging of rectal carcinoma by computed tomography and 0.15 T magnetic resonance imaging. Dis Colon Rectum 1986; 29:446.
19. McNicholas MMJ, Joyce WP, Dolan J, *et al.* Magnetic resonance imaging of rectal carcinoma: a prospective study. Br J Surg 1994; 81:911.
20. Thaler W, Watzka S, Martin F, *et al.* Preoperative staging of rectal cancer by endoluminal ultrasound vs. magnetic resonance imaging. Dis Colon Rectum 1994; 37:1189.
21. Hadfield MB, Nicholson AA, MacDonald AW, *et al.* Preoperative staging of rectal carcinoma by magnetic resonance imaging with a pelvic phased-array coil. Br J Surg 1997; 84:529.
22. Chan TW, Kressel HY, Milestone B, *et al.* Rectal carcinoma: staging at MR imaging with endorectal surface coil: work in progress. Radiology 1991; 181:461.
23. Anderson BO, Hann LE, Enker WE, *et al.* Transrectal ultrasonography and operative selection for early carcinoma of the rectum. J Am Coll Surg 1994; 179:513.
24. Boyce GA, Sivak MV Jr, Lavery IC, *et al.* Endoscopic ultrasound in the pre-operative staging of rectal carcinoma. Gastrointest Endosc 1992; 38:468.
25. Cohen JL, Grotz RL, Welch JP, Deckers PJ. Intrarectal sonography. A new technique for the assessment of rectal tumors. Am Surg 1991; 57:459.
26. Glaser F, Schlag P, Herfarth CH. Endorectal ultrasonography for the assessment of invasion of rectal tumours and lymph node involvement. Br J Surg 1990; 77:883.
27. Katsura Y, Yamada K, Ishizawa T, *et al.* Endorectal ultrasonography for the assessment of wall invasion and lymph node metastasis in rectal cancer. Dis Colon Rectum 1992; 35:362.
28. Konishi F, Muto T, Takahashi H, *et al.* Transrectal ultrasonography for the assessment of invasion of rectal carcinoma. Dis Colon Rectum 1985; 28:889.

29. Milsom JW, Graffner H. Intrarectal ultrasonography in rectal cancer staging and in the evaluation of pelvic disease. Ann Surg 1990; 212:602.

30. Rifkin MD, Marks GJ. Transrectal US as an adjunct in the diagnosis of rectal and extrarectal tumors. Radiology 1985; 157:499.

31. Saitoh N, Okui K, Sarashina H, et al. Evaluation of echographic diagnosis of rectal cancer using intra-rectal ultrasonic examination. Dis Colon Rectum 1986; 29:234.

32. Hildebrandt U, Feifel G, Scherr O. Endorectal ultrasound: instrumentation and clinical aspects. Int J Colorect Dis 1986; 1:203.

33. Beynon J, Foy DMA, Roe AM, et al. Endoluminal ultrasound in the assessment of local invasion in rectal cancer. Br J Surg 1986; 73:474.

34. Hildebrandt U, Feifel G. Preoperative staging of rectal cancer by intrarectal ultrasound. Dis Colon Rectum 1985; 28:42.

35. Kramann B, Hildebrandt U. Computed tomography versus endosonography in the staging of rectal carcinoma: a comparative study. Int J Colorect Dis 1986; 1:216.

36. Adams WJ, Wong WD. Endorectal ultrasonic detection of malignancy within rectal villous lesions. Dis Colon Rectum 1995; 38:1093.

37. Kusunoki M, Yanagi H, Gondoh N, et al. Use of transrectal ultrasonography to select type of surgery for villous tumors in the lower two thirds of the rectum. Arch Surg 1996; 131:714.

38. Hildebrandt U, Klein T, Feifel G, et al. Endosonography of pararectal lymph nodes. In vitro and in vivo evaluation. Dis Colon Rectum 1990; 33:863.

39. Jochem RJ, Reading CC, Dozois RR, et al. Endorectal ultrasonographic staging of rectal carcinoma. Mayo Clin Proc 1990; 65:1571.

40. Roubein LD, David C, DuBrow R, et al. Endoscopic ultrasonography in staging rectal cancer. Am J Gastroenterol 1990; 85:1391.

41. Glaser F, Kuntz C, Schlag P, Herfarth C. Endorectal ultrasound for control of preoperative radiotherapy of rectal cancer. Ann Surg 1993; 217:64.

42. Herzog U, von Flüe M, Tondelli P, Schuppisser JP. How accurate is endorectal ultrasound in the preoperative staging of rectal cancer? Dis Colon Rectum 1993; 36:127.

43. Orrom WJ, Wong WD, Rothenberger DA, et al. Endorectal ultrasound in the preoperative staging of rectal tumors. Dis Colon Rectum 1990; 33:654.

44. Beynon J, Mortensen NJMC, Foy DMA, et al. The detection and evaluation of locally recurrent rectal cancer with rectal endosonography. Dis Colon Rectum 1989; 32:509.

45. Charnley RM, Pyf G, Amar SS, Hardcastle JD. The early diagnosis of recurrent rectal carcinoma by rectal endosonography. Br J Surg 1988; 75:1232.

46. Mascagni D, Corbellini L, Urciuoli P, Di Matteo D. Endoluminal ultrasound for early detection of local recurrence of rectal cancer. Br J Surg 1989; 76:1176.

47. Napoleon B, Pujol B, Berger F, et al. Accuracy of endosonography in the staging of rectal cancer treated by radiotherapy. Br J Surg 1991; 78:785.

48. Romano G, de Rosa P, Vallone G, et al. Intrarectal ultrasound and computed tomography in the pre- and postoperative assessment of patients with rectal cancer. Br J Surg 1985; 72:117.

49. Zainea GG, Lee F, McLeary RD, et al. Transrectal ultrasonography in the evaluation of rectal and extrarectal disease. Surg Gynecol Obstet 1989; 169:153.

50. Solomon MJ, McLeod RS, Cohen EK, et al. Reliability and validity studies of endoluminal ultrasonography for anorectal disorders. Dis Colon Rectum 1994; 37:546.

51. Goldman S, Arvidsson H, Norming U, et al. Transrectal ultrasound and computed tomography in preoperative staging of lower rectal adenocarcinoma. Gastrointest Radiol 1991; 16:259.

52. Milsom JW, Lavery IC, Stolfi VM, et al. The expanding utility of endoluminal ultrasonography in the management of rectal cancer. Surgery 1992; 112:832.

53. Beynon J, Mortensen NJMC, Foy DMA, et al. Preoperative assessment of local invasion in rectal cancer: digital examination, endoluminal sonography or computed tomography? Br J Surg 1986; 73:1015.

54. Harnsberger JR, Charvat P, Longo WE, et al. The role of intrarectal ultrasound (IRUS) in staging of rectal cancer and detection of extrarectal pathology. Am Surg 1994; 60:571.

55. Romano G, Esercizio L, Santangelo M, et al. Impact of computed tomography vs. intrarectal ultrasound on the prognosis of locally recurrent rectal cancer. Dis Colon Rectum 1993; 36:261.

56. Waizer A, Powsner E, Russo I, et al. Prospective comparative study of magnetic resonance imaging versus transrectal ultrasound for preoperative staging and follow-up of rectal cancer. Preliminary report. Dis Colon Rectum 1991; 34:1068.

57. Fleshman JW, Myerson RJ, Fry RD, Kodner IJ. Accuracy of transrectal ultrasound in predicting pathologic stage of rectal cancer before and after preoperative radiation therapy. Dis Colon Rectum 1992; 35:823.

58. Kahn H, Alexander A, Rakinic J, et al. Preoperative staging of irradiated rectal cancers using digital rectal examination, computed tomography, endorectal ultrasound, and magnetic resonance imaging does not accurately predict T0, N0 pathology. Dis Colon Rectum 1997; 40:140.

59. Sentovich SM, Blatchford GJ, Falk PM, *et al.* Transrectal ultrasound of rectal tumors. Am J Surg 1993; 166:638.

60. Williamson PR, Hellinger MD, Larach SW, Ferrara A. Endorectal ultrasound of T3 and T4 rectal cancers after preoperative chemoradiation. Dis Colon Rectum 1996; 39:45.

61. Hünerbein M, Schlag PM. Three-dimensional endosonography for staging of rectal cancer. Ann Surg 1997; 225:432.

62. Ivanoc KD, Diacov CD. Three-dimensional endoluminal ultrasound. New staging techniques in patients with rectal cancer. Dis Colon Rectum 1997; 40:47.

63. Milsom JW, Czyrko C, Hull TL, *et al.* Preoperative biopsy of pararectal lymph nodes in rectal cancer using endoluminal ultrasonography. Dis Colon Rectum 1994; 37:364.

64. Reybard JF. Mémoire sur une tumeur cancéreuse affectant l'iliaque du colon; ablation de la tumeur et de l'intestin; réunion directe et immédiate des deux bouts de cet organe. Bull Acad Med Paris 1843–44; 9:1031.

65. Dixon CF. Anterior resection for malignant lesions of the upper part of the rectum and lower part of the sigmoid. Ann Surg 1948; 128:425.

66. Kirwan WO, O'Riordain MG, Waldron R. Declining indications for abdominoperineal resection. Br J Surg 1989; 76:1061.

67. Törnquist A, Ekelund G, Forsgren A, *et al.* Single dose doxycycline prophylaxis and preoperative bacteriological culture in elective colorectal surgery. Br J Surg 1981; 68:565.

68. Scott JR, Daneker G, Lumsden AB. Prevention of compartment syndrome associated with the dorsal lithotomy position. Am Surg 1997; 63:801.

69. Fowl RJ, Akers DL, Kempczinski RF. Neurovascular lower extremity complications of the lithotomy position. Ann Vasc Surg 1992; 6:357.

70. Schwenk W, Böhm B, Junghans T, *et al.* Intermittent sequential compression of the lower limb prevents venous stasis in laparoscopic and conventional colorectal surgery. Dis Colon Rectum 1997; 40:1056.

71. Pezim ME, Nicholls RJ. Survival after high or low ligation of the inferior mesenteric artery during curative surgery for rectal cancer. Ann Surg 1984; 200:729.

72. Surtees P, Ritchie JK, Phillips RKS. High versus low ligation of the inferior mesenteric artery in rectal cancer. Br J Surg 1990; 77:618.

73. Enker WE, Heilweil ML, Hertz RL, *et al.* En bloc pelvic lymphadenectomy and sphincter preservation in the surgical management of rectal cancer. Ann Surg 1986; 203:426.

74. Moreira LF, Hizuta A, Iwagaki H, *et al.* Lateral lymph node dissection for rectal carcinoma below the peritoneal reflection. Br J Surg 1994; 81:293.

75. Qinyao W, Weijin S, Youren Z, *et al.* New concepts in severe presacral hemorrhage during proctectomy. Arch Surg 1985; 120:1013.

76. Metzger PP. Modified packing technique for control of presacral pelvic bleeding. Dis Colon Rectum 1988; 31:981.

77. Zama N, Fazio VW, Jagelman DG, *et al.* Efficacy of pelvic packing in maintaining hemostasis after rectal excision for cancer. Dis Colon Rectum 1988; 31:923.

78. Stolfi VM, Milsom JW, Lavery IC, *et al.* Newly designed occluder pin for presacral hemorrhage. Dis Colon Rectum 1992; 35:166.

79. Cawthorn SJ, Parums DV, Gibbs NM, *et al.* Extent of mesorectal spread and involvement of lateral resection margin as prognostic factors after surgery for rectal cancer. Lancet 1990; 335:1055.

80. Hida J-I, Yasumoti M, Maruyama T, *et al.* Lymph node metastases detected in the mesorectum distal to carcinoma of the rectum by the clearing method: justification of total mesorectal excision. J Am Coll Surg 1997; 184:584.

81. Karanjia ND, Schache DJ, North WRS, Heald RJ. 'Close shave' in anterior resection. Br J Surg 1990; 77:510.

82. MacFarlane JK, Ryall RDH, Heald RJ. Mesorectal excision for rectal cancer. Lancet 1993; 341:457.

83. Reynolds JV, Joyce WP, Dolan J, *et al.* Pathological evidence in support of total mesorectal excision in the management of rectal cancer. Br J Surg 1996; 83:1112.

84. Heald RJ. Total mesorectal excision is optimal surgery for rectal cancer: a Scandinavian consensus. Br J Surg 1995; 82:1297.

85. Heald RJ, Smedh RK, Kald A, *et al.* Abdominoperineal excision of the rectum: an endangered operation. Dis Colon Rectum 1997; 40:747.

86. Beart R. Mesorectal excision for rectal carcinoma: the new standard? Adv Surg 1999; 199.

87. Hainsworth PJ, Egan MJ, Cunliffe WJ. Evaluation of a policy of total mesorectal excision for rectal and rectosigmoid cancers. Br J Surg 1997; 84:652.

88. Arbman G, Nilsson E, Hallböök O, Sjödahl R. Local recurrence following total mesorectal excision for rectal cancer. Br J Surg 1996; 83:375.

89. Enker WE, Thaler HT, Cranor ML, Polyak T. Total mesorectal excision of the operative treatment of carcinoma of the rectum. J Am Coll Surg 1995; 181:335.

90. Havenga K, Enker WE, McDermott K, *et al.* Male and female sexual and urinary function after total mesorectal excision with autonomic nerve preservation for carcinoma of the rectum. J Am Coll Surg 1996; 182:495.

91. Adam IJ, Mohamdee MO, Martin IG, *et al.* Role of circumferential margin involvement in the local recurrence of rectal cancer. Lancet 1994; 344:707.

92. Ng IOL, Luk ISC, Yuen ST, *et al.* Surgical lateral clearance in resected rectal carcinomas.

A multivariate analysis of clinicopathologic features. Cancer 1993; 71:1972.

93. Quirke P, Dixon MF, Durdey P, Williams NS. Local recurrence of rectal adenocarcinoma due to inadequate surgical resection: histopathological study of lateral tumour spread and surgical excision. Lancet 1986; 2:996.

94. Moriya Y, Hojo K, Sawada T, Koyama Y. Significance of lateral node dissection for advanced rectal carcinoma at or below the peritoneal reflection. Dis Colon Rectum 1989; 32:307.

95. Graham RA, Hohn DC. Management of inguinal lymph node metastases from adenocarcinoma of the rectum. Dis Colon Rectum 1990; 33:212.

96. Deen KI. Foley catheter-assisted sutured colorectal anastomosis. Br J Surg 1995; 82:324.

97. Goldsmith HS. Protection of low rectal anastomosis with intact omentum. Surg Gynecol Obstet 1977; 144:584.

98. Goldsmith HS. Use of the omentum in the presacral space. Dis Colon Rectum 1978; 21:405.

99. Lanter B, Mason RA. Use of omental pedicle graft to protect low anterior colonic anastomosis. Dis Colon Rectum 1979; 22:448.

100. McLachlin AD. Anastomotic leakage below the peritoneal reflection, a study in the dog. Dis Colon Rectum 1978; 21:400.

101. Sagar PM, Couse N, Kerin M, et al. Randomized trial of drainage of colorectal anastomosis. Br J Surg 1993; 80:769.

102. Sagar PM, Hartley MN, Macfie J, et al. Randomized trial of pelvic drainage after rectal resection. Dis Colon Rectum 1995; 38:254.

103. Scott H, Brown AC. Is routine drainage of pelvic anastomosis necessary? Am Surg 1996; 62:452.

104. Cohen Z, Myers E, Langer B, et al. Double stapling technique for low anterior resection. Dis Colon Rectum 1983; 26:231.

105. Griffen FD, Knight CD. Stapling technique for primary and secondary rectal anastomoses. Surg Clin North Am 1984; 64:579.

106. Julian TB, Ravitch MM. Evaluation of the safety of end-to-end (EEA) stapling anastomoses across linear stapled closures. Surg Clin North Am 1984; 64:567.

107. Knight CD, Griffen FD. An improved technique for low anterior resection of the rectum using the EEA stapler. Surgery 1980; 88:710.

108. Eisenstat TE, Rubin RJ, Salvati EP, Oliver GC. New method for low transection of the rectum. Dis Colon Rectum 1990; 33:346.

109. Ganchrow MI, Facelle TL. Double roticulator stapling technique for low-lying rectal tumors. Am J Surg 1993; 166:54.

110. Ravitch MM. Intersecting staple lines in intestinal anastomoses. Surgery 1985; 97:8.

111. Fazio VW. Cancer of the rectum – sphincter-saving operations. Surg Clin North Am 1988; 68:1367.

112. Karanjia ND, Corder AP, Holdsworth PJ, Heald RJ. Risk of peritonitis and fatal septicaemia and the need to defunction the low anastomosis. Br J Surg 1991; 78:196.

113. Grabham JA, Moran BJ, Lane RHS. Defunctioning colostomy for low anterior resection: a selective approach. Br J Surg 1995; 82:1331.

114. Goligher JC, Graham NG, DeDombal FT. Anastomotic dehiscence after anterior resection of rectum and sigmoid. Br J Surg 1970; 57:109.

115. Schrock TR, Deveney CW, Dunphy JE. Factors contributing to leakage of colonic anastomoses. Ann Surg 1973; 177:513.

116. Blomquist P, Jiborn H, Zederfeldt B. Effect of diverting colostomy on collagen metabolism in the colonic wall. Am J Surg 1985; 149:330.

117. Senagore A, Milsom JW, Walshaw RK, et al. Does a proximal colostomy affect colorectal anastomotic healing? Dis Colon Rectum 1992; 35:182.

118. Appleton GVN, Williamson RCN. Hypoplasia of defunctioned rectum. Br J Surg 1989; 76:787.

119. Mirelman D, Corman ML, Veidenheimer MC, Coller JA. Colostomies – indications and contraindications: Lahey clinic experience, 1973–1974. Dis Colon Rectum 1978; 21:172.

120. Gordon PH, Vasilevsky C. Experience with stapling in rectal surgery. Surg Clin North Am 1984; 64:555.

121. Leff EI, Hoexter B, Labow SB, et al. The EEA stapler in low colorectal anastomoses: initial experience. Dis Colon Rectum 1982; 25:704.

122. Manson PN, Corman ML, Coller JA, Veidenheimer MC. Anterior resection for adenocarcinoma: Lahey clinic experience from 1963 through 1969. Am J Surg 1976; 131:434.

123. Cirocco WC, Golub RW. Endoscopic treatment of postoperative hemorrhage from a stapled colorectal anastomosis. Am Surg 1995; 61:460.

124. Heald RJ, Leicester RJ. The low stapled anastomosis. Dis Colon Rectum 1981; 24:437.

125. Debas HT, Thomson FB. A critical review of colectomy with anastomosis. Surg Gynecol Obstet 1972; 135:747.

126. Hawley PR. Infection – the cause of anastomotic breakdown: an experimental study. Proc R Soc Med 1970; 63:752.

127. Sweeney WB, Deshmukh N. Modified Kraske approach for disease of the mid-rectum. Am J Gastroenterol 1991; 86:75.

128. Golub R, Golub RW, Cantu R Jr, Stein DH. A multivariate analysis of factors contributing to leakage of intestinal anastomoses. J Am Coll Surg 1997; 184:364.

129. Foster ME, Lancaster JB, Leaper DJ. Leakage of low rectal anastomosis: an anatomic explanation? Dis Colon Rectum 1984; 27:157.

130. Mileski WJ, Joehl RJ, Rege RV, Nahrwold DL. Treatment of anastomotic leakage following low anterior colon resection. Arch Surg 1988; 123:968.

131. Clark CG, Harris J, Elmasri S, *et al.* Polyglycolic acid sutures and catgut in colonic anastomosis. A controlled clinical trial. Lancet 1972; 2:1006.

132. Dunphy JE. The cut gut. Presidential address. Am J Surg 1970; 119:1.

133. Irvin TT, Goligher JC. Aetiology of disruption of intestinal anastomoses. Br J Surg 1973; 60:461.

134. Morgenstern L, Yamakawa T, Ben-Shashkan M, *et al.* Anastomotic leakage after low colonic anastomosis: clinical and experimental aspects. Am J Surg 1972; 123:104.

135. Sehapayak S, McNatt M, Carter HG, *et al.* Continuous sump-suction drainage of the pelvis after low anterior resection: a reappraisal. Dis Colon Rectum 1973; 16:485.

136. Cade D, Gallagher P, Schofield PF, Turner L. Complications of anterior resection of the rectum using the EEA stapling device. Br J Surg 1981; 68:339.

137. Carty NJ, Keating J, Campbell J, *et al.* Prospective audit of an extramucosal technique for intestinal anastomosis. Br J Surg 1991; 78:1439.

138. Chassin JL, Rifkind KM, Sussman B, *et al.* The stapled gastrointestinal tract anastomosis: incidence of postoperative complications compared with the sutured anastomosis. Ann Surg 1978; 188:689.

139. Heberer G, Denecke H, Pratschke E, Teichmann R. Anterior and low anterior resection. World J Surg 1982; 6:517.

140. Hunt TK. Anastomotic failure. In Simmons RL, ed. *Topics in intraabdominal surgical infection.* Norwalk, CT, Appleton-Century-Crofts, 1982, 101.

141. Max E, Sweeney WB, Bailey HR, *et al.* Results of 1,000 single-layer continuous polypropylene intestinal anastomoses. Am J Surg 1991; 162:461.

142. Beard JD, Nicholson ML, Sayers RD, *et al.* Intraoperative air testing of colorectal anastomoses: a prospective, randomized trial. Br J Surg 1990; 77:1095.

143. Goldstein M, Duff JH. Reconsideration of colostomy in elective left colon resection. Surg Gynecol Obstet 1972; 134:593.

144. Manz CW, LaTendresse C, Sako Y. The detrimental effects of drains on colonic anastomosis: an experimental study. Dis Colon Rectum 1970; 13:17.

145. Karanjia ND, Corder AP, Bearn P, Heald RJ. Leakage from stapled low anastomosis after total mesorectal excision for carcinoma of the rectum. Br J Surg 1994; 81:1224.

146. McGinn FP, Gartell PC, Clifford PC, Brunton FJ. Staples or sutures for low colorectal anastomoses: a prospective randomized trial. Br J Surg 1985; 72:603.

147. Beart RW Jr, Kelly KA. Randomized prospective evaluation of the EEA stapler for colorectal anastomoses. Am J Surg 1981; 141:143.

148. Everett WG, Friend PJ, Forty J. Comparison of stapling and hand-suture for left-sided large bowel anastomosis. Br J Surg 1986; 73:345.

149. Waxman BP. Large bowel anastomoses. II. The circular staplers. Br J Surg 1983; 70:64.

150. Fazio VW, Jagelman DG, Lavery IC, McGonagle BA. Evaluation of the proximate-ILS circular stapler: a prospective study. Ann Surg 1985; 210:108.

151. Vignali A, Fazio VW, Lavery IC, *et al.* Factors associated with the occurrence of leaks in stapled rectal anastomoses: a review of 1,014 patients. J Am Coll Surg 1997; 185:105.

152. Graffner H, Fredlund P, Olsson S-A, *et al.* Protective colostomy in low anterior resection of the rectum using the EEA stapling instrument – a randomized study. Dis Colon Rectum 1983; 26:87.

153. Luchtefeld MA, Milsom JW, Senagore A, *et al.* Colorectal anastomotic stenosis. Results of a survey of the ASCRS membership. 1989; 32:733.

154. Hood K, Lewis A. Dilator for high rectal strictures. Br J Surg 1986; 73:633.

155. Aston NO, Owen WJ, Irving JD. Endoscopic balloon dilatation of colonic anastomotic strictures. Br J Surg 1989; 76:780.

156. Banerjee AK, Walters TK, Wilkins R, Burke M. Wire-guided balloon coloplasty – a new treatment for colorectal strictures. J R Soc Med 1991; 84:136.

157. Bedogni G, Ricci E, Pedrazzoli C, *et al.* Endoscopic dilation of anastomotic colonic stenosis by different techniques: an alternative to surgery? Gastrointest Endosc 1987; 33:21.

158. McLean GK, Cooper GS, Hartz WH, *et al.* Radiologically guided balloon dilation of gastrointestinal strictures. Part I. Technique and factors influencing procedural success. Radiology 1987; 165:35.

159. Neufeld DM, Shemesh EI, Kodner IJ, Shatz BA. Endoscopic management of anastomotic colon strictures with electrocautery and balloon dilation. Gastrointest Endosc 1987; 33:24.

160. Oz MC, Forde KA. Endoscopic alternatives in the management of colonic strictures. Surgery 1990; 108:513.

161. Kingsley AN. Colonic strictures. Management by endoscopic balloon dilation. Contemp Surg 1991; 38:50.

162. Chia YW, Ngoi SS, Tung KH. Use of the optical urethrotome knife in the treatment of a benign low rectal anastomotic stricture. Dis Colon Rectum 1991; 34:717.

163. Shimada S, Matsuda M, Uno K, *et al.* A new device for the treatment of coloproctostomic stricture after double stapling anastomoses. Ann Surg 1996; 224:603.

164. Accordi F, Sogno O, Carniato S, *et al.* Endoscopic treatment of stenosis following stapler anastomosis. Dis Colon Rectum 1987; 30:647.

165. Woodward A, Tydeman G, Lewis MH. Eder Puestow dilatation of benign rectal stricture following anterior resection. Dis Colon Rectum 1990; 33:79.

166. Pagni S, McLaughlin CM. Simple technique for the treatment of strictured colorectal anastomosis. Dis Colon Rectum 1995; 38:433.

167. Salinas JC, Quintana J, De Gregorio MA, et al. Management of benign rectal stricture by implantation of a self-expanding prosthesis. Br J Surg 1997; 84:674.

168. Ovnat A, Peiser J, Avinoah E, Charuzi I. A new approach to rectal anastomotic stricture. Dis Colon Rectum 1989; 32:351.

169. Williams JG, Williams LA. Colonoscopy and brush cytology in the diagnosis of colonic strictures. J R Coll Surg Edinb 1988; 33:119.

170. Stone JM, Bloom RJ. Transendoscopic balloon dilatation of complete colonic obstruction. An adjunct in the treatment of colorectal cancer: report of three cases. Dis Colon Rectum 1989; 32:429.

171. Triadafilopoulos G, Sarkisian M. Dilatation of radiation-induced sigmoid stricture using sequential Savary–Guilliard dilators. A combined radiologic–endoscopic approach. Dis Colon Rectum 1990; 33:1065.

172. Johansson C. Endoscopic dilation of rectal strictures. A prospective study of 18 cases. Dis Colon Rectum 1996; 39:423.

173. Goligher JC. Further reflections on preservation of the anal sphincters in the radical treatment of rectal cancer. Proc R Soc Med 1962; 55:341.

174. Goligher JC, Hughes ESR. Sensibility of the rectum and colon: its role in the mechanism of anal continence. Lancet 1951; 1:543.

175. Farouk R, Drew PJ, Duthie GS, et al. Disruption of the internal anal sphincter can occur after transanal stapling. Br J Surg 1996; 83:1400.

176. Molloy RG, Moran KT, Coulter J, et al. Mechanism of sphincter impairment following low anterior resection. Dis Colon Rectum 1992; 35:462.

177. Hallböök O, Sjödahl R. Anastomotic leakage and functional outcome after anterior resection of the rectum. Br J Surg 1996; 83:60.

178. Pedersen IK, Hint K, Olsen J, et al. Anorectal function after low anterior resection for carcinoma. Ann Surg 1986; 204:133.

179. Nakahara S, Itoh H, Mibu R, et al. Clinical and manometric evaluation of anorectal function following low anterior resection with low anastomotic line using an EEATM stapler for rectal cancer. Dis Colon Rectum 1988; 31:762.

180. O'Riordain MG, Molloy RG, Gillen P, et al. Rectoanal inhibitory reflex following low stapled anterior resection of the rectum. Dis Colon Rectum 1992; 35:874.

181. Lewis WG, Holdsworth PJ, Stephenson BM, et al. Role of the rectum in the physiological and clinical results of coloanal and colorectal anastomosis after anterior resection for rectal carcinoma. Br J Surg 1992; 79:1082.

182. Lewis WG, Martin IG, Williamson MER, et al. Why do some patients experience poor functional results after anterior resection of the rectum for carcinoma? Dis Colon Rectum 1995; 38:259.

183. Manson PN, Corman ML, Coller JA, Veidenheimer MC. Anastomotic recurrence after anterior resection for carcinoma: Lahey clinic experience. Dis Colon Rectum 1976; 19:219.

184. Zollinger RM, Sheppard MH. Carcinoma of the rectum and the rectosigmoid: a review of 729 cases. Arch Surg 1971; 102:335.

185. Vernava AM III, Moran M, Rothenberger DA, Wong WD. A prospective evaluation of distal margins in carcinoma of the rectum. Surg Gynecol Obstet 1992; 175:333.

186. Deddish MR, Stearns MW Jr. Anterior resection for carcinoma of the rectum and rectosigmoid area. Ann Surg 1961; 154:961.

187. Durdey P, Williams NS. The effect of malignant and inflammatory fixation of rectal carcinoma on prognosis after rectal excision. Br J Surg 1984; 71:787.

188. Enker WE, Laffer UT, Block GE. Enhanced survival of patients with colon and rectal cancer is based upon wide anatomic resection. Ann Surg 1979; 190:350.

189. Gilbertsen VA. The results of surgical treatment of cancer of the rectum. Surg Gynecol Obstet 1962; 114:313.

190. Gilchrist RK, David VC. Consideration of pathological factors influencing five year survival in radical resection of large bowel and rectum for carcinoma. Ann Surg 1947; 126:421.

191. Gilchrist RK, David VC. Prognosis in carcinoma of bowel. Surg Gynecol Obstet 1948; 86:359.

192. Localio SA. Curative surgery of midrectal cancer with preservation of the sphincters. Surg Ann 1974; 6:213.

193. Lofgren EP, Waugh JM, Dockerty MB. Local recurrence of carcinoma after anterior resection of the rectum and the sigmoid: relationship with the length of normal mucosa excised distal to the lesion. Arch Surg 1957; 74:825.

194. Mayo CW, Schlicke CP. Carcinoma of the colon and rectum: a study of metastasis and recurrences. Surg Gynecol Obstet 1942; 74:83.

195. Miles WE. Cancer of the rectum. Trans Med Soc Lond 1923; 46:127.

196. Slanetz CA Jr, Herter FP, Grinnell RS. Anterior resection versus abdominoperineal resection for cancer of the rectum and rectosigmoid: an analysis of 524 cases. Am J Surg 1972; 123:110.

197. Stearns MW Jr. Surgical management of colo-rectal cancer. Proc Natl Cancer Conf 1973; 7:481.

198. Stearns MW Jr. Carcinoma of the rectum: results of abdominoperineal resection (symposium). Dis Colon Rectum 1974; 17:586.

199. Goligher JC, Dukes CE, Bussey HJR. Local recurrences after sphincter-saving excisions of carcinoma of rectum and rectosigmoid. Br J Surg 1951; 39:199.

200. Long JW, Mayo CW, Dockerty MB, *et al.* Recurrent versus new and independent carcinomas of the colon and rectum. Mayo Clin Proc 1950; 25:169.

201. Cohn I. Implantation in cancer of the colon. Surg Gynecol Obstet 1967; 124:501.

202. Cohn I. Cause and prevention of recurrence following surgery for colon cancer. Cancer 1971; 28:183.

203. Cole WH. Recurrence in carcinoma of colon and proximal rectum following resection for carcinoma. Arch Surg 1952; 65:264.

204. Cole WH, Packard D, Southwick W. Carcinoma of the colon with special reference to prevention of recurrence. JAMA 1954; 155:1549.

205. McGrew EA, Laws JF, Cole WH. Free malignant cells in relation to recurrence of carcinoma of colon. JAMA 1954; 154:1251.

206. Southwick HW, Harridge WH, Cole WH. Recurrence at the suture line following resection for carcinoma of the colon. Incidence following preventive measures. Am J Surg 1962; 103:86.

207. Umpleby HC, Fermor B, Symes MO, Williamson RCN. Viability of exfoliated colorectal carcinoma cells. Br J Surg 1984; 71:659.

208. Vink M. Local recurrence of cancer in large bowel: role of implantation metastases and bowel disinfection. Br J Surg 1954; 41:431.

209. Franklin R, McSwain B. Carcinoma of the colon, rectum, and anus. Ann Surg 1970; 171:811.

210. Buhre LMD, Mulder NH, DeRuiter AJ, *et al.* Effect of extent of anterior resection and sex on disease-free survival and local recurrence in patients with rectal cancer. Br J Surg 1994; 81:1227.

211. Herter FP, Slanetz CA Jr. Preoperative intestinal preparation in relation to the subsequent development of cancer at the suture line. Surg Gynecol Obstet 1968; 127:49.

212. Labow SB, Salvati EP, Rubin RJ. Suture-line recurrences in carcinoma of the colon and rectum. Dis Colon Rectum 1975; 18:123.

213. Morgan CN, Lloyd-Davies OV. Discussion on conservative resection in carcinoma of the rectum. Proc R Soc Med 1950; 43:701.

214. Pollett WG, Nicholls RJ. The relationship between the extent of distal clearance and survival and local recurrence rates after curative anterior resection for carcinoma of the rectum. Ann Surg 1983; 198:159.

215. Rosi PA, Cahill WJ, Carey J. A ten year study of hemicolectomy in the treatment of carcinoma of the left half of the colon. Surg Gynecol Obstet 1962; 114:15.

216. Turnbull RB Jr. Cancer of the colon: the five- and ten-year survival rates following resection utilizing the isolation technique. Ann R Coll Surg Engl 1970; 46:243.

217. Turnbull RB Jr, Kyle K, Watson FR, *et al.* Cancer of the colon: the influence of the no-touch isolation technic on survival rates. Ann Surg 1967; 166:420.

218. Norgren J, Svensson JO. Anal implantation metastasis from carcinoma of the sigmoid colon and rectum – a risk when performing anterior resection with the EEA stapler? Br J Surg 1985; 72:602.

219. Gertsch P, Baer HU, Kraft R, *et al.* Malignant cells are collected on circular staplers. Dis Colon Rectum 1992; 35:238.

220. Neville R, Fielding LP, Amendola C. Local tumor recurrence after curative resection for rectal cancer: a ten-hospital review. Dis Colon Rectum 1987; 30:12.

221. Rosen CB, Beart RW Jr, Ilstrup DM. Local recurrence of rectal carcinoma after hand-sewn and stapled anastomoses. Dis Colon Rectum 1985; 28:305.

222. Sauven P, Playforth MJ, Evans M, Pollock AV. Early infective complications and late recurrent cancer in stapled anastomoses. Dis Colon Rectum 1989; 32:33.

223. Leff EI, Hoexter B, Labow S, *et al.* Anastomotic recurrences after low anterior resection: stapled vs. hand-sewn. Dis Colon Rectum 1985; 28:164.

224. Malmberg M, Graffner H, Ling L, Olsson S. Recurrence and survival after anterior resection of the rectum using the end to end anastomotic stapler. Surg Gynecol Obstet 1986; 163:231.

225. Odou MW, O'Connell TX. Changes in the treatment of rectal carcinoma and effects on local recurrence. Arch Surg 1986; 121:1114.

226. Wolmark N, Gordon PH, Fisher B, *et al.* A comparison of stapled and handsewn anastomoses in patients undergoing resection for Dukes' B and C colorectal cancer. Dis Colon Rectum 1986; 29:344.

227. Akyol AM, McGregor JR, Galloway DJ, *et al.* Recurrence of colorectal cancer after sutured and stapled large bowel anastomoses. Br J Surg 1991; 78:1297.

228. Docherty JG, McGregor JR, Akyol AM, *et al.* Comparison of manually constructed and stapled anastomoses in colorectal surgery. Ann Surg 1995; 221:176.

229. Heald RJ, Ryall RDH. Recurrence and survival after total mesorectal excision for rectal cancer. Lancet 1986; 1:1479.

230. Heimann TM, Szporn A, Bolnick K, Aufses AH Jr. Local recurrence following surgical treatment of rectal cancer: comparison of anterior and abdominoperineal resection. Dis Colon Rectum 1986; 29:862.

231. Hojo K. Anastomotic recurrence after sphincter-saving resection for rectal cancer. Dis Colon Rectum 1986; 29:11.

232. Hughes TG, Jenevein EP, Poulos E. Intramural spread of colon carcinoma. Am J Surg 1983; 146:697.

233. Laxamana A, Solomon MJ, Cohen Z, *et al.* Long-term results of anterior resection using the double-stapling technique. Dis Colon Rectum 1995; 38:1246.

234. Madsen PM, Christiansen J. Distal intramural spread of rectal carcinomas. Dis Colon Rectum 1986; 29:279.

235. Phillips RKS, Hittinger R, Blesovsky L, *et al*. Local recurrence following 'curative' surgery for large bowel cancer. II. The rectum and rectosigmoid. Br J Surg 1984; 71:17.

236. Williams NS, Durdey P, Johnston D. The outcome following sphincter-saving resection and abdomino-perineal resection for low rectal cancer. Br J Surg 1985; 72:595.

237. Wolmark N, Fisher B. An analysis of survival and treatment failure following abdominoperineal and sphincter-saving resection in Dukes' B and C rectal carcinoma. Ann Surg 1986; 204:480.

238. Schlag P, Lehner B, Strauss LG, *et al*. Scar or recurrent rectal cancer. Positron emission tomography is more helpful for diagnosis than immunoscintigraphy. Arch Surg 1989; 124:197.

239. Strauss LG, Clorius JH, Schlag P, *et al*. Recurrence of colorectal tumor: PET evaluation. Radiology 1989; 170:329.

240. Segall MM, Nivatvongs S, Balcos E, *et al*. Abdominoperineal resection for recurrent cancer following anterior resection. Dis Colon Rectum 1981; 24:80.

241. Wanebo HJ, Gaker DL, Whitehill R, *et al*. Pelvic recurrence of rectal cancer: options for curative resection. Ann Surg 1987; 205:482.

242. Ricardo N, Beart R, Simons A, *et al*. Use of brachtherapy in management of locally recurrent rectal cancer. Dis Colon Rectum 1997; 1177.

243. Parks AG. Transanal technique in low rectal anastomosis. Proc R Soc Med 1972; 65:975.

244. Enker WE, Stearns MW Jr, Janov AJ. Perianal coloanal anastomosis following low anterior resection for rectal carcinoma. Dis Colon Rectum 1985; 28:576.

245. Paty PB, Enker WE, Cohen AM, Lauwers GY. Treatment of rectal cancer by low anterior resection with coloanal anastomosis. Ann Surg 1994; 219:365.

246. Castrini G, Toccaceli S. Cancer of the rectum – Sphincter-saving operation. A new technique of coloanal anastomosis. Surg Clin North Am 1988; 68:1383.

247. Cohen AM, Enker WE, Minsky BD. Proctectomy and coloanal reconstruction for rectal cancer. Dis Colon Rectum 1990; 33:40.

248. Hautefeuille P, Valleur P, Perniceni T, *et al*. Functional and oncologic results after coloanal anastomosis for low rectal carcinoma. Ann Surg 1988; 207:61.

249. Rudd WWH. The transanal anastomosis: a sphincter-saving operation with improved continence. Dis Colon Rectum 1979; 22:102.

250. Sweeney JL, Ritchie JK, Hawley PR. Resection and sutured peranal anastomosis for carcinoma of the rectum. Dis Colon Rectum 1989; 32:103.

251. Vernava AM III, Robbins PL, Brabbee GW. Restorative resection: coloanal anastomosis for benign and malignant disease. Dis Colon Rectum 1989; 32:690.

252. Paty PB, Enker WE, Cohen AM, *et al*. Long-term functional results of coloanal anastomosis for rectal cancer. Am J Surg 1994; 167:90.

253. Miller AS, Lewis WG, Williamson MER, *et al*. Factors that influence functional outcome after coloanal anastomosis for carcinoma of the rectum. Br J Surg 1995; 82:1327.

254. Huguet C, Harb J, Bona S. Coloanal anastomosis after resection of low rectal cancer in the elderly. World J Surg 1990; 14:619.

255. Lazorthes F, Fages P, Chiotasso P, *et al*. Resection of the rectum with construction of a colonic reservoir and colo-anal anastomosis for carcinoma of the rectum. Br J Surg 1986; 73:136.

256. Parc R, Tiret E, Frileux P, *et al*. Resection and colo-anal anastomosis with colonic reservoir for rectal carcinoma. Br J Surg 1986; 73:139.

257. Banerjee AK, Parc R. Prediction of optimum dimensions of colonic pouch reservoir. Dis Colon Rectum 1996; 39:1293.

258. Drake DB, Pemberton JH, Beart RW Jr, *et al*. Coloanal anastomosis in the management of benign and malignant rectal disease. Ann Surg 1987; 206:600.

259. Cavaliere F, Pemberton JH, Cosimelli M, *et al*. Coloanal anastomosis for rectal cancer. Long-term results at the Mayo and Cleveland Clinics. Dis Colon Rectum 1995; 38:807.

260. Benoist S, Panis Y, Boleslawski E, *et al*. Functional outcome after coloanal versus low colorectal anastomosis for rectal carcinoma. J Am Coll Surg 1997; 185:114.

261. Hida J-I, Yasutomi M, Fujimoto K, *et al*. Functional outcome after low anterior resection with low anastomosis for rectal cancer using the colonic J-pouch. Dis Colon Rectum 1996; 39:986.

262. Leo E, Belli F, Baldini MT, *et al*. New perspective in the treatment of low rectal cancer: total rectal resection and coloendoanal anastomosis. Dis Colon Rectum 1994; 37:S62.

263. Mortensen NJM, Ramirez JM, Takeuchi N, *et al*. Colonic J pouch-anal anastomosis after rectal excision for carcinoma: functional outcome. Br J Surg 1995; 82:611.

264. Ramirez JM, Mortensen NJM, Takeuchi N, *et al*. Colonic J-pouch rectal reconstruction: is it really a neorectum? Dis Colon Rectum 1996; 39:1286.

265. Seow-Choen F. Colonic pouches in the treatment of low rectal cancer. Br J Surg 1996; 83:881.

266. Wang J-Y, You Y-T, Chen H-H, *et al*. Stapled colonic J-pouch-anal anastomosis without a diverting colostomy for rectal carcinoma. Dis Colon Rectum 1997; 40:30.

267. Pélissier EP, Blum D, Bachour A, Bosset JF. Functional results of coloanal anastomosis with reservoir. Dis Colon Rectum 1992; 35:843.

268. Nicholls RJ, Lubowski DZ, Donaldson DR. Comparison of colonic reservoir and straight colo-anal reconstruction after rectal excision. Br J Surg 1988; 75:318.

269. Kusunoki M, Shoji Y, Yanagi H, *et al*. Function after anoabdominal rectal resection and colonic J pouch-anal anastomosis. Br J Surg 1991; 78:1434.

270. Hallböök O, Påhlman L, Krog M, *et al*. Randomized comparison of straight and colonic J pouch anastomosis after low anterior resection. Ann Surg 1996; 224:58.

Commentary

JOHN L ROMBEAU

In this commentary, I express my personal preferences concerning low anterior resection of the rectum in sphincter preservation.

FACTORS INFLUENCING THE CHOICE OF OPERATION

Fourteen factors are discussed in the choice of operation. The surgeon is often faced with a dilemma of evaluating a patient with several of these factors and 'weighting' each variable in terms of its potential effect on postoperative outcome. I agree with the authors of the chapter that the distance of the lower edge of the tumor from the anal verge is the most important variable in the decision about which operation to perform. Moreover, I concur that the use of a rigid proctosigmoidoscope is mandatory to correctly identify this distance. I have encountered numerous measurement inaccuracies when the level of the tumor was measured by using a flexible sigmoidoscope. Additionally, the authors note a very important measurement principle; namely, spreading the buttocks so the instrument can be measured from the side of the anus and not the buttock fat.

There is no universal agreement on preoperative testing in this patient population. The authors have carefully reviewed the many available tests, including their strengths and weaknesses. Clearly, the microscopic appearance of the tumor is an important variable. The authors correctly note that the more anaplastic the tumor, the more aggressive the resection and distal margin that is required for cure.

I believe transrectal ultrasound (TRUS) has provided a new and important advance in the decision-making process for these patients. Similar to other ultrasound examinations, its value is dependent upon the experience of the operator. As a result of the increased usage of preoperative radiation therapy, TRUS has become increasingly important in staging the tumor. In my practice, it is gaining importance, particularly in the identification of lymph nodal enlargement and penetration of the tumor through the bowel wall. Recently, I have noted it to be very helpful in assessing the depth of penetration within the bowel wall. I believe TRUS will continue to be used more frequently in the preoperative evaluation of patients with rectal cancer.

I obtain abdominal computerized axial tomography (CT scan) in every patient undergoing surgery for rectal cancer. I agree with the authors that the CT scan is not consistently effective in determining the depth of invasion of the rectal cancer; however, it is extremely valuable in identifying metastatic disease, particularly in the liver and extrahepatic soft tissues.

As noted, the positive emission tomography (PET) scan may be more sensitive and specific than CT scans in identifying preoperative metastatic disease. At our institution, this study is still in its experimental stage. Additionally, it is currently not cost-effective when compared to other modalities. Magnetic resonance imaging (MRI) with the use of the endorectal coil has not provided an additional advantage beyond the use of TRUS at our institution.

The authors briefly mention the patient's body habitus and gender as important variables in the decision-making process. Anastomoses can, indeed, be performed lower and more easily in women and thin patients.

In summary, many variables determine whether a sphincter-saving operation can be performed safely and effectively. The judgment and experience of the surgeon are extremely important factors in the decision-making process. Because of the many preoperative variables influencing clinical outcome, it is recommended that each patient be individualized rather than subjected exclusively to a 'cookbook' decision-making process.

LOW ANTERIOR RESECTION OF THE RECTUM

As mentioned, the most important determinant in performing this operation is the level of the inferior margin of the tumor. I believe that low anterior resection can be performed when the inferior level of the tumor is as low as 5 cm from the anal verge in women who are thin and in whom the tumor can be mobilized without considerable difficulty. The addition of a colonic J-pouch may improve the early functional outcome in these patients. Additionally, I perform a proximal diverting loop stoma in all patients with anastomoses within 5 cm from the anal verge.

Surgical technique is largely based upon training and personal experience. I believe the positioning of the patient is a very important and often underrated component of the operation. My preference is to begin the operation with the patient in the supine position, with repositioning into lithotomy following the rectal mobilization. I believe this reduces the possibility of a compartment syndrome secondary to prolonged positioning in lithotomy. Also, the primary surgeon, if right-handed, should be positioned on the left side of the patient. This position aids in manual dissection of the low rectum with the dominant right hand. If the surgeon is left-handed, the position is changed accordingly. My preference is to irrigate the rectum with saline prior to preparing the patient. Although I do not believe that this reduces the likelihood of spread of the cancer, it clearly leads to less fecal spillage in the event that the rectum is entered inadvertently during its dissection. Perhaps the most important reason for irrigating the rectum is so that the rectal tube can be left in place during the mobilization of the sigmoid colon and the upper rectum. This prevents residual colonic contents from pooling into the rectum, thereby aiding in the dissection. The rectal tube is then removed by the circulating nurse prior to mobilization of the low rectum.

As mentioned, there are no data to justify ligation of the inferior mesenteric artery at its origin. The decision about the extent and depth of the mesenteric dissection is often a difficult one, particularly in a young, thin, male. Permanent injury to the nervi erigentes may occur in these patients due to an overly extensive mesenteric resection. Moreover, it is estimated that at least 15–20 lymph nodes should be removed in order to adequately stage most rectal cancers. In young males, my tendency has been to err on the side of protecting the nerves in lieu of removing lymph nodes contiguous to the nerves.

Whether the complete sigmoid colon should be resected is also controversial. I tend to remove most of the sigmoid colon in order to facilitate the mesenteric resection of the upper rectum. This approach, in turn, requires mobilization of the splenic flexure in approximately 50% of patients to ensure a tension-free low colorectal anastomosis. I have a very low threshold for extending the midline incision and taking down the splenic flexure to prevent undue tension at the anastomosis.

As mentioned, the work by Heald and colleagues has popularized total mesorectal excision. Most importantly, this work has emphasized the need to widely resect the lateral margins of the perirectal tissue. I believe that the term 'total mesorectal excision' is a synonym for essentially the same resection that has been used by most well-trained colorectal and oncologic surgeons for many years.

I agree with the authors that there is no justification for removing the mesentery to the rectum distal to the anastomosis. I believe this is potentially dangerous and should not be performed due to the risk of ischemia.

My preference has been to use the double-stapled anastomotic technique, with the largest possible diameter of stapler. I rarely perform this operation with a stapler diameter less than 28 mm. The PI30 is particularly helpful in stapling across the lower rectum. If there is a question as to the initial placement of the stapler while the patient is supine, the stapler can be applied without firing. The patient is then placed into the lithotomy position and a rectal examination is performed to adequately assess the placement of the instrument. The stapler is then fired and a right-angle bowel clamp is placed proximal to the stapler, with the tumor and accompanying rectum and sigmoid colon removed en bloc. I agree with Fazio's 'truisms' concerning the stapling technique. I routinely check the circumferential nature of the excised 'doughnuts' and insufflate air into the rectum while the anastomosis is placed under water. If there is an anastomotic leak anteriorly, this can occasionally be 'patched' with interrupted 3-0 silk sutures. Occasionally, sutures can be placed transrectally, although this is often technically difficult. My preference has been to drain all of these low anastomoses.

I perform a diverting ostomy in all patients undergoing an anastomosis in the low rectum. My preference has been to use a diverting loop ileostomy rather than a colostomy, as this type of stoma is easier to close, less malodorous, and associated with fewer complications when compared to a transverse colostomy. Additionally, if the splenic flexure is taken down to reduce the likelihood of tension at the colorectal anastomosis, it is often more difficult to perform a proximal diverting colostomy because of the tension on the colonic mesentery.

My policy has been to place nasogastric tubes, for the first 24 h in most patients. Despite the absence of confirmatory data, I believe the tube reduces the amount of swallowed air and lessens the possibility of aspiration during the initial postoperative period. Our tendency has been to prescribe liquid diets at approximately 48 h postoperatively. I agree with leaving the indwelling urinary catheter for approximately 5 days after the operation. This practice reduces the discomfort due to impaired bladder emptying in these patients, who often have high urinary outputs during the first postoperative days.

Prevention is, indeed, the key to reducing postoperative complications. The time to prevent postoperative bleeding, tension-induced anastomotic leakage, and abdominal sepsis is at the time of the initial operation. The importance of spending more time at the initial operation to prevent these potentially major complications, rather than presuming that problems will not occur, cannot be emphasized enough.

A Hypaque enema is generally performed at approximately 6 weeks postoperatively. It is important to inform the radiologist as to the site of the anastomosis, in order that the enema catheter is not placed too proximally. If the x-ray is normal, the ileostomy is closed shortly thereafter. In patients in need of postoperative radiotherapy, the ileostomy is left in place for at least 6 weeks after the completion of chemoradiation therapy.

My results of reoperation in patients with pelvic recurrences have been discouraging. If the pelvic recurrence is extensive and the perineal pain significant, radiotherapy can occasionally lessen the pain.

As mentioned, the colonic J-pouch, when performed properly with limb lengths of 5 cm, will reduce the frequency of bowel movements during the first 2 years postoperatively. This benefit must be tempered against the potential for increased tension at the anastomosis by placing the anastomosis in the more proximal colon.

SUMMARY

In summary, sphincter-saving operations are being performed more frequently and efficaciously when compared to previous years. Similar to most types of surgery, the patients must be individualized, and clinical judgment remains an important determinant. When performed properly in well-selected patients, the operation, indeed, leads to improved quality of life and comparable survival when compared to abdominoperineal resections.

Editors' selected abstracts

Sexual dysfunction, informed consent and multimodality therapy for rectal cancer.

Chorost MI, Weber TK, Lee RJ, Rodriguez-Bigas MA, Petrelli NJ.

Department of Surgical Oncology, Roswell Park Cancer Institute, Buffalo, NY, USA.

American Journal of Surgery 179(4):271–4, 2000, April.

Background: This study assessed the presurgical and preradiation discussion of the risk of posttherapy sexual dysfunction among patients who underwent potentially curative therapy for rectal cancer. The incidence of sexual dysfunction after treatment for rectal cancer was then determined. *Methods:* A retrospective review of the medical records of 52 consecutive patients who underwent potentially curative procedures for rectal cancer within 15 cm from the anal verge was performed. *Results:* Presurgical discussion of the risk of sexual dysfunction was not documented in the consent in 37 of 52 patients (71%). Among the 5 males who underwent local excision, none reported posttherapy sexual dysfunction. Of the 6 males who were treated by low anterior resection, only 1 had a postoperative complaint of sexual dysfunction. Five of 15 males (33%) treated with abdominoperineal resection (APR) alone reported postprocedure sexual dysfunction, whereas 6 of 8 males (75%) treated with APR and radiation reported dysfunction. Of the entire female cohort, only 1 of the 16 reported sexual dysfunction posttherapy. *Conclusion:* A discussion of the risks of posttherapy sexual dysfunction was documented for fewer than one third of the patients. Among males after APR, the use of postoperative radiation showed a trend toward an increase in sexual dysfunction. Surgery and/or radiation therapy did not impact on sexual dysfunction in females.

Local excision of rectal cancer without adjuvant therapy: a word of caution.

Garcia-Aguilar J, Mellgren A, Sirivongs P, Buie D, Madoff RD, Rothenberger DA.

Department of Surgery, University of Minnesota Cancer Center, Minneapolis, MN, USA.

Annals of Surgery 231(3):345–51, 2000, March.

Objective: To evaluate the results of local excision alone for the treatment of rectal cancer, applying strict selection criteria. *Background data:* Several retrospective studies have demonstrated that tumor control in properly selected patients with rectal cancer treated locally is comparable to that observed after radical surgery. Although there is a consensus regarding the need for patient selection for local excision, the specific criteria vary among centers. *Methods:* The authors reviewed 82 patients with T1 (n = 55) and T2 (n = 27) rectal cancer treated with transanal excision only during a 10-year period. At pathologic examination, all tumors were localized to the rectal wall, had negative excision margins, were well or moderately differentiated, and had no blood or lymphatic vessel invasion, nor a mucinous component. End points were local and distant tumor recurrence and patient survival. *Results:* Ten of the 55 patients with T1 tumors (18%) and 10 of the 27 patients with T2 tumors (37%) had recurrence at 54 months of follow-up. Average time to recurrence was 18 months in both groups. Seventeen of the 20 patients with local recurrence underwent salvage surgery. The survival rate was 98% for patients with T1 tumors and 89% for patients with T2 tumors. Preoperative staging by endorectal ultrasound did not influence local recurrence or tumor-specific survival. *Conclusion:* Local excision of early rectal cancer, even in the ideal candidate, is followed by a much higher recurrence rate than previously reported. Although most patients in whom local recurrence develops can be salvaged by radical resection, the long-term outcome remains unknown.

Prospective trial of preoperative concomitant boost radiotherapy with continuous infusion 5-fluorouracil for locally advanced rectal cancer.

Janjan NA, Crane CN, Feig BW, Cleary K, Dubrow R, Curley SA, Ellis LM, Vauthey J, Lenzi R, Lynch P, Wolff R, Brown T, Pazdur R, Abbruzzese J, Hoff PM, Allen P, Brown B, Skibber J.

Department of Radiation Oncology, University of Texas, M.D. Anderson Cancer Center, Houston, TX, USA.

International Journal of Radiation Oncology, Biology, Physics 47(3):713–18, 2000, June 1.

Rationale: To evaluate the response to a concomitant boost given during standard chemoradiation for locally advanced rectal cancer. Methods and materials: Concomitant boost radiotherapy was administered preoperatively to 45 patients with locally advanced rectal cancer in a prospective trial. Treatment consisted of 45 Gy to the pelvis with 18 mV photons at 1.8 Gy/fraction using a 3-field belly board technique with continuous infusion 5FU chemotherapy (300 mg/m^2) 5 days per week. The boost was given during the last week of therapy with a 6-hour inter-fraction interval to the tumor plus a 2–3 cm margin. The boost dose equaled 7.5 Gy/5 fractions (1.5 Gy/fraction); a total dose of 52.5 Gy/5 weeks was given to the primary tumor. Pretreatment tumor stage, determined by endorectal ultrasound and CT scan, included 29 with T3N0 [64%], 11 T3N1, 1 T3Nx, 2 T4N0, 1 T4N3, and 1 with TxN1 disease. Mean distance from the anal verge was 5 cm (range 0–13 cm). Median age was 55 years (range 33–77 years). The population consisted of 34 males and 11 females. Median time of follow-up is 8 months (range 1–24 months). Results: Sphincter preservation (SP) has been accomplished in 33 of 42 (79%) patients resected to date. Three patients did not undergo resection because of the development of metastatic disease in the interim between the completion of chemoradiation (CTX/XRT) and preoperative evaluation. The surgical procedures included proctectomy and coloanal anastomosis ($n = 16$), low anterior resection ($n = 13$), transanal resection ($n = 4$). Tumor down-staging was pathologically confirmed in 36 of the 42 (86%) resected patients, and 13 (31%) achieved a pathologic CR. Among the 28 tumors (67%) located <6 cm from the anal verge, SP was accomplished in 21 cases (75%). Although perioperative morbidity was higher, toxicity rates during CTX/XRT were comparable to that seen with conventional fractionation. Compared to our contemporary experience with conventional CTX/XRT (45 Gy; 1.8 Gy per fraction), improvements were seen in SP (79% vs. 59%; $p = 0.02$), SP for tumors <6 cm from the anal verge (75% vs. 42%; $p = 0.003$), and down-staging (86% vs. 62%; $p = 0.003$). Conclusion: The SP rate with concomitant boost radiation has been highly favorable with rates of response which are higher than those previously reported for chemoradiation without administration of a boost. Further evaluation of this radiotherapeutic strategy appears warranted.

Anal sphincter conservation for patients with adenocarcinoma of the distal rectum: long-term results of Radiation Therapy Oncology Group Protocol 89-02.

Russell AH, Harris J, Rosenberg PJ, Sause WT, Fisher BJ, Hoffman JP, Kraybill WG, Byhardt RW.

Radiological Associates of Sacramento Medical Group, CA, USA.

International Journal of Radiation Oncology, Biology, Physics 46(2): 313–22, 2000, January 15.

Purpose: To assess the outcome of a multi-institutional, national cooperative group study attempting functional preservation of the anorectum for patients with limited, distal rectal cancer. Methods and materials: Between September 21, 1989 and November 1, 1992, a Phase II trial of sphincter-sparing therapy was conducted for patients with clinically mobile rectal cancers located below the pelvic peritoneal reflection. Protocol treatment was designed for patients who were, in the judgement of their attending surgeon, unsuitable for anal sphincter conservation in the context of anterior resection, and would have required abdominoperineal resection (APR) as conventional surgical therapy. Primary cancers were estimated to be 4 cm or less in largest clinical diameter, and occupied 40% or less of the rectal circumference. Chest radiography and computerized axial tomography (CT) of the abdomen and pelvis excluded patients with overt lymphatic or hematogenous metastases. Protocol surgery was intended to remove the primary cancer by en-bloc, transmural excision of an ellipse of rectal wall by transanal, transcoccygeal, or transsacral technique, while conserving the anal sphincter. Based on tumor size, T classification, grade, and adequacy of surgical margins, patients were allocated to one of three treatment assignments: observation, or adjuvant treatment with 5-fluorouracil (5-FU) and one of two different dose levels of local–regional radiation. After completion of protocol therapy, patients were observed with follow-up that included periodic general physical and rectal examination, determinations of CEA, abdominopelvic CT, chest radiography, and surveillance endoscopy. Sixty-five eligible and analyzable patients were registered. Results: With minimum follow-up of 5 years and median follow-up of 6.1 years, 11 patients have failed: 3 patients recurred local–regionally only, 3 patients had distant failure alone, and 5 patients manifested local–regional and distant failure. Eight patients died of intercurrent illness. Local–regional failure correlated with T-category revealed: T1 1/27 (4%), T2 4/25 (16%), and T3 3/13 (23%). Local–regional failure escalated with percentage involvement of the rectal circumference: 2/31 (6%) among patients with cancers involving 20% or less of the rectal circumference, and 6/34 (18%) among patients with cancers involving 21–40% of the circumference. Distant dissemination rose with T-category with 1/27 (4%) T1, 3/25 (12%) T2, and 4/13 (31%) T3 patients manifesting hematogenous spread. Eight patients (12%) required temporary or permanent colostomy. Five of 8 patients with local–regional recurrence achieved local–regional control with management including surgery, although 4 of these patients subsequently developed distant dissemination. Three patients (5%) had persistent, uncontrolled, local disease. Actuarial freedom from pelvic relapse at 5 years is 88% based on the entire study population, and 86% for the less favorable patients treated with adjuvant radiation and 5-FU. Conclusion: Conservative, sphincter-sparing therapy is a feasible alternative treatment for selected patients with limited cancer involving the middle and lower rectum. Risk of both local and distant failure appears to escalate with increasing T-category (depth of invasion). Results achieved in the multi-institutional, cooperative group setting approximate results reported from single institutions.

Functional and quality-of-life outcomes in patients with rectal cancer after combined modality therapy, intraoperative radiation therapy, and sphincter preservation.

Shibata D, Guillem JG, Lanouette N, Paty P, Minsky B, Harrison L, Wong WD, Cohen A.

Department of Surgery, Memorial Sloan-Kettering Cancer Center, New York, NY, USA.

Diseases of the Colon Rectum 43(6):752–8, 2000, June.

Purpose: Locally advanced primary and recurrent rectal cancers treated with external beam radiation therapy, intraoperative radiation therapy, and chemotherapy represent a complex group of patients in the setting of extensive pelvic surgery and sphincter preservation. We sought to define functional outcome and quality of life in this subset of patients. *Methods:* We retrospectively reviewed our experience with locally advanced primary and recurrent rectal cancer patients who underwent intraoperative radiation therapy with either low anterior resection ($n = 12$) or coloanal anastomosis ($n = 6$) between 1991 and 1998. Current functional outcome and quality of life were evaluated by a detailed questionnaire. *Results:* Median time from operation to assessment was 24 (range, 6–93) months. Using a standardized Sphincter Function Scale, incorporating the number of bowel movements per day and degree of incontinence, patients were graded as poor, fair, good, or excellent function. Of all patients, 56 percent reported unfavorable (poor or fair) function. Of the subset of patients with coloanal anastomosis or very low anterior resection, 88 percent had unfavorable function as compared with 30 percent with standard low anterior resection ($p = 0.02$; Fisher's exact probability test). A quality-of-life satisfaction score based on social, professional, and recreational restrictions demonstrated 56 percent of patients to be dissatisfied with their bowel function. *Conclusions:* The majority of patients with advanced rectal cancers who require external beam radiation therapy, extensive pelvic surgery, and intraoperative radiation therapy report unfavorable functional and quality-of-life outcomes after sphincter preservation. In this setting patients being considered for coloanal anastomosis or very low anterior resection may be better served by permanent diversion.

Impact of number of nodes retrieved on outcome in patients with rectal cancer.

Tepper JE, O'Connell MJ, Niedzwiecki D, Hollis D, Compton C, Benson AB 3rd, Cummings B, Gunderson L, Macdonald JS, Mayer RJ.

Department of Radiation Oncology, University of North Carolina, Chapel Hill, and Cancer and Leukemia Group B Statistical Office, Duke University Medical Center, Durham, NC, USA.

Journal of Clinical Oncology 19(1): 157–63, 2001, January 1.

Purpose: We postulated that the pathologic evaluation of the lymph nodes of surgical specimens from patients with rectal cancer can have a substantial impact on time to relapse and survival. *Patients and methods:* We analyzed data from 1,664 patients with T3, T4, or node-positive rectal cancer treated in a national intergroup trial of adjuvant therapy with chemotherapy and radiation therapy. Associations between the number of lymph nodes found by the pathologist in the surgical specimen and the time to relapse and survival outcomes were investigated. *Results:* Patients were divided into groups by nodal status and the corresponding quartiles of numbers of nodes examined. The number of nodes examined was significantly associated with time to relapse and survival among patients who were node-negative. For the first through fourth quartiles, the 5-year relapse rates were 0.37, 0.34, 0.26, and 0.19 ($p = 0.003$), and the 5-year survival rates were 0.68, 0.73, 0.72, and 0.82 ($p = 0.02$). No significant differences were found by quartiles among patients determined to be node-positive. We propose that observed differences are primarily related to the incorrect determination of nodal status in node-negative patients. Approximately 14 nodes need to be studied to define nodal status accurately. *Conclusion:* These results suggest that the pathologic assessment of lymph nodes in surgical specimens is often inaccurate and that examining greater number of nodes increases the likelihood of proper staging. Some patients who might benefit from adjuvant therapy are misclassified as node-negative due to incomplete sampling of lymph nodes.

25

Adjuvant and neoadjuvant therapy for colorectal carcinoma

GREGORY SARNA

INTRODUCTION

Whereas surgery is clearly the treatment modality with curative potential for locoregional colorectal carcinoma, there is a substantial failure rate of surgery alone in this setting.[1] Based upon SEER (*Surveillance, Epidemiology and End Results*) data[2] (1973–1987), 10-year survival for stage I (Dukes' A) colorectal cancer approximates 85%. For stage II (Dukes' B) it approximates 70%, and for stage III (Dukes' C) 40%. Five-year SEER survival figures,[2] broken down by colon versus rectal, are as follows: colon cancer: localized 92.5%, regional 62.9%; rectal cancer localized 86.6%, regional 52.5%. The latter figures are based on cases diagnosed from 1983 to 1990 and may reflect activity of adjuvant therapy in an undefined subset of patients. The 1983–1990 *overall* 5-year survival data (all stages) are superior to such data from 1974–1976 (preadjuvant therapy). Thus, 5-year survival has apparently improved with time, in colon cancer (all stages) moving from 50% to 60%, and in rectal cancer (all stages) moving from 48% to 58%. It is unclear how much of this improvement is due to adjuvant therapy, and how much is due to other factors (e.g., earlier diagnosis with lead time bias and change in stage mix, change in disease biology, change in surgical roles and techniques, change in staging with stage migration, change in treatment of advanced disease). Whereas the above figures suggest improvement in the survival of patients with colorectal cancer, there is still significant mortality for this disease, even in early stages. Colorectal cancer accounted for an estimated 55 000 deaths in the USA in 1995.[3] This was 10% of all cancer deaths, and second only to lung cancer. Five-year survival was estimated as 91% for localized disease (37% of cases) and 61% for regional disease (38% of cases). In addition to stage, other prognostic factors may identify patients with greater or lesser risk of recurrence, providing information of possible (but not proven) utility in assessing the indications for adjuvant therapy. Possible adverse risk factors would include, but are not limited to: aneuploidy and increased 'S' phase activity or increased proliferative index,[4,5] abnormal oncogene expression including p53[6,7] and loss of Bcl-2;[8] pathologic features including lymphatic invasion,[9] vascular invasion,[9] high histologic grade,[10] increasing numbers of involved lymph nodes,[11] thymidylate synthetase overexpression,[12] increased expression of CD44v6,[13] allelic loss of chromosome 18q (*DCC* gene),[14,15] high carcinoembryonic antigen (CEA)[16] level preoperatively, and bowel obstruction.[17]

ADJUVANT THERAPY: GENERAL CONSIDERATIONS

The term 'adjuvant therapy,' as applied to colorectal cancer, indicates the use of an additional non-surgical modality after surgical resection of all known disease. Such surgery would generally be resection of the primary tumor and of regional spread (if present). The term might be applied as well, however, after resection of all known metastases (e.g., hepatic). Adjuvant therapy would commonly be chemotherapy, but other modalities may also play roles. Radiation therapy would frequently be indicated in rectal cancer (but less commonly in colon cancer). Adjuvant therapy may, at least investigationally, be other therapy (e.g., immunotherapy). The logic of adjuvant therapy would be as follows:

1 The patient, based on clinical and pathologic findings, is determined to be at substantial risk of relapse, both locoregional and distant.
2 There exists non-surgical therapy which is active against metastatic, recurrent, or persistent cancer

(usually acting directly, possibly acting indirectly in the case of immunotherapy).

3 Such therapy may be more effective (and potentially curative) in a patient clinically disease free (but with undetected microscopic disease) than it would be in the setting of gross recurrence.

4 The adjuvant therapy is warranted on the basis of sufficient efficacy and acceptable toxicity. The benefits of treating those patients with occult disease outweigh the risks, costs, and other implications of treating those patients without occult disease.

There are abundant preclinical data and animal models supporting these concepts. There is a variety of biologic explanations for possible superior efficacy of a treatment modality in the setting of occult disease as compared to in the setting of gross recurrence.

These explanations include (but are not limited to) the following:

1 Less 'log kill' would be necessary to eradicate a small tumor burden or lower it to a threshold which can be controlled by host factors.

2 Early disease has had less time to acquire de novo drug (or radiation) resistance.

3 Early disease may have a higher growth fraction and be cytokinetically more sensitive to chemotherapy or radiation therapy.

4 Early disease may be better vascularized and better oxygenated, and may be more sensitive to chemotherapy or radiation therapy on those bases.

As a practical matter, in human tumors, there is a clear role for adjuvant therapy in a variety of malignancies including breast cancer, high-grade and intermediate-grade lymphomas, and ovarian carcinomas. There are increasing data supporting the role of adjuvant therapy in other cancers such as high-grade sarcomas and lung cancer.

NEOADJUVANT THERAPY: GENERAL CONSIDERATIONS

The term 'neoadjuvant therapy,' as applied to colorectal cancer, would indicate the use of treatment (usually chemotherapy and/or radiation therapy) prior to definitive surgery. As with adjuvant therapy (which may be part of a patient's regimen in addition to neoadjuvant therapy), this may have the goals of improving curability, disease-free survival or survival in a patient at high risk. It may also have the goal of facilitating surgery by shrinking tumors preoperatively, e.g., by improving operative exposure, by potentially improving margins, or perhaps by allowing a more conservative operation (for example avoiding an abdominoperineal resection in a patient with rectal cancer). The neoadjuvant approach is frequently employed in the treatment of head and neck and esophageal cancers, and sometimes in the treatment of

advanced lung and breast cancers. In general, however, survival benefit has not been clearly demonstrated with this approach (as compared to adjuvant therapy) and it is unclear whether or not margins or scope of surgery can, in fact, be properly modified.

EARLY ADJUVANT SYSTEMIC THERAPY STUDIES

Historically, attempts to treat resected colon carcinomas in the adjuvant setting have progressed from single-agent therapy, predominantly 5-fluorouracil (5-FU), also floxuridine (FUDR) and thiotepa, to combination therapy, usually based upon 5-FU. In early randomized controlled trials, single-agent studies of 5-FU generally showed a slight, perhaps clinically insignificant, benefit to therapy. Individual studies showed trends toward 'small' improvements in survival (e.g., 5% at 5 years),[18–23] which were generally not statistically significant taken singly. Early single-agent studies were also performed of thiotepa[21,24] and FUDR,[25,26] showing no benefit.

Early combination chemotherapy studies of both colon and rectal carcinoma using MOF – 5-FU plus vincristine plus methyl-CCNU (semustine) – showed a slight advantage to treatment. This, however, was associated with a small risk of iatrogenic myelodysplasia or acute leukemia atributable to methyl-CCNU,[27,28] and a subsequent study of radiation therapy and 5-FU plus or minus methyl-CCNU in rectal cancer showed no benefit to the methyl-CCNU group.[29] Early studies of immunotherapy, including BCG[27] and levamisole (alone),[30,31] showed no clear benefit.

In 1988, Buyse et al.[32] performed a meta-analysis of controlled trials of adjuvant treatment of colorectal cancer (published up to 1987). In that pooled analysis, they found that adjuvant chemotherapy with 5-FU alone or in combination decreased the odds of death by 10% and increased 5-year survival by 2.3–5.7%. When only long-term (>1 year) programs were considered, the odds of death were decreased by 17%, but 5-year survival was increased only by 3.4%. Overall, 5-FU-based therapy (as used up to the mid 1980s) can be viewed as being of small benefit, arguably not worth the risks and side-effects of treatment. More recent adjuvant chemotherapy, based upon 5-FU plus levamisole or 5-FU plus leucovorin, appears to be of greater value.

RECENT STUDIES OF ADJUVANT THERAPY IN COLON CANCER

5-Fluorouracil plus levamisole

Despite data indicating no advantage to levamisole as single-agent adjuvant therapy in colorectal cancer,[31] and

Table 25.1 *Data from intergroup study of adjuvant 5-FU/levamisole for stage III colon cancer*[33]

	Levamisole/5-FU	Levamisole	No therapy
Recurrence rate (observed) (%)	39	55	56
Recurrence rate (actuarial) (%)	41	58	65
Death rate (absolute) (%)	40	51	53
Death rate (actuarial) (%)	44	64	68

Table 25.2 *Adjuvant studies of 5-FU/leucovorin in colon cancer*

Study group	Number of patients	Control group Treatment	Follow-up (years)	Disease-free survival 5-FU/CF vs control (%)	Survival 5-FU/CF vs control (%)
NSABP[42]	1081 (292 B, 739 C)	MeCCNU, VCR, 5-FU	3	B: 87 vs 82 C: 67 vs 58	B: 95 vs 93 C: 79 vs 71
Intergroup[43]	309 (57 B, 252 C)	No therapy	5	74 vs 58	74 vs 63
Francini[44] (Italy)	239 (121 B2, 118 C)	No therapy	4.5	B2: 83 vs 77 C: 66 vs 41	B2: 89 vs 86 C: 69 vs 43
'IMPACT'[45,46]	1668 (1016 B2, 652 C)	No therapy	5 3	B2[a]: 76 vs 73 C[a]: 76 vs 64	B2: 82 vs 80 C: 62 vs 42

[a]Event-free survival.
Abbreviations: see text for explanations.

no advantage to adding levamisole to 5-FU in the therapy of advanced disease, 5-FU combined with levamisole appears to have value as an adjuvant treatment. The original postulated mechanism of action for levamisole was immunoaugmentation. It is not clear whether the putative role of levamisole in this therapy is due to such action or to an alternative mechanism such as pharmacologic modulation of 5-FU. The largest experience with 5-FU/levamisole comes from two large intergroup trials. Moertel *et al.* reported on an intergroup study of over 900 patients with stage III disease, followed for a median of 6.5 years.[33] In this study, adjuvant 5-FU plus levamisole was compared to levamisole alone or no therapy. The combined-therapy group had a substantial decrease in both recurrence rate (by approximately 40%) and death rate (by approximately 33%) as compared to no therapy, with levamisole alone showing little or no benefit (Table 25.1). These data confirmed a smaller but substantial study (401 patients including 21 with rectal cancer) from the North Central Cancer Treatment Group and the Mayo Clinic,[34] which showed comparable results (for Dukes' C disease, 50% recurrence and 45% death rate with 5-FU/levamisole versus 65% recurrence rate and 58% death rate with no therapy). It should be noted, however, that a smaller (185 patient) Italian study[35] recently showed no benefit for 5-FU plus levamisole as compared to 5-FU alone, raising issues as to the putative role of levamisole. In a second intergroup trial, a parallel study of stage II disease,[36] 318 patients were randomized to 5-FU/levamisole or no therapy. After a median follow-up of 7 years, relapse rate was decreased by about 31%, but

survival was not improved. While that study raises questions about the role of adjuvant chemotherapy in stage II disease, an analysis of over 1500 patients with Dukes' B colon cancer entered in four different National Surgical Adjuvant Breast and Bowel Project (NSABP) studies[37,38] had different results. That analysis suggested comparable benefits in Dukes' B colon cancer to that seen in Dukes' C disease. Pooled data, with a variety of regimens, indicated a 30% decrease in mortality in Dukes' B disease and an 18% decrease in mortality in Dukes' C disease. These results, however, are not supported by studies of 5-FU/leucovorin as adjuvant therapy for Dukes' B disease (see below). Toxicity of levamisole generally includes nausea, occasional emesis, rash, fatigue, arthralgias, dysgeuzia, and alcohol intolerance. In addition, rare neurotoxicity (dementia or leukoencephalopathy) has been reported.[39] It is also of note that one study comparing levamisole to placebo reported increased late mortality in the levamisole group.[31]

5-Fluorouracil plus leucovorin

Leucovorin (folinic acid, citrovorum factor) has been shown to biomodulate 5-FU and to improve response rates in metastatic disease,[40] although the impact on survival may be marginal.[41] In the adjuvant setting, leucovorin-modulated 5-FU, like 5-FU and levamisole, appears to be of value. Table 25.2 presents results of four pertinent studies.[42–46] All studies show improvement in both survival and disease-free survival in stage C disease;

benefit is not clearly demonstrated in stage B disease. Three of the four studies use a no-treatment control group; the NSABP study uses as the control an MOF regimen (see above).

5-Fluorouracil/levamisole versus 5-fluorouracil/leucovorin

The above-cited data indicate some benefit for both 5-FU/levamisole and 5-FU/leucovorin in the adjuvant setting (at least for Dukes' C disease). More recent studies compare (or combine) these two approaches. The NASBP[47] compared three regimens – 5-FU/leucovorin, 5-FU/levamisole, and 5-FU levamisole/leucovorin – in over 2000 patients with Dukes' B and C disease. In this study, preliminary data (median follow-up 5 years) show no advantage to levamisole and show possible superiority of the leucovorin-containing arms. The North Central Cancer Treatment Group and the National Cancer Institute (NCI) Canada entered approximately 900 patients in a study comparing 5-FU/levamisole to 5-FU/ levamisole/leucovorin and comparing 6 months to 12 months of therapy in each arm.[48] Survival with 6 months of 5-FU/levamisole was inferior to that with 6 months of 5-FU/levamisole/leucovorin, and there was no difference seen between the 6-month, three-drug regimen and either 12-month regimen. An intergroup study[49] of almost 4000 patients compared 5-FU/levamisole to 5-FU/high-dose leucovorin, compared 5-FU/high-dose leucovorin to 5-FU/low-dose leucovorin, and compared 5-FU/low-dose leucovorin to 5-FU/low-dose leucovorin plus levamisole. No differences were seen in these comparisons. Overall, it appears that 5-FU/leucovorin is as good as 5-FU/leucovorin/levamisole or 5-FU/levamisole. It may allow shorter therapy (e.g., 6 months) than the original levamisole regimen, and it may avoid levamisole toxicity.

Fluoropyrimidines by alternative routes

The approaches cited above use adjuvant therapy based upon intravenous 5-FU. Alternative routes of adjuvant therapy – intrahepatic arterial, intraportal vein, intraperitoneal – have also been studied. Intrahepatic arterial adjuvant therapy, primarily based upon FUDR rather than 5-FU, has been used as adjuvant therapy primarily following the resection of liver metastases. This has been used both with[50,51] and without[52–54] additional intravenous adjuvant therapy. The results of randomized studies are mixed. A German study of 226 patients found no benefit from adjuvant intrahepatic arterial 5-FU plus leucovorin after resection of liver metastases.[55] An Intergroup study of 109 patients found an improved recurrence-free rate (58% versus 34%) with adjuvant intrahepatic FUDR and systemic infusion of 5-FU as

compared to surgery alone.[56] Survival, however, was not significantly improved, although a trend existed. A Memorial Sloan-Kettering study compared adjuvant hepatic arterial FUDR plus infusional 5-FU/leucovorin to infusional 5-FU/leucovorin alone.[57] The combined intra-arterial and intravenous approach improved 2-year survival (85% versus 69%) and hepatic disease-free survival (86% versus 57%). Overall, these data argue in a preliminary fashion for a role for intra-arterial FUDR but not intra-arterial 5-FU, in this setting.

Portal vein adjuvant chemotherapy has been used, based upon the premise that newly established hepatic micrometastases may be preferentially vascularized by the portal system rather than the hepatic arterial system. A meta-analysis of approximately 3800 patients in nine randomized trials comparing portal vein therapy (generally perioperative 5-FU) with no therapy has been performed.[58] This analysis found a 13% decrease overall in 5-year death rate with treatment (24% versus 30% in Dukes' B, 47% versus 57% in Dukes' C). Disease-free survival and time to relapse were also shown to be improved. Not all studies, however, show benefit,[59–62] and it is not clear that hepatic metastases are decreased in frequency.[63,64] While there may be efficacy to adjuvant portal vein therapy as compared to no treatment, it is not clear that the portal vein route offers an advantage over systemic adjuvant therapy. An Italian study of 1199 patients, which compared intraportal adjuvant therapy to systemic adjuvant therapy to both intraportal and systemic adjuvant therapy, found no significant difference among the three arms. Intraperitoneal therapy (e.g., with 5-FU) is also being studied as an adjuvant. It is hoped that this would decrease the risk of peritoneal, mesenteric, and omental tumor seeding. This approach appears feasible.[65] Results of a randomized study[66] comparing intravenous 5-FU plus levamisole to intravenous and intraperitoneal 5-FU plus levamisole indicated a lower relapse rate with the intravenous/intraperitoneal approach in stage III but not in stage II disease. This should be interpreted, however, with consideration that 6 months of 5-FU plus levamisole may be an inadequate control. More data and longer follow-up are necessary to evaluate the role of this approach.

Immunotherapy

Immunotherapy in the adjuvant setting for colorectal cancer has been studied. Whereas levamisole may enhance the effects of adjuvant 5-FU, most studies of adjuvant levamisole alone have not shown benefit.[30,31,34] BCG, too, has failed to show clear benefit as adjuvant non-specific immunotherapy.[67,68] Tumor vaccines have also been studied as adjuvant therapy for colorectal cancer. Whereas data showing some benefit for this approach in colon, but not rectal, cancer have been reported,[69] those data are inconclusive,[70] and other trials

Table 25.3 *Adjuvant radiation in B3 and C3 colon cancer*[76]*

Stage	Surgery alone			Surgery + Radiation		
	Number of patients	5-year local relapse rate (%)	5-year relapse-free survival (%)	Number of patients	5-year local relapse rate (%)	5 year relapse-free survival (%)
B3	83	31	63	54	7	79
C3	49	53	38	39	28	53

*Historical data.

have been negative[71] or are at too early a stage for evaluation.[72] Monoclonal antibody therapy, using a '17-1A antibody' (Panorex), has been reported to be of benefit in Dukes' C colon cancer. Riethmuller *et al.*[73] studied monoclonal antibody 17-1 A adjuvant therapy versus no therapy in 189 such patients, and reported an approximately 30% decrease in both mortality and recurrence at 5 years. Further studies of this approach will be of interest. Interferon-alpha when combined with 5-FU, has received study in the adjuvant setting. No clear advantage is seen to this approach.[74,75]

Radiation therapy

Radiation therapy as an adjuvant therapy has received less study in colon cancer than in rectal cancer (see below), presumably because of the decreased importance of local recurrence (versus systemic recurrence) in colon cancer and the increased toxicity of wide-field abdominal radiation. Nevertheless, selected patients with locally advanced colon cancer have a high risk of local recurrence, and radiation may be reasonable in this setting. In a historically controlled study,[76] 173 patients with colon (not rectal) cancer were treated with adjuvant radiation therapy. Of these patients, 63 had chemotherapy as well, usually 5-FU daily × 3 in the first and last weeks of radiation. These groups were compared to a historical control of 395 patients. In the control groups, high local failure rates were seen in those with B3 and C3 disease (transmural with adherence to or invasion of adjacent structures, essentially T4). In the B3/C3 radiation group, local recurrence rate decreased and relapse-free survival improved (Table 25.3). Local recurrences were fewer with surgery alone in B2 (10%) and C2 patients (36%), and there was no clear benefit to radiation in those groups (9% and 30% local recurrences, respectfully). Pilot studies of adjuvant whole abdominal radiation plus infusional 5-FU have been performed by the Southwest Oncology Group (SWOG).[77] However, a randomized study (Intergroup 0130), comparing 5-FU/levamisole to 5-FU/levamisole plus radiation for B3 and C3 colon carcinomas, has recently reported negative results, with no significant improvement in relapses or death rates in the radiation therapy arm.[78]

Conclusions: colon cancer

1 Adjuvant chemotherapy is of value for Dukes' C colon cancer, with 5-FU/leucovorin for 6 months one of several reasonable choices.
2 Adjuvant chemotherapy may or may not be of value in Dukes' B colon cancer (or high-risk subsets thereof). Further studies and longer term analysis may be helpful in clarifying this issue.
3 Local irradiation may play a role in B3 and C3 disease (T4 tumors), but data supporting these are limited and historically controlled, while a randomized study is negative.

STUDIES OF ADJUVANT THERAPY IN RECTAL CANCER

Rectal carcinoma differs clinically from colon carcinoma in several ways. Survival and disease-free survival are poorer for rectal carcinoma both overall and stage for stage[79] (Table 25.4). Rectal carcinoma is more likely than colon cancer to recur locally, and the first site of distant metastasis for rectal cancer is less likely to be liver. These data would suggest, perhaps, that adjuvant chemotherapy might have a greater potential role in Dukes' B rectal cancer than in Dukes' B colon cancer, that radiation might play a greater role as adjuvant therapy in rectal cancer than colon cancer, and that there would be less rationale with rectal cancer for intrahepatic arterial or for intraportal vein therapy.

Adjuvant radiation therapy

Adjuvant radiation therapy by itself, preoperative[80,81] (neoadjuvant) or postoperative,[82–84] or both ('sandwich' technique), is of value in decreasing local recurrence rate by about 20–50%, albeit with little impact on survival (possibly more impact on survival with the sandwich approach).[85–88] It should be noted, however, that regardless of impact on mortality, the improvement in *morbidity* due to a lower local recurrence rate warrants the adjunctive use of radiation, at least in stage II (Dukes' B) or greater rectal cancer.

Table 25.4 *Outcome data after surgery alone*[79]

	Colon cancer (n = 279)	Rectal cancer (n = 293)
Overall 5-year survival (%)	80	60
Overall 5-year disease-free survival (%)	76	60
5-year disease-free survival (%)		
Dukes' A	92	84
Dukes' B	88	63
Dukes' C	54	39
First recurrence local (%)	16	31
First recurrence liver (%)	36	25

Adjuvant chemotherapy

Because of the accepted value of adjuvant radiation therapy in the treatment of rectal carcinoma, most modern adjuvant chemotherapy trials have focused on chemotherapy plus radiation therapy rather than chemotherapy alone. There are, however, some older studies of adjuvant treatment for rectal cancer which compare chemotherapy alone to no therapy. Examples would be an NSABP study of methyl-CCNU, vincristine and 5-FU[26] and a Gastrointestinal Tumor Study Group (GITSG) study of 5-FU and methyl-CCNU.[89] These studies tended to show modest improvement in disease-free and overall survival with chemotherapy as compared to no therapy. However, a more modern study from the Netherlands[90] of 5-FU/ levasimole failed to show benefits in rectal cancer.[90]

Adjuvant chemotherapy plus radiation therapy

Combined modality adjuvant therapy for resected rectal cancer has been the dominant approach in recent years. The definitive randomized studies comparing this approach to no adjuvant therapy come from the GITSG,[89,91] which compared 5-FU/methyl-CCNU/ radiation to 5-FU/methyl-CCNU alone, radiation alone, and no adjuvant therapy. Survival was best in the combined modality arm (59% versus 44% no therapy, 52% radiation therapy alone, 50% chemotherapy alone), as was local recurrence rate (11% versus 24% no therapy, 20% radiation alone, 27% chemotherapy alone). Subsequent studies, as previously discussed,[29,92] have shown that methyl-CCNU adds little to the regimen and, given its leukemogenic potential, generally should be avoided. Other large, randomized studies have compared the combined modality approach to either radiation alone or chemotherapy alone in rectal cancer. The North Central Cancer Treatment Group[93] studied 204 patients with rectal cancer and compared radiation therapy alone to a regimen of 5-FU/methyl-CCNU followed by further combined radiation/5-FU followed by 5-FU/methyl-CCNU.

The combined approach, when compared to radiation therapy alone, decreased 5-year recurrence rates from 63% to 42% and improved 5-year survival from approximately 37% to approximately 55%. How best to administer combined modality adjuvant therapy is uncertain. As mentioned above, methyl-CCNU does not appear to add meaningfully to 5-FU and probably can be avoided. Infusional 5-FU may be superior to bolus 5-FU,[92] but it requires an indwelling venous access and a pump for outpatient administration. Because 5-FU plus levamisole appears superior to (bolus) 5-FU as adjuvant therapy in colon cancer, and because 5-FU/leucovorin appears superior to (bolus) 5-FU for colon cancer in the adjuvant and advanced settings, it is logical to explore whether these approaches should be combined with radiation in rectal cancer. This issue is being addressed by Intergroup trial 0114,[94,95] which keeps radiation constant and compares four variants of adjuvant chemotherapy: bolus 5-FU alone; 5-FU plus leucovorin; 5-FU plus levamisole; and 5-FU plus leucovorin plus levamisole. In a preliminary report of approximately 1700 patients, the three-drug regimen resulted in more high-grade diarrhea, and more treatment-related deaths than 5-FU alone. There is to date no evidence of improved results with any combination regimen as compared to 5-FU alone.

Neoadjuvant therapy

Preoperative therapy, with radiation plus or minus chemotherapy, has conceptual appeal in the treatment of rectal carcinoma. Radiation prior to surgery should be less toxic to the small bowel as loops of small bowel would not be expected to be fixed in the pelvic radiation field. Preoperative therapy arguably may increase the resectability of locally advanced disease and may allow sphincter-saving procedures in otherwise marginal patients. With these benefits in mind, neoadjuvant radiation therapy and combined chemotherapy/radiation therapy have been studied. Frykholm *et al.*[96] have reported on 471 patients with rectal or rectosigmoid cancer randomized to preoperative versus postoperative radiation. With the preoperative approach, they found a lower local recurrence rate (13% versus 22%), and fewer episodes of small-bowel obstruction (5% versus 11%), but no differences in survival. Preoperative combined modality therapy, using 5-FU/leucovorin plus radiation, has been compared to the same regimen postoperatively in a synchronous but non-randomized trial.[97] The preoperative approach allowed greater dose intensity with less severe toxicity. Efficacy data were not evaluable. A mitomycin C, 5-FU, leucovorin plus radiation neoadjuvant regimen[98] has also been studied, with a 42% histologic response rate. A 5-FU/leucovorin plus cisplatin neoadjuvant regimen[99] has been compared with historical controls who received postoperative radiation therapy plus 5-FU. In this study, no differences were seen.

Conclusions: rectal cancer

1 Adjuvant chemotherapy/radiation therapy is of value for at least Dukes' B2 and C rectal cancer. Arguably, superior results have been reported with the North Central Cancer Treatment Group regimen[92] of bolus 5-FU on days 1–5, and days 36–40; 4500 cGy radiation therapy plus infusional 5-FU over 5 weeks starting on day 64, and further bolus 5-FU on days 134–138 and 169–173. Other regimens, such as 4140 cGy of radiation with bolus 5-FU on the first 3 days and last 3 days of treatment,[29] may be simpler and certainly acceptable. There is currently no need to use 5-FU/leucovorin or 5-FU/levamisole.

2 Neoadjuvant combined modality therapy appears at this point to be an acceptable alternative, perhaps preferable in those with bulky disease or borderline resectability via a low anterior approach.

FUTURE CONSIDERATIONS

As ongoing and future clinical trials evolve, data should emerge which better answer the following questions:

1 Who is a candidate for adjuvant or neoadjuvant therapy, based upon both stage and other independent prognostic factors (histologic, chromosomal, molecular biologic, etc.)?

2 Which approach is superior: adjuvant, neoadjuvant, or both?

3 Which regimen is preferable: 5-FU bolus, 5-FU infusion, 5-FU/levamisole, 5-FU/leucovorin, or other?

4 How best should radiation therapy be given with chemotherapy? Additionally, new chemotherapeutic agents are appearing with activity in colorectal cancer, either alone (e.g., irinotecan or CPT-11,[100,101] tomudex[102]), or in combination with 5-FU (e.g., oxaliplatin[103]). These drugs will probably merit study in the adjuvant setting, as will capecitabine, an oral prodrug of 5-FU.[104]

REFERENCES

1. Beahrs OH, Henson DE, Hutter RVP, Kennedy BJ (eds). *Manual for staging of cancer*, 4th edition. Philadelphia, JB Lippincott & Co, 1992, 76.

2. Gloeckler LA ed. *SEER cancer statistics review 1973–1991*. USDHHS, PHS, NIH, NIH publication No. 94–2789, 1994.

3. Wingo PA, Tong T, Bolden BA. Cancer statistics, 1995. CA A Cancer J Clin 1995; 45:8–30.

4. Moertel CG, Loprinzi CL, Witzig TE, *et al.* The dilemma of stage B2 colon cancer. Is adjuvant therapy justified? Proc Am Soc Clin Oncol 1990; 9:108.

5. Albe X, Vassilakos P, Helfer-Guarnori K, *et al.* Independent prognostic value of ploidy in colorectal cancer. Cancer 1990; 66:1168–75.

6. Zeng Z-S, Sarkis AS, Zhang ZF, *et al.* P53 nuclear overexpression: an independent prediction of survival in lymph node-positive colorectal cancer patients. J Clin Oncol 1994; 12:2043–50.

7. Bosari S, Viale G, Bossi P, *et al.* Cytoplasmic accumulation of P53 protein: an independent prognostic indicator in colorectal adenocarcinomas. J Natl Cancer Inst 1994; 86:681–7.

8. Ilyas M, Hao XP, Wilkinson K, *et al.* Loss of Bcl-2 expression correlates with tumor recurrence in colorectal cancer. Gut 1998; 43(3):383–7.

9. Minsky BD, Mies C, Rich TA, Recht A. Lymphatic vessel invasion is an independent prognostic factor for survival in colorectal cancer. Int J Radiat Oncol Biol Phys 1989; 17:311–18.

10. Chapuis PH, Dent OF, Fisher R, *et al.* A multivariate analysis of clinical and pathological variables in prognosis after resection of large bowel cancer. Br J Surg 1985; 72:698–702.

11. Willett CG, Tepper JE, Chen AM, *et al.* Failure patterns following curative resection of colonic carcinoma. Ann Surg 1984; 200:685–90.

12. Johnston PG, Fisher CR, Rockett HE, *et al.* The role of thymidylate synthetase expression in prognosis and outcome of adjuvant chemotherapy in patients with rectal cancer. J Clin Oncol 1994; 12:2640–7.

13. Mulder JW, Kruyt PM, Sewnath M, *et al.* Colorectal cancer prognosis and expression of exon-V6-containing CD44 proteins. Lancet 1994; 44:1470–2.

14. Jen J, Hoguen K, Piantadosi S, *et al.* Allelic loss of chromosome 18q and prognosis in colon cancer. N Engl J Med 1994; 331:213–21.

15. Shibata D, Reale MA, Lavin P, *et al.* The DCC protein and prognosis in colorectal cancer. N Engl J Med 1996; 335:1727–32.

16. Wolmark N, Fisher B, Wieland S, *et al.* The prognostic significance of preoperative carcinoembryonic antigen levels in colorectal cancer. Ann Surg 1984; 199:375–81.

17. Crucitti F, Sofo L, Doglietto GB, *et al.* Prognostic factors in colorectal cancer: current status and new trends. J Surg Oncol Suppl. 1991; 2:76–82.

18. Higgins GA, Dwight RW, Smith JV, *et al.* Fluorouracil as an adjuvant to surgery in carcinoma of the colon. Arch Surg 1971; 102:339–43.

19. Higgins GA Jr, Humphrey E, Juler GL, *et al.* Adjuvant chemotherapy in the surgical treatment of large bowel cancer. Cancer 1976; 38:1461–7.

20. Higgins GA, Dwight RW, Walsh WS, *et al.* Preoperative radiation therapy as an adjuvant to surgery for carcinoma of the colon and rectum. Am J Surg 1968; 115:241–6.

21. Higgins GA, Donaldson RC, Humphrey EW, *et al.* Adjuvant therapy for large bowel cancer. Update of

Veterans Administration Surgical Oncology Group trials. Surg Clin North Am 1981; 61:1311–20.

22. Grage TB, Hill GJ, Cornell GN, *et al*. Adjuvant chemotherapy in large bowel cancer – updated analysis of single agent chemotherapy. In: Jones SE, Salmon SE, eds. *Adjuvant therapy of cancer II*. New York, Grune & Stratton, 1979, 587–94.

23. Grage TB, Moss SE. Adjuvant chemotherapy in cancer of the colon and rectum: demonstration of effectiveness of prolonged 5-FU chemotherapy in a prospectively controlled, randomized trial. Surg Clin North Am 1981; 61:1321–9.

24. Dixon WJ, Longmire WP Jr, Holden WD. Use of triethylenethiophosphoramide as an adjuvant to the surgical treatment of gastric and colorectal carcinoma: ten-year follow-up. Ann Surg 1971; 173:26–39.

25. Veterans Administration Adjuvant Cancer Chemotherapy Cooperative Group. The use of 5-fluorodeoxyuridine (FUDR) as a surgical adjuvant in carcinoma of the stomach and colorectum. Arch Surg 1963; 86:926–31.

26. Dwight RW, Humphrey EW, Higgins GA, *et al*. FUDR as an adjuvant to surgery in cancer of the large bowel. J Surg Oncol 1973; 5:243–9.

27. Fisher B, Wolmark N, Rockette H, *et al*. Postoperative adjuvant chemotherapy or radiation therapy for rectal cancer. Results from NSABP protocol R-01. J Natl Cancer Inst 1988; 80:21–9.

28. Wolmark N, Fisher B, Rockette H, *et al*. Postoperative adjuvant chemotherapy or BCG for colon cancer: results from NSABP protocol C-01. J Natl Cancer Inst 1988; 80:30–6.

29. Gastrointestinal Tumor Study Group. Radiation therapy and fluorouracil with or without semustine for the treatment of patients with surgical adjuvant adenocarcinoma of the rectum. J Clin Oncol 1992; 10:549–57.

30. Arnaud JP, Buyse M, Nordlinger B, *et al*. Adjuvant chemotherapy of poor prognosis colon cancer with levamisole: results of an EORTC double-blind randomized clinical trial. Br J Surg 1989; 76:284–9.

31. Chlebowski RT, Lillington L, Nystrom JS, Sayre J. Late mortality and levamisole adjuvant therapy in colorectal cancer. Br J Cancer 1994; 69:1094–7.

32. Buyse M, Zeleniuch-Jacquotte A, Chalmers T. Adjuvant therapy of colorectal cancer. JAMA 1988; 259:3571–8.

33. Moertel CG, Fleming TR, MacDonald JS, *et al*. Fluorouracil plus levamisole as effective adjuvant therapy after resection of stage III colon carcinoma: a final report. Ann Int Med 1995; 122:321–6.

34. Laurie JA, Moertel CG, Fleming TR, *et al*. Surgical adjuvant therapy of large-bowel carcinoma: an evaluation of levamisole and the combination of levamisole and fluorouracil. J Clin Oncol 1989; 7:1447–56.

35. Cascinu S, Catalano L, Latini G, *et al*. A randomized trial of adjuvant therapy of stage III colon cancer: levamisole and 5-fluorouracil versus 5-fluorouracil alone. Proc Am Soc Clin Oncol 18:240 (Abstract 923).

36. Moertel CG, Fleming TR, MacDonald JS, *et al*. Intergroup study of fluorouracil plus levamisole as adjuvant therapy for stage II/Dukes' B2 colon cancer. J Clin Oncol 1995; 13:2936–43.

37. Mamounas EP, Rockette H, Jones J, *et al*. Comparative efficacy of adjuvant chemotherapy in patients with Dukes' B vs Dukes' C colon cancer: result from four NSABP adjuvant studies (C-01, C-02, C-03, C-04). Proc Am Soc Clin Oncol 1996; 15:205 (Abstract 461).

38. Mamounas E, Wieand S, Wolmark N, *et al*. Comparative efficacy of adjuvant chemotherapy in patients with Duke's B vs Duke's C colon cancer: results from four National Surgical Adjuvant Breast and Bowel Project adjuvant studies (C-01, C-02, C-03, C-04). J Clin Oncol 1999; 17:1349–55.

39. Figueredo AT, Fawcets E, Molloy DW, Dombranowski J, Paulseth JE. Disabling encephalopathy during 5-fluorouracil and levamisole adjuvant therapy for resected colorectal cancer: a report of two cases. Cancer Invest 1995; 13:608–11.

40. Advanced Colorectal Cancer Meta-Analysis Project. Modulation of fluorouracil by leucovorin in patients with advanced colorectal cancer: evidence in terms of response rate. J Clin Oncol 1992; 10:896–903.

41. Poon MA, O'Connel MJ, Wieand HS, *et al*. Biochemical modulator of fluorouracil with leucovorin: confirmatory evidence of improved therapeutic efficacy in advanced colorectal cancer. J Clin Oncol 1991; 9:1967–7.

42. Wolmark N, Rockette H, Fisher B, *et al*. The benefits of leucovorin – modulated fluorouracil as postoperative adjuvant therapy for primary colon cancer: results from National Surgical Adjuvant Breast and Bowel Protocol C-03. J Clin Oncol 1993; 11:1879–87.

43. O'Connell M, Mailliard J, Kahn MJ, *et al*. Controlled trial of fluorouracil and low-dose leucovorin given for 6 months as postoperative adjuvant therapy for colon cancer. J Clin Oncol 1997; 15:246–50.

44. Francini G, Petrioli R, Lorenzini L, *et al*. Folinic acid and 5 fluorouracil as adjuvant chemotherapy in colon cancer. Gastroenterology 1994; 106:899–906.

45. IMPACT Investigators. Efficacy of adjuvant fluorouracil and folinic acid in colon cancer. Lancet 1995; 345:939–44.

46. IMPACT B2 Investigators. Efficacy of adjuvant fluorouracil and folinic acid in B2 colon cancer. J Clin Oncol 1999; 17:1356–63.

47. Wolmark N, Rockette H, Mamounas EP, *et al*. The relative efficacy of 5-FU + leucovorin (FU-LV),

5-FU + levamisole (5-FU-LEV), and 5-FU leucovorin + levamisole (5-FU-LU–LEV) in patients with Dukes' B and C carcinoma of the colon: first report of NSABP C-04. Proc Am Soc Clin Oncol 1996; 15:205 (Abstract 460).

48. O'Connell MJ, Laurie JA, Kahn M, et al. Prospective randomized trial of postoperative adjunct chemotherapy in patients with high-risk colon cancer. J Clin Oncol 1998; 16:295–300.

49. Haller DG, Catalano PJ, MacDonald JS, Mayer RJ. Fluorouracil (FU) leucovorin (LV) and levamisole adjuvant therapy for colon cancer: preliminary result INT-0089. Proc Am Soc Clin Oncol 1996; 15:211 (Abstract 486).

50. Kemeny N, Conti JA, Sigurdson E, et al. A pilot study of hepatic artery floxuridine combined with systemic 5-fluorouracil and leucovorin. Cancer 1993; 71:1964–71.

51. Safi F, Hepp G, Link KH, Beger HG. Simultaneous adjuvant regional and systemic chemotherapy after resection of liver metastases of colorectal cancer. Proc Am Soc Clin Oncol 1995; 14:217 (Abstract 544).

52. Curley SA, Roh MS, Chase JL, Hohn DC. Adjuvant hepatic arterial infusion chemotherapy after curative resection of colorectal liver metastases. Am J Surg 1993; 166:743.

53. Frye JW, Venook AP, Stagg RJ, Warren RS. Adjuvant (Adj) hepatic intra-arterial (HIA) chemotherapy (CTR) in patients (pts) with liver metastases (mets) from colorectal cancer (CRC). Proc Am Soc Clin Oncol 1994; 13:218 (Abstract 657).

54. Lorenz M, Encke A. Adjuvant regional treatment after resection of colorectal liver metastases. Rev Oncol 1993; 3:24.

55. Lorenz M, Muller HH, Schramm H, et al. Randomized trial of surgery versus surgery followed by adjuvant hepatic arterial infusion with 5-fluorouracil and folinic acid for liver metastases (Arbeitsgruppe Lebermetastasen). Ann Surg 1998; 228(6):756–62.

56. Kemeny MM, Adak S, Lipsitz S, Gray B, MacDonald J, Benson AB III. Results of the Intergroup [Eastern Cooperative Oncology Group (ECOG) and Southwest Oncology Group (SWOG)] prospective randomized study of surgery alone versus continuous hepatic artery infusion of FUDR and continuous systemic infusion of 5 FU after hepatic resection for colorectal liver metastases. Proc Am Soc Clin Oncol 1999; 18:264a (Abstract 1012).

57. Kemeny N, Cohen A, Huang Y, et al. Randomized study of hepatic arterial infusion (HAI) and systemic chemotherapy (SYS) versus SYS alone as adjuvant therapy after resection of hepatic metastases from colorectal cancer. Proc Am Soc Clin Oncol 1999; 18:263a (Abstract 1011).

58. Piedbois P, Buyse M, Gray R, et al. Portal vein infusion is an effective adjuvant treatment for patients with colorectal cancer. Proc Am Soc Clin Oncol 1995; 14:192 (Abstract 444).

59. Beart RW, Moertel CG, Wieand HS, et al. Adjuvant therapy for resectable colorectal carcinoma with fluorouracil administered by portal vein infusion. Arch Surg 1990; 125:897–901.

60. Fielding L, Hittinger R, Grace R, et al. Randomized controlled trial of adjuvant chemotherapy by portal vein perfusion after curative resection for colorectal adenocarcinoma. Lancet 1992; 340:502–6.

61. Nitti D, Wils J, Sahmoud T, et al. Final results of a phase III clinical trial on adjuvant intraportal infusion with heparin and 5-fluorouracil (5-FU) in resectable colon cancer (EORTC GITCCG 1983–1987). Eur J Cancer 1997; 33:1209–15.

62. Rougier P, Sahmoud T, Nitti D, et al. Adjuvant portal-vein infusion of fluorouracil and heparin in colorectal cancer: a randomized trial. Lancet 1998; 352(9131): 910.

63. Wolmark N, Rockette H, Petrelli N, et al. Long-term results of the efficacy of perioperative portal vein infusion of 5-FU for treatment of colon cancer: NSABP C-02. Proc Am Soc Clin Oncol 1994; 13:194 (Abstract 561).

64. Labianca R, Boffi L, Marsoni S, et al. A randomized trial of intraportal (IP) versus IP + systemic (SY) versus IP + SY adjuvant chemotherapy in patients (pts) with resected Dukes B-C colon carcinoma (CC). Proc ASCO 1999; 18:264a (Abstract 1014).

65. Graf W, Westlin JE, Pahiman L, Glimelius B. Adjuvant intraperitoneal 5-fluorouracil and intravenous leucovorin after colorectal cancer surgery: a randomized phase II placebo-controlled study. Int J Colorectal Dis 1994; 9:35–9.

66. Scheithauer W, Kornek GV, Marczell A, et al. Combined intravenous and intraperitoneal chemotherapy with fluorouracil + leucovorin vs fluorouracil + levamisole for adjuvant therapy of resected colon carcinoma. Br J Cancer 1998; 77(8):1349–54.

67. Gastrointestinal Tumor Study Group. Prolongation of the disease-free interval in surgically treated rectal carcinoma. N Engl J Med 1985; 312:1465–72.

68. Wolmark N, Fisher B, Rockette H, et al. Postoperative adjuvant chemotherapy or BCG for colon cancer: results from NSABP Protocol C-01. J Natl Cancer Inst 1988; 80:30–6.

69. Hoover HC, Brandhorst JS, Peters LC, et al. Adjuvant active specific immunotherapy for human colorectal cancer: 6.5 year median follow-up of a phase III prospectively randomized trial. J Clin Oncol 1993; 11:390–9.

70. Moertel CG. Vaccine adjuvant therapy for colorectal cancer: 'very dramatic' or ho-hum? J Clin Oncol 1993; 11:385–6.

71. Schirrmacher V, Ockert D, Beck N, *et al.* Newcastle disease virus infected intact autologous tumor cell vaccine for adjuvant active specific immunotherapy of resected colorectal carcinoma. Proc Am Assoc Cancer Res 1995; 36:A1336.

72. Harris J, Ryan L, Adams G, Benson A, Haller D. Survival and relapse in adjuvant autologous tumor vaccine therapy for Dukes' B and C colon cancer – EST 5283. Proc Am Soc Clin Oncol 1994; 13:294 (Abstract 955).

73. Riethmuller G, Schneider-Gadicke E, Schlimok G, *et al.* Randomized trial of monoclonal antibody for adjuvant therapy of resected Dukes' C colorectal carcinoma. Lancet 1994; 343:1177–83.

74. Fountzilas G, Zisiadis A, Dafni U, *et al.* Fluorouracil (FU) and leucovorin (LV) with or without interferon α-2a (IFN) as adjuvant treatment in high risk colon cancer. Proc ASCO 1999; 18:239a (Abstract 916).

75. Gennatas C, Vlahonikolis J, Dardoufas C, *et al.* Surgical adjuvant therapy of rectal carcinoma: a controlled evaluation of fluorouracil, leucovorin and radiation therapy with or without interferon Alfa-2b. Proc ASCO 1999; 18:240a (Abstract 921).

76. Willett CG, Fung CY, Kaufman DS, Efird J, Shellito PC. Postoperative radiation therapy for high-risk colon carcinoma. J Clin Oncol 1993; 11:1112–17.

77. Fabian C, Giri S, Estes N, *et al.* Adjuvant continuous infusion 5-FU, whole abdominal radiation, and tumor-bed boost in high-risk stage III colon carcinoma: a Southwest Oncology Group study. Int J Radiat Oncol Biol Phys 1995; 32:457–64.

78. Martenson J, Willett C, Sargent D, *et al.* A phase III study of adjuvant radiation therapy (RT), 5-fluorouracil (5-FU), and levamisole (LEV) vs 5-FU and LEV in selected patients with resected, high risk colon cancer: initial results of Int 0130. Proc ASCO 1999; 18:235a (Abstract 904).

79. Tominaga T, Sakabe T, Koyama Y, *et al.* Prognostic factors for patients with colon or rectal carcinoma treated with resection only. Cancer 1996; 78:403–8.

80. Gerard A, Buyse M, Nordlinger B, *et al.* Preoperative radiotherapy as adjuvant treatment in rectal cancer: final results of a randomized study of the European Organization for Research and Treatment of Cancer (EORTC). Ann Surg 1988; 208:606–14.

81. Cedermark B, Johansson H, Rutqvist LE, *et al.* The Stockholm I Trial of Preoperative Short Term Radiotherapy in Operable Rectal Cancer: a prospective randomized trial. Cancer 1995; 75:2269–75.

82. Gastrointestinal Tumor Study Group. Survival after post-operative combination treatment of rectal cancer. N Engl J Med 1986; 315:1294–5.

83. Fisher B, Wolmark N, Rockette H, *et al.* Postoperative adjuvant chemotherapy for rectal cancer; results from NSABP protocol R-01. J Natl Cancer Inst 1988; 80:21–9.

84. Cedermark B, Theve NO, Rieger A, *et al.* Preoperative short term radiotherapy in rectal carcinoma: a preliminary report of a prospective study. Cancer 1985;55:1182–5.

85. Sause W, Martz K, Noyes D, *et al.* RTOG 81-15 ECOG 83-23 evaluation of preoperative radiation therapy in operable rectal carcinoma. Int J Radiat Oncol Biol Phys 1990; 19(S1):179 (Abstract).

86. Mohiuddin M, Derdel J, Marks G, *et al.* Results of adjuvant radiation therapy in cancer of the rectum. Thomas Jefferson University Hospital experience. Cancer 1985; 55:350–3.

87. Gunderson LL, Dosorety D, Blitzer DH, *et al.* Low dose preoperative irradiation for resectable rectal and rectosigmoid carcinoma. Cancer 1983; 52:446–51.

88. Shank B, Enker W, Santant J, *et al.* Local control with preoperative radiotherapy alone versus 'sandwich' radiotherapy for rectal carcinoma. Int J Radiat Oncol Biol Phys 1987; 13:111–15.

89. Douglass HO, Stablein DM, Mayer RJ. Ten years follow-up of first generation of surgical adjuvant rectal cancer studies of the gastrointestinal tumor study group. In Hamilton J, Elliot J, eds. *NIH Consensus Development Conference: adjuvant therapy for patients with colon and rectum cancer.* Bethesda, MD, National Institutes of Health, 1990; 35–40.

90. Zoetmulder FAN, Taal BG, Van Tinteren H. Adjuvant 5FU plus levamisole improves survival in stage II and III colonic cancer, but not in rectal cancer. Interim analysis of the Netherlands Adjuvant Colorectal Cancer Project (NACCP). Proc ASCO 1999; 18:266a.

91. Douglass HO Jr. Results of surgical adjuvant trials of the Gastrointestinal Tumor Study Group. In Wanebo HJ, ed. *Colorectal cancer.* St Louis, MO, Mosby-Year Book, 1993; 363–74.

92. O'Connell M, Martenson J, Wieand H, *et al.* Improving adjuvant therapy for rectal cancer by combining protracted-infusion fluorouracil with radiation therapy after curative surgery. N Engl J Med 1994; 331:502–7.

93. Krook JE, Moertel CG, Gunderson LL, *et al.* Effective surgical adjuvant therapy for high risk rectal carcinoma. N Engl J Med 1991; 324:709–15.

94. Tepper JE, O'Connell MJ, Petroni GR, *et al.* Adjuvant postoperative fluorouracil-modulated chemotherapy combined with pelvic radiation therapy for rectal cancer: initial results of Intergroup 0114. J Clin Oncol 1997; 15(5):2030–9.

95. Tepper J, O'Connell M, Petroni G, *et al.* Toxicity in the adjuvant therapy of rectal cancer: a preliminary report of Intergroup 0114 (CALGB9081). Proc Am Soc Clin Oncol 1996; 15:210 (Abstract 481).

96. Frykholm GJ, Glimelius B, Pahiman L. Preoperative or postoperative irradiation in adenocarcinoma of the rectum: final treatment results of a randomized trial and an evaluation of late secondary effects. Dis Colon Rectum 1993; 36:564–72.

97. Minsky BD, Cohen AM, Kemeny N, *et al.* Combined modality therapy of rectal cancer: decreased acute

toxicity with the preoperative approach. J Clin Oncol 1992; 10:1218–24.
98. Samuels B, Prasad L, Hooberman A, *et al.* Mitomycin, 5-fluorouracil (5-FU), leucovorin, & hyperfractionated radiation (MFL/HRT) as preoperative therapy for rectal carcinoma. Proc Am Soc Clin Oncol 1996; 15:205 (Abstract 462).
99. Roca E. Rectal carcinoma, adjuvant preoperative vs. postoperative concurrent chemoradiotherapy (CT-RT): a non randomized comparison. Proc Am Soc Clin Oncol 1996; 15:223 (Abstract 535).
100. Conti JA, Kemeny NE, Saltz LB, *et al.* Irinotecan is an active agent in untreated patients with metastatic colorectal cancer. J Clin Oncol. 1996; 14:709–15.
101. Rougier P, Bugat R, Douilland JY, *et al.* Phase II study of irinotecan in the treatment of advanced colorectal cancer in chemotherapy naive patients and patients pretreated with fluorouracil-based chemotherapy. J Clin Oncol 1997; 15:251–60.
102. Zalcberg Jr, Cunningham D, Van Cutsem R, *et al.* ZD 1694: a novel thymidylate synthase inhibitor with substantial activity in the treatment of patients with advanced colorectal cancer. J Clin Oncol 1996; 14:716–21.
103. Diaz-Rubio E, Marty M, Extra JM, *et al.* Multicentric phase II study with oxaliplatin (L-OHP®) in 5-FU refractory patients with advanced colorectal cancer (ACC). Proc Am Soc Clin Oncol 1995; 14:209 (Abstract 514).
104. Seitz JF. 5-Fluorouracil/leucovorin versus capecitabine in patients with stage III colon cancer. Semin Oncol 2001; 28(1 suppl.1):41–4.

Commentary

ROBERT W DECKER

INTRODUCTION

My colleague Dr Sarna has provided an excellent review of the adjuvant and neoadjuvant therapy of colorectal cancer. He has developed the rationale for this therapy, reviewed the incidence and natural history data for this type of cancer, and has summarized the evolution of studies addressing this topic in logical fashion. The conclusions reached are essentially in line with the recommendations of the National Cancer Institute, namely the routine use of adjuvant systemic chemotherapy in patients with stage III colon cancer, and the use of combined modality therapy in patients with stage II or III rectal cancer. The role of systemic adjuvant therapy in stage II colon cancer remains somewhat controversial, however, and additional discussion regarding therapy in these patients is warranted.

Estimates from Surveillance, Epidemiology and End Results (SEER) data[1] suggest that approximately 56 000 residents of the USA will die from colorectal cancer in the year 2000, underscoring the fact that much work remains to facilitate curative interventions in this disease. Several areas are worth pursuing in an attempt to improve outcomes:

1 We must employ more successful adjuvant therapy more specifically, i.e., we must identify and treat those patients within the various pathologically staged groups at the highest risk for recurrence and avoid treating those patients with relatively low risk.
2 We must continue to evaluate the role of novel surgical interventions, e.g., laparoscopic colectomy, total mesorectal excision/sharp dissection for low and mid-rectal cancers, and local resection for early rectal tumors, and apply these new techniques *only* in the appropriate patient groups.
3 Assuming that chemotherapy is *not* the entire solution, i.e., if fully effective therapy is not currently available, what novel therapies should be pursued in the future?
4 Early detection of malignant and/or premalignant disease needs to be a priority, i.e., optimization and utilization of screening studies is mandatory.

Let us now explore these areas in more detail.

ADJUVANT SYSTEMIC THERAPY FOR STAGE II CANCERS

The role of adjuvant systemic (chemo-) therapy in stage II colon cancer remains a controversial topic. The studies highlighted by Dr Sarna[2,3] were reviewed in an accompanying editorial,[4] with the author offering his perspective that ongoing trials of adjuvant therapy in stage II patients should include a 'no-treatment' control arm. The NSABP data pooled results from four different trials over a 13-year span, with two of them utilizing 'no-treatment' controls, and two comparing (apparently) less effective therapies (MOF or 5-FU plus levamisole).[2] Their analysis is difficult to interpret and accept, due to some unusual statistical methods. They have pooled the results according to the already determined outcomes, comparing the groups with better results to those with lesser results and concluding that the former do indeed have an improved outcome. A closer look at the data sets reveals a progressive improvement in outcome, with the 'no adjuvant treatment' group demonstrating improved 5-year survival from 72% to 76% from study C-01 to C-02 and the MOF treatment group improving from 75% to 84% (studies C-01 and C-03), even though the duration of adjuvant therapy was reduced by almost a half in the latter study. Results from C-03 appear to be better than those of most other comparable trials, and the 92% survival for 5-FU/LV-treated patients in C-03 is a 'high-water mark,' unable to be matched by the subsequent C-04 study's 85% survival for similarly treated patients. Additionally, these most impressive results represent data from subgroups of patients with less than 150 patients in either arm of the trial, a modest number from which to try to derive broad-ranging recommendations. The IMPACT study pooled five trials, all of which compared 5-FU and leucovorin, albeit at a (narrow) range of doses, and was unable to demonstrate a statistically significant benefit for those receiving treatment,[3] although a nearly significant trend in improved survival was noted for the treatment groups.

It is clearly preferable to attempt to improve upon the current long-term survival rate for patients with these lesions. Identification of a subgroup of stage II patients at higher risk or implementation of more effective therapies is likely to be necessary (see below). Alternatively, one might consider treating patients who might derive more benefit from such treatment, i.e., younger patients, a group with more years 'at risk' and able to tolerate therapy with less morbidity than their older counterparts.

The interpretation of trial results requires comparison with concurrent controls, as older studies may not have comparable surgical or pathologic staging. Prior 'understaging,' due to occult nodal or systemic metastases, may now be less common due to the development and application of higher resolution imaging and pathologic techniques. Hence, the prospect for 'no-treatment' control arms in trials of adjuvant therapy in stage II colon cancer remains a serious consideration; clearly, one must continue to attempt to enroll these patients in appropriate trials to help answer this important question.

IDENTIFICATION OF HIGH-RISK SUBGROUPS

A multitude of prognostic factors have been identified in colon cancer patients. The standard considerations used in assessing patient risk include tumor depth (T stage) and nodal involvement (N stage). Newer molecular prognostic markers continue to be recognized. Microsatellite instability of the DNA manifests as an increase in DNA repetitive sequences due to loss of a DNA mismatch repair gene. These mutations are found in 15–20% of colon cancers, predominantly in the right colon, and are associated with a better prognosis.[5] Loss of the *DCC* (deleted in colon cancer) gene,[6] deletion of the long arm of chromosome 18,[7] abnormalities of p53, HER-2-neu and other oncogenes, high preoperative carcinoembryonic antigen (CEA) values, etc., have all been described as additional factors to be considered in the prognosis of colorectal cancer. The questions of how and why patients with pathologically negative lymph nodes relapse approximately 20–25% of the time also warrant further understanding. Explanations include the possibility that the metastatic process may bypass the lymphatic system or, alternatively that micrometastatic disease may be missed by routine pathologic evaluation, and/or potentially involved nodes are not resected with the specimen. Liefers *et al.*[8] developed a method to allow for higher resolution analysis of resected lymph node specimens and found, in a small group of patients, that micrometastases were present in 54% of their 'stage II' patients; relapses occurred in 50% of those patients, but in only 9% of those with persistently negative nodes by their methodology. Although other studies of similar design had failed to demonstrate the relevance or worsening of prognosis associated with nodal micrometastases, this small study warrants further investigation. If these results can be confirmed in larger patient groups, then such methodology may allow for more accurate operative staging.

Another novel technique under investigation, also with parallels in other malignancies (breast cancer, melanoma) is the role of sentinel lymph node biopsy. The tumor site is injected with a tracer compound (e.g., isosulfan blue dye) and the primary nodal drainage area is specifically sampled and reviewed for involvement by metastatic disease. The high sensitivity and specificity of this technique have been demonstrated in axillary dissection for breast cancer.[9,10] Recent trials in colon cancer confirm a similar high rate of sensitivity and specificity for this technique.[11] The results may be utilized primarily to identify patients with lymph node-positive (stage III) disease so they may receive appropriate adjuvant therapy, rather than with the intent of limiting further nodal sampling, as is the case in breast cancer. The pathologist should utilize the highest sensitivity methods on the sentinel lymph node(s) if they appear negative for metastases by conventional review, thus minimizing the failure to identify patients with the earliest or most minimal stage III disease and allowing them to receive appropriate adjuvant therapy.

NEWER SURGICAL TECHNIQUES

The past 10–15 years have seen the development of new surgical techniques in treating colorectal cancer, recently reviewed by Guillem and Cohen.[12] The role of some of these, namely laparoscopic colectomy, local excision with sphincter preservation in early rectal cancers, and total mesorectal excision (TME) for rectal cancer treatment, is discussed briefly here. The first two novel approaches are important to discuss from the perspective of treating and attempting to cure malignant disease, as they have been popularized based on a presumed decrease in morbidity of the procedures. Long-term results are becoming available, with insights into applying these techniques in appropriate patient populations and taking care to avoid sacrificing long-term cure for short-term morbidity.

The utilization of the laparoscope in the surgical treatment of benign disease, e.g., cholecystectomy, has increased dramatically in the past decade on the basis of decreased morbidity and length of stay data. Broader applications followed, and patients with colorectal cancers have undergone laparoscopic, or laparoscopically assisted, colectomies subsequently without evidence to support the equivalence of long-term disease control by this method. Early studies demonstrated an increase in surgical morbidity and mortality which lessened with experience. Likewise, local recurrences at the trocar or port sites[13] and the potential for understaging due to inadequate nodal sampling were recognized as additional confounding factors. Recent studies have demonstrated a more acceptable result with this technique,[14] although it remains clear that this is operator dependent. With the answers not yet in hand, laparoscopic colectomy should still be considered experimental for cancer surgery, and prospective, randomized trials are warranted.

Rectal cancers may present earlier than their counterpart colon primaries on the basis of more apparent bleeding and alteration in bowel habits, thus earlier primaries (lower T stages) may be identified. Because low-lying tumors would preclude an adequate distal margin in most circumstances, hence necessitating an abdominoperineal resection (APR), attempts have been made to perform local excisions with sparing of the anal sphincter, to preserve organ function. This requires a full transanal excision of the tumor in selected patients for whom preoperative staging confirms the early nature of the tumor and the absence of obvious nodal or perirectal metastatic disease. Preoperative staging with rectal ultrasound and/or magnetic resonance imaging (MRI) are mandatory to exclude patients with locally advanced (T3 or N1) disease. Because this approach precludes adequate nodal sampling, it must be reserved for patients with T1 or early T2 lesions. Patients with T3 disease have a higher likelihood of regional nodal involvement and hence should be treated via more conventional techniques. Additional factors in selecting suitable patients for local excision include well-differentiated or moderately differentiated histology and tumor circumference of less than 25–40% of the lumen.[15,16]

Progress in local disease control has been made with the advent of the TME, a procedure designed to maintain the integrity of the visceral mesorectum and thus diminish the likelihood of tumor-cell spillage and thus local recurrence. A landmark pathologic study by Quirke et al.[17] in 1986 called attention to the prospect of tumor spillage when resection of rectal cancers is performed via blunt dissection along the visceral mesorectum. Taking a wider margin, with sharp dissection to the level of the parietal fascia and *en bloc* resection of the tumor, allows for clearer margins. The results of prospective studies have confirmed the benefits of this technique, with multiple studies demonstrating low rates of local recurrence ($<10\%$) *without* the use of adjuvant radiation therapy. This includes patients with up to T3 lesions and compares very favorably with historical controls and patients treated with adjuvant radiation therapy.[18]

PROSPECTS FOR NOVEL SYSTEMIC ADJUVANT THERAPY

Dr Sarna's review discusses the methodical evolution of adjuvant chemotherapy for colorectal cancer in the year 2000. Despite the demonstration of the benefit of such therapy, and its confirmed efficacy, the agents utilized are inherently weak in their antitumor activity and thus more dramatic improvements in cure rates have yet to be observed. Many studies have confirmed response rates with 5-FU and leucovorin (LV) in the 20–30% range, occasionally higher. It is to be hoped that the integration of irinotecan into adjuvant programs will parallel the improvements in adjuvant treatment prospects as the introduction of taxanes for breast cancer has done, namely by providing more options for combination therapy, as well as offering the hope that sequential or combination therapy with active agents will result in some further improvement in long-term results. Unfortunately, irinotecan also suffers from relatively low (20–25%) response rates and additional gastrointestinal toxicity in the form of severe diarrheal complications. The true *cure* of the disease, therefore, will require the utilization of other types of therapies (Table 1).

Table 1 *Systemic therapies for colorectal cancer*

Chemotherapy
  5-flourouracil ± leucovorin
  Irinotecan (CPT-11)
  Oxaliplatin
  Capecitabine
  Raltitrexed
  Mitomycin C
  Nitrosoureas

Non-chemotherapeutic
  Monoclonal antibodies
  Tumor vaccines
  Antisense therapy
  Anti-angiogenesis agents
  Signal transduction inhibitors

Monoclonal antibodies have been developed as part of our therapeutic armamentarium in other malignant diseases, with the first clinically available therapy being utilized in breast cancer patients whose tumors demonstrate amplification of the her-2-neu oncogene. Subsequently, we have seen the development of effective agents for the treatment of malignant B-cell lymphomas (anti-CD20 antibodies), cutaneous T-cell lymphomas, acute myeloid leukemia, and other diagnoses where tumor-specific or disease-specific antigens can be identified. Typical therapeutic antibodies are 'humanized,' i.e., hybridized to human antibody Fc fragments to diminish immunogenicity and thus maximize clinical effect. Researchers in colon cancer have developed antibodies to CEA, and more recent trials have utilized antibodies to vascular endothelial growth factor (VEGF)[19] and surface antigens 17-1A or A33 as therapeutic agents, with clinical trials ongoing. One can envision a combination of chemotherapeutic agents and monoclonal antibodies as a more effective therapy, although clinical trial results will not be available for some time yet. Likewise, the use of other novel therapies is being studied in early-phase trials, their clinical usefulness not yet having been demonstrated.

SCREENING AND PREVENTION/EARLY DETECTION

Current recommendations from the National Cancer Institute (NCI) for screening for colorectal cancer include testing the stool for occult blood, and visualization of the lower gastrointestinal tract, either directly (colonoscopy) or radiographically (barium enema). Patients without a first-degree relative affected with these cancers begin screening at the age of 50, whereas patients with first-degree relatives with these diagnoses enter the system earlier, with screening beginning at 35 or 40 years of age. Families carrying the *FAP* gene (familial adenomatous polyposis) should have children screened, while those with hereditary non-polyposis cancers fall into the young adult age range at screening onset. Other factors, e.g., inflammatory bowel disease, etc., will also result in more individualized and earlier screening studies. Unfortunately, the utilization of, or compliance with recommendations for routine screening studies has been quite poor.

Fecal occult blood testing, while shown to be effective as a screening tool in reducing mortality in colorectal cancer,[20] is fraught with several problems, including many false-positive tests due to dietary non-compliance during the testing period, false negatives due to improper testing of the specimen (without rehydrating), and generally the difficulty in methodically having all patients screened. More specific reagents may be required to optimize this test to allow it to achieve significant benefit, although several studies have confirmed the efficacy of currently available kits.

The role of colonoscopy as a screening test has been impeded by the substantial preparative procedures and the ardors of testing a large patient population. While this is undoubtedly the 'gold-standard' screening test at the present, the cost and preparation required probably preclude its maximal utilization. Newer radiographic procedures such as 'virtual endoscopy' may ultimately replace the more invasive studies and allow for more successful mass screening, perhaps paralleling the evolving role of electron beam computerized tomography in screening for coronary artery disease and similar studies to screen long-term smokers for early lung cancers.

Chemoprevention trials continue with a variety of agents. Early observations derived from population-based studies suggested lower risks of colon cancers in patients taking aspirin and non-steroidal anti-inflammatory drugs.[21] Non-specific cyclo-oxygenase inhibitors such as sulindac have been found to induce a marked regression of adenomas in patients with familial adenomatous polyposis. Speculation remains as to whether such responses are due solely to inhibition of cyclo-oxygenase-2 (cox-2) or of other pathways as well. Neoplastic colonic tissue demonstrates an 'up-regulation' of cox-2, and studies with the newer cox-2 inhibitors, e.g., celecoxib, demonstrate reductions in the range of 30% in the development of colonic neoplasia and the regression of adenomatous lesions.[22]

SUMMARY

Our goal as oncologists and physicians early in the twenty-first century is clear: the eradication of malignant disease. This will be accomplished by a fuller understanding of the molecular pathogenesis of these diseases and our ability to intercede in carcinogenesis. We will need to continue to develop more effective and specific, and less toxic, therapies and apply these modalities in patients whose risk (and benefit) can be more specifically quantitated. We will need to identify patients at risk for these diseases prior to their development and apply simple, inexpensive, and non-invasive screening modalities to achieve this goal.

REFERENCES

1. Greenlee R, Murray T, Bolden S, Wingo P. Cancer statistics, 2000. CA Cancer J Clin 2000; 50:7–33.
2. Mamounas E, Wieand S, Wolmark N, *et al*. Comparative efficacy of adjuvant chemotherapy in patients with Dukes' B versus Dukes' C colon cancer: results from four National Surgical Adjuvant Breast

and Bowel Project Adjuvant Studies (C-01, C-02, C-03 and C-04). J Clin Oncol 1999; 17:1349–55.

3. International Multicentre Pooled Analysis of B2 Colon Cancer Trials (IMPACT B2) Investigators. Efficacy of adjuvant fluorouracil and folinic acid in B2 colon cancer. J Clin Oncol 1999; 17:1356–63.

4. Harrington D. The tea leaves of small trials. J Clin Oncol 1999; 17:1336–8.

5. Gryfe R, Kim H, Hsieh E, *et al.* Tumor microsatellite instability and clinical outcome in young patients with colorectal cancer. N Engl J Med 2000; 342:69–77.

6. Shibata D, Reale M, Lavin P, *et al.* The DCC protein and prognosis in colorectal cancer. N Engl J Med 1996; 335:1727–32.

7. Jen J, Kim H, Piantadosi S, *et al.* Allelic loss of chromosome 18q and prognosis in colorectal cancer. N Engl J Med 1994; 331:213–21.

8. Liefers G, Cleton-Jansen A, Van de Velde C, *et al.* Micrometastases and survival in stage II colorectal cancer. N Engl J Med 1998; 339:223–8.

9. Giuliano A, Jones R, Brennan M, Statman R. Sentinel lymphadenectomy in breast cancer. J Clin Oncol 1997; 15:2345–50.

10. Krag D, Weaver D, Ashikaga T, *et al.* The sentinel node in breast cancer – a multicenter validation study. N Engl J Med 1998; 339:941–6.

11. Saha S, Bilchik A, Wiese D, *et al.* Phase II study for upstaging of colorectal cancer (CRCA) by sentinel lymph node mapping (SLNM) technique – a multicenter trial. Proc ASCO 2000; 19:239a.

12. Guillem J, Cohen A. Current issues in colorectal cancer surgery. Semin Oncol 1999; 26:505–13.

13. Johnstone P, Rohde D, Swartz S, *et al.* Port site recurrences after laparoscopic and thoracoscopic procedures in malignancy. J Clin Oncol 1996; 14:1950–6.

14. Franklin M, Rosenthal D, Abrego-Medina D, *et al.* Prospective comparison of open vs. laparoscopic colon surgery for carcinoma: five-year results. Dis Colon Rectum 1996; 39:S35–46.

15. Ng A, Recht A, Busse P. Sphincter preservation therapy for distal rectal carcinoma: a review. Cancer 1997; 79:671–83.

16. Bleday R, Breen E, Jessup M, *et al.* Prospective evaluation of local excision for small rectal cancers. Dis Colon Rectum 1997; 40:388–92.

17. Quirke P, Durdey P, Dixon M, *et al.* Local recurrence of rectal adenocarcinoma due to inadequate surgical resection. Histopathologic study of lateral tumor spread and surgical excision. Lancet 1986;1:996–9.

18. Enker W, Thaler H, Cranor M, Polyak T. Total mesorectal excision in the operative treatment of carcinoma of the rectum. J Am Coll Surg 1995; 181:335–46.

19. Bergsland E, Hurwitz H, Fehrenbacher L, *et al.* A randomized phase II trial comparing rhuMAb VEGF (recombinant humanized monoclonal antibody to vascular endothelial cell growth factor) plus 5-fluorouracil/leucovorin (FU/LV) to FU/LV alone in patients with metastatic colorectal cancer. Proc ASCO 2000; 19:242a.

20. Mandel J, Bond J, Church T, *et al.* Reducing mortality from colorectal cancer by screening for fecal occult blood. N Engl J Med 1993; 328:1365–71.

21. Thun M, Namboodiri B, Heath C. Aspirin use and reduced risk of fatal colon cancer. N Engl J Med 1991; 325:1593–6.

22. Steinbach G, Lynch P, Phillips R, *et al.* The effect of celecoxib, a cyclooxygenase-2 inhibitor, in familial adenomatous polyposis. N Engl J Med 2000; 342:1946–52.

Editors' selected abstracts

Preoperative radiotherapy for resectable rectal cancer: a meta-anlaysis.

Camma C, Giunta M, Fiorica F, Pagliaro L, Crax A, Cottone M.

Istituto di Clinica Medica, Palermo, Italy.

Journal of the American Medical Association 284:1008–15, 2000, August 23/30.

Context: The benefit of adjuvant radiotherapy for resectable rectal cancer has been extensively studied, but data on survival are still equivocal despite a reduction in the rate of local recurrence. *Objective:* To assess the effectiveness of preoperative radiotherapy followed by surgery in the reduction of overall and cancer-related mortality and in the prevention of local recurrence and distant metastases. *Data sources:* Computerized bibliographic searches of MEDLINE and CANCERLIT (1970 to December 1999), including non-English sources, were supplemented with hand searches of reference lists. The medical subject headings used were *rectal cancer, radiotherapy, surgery, RCT, randomized,* and *clinical trial. Study selection:* Studies were included if they were randomized controlled trials (RCTs) comparing preoperative radiotherapy plus surgery with surgery alone and if they included patients with resectable histologically proven rectal adenocarcinoma, without metastatic disease. Fourteen RCTs were analyzed. *Data extraction:* Data on population, intervention, and outcomes were extracted from each RCT according to the intention-to-treat method by 3 independent observers and combined using the DerSimonian and Laird method. *Data synthesis:* Radiotherapy plus surgery compared with surgery alone significantly reduced the 5-year overall mortality rate (odds ratio [OR] 0.84; 95% confidence interval [CI],

0.72–0.98; $p = 0.03$), cancer-related mortality rate (OR, 0.71; 95% CI, 0.61–0.82; $p < 0.001$), and local recurrence rate (OR, 0.49; 95% CI, 0.38–0.62; $p < 0.001$). No reduction was observed in the occurrence of distant metastases (OR, 0.93; 95% CI, 0.73–1.18; $p = 0.54$). *Conclusions:* In patients with resectable rectal cancer, preoperative radiotherapy significantly improved overall and cancer-specific survival compared with surgery alone. The magnitude of the benefit is relatively small and criteria are needed to identify patients most likely to benefit from adjuvant radiotherapy.

Fluorouracil and leucovorin with or without interferon alfa-2a as adjuvant treatment, in patients with high-risk colon cancer: a randomized phase III study conducted by the Hellenic Cooperative Oncology Group.

Fountzilas G, Zisiadis A, Dafni U, Konstantaras C, Hatzitheoharis G, Papavramidis S, Bousoulegas A, Basdanis G, Giannoulis E, Dokmetzioglou J, Katsohis C, Nenopoulou E, Karvounis N, Briassoulis E, Aravantinos G, Kosmidis P, Skarlos D, Pavlidis N.

1st Department of Internal Medicine, Oncology Section, AHEPA Hospital, Aristotle University of Thessaloniki Medical School, Thessaloniki, Greece.

Oncology 58(3):227–36, 2000, April.

Background: It has been shown in randomized studies that adjuvant treatment with the combination of fluorouracil (FU) and levamisole reduced the risk of recurrence and deaths of patients with stage III colon cancer. Pharmacological studies of FU led to its use in combination with a number of modulating agents including interferon-alpha and leucovorin (LV) that appear to enhance its activity in vitro. Furthermore, a meta-analysis suggested that the combination of FU with LV increased the response rate as compared to FU monotherapy in patients with advanced colorectal cancer. *Purpose:* To evaluate the impact of adjuvant treatment with the combination of FU and LV with or without interferon alfa-2a (IFN) on disease-free survival (DFS) and overall survival (OS) for patients with stage II or III colon cancer. *Patients and methods:* From August 1989 to July 1997, 280 pateints with stage II and III colon cancer entered the study and were randomly assigned to receive either the combination of FU (600 mg/m^2/week × 6, followed by a 2-week rest) and LV (500 mg/m^2/week × 6 as a 2-hour infusion, followed by a 2-week rest) for 4 cycles (group A, 139 patients), or the same chemotherapy plus recombinant IFN (3 MU subcutaneously 3 times a week) for 1 year (group B, 141 patients). *Results:* A total of 109 patients (78.9%) of group A and 119 (84.4%) of group B completed four cycles of chemotherapy. Also, 51.4% of patients of group A and 53.9% of group B received ⩾80% of the planned dose of FU. One patient (group A) was found to be ineligible and was not included in the analysis. The median relative dose intensity of FU in the two groups was 0.90 and 0.85, respectively. As of August 1998, after a median follow up of 4 years, there was no significant difference in either 3-year DFS (group A, 83.1%; group B, 75.9%, $p = 0.14$) or OS (group A, 84.5%; group B, 80.0% $p = 0.27$). In the Cox model, stage of disease, number of infiltrated nodes, tumor grade and presence of regional implants were identified as significant prognostic factors for OS. Grade 3–4 toxicities, mainly

diarrhea, were observed in 26.1% of patients of group A and in 24.8% of group B. There were no treatment-related deaths. *Conclusions:* The addition of IFN to the combination of FU with LV postoperatively does not improve DFS and OS of patients with stage II or III colon cancer.

Adjuvant active specific immunotherapy for stage II and III colon cancer with an autologous tumor cell vaccine: Eastern Cooperative Oncology Group Study E5283.

Harris JE, Ryan L, Hoover HC Jr, Stuart RK, Oken MM, Benson AB 3rd, Mansour E, Haller DG, Manola J, Hanna MG Jr.

Rush-Presbyterian–St Luke's Medical Center, Chicago, IL, USA.

Journal of Clinical Oncology 18(1):148–57, 2000, January.

Purpose: A randomized phase III clinical trial of adjuvant active specific immunotherapy (ASI) with an autologous tumor cell-bacillus Calmette–Guerin (BCG) vaccine was conducted to determine whether surgical resection plus ASI was more beneficial than resection alone in stage II and III colon cancer patients. *Patients and methods:* Patients ($n = 412$) with colon cancer (297 with stage II disease, 115 with stage III disease) were randomly allocated to an observation arm or to a treatment arm in which they received three weekly intradermal vaccine injections of 10^7 irradiated autologous tumor cells beginning approximately 4 weeks after surgery. The first two weekly injections also contained 10^7 BCG organisms. Patients were observed for determination of time to recurrence and disease-free and overall survival. *Results:* This was a negative study in that after a 7.6-year median follow-up period, there were no statistically significant differences in clinical outcomes between the treatment arms. However, there were disease-free survival ($p = 0.078$) and overall survival ($p = 0.12$) trends in favor of ASI when treatment compliance was evaluated, i.e., patients who received the intended treatment had a delayed cutaneous hypersensitivity (DCH) response to the third vaccination (induration ⩾5 mm). Also, the magnitude of the DCH response correlated with improved prognosis. The 5-year survival proportion was 84.6% for those with indurations greater than 10 mm, compared with 45.0% for those with indurations less than 5 mm. *Conclusions:* When all randomized patients were evaluated, no significant clinical benefit was seen with ASI in surgically resected colon cancer patients with stage II or III colon cancer. However, there was an indication that treatment compliance with effective immunization results in disease-free and overall survival benefits.

Randomized trial of postoperative adjuvant chemotherapy with or without radiotherapy for carcinoma of the rectum: National Surgical Adjuvant Breast and Bowel Project Protocol R-02.

Wolmark N, Wieand HS, Hyams DM, Colangelo L, Dimitrov NV, Romond EH, Wexler M, Prager D, Cruz AB Jr, Gordon PH, Petrelli NJ, Deutsch M, Mamounas E, Wickerham DL, Fisher ER, Rockette H, Fisher B.

N. Wolmark, D.L. Wickerham, E.R. Fisher, B. Fisher, National Surgical Adjuvant Breast and Bowel Project (NSABP) Operations Center, Pittsburgh, PA, USA.

Journal of the National Cancer Institute 92(5):388–96, 2000, March 1.

Background: The conviction that postoperative radiotherapy and chemotherapy represent an acceptable standard of care for patients with Dukes' B (stage II) and Dukes' C (stage III) carcinoma of the rectum evolved in the absence of data from clinical trials designed to determine whether the addition of radiotherapy results in improved disease-free survival and overall survival. This study was carried out to address this issue. An additional aim was to determine whether leucovorin (LV)-modulated 5-fluorouracil (5-FU) is superior to the combination of 5-FU, semustine, and vincristine (MOF) in men. *Patients and methods:* Eligible patients ($n = 694$) with Dukes' B or C carcinoma of the rectum were enrolled in National Surgical Adjuvant Breast and Bowel Project (NSABP) Protocol R-02 from September 1987 through December 1992 and were followed. They were randomly assigned to receive either postoperative adjuvant chemotherapy alone ($n = 348$) or chemotherapy with postoperative radiotherapy ($n = 346$). All female patients ($n = 287$) received 5-FU plus LV chemotherapy; male patients received either MOF ($n = 207$) or 5-FU plus LV ($n = 200$). Primary analyses were carried out by use of a stratified log-rank statistic; p values are two-sided. *Results:* The average time on study for surviving patients is 93 months as of September 30, 1998. Postoperative radiotherapy resulted in no beneficial effect on disease-free survival ($p = 0.90$) or overall survival ($p = 0.89$), regardless of which chemotherapy was utilized, although it reduced the cumulative incidence of locoregional relapse from 13% to 8% at 5-year follow-up ($p = 0.02$). Male patients who received 5-FU plus LV demonstrated a statistically significant benefit in disease-free survival at 5 years compared with those who received MOF (55% versus 47%; $p = 0.009$) but not in 5-year overall survival (65% versus 62%; $p = 0.17$). *Conclusions:* The addition of postoperative radiation therapy to chemotherapy in Dukes' B and C rectal cancer did not alter the subsequent incidence of distant disease, although there was a reduction in locoregional relapse when compared with chemotherapy alone.

26

Surgical management of metastatic liver disease

LINDA S CALLANS AND JOHN M DALY

INTRODUCTION

The liver is a common site of metastatic disease for many different malignancies. This chapter focuses on the surgical approaches to the treatment of hepatic metastases from colorectal carcinoma, including hepatic resection, cryosurgery, and infusional therapy. Colorectal carcinoma is diagnosed in more than 130 000 people in the USA each year and an estimated 56 000 die of recurrent disease.[1] While many of these patients develop liver metastases in the course of their disease, the liver is the only site of recurrence in 23%.[2] These patients are potential candidates for surgical management. Without resection, the median survival of patients with liver metastases ranges from 6 to 20 months, depending on tumor burden, and 5-year survival of patients with even solitary liver metastases is rare.[2–4]

EVALUATION OF THE PATIENT WITH LIVER METASTASES

The initial evaluation of a patient with liver metastases from colorectal cancer should include a chest radiograph as well as computerized tomography (CT) scans of the chest, abdomen, and pelvis to identify other sites of metastatic disease. Evidence of local recurrence can be assessed by a barium enema or colonoscopy. A bone scan is of limited value and should only be done if symptoms suggestive of a bony metastasis are present. Of a group of 132 patients felt to have isolated liver metastases, 25 patients had other sites of distant spread (primarily lung metastases) on their preoperative evaluation.[5] Even when all preoperative studies were negative, 26% of the remaining 107 patients had extrahepatic disease discovered at exploratory laparotomy. The most common sites of intra-abdominal extrahepatic disease were the celiac and porta hepatis lymph nodes.[5,6] Other studies have shown similar unresectability rates at laparotomy ranging from 21% to 54%.[7–10]

In addition to identifying extrahepatic disease, preoperative studies are aimed at assessing the extent and resectability of the hepatic disease (Table 26.1). The number, size, and location of liver lesions as well as their proximity to major vascular or biliary structures need to be determined. The standard CT scan tends to be a poor predictor of resectability (Table 26.2). In one study of

Table 26.1 *Factors determining resectability of hepatic lesions*

Factor	Consideration
Number of lesions	3–4 or fewer lesions
Location of lesions	1. Proximity to major vascular structures
	2. Type of resection required
	3. Ability to obtain clear margins (≥ 1 cm)
Extrahepatic disease	Presence precludes hepatic resection for cure

Table 26.2 *Radiologic evaluation of liver metastases*

Modality	Sensitivity (%)	Specificity (%)
Ultrasound	20–88	60–70
Computed tomography (CT)	38–91	80–90
CT portogram	83–94	80–90
Magnetic resonance imaging	57–82	80–90
Intraoperative ultrasound	82–98	70–80

Adapted from Daly JM, Kemeny NE. Metastatic cancer to the liver. In DeVita VT, Hellman S, Rosenberg SA, eds. *Cancer: principles and practice of oncology*, 5th edn. Philadelphia, J.B. Lippincott Co., 1997, 2554.

139 patients, Benotti and Steele reported that the number of liver lobes involved was underestimated in 33% and overestimated in 4%. Further, extrahepatic disease was not identified in 12%.[11] In various studies, the detection rate of hepatic metastases using CT ranged from 38% to 91%.[12–15]

Magnetic resonance imaging (MRI) with gadolinium enhancement and CT portography are used frequently to image the liver in patients with liver metastases. The sensitivity of MRI in the detection of liver metastases ranges from 57% to 82%.[13–15] CT portography demonstrated improved sensitivity ranging from 83% to 94%,[12,16,17] with a false-positive rate of 15%.[16–18] The CT portogram can accurately detect small lesions or additional metastases that alter the surgical approach or preclude resection.[12] False positives have been seen in the setting of fatty infiltration, cirrhosis, portal perfusion defect, hemangiomas, granulomas, and cysts.[16,18] CT portography can be performed in conjunction with arteriography to define the hepatic arterial anatomy, which is particularly useful if hepatic infusion pump placement is considered for disease found to be unresectable at the time of laparotomy.

The resectability rate of liver metastases from colorectal cancer is only 50–70%, despite extensive preoperative studies. Gibbs and colleagues have assessed the intraoperative factors determining unresectability in 62 patients.[6] The most common factor was extrahepatic disease, found in 40% of patients, primarily in the porta hepatis and celiac lymph nodes, and they advocate routine biopsy of these nodes at the time of exploration. Other factors include the prohibitive extent of liver resection required (31%), more than four metastatic lesions (13%) or satellitosis (10%), and extensive hepatic parenchymal disease (6%).

Clearly, the evaluation at lapartomy is critical and should include exploration of the abdomen and pelvis, with particular attention to the porta hepatis and celiac lymph nodes, as well as assessment of the liver itself. In addition to palpation of the liver, intraoperative ultrasound (IOUS) should be used to confirm the number of hepatic lesions and identify unsuspected metastases. The sensitivity of IOUS reported in several studies ranges from 82% to 98% and has been shown to be superior to that of preoperative ultrasonography, conventional or dynamic CT scanning, CT portogram, and palpation alone.[19–23] IOUS is able to detect smaller lesions (0.5–1.5 cm), often missed by CT scan, and deep lesions not identified by palpation.[19–21] Five to ten percent of liver metastases are only detectable by IOUS.[19,20,23] Further, IOUS can define venous anatomy and evaluate the adequacy of resection margin. In one series, information obtained by IOUS changed the operative management in 49% of cases.[22]

Radioimmunoguided surgery (RIGS) is currently being studied as a means of detecting occult disease for more accurate staging and selection of patients. RIGS has been performed using 125I-labeled B72.3 antibody[24–26] and CC49 antibody[27–29] directed against the TAG-72 antigen. Surgery is typically performed an average of 20 days after intravenous infusion of the labeled antibody, and the abdomen and pelvis are scanned using a hand-held gamma detection probe. Any tissue with signals greater than 1.5 times the background is assumed to contain occult metastases and treatment plans are adjusted accordingly. In these studies, the false-negative rate (clinically positive, RIGS-negative) has ranged from 16% to 38% for B72.3 and from 11% to 17% for CC49. In initial studies, RIGS detected histologically confirmed occult metastases in only 9–11%. The majority of the grossly normal, RIGS-positive tissue was histologically negative. In subsequent analyses, tumor cells have been confirmed in an additional percentage of this tissue using more sensitive techniques such as immunohistochemical staining, autoradiography, and lymph node dissociation with gradient centrifugation. Still, the overall false-positive rate varies between 45% and 60%.

RIGS had mostly been used in patients with primary colorectal carcinomas. In these studies, the detection of RIGS-positive tissue altered management in 21–50% of patients. More extensive resection was performed in 11–37%, and planned procedures were precluded by the discovery of additional foci in approximately 10–20%. The impact of these altered interventions based on RIGS data is unclear because there is little long-term follow-up available regarding disease-free or overall survival. RIGS is an exciting modality of unclear clinical significance that should be studied further in prospective, controlled, multicenter trials.

HEPATIC RESECTION FOR COLORECTAL METASTASES

Patients with isolated hepatic metastases may be candidates for liver resection, cryosurgery, or hepatic artery infusional therapy, depending on the extent of their disease (Table 26.3) and host factors such as comorbid disease.

Table 26.3 *Approaches to the management of hepatic metastases from colorectal cancer*

Presentation	Management option
Liver and extrahepatic disease	Systemic chemotherapy
Liver disease only	
few lesions, any size, favorable anatomy	Hepatic resection
multiple bilobar lesions, unfavorable anatomy	Cryosurgery combined with resection
numerous or diffuse liver disease	Hepatic artery infusion or systemic chemotherapy

Patient selection

Many clinical, operative, and pathologic factors have been evaluated in the attempt to improve the selection of patients for hepatic resection (Table 26.4).[8,9,30–46] Age and gender are not important factors, though comorbid disease may be limiting in the elderly patient. The location and stage of the primary colon or rectal cancer have been studied, including invasion of the serosa and involvement of mesenteric lymph nodes. Adson and coworkers demonstrated a clear relationship between Dukes' stage and overall survival following resection of liver metastases.[39] Others, however, have not confirmed these findings and the literature is fairly divided on the prognostic significance of primary tumor stage. Similarly, the influence of synchronous versus metachronous presentation and disease-free interval has been variable. The time intervals evaluated differ in various series, perhaps accounting for the lack of consensus and difficulty comparing studies. Preoperative carcinoembryonic antigen (CEA) levels have been predictive in several models but not in others. Clearly, a patient with resectable disease should not be excluded on the basis of these clinical factors.

Most series have assessed the characteristics of the metastatic disease, including size, number, and distribution of liver metastases, and the presence or absence of extrahepatic disease. Many series have used 5 cm as a cut-off for the largest lesion in determining prognostic significance, though some have used 3 cm[43] or 4 cm[31] and Doci and coworkers found the extent of liver involvement to be predictive.[37] There does not appear to be a consistent size limitation if the lesion can be resected with negative margins. Similarly, there is surprising variability in the results regarding number of liver lesions, though their location in one or both lobes does not seem important. Cady et al.[36] and Fortner et al.[40] have found that one versus two or more lesions (single versus multiple) are significant factors for overall survival. Several studies[30,32,33,42] report significantly better prognosis with three or fewer nodules as opposed to four or more, though the results from Scheele and associates do not confirm this finding.[38] Others have evaluated four or fewer compared with five or more metastases, with variable results.[9,10,47] Moreover, several authors report long-term survival in patients with up to ten nodules.[9,38,47] Although the results regarding the absolute number of lesions to be resected are inconsistent, there is general agreement that patients with few lesions have a significantly better prognosis and that those with more than three or four lesions should be considered poor candidates for hepatic resection.

The most consistent and significant factors predicting poor outcome are the presence of extrahepatic disease and positive margins. Patients with clear margins of 1 cm or more have a significantly improved survival, whereas those with less than 1 cm or histologically positive margins have a similar poor prognosis.[38]

In summary, patients with three or four lesions and no evidence of extrahepatic disease are candidates for hepatic resection of their metastases, either by wedge or anatomic resection, as long as there is a reasonable expectation of obtaining at least 1-cm margins around the lesions (see Table 26.3). The preoperative evaluation should be detailed and sensitive enough to exclude those with extrahepatic disease. Evaluation of the liver should include an assessment of the number of lesions as well as the anatomy to determine resectability and the ability to obtain clear margins. Patients with extrahepatic disease should be considered for systemic chemotherapy, whereas those with numerous bilateral lesions and no extrahepatic disease may be candidates for hepatic artery infusional therapy. Cryosurgery or radiofrequency ablation with or without resection may be an option for patients with

Table 26.4 *Prognostic factors for survival following hepatic resection for colorectal metastases*

Prognostic factor	Reference number	
	Significant	Non-significant
Age	33	30,31,34,36,37,38,40,41,42,44
Gender	37	30,31,33,34,35,38,39,40,41,42
Dukes' stage	34,37,38,39,40,41,42	8,30,31,33,35,36,44,46,53
Synchronous/metachronous	8,34,38,41	30,31,40,46
Disease-free interval	33,38,42,53	9,30,31,34,36,37,40,44
Preoperative carcinoembryonic antigen	36,41,42,44,	8,35,37,40,53
Size of metastases	30,32,41,42,43,44,46	8,9,30,33,34,35,36,38,39
Number of metastases	9,30,32,33,36,42,44	8,31,34,35,37,38,40,43,46,53
Unilobar versus bilobar	30,33,37	8,9,32,36,38,41,42,44,46,53
Extrahepatic disease	31,33,34,35,38,39,40,41,53	
Type of liver resection	30,36,37,41	8,9,32,33,34,35,38,39,42,44
Blood loss	34,36,43,44,45	30,33
Surgical margin	8,31,32,33,35,36,38,41,42,46,53	
Satellite lesions	34,38,41	
Ploidy	32,36	

multiple lesions with bilobar distribution or lesions excluded from resection due to anatomic considerations.

Operative procedure

The type of hepatic resection does not influence prognosis.[8,32–35,38,39,42,44] Rather, the operative approach should be guided by the anatomy of the liver disease, with the goals of obtaining adequate margins and minimizing the incidence of postoperative liver failure by preserving normal liver tissue (Table 26.5).

Another consideration is the management of synchronous versus metachronous metastases. Synchronous liver metastases are found in 15–25% of patients with primary colorectal cancer.[4] When resectable liver metastases are identified preoperatively in a good candidate, either a combined procedure or a staged approach can be employed. Resection of hepatic metastases discovered at the time of exploratory laparotomy for resection of a colorectal primary should be addressed at a second operation unless there is minimal disease that can be resected with a straightforward wedge resection. Major anatomic resections performed in this setting are associated with a significant risk of septic and gastrointestinal complications, including anastomotic dehiscence, small-bowel obstruction, perforation, and ischemic colitis.[10,48,49]

The liver is exposed through an extended right subcostal incision and detailed abdominal and pelvic exploration is performed to confirm the absence of extrahepatic disease, with particular attention to the porta hepatis. RIGS may increase the sensitivity of this exploration and improve the selection of candidates for curative resection, though this needs to be further evaluated.[27] Any suspicious extrahepatic lesions should be biopsied, with frozen-section analysis done; hepatic resection should be aborted if metastatic disease is identified in these extrahepatic tissues. In this situation, a decision can be made regarding the placement of a hepatic infusion pump. In the absence of extrahepatic disease, the liver is fully mobilized and examination is performed using IOUS. The number and location of the lesions are confirmed and the vascular anatomy is defined. A final decision is made regarding resectability and the type of resection to be performed (Table 26.5; Figure 26.1). If the lesions are unresectable, cryosurgery or placement of a hepatic infusion pump can be considered (see Table 26.3).

Resection is performed using the continuous ultrasonic surgical aspirator (CUSA) or finger-fracture of the hepatic parenchyma after scoring Glisson's capsule. Small vessels and biliary radicals are clipped as they are encountered and larger branches are ligated or suture ligated (Figure 26.2). In formal resections, the hepatic vein is oversewn. The argon beam laser can be helpful to attain hemostasis of the raw surface of the liver. Temporary vascular occlusion can be performed using the Pringle maneuver, applying a vascular clamp to the porta hepatis. Vascular inflow can be occluded for up to 45 min at a time, but should be minimized to decrease the incidence of hepatic failure postoperatively. Usually, total hepatic isolation is not necessary. At the completion of the procedure, the surface is examined and any biliary radicals identified are clipped or oversewn; a drain may or may not be necessary.

Postoperatively, patients are initially observed for signs of clotting abnormalities and bleeding. The administration of vitamin K and fresh frozen plasma is begun if the prothrombin time exceeds 18 s or if non-surgical bleeding develops. After major lobectomy, patients are given 50 mmol per day of phosphorus (usually as K-acid phosphate) to maintain normal serum phosphorus levels. If a nasogastric tube has been placed, it is removed quickly to improve pulmonary function.

Clinical monitoring of liver function is performed. If persistent or increasing hyperbilirubinemia occurs, a nuclear medicine scan can be used to evaluate for the presence of biliary obstruction. Alternatively, endoscopic retrograde cholangiopancreatography (ERCP) can be done if this is inconclusive or if a persistent bile leak occurs. Generally, the postoperative length of stay after major resection is in the range of 6–9 days.

Results

The perioperative mortality for hepatic resection for colorectal metastases with curative intent ranges from 0% to 9% in recent series, with the majority less than 5% (Table 26.6).[8,10,30,31,33–35,38,45,49–58] The major operative morbidity ranges from 13% to 35% with an average of 23%, reviewing the series listed in Table 26.7. The complications

Table 26.5 *Operative approaches to hepatic resection based on pattern of disease*

Operative approach	Pattern of disease
Wedge resections	Single or multiple superficial nodules Unilobar or bilobar
Anatomic resection (lobectomy, extended lobectomy, trisegmentectomy)	Multiple, unilobar metastases Bilobar lesions amenable to trisegmentectomy Large, bulky lesion Deep or central nodule
Anatomic plus wedge resection (or anatomic resection with cryoablation)	Large or deep lesion with smaller, superficial metastasis in contralateral lobe Multiple unilobar metastases with single lesion in contralateral lobe

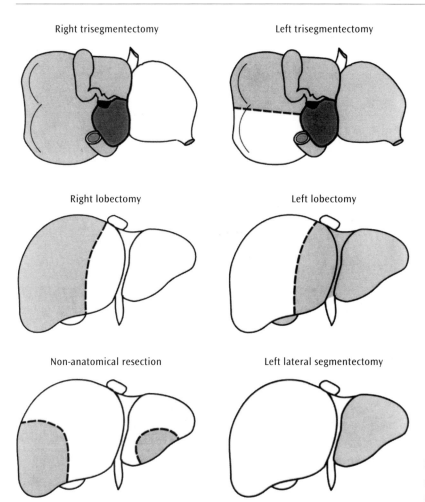

Right trisegmentectomy

Left trisegmentectomy

Right lobectomy

Left lobectomy

Non-anatomical resection

Left lateral segmentectomy

Figure 26.1 *Types of hepatic resection. (Reproduced with permission from Iwatsuki and Starzl, 1993.[121])*

most often contributing to operative mortality are hepatic failure and hemorrhage;[38,42] the major sources of non-fatal morbidity are hepatic failure, bleeding, abscess, and bile leak resulting in fistula or biloma. In addition to the careful selection of patients with adequate hepatic reserve, precise and rapid dissection with judicious use of vascular occlusion are critical to minimize these complications. Also, specific attention should be directed at oversewing small biliary radicals and securing the major bile duct at the completion of the resection. Most bile collections and abscesses can be drained percutaneously. Significant bleeding requires reoperation.

The 5-year survival for patients undergoing curative hepatic resection for colorectal metastases ranges from 21% to 48% (Tables 26.6 and 26.8). The survival data in these tables reflect patients undergoing complete resection of all metastases with clear surgical margins. The data from several of these series underscore the significance of obtaining adequate surgical margins. Scheele and coworkers[38] report a 37% 5-year survival in 207 of 219 patients resected for cure with negative surgical margins. The 10-year survival in this group was 25%. In this same series, 44 patients underwent curative resection but had histologically positive margins. None of these

patients survived more than 4 years. Similarly, Savage and Malt[35] report a 27% 5-year survival for patients resected with margins more than 5 mm, as opposed to 9% if the margin was 5 mm or less. The 5-year survival for all patients in their series was 18%. More recent studies have confirmed these findings, emphasizing the importance of obtaining a minimum clear surgical margin.[46,59]

A number of clinical and pathologic factors are thought to influence the prognosis following liver resection for colorectal metastases (see Table 26.4). By far the most significant factors determining outcome are the absence of extrahepatic disease and clear surgical margins (≥ 1 cm). The type of resection, comparing formal lobectomy to wedge resection, does not appear important as long as adequate margins can be obtained. Although only a few studies have included an evaluation of intraoperative blood loss, several have found a correlation between blood loss or the use of perioperative transfusion and survival.[34,36,43–45] Further, Doci *et al.* also found a significant correlation between blood transfusion and postoperative complications.[49] Pathologic factors such as satellite lesions[34,38] or aneuploid tumors[32,36] are associated with a poorer prognosis. Yamaguchi and

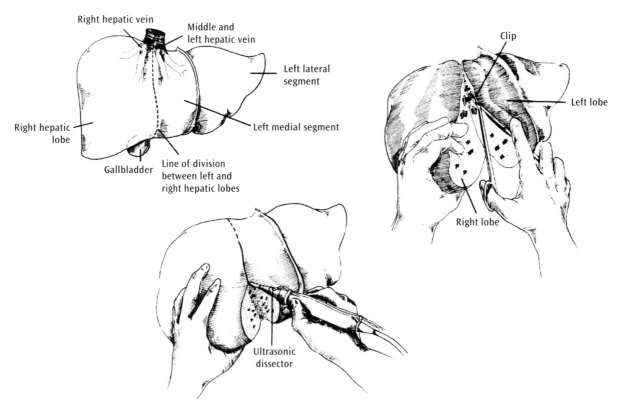

Figure 26.2 *Technique of hepatic lobectomy. The branches of the hepatic artery, hepatic duct, and portal vein are divided. Glisson's capsule is scored along the line of demarcation and the resection is performed using the continuous ultrasonic surgical aspirator (CUSA). Vessels and biliary radicals are either clipped or ligated as they are encountered. (Reproduced with permission from Daly, 1993.[122])*

Table 26.6 *Survival after curative hepatic resection[a] for colorectal metastases, 1990–1999*

Series	Number of patients	Operative mortality (%)	5-year survival (%)
Bradley *et al.* (1999)[50]	134	4	36 (23% 10-year)
Nakamura *et al.* (1999)[51]	79	–	49 (33% 10-year)
Rees *et al.* (1997)[46]	89	0.9	37
Fong *et al.* (1997)[53]	456	4	38
Pinson *et al.* (1996)[52]	95	4	32
Wanebo *et al.* (1996)[30]	74	7	24
Scheele *et al.* (1995)[41]	434	4.4	33 (20% 10-year)
Pedersen *et al.* (1994)[31]	50	7.5	36 (3-year)
Gayowski *et al.* (1994)[33]	204	0	32
Sugihara *et al.* (1993)[8]	109	1.8	48
Bozzetti *et al.* (1993)[54]	39	–	47 (3-year)
Rosen *et al.* (1992)[34]	280	1.4	28
Savage and Malt (1992)[35]	104	4.8	27
Lind *et al.* (1992)[55]	50	9	28
van Ooijen *et al.* (1992)[45]	118	7.6	21
Hodgson *et al.* (1992)[56]	22	0	35
Doci *et al.* (1991)[37]	100	5	30
Steele *et al.* (1991)[10]	69	2.7	Median survival 37 months
Fegiz *et al.* (1991)[57]	859	6.8	33
Scheele *et al.* (1991)[38]	219	5.5	37 (25% 10-year)
Lise *et al.* (1990)[58]	39	5	32

[a]Where possible, only patients with absence of extrahepatic disease and negative resection margins (minimum of 0.5–1.0 cm as defined by author) were included from each series for survival data in this table.
– Not available.

Table 26.7 *Complications following hepatic resection for colorectal metastases*

	Reference number							Total number, all series
	10	30	38	40	42	49	60	
Year of study	1991	1996	1991	1984	1996	1995	1992	–
Number of patients in series	142	74	266	65	1568	208	43	2366
Number of patients with morbidity	19	26	55	18	345	72	10	545
Overall major morbidity (%)	(13)	(26)	(22)	(27)	(23)	(35)	(23)	(23)
Complication								
Liver failure	–	6	14	–	43	2	1	66 (13)
Hemorrhage	2	–	8	1	28	4	–	43 (8)
Subphrenic abscess	4	5	4	5	–	13	–	26 (14)
Bile leak/fistula	3	2	8	–	48	10	1	72 (14)
Sepsis	1	3	–	–	105	–	–	109 (28)
All pulmonary complications	3	9	16	9	–	23	3	63 (31)
Pulmonary embolus	1	1	1	–	–	–	–	3 (3)
Pleural effusion	1	5	12	6	–	–	–	24 (20)
Cardiac complications	1	2	2	–	–	1	–	6 (3)
Wound infection/dehiscence	1	3	2	1	–	3	3	13 (6)
Acute renal failure	1	2	1	–	–	–	–	4 (4)
Deep venous thrombosis	–	–	2	1	–	–	2	5 (6)
Gastrointestinal complications	1	–	12	–	–	8	–	21 (14)

– None reported. Numbers in parentheses are percentages.

Table 26.8 *Survival after curative hepatic resection[a] for colorectal metastases, 1980–1989*

Series	Number of patients	Operative mortality (%)	5-year survival (%)
Hughes *et al.* (1989)[61]	800	–	32
Iwatsuki *et al.* (1989)[62]	86	0	38
Sesto *et al.* (1987)[63]	61	7	28
Nordlinger *et al.* (1987)[48]	80	5	25
Butler *et al.* (1986)[64]	62	10	34
Adson *et al.* (1984)[39]	141	2	25
Fortner *et al.* (1984)[40]	65	7	40
Foster and Lundy (1981)[65]	231	5	23

[a]Where possible, only patients with absence of extrahepatic disease and negative resection margins (minimum of 0.5–1.0 cm as defined by author) were included from the series for survival data in this table.
– Not available.

coworkers[32] found that aneuploid tumors had a recurrence rate of 56%, compared to diploid tumors with an 18% recurrence rate.

Recurrence of colorectal carcinoma occurs in 60–80% of patients following hepatic resection. The lung is the most common site of recurrent extrahepatic disease, found in over 50% of patients with recurrence, followed by other intra-abdominal sites such as porta hepatis or retroperitoneal lymph nodes and the adrenal.[8,66] Approximately 40–50% of patients have a recurrence in the liver, and 20–40% have disease limited to the liver.[8,42,50,53,66,67] Most commonly, hepatic recurrence occurs at sites other than the resection bed. Resection-bed recurrence is found in only 15–30% of patients with liver-only disease, though this clearly relates to the surgical margin obtained at the original resection.[8,38,66]

In their series of 109 patients, Sugihara and coworkers report 64 patients with recurrence and 91% of liver recurrences were detected within the first 18 months.[8]

REPEAT HEPATIC RESECTION

As a generalization, approximately one-third of patients undergoing resection for hepatic metastases will have long-term survival. Of patients that recur, about 30–40% recur in the liver only,[50,53] and the remainder develop disseminated disease. Because resection is the only modality offering a chance of cure, patients who have recurrent disease limited to the liver should be considered for repeat hepatic resection. There have been numerous

Table 26.9 *Repeat hepatic resection for colorectal metastases*

Series	Number of patients	Operative mortality (%)	Morbidity (%)	Median survival (months)	Overall survival (%)
Fong et al. (1994)[69]	25	0	28	30	–
Que and Nagorney (1994)[70]	21	5	Low	40	43 (4 years)
Nordlinger et al. (1994)[71]	116	0.9	25	30	33 (3 years)
Fernandez-Trigo et al. (1995)[72]	170	–	19	34	45 (3 years) 32 (5 years)
Tuttle et al. (1997)[73]	23	0	22	40	32 (5 years) 13 (>5 years)

– Not available.

small, single-institution series, reviewed by Wanebo and coworkers,[68] that demonstrate the technical feasibility of repeat hepatic resection. Several larger single and multi-institutional series confirm that the operative mortality is low and the morbidity is similar to that reported for initial resections (Table 26.9).[51,69–73] To minimize complications, patients should be carefully selected for repeat liver resection, especially with regard to hepatic reserve. Tests of hepatic reserve such as indocyanin green or galactose tolerance tests can be helpful.

The median survival following second hepatectomy ranges from 30 to 40 months. The overall survival following second liver resection approximates the results seen following initial resection. The 3-year survival is reported as 33–45% and one group reports a 5-year survival of 32%.[70–72] Nordlinger and associates report recurrence in 66% of 116 patients undergoing second resection for colorectal metastases. Eighty-four percent of these recurrences involved the liver.[71] The prognostic factors for outcome are similar for the first and second resections. In the series of 170 patients from the Registry of Repeat Resection of Hepatic Metastasis, the absence of extrahepatic disease and negative surgical margins were important factors in predicting long-term survival after second hepatic resection for colorectal metastases. The interval between first and second resection, the type of resection, and the number of liver lesions did not impact significantly on outcome.[72]

CRYOTHERAPY

Cryotherapy provides an adjunct to hepatic resection for the treatment of liver metastases.[74–77] The main indications for cryosurgery include unresectable lesions due to multiplicity, bilobar distribution, or anatomic limitations and patient comorbid conditions or limited hepatic reserve that prohibit hepatic resection (Table 26.10). Additionally, cryoablation may be used in the setting of cryo-assisted resection[78] or in conjunction with resection in the treatment of contralateral lobe lesions in a patient undergoing hepatic lobectomy. In general, however,

Table 26.10 *Indications for cryoablation: unresectable disease*

	Indication for cryosurgery
Tumor characteristics	Multiple bilateral lesions Central lesion not amenable to anatomic resection Contralateral nodules in patient undergoing hepatic lobectomy
Host factors	Comorbid disease precluding resection Limited hepatic reserve Cirrhosis Prior liver resection
Technical considerations	Cryo-assisted resection

hepatic resection is the treatment of choice for liver metastases and is the only proven effective modality.

Cryotherapy ablates tumor tissue along with a margin of adjacent normal liver tissue using a probe cooled with liquid nitrogen inserted directly into the metastasis. The subzero temperatures result in the formation of intracellular ice crystals, denaturation of cellular proteins, reduction of cell volume, and destruction of tumor vasculature.[79,80] In a small phase I trial, cryoablated lesions were immediately resected, showing that the IOUS findings correlated well with the histologic findings and confirming adequate margins.[76] Most patients treated with cryosurgery, however, have been followed clinically with CT scans and serum CEA levels and cryoablated lesions persist as abnormal densities on serial CT scans. Few patients have had subsequent histologic confirmation of disease control; biopsy of the persistent cryoablated site usually shows scar tissue.[74,77]

Operative technique

The operative approach is quite similar to that for hepatic resection. Use of the Bair Hugger warming device has been shown to minimize hypothermia.[81] The liver is exposed through an extended right subcostal incision and is mobilized by dividing the hepatic ligaments. A thorough exploration of the abdomen and pelvis is performed to assess the liver and confirm the absence of extrahepatic disease. IOUS is used to identify additional hepatic metastases to be treated and to define the anatomy of the lesions in relation to major vascular and biliary structures. Any resectable lesions are excised. Prior to the first freeze, the patient is given mannitol and sodium bicarbonate to minimize complications from myoglobinuria. Glisson's capsule is incised with cautery over the lesion to be cryoablated and IOUS is used to guide the needle and sheath introducer and probe placement. IOUS is also used to monitor the progress of the freeze process. Different-sized probes can be used, depending on the size of the ice ball to be achieved. Large lesions require the placement of multiple probes and lesions as large as 10–12 cm have been treated successfully. Freezing is continued until the freeze front extends 1–2 cm beyond the edges of the lesion, usually for a median of 8 min. By IOUS, the metastasis remains hyperechoic while the frozen adjacent liver appears hypoechoic. The period of thawing is of approximately the same duration as the freeze cycle and a minimum of two freeze–thaw cycles is recommended, based on experimental animal data.[82] After removal, bleeding from the probe site is controlled by packing with Surgicel or Gelfoam.

Polk and coworkers[78] have described a technique of cryo-assisted hepatic resection, maintaining an ice ball with alternating freeze and thaw cycles every minute during the hepatic dissection. The plane of dissection is on or near the ice ball and the probe can be used as a handle to facilitate exposure. This approach is felt to improve the likelihood of obtaining clear margins during wedge resection, to facilitate resection in anatomically difficult areas, and to allow minimal resection of normal parenchyma in patients with limited hepatic reserve.

Results

The operative mortality is less than 5%, though there were no operative deaths reported in combined series of 250 patients.[76] The major morbidity rate ranges from 6% to 38%[74,77] and includes the cryoshock phenomenon of disseminated intravascular coagulation and multisystem organ failure, severe coagulopathy, hepatic hemorrhage requiring reoperation, biliary fistula, subphrenic or hepatic abscess, and acute tubular necrosis (Table 26.11). Myoglobinuria and asymptomatic right pleural effusions are common minor complications that are seen in most patients.

Ravikumar et al.[74] reported a series of 32 patients with colorectal, neuroendocrine, and 'other' metastases or hepatocellular carcinoma that were treated with cryosurgery between 1985 and 1990. Only 75% could be rendered free of disease. The disease-free survival in

Table 26.11 *Complications of cryosurgery*

Major complications	Minor complications
Cryoshock phenomenon	Pleural effusions
Severe coagulopathy	Myoglobinuria
Hepatic hemorrhage	Fever
Biliary fistula	Increased PT, decreased
Subphrenic or hepatic abscess	platelets
Acute tubular necrosis	Transient increased LFTs
Wound dehiscence	Leukocytosis

PT, prothrombin time; LFTs, liver function tests.

patients with colorectal metastases was 29%, with a median follow-up of 24 months. Fifty-nine percent of recurrences occurred in both the liver and extrahepatic sites; there were local recurrences at the cryoablated site in two patients. Similar results were reported by Onik and coworkers in a series of 18 patients treated with hepatic cryosurgery, four of whom were left with residual disease. After a median follow-up of 28.8 months, 22% were in complete remission (four patients).[75] Another series of 136 patients with otherwise unresectable disease underwent cryosurgery, with a median survival of 30 months and an operative mortality of 3.6%.[77] Morris and Ross report 92 patients with unresectable colorectal hepatic metastases treated with cryosurgery who had a median survival of 23 months. Analysis of those patients whose serum CEA level normalized after treatment revealed a median survival of 33 months, compared with 13 months for those whose CEA levels remained elevated.[83] When updating their series to 116 patients, Seifert and Morris reported that low preoperative CEA, size of the lesions treated (≤ 3 cm), absence of untreated extrahepatic disease at laparotomy, synchronous development of metastases, stage (no nodes) and low or moderate differentiation of the primary tumor, and completeness of cryoablation were independent prognostic factors for outcome.[84] Steele highlights the impact of residual disease on survival following cryosurgery, showing that survival in patients who can be rendered disease free by cryosurgery approximates that of the Gastrointestinal Tumor Study Group (GITSG).[76] However, no direct comparison can be made between patients undergoing resection and those treated with cryosurgery, and the current cryosurgery series are small with limited follow-up.

HEPATIC ARTERY INFUSION

Hepatic artery infusion (HAI) of chemotherapeutic agents using an implantable pump is an option for patients with unresectable liver metastases from colorectal carcinoma. The basis of regional therapy using HAI is the fact that tumor deposits in the liver are selectively perfused by branches of the hepatic artery while the

Table 26.12 *Hepatic artery infusion pump: toxicities associated with FUDR infusion*

Series	Number of patients	Complication (%)					
		Gastritis	Ulcer	SGOT	Bilirubin	Diarrhea	Biliary sclerosis
Niederhuber et al. (1984)[88]	70	56	8	32	24	–	–
Balch and Urist (1986)[89]	50	–	6	23	23	0	–
Kemeny N, et al. (1984)[90]	41	29	29	71	22	0	5
Shepard et al. (1985)[91]	53	–	20	49	24	–	–
Cohen et al. (1983)[92]	50		–	40	10	25	–
Weiss et al. (1983)[93]	17	50	11	80	23	23	–
Schwartz et al. (1985)[94]	23	53	–	77	20	10	–
Johnson et al. (1983)[95]	40	40	8	50	13	0	5
Kemeny MM, et al. (1986)[96]	31	17	6	47	–	8	19
Hohn et al. (1987)[97]	6	35	2	0	78	11	29

SGOT, serum alanine aminotransferase.
Reprinted with permission from Kemeny NE, Younes A. Chemotherapeutic liver infusion. In Wanebo HJ, ed. *Colorectal cancer.* Philadelphia, Mosby, 1993, 422.

primary blood supply to the normal liver is through the portal vein.[85] Thus, chemotherapeutic agents administered through the hepatic artery are targeted to the metastases. Further, Sigurdson and coworkers showed that ^{3}H-FUDR (5-fluro-2-deoxyuridine) is concentrated 15-fold in tumor cells when injected via the hepatic artery when compared with portal vein delivery, whereas the drug was uniformly distributed in the normal parenchyma when infused through either route.[86]

Regional hepatic chemotherapy also maximizes local drug exposure while minimizing systemic toxicities by using agents primarily cleared by the liver. FUDR, the primary drug used for HAI of colorectal metastases, is an antimetabolite that is catabolized to 5-fluorouracil (5-FU) when given intra-arterially. FUDR is cleared primarily by the liver on first pass (94–99% of FUDR[87] compared to 19–55% of 5-FU), and much higher effective doses can be delivered locally with limited systemic effects. The main toxicities of HAI are related to local effects on the liver and upper gastrointestinal tract (Table 26.12).[88–97] The liver function tests should be monitored closely. Hepatic toxicity is initially manifested by an elevation in serum aspartate aminotransferase, with elevations in alkaline phosphatase and finally bilirubin reflecting more severe toxicity. Initially, these changes are reversible and liver function tests return to normal when the FUDR is withheld. A certain percentage of patients, however, develop irreversible biliary strictures or more diffuse biliary sclerosis with findings similar to those of idiopathic sclerosing cholangitis.[98] For more focal strictures, ductal drainage can be accomplished using ERCP or a percutaneous transhepatic route. External compression of the ducts by bulky metastatic porta hepatis lymph nodes can be excluded by CT scan.

Gastritis and ulcer disease associated with HAI are felt to be due to chemotherapy perfusion of branches to the stomach and duodenum. Careful dissection and ligation of all branches to the stomach, duodenum, pancreas, and bile ducts distal to the cannulation site are necessary to prevent these complications.

Surgical considerations

All patients who are candidates for pump placement should have a preoperative celiac and superior mesenteric arteriogram to define the vascular anatomy. The option of hepatic infusion pump placement should be discussed with patients for whom hepatic resection is planned should the liver disease prove unresectable. Patients with extensive extrahepatic disease on exploration are not candidates for an infusion pump, but rather should be considered for systemic chemotherapy.

The hepatic infusion pump may be placed using either a right subcostal or upper midline incision. After exploration, cholecystectomy is performed to prevent chemical cholecystitis. Most commonly, the catheter is placed in the gastroduodenal artery (GDA) to the junction of the common hepatic and proper hepatic arteries and the GDA is ligated distal to the insertion site (Figure 26.3). Vascular anomalies, however, are common and require adjustment of the surgical approach (Table 26.13). In the usual situation, the junction of the common hepatic, proper hepatic, and gastroduodenal arteries is exposed and the GDA is dissected for 2 cm to the first portion of the duodenum. The right gastric artery is ligated, as are all branches distal to the infusion site that feed the stomach, duodenum, pancreas, or bile duct. Particular attention should be paid to the supraduodenal or the posterior pancreaticoduodenal artery arising from the posterior aspect of the GDA. After creating the subcutaneous pocket for the pump, the catheter is passed through the abdominal wall. The GDA is ligated distally and the catheter is advanced retrogradely through the GDA and secured at the junction with the common hepatic artery (Figure 26.3). Protrusion

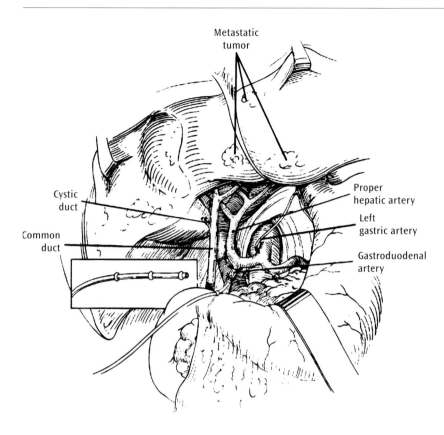

Cystic duct

Common duct

Metastatic tumor

Proper hepatic artery

Left gastric artery

Gastroduodenal artery

Figure 26.3 *Hepatic artery infusion pump placement. Cholecystectomy is performed to avoid the risk of chemical cholecystitis. The catheter is ligated in place in the gastroduodenal artery (GDA) with the tip just at the junction of the GDA and the proper hepatic artery. The right gastric artery and branches of the proximal GDA are divided. (Reproduced with permission from Niederhuber, 1993.[123])*

Table 26.13 *Hepatic artery infusion pump: altered surgical approach based on vascular supply*

Vascular supply	Incidence (%)	Surgical approach
(R) and (L) hepatic a. from proper hepatic a.	50	Single catheter via GDA to junction with proper hepatic a. (see text)
(R) and (L) hepatic a. at take-off of GDA	16	Single catheter via splenic a. to junction with common hepatic, ligate GDA
Accessory (L) hepatic a.	5	Single catheter via GDA, ligate accessory (L) hepatic a.
Accessory (R) hepatic a.	–	Single catheter via GDA, ligate accessory (R) hepatic a.
Replaced (L) hepatic a. from (L) gastric a.	5–6	Two catheters: (1) via GDA; (2) retrograde via (L) gastric a. to junction with (L) hepatic a.
Replaced (R) hepatic a. from SMA	16	Two catheters: (1) via GDA; (2) non-occluding 1.57 mm O.D. catheter into replaced (R) hepatic a.
Celiac a. stenosis with retrograde perfusion of proper hepatic a. via SMA to GDA	–	Single catheter via common hepatic a. to GDA junction, GDA *not* ligated

(R), right; (L), left; a., artery; GDA, gastroduodenal artery; SMA, superior mesenteric artery; O.D., outside diameter.

of the catheter into the common hepatic artery may result in turbulent flow, with unequal distribution of the chemotherapy drug or thrombosis of the vessel itself. Uniform perfusion of the liver can be confirmed at the completion of the procedure by injecting half-strength fluorescein through the sideport and viewing with the Wood's lamp. If operative flow to both lobes is

confirmed, a technetium perfusion scan postoperatively may not be required.

Apart from the hepatotoxicity already mentioned, most complications are related to technical considerations (Table 26.14). Dissection of side branches of the GDA and proper hepatic arteries must be complete. Care must be taken in the exact placement of the tip of the catheter at

Table 26.14 *Hepatic artery infusion: complications related to pump placement*

Complication	Causes	Treatment
Incomplete hepatic perfusion	Missed accessory or replaced (L) hepatic a. Short proper hepatic a. with incomplete mixing	May attempt embolization of (L) hepatic a. or ligation of (L) gastric a. to allow collateral flow
Extrahepatic perfusion (includes epigastric pain, ulcers, gastritis)	Perfusion of stomach, duodenum, etc. with chemotherapy agent Incomplete dissection intraoperatively	May be able to embolize small vessels to stomach or duodenum
Arterial thrombosis	Catheter advanced into common hepatic too far Catheter too far back in GDA with chemical vasculitis	Rarely, urokinase works
Catheter thrombosis	Backbleeding with improper flushing of sideport Incomplete or infrequent filling of pump	Rarely, urokinase works
Intra-abdominal bleeding	Pump catheter dislodges Clip dislodged from side branch	Immediate embolization or ligation of the artery
Infected pump pocket	Seroma with secondary infection Direct infection during pump manipulation	Removal of pump (antibiotics rarely work)

(L), left; a., artery; GDA, gastroduodenal artery.

Table 26.15 *Randomized studies of intrahepatic versus systemic chemotherapy for hepatic metastases*

Group	Number of patients	Response (%)			Survival (months)	
		HAI	Systemic	*p* value	HAI	Systemic
MSKCC[99]	162	52	20	0.001	18[a]	12
NCOG[96]	143	42	10	0.0001	16.6	16
NCI[100]	64	62	17	0.003	20[b]	11
Consortium[101]	43	58	38	–	–	–
City of Hope[102]	41	56	0	–	–	–
Mayo Clinic[103]	69	48	21	0.02	12.6	10.5
French[104]	163	49	14	–	15	11
English[105]	100	50	0	0.001	13	6.3

– Not stated; HAI, hepatic artery infusion; MSKCC, Memorial Sloan-Kettering Cancer Center; NCI, National Cancer Institute; NCOG, Northern California Oncology Group.
[a]Updated.
[b]*p*, 0.03 for patients with negative hepatic lymph nodes.
Reprinted with permission from Daly JM, Kemeny NE. Metastatic cancer to the liver. In DeVita VT, Hellman S, Rosenberg SA, eds. *Cancer: principles and practice of oncology*, 5th edn. Philadelphia, J.B. Lippincott, Co., 1997, 2562.

the junction of the GDA and the common hepatic artery. Uniform perfusion of the liver should be confirmed at the completion of the procedure. Special attention must be given to pump filling and manipulation of the sideport to avoid catheter thrombosis and pocket infection.

Results

There have been a number of randomized, clinical trials reviewed elsewhere[99] that have studied HAI versus systemic chemotherapy in patients with unresectable metastatic disease isolated to the liver.[97,100–106] Essentially, all have demonstrated a significantly higher response rate in patients treated with HAI (42–62%) compared with those treated with systemic chemotherapy (10–38%), though the difference in survival was not statistically significant (Table 26.15). These trials, however, were limited by small numbers of patients and cross-over design. A recent study by the Cancer and Leukemia Group B (CALGB) was designed to clarify the role of HAI versus systemic chemotherapy in patients with isolated hepatic metastases.

A few patients with initially unresectable disease may become operative candidates following treatment with HAI, though these patients are rare. Alternatively, some consideration has been given to HAI as an adjunct to hepatic resection, with an infusion pump placed at the time of resection. Several trials are underway to assess this issue. Trials reported to date have shown mixed results, with two trials supporting the implantation of hepatic artery pumps at the time of resection.[107–112] Most patients, however, recur in extrahepatic sites[8,66,67] and would require systemic chemotherapy. Patients with isolated liver recurrence after resection may be candidates for repeat hepatic resection (see above) or for HAI at that time.

FUTURE APPROACHES

New approaches to the management of colorectal metastases to the liver are being developed and studied for efficacy. These fall into three broad categories:

1 local ablative approaches;
2 chemotherapy administration;
3 regional gene therapy.

Cryosurgery of liver metastases is currently performed as an open surgical procedure using IOUS guidance. With the development of laparoscopic IOUS[113] and cryosurgical probes, laparoscopic approaches are being studied. Also, intraoperative MRI is being assessed for monitoring of the freeze process to improve the accuracy of margins around the lesion.

Alternatives to cryosurgery, such as radiofrequency ablation, are also being evaluated for patients with limited but unresectable liver metastases. Radiofrequency ablation destroys tissue by direct thermal necrosis, heating the cells to temperatures above 50 °C, denaturing intracellular proteins, and completely disrupting the cell membranes. Using IOUS, a monopolar array needle electrode is placed directly into the tumor nodule and allows treatment of single lesions less than 3 cm. Larger lesions require repeated applications to span the area. Selected patients with small peripheral lesions may be treated percutaneously, though general anesthesia may still be required to alleviate the pain associated with application.[114] Curley and associates recently reported a series of 123 patients with unresectable liver tumors (61 with colorectal metastases) treated with radiofrequency ablation, with no deaths and an overall complication rate of 2.4%. After 15 months' follow-up, the tumor has recurred at the site of treatment in 3 of 169 lesions treated (1.8% local failure rate) and new disease has developed in 28%.[114]

Because many patients recur in extrahepatic sites following 'curative' resection, it is clear that the potential benefit of adjuvant systemic chemotherapy following liver resection needs to be addressed. Efforts are ongoing to identify the significant prognostic variables and to determine which patients are most at risk for recurrence. In addition to using HAI following resection to minimize local recurrence, the combination of systemic and hepatic artery infusion of chemotherapy post-resection is being evaluated in clinical trials.

Approaches to the management of unresectable hepatic disease from colorectal or other cancers are also under investigation. Isolated hepatic perfusion allows the infusion of chemotherapy directly to the metastatic disease in much higher doses because there is no systemic perfusion with the associated dose-limiting toxicity. Fraker and coworkers[115] use an open technique of isolated hepatic perfusion based on their experience with isolated limb perfusion for melanoma. In their current phase I/II trial, melphalan with tumor necrosis factor are infused through the hepatic artery at escalating doses. Venous bypass is used, shunting portal and infrahepatic inferior vena cava blood to the axillary vein. Several groups have developed a catheter-based technique of isolated hepatic perfusion using a dual-balloon vena cava catheter.[116,117] Ravikumar et al. report a phase I/II clinical trial that included eight patients with colorectal cancer treated with escalating doses of 5-FU and all progressed on treatment.[117]

Regional gene therapy is being applied to the treatment of primary and metastatic liver tumors.[118] Issues of the optimal vector for delivery and expression, route of administration, and specific transgene delivered are under investigation. Retrovirus or adenovirus can be administered by intratumoral injection, intra-arterially using a percutaneous catheter or HAI pump, or intravenously through the portal vein or a peripheral vein. Different types of genes are being studied, including suicide genes such as thymidine kinase (TK) or cytosine deaminase; immunostimulatory molecule or cytokine genes; and tumor suppressor genes such as p53. Animal studies have been reported using rat or murine models, with subcapsular colon cancer liver nodules injected with HSV1-TK retroviral producer cells[119] or adenovirus with the IL2 and/or TK transgenes,[120] with evidence of regression. Antisense therapy remains another alternative. Gene therapy is an exciting modality under active investigation that can be applied to the treatment of colorectal liver metastases.

REFERENCES

1. Greenlee RT, Murray T, Bolden S, Wingo PA. Cancer statistics, 2000. CA Cancer J Clin 2000; 50:7–26.
2. Scheele J, Stangl R, Altendorf-Hofmann A. Hepatic metastases from colorectal carcinoma: impact of surgical resection on the natural history. Br J Surg 1990; 77:1241–6.

3. Wood CB, Gillis CR, Blumgart LH. A retrospective study of the natural history of patients with metastases from colorectal cancer. Clin Oncol 1976; 2:285–8.

4. Ballantyne GH, Quin J. Surgical treatment of liver metastases in patients with colorectal cancer. Cancer 1993; 71:4252–66.

5. Lefor AT, Hughes KS, Shiloni E, et al. Intra-abdominal extrahepatic disease in patients with colorectal hepatic metastases. Dis Col Rect 1988; 31:100–3.

6. Gibbs JF, Weber TK, Rodriguez-Bigas MA, Driscoll DL, Petrelli NJ. Intraoperative determinants of unresectability for patients with colorectal hepatic metastases. Cancer 1998; 82:1244–9.

7. Jarnagin WR, Fong Y, Ky A, et al. Liver resection for metastatic colorectal cancer: assessing the risk of occult irresectable disease. J Am Coll Surg 1999; 188:33–42.

8. Sugihara K, Hojo K, Moriya Y, Yamasaki S, Kosuge T, Takayama T. Pattern of recurrence after hepatic resection for colorectal metastases. Br J Surg 1993; 80:1032–5.

9. Kemeny MM. Hepatic resection: when, what kind, and for which patients. J Surg Oncol 1991; 2:54–8.

10. Steele G Jr, Bleday R, Mayer RJ, Lindblad A, Petrelli N, Weaver D. A prospective evaluation of hepatic resection for colorectal carcinoma metastases to the liver: Gastrointestinal Tumor Study Group Protocol 6548. J Clin Oncol 1991; 9:1105–12.

11. Benotti P, Steele G Jr. Patterns of recurrent colorectal cancer and recovery surgery. Cancer 1992; 70:1409–13.

12. Soyer P, Levesque M, Elias D, Zeitoun G, Roche A. Preoperative assessment of resectability of hepatic metastases from colonic carcinoma: CT portography vs. sonography and dynamic CT. Am J Roentgenol 1992; 159:741–4.

13. Wernecke K, Rummeny E, Bongartz G, et al. Detection of hepatic masses in patients with carcinoma: comparative sensitivities of sonography, CT, and MR imaging. Am J Roentgenol 1991; 157:731–9.

14. Heiken JP, Weyman PJ, Lee JK, et al. Detection of focal hepatic masses: prospective evaluation with CT, delayed CT, CT during arterial portography, and MR imaging. Radiology 1989; 171:47–51.

15. Nelson RC, Chezmer JL, Sugarbaker PH, Bernardino ME. Hepatic tumors: comparison of CT during arterial portography, delayed CT, and MR imaging for preoperative evaluation. Radiology 1989; 172:27–34.

16. Vogel SB, Drane WE, Ros PR, Kerns SR, Bland KI. Prediction of surgical resectability in patients with hepatic colorectal metastases. Ann Surg 1994; 219:508–14.

17. Soyer P, Bluemke DA, Hruban RH, Sitzmann JV, Fishman EK. Hepatic metastases from colorectal cancer: detection and false-positive findings with helical CT during arterial portography. Radiology 1994; 193:71–4.

18. Soyer P, Lacheheb D, Levesque M. False-positive CT portography: correlation with pathologic findings. Am J Roentgenol 1993; 160:285–9.

19. Machi J, Isomoto H, Kurohiji T, et al. Accuracy of intraoperative ultrasonography in diagnosing liver metastasis from colorectal cancer: evaluation with postoperative follow-up results. World J Surg 1991; 15:551–6.

20. Russo A, Sparacino G, Plaja S, et al. Role of intraoperative ultrasound in the screening of liver metastases from colorectal carcinoma: initial experiences. J Surg Oncol 1989; 42:249–55.

21. Knol JA, Marn CS, Francis IR, Rubin JM, Bromberg J, Chang AE. Comparisons of dynamic infusion and delayed computed tomography, intraoperative ultrasound, and palpation in the diagnosis of liver metastases. Am J Surg 1993; 165:81–8.

22. Parker GA, Lawrence W Jr, Horsley JS III, et al. Intraoperative ultrasound of the liver affects operative decision making. Ann Surg 1989; 209:569–76.

23. Soyer P, Levesque M, Elias D, Zeitoun G, Roche A. Detection of liver metastases from colorectal cancer: comparison of intraoperative US and CT during arterial portography. Radiology 1992; 183:541–4.

24. Cohen AM, Martin EW Jr, Lavery I, et al. Radioimmunoguided surgery using iodine 125 B72.3 in patients with colorectal cancer. Arch Surg 1991; 126:349–52.

25. Martin EW Jr, Carey LC. Second-look surgery for colorectal cancer. The second time around. Ann Surg 1991; 214:321–5.

26. DiCarlo V, Badellino F, Stella M, et al. Role of B72.3 iodine 125-labeled monoclonal antibody in colorectal cancer detection by radioimmunoguided surgery. Surgery 1994; 115:190–8.

27. Arnold MW, Schneebaum S, Berens A, et al. Intraoperative detection of colorectal cancer with radioimmunoguided surgery and CC49, a second-generation monoclonal antibody. Ann Surg 1992; 216:627–32.

28. Arnold MW, Schneebaum S, Berens A, Mojzisik C, Hinkel G, Martin EW Jr. Radioimmunoguided surgery challenges traditional decision making in patients with primary colorectal cancer. Surgery 1992; 112:624–30.

29. Triozzi PL, Kim JA, Aldrich W, Young DC, Sampsel JW, Martin EW Jr. Localization of tumor-reactive lymph node lymphocytes in vivo using radiolabeled monoclonal antibody. Cancer 1994; 73:580–9.

30. Wanebo HJ, Chu QD, Vezeridis MP, Soderberg C. Patient selection for hepatic resection of colorectal metastases. Arch Surg 1996; 131:322–9.

31. Pedersen IK, Burcharth F, Roikjaer O, Baden H. Resection of liver metastases from colorectal cancer. Indications and results. Dis Col Rect 1994; 37:1078–82.

32. Yamaguchi A, Kurosaka Y, Kanno M, *et al*. Analysis of hepatic recurrence of colorectal cancer after resection of hepatic metastases. Int Surgery 1993; 78:16–19.

33. Gayowski TJ, Iwatsuki S, Madariaga JR, *et al*. Experience in hepatic resection for metastatic colorectal cancer: analysis of clinical and pathologic risk factors. Surgery 1994; 116:703–11.

34. Rosen CB, Nagorney DM, Taswell HF, *et al*. Perioperative blood transfusion and determinants of survival after resection for metastatic colorectal carcinoma. Ann Surg 1992; 216:493–504.

35. Savage AP, Malt RA. Survival after hepatic resection for malignant tumours. Br J Surg 1992; 79:1095–101.

36. Cady B, Stone MD, McDermott WV Jr, *et al*. Technical and biological factors in disease-free survival after hepatic resection for colorectal cancer metastases. Arch Surg 1992; 127:561–8.

37. Doci R, Gennari L, Bignami P, Montalto F, Morabito A, Bozzetti F. One hundred patients with hepatic metastases from colorectal cancer treated by resection: analysis of prognostic determinants. Br J Surg 1991; 78:797–801.

38. Scheele J, Stangl R, Altendorf-Hofmann A, Gall FP. Indicators of prognosis after hepatic resection for colorectal secondaries. Surgery 1991; 110:13–29.

39. Adson MA, van Heerden JA, Adson MH, Wagner JS, Ilstrup DM. Resection of hepatic metastases from colorectal cancer. Arch Surg 1984; 119:647–51.

40. Fortner JG, Silva JS, Golbey RG, Cox EB, MacLean BJ. Multivariate analysis of a personal series of 247 consecutive patients with liver metastases from colorectal cancer. I. Treatment by hepatic resection. Ann Surg 1984; 199:306–16.

41. Scheele J, Stang R, Altendorf-Hofmann A, Paul M. Resection of colorectal liver metastases. World J Surg 1995; 19:59–71.

42. Nordlinger B, Guiguet M, Vaillant J-C, *et al*. Surgical resection of colorectal carcinoma metastases to the liver: a prognostic scoring system to improve case selection, based on 1568 patients. Cancer 1996; 77:1254–62.

43. Stephenson KR, Steinberg SM, Hughes KS, Vetto JT, Sugarbaker PH, Chang AE. Perioperative blood transfusions are associated with reduced time to recurrence and decreased survival after resection of colorectal liver metastases. Ann Surg 1988; 208:679–87.

44. Younes RN, Rogatko A, Brennan MF. The influence of intraoperative hypotension and perioperative blood transfusion on disease-free survival in patients with complete resection of colorectal liver metastases. Ann Surg 1991; 214:107–13.

45. van Ooijen B, Wiggers T, Meijer S, *et al*. Hepatic resections for colorectal metastases in the Netherlands. A multi-institutional 10-year study. Cancer 1992; 70:28–34.

46. Rees M, Plant G, Bygrave S. Late results justify resection for multiple hepatic metastases from colorectal cancer. Br J Surg 1997; 84:1136–40.

47. Iwatsuki S, Esquivel CO, Gordon RD, Starzl TE. Liver resection for metastatic colorectal cancer. Surgery 1986; 100:804–10.

48. Nordlinger B, Quilichini MA, Parc Rannoun L, Delva E, Huguet C. Hepatic resection for colorectal liver metastases: influence on survival of preoperative factors and surgery for recurrence in 80 patients. Ann Surg 1987; 205:256–63.

49. Doci R, Gennari L, Bignami P, *et al*. Morbidity and mortality after hepatic resection of metastases from colorectal cancer. Br J Surg 1995; 82:377–81.

50. Bradley AL, Chapman WC, Wright JK, *et al*. Surgical experience with hepatic colorectal metastasis. Am Surg 1999; 65:560–6.

51. Nakamura S, Suzuki S, Konno H. Resection of hepatic metastases of colorectal carcinoma: 20 years' experience. J Hepatobiliary Pancreat Surg 1999; 6:16–22.

52. Pinson CW, Wright JK, Chapman WC, Garrard CL, Blair TK, Sawyers JL. Repeat hepatic surgery for colorectal cancer metastasis to the liver. Ann Surg 1996; 223:765–76.

53. Fong Y, Cohen AM, Fortner JG, *et al*. Liver resection for colorectal metastases. J Clin Oncol 1997; 15:938–46.

54. Bozzetti F, Cozzaglio L, Borracchi P, *et al*. Comparing surgical resection of limited hepatic metastases from colorectal cancer to non-operative treatment. Eur J Surg Oncol 1993; 19:162–7.

55. Lind DS, Parker GA, Horsley JS III, *et al*. Formal hepatic resection of colorectal liver metastases. Ploidy and prognosis. Ann Surg 1992; 215:677–83.

56. Hodgson WJ, Morgan J, Byrne D, Delguercio LR. Hepatic resections for primary and metastatic tumors using the ultrasonic dissector. Am J Surg 1992; 163:246–50.

57. Fegiz G, Romacciato G, Gennari L, *et al*. Hepatic resections for colorectal metastases: the Italian multicenter experience. J Surg Oncol 1991; Suppl. 2:144–54.

58. Lise M, DaPian PP, Nitti D, Pilati PL, Previdi C. Colorectal metastases to the liver: present status of management. Dis Colon Rectum 1990; 33:688–94.

59. Nuzzo G, Giuliante F, Giovannini I, Tebala, Clemente G, Vellone M. Resection of hepatic metastases from colorectal cancer. Hepato-Gastroenterology 1997; 44:751–9.

60. Cole DJ, Ferguson CM. Complications of hepatic resection for colorectal carcinoma metastasis. Am Surg 1992; 58:88–91.

61. Hughes K, Scheele J, Sugarbaker PH. Surgery for colorectal cancer metastatic to the liver. Surg Clin North Am 1989; 69:339–59.

62. Iwatsuki S, Sheahan DG, Starzl TE. The changing face of hepatic resection. Curr Probl Surg 1989; 26:283–379.

63. Sesto ME, Vogt DP, Hermann RE. Hepatic resection in 128 patients: a 24-year experience. Surgery 1987; 102:846–51.

64. Butler J, Attiyeh FF, Daly JM. Hepatic resection for metastatic colon and rectum. Surg Gynecol Obstet 1986; 162:109–13.

65. Foster JH, Lundy J. Liver metastases. Curr Probl Surg 1981; 18:157–202.

66. Harned II RK, Chezmar JL, Nelson RC. Recurrent tumor after resection of hepatic metastases from colorectal carcinoma: location and time of discovery as determined by CT. Am J Roentgenol 1994; 163:93–7.

67. Hughes KS, Simon R, Songhorabodi S, et al. Resection of the liver for colorectal carcinoma metastases: a multi-institutional study of patterns of recurrences. Surgery 1986; 100:278–84.

68. Wanebo HJ, Chu QD, Avradopoulos KA, Vezeridis MP. Current perspectives on repeat hepatic resection for colorectal carcinoma: a review. Surgery 1996; 119:361–71.

69. Fong Y, Blumgart LH, Cohen A, Fortner J, Brennan MF. Repeat hepatic resections for metastatic colorectal cancer. Ann Surg 1994; 220:657–62.

70. Que FG, Nagorney DM. Resection of 'recurrent' colorectal metastases to the liver. Br J Surg 1994; 81:255–8.

71. Nordlinger B, Vaillant J-C, Guiget M, et al. Survival benefit of repeat liver resections for recurrent colorectal metastases: 143 cases. J Clin Oncol 1994; 12:1491–6.

72. Fernandez-Trigo V, Shamsa F, Sugarbaker PH, et al. Repeat liver resections from colorectal metastases. Surgery 1995; 117:296–304.

73. Tuttle TM, Curley SA, Roh MS. Repeat hepatic resection as effective treatment of recurrent colorectal liver metastases. Ann Surg Oncol 1997; 4:125–30.

74. Ravikumar TS, Kane R, Cady B, Jenkins R, Clouse M, Steele G. A 5-year study of cryosurgery in the treatment of liver tumors. Arch Surg 1991; 126:1520–4.

75. Onik G, Rubinsky B, Zemel R, et al. Ultrasound-guided hepatic cryosurgery in the treatment of metastatic colon carcinoma. Cancer 1991; 67:901–907.

76. Steele G Jr. Cryoablation in hepatic surgery. Semin Liver Dis 1994; 14:120–5.

77. Weaver ML, Ashton JG, Zemel R. Treatment of colorectal liver metastases by cryotherapy. Semin Surg Oncol 1998; 14:163–70.

78. Polk W, Fong Y, Karpeh M, Blumgart LE. A technique for the use of cryosurgery to assist hepatic resection. J Am Coll Surg 1995; 180:171–6.

79. Farrant J, Walter C. The cryobiological basis for cryosurgery. J Dermatol Surg Oncol 1977; 3:403–7.

80. Rubinsky B, Lee CY, Batacky J, Onik G. The process of freezing and the mechanism of damage during hepatic cryosurgery. Cryobiology 1990; 27:85–7.

81. Onik GM, Chambers N, Chernus SA, Zamel R, Atkinson D, Weaver ML. Hepatic cryosurgery with and without the Bair Hugger. J Surg Oncol 1993; 52:185–7.

82. Ravikumar TS, Steele G Jr, Kane R, King V. Experimental and clinical observations on hepatic cryosurgery for colorectal metastases. Cancer Res 1991; 51:6323–7.

83. Morris DL, Ross WB. Australian experience of cryoablation of liver tumors: metastases. Surg Oncol Clin North Am 1996; 5:391–7.

84. Seifert JK, Morris DL. Prognostic factors after cryotherapy for hepatic metastases from colorectal cancer. Ann Surg 1998; 228:201–8.

85. Breedis C, Young C. The blood supply of neoplasms in the liver. Am J Pathol 1954; 30:969.

86. Sigurdson ER, Ridge JA, Kemeny N, Daly JM. Tumor and liver drug uptake following hepatic artery and portal vein infusion. J Clin Oncol 1987; 5:1836–40.

87. Ensminger WD, Rosowsky A, Raso V. A clinical pharmacological evaluation of hepatic arterial infusions of 5-fluoro-2-deoxyuridine and 5-fluorouracil. Cancer Res 1978; 38:3784–92.

88. Niederhuber JE, Ensminger W, Gyves J, Thrall J, Walker S, Cozzi E. Regional chemotherapy of colorectal cancer metastatic to the liver. Cancer 1984; 53:1336–43.

89. Balch CM, Urist MM. Intraarterial chemotherapy for colorectal liver metastases and hepatomas using a totally implantable drug infusion pump. Recent Results Cancer Res 1986; 100:234–47.

90. Kemeny N, Daly J, Oderman P, et al. Hepatic artery pump infusion toxicity and results in patients with metastatic colorectal carcinoma. J Clin Oncol 1984; 2:595–600.

91. Shepard KV, Levin B, Karl RC, et al. Therapy for metastatic colorectal cancer with hepatic artery infusion chemotherapy using a subcutaneous implanted pump. J Clin Oncol 1985; 3:161–9.

92. Cohen AM, Kaufman SD, Wood WC, Greenfield AJ. Regional hepatic chemotherapy using an implantable drug infusion pump. Am J Surg 1983; 145:529–33.

93. Weiss GR, Garnick MB, Osteen RT, et al. Long-term arterial infusion of 5-fluorodeoxyuridine for liver metastases using an implantable infusion pump. J Clin Oncol 1983; 1:337–44.

94. Schwartz SI, Jones LS, McCune CS. Assessment of treatment of intrahepatic malignancies using chemotherapy via an implantable pump. Ann Surg 1985; 201:560–7.

95. Johnson LP, Wassermann PB, Rivkin SE. FUDR hepatic arterial infusion via an implantable pump for treatment of hepatic tumors. Proc Am Soc Clin Oncol 1983; 2:119.

96. Kemeny MM, Goldberg D, Beatty JD, *et al.* Results of prospective randomized trial of continuous regional chemotherapy and hepatic resection as treatment of hepatic metastases from colorectal primaries. Cancer 1986; 57:492–8.

97. Hohn DC, Stagg RJ, Friedman MA, *et al.* The NCOG randomized trial of intravenous (IV) vs. hepatic arterial (IA) FUDR for colorectal cancer metastatic to the liver. Proc Am Soc Clin Oncol 1987; 6:85.

98. Kemeny M, Battifora H, Blayney D, *et al.* Sclerosing cholangitis after continuous hepatic artery infusion of FUDR. Ann Surg 1985; 202:176–81.

99. Daly JM, Kemeny NE. Metastatic cancer to the liver. In DeVita VT, Hellman S, Rosenberg SA, eds. *Cancer: principles and practice of oncology*, 5th edn. Philadelphia, J.B. Lippincott Co., 1997; 2551–70.

100. Kemeny N, Daly J, Reichman B, Geller N, Botet J, Oderman P. Intrahepatic or systemic infusion of fluorodeoxyuridine in patients with liver metastases from colorectal carcinoma. Ann Intern Med 1987; 107:459–65.

101. Chang AE, Schneider PD, Sugerbaker PH. A prospective randomized trial of regional versus systemic continuous 5-fluorodeoxyuridine chemotherapy in the treatment of colorectal liver metastases. Ann Surg 1987; 206:685–93.

102. Grage T, Vassilopoulos P, Shingleton W, *et al.* Results of a prospective randomized study of hepatic artery infusion versus intravenous 5-fluorouracil in patients with hepatic metastases from colorectal cancer: a central oncology group study. Surgery 1979; 86:550–5.

103. Wagman LD, Kemeny MM, Leong L, *et al.* A prospective randomized evaluation of the treatment of colorectal cancer metastatic to the liver. J Clin Oncol 1990; 8:1885–93.

104. Martin JK Jr, O'Connell MJ, Wieand HS, *et al.* Intra-arterial floxuridine vs. systemic fluorouracil for hepatic metastases from colorectal liver metastases. A randomized trial. Arch Surg 1990; 125:1022–7.

105. Rougier PH, Hay JM, Ollivier JM, *et al.* A controlled multicenter trial of intrahepatic chemotherapy (IHC) vs. standard palliative treatment for colorectal liver metastases. Proc Am Soc Clin Oncol 1990; 9:104.

106. Allen-Mersh TG, Earlam S, Fordy C, Abrmas K, Houghton J. Quality of life and survival with continuous hepatic-artery floxuridine infusion for colorectal liver metastases. Lancet 1994; 344:1255–60.

107. Kemeny N, Huang Y, Cohen A, *et al.* Hepatic arterial infusion chemotherapy after resection of metastases from colorectal cancer. N Engl J Med 1999; 341:2039–48.

108. Berlin J, Merrick HW, Smith TJ, Lerner. Phase II evaluation of treatment of complete resection of hepatic metastases from colorectal cancer and adjuvant hepatic arterial infusion of floxuridine: an Eastern Cooperative Oncology Group study (PB083). Am J Clin Oncol 1999; 22:291–3.

109. Ambiru S, Miyazaki M, Ito H, Nakagawa K, Shimizu H, Nakajuma N. Adjuvant regional chemotherapy after hepatic resection for colorectal metastases. Br J Surg 1999; 86:1025–31.

110. Lorenz M, Staib-Sebler E, Koch B, Gog C, Waldeyer M, Encke A. The value of postoperative hepatic arterial infusion following curative liver resection. Anticancer Res 1997; 17:3825–33.

111. Rudroff C, Altendorf-Hoffmann A, Stangl R, Scheele J. Prospective randomised trial on adjuvant hepatic-artery infusion chemotherapy after R0 resection of colorectal liver metastases. Langenbecks Arch Surg 1999; 384:243–9.

112. Lorenz M, Muller HH, Schramm H, *et al.* Randomized trial of surgery versus surgery followed by hepatic arterial infusion with 5-fluorouracil and folinic acid for liver metastases of colorectal cancer. German Cooperative on Liver Metastases (Arbeitsgruppe Lebermetastasen). Ann Surg 1998; 228:756–62.

113. Goletti O, Celoma G, Galatioto C, *et al.* Is laparoscopic sonography a reliable and sensitive procedure for staging colorectal cancer? A comparative study. Surg Endosc 1998; 12:1236–41.

114. Curley SA, Izzo F, Delrio P, *et al.* Radiofrequency ablation of unresectable primary and metastatic hepatic malignancies: results in 123 patients. Ann Surg 1999; 230:1–8.

115. Fraker DL, Alexander HR, Thom AK. Use of tumor necrosis factor in isolated hepatic perfusion. Circulatory Shock 1994; 44:45–50.

116. Lowy AM, Curley SA. Clinical and preclinical trials of isolated liver perfusion for advanced liver tumors. Primary liver tumors. Surg Oncol Clin North Am 1996; 5:429–41.

117. Ravikumar TS, Pizzorno G, Bodden W, *et al.* Percutaneous hepatic vein isolation and high dose hepatic arterial infusion chemotherapy for unresectable liver tumors. J Clin Oncol 1994; 12:2723–36.

118. Panis Y, Rad ALK, Boyer O, Houssin D, Salzmann JL, Klatzmann D. Gene therapy for liver tumors. Surg Oncol Clin North Am 1996; 5:461–73.

119. Caruso M, Panis Y, Gagandeep S, Houssin D, Salzmann JL, Klatzmann D. Regression of established macroscopic liver metastases after in situ transduction of a suicide gene. Proc Natl Acad Sci USA 1993; 90:7024–8.

120. Chen SH, Chen XH, Wang Y, *et al.* Combination gene therapy for liver metastasis of colon carcinoma in vivo. Proc Natl Acad Sci USA 1995; 92:2577–81.

121. Iwatsuki S, Starzl TE. Right and left hepatic trisegmentectomy. In Daly JM, Cady B, eds. *Atlas of surgical oncology*. Philadelphia, Mosby, 1993.

122. Daly JM. Right hepatic lobectomy. In Daly JM, Cady B, eds. *Atlas of surgical oncology*. Philadelphia, Mosby, 1993.

123. Niederhuber JE. Hepatic infusion. In Daly JM, Cady B, eds. *Atlas of surgical oncology*. Philadelphia, Mosby, 1993.

ANNOTATED BIBLIOGRAPHY

Curley SA, Izzo F, Delrio P, *et al*. Radiofrequency ablation of unresectable primary and metastatic hepatic malignancies: results in 123 patients. Ann Surg 1999; 230:1–8.

Curley and coworkers present results of a prospective, non-randomized study of 123 patients with liver lesions treated with radiofrequency ablation (RFA) from two institutions (University of Texas M.D. Anderson Cancer Center and the G. Pascale National Cancer Institute of Naples, Italy). Forty-eight of 123 patients had primary hepatocellular carcinoma, and 75 patients had metastatic disease (61 with metastases from colorectal cancer); 95 patients (77%) had single lesions. The details of RFA and the needle array probe are described. There were no operative deaths and the overall morbidity was 2.4% (compared with a 25–30% complication rate for cryotherapy), including two abscesses in patients who had combined resections and one post-treatment hemorrhage requiring embolization. With a median follow-up of 15 months, 27.6% have recurred (80% of these involving the liver, but only 6% in the liver only). Of the 169 lesions treated with RFA, 3 (1.8%) have recurred at the site.

Nordlinger B, Guiguet M, Vaillant J-C, *et al*. Surgical resection of colorectal carcinoma metastases to the liver: a prognostic scoring system to improve case selection, based on 1568 patients. Cancer 1996; 77:1254–62.

This article reports data collected by the Association Française de Chirurgie regarding 1568 patients from 85 institutions who responded to a questionnaire. Univariate analysis was performed on numerous factors, including demographics, characteristics of the primary and metastatic lesions, pathology, morbidity, mortality, and overall and disease-free survival. In the final Cox's model, age, extension into the serosa and lymph node involvement of the primary cancer, disease-free interval, preoperative CEA levels, size and number of metastases, and surgical margin were predictive of survival. Using these factors, the authors describe a scoring system defining low-risk, intermediate-risk, and high-risk patients. Also included in this article is a review of the literature in tabular form that indicates the predictive value of numerous factors evaluated in univariate or multivariate analysis from the various series.

Panis Y, Rad ALK, Boyer O, Houssin D, Salzmann JL, Klatzmann D. Gene therapy for liver tumors. Surg Oncol Clin North Am 1996; 5:461–73.

Panis and coworkers present a concise review of the current status of gene therapy for colorectal metastases and hepatomas in experimental systems. They summarize different approaches to gene therapy of cancer including viral and non-viral vectors as well as the potential gene strategies. Data are presented regarding the use of suicide genes, immunomodulation, tumor suppressor genes, and antisense approaches.

Ravikumar TS, Steele G Jr, Kane R, King V. Experimental and clinical observations on hepatic cryosurgery for colorectal metastases. Cancer Res 1991; 51:6323–7.

Ravikumar *et al*. evaluate the use of cryoablation in a rat model by measuring subcutaneous syngeneic colon cancer tumor nodules and using light microscopy to assess viability of the cells. The treatment of subcapsular liver implants was also evaluated. Two freeze–thaw cycles seemed as effective as three cycles but better than one cycle. Using these experimental guidelines, they report a clinical series of 24 patients with liver metastases treated with cryosurgery using three or two freeze–thaw cycles. The operative complications, survival, recurrence rate and patterns are described.

Scheele J, Stangl R, Altendorf-Hofmann A, Gall FP. Indicators of prognosis after hepatic resection for colorectal secondaries. Surgery 1991; 110:13–29.

These authors report results from a prospective database of a single-institution experience with 219 patients who underwent curative hepatic resections for colorectal metastases between 1960 and 1988. Actual 5-year survival and tumor-free survival were 31% and 23% ($n = 84$); actuarial 5-year, 10-year, and 20-year survivals were 37%, 25%, and 17%, respectively ($n = 219$). The prognostic importance of numerous factors impacting on overall and disease-free survival was analysed. Clear surgical margins (≥ 10 mm), mesenteric lymph node status of the primary tumor, and the presence or absence of satellite lesions were statistically significant factors. Disease-free interval and the size, number, and lobar distribution of the metastases did not impact on prognosis. The authors discuss their findings for each factor relative to other series in the literature.

Seifert JK, Morris DL. Prognostic factors after cryotherapy for hepatic metastases from colorectal cancer. Ann Surg 1998; 228:201–8.

Seifert and Morris report 116 patients with colorectal liver metastases treated with cryoablation at the University of New South Wales, Sydney, Australia, over a 7-year period. Hepatic artery infusion pumps were routinely placed and 90% received at least one cycle of intra-arterial 5-FU. The operative mortality was 0.9% and morbidity was 27.6%, including liver failure, hemorrhage, abscess, bile leaks, and pulmonary complications. Median survival was 26 months, with a 5-year survival rate of 13%. Univariate and multivariate analysis of multiple variables was performed to assess prognostic significance following cryosurgery. Multivariate analysis indicated that stage and differentiation of the primary tumor, synchronous versus metachronous presentation, serum CEA level prior to liver resection, small size of liver lesions (≤3 cm), absence of extrahepatic disease, and adequacy of cryotherapy were independent prognostic factors. Numbers of lesions treated, age at diagnosis, and blood transfusions during surgery were not independent factors.

Steele G Jr, Bleday R, Mayer RJ, Lindblad A, Petrelli N, Weaver D. A prospective evaluation of hepatic resection for colorectal carcinoma metastases to the liver: Gastrointestinal Tumor Study Group Protocol 6548. J Clin Oncol 1991; 9:1105–12.

The aims of this multi-institutional surgical trial were to assess the accuracy of the preoperative staging of patients considered candidates for hepatic resection for colorectal cancer metastases, to identify prognostic variables, and to determine the surgical morbidity, mortality, and overall survival for hepatic resection. Of 150 evaluable patients, 46% underwent curative resection, 12% underwent non-curative resection with residual tumor or positive histologic margins, and 42% were unresectable due to anatomy of the hepatic metastases (two-thirds) or extrahepatic disease (one-third). The operative mortality was 2.7% and the surgical morbidity was 13%. The median survival for the curative resection group was 37.1 months, compared with 21.2 months or 16.5 months for the non-curative or the unresected group, respectively ($p < 0.01$). Of note, the median survival of the non-curatively resected group was not statistically different from that of the unresected group. There were no statistically significant factors predicting resectability, including age, disease-free interval from the colorectal primary, various preoperative blood studies including CEA levels, and number of hepatic metastases. Of patients that recurred, 75% recurred in the liver (65% liver only).

Sugihara K, Hojo K, Moriya Y, Yamasaki S, Kosuge T, Takayama T. Pattern of recurrence after hepatic resection for colorectal metastases. Br J Surg 1993; 80:1032–5.

Sugihara and coworkers reviewed 159 patients, 107 of whom underwent curative resection of colorectal metastases to the liver. Sixty percent (64 of 107 patients) had recurrence. Fifty-three percent of these recurred in the liver, 31% in the lung, and 19% in the abdominal cavity. All liver recurrences were detected within 18 months of resection and one-third were in the liver bed. Data regarding 17 patients who had resection of five or more metastases are detailed in the article.

Wanebo HJ, Chu QD, Avradopoulos KA, Vezeridis MP. Current perspectives on repeat hepatic resection for colorectal carcinoma: a review. Surgery 1996; 119:361–71.

Wanebo and coworkers review 28 major series of initial or repeat hepatic resection for colorectal metastases, focusing on the patients who underwent second liver resection for liver-only recurrence. They discuss the incidence of isolated liver recurrence after initial resection for colorectal metastases and the indications for repeat hepatectomy. The morbidity rate approximates that of initial liver resections, with an average of 26% from 11 series. The operative mortality ranged from 0% to 11%. Reviews of the two largest series of repeat hepatectomy show a long-term survival rate similar to that following initial resection. Also included in this article is a tabular review of series that report patients undergoing third hepatic resections.

Commentary

LAWRENCE D WAGMAN

Surgical options for patients with tumors in the liver, whether they are primary or metastatic, have expanded. This expansion has been the result of improvements in surgical techniques, intraoperative and perioperative support, multimodality therapies, stimulating and aggressive adjuvant interventions, an increase in the number of surgeons skilled at hepatic resection, and a clarification of the definition of those patients who will be the best surgical candidates. Thus far, little has been studied in a prospective, randomized fashion documenting how each of these elements of patient care has improved outcomes. The primary objective for surgeons caring for patients with colorectal metastases should be to address the absence of scientific studies. Such activities would potentially explain the value of various techniques for parenchymal division (comparing the ultrasonic dissector to the finger-fracture technique), vascular control (total vascular exclusion versus segmental exclusion), or the use of blood products (number of transfusions as an independent predictor of survival). Even if studies showed an equivalence of these alternative procedures, the field would benefit by them becoming accessible, reasonable, and interchangeable alternatives. The area that requires the greatest amount of study in the prospective, randomized format is the use of adjuvant therapies following complete resection of metastases. This would include the use of a variety of adjuvant chemotherapeutic agents, radioimmunotherapeutic agents, and gene therapy products. Furthermore, the delivery routes (intrahepatic, intraportal, isolated perfusion preparations) and intervals of administration (bolus, infusional) should be explored. Single-institution trials have shown exciting and encouraging results in several of these clinical scenarios and are now awaiting confirmation as valuable tools for their general use in larger, prospective, randomized, multi-institutional clinical trials.

SELECTION

If any particular element of the successful surgical treatment of patients with metastases has emerged, it is the careful selection of patients for operation. As the indications for surgery remain varied and inclusive, a few absolutes have been identified as such poor prognostic features that they form the basis for patient exclusion as a resection candidate. The two absolute contraindications for exclusion from surgical candidacy are multiple extrahepatic sites of disease and/or liver metastases with biopsy-positive portal node involvement. The unerring biologic consistency of failure has kept even the most aggressive and optimistic surgeon from attempting to surgically cure these patients. Unlike the dismal scenario of multiple metastases outside the liver, additional single-organ or primary-site recurrence is not linked with such unsuccessful outcomes. This scenario has been best studied in patients with disease limited to the liver and lung, usually with a solitary lesion in the lung. With curative resection rates of solitary lesions of the lung metastatic from colorectal cancer reported in highly selected series of approximately 35%, liver surgeons can anticipate similar outcomes with combinations of resection of small-volume disease in these two organs, either synchronously or metachronously.

The elements of patient selection begin long before the surgeon and patient interact. The postoperative care of the patient with colon or rectal cancer is often transferred to, although ideally shared with, the medical oncologist or primary-care physician. In the setting in which the medical oncologist or primary-care physician is responsible for patient follow-up, the patient in whom liver metastases are identified will only be 'selected' for referral to the surgeon by a medical oncologist or primary-care physician who has knowledge of the surgical options available to treat such patients. This area represents an opportunity for professional education that has thus far not received adequate emphasis. Further efforts in this area of education will improve the initial selection of surgical candidates and increase the number of patients given an opportunity to undergo surgical resection. Local

referral patterns and biases can be dealt with by providing critical information regarding methods and interval for follow-up, basic elements of operability and resectability, and anticipated outcome (disease-free, symptom-free and overall survival patterns). The patient who gets over this first hurdle in the selection process and is referred to the surgical oncologist or hepatic surgeon begins another series of selection evaluations. These are designed to identify multiple sites of disease outside the liver, to clarify the disease within the liver, and to assess the patient's overall ability to tolerate operative and/or ablative procedures.

Studies to evaluate extrahepatic disease may include computerized tomography (CT) scans of the chest, abdomen, and pelvis and, rarely, bone scans for symptomatic patients. The value of chest CT versus chest radiograph lies with the likelihood of finding synchronous lung metastases and the overall analysis of risk and benefit. The CT scan of the abdomen will define the hepatic lesions and also evaluate the portal and retroperitoneal nodes. New functional studies, particularly positron emission spectroscopy (PET) scans, and older radioimmunoimaging against specific colon cancer and carcinoembryonic antigen (CEA) proteins may also be performed to define the full extent of the metastatic disease.

Assuming adequate pulmonary, cardiac, and renal function exists to tolerate a general anesthesia, a 3–4-h operation, and blood loss of 1–2 units, the surgeon must focus on the issue of the hepatic reserve as a predictor of postoperative hepatic failure. The surgeon has two simple and readily available tools: (1) the Childs–Pugh hepatic function classification, and (2) the estimate of liver to tumor ratio. The Childs–Pugh classification takes in elements of liver metabolic and synthetic function (bilirubin level, albumin level, and prothrombin time) and the impact of liver failure on the individual patient (encephalopathy). Utilizing preoperative scanning, including contrast enhanced magnetic resonance imaging (MRI) and rapid infusion CT scans, the surgeon must make an estimate of the final hepatic volume after the completion of surgical resection or ablation. These estimates are influenced by the amount of normal liver and that portion replaced by tumor, i.e., the area of tumor does not represent functioning liver tissue and its loss will not impact on hepatic function. A minimum prerequisite of 25% of the total hepatic volume at the end of the surgical procedure is required to have a 90% expectation of adequate liver function for perioperative survival. This volume estimate can be prepared by careful examination of the scans. Of course, this represents a significant art, as well as measurable science. Patients with underlying liver disease, primarily cirrhosis but also steatosis, will have less function despite equivalent volume. Anatomic variations in liver blood supply will impact on the amounts of devascularized and hence defunctionalized liver at the end of a resection. To re-emphasize, these elements of selection based on rough functional estimates and surgeon confidence and experience will have bottom-line impacts on surgical success and disease control.

SURGICAL INTERVENTION

The selection process continues intraoperatively. Here again, surgeon's experience, confidence and multidisciplinary support (blood bank, ultrasound, anesthesia, and other technologies) impact on resectability. The careful examination of the abdomen is the surgeon's initial obligation and must be completed in an aggressive fashion. The initial exploration may be performed through a limited incision in the right upper quadrant, allowing palpation of the liver, diaphragm, porta hepatis, and celiac axis areas. Occasionally, numerous miliary lesions in the liver, a node in the porta or celiac areas, or diaphragmatic implant will be palpated, requiring only biopsy confirmation, precluding further exploration, and negating the value of a liver resection. In some situations and in the hands of skilled laparoscopic surgeons, an initial laparoscopy can identify lesions that would make laparotomy unnecessary. Examples include borderline resectable lesions on preoperative scans, numerous intrahepatic metastases suggesting more extensive disease, suspicious but percutaneously inaccessible lymph nodes or other lesions on preoperative studies that require biopsy. One caveat regarding portal lymph nodes regards their size and consistency. Large, firm, not hard, nodes are usually negative for malignancy. The operating surgeon should not conclude the patient has metastases to nodes except by histologic confirmation. This feature of normal-sized lymph nodes that contain metastatic disease is important to remember when reviewing treatment trials of liver metastases that include a treatment arm without exploration. Assuming the laparoscopy and/or initial limited laparotomy do not reveal any disease outside of the liver, the incision is enlarged in accordance with the size and location of the lesion or lesions and the planned ablation or resection. The hallmark of safe and successful liver surgery is adequate exposure and mobilization of the liver, biliary tree, and vascular supplies. In the setting of metastatic disease, this can often be challenging, due to adhesions from the primary resection and liver biopsies. Patients whose metastatic disease is defined synchronously with the primary can have combined colorectal resections and liver resection. This avoids the repeat surgery and attendant repeat anesthesia, duplicative hospitalization, additive morbidity (preparation, pain, anxiety), and adhesive disease. Although some surgeons cite a potential risk of increased infection rates, particularly in the setting in which adjuvant hepatic-directed therapy is planned via implanted pump systems, this increased rate of complications has not been the experience of those who regularly perform the procedures simultaneously.

The anatomy of the inflow and outflow blood supply to the liver lends itself to control at several levels. The highest volume and most anatomically consistent of the blood supplies is the nutrient-containing portal system. Proximal control of the main portal vein is easily accomplished with the Pringle maneuver. Control or division of the main right or left branch can be done in the extrahepatic portion of the porta. The oxygen-rich blood supply from the hepatic artery is anatomically consistent in only 60% of cases. The main variation is a replaced right hepatic artery originating from the superior mesenteric artery and travelling parallel and in a posterolateral position to the common bile duct. It is identified by gently pinching the right side of the porta about 2–3 cm above the duodenal sweep. Time and effort can be saved by doing this early in the examination of the porta, as the operating surgeon will be apprised of a series of expected arterial variations, including those associated with the left hepatic and cystic artery locations. Also, the strategies for pump placement (dual catheters, two pumps, and arterial ligation) in those patients who are candidates for arterial, hepatic-directed therapies can be planned.

Surgeons are very familiar with the anatomy and techniques required for identification, dissection, and manipulation of the common and proper bile duct, i.e., the bile duct below the bifurcation into left and right branches. At and above the level of the bifurcation, the bile ducts become much smaller, have several lobar and segmental branches, and are surrounded by heavy, fibrous tissue. This increases the chances for damage to very small side branches and complicates the dissection. Furthermore, the bile duct is the most challenging of the portal structures to repair, requiring duct-to-bowel anastomosis and stenting and carrying a high risk of stenosis and long-term complications. For this reason, identification, mobilization, and division of the left or right duct should be performed prior to parenchymal division when performing a lobectomy.

The hepatic venous drainage is reasonably consistent with the three main outflow veins, the right, middle, and left, present at the most cephalad portion of the liver, and distributed on the anterior surface of the vena cava 1–2 cm below the diaphragm. A series of under-appreciated 1–3-mm hepatic veins exit the posterior aspect of the liver directly into the vena cava. They are best addressed after the entire right triangular ligament has been released in the loose areolar plane that is identified with firm but gentle retraction of the diaphragm away from the hepatic surface. This meticulous separation will also allow the liver to be dissected away from the adrenal gland and retroperitoneal fat and avoid injury to the small, high-flow venous outflow of the right adrenal to the cava. When addressing the main hepatic veins, care is taken to avoid injury to early branches. The extrahepatic portion of these veins is often short and the use of the stapling device (endovascular GIA) that places three lines of staples on each side of the vessel division has reduced the time necessary for vessel division and control. Because of the significant intrahepatic venous flow, one or two hepatic veins can be divided without resecting the lobe being drained. Division of the right hepatic vein is extremely helpful in the mobilization of the right lobe in preparation for segments VI, VII, and/or VIII resection. The surgeon will appreciate an increased turgor in the liver with division of the major draining vein and should be prepared for a possible increase in bleeding due to back-pressure on the tributary hepatic veins.

Special considerations for cryoablation and resection should be mentioned. Cryoablation requires volume expansion and high output of alkalinized urine to prevent cryoshock and renal failure. Resection is best done with the patient's volume status normal to low to reduce pressure in the hepatic veins and reduce backbleeding. The operative surgeon must sequence these procedures to keep the patient in the best volume status throughout the surgery. Close collaboration with the anesthesiologist is essential.

The ablative techniques of cryosurgery and radiofrequency ablation have garnered the attention of the surgical community because they provide two important options. The first is a method of destroying tumors that would otherwise be unresectable because of their location and the subsequent loss of hepatic tissue, and the second is the potential for tissue ablation percutaneously. Initially, cryoablation was performed in patients deemed unresectable due to numerous and poorly located tumors. The observation from this experience was that excellent control of treated lesions was achieved. Early difficulties with hypothermia, coagulopathy, and myoglobinuria-induced renal failure were anticipated and successfully prevented. Now, two-cycle cryoablation with ultrasound control of trocar placement and freeze margins challenges the results of resection. The technique of radiofrequency ablation is joining cryoablation as a potentially equivalent method for lesion ablation. The strong points of the radiofrequency ablation are the smaller needle and wire array, absence of the cryoshock syndrome, no surface cracking, and, currently, a greater likelihood of having percutaneous application. The drawbacks are the limited size of the ablation for each application of the probe array, the measurement of the ablation zone within the wire array, less control due to the thermodynamics of the ablation/feedback loops in the radiofrequency ablation apparatus, and the lack of a measurable tissue destruction zone. Focusing specifically on the last element, with cryoablation the ultrasound identifies a hyperechoic advancing edge of the iceball where all tissues within that perimeter are frozen. The ultrasound image can be reproduced in hard copy documenting the successful ablation. Although the ultrasonogram will show the deployed radio frequency ablation arrays within the tumor and the development of bubbles along the wires, there is no feature such as the hyperechoic line. Even pathologic biopsy is inadequate to document the kill zone at the time of ablation with radiofrequency ablation, as the histologic changes have not yet developed and the biochemical measurements utilizing an NADPH stain cannot be done as a frozen-section analysis. Alcohol injection has been associated with significant success in the treatment of hepatoma, but thus far has been rarely tried in metastatic colorectal cancers.

ADJUVANT THERAPIES

The recurrence rates following curative resection of hepatic metastases are between 60% and 100%. Estimates of the likelihood of recurrence can be made following the surgical procedure utilizing preoperative, intraoperative, and postoperative aspects of the patient, pathology, and surgical findings. The pattern of recurrence is hepatic only (40%), extrahepatic only (40%), or a combination (20%). This high recurrence rate and dispersed pattern of recurrence have led to the recommendations of adjuvant chemotherapy delivered both systemically and regionally. The concept of regional chemotherapy is attractive in hepatic disease because of the availability of inflow and the high percentage, first-pass extraction of some of the agents used. Floxuridine is the most commonly used intrahepatic agent and it has a 95–99% first-pass extraction, limiting its systemic toxicity and efficacy. The drug can be delivered through the hepatic artery or portal vein via an implanted catheter attached to a subcutaneously implanted, controlled delivery pump or a port that is percutaneously accessed and attached to an external drug-delivery pump system. The advantage of the hepatic artery is the perfusion of both large and small metastases. This is important in patients who have residual macroscopic disease at the end of a surgical therapy. The portal vein perfuses microscopic metastases and may be a valuable route for the post-complete resection regional infusion. Recent studies have been reported showing similar results in hepatic disease control when the portal vein access is used. The main difference in toxicity between the hepatic artery and portal vein routes is the presence of significant chemical hepatitis and sclerosing cholangitis in patients with arterial infusions. Because of the variability in hepatic arterial anatomy, many surgeons require preoperative vascular imaging (angiography, MRI angiography) to prevent intraoperative delays in defining the location of the hepatic artery or arteries. This is in contrast to the portal vein, which is highly consistent and easily accessed from the small-bowel or large-bowel mesentery, splenic branch, or directly. Studies of adjuvant hepatic artery or portal vein regional infusion combined with systemic therapy suggest a benefit to the combined treatment in controlling hepatic disease and systemic failures over no treatment or systemic therapy alone. A randomized, prospective study carefully controlling for prognostic indicators will be required to resolve the question of combined therapy and optimal route of administration. Other important questions concern the length of treatment, dose requirements, and best agents for the regional and systemic treatments.

FUTURE CONSIDERATIONS

Several areas of opportunity exist for the future. There is a need for a simple, low-cost, reliable test for colorectal cancer recurrence. The current use of CEA as follow-up for patients with initial elevations of CEA is a valuable tool in documenting potentially curable liver-only disease. The scanning remains time and dollar intensive and newer techniques of PET scanning and radio-immune techniques offer theoretic benefit. The development of surgical stapling instrumentation that will allow hemostatic division of full-thickness portions of the liver would decrease blood loss, shorten operative time, and potentially allow for laparoscopic techniques. Strategies other than hydration and alkalinization of the urine to offset the effects of cryoablation would increase the applicability and ease of administration of that modality. A technique to visualize and quantify the radiofrequency ablation of intrahepatic tumors is required to increase its acceptance as an ablative technique. Finally, the specifics of adjuvant drug delivery and neoadjuvant approaches to turn unresectable patients into resectable ones should command our interest and research attention.

Editors' selected abstracts

Two-stage hepatectomy: a planned strategy to treat irresectable liver tumors.

Adam R, Laurent A, Azoulay D, Castaing D, Bismuth H.

Centre Hepato-Biliaire, Hopital Paul Brousse, Villejuif, and Universite Paris-Sud, France.

Annals of Surgery 232(6):777–85, 2000, December.

Objective: To assess feasibility, risks, and patient outcomes in the treatment of colorectal metastases with two-stage hepatectomy. *Summary background data:* Some patients with multiple hepatic colorectal metastases are not candidates for a complete resection by a single hepatectomy, even when downstaged by chemotherapy, after portal embolization, or combined with a locally destructive technique. In two-stage hepatectomy, the highest possible number of tumors is resected in a first, noncurative intervention, and the remaining tumors are resected after a period of liver regeneration. In selected patients with irresectable multiple metastases not amenable to a single hepatectomy procedure, two-stage hepatectomy might offer a chance of long-term remission. *Methods:* Of consecutive patients with conventionally irresectable colorectal metastases treated by chemotherapy, 16 of 398 (4%) became eligible for curative two-stage hepatectomy combined with chemotherapy and adjuvant nonsurgical interventions as indicated. *Results:* Two-stage hepatectomy was feasible in 13 of 16 patients (81%). There were no surgical deaths. The postoperative death rate (2 months or less) was 0% for the first-stage procedure and 15% for the second-stage one. Postoperative complication rates were 31% and 45%, respectively, with only one complication leading to reoperation. The 3-year survival rate was 35%, with four patients (31%) disease-free at 7, 22, 36, and 54 months. Median survival was 31 months from the second hepatectomy and 44 months from the diagnosis of metastases. *Conclusions:* Two-stage hepatectomy combined with chemotherapy may allow a long-term remission in selected patients with irresectable multiple metastases and increases the proportion of patients with resectable disease.

Resection of nonresectable liver metastases from colorectal cancer after percutaneous portal vein embolization.

Azoulay D, Castaing D, Smail A, Adam R, Cailliez V, Laurent A, Lemoine A, Bismuth H.

Centre Hepato-Biliaire, Hopital Paul Brousse, Villejuif, France.

Annals of Surgery 231(4):480–6, 2000, April.

Objective: To assess the influence of preoperative portal vein embolization (PVE) on the long-term outcome of liver resection for colorectal metastases. *Summary background data:* Preoperative PVE of the liver induces hypertrophy of the remnant liver and increases the safety of hepatectomy. *Methods:* Thirty patients underwent preoperative PVE and 88 patients did not before resection of four or more liver segments. PVE was performed when the estimated rate of remnant functional liver parenchyma (ERRFLP) assessed by CT scan volumetry was less than 40%. *Results:* PVE was feasible in all patients. There were no deaths. The complication rate was 3%. The post-PVE ERRFLP was significantly increased compared with the pre-PVE value. Liver resection was performed after PVE in 19 patients (63%), with surgical death and complication rates of 4% and 7% respectively. PVE increased the number of resections of more than four segments by 19% (17/88). Actuarial survival rates after hepatectomy with or without previous PVE were comparable: 81%, 67%, and 40% versus 88%, 61%, and 38% at 1, 3, and 5 years respectively. *Conclusions:* PVE allows more patients with previously unresectable liver tumors to benefit from resection. Long-term survival is comparable to that after resection without PVE.

Survival after resection of multiple bilobar hepatic metastases from colorectal carcinoma.

Bolton JS, Fuhrman GM.

Department of General Surgery, Alton Ochsner Medical Institutions, New Orleans, LA, USA.

Annals of Surgery 231(5):743–51, 2000, May.

Objective: To define the long-term outcome and treatment complications for patients undergoing liver resection for multiple, bilobar hepatic metastases from colorectal cancer. *Methods:* A retrospective analysis of 165 consecutive patients undergoing liver resection for metastatic colorectal cancer was performed. Patients were divided into a simple hepatic metastasis group, consisting of patients with three or fewer metastases in a unilobar distribution, and a complex hepatic metastases group, consisting of patients with four or more unilobar metastases or at least two bilobar metastases. *Results:* The 5-year survival rate was 36% for the simple group and 37% for the complex group. Multivariate analysis revealed that the number of hepatic segments involved by tumor and the maximum diameter of the largest metastasis correlated significantly with the 5-year survival rate. The surgical death rate was 4.9% for the simple group and 9.1% for the complex group; this difference was not significant. Multivariate analysis revealed that extended lobar resection and concomitant colon and hepatic resection were significant and independent predictors of surgical death. The combination of extended lobar resection and concomitant colon resection was used significantly more frequently in the complex group than in the simple group. *Conclusions:* Resection of complex hepatic metastases, as defined in this study, results in a 5-year survival rate of 37% and confers the same survival benefit as does resection of limited hepatic metastases. The surgical death rate for this aggressive approach is significantly higher if extended lobar resections are necessary and if concomitant colorectal resection is performed. Patients who have complex hepatic metastases at the time of diagnosis of the primary colorectal cancer and who would require extended hepatic lobectomy should have hepatic resection delayed for at least 3 months after colon resection.

Anatomic segmental hepatic resection is superior to wedge resection as an oncologic operation for colorectal liver metastases.

DeMatteo RP, Palese C, Jarnagin WR, Sun RL, Blumgart LH, Fong Y.

Hepatobiliary Service, Department of Surgery, Memorial Sloan-Kettering Cancer Center, New York, NY, USA.

Journal of Gastrointestinal Surgery 4(2):178–84, 2000, March–April.

Hepatic wedge resection for colorectal liver metastasis has been reported to have a high incidence of positive surgical margins. Anatomic segmental resection is now widely practiced, although there are few data comparing segmental and wedge resection in terms of tumor clearance or long-term outcome. There were 267 patients who underwent liver resection for metastatic colorectal cancer between July 1985 and October 1998 at our institution who had either a wedge ($n = 119$) or segmental ($n = 148$) resection. Patient, tumor, and treatment data were compared, actuarial survival was determined, and prognostic factors were analyzed. Anatomic segmental resection was associated with similar blood loss, operative time, and complications as wedge resection. Segmental resection had a significantly lower rate of positive margins (2% vs. 16%) compared to

wedge hepatectomy ($p < 0.001$). On univariate analysis, segmentectomy resulted in longer survival with a median of 53 months vs. 38 months for wedge hepatectomy ($p = 0.015$). Preoperative carcinoembryonic antigen level, positive margin of resection, and the presence of extrahepatic disease independently predicted survival on multivariate analysis. Anatomic segmental resection is a safe procedure and is superior to wedge resection as an oncologic operation for colorectal liver metastasis because it results in better tumor clearance and improved survival.

Hepatic arterial infusion of chemotherapy after resection of hepatic metastases from colorectal cancer.

Kemeny N, Huang Y, Cohen AM, Shi W, Conti JA, Brennan MF, Bertino JR, Turnbull AD, Sullivan D, Stockman J, Blumgart LH, Fong Y.

Department of Medicine, Memorial Sloan-Kettering Cancer Center, New York, NY, USA.

New England Journal of Medicine 341(27):2039–48, 1999, December 30.

Background: Two years after undergoing resection of liver metastases from colorectal cancer, about 65 percent of patients are alive and 25 percent are free of detectable disease. We tried to improve these outcomes by treating patients with hepatic arterial infusion of floxuridine plus systemic fluorouracil after liver resection. *Methods:* We randomly assigned 156 patients at the time of resection of hepatic metastases from colorectal cancer to receive six cycles of hepatic arterial infusion with floxuridine and dexamethasone plus intravenous fluorouracil, with or without leucovorin, or six weeks of similar systemic therapy alone. Patients were stratified according to previous treatment and the number of liver metastases identified at operation. The study end points were overall survival, survival without recurrence of hepatic metastases, and survival without any metastases at two years. *Results:* The actuarial rate of overall survival at two years was 86 percent in the group treated with local plus systemic chemotherapy and 72 percent in the group given systemic therapy alone ($p = 0.03$). The median survival was 72.2 months in the combined-therapy group and 59.3 months in the monotherapy group, with a median follow-up of 62.7 months. After two years, the rates of survival free of hepatic recurrence were 90 percent in the monotherapy group and 60 percent in the monotherapy group ($p < 0.001$), and the respective rates of progression-free survival were 57 percent and 42 percent ($p = 0.07$). At two years, the risk ratio for death was 2.34 among patients treated with systemic therapy alone, as compared with patients who received combined therapy (95 percent confidence interval, 1.10 to 4.98; $p = 0.027$), after adjustment for important variables. The rates of adverse effects of at least moderate severity were similar in the two groups, except for a higher frequency of diarrhea and hepatic effects in the combined-therapy group. *Conclusions:* For patients who undergo resection of liver metastases from colorectal cancer, postoperative treatment with a combination of hepatic arterial infusion of floxuridine and intravenous fluorouracil improves the outcome at two years.

Interval hepatic resection of colorectal metastases improves patient selection.

Lambert LA, Colacchio TA, Barth RJ Jr.

Section of General Surgery, Dartmouth-Hitchcock Medical Center and Norris Cotton Cancer Center, Lebanon, NH, USA.

Archives of Surgery 135(4):473–9; discussion 479–80, 2000, April.

Hypothesis: Interval reevaluation for resectability of hepatic colorectal metastases aids patient selection. *Design:* A retrospective review. *Setting:* A tertiary care medical center. *Patients and methods*: From January 1, 1985, to July 1, 1998, 318 patients with colorectal hepatic metastases were identified. Resectable lesions (*n* = 73) were divided into synchronous (*n* = 36) or metachronous (*n* = 37) and retrospectively reviewed for immediate resection or interval reevaluation. Kaplan–Meier survival curves of treatment groups were compared by the log-rank test. *Results:* Survival curves of patients with synchronous and metachronous lesions undergoing interval reevaluation vs. immediate resection were not significantly different (*p* = 0.74 and *p* = 0.65, respectively). No lesions from patients who underwent interval reevaluation became unresectable due to growth of the initial metastases. After interval reevaluation, 8(29%) of 28 patients with synchronous metastases were spared the morbidity of laparotomy because of distant or an increased number of metastases and 10(36%) of 28 patients were spared the morbidity of hepatic resection at the time of interval laparotomy. Actuarial median and 5-year survival of patients after delayed hepatic resection (51 months and 45%, respectively) were significantly improved compared with those of all other patients with resectable metastases (23 months and 7%, respectively) (*p* = 0.02). For patients with metachronous lesions who underwent interval reevaluation, 4(29%) of 14 patients were spared the morbidity of laparotomy because of an increased number of hepatic or distant metastases. *Conclusions:* Delaying hepatic resection for metastatic colorectal cancer does not impair survival. Potentially, two thirds of patients can avoid major hepatic surgery. For synchronous metastases, delaying hepatic resection appears to select patients who will benefit from hepatic resection.

Curative liver resection for metastatic breast cancer.

Maksan SM, Lehnert T, Bastert G, Herfarth C.

Departments of Surgery, University of Heidelberg, Heidelberg, Germany.

European Journal of Surgical Oncology 26(3):209–12, 2000, April.

Aims: Hepatic resection is a standard procedure in the treatment of colorectal liver metastases. Liver metastases are frequent in breast cancer, but resectional treatment is rarely possible and few reports have addressed the results of surgical treatment for metastatic breast cancer. The aim of our study was to analyse the outcome of patients with metastatic breast cancer after resection of isolated hepatic secondaries and possibly to identify selection criteria for patients who may benefit from surgery. *Methods:* Between

1984 and 1998, 90 patients with a history of breast cancer and suspected liver metastases were referred for surgical evaluation. Fifty-four patients also had extrahepatic disease or metastases from another primary tumour; multiple liver metastases were not amenable to surgical treatment in 20 patients. Five patients were treated by regional chemotherapy via an intra-arterial port catheter; after liver resection two patients were found to have liver metastases from intercurrent colorectal cancer. Thus only nine liver resections for metastatic breast cancer could be performed with curative intent. *Results:* No patient died postoperatively after liver resection. In the follow-up period, four of the nine patients who were treated with curative intent received systemic chemotherapy. At a median follow-up of 29 months, four patients died from tumour recurrence. Five patients are currently alive. Five-year survival in the resection group was calculated as 51% (Kaplan–Meier estimate). Node-negative primary breast cancer and a long interval between treatment of the primary and liver metastases appeared to be associated with long survival after liver resection. *Conclusions:* These observations suggest that careful follow-up and adequate patient selection could offer some patients with isolated liver metastases from breast cancer a chance of long-term survival.

Extended hepatic resection: a 6-year retrospective study of risk factors for perioperative mortality.

Melendez J,[a] Ferri E,[a,d] Zwillman M,[a] Fischer M,[a] DeMatteo R,[b] Leung D,[c] Jarnagin W,[b] Fong Y,[b] Blumgart LH.[b]

[a]Department of Anesthesiology and Critical Care Medicine, Memorial Sloan-Kettering Cancer Center, New York, NY, USA; [b]Hepatobiliary Service, Department of Surgery, Memorial Sloan-Kettering Cancer Center, New York, NY, USA; [c]Department of Epidemiology and Biostatistics, Memorial Sloan-Kettering Cancer Center, New York, NY, USA; [d]Department of Anesthesiology and Intensive Care at University of Ferrara, Ferrara, Italy.

Journal of the American College of Surgeons 192:47–53, 2001.

Background: Extended hepatic resection (more than four liver segments) is a major operative procedure that is associated with significant risk. The purpose of this study was to assess the impact of perioperative variables on in-hospital mortality after extended hepatectomy. *Study design:* Consecutive patients who underwent extended hepatic resection were studied. The prognostic value of 29 perioperative variables was evaluated using in-hospital mortality as the endpoint. For each variable, the odds ratio (95% confidence interval) for in-hospital mortality was calculated. Those variables with a lower confidence limit >1 were considered important risk factors. The population was stratified into categories of patients having the same number of risk factors, and mortality was estimated for each group. These data were used to develop a risk assessment algorithm. *Results:* There were 14 deaths (6%) in 226 patients. Three preoperative variables (cholangitis, creatinine >1.3 mg/dL, and total bilirubin >6 mg/dL) and two operative variables (blood loss >3 L and vena caval resection) appear to be important factors for in-hospital mortality. The mortality associated with the presence of any two of the five factors was 100% (5 of 5), and the mortality associated with the absence of these factors was 3% (6 of 191). *Conclusions:* Perioperative evaluation of patients undergoing extended hepatic resection should include the quantitation of mortality risk factors. The combination of any two factors among preoperative cholangitis, elevated serum creatinine, elevated serum bilirubin, high operative blood loss, and vena cava resection may carry a high mortality risk. These results require prospective validation.

Surgery after downstaging of unresectable hepatic tumors with intra-arterial chemotherapy.

Meric F, Patt YZ, Curley SA, Chase J, Roh MS, Vauthey JN, Ellis LM.

Department of Surgical Oncology, The University of Texas M.D. Anderson Cancer Center, Houston, TX, USA.

Annals of Surgical Oncology 7(7):490–5, 2000, August.

Background: This retrospective study was performed to assess the outcome among patients who underwent hepatic resection or tumor ablation after hepatic artery infusion (HAI) therapy down-staged previously unresectable hepatocellular carcinoma (HCC) or liver metastases from colorectal cancer (CRC). *Methods:* Between 1983 and 1998, 25 patients with HCC and 383 patients with hepatic CRC metastases were treated with HAI therapy for unresectable liver disease. We retrospectively reviewed the records of 26(6%) of these patients who underwent subsequent surgical exploration for tumor resection or ablation. *Results:* At a median of 9 months (range 7–12 months) after HAI treatment, for patients (16%) with HCC underwent exploratory surgery; two underwent resection with negative margins, and the other two were given radiofrequency ablation (RFA) because of underlying cirrhosis. At a median postoperative follow-up of 16 months (range 6–48 months), all four patients were alive with no evidence of disease. At a median of 14.5 months (range 8–24 months) after HAI therapy, 22 patients with hepatic CRC metastases underwent exploratory surgery; 10 underwent resection, 6 underwent resection and RFA or cryotherapy, and 2 underwent RFA only. At a median follow-up of 17 months, 15(83%) of the 18 patients with CRC who had received surgical treatment had developed recurrent disease; the other 3 died of other causes (1 of postoperative complications) within 7 months of the surgery. One patient in whom disease recurred underwent a second resection and was disease-free at 1 year follow-up. *Conclusions:* Hepatic resection or ablation after tumor downstaging with HAI therapy is a viable option for patients with unresectable HCC. However, given the high rate of recurrence of metastases from CRC, hepatic resection or ablation after downstaging with HAI should be used with caution.

Extension of the frontiers of surgical indications in the treatment of liver metastases from colorectal cancer: long-term results.

Minagawa M, Makuuchi M, Torzilli G, Takayama T, Kawasaki S, Kosuge T, Yamamoto J, Imamura H.

Department of Hepato-Biliary-Pancreatic Surgery, Graduate School of Medicine, University of Tokyo, Tokyo, Japan.

Annals of Surgery 231(4):487–99, 2000, April.

Objective: To evaluate retrospectively the long-term results of an approach consisting of performing surgery in every patient in whom radical removal of all metastatic disease was technically feasible. *Summary background data:* The indications for surgical resection for liver metastases from colorectal cancer remain controversial. Several clinical risk factors have been reported to influence survival. *Methods:* Between March 1980 and December 1997, 235 patients underwent hepatic resection for metastatic colorectal cancer. Survival rates and disease-free survival as a function of clinical and pathologic determinants were examined retrospectively with univariate and multivariate analyses. *Results:* The overall 3-, 5-, 10-, and 15-year survival rates were 51%, 38%, 26%, and 24%, respectively. The stage of the primary tumor, lymph node metastasis, and multiple nodules were significantly associated with a poor prognosis in both univariate and multivariate analyses. Disease-free survival was significantly influenced by lymph node metastasis, a short interval between treatment of the primary and metastatic tumors, and a high preoperative level of carcinoembryonic antigen. The 10-year survival rate of patients with four or more nodules (29%) was better than that of patients with two or three nodules (16%), and similar to that of patients with a solitary lesion (32%). *Conclusions:* Surgical resection is useful for treating liver metastases from colorectal cancer. Although multiple metastases significantly impaired the prognosis, the life expectancy of patients with four or more nodules mandates removal.

Liver metastases from breast cancer: long-term survival after curative resection.

Selzner M, Morse MA, Vredenburgh JJ, Meyers WC, Clavien PA.

Department of Surgery, Duke University Medical Center, Durham, NC, USA.

Surgery 127(4):383–9, 2000, April.

Background: Liver metastases from breast cancer are associated with a poor prognosis (median survival <6 months). A subgroup of these patients with no dissemination in other organs may benefit from surgery. Available data in the literature suggest that only in exceptional cases do these patients survive more than 2 years when given chemohormonal therapy or supportive care alone. We report the results of liver resection in patients with isolated hepatic metastases from breast cancer and evaluate the rate of long-term survival, prognostic factors, and the role of neoadjuvant high-dose chemotherapy. *Patients and methods:* Over the past decade, 17 women underwent hepatic metastectomy with curative intent for metastatic breast cancer. The follow-up was complete in each patient. The median age at the time breast cancer was diagnosed was 48 years. Neoadjuvant high-dose chemotherapy (HDC) with hematopoietic progenitor support was used in 10 patients before liver resection. Perioperative complications, long-term outcome, and prognostic factors were evaluated. *Results:* Seven of the 17 patients are currently alive, with follow-up of up to 12 years. Four of these patients are free of tumors after 6 and 17 months and 6 and 12 years. The actuarial 5-year survival rate is 22%. One patient died postoperatively (mortality rate, 6%) of carmustine-induced fibrosing pneumonitis. There was no further major morbidity in the other patients. The liver was the primary site of recurrent disease after liver resection in 67% of the patients. Patients in whom liver metastases were found more than 1 year after resection of the primary breast cancer had a significantly better outcome than those with early (<1 year) metastatic disease ($p = 0.04$). The type of liver resection, the lymph node status at the time of the primary breast cancer resection, and HDC had no significant impact on patient survival in this series. *Conclusions:* Favorable 22% long-term survival can be achieved with metastasectomy in this selected group of patients. Careful evaluation of pulmonary toxicity from carmustine and exclusion of patients with extrahepatic disease are critical. Improved survival might be achieved with better selection of patients and the use of liver-directed adjuvant therapy.

Survival after resection of multiple hepatic colorectal metastases.

Weber SM, Jarnagin WR, DeMatteo RP, Blumgart LH, Fong Y.

Hepatobiliary Service, Memorial Sloan-Kettering Cancer Center, New York, NY, USA.

Annals of Surgical Oncology 7(9):643–50, 2000, October.

Background: Hepatic resection is potentially curative in selected patients with colorectal metastases. It is a widely held practice that multiple colorectal hepatic metastases are not resected, although outcome after removal of four or more metastases is not well defined. *Methods:* Patients with four or more colorectal hepatic metastases who submitted to resection were identified from a prospective database. Number of metastases was determined by serial sectioning of the gross specimen at the time of resection. Demographic data, tumor characteristics, complications, and survival were analyzed. *Results:* From August 1985 to September 1998, 155 patients with four or more metastatic tumors (range 4–20) underwent potentially curative resection by extended hepatectomy (39%), lobectomy (42%), or multiple segmental resections (19%). Operative morbidity and mortality were 26% and 1%, respectively. Actuarial 5-year survival was 23% for the entire group (median = 32 months) and there were 12 actual 5-year survivors. On multivariate analysis, only number of hepatic tumors ($p = 0.005$) and the presence of a positive margin ($p = 0.003$) were independent predictors of poor survival. *Conclusions:* Hepatic resection in patients with four or more colorectal metastases can achieve long-term survival although the results are less favorable as the number of tumors increases. Number of hepatic metastases alone should not be used as a sole contraindication to resection, but it is clear that the majority of patients will not be cured after resection of multiple lesions.

27

Non-operative treatment of hepatic metastasis from colorectal carcinoma

SHERRY M WREN

INTRODUCTION

Colorectal carcinoma is one of the most common malignancies in the USA. It was predicted that 155 000 new patients would be diagnosed in 2000. Currently, colorectal carcinoma accounts for 11% of all new cancer diagnoses, with an incidence of 44 cases per 100 000 people. Of these, approximately 50 000 will have disseminated disease at the time of diagnosis, with 60% of these having disease within the liver. The liver is the sole site of metastasis in only 25–35% of cases. Many series have demonstrated that surgical resection of metastases confined to the liver offers the only real chance of long-term survival for these patients. The overall 5-year survival of patients undergoing resection for isolated hepatic metastases ranges from 25% to 40%.[1,2] Even more encouraging is a recent report from the Mayo Clinic (Rochester, MN) demonstrating that disease-free patient survival beyond 5 years from surgical resection represents patient cure in nearly all instances.[3] Liver resection should be considered standard therapy for all patients with colorectal metastases isolated to the liver.[2] The selection of patients for hepatic resection is limited by the patient's overall medical status, confirmation that the liver is the only site of metastatic disease, and anatomic location and number of hepatic lesions. Unfortunately, only 5–10% of patients fall into the category of being potentially curable by liver resection,[1,4,5] due to extrahepatic involvement or numerous hepatic lesions. The goal of this chapter is to examine the non-surgical therapeutic modalities employed in the treatment of metastatic colorectal cancer not amenable to surgical resection.

ABLATIVE NON-RESECTION THERAPY

Cryosurgery and radiofrequency ablation of hepatic metastases are two regional techniques that offer patients ineligible for hepatic resection potentially beneficial treatment. Both of these treatments provide direct tumor kill *in situ* within the hepatic parenchyma. Cryosurgery causes cellular death by freezing of tumor cells and radiofrequency ablation causes hyperthermic tumor-cell lysis. Both treatments fall into the category of directed cytotoxic regional treatment. They offer the advantage of directed tumor kill with a margin of normal liver tissue combined with the preservation of maximal hepatic parenchyma. The majority of experience has been with cryoablation of lesions metastatic to the liver.[6–9] Initial results suggest that the overall 5-year survival approaches the overall survival seen with hepatic resection. Cryosurgery also has the advantage of lower morbidity and mortality rates when compared to major hepatic resection.[8] A recent review by Tanden of the published series in the literature compared long-term survival after hepatic cryosurgery versus surgical resection for colorectal carcinoma metastatic to the liver.[10] There were a total of four cryosurgery and nine resection reports that met study criteria (patient number and follow-up). The authors state that a valid determination could not be made on the 5-year survival rate following cryosurgery.[10] They conclude that the data published to date did not support the use of cryosurgery on patients with potentially resectable disease outside the confines of a controlled trial.[10] The experience with radiofrequency ablation is even more anecdotal. This treatment offers potential benefits of being able to be performed laparoscopically or percutaneously under ultrasound or open magnet magnetic resonance imaging (MRI) guidance.[11–14] Currently, there are no long-term studies with sufficient numbers of patients to comment on the efficacy of this treatment regimen. One disturbing finding in the series reported by Solbiati *et al.* is that viable cancer cells were identified in radiofrequency-ablated tumors that were subsequently surgically resected.[11] This illustrates a persistent and nagging problem with the *in-situ* regional treatments of hepatic lesions, those of adequacy of margin and complete tumor lysis of the entire three-dimensional tumor volume. It is hoped that rapidly evolving technology to address these concerns in treatment regimens and imaging capabilities will make ablative treatments a more viable treatment choice in the near future.

An additional regional therapy, percutaneous alcohol ablation, has been widely practiced in Europe and Asia. The majority of series have been in patients with primary hepatocellular cancers (HCC). The limitation to this treatment has primarily been related to lesion size. In a series from Barcelona, complete response to treatment was only observed in patients with tumors less than 2 cm.[15] Patients with lesions 3 cm or greater had significantly worse results, with only 1 of 11 cases having a complete response.[15] The size constraints are due in part to the pain induced by injections of alcohol greater than 2 mL and the limited diffusion of such small volumes through the cancer.[16] This limitation was overcome in a subsequent study by treatment under general anesthesia. In this series, patients with HCC or metastatic colon cancer with lesions up to 8 cm in size were ablated with alcohol, with encouraging results. Complete responses were more often observed in patients with HCC versus colorectal lesions.[17]

CHEMOTHERAPEUTIC TREATMENT OF HEPATIC METASTASES

5-Fluoropyrimidines: mechanism of action

Because only small subsets, 5–10% of patients with hepatic lesions, are amenable to resection, the majority of patients are offered chemotherapy as the primary treatment.[4,5] The most well studied and widely used chemotherapeutic agent in metastatic colorectal carcinoma is 5-fluorouridine (5-FU), a fluoropyrimidine compound. Floxuridine (FUDR), the agent primarily used in hepatic artery infusion therapy, is also a fluoropyrimidine compound. 5-FU was introduced in 1957 and thousands of patients have been treated.[18] 5-FU causes cytotoxic effects through its interference with DNA synthesis and repair and its incorporation into RNA instead of uracil. 5-FU enters the cell through a uracil transport mechanism. It is then converted to FUDR by enzymatic action. Further phosphorylation by thymidine kinase forms the active metabolite, fluorodeoxyuridine monophosphate (F-dUMP). F-dUMP, in the presence of a reduced folate cofactor, forms a stable complex with the important enzyme thymidylate synthase (TS). The TS enzyme usually catabolizes the formation of deoxyuridine monophosphate (dUMP) to thymidine monophosphate (dTMP). The complex of TS and F-dUMP results in a decreased level of available thymidine triphosphate (dTTP), a key molecule in DNA

synthesis and repair.[19] 5-FU may also be metabolized to fluorouridine monophosphate (FUMP). FUMP is further phosphorylated to the diphosphate and triphosphate compounds FUDP and FUTP. FUTP can be directly incorporated into RNA in place of the natural uracil.[19] The 5-FU incorporation into RNA interferes with normal RNA processing and function. It is uncertain exactly how these effects on RNA result in cytotoxicity.

A principal and important component of 5-FU-directed cytotoxicity is its metabolite that complexes with TS. Because a folate cofactor is required for the formation of the complex, depletion of intracellular folate stores can interfere with this process and decrease the efficacy of 5-FU. The addition of supplementary folate by administering pharmacologic doses of leucovorin (folinic acid) can expand the intracellular folate pool and increase the extent of TS inhibition. Recently, TS levels have been recognized in clinical studies to correlate with responsiveness to 5-FU.[20] TS levels have also been shown to be a prognostic factor of survival in rectal cancer.[21] Gastrointestinal tumor levels of TS messenger RNA have been able to predict tumor responsiveness and overall survival.[22–25] It has been suggested that the determination of intratumoral levels of TS should be used to determine the responsiveness to fluoropyrimidine therapy prior to initiation.[26]

Pharmacokinetics and toxicity

5-FU can be administered by either bolus or continuous infusion. Each of these routes is associated with different toxicities due to the pharmacokinetics of 5-FU metabolism. 5-FU readily penetrates into tissues, ascitic fluid, and pleural effusions. After a bolus injection, the peak concentration is rapidly reached and subsequent elimination is rapid, with a primary half-life of 8–14 min.[27] Plasma drug levels fall below the cytotoxic range usually within 2 h after the bolus. Elimination occurs by enzymatic inactivation to dihydrofluorouracil (DHFU) by the enzyme dihydropyrimidine dehydrogenase (DPD). The liver has the highest concentration of the DPD enzyme, but it is widely distributed amongst other tissues. Further enzymatic pathways lead to catabolic products being excreted in the biliary secretions. It should be noted that there are rare patients with an inherited DPD deficiency who can have life-threatening or fatal events if treated with the fluoropyrimidines.[28]

Colorectal metastatic implants in the liver derive their blood supply initially from the portal venous circulation. Then the supply is derived from the hepatic artery. This anatomic set-up makes directed delivery of drugs to the hepatic circulation an attractive option. Hepatic first-pass extraction of 5-FU is only 20–50% of the dose, with the remainder reaching the systemic circulation.[29] This is in stark contrast to FUDR, which has a 95% first-pass extraction within hepatic parenchyma. Therefore, higher doses of regional FUDR can be given because there is less spill into the systemic circulation.

The toxicities associated with this family of chemotherapy agents primarily affect the gut mucosa and bone marrow. Toxicity varies greatly, depending on the dose, schedule, bolus versus continuous infusion, and route of administration. Ulceration of the mucosa can result in limitation of therapy due to severe diarrhea and/or mucositis in the oral cavity. In the bone marrow, the effect of myelosuppression is greatest on the granulocyte lineage. The bone-marrow toxicity appears to be greatest in those patients receiving bolus versus continuous infusion. Another significant syndrome is painful erythroderma of the hands and feet. Regional infusion into the hepatic circulation can result in significant toxicities, including chemical hepatitis, biliary sclerosis, and duodenal ulceration and hemorrhage.[30–35] The addition of dexamethasone to the hepatic infusion of FUDR has been shown to reduce the incidence of biliary sclerosis and improve the antitumor response.[36,37]

Clinical trial results

The response to 5-FU in colorectal carcinoma has ranged from a low of 8% to a high of 85%.[38] Many variables can affect the response rate, but one of the most important is dose intensity. An important caveat to remember while reading all of the trial results is stated by a standard textbook of oncology: 'Even after three decades of use, no single schedule or dose scheme has been shown to be ideal.'[38]

Unfortunately, 5-FU does not increase the survival of all patients with metastatic colorectal cancer. Median survival is only 6–8 months overall. If patients are stratified to those with objective response (measurable decrease in metastatic lesion size), median survival is increased to the 12–18-month range.[38] One of the most difficult questions to answer in clinical studies is whether continuous infusion is superior to bolus administration. In a prospective trial directed by the Mid-Atlantic Oncology Program, chemotherapy-naïve patients ($n = 179$) with measurable advanced colorectal carcinoma (many with hepatic metastases) were randomized to receive either bolus or continuous infusion of 5-FU. The results demonstrated a significant difference ($p < 0.001$) in objective tumor response rate of 30% in the continuous-infusion group as compared to 7% in those who received bolus therapy. However, overall survival in the two treatment groups was nearly identical.[39] Two other major studies, one by the National Cancer Institute of Canada and the other by the Southwestern Oncology Group (SWOG) have confirmed no difference in overall survival when bolus versus continuous infusion is compared.[40,41] Overall response rate is from 11% to 29% with median survival being 11–14 months.[40,41] More recently, the final results were published of a report from France of a randomized phase III trial comparing continuous infusion to bolus in previously non-treated patients, with 70% of the patients having measurable hepatic lesions. This trial also showed a statistically significant difference ($p < 0.04$) in response rate (26% in the continuous infusion group versus 13% in the bolus-treated arm). Once again, there was no difference in median survival (10 versus 9 months) or 1-year survival (42% versus 40%), confirming the results from other trials.[42] Currently, therapeutic regimens of bolus versus continuous infusion are based on individual patients' needs and lifestyles.

Modulation of 5-FU with other agents

The combination of 5-FU with a wide variety of other agents has been and is currently being investigated in an attempt to improve patient survival seen with 5-FU infusion alone. The addition of interferon, leucovorin, cisplatin, methotrexate and an ever-increasing list of agents have been used in clinical trials. There are many trials that show increased response rates to combination agents, but few that are well controlled demonstrate an improvement in overall survival. One of the best-studied modulating agents is leucovorin, a tetrahydrofolate compound used to help expand the intracellular folate pool to maximize the TS suppression, as discussed previously.

There have been 12 prospective randomized trials evaluating the addition of leucovorin to 5-FU. There have been both high-dose and low-dose ranges of leucovorin utilized in these trials. The results demonstrate a significantly higher response rate in patients treated with 5-FU and leucovorin in nine of the studies. In two of the studies, there was a statistically significant increase in overall survival rate for those patients treated with the combination 5-FU and leucovorin.[43–51] In 1992, the Advanced Colorectal Cancer Meta-Analysis Project reviewed 1381 treated patients and reported an overall response rate of 11% for 5-FU treatment alone versus 23% for the combination of 5-FU and leucovorin. However, the median survivals for these groups were not clinically different (11 versus 11.5 months, respectively) and the authors concluded that overall tumor response should not be considered a valid end-point in the design of future trials.[52] The determination of statistical odd ratios for survival did not demonstrate a survival advantage to the combination treatment.[52]

As the majority of studies do not demonstrate an significant improvement in patient survival with the combination of 5-FU and leucovorin, why is this combination the most frequently prescribed regimen? Two important studies that focused on quality-of-life issues compared performance status, weight gain, and symptomatic relief. The first report by Poon et al. compared six treatment regimens (5-FU alone, 5-FU/cisplatin, 5-FU/methotrexate, 5-FU/methotrexate/leucovorin rescue, 5-FU/high-dose leucovorin, and 5-FU/low-dose leucovorin) in

429 patients. The treatment associated with the greatest improvement of quality-of-life issues was the 5-FU and low-dose leucovorin regimen.[53] The 5-FU plus high-dose or low-dose leucovorin were directly compared by Buroker et al. in a 1994 report.[54] Symptomatic improvement was again statistically greatest in the low-dose leucovorin treatment arm (44% versus 31%). The high-dose leucovorin treatment arm had an increased gastrointestinal toxicity, with an increase in hospitalizations to manage the diarrhea.[54]

In summary, 5-FU has been demonstrated to increase overall survival, although the optimal treatment regimen has not been determined. The addition of leucovorin increases objective response rates and symptomatic improvement but does not improve survival. The combination of other agents with 5-FU has not been conclusively or reproducibly demonstrated to result in increased overall survival. There are currently trials in progress with 5-FU with other chemotherapy agents to try to increase its overall effectiveness. One of these new agents Tomudex, a TS inhibitor, has shown promise in a recent phase II trial in Europe.[55] Another development in Japan has been UFT, an oral combination treatment regimen of tetrahydrofuryl-5-FU (tegafur) and uracil.[56] This treatment offers the advantage of the inhibition by uracil of the DPD-mediated degradation of 5-FU, thereby augmenting the 5-FU effects on cytotoxicity. A preliminary report of a phase II trial in Spain using the oral regimen of UFT and leucovorin on elderly patients (≥ 72 years) had an overall median survival of 14.4 months with acceptable toxicities, allowing for further trials of this oral-based treatment.[57] Lastly, there is a report by Bismuth et al. that offers hope to patients with inoperable hepatic metastases. The French group aggressively treated 330 patients with unresectable lesions due to location, number, or extrahepatic disease with a regimen of 5-FU, leucovorin, and oxaliplatin (a new platinum-based agent). Fifty-three patients had sufficient response to treatment so that subsequent resections could be performed. The results from these 53 patients are summarized in Table 27.1. This paper demonstrates that aggressive chemotherapy with re-evaluation of patients for hepatic resection offers a significant chance to improve long-term survival substantially by increasing the number of patients undergoing hepatic resection.[58]

HEPATIC ARTERIAL INFUSION THERAPY

The anatomic blood supply of the liver makes direct infusion of chemotherapy drugs a logical strategy. As discussed previously, the pharmacokinetics of FUDR make it an attractive agent due to near complete first-pass extraction in the liver, allowing for very high intrahepatic drug levels and low systemic leakage. Initial phase II results demonstrating response rates as high as 80% generated even more interest in this treatment modality.[59–63] To date, there have been seven trials that have been completed comparing intra-arterial FUDR to systemic 5-FU-based treatment or supportive care. In 1996, the Meta-analysis Group in Cancer reported their findings on hepatic artery infusion (HAI) in the treatment of colorectal metastases.[64] In five of the seven studies, there was a comparison of HAI to conventional systemic treatment, which demonstrated a significant increase in tumor response in those patients with HAI treatment (41% versus 14%), but no statistically significant survival advantage.[65–69] There was also a sizable number of hepatic toxicities, including chemical hepatitis and biliary sclerosis. Kemeny et al. demonstrated that the addition of dexamethasone to the arterial infusion reduced the chemotherapy-related toxicities and diminished the need for dose reduction over the course of treatment.[36] Modulation of HAI with FUDR, leucovorin, and dexamethasone resulted in response rates of 78% and a median survival of 24 months in chemotherapy-naïve patients with metastatic liver disease.[70] Unfortunately, in these studies, about 55% of the patients went on to develop extrahepatic disease. The strategy of high intrahepatic and low systemic drug levels may need to be altered to treat both intrahepatic and extrahepatic sites simultaneously. This philosophy of treatment has recently been reported by Howell et al. A phase II trial of 5-FU via HAI and intravenous leucovorin was initiated with the intention of allowing 5-FU 'spillover' into the systemic circulation. Median survival was 19 months. They are proceeding to a prospective, randomized trial directly comparing HAI versus systemic 5-FU to see if a significant survival advantage is obtained.[71] HAI continues to be an attractive strategy for the regional treatment of unresectable hepatic disease and there may be a trend toward increased median survival.

Table 27.1 *Results of hepatic resection after chemotherapy*[58]

Non-resectable reason	Size	Location	Multiple lesions	Extrahepatic disease
Patient number	8	8	24	13
3-year survival (%)	62	75	54	43
5-year survival (%)	62	48	40	14
Hepatic recurrence[a]	6	5	17	6
Extrahepatic recurrence	2	1	15	7

[a]Repeat liver resections for hepatic recurrence were performed in 15 of 34 patients.

A surgical extension of HAI is based on the experience with isolated limb perfusion to treat other malignancies. Isolated hepatic perfusion in 12 patients was recently reported by Oldhafer et al.[72] In this paper, extensive isolation of all hepatic arterial and venous inflow and outflow pathways was performed. Veno-venous bypass was achieved via the femoral and portal veins with the axillary vein. The liver was then isolated on an extracorporeal circuit via cannulation of the retrohepatic cava and hepatic artery. The hepatic perfusion circuit was able to raise the intrahepatic temperature to 41 °C. Mitomycin was infused in the first six patients and the last six received tumor necrosis factor and melphalan. The 12 patients had a range of primary tumors, but 50% were colorectal in origin. Tumor biopsy specimens were taken in a second-look operation on the first day after surgery and histologically examined for the percentage of tumor necrosis. Significant complications were seen in the patients who received mitomycin, ranging from the development of ascites in two-thirds of the patients to death in two patients from veno-occlusive disease. Fifty percent of the patients had significant tumor necrosis on biopsy; seven of the patients are still alive, with one having a complete response. This is a preliminary report and no long-term survival data are available.[72] This experience reflects other groups' difficulty with mitomycin, suggesting this agent should not be used in isolated hepatic perfusion.[72,73] In a recent review, Vahrmeijer et al. ask whether this technically difficult, expensive, resource-intense procedure will be significantly better than simpler treatment regimens.[74] They report that a phase II trial with melphalan (L-PAM) as the administered agent now has a median survival of 17 months, and survival data from the end of the study should be available in 1998.[74] There are a number of European and USA phase II trials that have not yet published results, so a final verdict would be premature. Subsequent reporting on this complicated regimen has shown no added benefit, leading to the conclusion of the authors that 'because of the complexity of this treatment modality, intrahepatic perfusion (with melphalan) has at present no place in routine clinical practice.'[75]

Increased local cytostatic drug exposure by isolated hepatic perfusion: a phase I clinical and pharmacologic evaluation of treatment with high-dose melphalan in patients with colorectal cancer confined to the liver.

One interesting application of this technique may be for directed gene therapy against intrahepatic cancers.

CHEMOEMBOLIZATION OF HEPATIC METASTASES

Direct hepatic arterial injection of chemotherapy in combination with particulate embolic material allows for both a hypoxic injury to tumor cells from the cessation of blood flow and increased cytotoxicity due to prolonged contact time with drugs.[76] Suspensions of drugs with embolic agents such as collagen particles, polyvinyl alcohol, or Gelfoam have been employed.[77–79] There has been a significant amount of experience with this modality of treatment, especially in HCC or neuroendocrine tumors metastatic to the liver. There have been only a few trials examining the role of embolization in colorectal hepatic metastases. In a series of 24 patients who failed systemic chemotherapy, half were treated with the particulate polyvinyl alcohol alone and the other half with 5-FU and interferon with particulate matter. There was no significant difference in the two treatments, with overall response rates of 25% and a median survival of 9 months.[79] At this time, there is no evidence to suggest that this therapy offers any advantage over conventional systemic treatment regimens.

IRINOTECAN (CPT-11)

CPT-11, commercially available under the name of Irinotecan, is a promising new antineoplastic agent that appears to be effective in colorectal carcinoma. It is in a totally different class of drugs from 5-FU, that of DNA topoisomerase enzyme inhibition. The topoisomerase enzyme family is responsible for relaxation of the double-stranded DNA molecule so replication and transcription can proceed.[80] CPT-11 stabilizes the formation of cleavage complexes between topoisomerase I and DNA. This complex leads to the arrest of DNA replication and ultimately cellular death.[80,81] Colon cancer cells have been found to have an approximately 15-fold increase in levels of topoisomerase I, making it an attractive target in new regimen development.[82] Phase 1 trials demonstrated that neutropenia and diarrhea are the two main dose-limiting toxicities of CPT-11.[83,84] Rougier et al. reported the results of a phase II trial from France.[85] A total of 213 patients were enrolled, only 48 of whom were chemotherapy naïve. Toxicities were primarily hematologic, diarrhea, or a cholinergic-like syndrome with diaphoresis, abdominal cramps, and diarrhea. The overall response rate was 18%, with four complete responses occurring in patients in whom hepatic metastases were the only sites of measurable disease. The 1-year survival rate was 43%, with median survivals of 12 months in the chemotherapy-naïve group and 10 months in the previously treated cohort. These results were further interpreted to demonstrate no cross-resistance between 5-FU and CPT-11, which may make this agent an important salvage drug in patients failing 5-FU-based regimens.[85] Further trials of CPT-11 alone and in combination with 5-FU will establish its role in the armamentarium against metastatic colorectal carcinoma.

NOVEL THERAPIES: MONOCLONAL ANTIBODY AND GENE THERAPY

If tumor-specific markers can be isolated, monoclonal antibodies can be generated to bind these proteins. Cytotoxic agents such as drugs or radiopharmaceuticals can be joined to the monoclonal antibodies to provide efficient and targeted anticancer agents.[86–88] There have been small trials examining the effectiveness of this treatment with ^{131}I-anti-carcinoembryonic antigen (CEA) or tumor-associated glycoprotein (TAG72) which have failed to demonstrate a role for monoclonal antibodies as primary therapy.[89,90] A recent phase I/II trial in France used ^{131}I-anti-CEA in ten patients with non-resectable hepatic colorectal metastases. Hematologic toxicity, from radiation, requiring autologous bone marrow transplant was seen in 50% of the cases. Unfortunately, there was not any objective tumor response.[86] Perhaps the development of antibodies to newly described tumor-associated antigens will make this a more clinically relevant treatment in the future, but at the present time there is no proven role for this treatment in metastatic colon cancer.

Gene therapy is currently being intensively examined as a potential anticancer treatment. Gene transfer strategies include:

1 transfer of tumor suppressor genes,
2 suicide genes that convert drugs into cytotoxic products,
3 genes to encode for cytokines and other soluble factors that promote tumor destruction via immune modulation,
4 genes to increase resistance to chemotherapy drugs in non-cancer tissue.[91,92]

Suicide genes that have been developed thus far are herpes simplex virus thymidine kinase that converts the antiviral drug ganciclovir into the active drug form, which is a powerful inhibitor of DNA synthesis,[93,94] and the *Escherichia coli* cytosine deaminase gene, which converts a fluorouracil prodrug into the active FU metabolite.[95] Another strategy transfers histocompatibility antigens to tumor cells to elicit a rejection response. This has been recently reported by the Mayo Clinic in a phase I human trial in which HLA-B7 was transferred by directed injection into colorectal hepatic metastases. This was only a feasibility study to demonstrate successful transfer of the protein in 63% of the patients without any serious morbidity.[96] No data are yet available concerning the clinical relevance of these treatments.

CONCLUSIONS

Patients with isolated hepatic disease should be considered first and foremost as candidates for resection because this offers the greatest chance for long-term survival. For those patients who are not resection candidates, ablation with cryosurgery or radiofrequency may be the best second-line therapy. Aggressive downstaging with chemotherapy should be considered to increase the number of patients amenable to resection. Intrahepatic recurrences and the development of extrahepatic disease will continue to be the primary reasons for treatment failures. Therefore, consideration of any regional treatment including resection without systemic treatment is going to be inadequate in the majority of cases. Unfortunately, present chemotherapy regimens have limited efficacy, but new modalities may offer hope for the future.

REFERENCES

1. Blumgart LH, Fong Y. Surgical options in the treatment of hepatic metastases from colorectal cancer. Curr Prob Surg 1995; 32:336–421.

2. Fong Y, Cohen AM, Fortner JG, *et al*. Liver resections for colorectal metastases. J Clin Oncol 1997; 15(3):938–46.

3. Jamison RL, Donohue JH, Nagorney DM, Rosen CB, Harmsen WS, Ilstrup DM. Hepatic resection for metastatic colorectal cancer results in cure for some patients. Arch Surg 1997; 132(5):505–10.

4. Steele G Jr, Ravikumar TS. Resection of hepatic metastases from colorectal carcinoma: biological perspectives. Ann Surg 1989; 210:127–38.

5. Zavadsky KE, Lee YT. Liver metastases from colorectal carcinoma: incidence, resectability, and survival results. Am Surg 1994; 60:929–33.

6. Ravikumar XD, Tang ZY, Yu YQ, Ma ZC. Clinical evaluation of cryosurgery in the treatment of primary liver cancer: report of 60 cases. Cancer 1988; 61:1889–92.

7. Ravikumar TS, Steele G Jr, Kane R, King V. Experimental clinical observations on hepatic cryosurgery for colorectal metastases. Cancer Res 1991; 51:6323–7.

8. Onik GM, Atkinson D, Zemel R, Weaver LM. Cryosurgery of liver cancer. Semin Surg Oncol 1993; 9:309–17.

9. Zhou XD, Tang ZY, Yu YQ, *et al*. The role of cryosurgery in the treatment of hepatic cancer: a report of 113 cases. J Can Res Clin Oncol 1993; 120:100–2.

10. Tanden VR, Harmantas A, Gallinger S. Long-term survival after hepatic cryosurgery versus surgical resection for metastatic colorectal carcinoma: a critical review of the literature. Can J Surg 1997; 40(3):175–81.

11. Solbiati L, Ierace T, Goldberg SN, *et al*. Percutaneous US guided radiofrequency tissue ablation of liver metastases: treatment and follow-up in 16 patients. Radiology 1997; 202(1):195–203.

12. Rossi S, Buscarini E, Garbagnati F, *et al.* Percutaneous treatment of small hepatic tumors by an expandable RF needle electrode. Am J Roentgenol 1998; 170(4):1015–22.

13. Solbiati L, Goldberg SN, Ierace T, *et al.* Hepatic metastases: percutaneous radiofrequency ablation with cooled tip electrodes. Radiology 1997; 205(2):367–73.

14. Siperstein AE, Rogers SJ, Hansen PD, Gitomirsky A. Laparoscopic thermal ablation of hepatic neuroendocrine metastases. Surgery 1997; 122(6):1147–54.

15. Vilana R, Briux J, Bru C, Ayuso C, Sole M, Rodes J. Tumor size determines the efficacy of percutaneous ethanol injection for the treatment of small hepatocellular carcinoma. Hepatology 1992; 16:353–7.

16. Livraghi T, Bolondi L, Lazzaroni S, *et al.* Percutaneous ethanol injection in the treatment of hepatocellular carcinoma in cirrhosis: a study on 207 patients. Cancer 1992; 69:925–9.

17. Livraghi T, Lazzaroni S, Pellicano S, Ravasi S, Torzilli G, Vettori C. Percutaneous ethanol injection of hepatic tumors: single-session therapy with general anesthesia. Am J Roentgenol 1993; 61:1065–9.

18. Heidelberger CG, Chandhari NK, Dannenberg P, *et al.* Fluorinated pyrimidines: a new class of tumor inhibitory compounds. Nature 1969; 1279:665.

19. Rustrum YM, Harstrick A, Cao S, *et al.* Thymidylate synthase inhibitors in cancer therapy: direct and indirect inhibitors [review]. J Clin Oncol 1997; 15:389–400.

20. Johnston PG, Allegra CJ. Colorectal cancer biology: clinical implications. Semin Oncol 1995; 22:418–32.

21. Johnston PG, Fisher ER, Rockette HE, *et al.* The role of thymidylate synthase expression in the prognosis and outcome of adjuvant chemotherapy in patients with rectal cancer. J Clin Oncol 1994; 12:2640–7.

22. Leichman L, Lenz HJ, Leichman CJ, *et al.* Quantitation of intratumoral thymidylate synthase expression predicts resistance to protracted infusion of 5-FU and weekly leucovorin in disseminated colorectal cancers: preliminary report from an ongoing trial. Eur J Cancer 1995; 31:1306–10.

23. Lenz HJ, Leichman CG, Danenberg KD, *et al.* Thymidylate synthase mRNA level in adenocarcinoma of the stomach: predictor for primary tumor response and overall survival. J Clin Oncol 1996; 14:176–82.

24. Peters GJ, Van der Wilt CL, Van Groenongen CJ, *et al.* Thymidylate synthase inhibition after administration of fluorouracil with or without leucovorin in colon cancer patients: implications for treatment with fluorouracil. J Clin Oncol 1994; 12:2035–42.

25. Link KH, Kornmann M, Leder GH, *et al.* Regional chemotherapy directed by individual chemosensitivity testing in vitro: prospective decision aiding trial. Clin Cancer Res 1996; 2:1469–74.

26. Kornmann M, Link KH, Lenz HJ, *et al.* Thymidylate synthase is a predictor for response and resistance in

27. Heggie GD, Sommadossi JP, Cross DS, Huster WJ, Diasio RB. Clinical pharmacokinetics of 5-FU and its metabolites in plasma, urine, and bile. Cancer Res 1987; 47:2203.

28. Diasio RB, Beavers TL, Carpenter T. Familial deficiency of dihydropyrimidine dehydrogenase biochemical basis for familial pyrimidinemia and severe 5-fluorouracil-induced toxicity. J Clin Invest 1988; 81:47.

29. Ensminger WD, Rosowsky A, Raso VO, *et al.* A clinical pharmacological evaluation of hepatic arterial infusion of 5-fluoro 2'-deoxyuridine and 5-fluorouracil. Cancer Res 1978; 38:3784.

30. Hohn DC, Melnick J, Stagg R, *et al.* Biliary sclerosis in patients receiving hepatic arterial infusions of floxuridine. J Clin Oncol 1985; 3:98.

31. Shepard KV, Levin B, Faintuch J, *et al.* Hepatitis in patients receiving intra-arterial chemotherapy for metastatic colorectal cancer. Am J Clin Oncol 1987; 10:36.

32. Chuang VP, Wallace S, Stroehlein J, *et al.* Hepatic artery infusion chemotherapy: gastroduodenal complications. Am J Radiol 1981; 137:347.

33. Hike M, Scott-Gillin J, Kemeny N, *et al.* Severe gastroduodenal ulcerations complicating hepatic artery infusion chemotherapy for metastatic colon cancer. Am J Gastroenterol 1986; 81:176.

34. Doria MI, Shepard KV, Levin B, Riddell R. Liver pathology following hepatic arterial infusion chemotherapy. Cancer 1986; 58:855.

35. Shea WJ, Demas BE, Goldberg HI, *et al.* Sclerosing cholangitis associated with hepatic arterial FUDR chemotherapy: radiographic–histologic correlation. Am J Roentgenol 1986; 146:717.

36. Kemeny N, Seiter K, Niedzwiecki D, *et al.* A randomized trial of intrahepatic infusion of fluorodeoxyuridine with dexamethasone versus fluorodeoxyuridine alone in the treatment of metastatic colorectal cancer. Cancer 1992; 69:327.

37. Kemeny N, Seiter K, Conti J, *et al.* Hepatic arterial floxuridine and leucovorin for unresectable liver metastases from colorectal carcinoma: new dose schedules and survival update. Cancer 1994; 73:1134.

38. Cohen AM, Minsky BD, Schilsky RL. Cancer of the colon. In DeVita VT, Hellman S, Rosenberg SA, eds. *Cancer principles and practice of oncology*, 5th edition. Lippincott-Raven Publishers, 1997.

39. Lokich JJ, Ahlgren JD, Gullo JJ, Phillips JA, Frver JG. A prospective randomized comparison of continuous infusion fluorouracil with a conventional bolus schedule in metastatic colorectal carcinoma: a mid-Atlantic oncology program study. J Clin Oncol 1989; 7:425.

40. Weinerman B, Shah A, Fields A, *et al.* A randomized trial of continuous systemic infusion versus bolus

therapy with 5-fluorouracil in metastatic measurable colorectal cancer. Proc Am Soc Clin Oncol 1990; 9:103.

41. Leichman CG, Fleming TR, Muggia FM, *et al.* Phase II study of fluorouracil and its modulation in advanced colorectal cancer: a Southwestern Oncology Group study. J Clin Oncol 1995; 13:1303–11.

42. Rougier P, Paillot B, LaPlanche A, *et al.* 5 Fluorouracil continuous intravenous infusion compared with bolus administration. Final results of a randomized trial in metastatic colorectal cancer. Eur J Cancer 1997; 33:1789–93.

43. Leyland-Jones B, Burdette-Radoux S. Management of hepatic metastases from colorectal cancer: systemic chemotherapy. J Gastro Surg 1997; 6:576–82.

44. Poon MA, O'Connell MJ, Moertel CG, *et al.* Biochemical modulation of fluorouracil: evidence of significant improvement of survival and quality of life in patients with advanced colorectal carcinoma. J Clin Oncol 1989; 7:1407.

45. Valone FH, Friedman MA, Wittlinger PS, *et al.* Treatment of patients with advanced colorectal carcinomas with fluorouracil alone, high-dose leucovorin plus fluorouracil, or sequential methotrexate, fluorouracil and leucovorin: a randomized trial of the Northern California Oncology Group. J Clin Oncol 1989; 7:1427.

46. Petrelli N, Herrera L, Rustum Y, *et al.* A prospective randomized trial of 5-fluorouracil versus 5-fluorouracil and high dose leucovorin versus 5-fluorouracil and methotrexate in previously untreated patients with advanced colorectal carcinoma. J Clin Oncol 1987; 5:1559.

47. Petrelli N, Douglass HO Jr, Herrera L, *et al.* The modulation of fluorouracil with leucovorin in metastatic colorectal carcinoma; a prospective randomized phase III trial. J Clin Oncol 1989; 7:1419.

48. Nordic Gastrointestinal Tumor Adjuvant Therapy Group. Superiority of sequential methotrexate, fluorouracil and leucovorin to fluorouracil alone in advanced symptomatic colorectal carcinoma: a randomized trial. J Clin Oncol 1989; 7:1437.

49. Doroshaw JH, Multhauf P, Leong L, *et al.* Prospective randomized comparison of fluorouracil versus fluorouracil and high dose continuous infusion leucovorin calcium for the treatment of advanced measurable colorectal cancer in patients previously unexposed to chemotherapy. J Clin Oncol 1990; 8:491.

50. Erlichman C, Fine S, Wong A, Elhakim T. A randomized trial of fluorouracil and folinic acid in patients with metastatic colorectal carcinoma. J Clin Oncol 1988; 6:469.

51. DiCostanzo FB, Calabresi F. Fluorouracil alone versus high dose folinic acid and fluorouracil in advanced colorectal cancer: a randomized trial of the Italian Oncology Group for Clinical Trials. Ann Oncol 1992; 3:371.

52. Advanced Colorectal Cancer Meta-Analysis Project. Modulation of fluorouracil by leucovorin in patients with advanced colorectal cancer: evidence in terms of response rate. J Clin Oncol 1992; 10:896–903.

53. Poon M, O'Connell M, Wieand H, *et al.* Biochemical modulation of fluorouracil with leucovorin: confirmatory evidence of improved therapeutic efficacy in advanced colorectal cancer. J Clin Oncol 1991; 9:1967–72.

54. Buroker TR, O'Connell MJ, Wieand HS, *et al.* Randomized comparison of two schedules of fluorouracil and leucovorin in the treatment of advanced colorectal cancer. J Clin Oncol 1994; 1:14–20.

55. Cunningham D, Zalcberg JR, Rath U, *et al.* Tomudex (ZD1694): results of a randomized trial in advanced colorectal cancer demonstrate efficacy and reduced mucositis and leucopenia. The Tomudex Colorectal Cancer Study Group. Eur J Cancer 1995; 31A:1945–54.

56. Maehara Y, Kakeji Y, Ohno S, *et al.* Scientific basis for the combination of tegafur with uracil. Oncology 1997; 11(Suppl. 10):14–21.

57. Abad A, Navarro M, Sastre J, *et al.* UFT plus oral folinic acid as therapy for metastatic colorectal cancer on older patients. Oncology 1997; 11(Suppl. 10):53–7.

58. Bismuth H, Adam R, Levi F, *et al.* Resection of nonresectable liver metastases from colorectal cancer after neoadjuvant chemotherapy. Ann Surg 1996; 224:509–22.

59. Niederhuber JE, Ensminger W, Gyves J, Thrall J, Walker S, Cozzi E. Regional chemotherapy of colorectal cancer metastatic to the liver. Cancer 1984; 53:1336.

60. Balch CM, Urist MM, Soong SJ, Megregor M. A prospective phase II clinical continuous FUDR regional chemotherapy colorectal metastases to the liver using a totally implantable pump. Ann Surg 1983; 198:567.

61. Kemeny N, Daly J, Oderman P, *et al.* Hepatic artery pump infusion toxicity and results in patients with metastatic colorectal carcinoma. J Clin Oncol 1984; 2:595.

62. Weiss GR, Barneck MB, Osteen RT, *et al.* Long term hepatic arterial infusion of fluorodeoxyuridine for liver metastases using an implantable infusion pump. J Clin Oncol 1983; 1:337.

63. Shepard KV, Levin B, Karl RC, *et al.* Therapy for metastatic colorectal cancer with hepatic artery infusion chemotherapy using a subcutaneous implanted pump. J Clin Oncol 1985; 3:161.

64. Meta-analysis Group in Cancer. Reappraisal of hepatic arterial infusion in the treatment of nonresectable liver metastases from colorectal cancer. J Natl Cancer Inst 1996; 88:252–8.

65. Chang AE, Schneider PD, Sugarbaker PH, *et al.* A prospective randomized trial of regional versus systemic continuous 5-FU chemotherapy in the treatment of colorectal liver metastases. Ann Surg 1987; 206:685–93.

66. Hohn DC, Stagg RJ, Freidman MA, *et al.* A randomized trial of continuous intravenous versus hepatic intraarterial floxuridine in patients with colorectal cancer metastatic to the liver: the Northern California Oncology Group trial. J Clin Oncol 1989; 7:1646–54.

67. Kemeny MM, Goldberg D, Beatty JD, *et al.* Results of a prospective randomized trial of continuous regional chemotherapy and hepatic resection as treatment of hepatic metastases from colorectal cancer. Cancer 1986; 57:492–8.

68. Kemeny N, Daly J, Reichman B, *et al.* Intrahepatic or systemic infusion of floxuridine in liver metastases from colorectal carcinoma. Ann Intern Med 1987; 107:459–65.

69. Martin JK, O'Connell MJ, Wieand HS, *et al.* Intra-arterial floxuridine vs systemic fluorouracil for hepatic metastases from colorectal cancer. A randomized trial. Arch Surg 1990; 125:1022–7.

70. Kemeny N, Seiter K, Niedzwiecki D, *et al.* A randomized trial of intrahepatic infusion of fluorodeoxyuridine with dexamethasone versus fluorodeoxyuridine alone in the treatment of metastatic colorectal cancer. Cancer 1992; 69:327–34.

71. Howell JD, McArdle CS, Kerr DJ, *et al.* A Phase II trial of regional 2 weekly 5-fluorouracil infusion with intravenous folinic acid in the treatment of colorectal liver metastases. Br J Cancer 1997; 76:1390–3.

72. Oldhafer KJ, Lang H, Frerker M, *et al.* First experience and technical aspects of isolated liver perfusion for extensive liver metastasis. Surgery 1998; 123:622–31.

73. Marinelli A, de Brauw LM, Beerman H, *et al.* Isolated liver perfusion with mitomycin C in the treatment if colorectal cancer metastases confined to the liver. Jpn J Clin Oncol 1996; 26:341–50.

74. Vahrmeijer AL, Van der Eb MM, van Dieredonck JH, Kuppen PJK, van de Velde C. Delivery of anticancer drugs via isolated hepatic perfusion: a promising strategy in the treatment of irresectable liver metastases. Semin Surg Oncol 1998; 14:262–8.

75. Vahrmeijer AL, van Dierendonck JH, Keizer HJ, *et al.* Increased local cytostatic drug exposure by isolated hepatic perfusion: a phase I clinical and pharmacologic evaluation of treatment with high dose melphalan in patients with colorectal cancer confined to the liver. Br J Cancer 2000; 82:1539–46.

76. Kruskal JB, Hlatky L, Hahnfeldt P, Teramoto K, Stokes K, Clouse ME. *In vivo* and *in vitro* analysis of the effectiveness of doxorubicin combined with temporary occlusion in liver tumors. J Vasc Interv Radiol 1993; 4:741–7.

77. Coldwell DM, Stokes KR, Yakes WF. Embolotherapy: agents, clinical applications and techniques. RadioGraphics 1994; 14:623–43.

78. Daniels JR, Karian R, Dodds L, *et al.* Peripheral hepatic arterial embolization with cross-linked collagen fibrils. Invest Radiol 1987; 22:126–31.

79. Martinelli DJ, Wadler S, Bakal CW, *et al.* Utility of embolization or chemoembolization as second-line treatment in patients with advanced or recurrent colorectal carcinoma. Cancer 1994; 74:1706–12.

80. Chen AY, Liu LF. DNA topoisomerases: essential enzymes and lethal targets. Annu Rev Pharmacol Toxicol 1994; 34:191–218.

81. Creemers GJ, Lund B, Verweij J. Topoisomerase I inhibitors: topotecan and irinotecan. Cancer Treat Rev 1994; 20:73–96.

82. Giovanella BC, Stehlin JS, Wall ME, *et al.* DNA topoisomerase I-targeted chemotherapy of human colon cancer in xenografts. Science 1989; 246:1046–8.

83. De Forni M, Bugat R, Chabot GG, *et al.* Phase I and pharmacokinetic study of the camptothecin derivative irinotecan, administered on a weekly schedule in cancer patients. Cancer Res 1994; 54:4347–54.

84. Abigerges D, Chabot GG, Armand J, *et al.* Phase I and pharmacologic studies of the camptothecin analogue irinotecan administered every 3 weeks in cancer patients. J Clin Oncol 1995; 13:210–21.

85. Rougier P, Bugat R, Douillard S, *et al.* Phase II study of irinotecan in the treatment of advanced colorectal cancer in chemotherapy naïve patients and patients pretreated with fluorouracil based chemotherapy. J Clin Oncol 1997; 15:251–60.

86. Ychou M, Pelegrin A, Faurous P, *et al.* Phase I/II radio-immunotherapy study with iodine-131-labeled anti-CEA monoclonal antibody F6 F(ab')2 in patients with non-resectable liver metastases from colorectal cancer. Int J Cancer 1998; 75:615–19.

87. Van Wussow P, Spitler L, Block B, Deicher H. Immunotherapy in patients with advanced malignant melanoma using an anti melanoma antibody ricin A immunotoxin. Eur J Cancer Clin Oncol 1988; 24:S69–73.

88. Steplewski Z. Wistar symposium on immunodiagnosis and immunotherapy with CO17-1A Mab in gastrointestinal cancer. Hybridoma 1986; 5(Suppl.):1.

89. Order SE, Klein JL, Leichner PK, Frincke J, Lollo C, Carlo DJ. [90]Yttrium antiferritin – a new therapeutic radiolabelled antibody. Int J Radiat Oncol Biol Phys 1986; 12:277–81.

90. Ychou M, Richard M, Lumbroso J, *et al.* Potential contribution of ^{131}I-labelled monoclonal anti-CEA antibodies in the treatment of liver metastases from colorectal carcinomas: pretherapeutic study with dose recovery in resected tissues. Eur J Cancer 1993; 29A:1111–14.

91. Davis BM, Koc OC, Lee K, Gersoon SL. Current progress in the gene therapy of cancer [review]. Curr Opin Oncol 1996; 8:499–508.

92. Roth JA, Cristiano RJ. Gene therapy for cancer: what have we done and where are we going [review]? J Natl Cancer Inst 1997; 89:21–39.

93. Culver KW, Ram Z, Wallbridge S, *et al.* In vivo gene transfer with retroviral vector-producer cells for treatment of experimental brain tumors. Science 1992; 256:1550–2.

94. Smythe WR, Hwang HC, Amin KM, *et al.* Use of recombinant adenovirus to transfer the herpes simplex virus thymidine kinase (*HSVtk*) gene to thoracic neoplasms: an effective in vitro drug sensitization system. Cancer Res 1994; 54:2055–9.

95. Hirschowitz EA, Ohwada A, Pascal WR, *et al.* In vivo adenovirus-mediated gene transfer of the *Escherichia* *coli* cytosine deaminase gene to human colon carcinoma derived tumors induces chemosensitivity to 5-fluorocytosine. Hum Gene Ther 1995; 6:1055–63.

96. Rubin J, Galanis E, Pitot HC, *et al.* Phase I immunotherapy of hepatic metastases of colorectal carcinoma by direct gene transfer of an allogeneic histocompatibility antigen, HLA-B7. Gene Ther 1997; 4:419–25.

Commentary

NANCY E KEMENY

For patients with resectable metastatic colorectal disease, I agree with Dr Sherry Wren that liver resection offers the best results. In the past, patients with only one to four metastases were resected. However, I believe that we can enlarge this number because we now have better methods of controlling undetected disease.

I also agree that ablative techniques, such as cryosurgery or radiofrequency ablation, should be considered as secondary techniques. Currently, we should only use these techniques when liver resection is not possible. With ablative techniques, viable cancer cells can remain behind and are difficult to detect at the time of ablation. We have demonstrated that viable tumor cells may be detected by positron emission tomography (PET) after ablative techniques[1] and not detected by magnetic resonance imaging (MRI) or computerized tomography (CT).

The review of systemic chemotherapy extensively covers 5-fluorouracil (5-FU), but does not describe the outcome of new randomized trials using 5-FU plus leucovorin (LV) with new agents versus 5-FU plus LV alone. CPT-11, a topoisomerase inhibitor,[2] and Oxaliplatin,[3] a new platinum derivative, when given in combination with 5-FU and LV, produce response rates higher than those with 5-FU and LV alone. Randomized studies of CPT-11, 5-FU, LV versus 5-FU and LV have significantly increased survival with the three drugs. The median survival increased from 12.8 to 14.8 months in one study[4] and from 14 to 16 months in the other.[5] However, even with all three agents, the 2-year survival for systemic chemotherapy is still only 25–30%, versus 20% for 5-FU and LV alone.

In the discussion of hepatic arterial infusion (HAI) therapy, Dr Wren mentions a meta-analysis of HAI therapy versus systemic chemotherapy. She states that the analysis demonstrated a significant increase in response rates, but not in survival rates. This is inaccurate. When all seven randomized studies are reviewed, there is a significant increase in survival with the HAI therapy (16 versus 12 months).[6] If the two larger studies (which did not use appropriate systemic chemotherapies) are excluded, then there is no increase in survival. However, by excluding these two larger studies, the power of analysis is vastly diminished. Dr Wren mentions that there were a sizable number of hepatic toxicities. The meta-analysis did not address this. Table 1 summarizes the

Table 1 *Toxicity of hepatic arterial therapy*

Group	Hepatic toxicity	Systemic toxicity (grade 3 or 4)	
	Grade 3 bilirubin elevation[a] (%)	Diarrhea[b] (%)	Stomatitis[c] (%)
MSKCC[7]	18	70	–
NCOG[8]	16	18	18
NCI[9]	33	59	–
Mayo[10]	26	18	30
French[11]	35	–	–

[a]Bilirubin 1.5–3.0 × normal.
[b]Grade 3 diarrhea – increase of 7–9 stools/day, or incontinence, or severe cramping.
 Grade 4 diarrhea – increase of >9 stools/day or grossly bloody diarrhea, or need for parenteral support.
[c]Grade 3 stomatitis – painful erythema, edema, or ulcers, and cannot eat.
 Grade 4 stomatitis – requires parenteral or enteral support.
 MSKCC, Memorial Sloan-Kettering Cancer Center; NCOG, North Central Oncology Group; NCI, National Cancer Institute.

major toxicities from these trials. An increase in bilirubin was seen, on average, in 25% of cases. In most patients, bilirubin returns to normal after stopping the HAI therapy. In the systemic arm, the major toxicity was diarrhea, occurring, on average, in 41% of cases.

In Dr Wren's review, there was no mention of newer trials of HAI using either combinations of floxuridine (FUDR) plus LV or FUDR plus dexamethasone, or the incorporation of all three drugs. The response rates for these three trials of HAI therapy, using FUDR plus LV,[12] FUDR plus dexamethasone,[13] and FUDR plus LV plus dexamethasone,[14] were 66%, 71%, and 78%, respectively. The median survivals were 24, 23, and 22 months. The 2-year survivals were 64%, 55%, and 53%, respectively. Hence, these three studies demonstrate median survivals that are almost double those seen with systemic chemotherapy, with an average 2-year survival of 57%.

Dr Wren makes the comment that 55% of patients on HAI therapy develop extrahepatic disease. While this may be true of patients on HAI therapy, patients with systemic chemotherapy also develop extrahepatic disease. Nonetheless, if a patient is alive at 24 months with HAI versus 12 months with systemic therapy, the development of extrahepatic metastases assumes less importance.

Newer studies suggest that a combination of chemotherapy and surgery may be useful. Dr Wren mentions the French studies,[15] in which chemotherapy is given first, followed by resection of liver metastases in patients who were originally thought to be non-resectable. Another approach is to resect all disease, even in patients with more than four metastases, and then administer HAI and systemic therapy.[16] Two-year survival with this method was 79% for patients with four lesions or more, and 86% for the entire group receiving both HAI and systemic therapy.[16]

As Dr Wren points out, alcohol injections are more useful in smaller lesions. However, she does not mention that their use for colorectal cancer is much less effective than for hepatocellular cancer, due to the fact that colon cancers are hard lesions, whereas hepatocellular lesions are soft and therefore easier to penetrate.

Promising aspects of treating liver metastases now are the development of new active drugs, the good results observed with a combination of systemic and HAI therapy, and the development of multidisciplinary teams of physicians including surgeons, medical oncologists, and interventional radiologists, working together to further improve results.

REFERENCES

1. Kemeny N, Gonen M, Sullivan D, et al. A Phase I study of hepatic arterial infusion (HAI) of floxuridine (FUDR) and dexamethasone with systemic irinotecan for unresectable hepatic metastases from colorectal cancer. J Clin Oncol 2001; 19:2687–95.

2. Rotheberg M, Eckardt J, Kuhn J, et al. Phase II trial of irinotecan in patients with progress of rapidly recurrent colorectal cancer. J Clin Oncol 1996;14:1128–35.

3. De Gramont A, Vignoud J, Tournigand C, et al. Oxaliplatin with high-dose leucovorin and 5-fluorouracil 48-hour continuous infusion in pretreated metastatic colorectal cancer. Eur J Cancer 1997; 3:214–19.

4. Saltz L, Locker K, Pirotta N, et al. Weekly irinotecan (CPT-11), leucovorin (LV), and fluorouracil (FU) is superior to daily × 5 LV/FU in patients with previously untreated metastatic colorectal cancer. Proc Am Soc Oncol 1999; 18:233.

5. Douillard J, Cunningham D, Roth A, et al. Irinotecan combined with fluorouracil compared with fluorouracil alone as first-line treatment for metastatic colorectal cancer: a multicentre randomised trial. Lancet 2000; 35:1041–7.

6. Meta-analysis Group in Cancer. Reappraisal of hepatic arterial infusion in the treatment of nonresectable liver metastases from colon cancer. J Natl Cancer Inst 1996; 88:252–7.

7. Kemeny N, Daly J, Oderman P, et al. Randomized study of intrahepatic versus systemic infusion of fluorodeoxyuridine in patients with liver metastases from colorectal carcinoma. Ann Int Med 1987; 107:459–65.

8. Hohn D, Stagg R, Friedman M, et al. A randomized trial of continuous intravenous versus hepatic intra-arterial floxuridine in patients with colorectal cancer metastatic to the liver: the Northern California Oncology Group Trial. J Clin Oncol 1989; 7:1646–54.

9. Chang AE, Schneider PD, Sugarbaker PH. A prospective randomized trial of regional versus systemic continuous 5-fluorodeoxyuridine chemotherapy in the treatment of colorectal liver metastases. Ann Surg 1987; 206:685–93.

10. Martin J, O'Connell J, Wieland H, et al. Intra-arterial floxuridine vs systemic fluorouracil for hepatic metastases from colorectal cancer. A randomized trial. Arch Surg 1990; 125:1022–7.

11. Rougier P, Laplanche A, Huguier M, et al. Hepatic arterial infusion of floxuridine in patients with liver metastases from colorectal carcinoma: long-term results of a prospective randomized trial. J Clin Oncol 1992; 10:1112–18.

12. Kemeny N, Cohen A, Bertino JR, et al. Continuous intrahepatic infusion of floxuridine and leucovorin through an implantable pump for the treatment of hepatic metastases from colorectal carcinoma. Cancer 1990; 65:2446–50.

13. Kemeny N, Seiter K, Niedzwiecki D, et al. A randomized trial of intrahepatic infusion of fluorodeoxyuridine (FUDR) with dexamethasone versus fluorodeoxyuridine alone in the treatment of metastatic colorectal cancer. Cancer 1992; 69:327–34.

14. Kemeny N, Conti J, Cohen A, *et al.* A Phase II study of hepatic arterial FUDR, leucovorin, and dexamethasone for unresectable liver metastases from colorectal carcinoma. J Clin Oncol 1994; 12:2288–95.

15. Giachetti S, Itzhaki M, Grula G, *et al.* Long term survival of patients with unresectable colorectal cancer liver metastases following infusional chemotherapy with 5-fluorouracil, leucovorin, oxaliplatin, and surgery. Ann Oncol 1999; 10:663–9.

16. Kemeny N, Huang Y, Cohen A, *et al.* Hepatic arterial infusion of chemotherapy after resection of hepatic metastases from colorectal cancer. N Engl J Med 1999; 341:2039–48.

Editors' selected abstracts

Cryosurgical ablation and radiofrequency ablation for unresectable hepatic malignant neoplasms: a proposed algorithm.

Bilchik AJ, Wood TF, Allegra D, Tsioulias GJ, Chung M, Rose DM, Ramming KP, Morton DL.

John Wayne Cancer Institute at Saint John's Health Center, Santa Monica, CA, USA.

Archives of Surgery 135(6):657–62, 2000, June.

Background: Thermal ablation of unresectable hepatic tumors can be achieved by cryosurgical ablation (CSA) or radiofrequency ablation (RFA). The relative advantages and disadvantages of each technique have not yet been determined. *Hypothesis:* Radiofrequency ablation of malignant hepatic neoplasms can be performed safely, but is currently limited by size. Cryosurgical ablation, while associated with higher morbidity, is more effective for larger unresectable hepatic malignant neoplasms. *Design:* Retrospective analysis of prospective patient database. *Patients and methods:* Between July 1992 and September 1999, 308 patients with liver tumors not amenable to curative surgical resection were treated with CSA and/or RFA (percutaneous, laparoscopic, celiotomy). No patient had preoperative evidence of extrahepatic disease. All patients underwent laparoscopy with intraoperative ultrasound if technically possible. Both RFA and CSA were performed under ultrasound guidance. Resection, as an adjunctive procedure, was combined with ablation in certain patients. *Results:* Laparoscopy identified extrahepatic disease in 12% of patients, and intraoperative hepatic ultrasound identified additional lesions in 33% of patients, despite extensive preoperative imaging. Radiofrequency ablation alone or combined with resection or CSA resulted in reduced blood loss ($p < 0.05$), thrombocytopenia ($p < 0.05$), and shorter hospital stay compared with CSA alone ($p < 0.05$). Median ablation times for lesions greater than 3 cm were 60 minutes with RFA and 15 minutes with CSA ($p < 0.001$). Local recurrence rates for lesions greater than 3 cm were also greater with RFA (38% vs 17%). *Conclusions:* Laparoscopy and intraoperative ultrasound are essential in staging patients with hepatic malignant neoplasms. Radiofrequency ablation when combined with CSA reduces the morbidity of multiple freezes. Although RFA is safer than CSA and can be performed via different approaches (percutaneously, laparoscopically, or at celiotomy), it is limited by tumor size (< 3 cm). Percutaneous RFA should be considered in high-risk patients or those with small local recurrences.

Radiofrequency ablation of hepatocellular cancer in 110 patients with cirrhosis.

Curley SA, Izzo F, Ellis LM, Nicolas Vauthey J, Vallone P.

Department of Surgical Oncology, The University of Texas M.D. Anderson Cancer Center, Houston, Texas, USA.

Annals of Surgery 232(3):381–91, 2000, September.

Objective: To determine the treatment efficacy, safety, local tumor control, and complications related to radiofrequency ablation (RFA) in patients with cirrhosis and unresectable hepatocellular carcinoma (HCC). *Summary background data:* Most patients with HCC are not candidates for resection because of tumor size, location, or hepatic dysfunction related to cirrhosis. RFA is a technique that permits in situ destruction of tumors by means of local tissue heating. *Methods:* One hundred ten patients with cirrhosis and HCC (Child class A, 50; B, 31; C, 29) were treated during a prospective study using RFA. Patients were treated with RFA using an open laparotomy, laparoscopic, or percutaneous approach with ultrasound guidance to place the RF needle electrode into the hepatic tumors. All patients were followed up at regular intervals to detect treatment-related complications or recurrence of disease. *Results:* All 110 patients were followed up for at least 12 months after RFA (median follow-up 19 months). Percutaneous or intraoperative RFA was performed in 76 (69%) and 34 patients (31%), respectively. A total of 149 discrete HCC tumor nodules were treated with RFA. The median diameter of tumors treated percutaneously (2.8 cm) was smaller than that of lesions treated during laparotomy (4.6 cm). Local tumor recurrence at the RFA site developed in four patients (3.6%); recurrent HCC subsequently developed in other areas of the liver in all four. New liver tumors or extrahepatic metastases developed in 50 patients (45.5%), but 56 patients (50.9%) had no evidence of recurrence. There were no treatment-related deaths, but complications developed in 14 patients (12.7%) after RFA. *Conclusions:* In patients with cirrhosis and HCC, RFA produces effective local control of disease in a significant proportion of patients and can be performed safely with minimal complications.

Escalated focal liver radiation and concurrent hepatic artery fluorodeoxyuridine for unresectable intrahepatic malignancies.

Dawson LA, McGinn CJ, Normolle D, Ten Haken RK, Walker S, Ensminger W, Lawrence TS.

Departments of Radiation Oncology, Internal Medicine, and Pharmacology, University of Michigan, Ann Arbor, MI, USA.

Journal of Clinical Oncology 18(11):2210–18, 2000, June.

Purpose: To evaluate the response, time to progression, survival, and impact of radiation (RT) dose on survival in patients with intrahepatic malignancies treated on a phase I trial of escalated focal liver RT. *Patients and methods:* From April 1996 to January 1998, 43 patients with unresectable intrahepatic hepatobiliary cancer (HB; 27 patients) and colorectal liver metastases (LM; 16 patients) were treated with high-dose conformal RT. The median tumor size was $10 \times 10 \times 8$ cm. The median RT dose was 58.5 Gy (range, 28.5 to 90 Gy), 1.5 Gy twice daily, with concurrent continuous-infusion hepatic arterial fluorodeoxyuridine (0.2 mg/kg/d) during the first 4 weeks of RT. *Results:* The response rate in 25 assessable patients was 68% (16 partial and one complete response). With a median potential follow-up period of 26.5 months, the median times to progression for all tumors, LM, and HB were 6, 8, and 3 months, respectively. The median survival times of all patients, patients with LM, and patients with HB were 16, 18, and 11 months, respectively. On multivariate analyses, escalated RT dose was independently associated with improved progression-free and overall survival. The median survival of patients treated with 70 Gy or more has not yet been reached (16.4+ months), compared with 11.6 months in patients treated with lower RT doses ($p = 0.0003$). *Conclusion:* The excellent response rate, prolonged intrahepatic control, and improved survival in patients treated with RT doses of 70 Gy or more motivate continuation of dose-escalation studies for patients with intrahepatic malignancies.

Resection with cryotherapy of colorectal hepatic metastases has the same survival as hepatic resection alone.

Finlay IG, Seifert JK, Stewart GJ, Morris DL.

The UNSW Department of Surgery, St George Hospital, Sydney, Australia.

European Journal of Surgical Oncology 26(3):199–202, 2000, April.

Background: Hepatic resection is well established as a potentially curative treatment for hepatic colorectal cancer metastases. However, only a small proportion of patients with liver metastases are suitable for resection because they either have extrahepatic disease, or the extent and/or the distribution of their hepatic disease would make excision impossible. We have previously described the use of cryotherapy for inadequate resection margins and lesions in the remaining lobe of the liver. Combining such cryo-destructive techniques with resection offers the possibility of increasing the proportion of patients to whom potentially curative treatment can be offered. The aim of this study was to compare survival in patients treated with resection and cryotherapy against those of patients treated with resection alone. Potential prognostic variables were also examined. *Method:* Patients undergoing a hepatic resection with or without cryotherapy at our unit between April 1990 and July 1997 were identified from our database and their notes reviewed. Survival was estimated using the Kaplan–Meier method and compared using the log rank test. *Results:* One hundred and seven patients were treated in total: 32 underwent resection alone, and 75 underwent resection combined with cryotherapy. There was no significant difference between the survival of patients treated with resection alone and those treated with resection and cryotherapy. *Conclusions:* Edge and contralobe cryotherapy can be combined with hepatic resection to allow a greater proportion of patients with hepatic colorectal metastases to be offered treatment, and results in similar survival figures comparable to hepatic resection for at least 3 years.

Survival after percutaneous, image-guided, thermal ablation of hepatic metastases from colorectal cancer.

Gillams AR, Lees WR.

Department of Medicine, University College London Medical School and The Middlesex Hospital, London, UK.

Diseases of the Colon and Rectum 43(5):656–61, 2000, May.

Purpose: One-year, two-year, three-year, and four-year survival rates and median survival time for patients with inoperable liver metastases from colorectal cancer is 32, 10, and 3 percent and 7.4 to 11 months, respectively. Systemic chemotherapy produces a modest improvement to 48, 21, and 3 percent and 12 months, respectively. Regional chemotherapy produces a further improvement to 64, 25, and 5 percent and 15 to 17 months, respectively. For those with operable disease, hepatic resection survival rates are 90, 62, 48, and 40 percent, respectively, and survival time is 33 months. Thermal ablation is effective in producing necrosis in liver metastases. We report the impact on survival in 69 patients treated from 1993 to 1997, with follow-up to 1998. *Methods:* Sixty-nine patients, 50 male, mean age 60 (range, 33–87) years were treated. Liver resection was not feasible because of disease extent in the liver, extrahepatic disease or concurrent medical conditions. The average number of liver metastases was 2.9 (range, 1–16), the mean maximal diameter was 3.9 (range, 1–8) cm, and the mean initial total liver tumor volume was 47 (range, 1–371) ml. Eighteen (26 percent) had undergone previous hepatic resection. Sixty-two of 67 (93 percent) received chemotherapy at some stage. Twenty (29 percent) had extrahepatic disease. *Results:* One-year, two-year, three-year, and four-year survival rates and median survival time from liver metastasis diagnosis was 90, 60, 34, and 22 percent 27 months, respectively. Forty of 69 (58 percent) developed new liver metastases, and 23 of 69 (33 percent) developed new extrahepatic disease. Of a subgroup of 24 patients with less than four metastases, <5 cm diameter, treated after January 1995, the median survival time was 33 months from first thermal ablation vs. 15 months for the remainder ($p = 0.0004$). Major morbidity occurred in 3.2 percent, minor morbidity occurred in 12 percent, and there was one periprocedural death. *Conclusions:* Thermal ablation therapy improves survival in patients with inoperable but limited liver metastases. This is an improvement on the natural history of the disease and published chemotherapy results. Recent and ongoing technical refinements, not reflected in these results, are expected to further improve survival.

Radiofrequency ablation of 231 unresectable hepatic tumors: indications, limitations, and complications.

Wood TF, Rose DM, Chung M, Allegra DP, Foshag LJ, Bilchik AJ.

Department of Surgical Oncology, John Wayne Cancer Institute, Santa Monica, CA, USA.

Annals of Surgical Oncology 7(8):593–600, 2000, September.

Background: Radiofrequency ablation (RFA) is increasingly used for the local destruction of unresectable hepatic malignancies. There is little information on its optimal approach or potential complications. *Methods:* Since late 1997, we have undertaken 91 RFA procedures to ablate 231 unresectable primary or metastatic liver tumors in 84 patients. RFA was performed via celiotomy ($n = 39$), laparoscopy ($n = 27$), or a percutaneous approach ($n = 25$). Patients were followed with spiral computed tomographic (CT) scans at 1 to 2 weeks postprocedure and then every 3 months for 2 years. *Results:* Intraoperative ultrasound (IOUS) detected intrahepatic disease not evident on the preoperative scans of 25 of 66 patients (38%) undergoing RFA via celiotomy or laparoscopy. In 38 of 84 patients (45%), RFA was combined with resection or cryosurgical ablation (CSA), or both. RFA was used to treat an average of 2.8 lesions per patient, and the median size of treated lesions was 2 cm (range, 0.3–9 cm). The average hospital stay was 3.6 days overall (1.8 days for percutaneous and laparoscopic cases). Ten patients underwent a second RFA procedure (sequential ablations) and, in one case, a third RFA procedure for large (one patient), progressive (seven patients), and/or recurrent (three patients) lesions. Seven (8%) patients had complications: one skin burn; one postoperative hemorrhage; two simple hepatic abscesses; one hepatic abscess associated with diaphragmatic heat necrosis following sequential percutaneous ablations of a large lesion; one postoperative myocardial infarction; and one liver failure. There were three deaths, one (1%) of which was directly related to the RFA procedure. Three of the complications, including one RFA-related death, occurred after percutaneous RFA. At a median follow-up of 9 months (range, 1–27 months), 15 patients (18%) had recurrences at an RFA site, and 36 patients (43%) remained clinically free of disease. *Conclusions:* Celiotomy or laparoscopic approaches are preferred for RFA because they allow IOUS, which may demonstrate occult hepatic disease. Operative RFA also allows concomitant resection, CSA, or placement of a hepatic artery infusion pump, and isolation of the liver from adjacent organs. Percutaneous RFA should be reserved for patients at high risk for anesthesia, those with recurrent or progressive lesions, and those with smaller lesions sufficiently isolated from adjacent organs. Complications may be minimized when these approaches are applied selectively.

28

Surgical options for malignant biliary obstruction

KIM U KAHNG AND JOEL J ROSLYN*

INTRODUCTION

The diagnosis and treatment of patients with malignant biliary obstruction are often two of the more challenging problems that confront the surgeon. Confirmation of a precise histologic diagnosis may be elusive, clinical staging inexact, and the role of surgical intervention a matter of debate. During the last two decades, remarkable advances have been made in related fields which have facilitated our ability to image the biliary tract and intervene, when appropriate, in a minimally invasive way. In addition, we have acquired new knowledge regarding the interrelationships between biliary obstruction and its systemic effects on renal function, immunologic status, and bleeding diatheses. The challenge is to integrate these technical advances and new insights regarding the systemic effects of biliary obstruction into a rational approach for the management of this complex clinical problem.

Obstruction of the biliary tract due to malignancy can occur at any level as a consequence of either metastatic cancer or a primary neoplasm. Regardless of the etiology or pathology, most of these patients will suffer with some degree of jaundice. The factors to consider in determining the appropriate palliative or curative intervention include not only the nature of the malignant process and specific anatomic considerations, but also the patient's overall status in terms of comorbid conditions. The proximity of biliary tract malignancies to the liver and to such major vascular structures as the portal vein and hepatic artery contributes to the challenge of achieving curative resection in this clinical setting. Many patients with malignant biliary obstruction are elderly and will have concomitant cardiovascular or pulmonary disease. These associated diseases increase the perioperative risk and need to be considered in the decision-making

process. In addition, biliary obstruction is often associated with impaired renal and immune function, causing these patients to be susceptible to renal failure and sepsis. The surgeon, gastroenterologist, and interventional radiologist must be cognizant of these risk factors and carefully consider them when evaluating the therapeutic options. Biliary obstruction that is longstanding, as is often the case with tumors, is associated with specific morphologic changes within the liver, including bile plugging within the intrahepatic biliary canaliculi, centrilobular bile stasis, and periductular extravasation of bile with reactive edema and infiltration of polymorphonuclear leukocytes. Of much greater significance than these morphologic derangements, however, are the alterations in renal, immune, and hematologic function that occur in patients with obstructive jaundice.

SYSTEMIC COMPLICATIONS OF HYPERBILIRUBINEMIA

Renal failure

The clinical relationship between obstructive jaundice and renal failure was recognized over 50 years ago.[1,2] Contemporary reports suggest that the incidence of renal failure in patients undergoing surgical procedures for the relief of obstructive jaundice is approximately 10%.[3] The mortality rate in this subset of patients is extremely high, ranging from 32% to 100%.[4,5] The level of hyperbilirubinemia correlates with the postoperative decrease in creatinine clearance. The etiology of acute renal failure in the presence of obstructive jaundice is almost certainly multifactorial, including renal ischemia, prostaglandin-mediated alterations in renal microcirculation, myocardial depression, reduction of intravascular volume, and sepsis. The primary event leading to renal failure appears to be a decrease in renal blood flow, for which there may

---

be several mechanisms. Decreased renal perfusion may be secondary to changes in systemic hemodynamics. Decreased peripheral vascular resistance has been documented to occur in animal models of obstructive jaundice. In addition to lower blood pressure under basal conditions, the hypotensive response to hemorrhage is greater in the presence of jaundice. Both the decrease in basal peripheral vascular resistance and the exaggerated hypotensive response to hemorrhage may be related to attenuated vasoconstrictor responses of the systemic vasculature to catecholamines and angiotensin II. These changes in systemic hemodynamics may be accentuated by volume depletion, which may be due to decreased oral intake and impaired renal concentrating ability.

Decreased renal perfusion may also be related to specific alterations in renal vascular reactivity. The distribution of renal blood flow away from the cortex appears to be mediated by α-adrenergic activity. In contrast to the decreased peripheral vascular responses to catecholamines, the responses of the renal vasculature have been shown to be increased after bile-duct ligation. Renal vasoconstriction is enhanced by the inhibition of prostaglandin synthesis, indicating that renal prostaglandins may have a protective role in preserving renal blood flow by modulating changes in local vascular tone. Although the exact mechanism remains unclear, both bilirubin and bile salts have been implicated as agents causing sensitization of the kidney to ischemia in patients with jaundice.

Endotoxemia appears to have a central role in the development of acute renal failure. The absence of bile salts from the lumen of the gastrointestinal tract facilitates the absorption of endotoxin from the gastrointestinal tract into the portal circulation. The reticuloendothelial system (RES) is suppressed in patients with biliary obstruction, and impaired clearance of endotoxin results in spillover into the systemic circulation, and thus endotoxemia.[6] The importance of this factor to the development of renal failure in patients with obstructive jaundice is underscored by a recent report suggesting that the prevention of endotoxemia in this setting preserves renal function.[7]

Sepsis

In the presence of obstructive jaundice, sepsis is often associated with two distinct clinical syndromes: cholangitis and a generalized impairment of host defense mechanisms. Cholangitis, as classically described over 100 years ago by Charcot, is characterized by the triad of fever, right upper quadrant pain, and jaundice. Although most often associated with common bile duct stones, cholangitis is being reported with increasing frequency in patients with malignant strictures, particularly after instrumentation via trans-hepatic percutaneous cholangiography or endoscopic retrograde cholangiopancreatography (ERCP). Traditional teaching suggests that

both biliary stasis and bactibilia must be present in order for cholangitis to occur (Figure 28.1). While bactibilia is clearly a factor in the high rate of septic complications observed in jaundiced patients undergoing surgery, considerable evidence indicates that there are specific alterations in the host defense mechanisms that are responsible for the jaundice-associated sepsis syndrome. Neutrophil chemotaxis and phagocytosis, RES function, and cell-mediated immunity are compromised in the setting of biliary obstruction.[8] The absence of bile from the gut has been proposed as an initiator of a cascade of events leading to altered phagocytic function and changes in the RES. It is generally believed that the absence of bile from the gut results in an increase in the intraluminal bacterial count and mucosal atrophy with a concomitant intestinal barrier dysfunction.[9] The net effect of these structural changes is enhanced bacterial

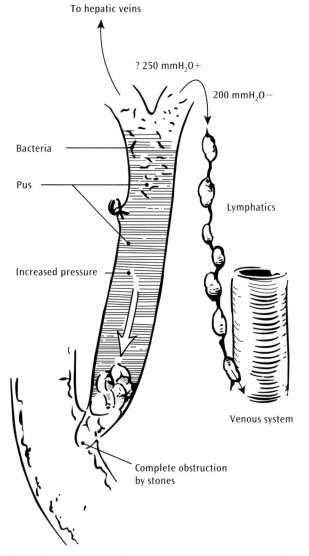

Figure 28.1 *Diagram of the pathophysiology of cholangitis. The presence of bacteria and biliary stasis are essential for the development of cholangitis. (Reproduced with permission from Lipsett and Pitt, 1990.[86])*

translocation and increased transport of lipopolysac-charides (LPS) to the liver. LPS induces the release of cytokines and cellular mediators, which may be responsible for the observed inhibition and reduction of phagocytic function.[10,11]

Bleeding

The anatomic and physiologic relationships of the biliary tract to the liver and the portal circulation make hemorrhage a critical factor in the decision-making process and operative management for patients with obstructive jaundice. Although clinical experience suggests that excessive bleeding due to coagulopathy is common in jaundiced patients undergoing biliary tract surgery, other important causes of bleeding in the setting include inadequate hemostasis or injury to a local vessel, hemobilia as a result of instrumentation through the liver, and portal hypertension. Jaundice-associated coagulopathy is often due to a combination of hepatocellular dysfunction and vitamin K deficiency. Normal hepatic function is essential for the synthesis of specific coagulation factors II, VII, IX, and prothrombin. Severe liver dysfunction leads to reduced synthesis of these factors and results in hypoprothrombinemia. Vitamin K is the fat-soluble vitamin that is a critical cofactor in the synthesis of coagulation proteins by the liver. In the setting of biliary obstruction, reduction in intestinal bile salt concentration decreases vitamin K absorption and may further impair the clotting mechanism in patients with compromised hepatic function on the basis of cholestasis and/or sepsis.

PRINCIPLES OF SURGICAL MANAGEMENT

The management of patients with obstructive jaundice secondary to carcinoma should focus on diagnosis, amelioration of symptoms, relief of biliary obstruction, and resection of the neoplastic process, if cure is possible. In the planning of interventional strategy, the surgeon must consider the impact of risk for renal failure, sepsis, and bleeding tendencies on non-operative or operative outcomes. A series of reports suggested that the perioperative morbidity and mortality for surgery in patients with obstructive jaundice approached 50% and 25%, respectively.[12,13] These outcomes were largely influenced by the status of renal and hepatic synthetic function, and the presence of biliary sepsis and malnutrition. The mortality rate in this group of patients is directly linked to the number of factors present, with death often occurring as a result of renal failure, sepsis, or multisystem organ failure. Recognition of the critical relationship between hyperbilirubinemia and surgical outcome led to the hypothesis in the 1970s that alleviation of the biliary obstruction would reduce perioperative morbidity and

mortality in jaundiced patients undergoing surgical intervention. Although relief of biliary obstruction results in a prompt choleretic response, the degree to which serum bilirubin levels return toward normal is less predictable. There appears to be little correlation between the duration of obstruction and the rate of return of serum bilirubin levels to normal. Experience indicates that an 8–10% per day decline in serum bilirubin can be anticipated in patients undergoing some form of biliary decompression.

A number of retrospective and uncontrolled studies suggested that preoperative percutaneous trans-hepatic biliary drainage (PTD) was not only safe and easily performed, but would also improve subsequent surgical outcome in patients with biliary obstruction.[14–16] Ultimately, three independently performed prospective, randomized, controlled studies all failed to demonstrate any significant benefit from the routine use of preoperative biliary drainage in patients with obstructive jaundice (Figure 28.2).[17–19] These studies and others suggest that any benefit from preoperative drainage is offset by catheter-related complications.[20] Endoscopic biliary drainage may avoid some of the complications associated with a percutaneous approach; however, the bactibilia that occurs in the presence of a biliary stent appears to result in a higher incidence of postoperative infectious complications.[21] Although preoperative biliary drainage cannot be recommended on a routine basis for patients with obstructive jaundice, it may be of benefit in selected patients who, for whatever reason, require some delay in carrying out definitive management. A specific benefit of PTD is to facilitate the intraoperative identification of the bile ducts in the presence of proximal biliary obstruction.

In patients with malignant biliary obstruction, the goals of intervention focus on achieving biliary drainage,

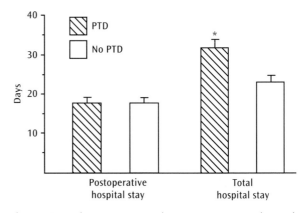

Figure 28.2 *Histogram comparing mean postoperative and total hospital stay for patients with obstructive jaundice managed either by surgery alone (No PTD) or surgery following percutaneous biliary drainage (PTD). Total hospital stay was significantly longer (*p < 0.005) in the PTD group. (Reproduced with permission from Pitt* et al.*, 1985.[17])*

accurate diagnosis and staging of the neoplastic process, and possible curative resection. The ideal situation is to be able to provide internal biliary drainage and avoid an external biliary fistula. Current therapeutic options to accomplish this specific goal include surgery, percutaneous management using radiologic guidance, and endoscopic intubation. The decision about how to proceed for an individual patient is best made in the setting of a multidisciplinary discussion amongst the surgeon, interventional radiologist, and endoscopist. An appropriate course of action can only be established after data regarding the level and nature of obstruction, the status of hepatic and renal function, and the likelihood of cure are all considered. In many patients with malignant biliary obstruction, optimal management may include utilization of multiple modalities, each designed to accomplish a specific goal. The responsible physicians must have a clear vision of whether they are attempting to achieve palliation or cure. Surgery, whether it be for palliation or cure, continues to be the mainstay of therapy for many patients with malignant biliary obstruction.

Obstruction of the bile duct can result from a number of benign or malignant causes. These include non-neoplastic strictures from calculus disease, iatrogenic injury during cholecystectomy, chronic pancreatitis, post-irradiation, Mirizzi's syndrome, trauma, chronic pancreatitis, hepatic infusion chemotherapy, sclerosing cholangitis, and autoimmune deficiency syndrome (AIDS). Benign tumors of the bile duct or pancreas can occur and should be considered in any differential diagnosis for biliary obstruction, but unfortunately are much less common than malignant lesions. The role of surgical intervention and of specific surgical strategies for patients with malignant biliary obstruction is best viewed from the perspective of metastatic disease versus primary tumor involvement, as occurs with carcinomas of the gallbladder, bile duct, periampullary region, and pancreas. A discussion of biliary obstruction secondary to tumors of the periampullary region and pancreas is beyond the scope of this chapter.

METASTATIC DISEASE AND BILIARY OBSTRUCTION

Jaundice is a common late manifestation in patients with extensive tumor involvement of the liver. In most situations, this is due to diffuse parenchymal disease and the clinical course is characterized by rapid progression of jaundice and hepatic deterioration culminating in death. Surgery has very little part to play for patients with extensive parenchymal disease other than, on occasion, to confirm the histologic diagnosis. In a smaller subset of patients with metastatic disease, progressive jaundice may result from tumor-containing lymph nodes located adjacent to the bile duct causing extrinsic compression or intraductal tumor or tumor debris free-floating in the

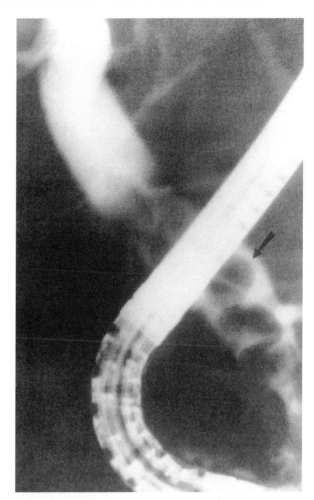

Figure 28.3 *Cholangiogram demonstrating biliary obstruction in a man with metastatic colon carcinoma with tumor debris in the bile duct.*

biliary ductal system. Extrinsic compression of the bile duct in the porta hepatis has been reported in patients with cancer of the lung,[22] colon,[23] and breast,[24] and leukemia.[25] Curative resection in these patients would be extremely unlikely, and satisfactory palliation in most of them can be accomplished either percutaneously or endoscopically. In the absence of demonstrable tumor progression, episodic jaundice and/or cholangitis in patients with known malignancy may be a consequence of intrabiliary tumor debris (Figure 28.3). This unusual entity has been described in patients with metastatic colon carcinoma[26] and hepatoma.[27] Safe and effective palliation can be achieved with appropriately selected surgical procedures.[23,24,28] Depending on the underlying disease and anatomic considerations, therapy may include either biliary-enteric bypass or resection.

GALLBLADDER CANCER

Carcinoma of the gallbladder is the most common cancer involving the hepatobiliary tract. The diagnosis

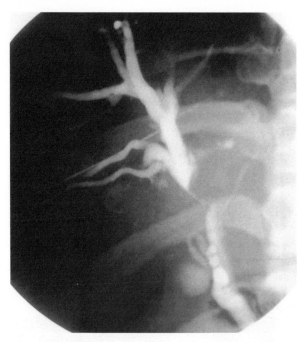

Figure 28.4 *Trans-hepatic cholangiogram demonstrating biliary obstruction in a patient with locally advanced carcinoma of the gallbladder.*

of carcinoma of the gallbladder is typically made at operation during cholecystectomy being performed for symptomatic cholelithiasis. Up to one-third of cases are identified during microscopic examination by the pathologist. Jaundice is usually an ominous sign in patients with gallbladder cancer, as it often denotes locally advanced disease with extension into the common bile duct (Figure 28.4). Many data suggest that the only curable lesions are those that are removed incidentally during cholecystectomy. In patients with gallbladder cancer who present with jaundice, surgical extirpation for cure would be extremely unlikely. Palliation can generally be accomplished non-operatively with either percutaneous or endoscopic techniques, although acute cholecystitis is a potential complication which must be considered. Operative palliation may include a segment III bypass with Roux-en-Y hepaticojejunostomy, although this should be considered only in selected patients.

CARCINOMA OF THE EXTRAHEPATIC BILE DUCTS

Incidence

Carcinomas of the bile duct are uncommon malignancies in the USA. Extrahepatic bile duct malignancies are present in 0.01–0.46% of all autopsies, and account for 1% of all biliary operations. These lesions account for one-third of all malignant tumors of the biliary tract. Carcinoma of the bile duct tends to be a disease of the elderly, with the mean age at presentation being 70 years.[29] In a recent report of 186 patients from the University of California at Los Angeles with documented bile duct cancers, 23% were older than 70 years.[30] It is important to recognize, however, that a subset of young patients with this disease has been identified,[31] and that the diagnosis of carcinoma of the bile duct must be included in the differential diagnosis for obstructive jaundice in young age groups. There is some evidence that the incidence of this disease may be increasing, although such trends may be artificial, due to changing demographics, advances in identification, and triage of these patients to referral centers.

Epidemiology/risk factors

Although up to 50% of patients with bile duct cancers have gallstones, there are few data to support an etiologic role for cholelithiasis in the pathogenesis of biliary tract malignancies. In contrast, however, hepatolithiasis does appear to be a significant risk factor for bile duct carcinoma.[32] The major risk factor for malignant tumors of the bile duct appears to be chronic inflammation. This premise is supported by a number of clinical observations. The incidence of biliary cancer is greatest in regions of the world where there is a high prevalence of infestation with liver flukes.[33] There is also a high incidence of cholangiocarcinoma (approximately 10%) in the presence of hepatolithiasis or Caroli's disease.[34,35] There is some preliminary information which suggests that certain toxins and other environmental factors may increase the risk of bile duct tumors.[36] The strongest evidence of the etiologic importance of chronic inflammation is the relationship between cholangiocarcinoma and inflammatory bowel disease. In patients with ulcerative colitis, the incidence of cholangiocarcinoma is somewhat less than 1%. In the presence of sclerosing cholangitis, the risk of developing cholangiocarcinoma increases tremendously. In these patients, cholangiocarcinoma is found in 9% of individuals at the time of liver transplantation and in 33–42% at autopsy.[37,38]

Classification and staging

Tumors of the bile duct can arise anywhere in the biliary tree and are classified according to site. Extrahepatic bile duct carcinoma, by definition, does not include peripheral or intrahepatic cholangiocarcinomas, which occur in the liver parenchyma proximal to the right and left hepatic ducts. In addition, gallbladder carcinoma and ampullary carcinoma are considered separately from extrahepatic biliary carcinomas. An understanding and appreciation of the clinical stage and pathologic stage are essential to the development of an organized and appropriate strategy for the management of patients with bile duct tumors. The traditional system for classifying extrahepatic biliary cancers is by location, as described by Longmire *et al.* in 1973.[39] According to this system, extrahepatic bile duct cancers are subdivided into upper-third, middle-third, and lower-third lesions. Based on various reports, approximately 60% of these lesions are in the upper third, 15% in the middle third, 15% in the distal third, and 10% diffuse (Figure 28.5).[40–42] The critical relationship between upper-third lesions and the vascular anatomy of the liver, especially with respect to surgical resection, has led to the development of the Bismuth system to further classify the perihilar extrahepatic biliary carcinomas. This system has been particularly useful for planning the extent of surgical resection required to achieve negative margins (Figure 28.6):[43]

Type I: lesion is in common hepatic duct below bifurcation.

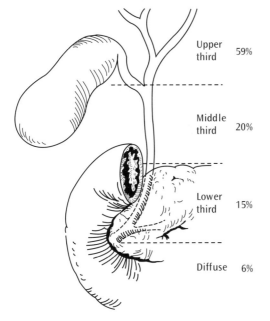

Figure 28.5 *Diagram showing the relative frequency of bile duct tumors based on location. Data represent 186 patients evaluated at UCLA between 1954 and 1988. (Reprinted with permission from Tompkins* et al.*, 1990.[40])*

Type II: lesion extends to the confluence of the hepatic ducts.

Type III: lesions extend up into the right (IIIA) or left duct (IIIB).

Type IV: lesions extend into both right and left ducts.

This schema has allowed surgeons to develop a more rational approach to the management of patients with proximal or hilar tumors.

Histologically, more than 90% of extrahepatic biliary tumors are adenocarcinomas, the majority of which are characterized as sclerosing. Papillary adenocarcinomas, which comprise only 7% of cases, are associated with a better prognosis than the sclerosing type.[36] Adjacent areas of dysplasia are typical, and multifocal carcinoma has been reported in 42% of cases.[44] Approximately 30–40% of all cases of bile duct carcinoma are associated with direct extension into the liver and/or regional nodes at the time of diagnosis.[45]

The TNM staging system for extrahepatic biliary duct cancers is based on the depth of penetration of the primary, lymph node involvement, and distant metastases (Table 28.1). This system, while enormously helpful in decision-making regarding postoperative therapy and outcome, does little to guide the surgeon in the operating room faced with intraoperative challenges and decisions.

Clinical presentation/clinical staging

Most patients with bile duct tumors present with jaundice. Because biliary obstruction tends to occur early in the course, other constitutional symptoms such as pain, anorexia, weight loss, and fatigability tend to be less prominent. Other than showing evidence of scleral icterus and jaundice, the physical examination is often unrevealing. Occasionally, patients with distal bile duct tumors will have a palpable, distended gallbladder. Laboratory evaluation will typically reveal hyperbilirubinemia, elevated alkaline phosphatase, and mild abnormalities of the transaminases. Serum tumor markers,

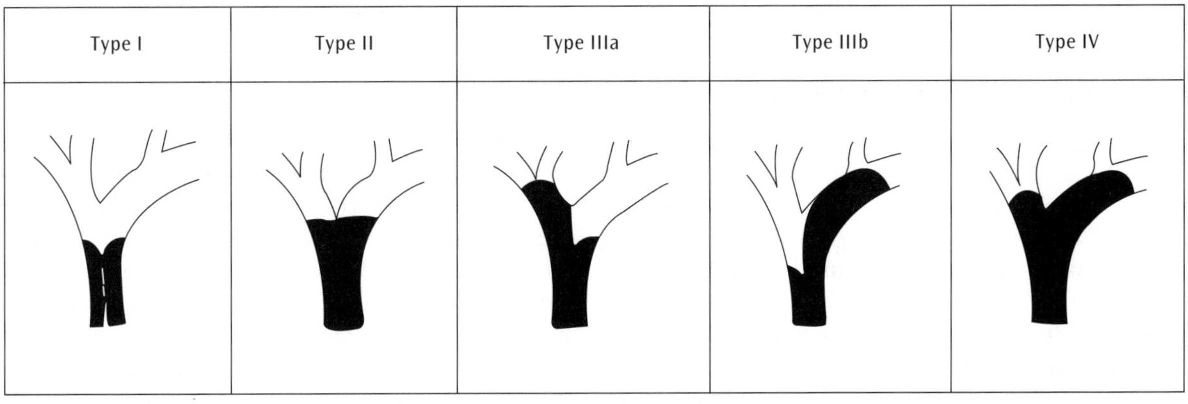

Type I	Type II	Type IIIa	Type IIIb	Type IV

Figure 28.6 *Diagram of the Bismuth system for classifying hilar biliary tumors.*

Table 28.1 *Extrahepatic bile duct tumors: TNM staging system*

Definitions	
Primary tumor (T)	
TX	Primary tumor cannot be assessed
T0	No evidence of primary tumor
Tis	Carcinoma *in situ*
T1	Tumor invades subepithelial connective tissue or fibromuscular layer
T1a	Tumor invades subepithelial connective tissue
T1b	Tumor invades fibromuscular layer
T2	Tumor invades perifibromuscular connective tissue
T3	Tumor invades adjacent structure(s), liver, pancreas, duodenum, gallbladder, colon, stomach
Regional lymph nodes (N)	
NX	Regional lymph nodes cannot be assessed
N0	No regional lymph node metastasis
N1	Metastasis in cystic duct, pericholedochal and/or hilar lymph nodes (i.e., in the hepatoduodenal ligament)
N2	Metastasis in peripancreatic (head only), periduodenal, periportal, celiac, and/or superior mesenteric and/or posterior pancreatic duodenal lymph nodes
Distant metastasis (M)	
MX	Distant metastasis cannot be assessed
M0	No distant metastasis
M1	Distant metastasis

Stage grouping

0	Tis	N0	M0
I	T1	N0	M0
II	T2	N0	M0
III	T1	N1	M0
	T1	N2	M0
	T2	N1	M0
	T2	N2	M0
IVA	T3	Any N	M0
IVB	Any T	Any N	M1

including CA 19-9 and carcinoembryonic antigen (CEA), have a limited role in the diagnosis of cholangiocarcinoma because of low specificity.[46] Recent studies suggest, however, that examining bile for tumor markers may be useful for diagnosis and monitoring disease progression. Biliary CEA has been detected in the bile of patients with cholangiocarcinoma,[47] and point mutations of K-ras detected by gene amplification techniques correlate highly with the presence of cholangiocarcinoma.[48]

The diagnosis of extrahepatic bile duct cancer is often suggested by radiologic studies, such as percutaneous transhepatic cholangiography or ERCP. However, these studies may be misleading and at least one report suggests that up to 10% of radiographically diagnosed malignant lesions may be incorrect as these lesions are ultimately proven to be benign in nature.[49] For this reason, it is generally recommended that a definitive

tissue diagnosis be established prior to the initiation of radiation or chemotherapy. Establishing a tissue diagnosis by non-operative means, however, is not always readily achieved. Available techniques include cytology of endoscopically obtained brushings and percutaneous computerized tomography (CT)-guided needle biopsy. Biliary cytology may not be accurate because of both false-positive and false-negative results. False positives occur as a result of chronic inflammation, which can be due to hepatolithiasis, cholangitis, or the presence of biliary stents. The false-negative rate is dependent on the adequacy of sampling and decreases with multiple negative brushings, and is reported to be less than 6% after three sequential negative cytological brushings.[50] A useful adjunct to cytology may be determining the presence of telomerase RNA by *in-situ* hybridization.[51] Percutaneous biopsy may not be feasible in the absence of a discernible mass lesion. For these reasons, open biopsy or actual resection may be required to establish a tissue diagnosis.

Cholangiography, CT, and angiography have been the standard radiologic studies used to assess clinical stage and resectability. CT findings of hepatic metastases or peritoneal metastases, cholangiographic findings of extensive bilobar intrahepatic duct involvement, or angiographic findings of vessel encasement or occlusion of the common hepatic artery or portal vein (Figure 28.7) are generally indications that curative resection is not feasible. The role of routine preoperative angiography for assessing vascular involvement continues to be controversial. Although many surgeons feel that resectability can be judged at the time of laparotomy, other experienced surgeons believe that precise preoperative knowledge of the arterial anatomy is advantageous. Endoscopic ultrasound is being used with increasing frequency to gauge the local extent of tumor involvement, including vascular invasion (Figure 28.8). Magnetic resonance (MR) cholangiography and MR arteriography have already proven to be of significant benefit in the evaluation of patients with pancreatic cancer and may render conventional angiography obsolete in the routine evaluation of patients with biliary obstruction (Figure 28.9). Several centers are advocating laparoscopy with ultrasonography as a reasonable modality to assess resectability. Correlation with standard techniques and operative findings and improved understanding of cost-effectiveness will be critical to assess fully the utility of these new and emerging technologies.

For patients who are candidates for resection, definition of the proximal extent of tumor within the bile duct is crucial. Cholangiography is the primary imaging study for this determination. Although cholangiography can be performed either endoscopically or percutaneously, transhepatic cholangiography (THC) has several advantages. The proximal extent of a totally obstructing lesion is best identified by THC (Figure 28.10). Furthermore, at the time of THC, biliary stents can be placed, which are often

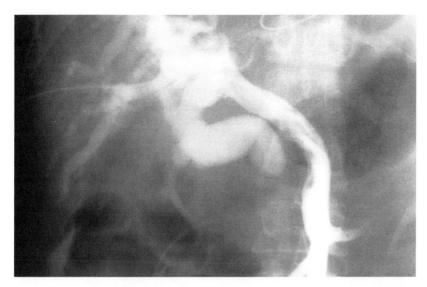

Figure 28.7 *Angiogram showing involvement of the superior mesenteric vein with tumor.*

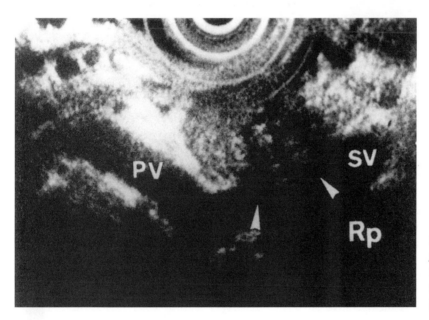

Figure 28.8 *Endoscopic ultrasound from a patient with distal bile duct tumor. PV, portal vein; SV, superior mesenteric vein; Rp, renal parenchyma.*

useful intraoperatively to facilitate the identification of the proximal ducts. However, cholangiography has limited accuracy. Cholangioscopy has been described as a more accurate technique for mapping the proximal extent of tumor,[52] but this has not been a uniform experience.[53] Helical CT is no more accurate than cholangiography in determining proximal tumor extent.[54]

Non-operative treatment of extrahepatic biliary tract cancer

Satisfactory palliation can usually be achieved by non-operative means for patients with widely metastatic disease. Endoscopically or percutaneously placed biliary catheters have been shown to be effective in relieving jaundice due to malignant biliary obstruction. These

therapeutic options have been greatly enhanced by technologic advances which permit internal drainage to be accomplished. Avoidance of an external biliary fistula reduces the nutritional and infectious complications. Although the development of new and improved expandable metal stents has provided a very good alternative to standard drainage catheters, limiting factors in the use of these devices continue to be the small caliber of the tubes and the associated incidence of cholangitis. Larger-bore stents and prophylactic exchange of the stents have been advocated in order to reduce the morbidity associated with the management of malignant biliary obstruction with endoscopic or percutaneously placed stents. Most recently, photodynamic therapy using cholangioscopy for intraluminal photo-activation has been used to successfully establish biliary drainage.[55]

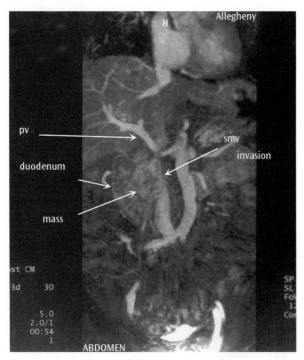

Figure 28.9 *Magnetic resonance imaging study in a patient with distal bile duct tumor. The study shows the relationship of mass to superior mesenteric artery and vein. PV, portal vein; SMV, superior mesenteric vein.*

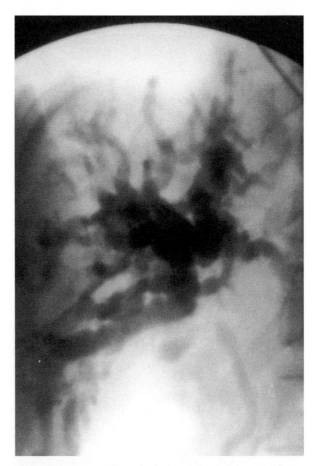

Figure 28.10 *Trans-hepatic cholangiogram demonstrating complete biliary obstruction in a patient with hilar cholangiocarcinoma.*

Surgical considerations

Surgery, whether it be for palliation or cure, continues to be the mainstay of therapy for patients with bile duct tumors. The decision to recommend surgery depends on a number of factors. Of primary importance is the extent of comorbid diseases; this is particularly true in this setting because so many of these patients are elderly. According to data reported by Pitt *et al.*,[12] the operative risk of biliary tract surgery can be further assessed by analysis of specific factors. Age, underlying disease process, presence of biliary sepsis, degree of malnutrition, and the status of renal and hepatic function have been shown to be predictive of outcome and to correlate directly with the hospital mortality rate (Figure 28.11).

Assuming that operative intervention is feasible based on the patient's overall condition, the main indications for laparotomy include establishing a tissue diagnosis, assessment for curative resection, and relief of biliary obstruction. As discussed above, a tissue diagnosis may be impossible to establish by non-operative means. Although malignancy may be strongly suggested by radiographic studies, cytology, and the detection of tumor markers within bile, exploration and open biopsy may be required to obtain sufficient tissue for pathologic confirmation of the diagnosis.

In the absence of demonstrable metastatic disease or unresectable local disease, exploration should be

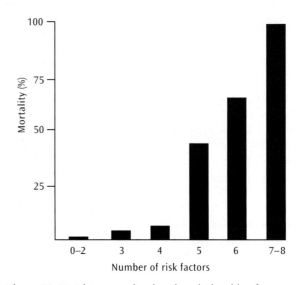

Figure 28.11 *Histogram showing the relationship of comorbid factors and hospital mortality in 155 consecutive patients undergoing bile duct surgery. (Reprinted with permission from Pitt et al., 1981.[12])*

considered, because surgical resection is the only potentially curative therapeutic modality. The overall rate of resectability for extrahepatic bile duct carcinoma is approximately 50%. Unfortunately, less than 30% of patients with proximal-third lesions will be resectable. The type of resection is predicated on the site and extent of ductal involvement. If, at the time of exploration, unsuspected metastatic disease or unresectable disease is found, palliation of biliary obstruction can be achieved in a number of ways.

Intraoperative definition of resectability

Several steps and concepts are critical to the intraoperative assessment and staging of patients with bile duct tumors. Resectability is best determined by an experienced biliary surgeon. The criteria for unresectability include metastatic disease, extensive vascular invasion, tumor within the secondary biliary radicals, and tumor involvement of both right and left hepatic lobes. Laparoscopy and laparoscopic ultrasonography are being used with increasing frequency to determine the presence of metastatic disease that could preclude resection. In the absence of metastatic disease or direct tumor extension into both lobes of the liver, the surgeon needs to carefully assess the relationship of the tumor to the portal vein and hepatic artery. This is facilitated by dissection of the hilar plate and direct palpation of the duct and continuous structures (Figure 28.12). Based on information obtained preoperatively and a careful intraoperative assessment, the surgeon can now proceed with the appropriate management of the bile duct tumor: palliation versus curative resection, or local versus extensive resection.

Surgical resection: goals and concepts

The most crucial factor in achieving long-term survival is complete resection. The type of resection is predicated on the site and extent of ductal involvement. For hilar tumors, curative resection is infrequent because of the locally invasive nature of these tumors and their proximity to major vascular structures. There continues to be controversy over limited versus extended resection that includes hepatectomy. Because many of these tumors directly invade the liver, a rational approach to the management of these patients has been proposed based on the Bismuth classification (see Figure 28.6):

Type I tumors: can be managed with local resection of the bile duct and surrounding tissues.

Type II tumors: often require local resection plus resection of liver segment I (caudate lobe).

Types IIIa and IIIb: require local excision plus right or left hepatectomy, respectively.

Type IV tumors: if considered resectable, require total hepatectomy and transplantation.

These procedures should only be undertaken in centers with significant experience in major hepatic resections.

As stated above, the intraoperative management of hilar or Klatskin tumors is greatly facilitated by the preoperative placement of bilateral trans-hepatic biliary stents. Careful palpation of the lesion should be carried out to assess resectability. This procedure should include dissection of the hilar plate and visualization of the right and left hepatic ducts. If normal duct is palpated above the tumor, an attempt to perform a local resection

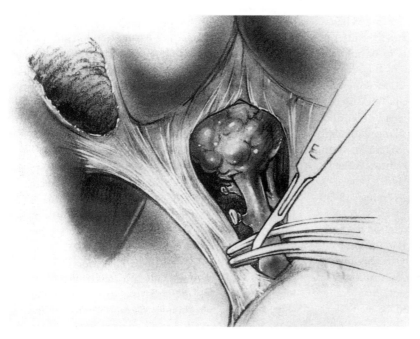

Figure 28.12 *Diagram showing the operative approach to a patient with a hilar tumor.*

should proceed. The distal duct is divided and oversewn. The mid and proximal bile ducts are next reflected off the portal vein and dissection is carried proximally up to the liver hilum. Although it is difficult to obtain a 1-cm margin beyond the tumor, every attempt should be made to carry the dissection until the surgeon palpates normal, non-fibrotic bile duct. Both ducts are then divided and a frozen section performed on the proximal margin. Resection of the caudate lobe has been advocated, but continues to be controversial.[56] Whether or not the caudate lobe is resected, reconstruction is done with bilateral Roux-en-Y hepaticojejunostomies over the biliary stents. For Bismuth types IIIa and IIIb, this procedure is modified to include right or left hepatic lobectomy based on the tumor location. Operative mortality is reported to be 5–8% for local resection alone and increases to 15% with the addition of major liver resection. Growing evidence suggests that long-term survival in the range of 15–30% can be achieved with this type of aggressive surgical approach.[56–63]

Carcinomas of the middle and distal third of the bile duct are traditionally managed, when resectable, with pancreaticoduodenectomy. Pylorus-preserving pancreaticoduodenectomy may be considered in selected patients because this procedure provides adequate margins for bile duct cancers, and may result in less alteration in digestive function as compared to the standard Whipple procedure. The location of these distal lesions results in greater resectability with easier adherence to basic oncologic principles. It is therefore not surprising that resectability rates are higher than those of proximal lesions, and 5-year survival is reported to be 30–50%.

Because complete surgical resection provides the only opportunity for cure in patients with bile duct cancers, surgeons continue to explore the possibility of more aggressive surgical approaches. In an effort to minimize the risk of hepatic failure after extended hepatectomy, preoperative embolization of either the arterial or portal vein branches to the segments to be resected has been used to promote hypertrophy of the remaining hepatic segments.[64,65] Hepatic resection combined with pancreaticoduodenectomy has been done successfully for localized but extensive extrahepatic bile duct cancers. In a series of ten such cases done with preoperative portal vein embolization, the operative mortality was 0%. The mean survival for these patients, who had either locally advanced gallbladder cancer or diffuse bile duct cancer, was 31.8 months (range: 18–59 months).[66]

Total hepatectomy with liver transplantation has been advocated by some for unresectable hilar tumors.[67–69] Long-term survival has been extremely disappointing, with local recurrence being exceedingly common. Given these realities and the scarcity of organs, liver transplantation for bile duct cancers should be viewed as experimental at the present time.

Surgical palliation

Because the majority of patients with bile duct cancers are unresectable based on conventional criteria, the role of palliation assumes major importance. Recent studies have advocated the non-operative palliation of all malignant biliary strictures using biliary endoprotheses placed either endoscopically or percutaneously.[70,71] The advantages of non-operative management include a shorter initial hospital stay, a lower incidence of procedure-related morbidity, and a 30-day mortality rate of 9–15%. A non-operative approach has several potential disadvantages that must be considered. In approximately 70% of patients, a definitive histologic or cytologic diagnosis cannot be established without an open procedure. Furthermore, the evaluation of resectability of these often small lesions by radiographic means may be unreliable. In addition, two studies suggest that non-operative decompression may be associated with poorer quality of life than operative decompression when factors such as frequency of hospital re-admissions, incidence of catheter-related problems, and post-procedural pain and jaundice are taken into account.[72,73]

If, at the time of exploration, unsuspected metastatic disease or unresectable disease is found, palliation of the biliary obstruction can be accomplished based on anatomic and pathologic considerations. In the presence of metastatic disease, preoperatively placed biliary stents are probably adequate therapy given the short life expectancy. In the presence of localized, but unresectable mid or distal cancers, palliation of biliary obstruction can be achieved by either cholecystojejunostomy or Roux-en-Y choledochojejunostomy. In patients with unresectable perihilar tumors, palliation with placement of trans-hepatic trans-tumoral tubes may be appropriate. If, at the time of laparotomy, operative findings suggest that resection is not feasible, a biliary drainage procedure should be performed. In 1963, Praderi[74] described a technique of placing a tube through the abdominal wall, hepatic parenchyma, bile duct, and back through the abdominal wall that would allow for biliary decompression in patients with hilar tumors. The U-tube technique was further popularized by Terblanche.[75] Today, most surgeons who utilize this technique for palliation perform trans-tumoral dilatation and place the end of the tube in a jejunal limb through a Roux-en-Y hepaticojejunostomy.[76] Retrospective studies suggest that the quality of life as defined by episodes of recurrent cholangitis may be less with this operative approach versus non-operative intubation.[68] Longmire introduced a palliative procedure in which the left lateral segment of the liver is transected and a Roux-en-Y limb is anastomosed to the dilated left duct. This procedure is now performed only occasionally and has few indications. Blumgart[77] has popularized an alternative approach in which the left ductal system is exposed through division of the ligamentum teres and an anastomosis is created to a limb of jejunum. There appears to be little role for palliative resection in patients with unresectable or metastatic bile duct tumors.

NEW HORIZONS

The issue of early diagnosis continues to be the focus of ongoing investigation. In addition to tumor markers such as CEA and CA 19-9, recent studies have suggested that human cholangiocarcinomas express somatostatin receptors.[78] This preliminary observation suggests that somatostatin analogues may be useful for the diagnostic localization and perhaps even treatment of biliary tract malignancies.[79] Although anecdotal reports have suggested that radiotherapy may improve survival, a report from Pitt et al.[80] failed to demonstrate any beneficial effect beyond surgical resection for radiotherapy on either length or quality of survival. An in-depth discussion of the role of radiotherapy in the management of patients with bile duct cancers is beyond the scope of this chapter. Interstitial or intraluminal brachytherapy[81,82] and intraoperative radiotherapy[83,84] have been hailed as major advances in the treatment of patients with bile duct cancers. To date, the results have been variable and there is no consensus on the benefit of these therapies. The efficacy of combined modality treatment is actively being investigated.[85]

REFERENCES

1. Helwig FC, Schultz CB. A liver kidney syndrome. Clinical pathological and experimental studies. Surg Gynecol Obstet 1930; 55:570.
2. Heyd CG. 'Liver deaths' in surgery of the gallbladder. JAMA 1931; 97:1847.
3. Wait RB, Kahng KU. Renal failure complicating obstructive jaundice. Am J Surg 1989; 157:256–63.
4. Dawson JL. The incidence of postoperative renal failure in obstructive jaundice. Br J Surg 1965; 52:663.
5. Bouillot J-L, Ledorner G, Alexandre J-HL. Facteurs de risque de la chirurgie des icteres obstructifs. Etude retrospective a propos de 176 patients. Gastroenterol Clin Biol 1985; 9:238–43.
6. Katz S, Grosfeld JL, Gross K, et al. Impaired bacterial clearance and trapping in obstructive jaundice. Ann Surg 1984; 199:14–20.
7. Pain JA, Cahill CJ, Gilbert JM, Johnson CD, Trapnell JE, Bailey ME. Prevention of postoperative renal dysfunction in patients with obstructive jaundice: a multicenter study of bile salts and lactulose. Br J Surg 1991; 78:467–9.
8. Scott-Conner CE, Grogan JB. The pathophysiology of biliary obstruction and effects on phagocytic and immune function. J Surg Res 1994; 57: 316–36.
9. Parks RW, Clements WD, Smye MG, Pope C, Rowlands BJ, Diamond T. Intestinal barrier dysfunction in clinical and experimental obstructive jaundice and its reversal by internal biliary drainage. Br J Surg 1996; 83:1345–9.
10. Tanaka N, Ryden S, Berqvist L, Christensen P, Bengmark S. Reticulo-endothelial function in rats with obstructive jaundice. Br J Surg 1985; 72:946–9.
11. Greve JW, Gouma DJ, Soeters PB, Buurman WA. Suppression of cellular immunity in obstructive jaundice is caused by endotoxins: a study with germ-free rats. Gastroenterology 1990; 98:478–85.
12. Pitt HA, Cameron JL, Postier RG, Gadacz TR. Factors affecting mortality in biliary tract surgery. Am J Surg 1981; 141:66–72.
13. Dixon JM, Armstrong CP, Duffy SW, Davies GC. Factors affecting morbidity and mortality after surgery for obstructive jaundice. A review of 373 patients. Gut 1983; 24:845–52.
14. Nakayama T, Ikeda A, Okuda K. Percutaneous transhepatic drainage of the biliary tract. Gastroenterology 1978; 74:554–9.
15. Hansson JA, Hoevels J, Simert G, Tylen U, Vang J. Clinical aspects of nonsurgical percutaneous transhepatic drainage in obstructive lesions of the extrahepatic bile ducts. Ann Surg 1979; 189:58–61.
16. Ferrucci JT Jr, Mueller PR, Harbin WP. Percutaneous transhepatic biliary drainage: technique, results, and applications. Radiology 1980; 135:1–13.
17. Pitt HA, Gomes AS, Lois JF, Mann LL, Deutsch LS, Longmire WP Jr. Does preoperative percutaneous biliary drainage reduce operative risk or increase hospital cost? Ann Surg 1985; 201:545–53.
18. Hatfield ARW, Tobias R, Terblanche J, et al. Preoperative external biliary drainage in obstructive jaundice: a prospective controlled clinical trial. Lancet 1982; II:896–9.
19. McPherson GAD, Benjamin IS, Hodgson HJF, et al. Preoperative percutaneous transhepatic biliary drainage: the results of a controlled trial. Br J Surg 1984; 71:371–5.
20. Smith RC, Pooley M, George CRP, Faithful GR. Preoperative percutaneous transhepatic internal drainage in obstructive jaundice: a randomized, controlled trial examining renal function. Surgery 1985; 97:641–8.
21. Hochwald SN, Burke EC, Jarnagin WR, Fong Y, Blumgart LH. Association of preoperative biliary stenting with increased postoperative infectious complications in proximal cholangiocarcinoma. Arch Surg 1999; 134:261–6.
22. Berkowitz D, Gambescia J, Thompson CM. Jaundice with signs of extra-hepatic obstruction as the presenting symptom of bronchogenic carcinoma. Gastroenterology 1952; 20:653–7.

23. Warshaw AL, Welch JP. Extrahepatic biliary obstruction by metastatic colon carcinoma. Ann Surg 1978; 188:593–7.

24. Popp JW Jr, Schapiro RH, Warshaw AL. Extrahepatic biliary obstruction caused by metastatic breast carcinoma. Ann Intern Med 1979; 91:568–71.

25. Lillicrap DP, Ginsburg AD, Corbett WEN. Relapse of acute myelogenous leukemia presenting with extrahepatic obstruction of the biliary tract. Can Med Assoc J 1981;127:1000–1.

26. Roslyn JJ, Kuchenbecker S, Longmire WP Jr, Tompkins RK. Floating tumor debris: a cause of intermittent biliary obstruction. Arch Surg 1984; 119:1312–15.

27. Tsuzuki T, Ogata Y, Iida S, et al. Hepatoma with obstructive jaundice due to the migration of a tumor mass in the biliary tract: report of a successful resection. Surgery 1979; 85:593–8.

28. Levine AW, Donegan WL, Irwin M. Adenocarcinoma of the colon with hepatic metastases: fifteen-year survival. JAMA 1982; 247:2809–10.

29. Henson DE, Albores-Saavedra J, Corle D. Carcinoma of the extrahepatic bile ducts. Histologic types, stage of disease, grade, and survival rates. Cancer 1992; 70:1498–501.

30. Saunders K, Tompkins R, Longmire WP Jr, Roslyn JJ. Bile duct carcinoma in the elderly: a rationale for surgical management. Arch Surg 1991; 126:1186–91.

31. Saunders K, Tompkins RK, Cates JA, Longmire WP Jr, Roslyn JJ. The natural history of bile duct cancer in patients less than 45 years of age. Surg Gynecol Obstet 1992; 174:1–6.

32. Chijiiwa K, Ichimiya H, Kuroki S, et al. Late development of cholangiocarcinoma after treatment of hepatolithiasis: immunohistochemical study of mucin carbohydrates and core proteins in hepatolithiasis and cholangiocarcinoma. Int J Cancer 1993; 55:82–91.

33. Srivatanakul P, Parkin DM, Jiang Y, et al. The role of infection by Opistorchis viverrini, hepatitis B virus, and aflatoxin exposure in the etiology of liver cancer in Thailand. Cancer 1991; 68:2417.

34. Chen MF, Jan YY, Wang CS, et al. Clinical experience in 20 hepatic resections for peripheral cholangiocarcinoma. Cancer 1989; 64:2226–32.

35. Tsunoda T, Furui J, Yamada M, Eto T, et al. Caroli's disease associated with hepatolithiasis: a case report and review of the Japanese literature. Gastroenterol Jpn 1991; 26:74–9.

36. Gallinger S, Gluckman D, Langer B. Proximal bile duct cancer. Adv Surg 1990; 23:89.

37. Marsh JW, Iwatsuki S, Makowka L, et al. Orthotopic liver transplantation for primary sclerosing cholangitis. Ann Surg 1988; 207:21–5.

38. Rosen CB, Nagorney DM, Wiesner RH, et al. Cholangiocarcinoma complicating primary sclerosing cholangitis. Ann Surg 1991; 213:21–5.

39. Longmire WP Jr, McArthur MS, Bastounis EA, Hiatt JA. Carcinoma of the extrahepatic biliary tract. Ann Surg 1973; 178:333–45.

40. Tompkins RK, Saunders K, Roslyn JJ, Longmire WP Jr. Changing patterns in diagnosing and management of bile duct cancer. Ann Surg 1990; 211:614–21.

41. Chao TC, Greager JA. Carcinoma of the extrahepatic bile ducts. J Surg Oncol 1991; 46:145–50.

42. Reding R, Buard JL, Lebeau G, et al. Surgical management of 552 carcinomas of the extrahepatic bile ducts (gallbladder and periampullary tumors excluded): results of the French Surgical Association Survey. Ann Surg 1991; 213:326–41.

43. Bismuth H, Nakache R, Diamond T. Management strategies in resection for hilar cholangiocarcinoma. Ann Surg 1992; 215:31–8.

44. Suzuki M, Takahashi T, Ouchi K, Matsuno S. The development and extension of hepatohilar bile duct carcinoma: a three dimensional tumor mapping in the intrahepatic biliary tree visualized with the aid of a graphics computer system. Cancer 1989; 64:658–66.

45. Kopelson G, Harisiadis L, Tretter P. The role of radiation therapy in cancer of the extrahepatic biliary system: an analysis of thirteen patients and a review of the literature on the effectiveness of surgery, chemotherapy, and radiotherapy. Int J Radiat Oncol Biol Phys 1977; 2:883–94.

46. Hultcrantz R, Olsson R, Danielsson A, et al. A 3-year prospective study on serum tumor markers used for detecting cholangiocarcinoma in patients with primary sclerosing cholangitis. J Hepatol 1999; 30:669.

47. Nakeeb A, Lipsett PA, Lillemoe KD, et al. Biliary carcinoembryonic antigen levels are a marker for cholangiocarcinoma. Am J Surg 1996; 171:147–53.

48. Ito R, Tamura K, Ashida H, et al. Usefulness of K-ras gene mutation at codon 12 in bile for diagnosing biliary strictures. Int J Oncol 1998; 12:1019–23.

49. Wetter LA, Ring EJ, Pellegrini CA, Way LW. Differential diagnosis of sclerosing cholangiocarcinomas of the common hepatic duct (Klatskin tumors). Am J Surg 1991; 161:57–63.

50. Rabinovitz M, Zajko AB, Hassnein T, Shetty B, et al. Diagnostic value of brush cytology in the diagnosis of bile duct carcinoma: a study in 65 patients with bile duct strictures. Hepatology 1990; 12:747–52.

51. Morales CP, Burdick JS, Saboorian MH, Wright WE, Shay JW. In situ hybridization for telomerase RNA in routine cytologic brushings for the diagnosis of pancreaticobiliary malignancies. Gastrointest Endosc 1998; 48:4022–5.

52. Tamada K, Yasuda Y, Nagi H, et al. Limitation of cholangiography in assessing longitudinal spread of extrahepatic bile duct carcinoma to the hepatic side. J Gastroenterol Hepatol 1999; 14:691–8.

53. Sato M, Inoue H, Ogawa S, et al. Limitations of percutaneous transhepatic cholangioscopy for the

diagnosis of the intramural extension of bile duct carcinoma. Endoscopy 1998; 30:281–8.

54. Tillich M, Mischinger HJ, Preisegger KH, Rabl H, Szolar DH. Multiphasic helical CT in diagnosis and staging of hilar cholangiocarcinoma. Am J Roentgenol 1998; 171:651–8.

55. Ortner MA, Liebetruth J, Schreiber S, et al. Photo-dynamic therapy of nonresectable cholangiocarcinoma. Gastroenterol 1998; 114:536–42.

56. Nagino M, Numura Y, Kamiya J, et al. Segmental liver resections for hilar cholangiocarcinoma. Hepatogastroenterology 1998; 45:7–13.

57. Langer JC, Langer B, Taylor BR, Zeldin R, Cummings B. Carcinoma of the extrahepatic bile ducts: results of an aggressive surgical approach. Surgery 1985; 98:752–9.

58. Beazley RM, Hadjis N, Benjamin IS, Blumgart LH. Clinicopathological aspects of high bile duct cancer: experience with resection and bypass surgical treatments. Ann Surg 1984; 199:623–36.

59. Pinson CW, Rossi RL. Extended right hepatic lobectomy, left hepatic lobectomy and skeletonization resection for proximal bile duct cancer. World J Surg 1988; 12:52–9.

60. Cameron JL, Pitt HA, Zinner MJ, Kaufman SL, Coleman J. Management of proximal cholangiocarcinomas by surgical resection and radiotherapy. Am J Surg 1990; 159:91–7.

61. Washburn WK, Lewis WD, Jenkins RL. Aggressive surgical resection for cholangiocarcinoma. Arch Surg 1995; 130:270–6.

62. Miyazaki M, Ito H, Nakagawa K, et al. Aggressive surgical approaches to hilar cholangiocarcinoma: hepatic or local resection? Surgery 1998; 123:131–6.

63. Launois B, Terblanche J, Lakehal M, et al. Proximal bile duct cancer: high resectability rate and 5-year survival. Ann Surg 1999; 230:266–75.

64. Nagino M, Nimura Y, Kamiya J, et al. Right or left trisegment portal vein embolization before hepatic trisegmentectomy for hilar bile duct carcinoma. Surgery 1995; 117:677–81.

65. Vogl TJ, Balzer JO, Dette K, et al. Initially unresectable hilar cholangiocarcinoma; hepatic regeneration after transarterial embolization. Radiology 1998; 208:217–22.

66. Miyagawa S, Makuuchi M, Kawasaki S, et al. Outcome of major hepatectomy with pancreatoduodenectomy for advanced biliary malignancy. World J Surg 1996; 20:77–80.

67. Haug LE, Jenkins RL, Rohrer RJ, et al. Liver transplantation for primary hepatic cancer. Transplantation 1992; 53:376–82.

68. Olthoff KM, Millis JM, Rosove MH, Goldstein LI, Ramming KP, Busuttil RW. Is liver transplantation justified in the treatment of hepatic malignancies? Arch Surg 1990; 125:1261–8.

69. Goldstein RM, Stone M, Tillery AW, et al. Is liver transplantation indicated for cholangiocarcinoma? Am J Surg 1993; 166:768–72.

70. Speer AG, Cotton PB, Russell RCG, et al. Randomized trial of endoscopic versus percutaneous stent insertion in malignant obstructive jaundice. Lancet 1987; 2:57–62.

71. Gray R. Percutaneous biliary drainage with emphasis on hilar lesions. Can J Gastroenterol 1990; 4:579.

72. Lai ECS, Tompkins RK, Mann LL, Roslyn JJ. Proximal bile duct cancer: quality of survival. Am J Surg 1987; 205:111–18.

73. Lai ECS, Chur KM, Lo CY, Fan ST, Lo CM, Wong J. Choice of palliation for malignant hilar biliary obstruction. Am J Surg 1992; 163:208–12.

74. Praderi R. El drenaje biliar externo o interno per el hepatico izquierdo. Rev Assoc Med Bras 1963; 9:401–3.

75. Terblanche J, Saunders SG, Louw JW. Prolonged palliation in carcinoma of the main hepatic duct junction. Surgery 1972; 71:720–31.

76. Tompkins RK, Saunders K, Roslyn JJ, Longmire WP Jr. Changing patterns in diagnosis and management of bile duct cancer. Ann Surg 1990; 211:614–21.

77. Blumgart LH, Kelley CJ. Hepaticojejunostomy in benign and malignant high bile duct stricture: approaches to the left hepatic ducts. Br J Surg 1984; 71:57.

78. Tan CK, Podila PV, Taylor JE, et al. Human cholangiocarcinomas express somatostatin receptors and respond to somatostatin with growth inhibition. Gastroenterology 1995; 108:1908–16.

79. Sulkowski U, Dinse P, Hans U, Collins W. Regression of a distal bile duct carcinoma after treatment with octreotide for 6 months. Digestion 1997; 58:207–9.

80. Pitt HA, Nakeeb A, Abrams RA, et al. Perihilar cholangiocarcinoma. Postoperative radiotherapy does not improve survival. Ann Surg 1995; 221:788–98.

81. Dobelbower RR, Merrick HW, Ahuja RK, Skeel RT. [125]I interstitial implant, precision high-dose external beam therapy and 5-FU for unresectable adenocarcinoma of pancreas and extrahepatic biliary tree. Cancer 1986; 58:2185–95.

82. Montemaggi P, Costamagna G, Dobelbower R, et al. Intraluminal brachytherapy in the treatment of pancreas and bile duct carcinoma. Int J Radiat Oncol Biol Phys 1995; 32:437–43.

83. Todoroki T, Iwasaki Y, Okamura T, et al. Intraoperative radiotherapy for advanced carcinoma of the biliary system. Cancer 1979; 46:2179–84.

84. Iwasaki Y, Todoroki T, Fukao K, Ohara K, Okamura T, Nishimura A. The role of intraoperative radiation therapy in the treatment of bile duct cancer. World J Surg 1988; 12:91–8.

85. Urego M, Flickinger JC, Carr BI. Radiotherapy and multimodality management of cholangiocarcinoma. Int J Radiat Oncol Biol Phys 1999; 44:121–6.

86. Lipsett PA, Pitt HA. Acute cholangitis. Surg Clin North Am 1990; 70:1297.

29

Radiological intervention in malignant biliary obstruction

MARC L FRIEDMAN

INTRODUCTION

Malignant biliary obstruction accounts for approximately 90% of biliary strictures seen at percutaneous transhepatic cholangiography.[1] The most common cause is pancreatic carcinoma, which is the fourth leading cause of cancer death in the USA. Cholangiocarcinoma, gallbladder carcinoma, ampullary carcinoma, lymphoma, hepatoma, and metastases can produce malignant biliary obstruction. It is generally an unfavorable prognostic sign when jaundice appears in patients with malignancy. The pruritus that accompanies the jaundice is miserable for the patient. Surgical intervention for the construction of a biliary-enteric bypass imposes a significant recuperative period on an individual whose life expectancy may already be limited. This chapter focuses on numerous percutaneous techniques that enable the radiologist not only to image but also to biopsy and treat patients with malignant biliary obstruction.

Although the technique of transhepatic cholangiography was originally described by Burckhardt and Muller in 1921,[2] it was not until several decades later that percutaneous biliary intervention gained momentum. The Seldinger arteriographic technique[3] was modified for use in the biliary tract. In 1964, Weichel published his work with biliary catheters that were inserted by a percutaneous transhepatic approach.[4] Decompression of obstructed bile ducts by transhepatically placed catheters was first reported by Molnar and Stockum in 1974.[5] This coincided with the demonstration that modified angiographic catheters could be manipulated through the biliary tree and across obstructing lesions.[6]

Early reports suggested that preoperative biliary drainage improved hepatic function while diminishing surgical morbidity and mortality.[7,8] This has never been substantiated. Furthermore, cancer patient survival is not affected by surgical or non-surgical biliary drainage.[9]

Preoperative biliary decompression is currently being performed only in selected patients. Most commonly, this occurs in patients with cholangitis who require medical management prior to elective surgery. Some surgeons prefer a catheter in the bile duct as a landmark to guide the anatomical identification in the porta hepatis, which can be difficult when extensive scarring from previous surgery is present. Following choledochoenterostomy, the transhepatic catheter can be used to stent the anastomosis and allow for postoperative cholangiography. Today, the overwhelming majority of percutaneous biliary drainage procedures are performed for the palliative treatment of malignant biliary obstruction. Many investigators have published their work using a variety of catheters and stents and accompanying techniques for placing them into the biliary tree.[10–16] Although percutaneous transhepatic cholangiography and biliary drainage are technically demanding procedures, the low risk/benefit ratio is extremely desirable for the quality of life and sense of well-being of the jaundiced cancer patient.

PRE-PROCEDURE EVALUATION

Malignant biliary obstruction classically presents with painless jaundice. This can be associated with weight loss, anorexia, acholic stools, dark urine, abnormal liver function tests, and pruritus. The diagnosis is usually suspected before the interventionalist is consulted. Prior to intervention, it is incumbent upon the radiologist to review all imaging studies as these may provide anatomical information that might alter the percutaneous approach, convey the potential need for multiple drainage catheters, or even contraindicate the procedure. The demonstration of dilated intrahepatic ducts by cross-sectional imaging techniques including ultrasound, computerized tomography (CT), and magnetic resonance imaging (MRI) confirms bile duct obstruction. These studies often demonstrate the level of the obstruction as evidenced by an abrupt change in duct caliber. In addition, the presence of a mass at the level of obstruction or ascites in the planned percutaneous access route is easily delineated.

A large amount of perihepatic ascites is a relative contraindication to percutaneous biliary drainage. Catheters and guidewires tend to buckle in the easily compressible fluid-filled space between the abdominal wall and liver. This can result in dislodgement during stent placement, especially when catheter advancement across a tight obstruction is attempted. If dislodgement occurs, percutaneous access to a decompressed system can become difficult or impossible. The risk of intra-procedural catheter dislodgement can be reduced by several factors. Pre-procedure paracentesis can significantly decrease the size of the perihepatic fluid-filled space. Puncturing an intrahepatic duct that ultimately limits the degree of tortuosity of the transhepatic catheter course is crucial. In addition, maximum stiffness of the working guidewire and the presence of a safety guidewire are recommended. Perihepatic ascites also tends to leak around a transhepatic catheter and can present an annoying clinical problem for the patient as the skin becomes irritated and prone to infection.

Review of the cross-sectional imaging studies is also important for the evaluation of hepatic parenchymal disease. The presence of liver masses can alter the planned access route. For example, the risk of secondary infection of liver cysts by a transhepatic catheter and anaphylaxis from puncture of hydatid cysts must be avoided.[17] In patients with extensive hepatic metastases, percutaneous biliary drainage may not significantly lower the level of jaundice. In addition, multifocal obstruction with isolation of hepatic segments often requires multiple procedures to place several drainage catheters. This may not be advantageous for a patient with limited life expectancy. Incomplete drainage of the biliary tree can reduce jaundice; however, there is a significant risk of cholangitis in the undrained segments.

Pre-procedure laboratory evaluation is essential prior to percutaneous biliary intervention. This includes a complete blood count, coagulation profile, and blood chemistries. A baseline hematocrit allows the evaluation of any subsequent bleeding complication. Although a bleeding diathesis is the only absolute contraindication to percutaneous biliary drainage, coagulation disorders can usually be corrected by the administration of various blood products. If the platelet count is less than 50 000/UL platelet transfusions are performed. If the coagulation profile is abnormal, the administration of vitamin K, fresh frozen plasma or specific blood coagulation products will usually allow the procedure to be performed. Post-procedure metabolic abnormalities can occur, especially when external biliary drainage is fashioned, and therefore baseline electrolyte evaluation is essential.

Patients receive intravascular contrast media during needle interrogation of the liver through various hepatic venous and portal venous radicals, especially in patients with minimally dilated intrahepatic ducts. Therefore, baseline blood urea nitrogen and creatinine should be documented. Lastly, pre-procedure liver function tests provide a reference for chemical monitoring of the post-procedure effects of biliary drainage.

Antibiotic prophylaxis is mandatory during percutaneous transhepatic biliary drainage. There is a relatively high risk of infectious complications from manipulation in the biliary tree secondary to the likelihood of bacterial pathogens in an obstructed system.[18] For patients who are at low or moderate risk of infection, single-agent prophylaxis is recommended.[19] Cefazolin is commonly used because it has both well-established efficacy and the lowest cost of the parenteral cephalosporins. For patients at high risk and for those who have signs of clinical infection, ampicillin and gentamycin are recommended. For patients who are allergic to penicillin, cefazolin may be substituted for ampicillin. Cross-reactivity to cephalosporin in penicillin-allergic patients is rare. Vancomycin is another alternative, but this must be given with gentamycin as it has virtually no Gram-negative coverage. Antibiotics must be started 30–60 min prior to the procedure. Single-dose therapy is usually sufficient, assuming that successful drainage is accomplished. Of course, consultation with an infectious disease specialist may be helpful in choosing the best regime for an individual patient.

The patient is carefully informed of the methods and expectations from percutaneous biliary drainage. The risks, benefits, and therapeutic alternatives are discussed. The principal risks include bleeding, infection (e.g., peritonitis and septicemia), the possible need for emergency surgery of intervention (e.g., transcatheter embolotherapy for significant hemobilia), and possible loss of life.[17] The patient must understand the potential need for multiple procedures and the possible requirement for an externally draining catheter. Drainage is associated with transhepatic catheter-related pain, which often requires intravenous or intramuscular analgesia following the procedure. If drainage is not internalized, transhepatic catheter-related pain diminishes daily and usually resolves within 7–10 days.

Intravenous sedation and analgesia are important factors in accomplishing successful percutaneous biliary drainage because percutaneous access, tract dilatation, and manipulation within the biliary system can be extremely painful for the patient. It is not possible for the interventional radiologist to administer medication and monitor conscious sedation while concurrently performing percutaneous transhepatic biliary drainage. Therefore, it is essential that an anesthesiologist or trained interventional nurse specialist be present. The vital signs, electrocardiogram, and pulse oximetry are routinely monitored. We usually administer a benzodiazepine and an opiate derivative.

Midazolam produces amnesia, anxiolysis, and sedation. Fentanyl, which is 100 times more potent than morphine, provides analgesia while blunting the automatic response to painful stimulation.[20] Our anesthesiologists typically use a continuous infusion of propofol. This short-acting sedative/hypnotic demonstrates modest respiratory effects if doses are kept low. It has a much shorter recovery time than benzodiazepines or barbiturates and has a low incidence of post-procedure nausea and vomiting. Celiac plexus block[21] and pleural block[22] have been used to accomplish analgesia for deep visceral pain sensation transmitted from the liver. Ultimately, the choice depends upon the condition of the patient and the experience of the interventionalist.

TECHNIQUE

Percutaneous transhepatic biliary drainage is initiated by opacifying the intrahepatic ducts using a fine needle (22 gauge). The interventionalist must decide whether a right-sided or left-sided approach to the biliary tree is appropriate. When the obstruction involves the extrahepatic duct, a branch of the right hepatic duct is usually chosen as the entry site (Figure 29.1). If the obstruction is in the porta hepatis, as with cholangiocarcinoma involving the junction of the right and left hepatic ducts or metastatic disease to the liver hilum, multiple duct stenoses are more likely to occur on the right.[23] Consequently, left hepatic duct drainage is preferred because one catheter is more likely to drain a larger percentage of the biliary tree. The left lobe must not be atrophic or in a high position under the costal margin, which can make duct puncture from a subxyphoid approach technically difficult. Ultrasound guidance allows puncture of the segment II or III duct (Figure 29.2), which is preferred because of the extrahepatic position of the left hepatic duct medial to the falciform ligament. Extrahepatic duct puncture increases the risk of bile leakage.[24] In addition, the lung, stomach, and transverse colon can be avoided using ultrasound guidance. The subcostal location of an anterior left hepatic duct catheter is often better tolerated by the patient than the intercostal position of a lateral right hepatic duct catheter. The left-sided approach can be more technically demanding because of the tendency of the fluoroscopic field to include the hands of the interventionalist.

The right-sided approach is more commonly used. The puncture site is selected at an intercostal space caudal to the costophrenic angle but cephalad to the colon. Although a more cephalic entry point is desirable as this typically allows a less angled path to the extrahepatic duct, the risk of pleural transgression increases with a more cephalic entry. A mid-axillary or slightly anterior to mid-axillary entry point, typically in the tenth intercostal space, tends to avoid the posteriorly deepening pleural space. Under fluoroscopic guidance, the needle is generally aimed toward the upper 12th vertebral body along a coronal plane which is typically parallel to the table top. Needle excursion stops approximately 2 cm from the lateral spinal margin. The needle is then slowly withdrawn, while small dilute contrast pulses are administered under fluoroscopy. Entry into a bile duct is recognized by slow flow away from the needle tip within a tubular structure. Hepatic vein and portal vein opacification is recognized by faster tubular flow, with washout directed toward the right atrium and liver periphery respectively. Periportal lymphatic opacification appears as a delicate network of tubular channels extending toward the porta hepatis. Once a bile duct is entered, opacification of the biliary tree is accomplished and multiple spot films are obtained. A tilting table is advantageous in this regard as it allows dependent maneuvering of the contrast material to define the level of obstruction. Attempts are made to limit the amount of ductal distension with contrast material. This lessens the risk of septicemia caused by manipulation within the infected biliary tree.

The suitability of the initially punctured duct for the establishment of percutaneous drainage depends on several factors. A peripheral rather than central duct entry is preferred as this reduces the risk of venous or arterial injury and subsequent hemobilia. Peripheral puncture also provides more room for drainage catheter sideholes above an obstruction. Maximizing a straight-line course from the skin to the level of obstruction facilitates subsequent manipulation, including crossing the obstruction and placing a stent. If the entered bile duct is suboptimal, c-arm fluoroscopic guidance is used to directly puncture a suitable duct using a second 21-gauge needle.

Once a suitable duct has been entered, a 0.018-inch guidewire with a steerable radio-opaque tip is advanced through the fine needle into the biliary tree. A coaxially tapered dilator/stiffening cannula/sheath assembly is then directed over the fine guidewire into the biliary tree. The dilator/stiffening cannula is removed, leaving a working sheath and 0.018-inch safety guidewire. Following advancement of a standard 0.035-inch working guidewire into the bile duct, the tract is dilated and one of several options is pursued.

If the patient is unstable or there is evidence of grossly purulent bile or clinical septicemia, simple external drainage is established by leaving a catheter positioned proximal to the obstruction and connecting the external hub to a bile drainage bag. A Cope loop design[25] anchoring mechanism is recommended to prevent catheter withdrawal, which may occur as a result of normal respiratory motion. The external portion of the drainage catheter is fixed to the skin by an adhesive device or suture. Further percutaneous manipulation is delayed until the patient's condition stabilizes.

In most patients with an apparently complete obstruction, a torquing guidewire and catheter can usually be

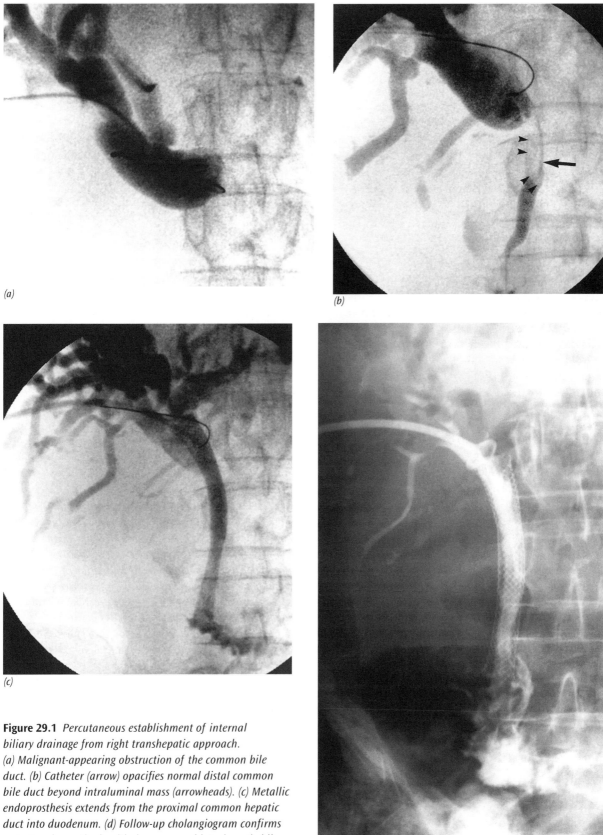

(a)

(b)

(c)

(d)

Figure 29.1 *Percutaneous establishment of internal biliary drainage from right transhepatic approach. (a) Malignant-appearing obstruction of the common bile duct. (b) Catheter (arrow) opacifies normal distal common bile duct beyond intraluminal mass (arrowheads). (c) Metallic endoprosthesis extends from the proximal common hepatic duct into duodenum. (d) Follow-up cholangiogram confirms patent endoprosthesis with decompressed intrahepatic bile ducts. The external drain was removed.*

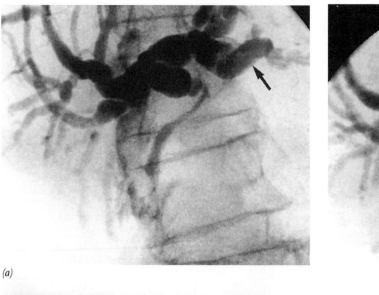

(a)

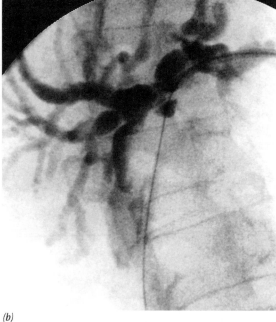

(b)

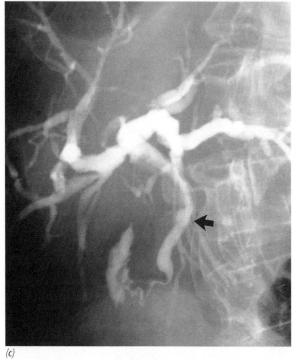

(c)

Figure 29.2 *Percutaneous establishment of internal biliary drainage from left transhepatic approach. CT scan suggested proximal common hepatic duct obstruction. (a) Needle puncture of segment III duct (long arrow). Note incomplete obstruction and marked deviation of the common bile duct course by metastatic gastric cancer. (b) Stiff guidewire advanced across obstruction and into duodenum. (c) Metallic endoprosthesis is positioned in common duct so that distal end (short arrow) is just below the level of obstruction. Sphincter function is preserved.*

negotiated through the narrowed ductal lumen into the distal common bile duct and duodenum. If the narrowed lumen cannot be traversed initially, a repeat attempt after 2 or 3 days of biliary drainage is almost always successful as the edema that is associated with high-grade obstruction resolves.

TRANSCATHETER BILIARY BIOPSY

Although the cholangiographic appearance of a malignant biliary obstruction is characteristic (abruptly tapered, shouldered, irregular, rounded, etc.), morphological distinction between malignant and benign disease is not entirely reliable. If a malignant etiology has not been established, several transcatheter biopsy methods are available once a stable guidewire has been advanced into the duodenum. Simple bile aspiration has a low sensitivity (34%).[26] Brush biopsy can be performed by advancing a 9 French peel-away sheath just beyond the obstruction (Figure 29.3). The sheath dilator is removed and a cytological biopsy brush is then advanced to the level of the obstruction. The tip of the sheath is withdrawn so that the brush is uncovered at the level of obstruction, and brush biopsy is performed by moving the brush across the stricture multiple times. The brush is then removed from the sheath and cut from the

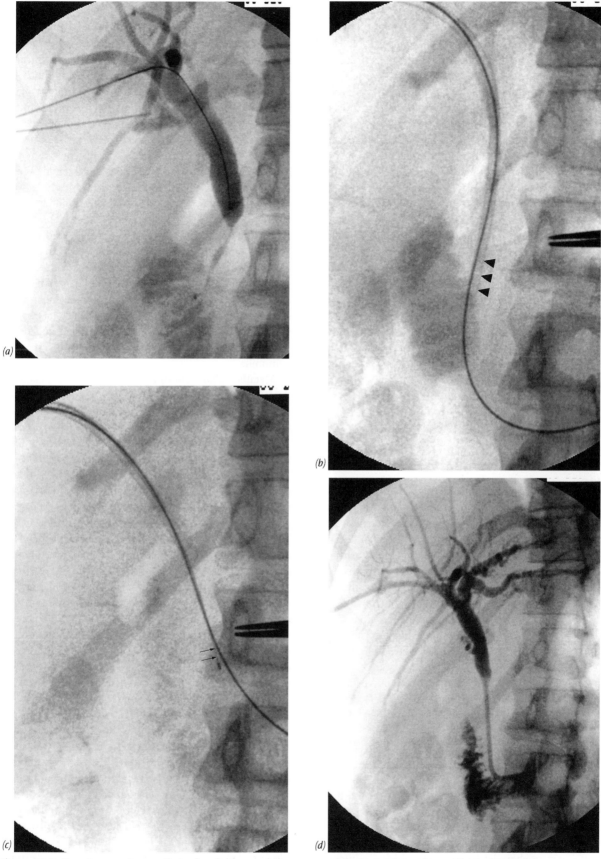

Figure 29.3 *Percutaneous transcatheter brush biopsy of the common bile duct stricture in a patient with chronic pancreatitis. (a) Initial needle puncture of caudal branch of right hepatic duct is suboptimal for transhepatic drainage. A more suitable duct entry is accomplished. Distal common bile duct stricture is demonstrated. (b) Following placement of a stiff guidewire into duodenum, a 9-French sheath (arrowheads) is situated across the stricture. (c) Once the brush (arrows) is in position, the sheath is withdrawn and brush biopsy is completed. Three specimens demonstrated no malignant cells. (d) Internal/external drainage is established. Subsequent biliary-enteric bypass was performed. No tumor was found.*

remainder of the instrument. It is placed in saline and sent for cytological examination. The procedure is typically repeated three times as it has been shown that the probability of having bile duct carcinoma after three sequential negative cytological brushings is less than 6%.[27]

Scrape biopsy has also been described in which the biopsy instrument is a dilator into which four to six flaps are fashioned with an 11 scalpel blade. This is positioned through a sheath in collapsed form at the level of the obstruction. The sheath is withdrawn to expose the flaps and a back-and-forth motion collects the specimen. A sensitivity of 60% and a false-negative rate of 13% have been demonstrated with this technique.[28]

Transcatheter needle biopsy can also be performed through a guiding sheath with the needle tip positioned using c-arm fluoroscopy.[29] This technique is limited by the rigid nature of the needle and the often tortuous course of the transhepatic tract. However, it can produce histological core specimens using a variety of automated biopsy devices.[30] Transcatheter tissue biopsy specimens can also be obtained with an atherectomy device[31] and a flexible biopsy forceps.[32]

RADIOTHERAPEUTIC APPLICATIONS

Once unresectable malignant bile duct obstruction has been confirmed and transhepatic internal/external drainage has been established, palliative internal radiotherapy using iridium-192 or other source can be instituted.[33–38] The iridium wire is placed into the transhepatic catheter using a modified angiographic guidewire. The length of active iridium wire is positioned directly at the level of the tumor under fluoroscopic control and fixed at the catheter hub. A high radiotherapeutic dose can be delivered directly to the tumor bed while limiting radiation damage to surrounding organs. Depending on the isodose distribution, the radionuclide source may be used as the only source of radiation or may be supplemented by external-beam therapy.

BILIARY ENDOPROSTHESIS PLACEMENT

Endoprosthesis placement for biliary drainage was introduced by Pereiras et al. in 1978 when they described a method to place a completely detached internal tube.[39] Over the years, several different designs of plastic and metallic stents have been developed which are intended to insure antegrade bile flow without the disadvantages of external drainage. These include the need for regular catheter flushing and dressing, possible bile and peritoneal fluid leakage, infection and pain at the catheter entry site, and the psychological problems associated with an external drainage tube. The patient's emotional attachment to the catheter and the catheter's significance as a reminder of impending death tend to diminish the patient's quality of life. Occlusion or migration of an indwelling endoprosthesis is its major disadvantage because a repeat percutaneous and/or endoscopic procedure to re-establish drainage is required.

Biliary endoprostheses were initially constructed of plastic. These stents were prone to migration and premature occlusion.[40] Plastic tubes typically occlude with debris, which may be triggered by bacterial adherence to the tube surface. This is followed by the deposition of glycoproteins, deconjugation of bilirubin, and deposition of calcium bilirubinate crystals. Attempts to prolong patency led to the development of larger-bore plastic stents, which are typically 12–14 F in diameter. These are best inserted a few days after drainage has been established, when a biliary-cutaneous tract has begun to form. This tends to make insertion easier and probably reduces the incidence of complications such as hemobilia.[40]

Metallic biliary endoprostheses became available in the late 1980s. These self-expandable or balloon-expandable stents are delivered through small-caliber sheaths (7 F or 8 F) and attain internal diameters up to 10 mm. The small introducer allows placement of the endoprostheses during the initial percutaneous intervention. Typically, an external biliary drainage catheter is left in place overnight. On the following day, if cholangiography confirms satisfactory stent position, distal integrade flow, and absence of significant clot or debris above the endoprosthesis, the external catheter is removed (see Figures 29.1 and 29.2). Unfortunately, metallic endoprostheses tend to develop ingrowth or marginal overgrowth of tumor and/or granulation tissue, which ultimately leads to occlusion. Although it is difficult to determine long-term patency rates in patients with median survival of 6 months,[41] the small number of randomized, prospective, comparative studies have confirmed that metallic stents are associated with fewer complications and probably have a lower rate of occlusion than their plastic counterparts.[42–46] Although metallic stents are significantly more expensive, cost–effectiveness analyses have shown that the cost of treatment of each patient was lower when Wallstents were used because of the lower rate of re-intervention.[43,44] Plastic (removable) endoprostheses and internal/external drainage catheters are preferred in patients with obstruction secondary to compression by lymphomatous nodes as successful chemotherapy treatment will often resolve jaundice and eliminate the need for percutaneous drainage. Metallic endoprostheses cannot be removed and will eventually occlude with granulation tissue.

Endoscopic placement of an endoprosthesis represents a compelling alternative to percutaneous biliary drainage in many patients. The advantages include direct

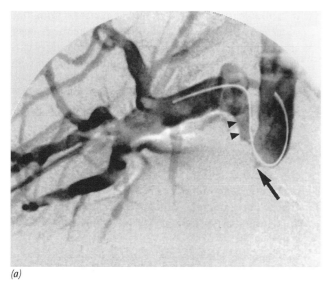

(a)

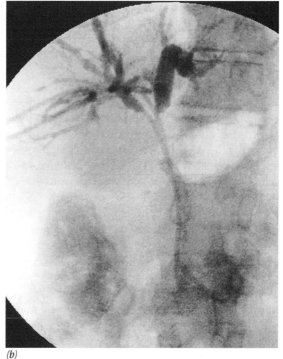

(b)

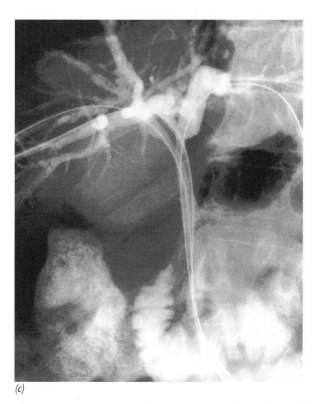

(c)

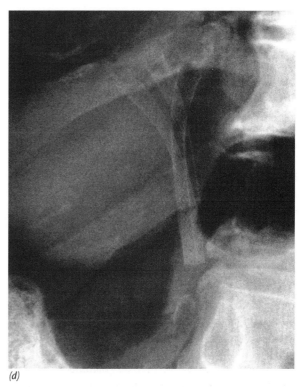

(d)

Figure 29.4 *Percutaneous internal biliary drainage in a patient with hilar cholangiocarcinoma. (a) Initial transhepatic cholangiogram demonstrates malignant obstruction at the confluence of the left hepatic duct (arrow) and posterior sector right hepatic duct (arrowheads). Anterior sector right hepatic duct is not opacified. (b) Following needle puncture of isolated anterior sector duct, complete internal/external drainage is established with two catheters. However, left hepatic duct obstruction appears imminent. (c) Left hepatic direct drainage is accomplished from subxyphoid approach. Three metallic endoprostheses are placed and appear widely patent. (d) Plain film appearance of endoprostheses. The patient died 8 months later with no evidence of recurrent biliary obstruction.*

visualization of the periampullary region, controlled sphincterotomy, and biopsy of distal lesions. These procedures tend to be well tolerated by the patient and require only a brief period of recuperation. Patients with ascites are also better suited for endoscopic placement because of the tendency for peritoneal fluid to leak externally around the transhepatic catheter. Endoscopic stenting of hilar lesions is less successful as it is often difficult for the endoscopist to direct the endoprosthesis into a particular hepatic lobe or segment. Therefore, hilar lesions are best managed by the interventional radiologist, who can use one or more access routes to gain maximum drainage of the biliary tree (Figure 29.4). In addition, patients who have had prior gastroenteric reconstruction are better suited for percutaneous manipulation because of altered retrograde access to the choledocho-enteric junction. The decision about which drainage technique to use may be ultimately determined by the availability of a physician with the appropriate skills.

COMPLICATIONS

Major complications of percutaneous biliary drainage include hemorrhage, septic shock, and death. A literature review indicates that the incidence of major complications is 4.6–25%, and the incidence of procedure-related deaths is 0–5.6%.[17] With careful technique, major complications are infrequent but unavoidable, especially when considering the often debilitated condition of the patient with malignant biliary obstruction. Fever and chills may occur in 5–26% of patients undergoing biliary drainage. If frank septicemia is apparent (fever spike, chills, tachycardia, etc.), fluid administration and antibiotic therapy are initiated. Simple establishment of external biliary drainage is expedited and further manipulation is avoided.

Hemobilia occurs in 2.6–9.6% of cases.[17] Bleeding is the most common cause of serious morbidity, but it is rarely a cause of death. Venous bleeding into the bile ducts occurs frequently during the procedure but is of no consequence if clotting function is adequate. On follow-up cholangiography, clotted blood usually clears completely within 24–48 h. It is important to make sure that catheter side holes have not migrated into the intraparenchymal tract, where they can communicate with hepatic or portal veins. Advancement of the catheter side holes into the biliary tree should resolve the hemobilia. Occasionally, upsizing the catheter to tamponade the bleeding is necessary. With biliary-cutaneous tract maturation, venous bleeding typically resolves.

Arterial bleeding is much more serious. A thrombus caste of the biliary tree associated with poor drainage of sanguinous bile is usually noted at the initial procedure.

If pulsatile, bright red blood emanates from the transhepatic tract, especially during catheter exchanges, arterial injury should be suspected. This typically occurs from a traumatic hepatic artery pseudo-aneurysm with an arterial biliary fistula (Figure 29.5). This can be successfully treated with arterial embolization techniques.[47] A hepatic arteriogram performed while the transhepatic biliary drainage catheter has been withdrawn over a guidewire will usually delineate the bleeding source. The hepatic artery branch is then embolized with Gelfoam (Upjohn, Kalamazoo, MI) or embolic coils. The incidence of arterial trauma can be minimized by avoiding central duct puncture. Patients with cirrhosis who have an increased arterial blood flow are at increased risk for arterial injury.

Significant bile leakage occurs rarely. In the case of a transhepatic catheter, this usually occurs because a side hole is positioned within the biliary-cutaneous tract. Bile can accumulate in the subcapsular space, intraperitoneal cavity, or at the skin entrance site. Biliary ascites can occur following acute occlusion or migration of a percutaneously placed endoprosthesis. Repeat cholangiography should identify the cause of leakage and enable tube repositioning or appropriate placement of a drainage catheter.

Late complications are related to occlusion and migration of the transhepatic catheter or endoprosthesis. Stent occlusion is inevitable; however, its occurrence depends on the length of patient survival. Recurrent obstruction typically presents with cholangitis (fever, chills, etc.), right upper quadrant pain, jaundice, or bile leak around an external drainage tube. If a transhepatic biliary drainage tube occludes, it is easily and safely replaced over a guidewire in the outpatient setting. Recurrent biliary obstruction in a patient with an indwelling endoprosthesis requires a new interventional procedure. If the endoprosthesis protrudes into the duodenum, endoscopic replacement is recommended as this procedure is better tolerated by the patient. Occluded plastic stents are typically removed and replaced with a new endoprosthesis. If a metallic stent has occluded, a second endoprosthesis is placed which overlaps the first and restores antegrade bile flow into the duodenum. If the occluded endoprosthesis does not extend into the duodenum, or if the site of obstruction is at the level of the liver hilum, repeat percutaneous intervention is recommended.

CONCLUSION

Percutaneous biliary drainage remains an important method of non-surgical palliation in malignant biliary obstruction. The technique allows relief of cholestasis and its clinical sequelae, with low risk for the patient.

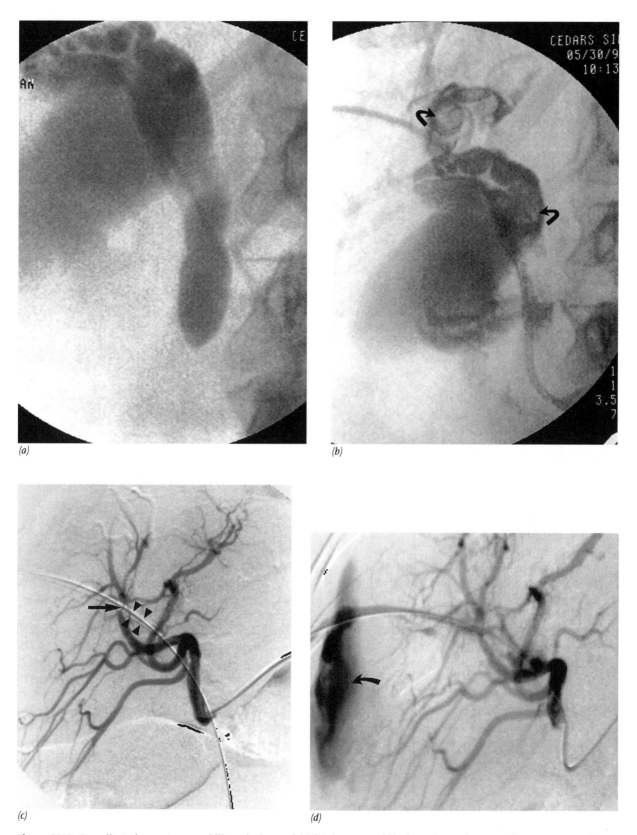

Figure 29.5 *Complicated percutaneous biliary drainage. (a) Distal common bile duct obstruction secondary to pancreatic cancer. (b) Thrombus caste (hooked arrows) seen in the common bile duct and intrahepatic ducts. Brisk pulsatile bleeding was noted from the tract during catheter exchanges. (c) Right hepatic arteriogram demonstrates focal narrowing of artery (closed arrow) at the crossing of the transhepatic catheter tract. The introducer sheath (arrowheads) tamponades the bleeding. (d) Repeat arteriogram following sheath removal confirms arterial–biliary fistula with blood collecting on patient's skin (curved arrow).*

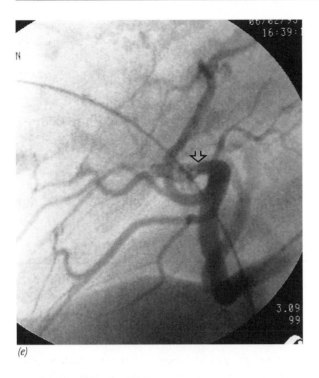

(e)

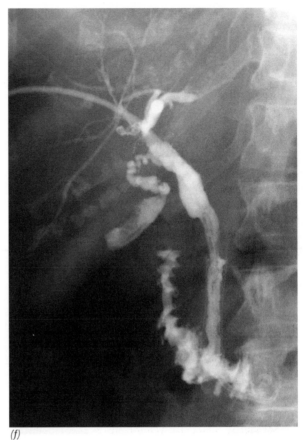

(f)

Figure 29.5 *(Continued) (e) Successful embolic occlusion (open arrow) of right hepatic artery branch with no further extravasation seen. (f) Follow-up cholangiogram demonstrates widely patent endoprosthesis and decompressed ducts. The external drain was removed uneventfully.*

REFERENCES

1. Soulen MC. Treatment of biliary strictures. In LaBerge JM, Venbrux AC, eds. *Biliary interventions.* Fairfax, VA, Society of Cardiovascular and Interventional Radiology, 1995, 221–32.

2. Burckhardt H, Muller W. Versuche uber die Punktion der Gallenblase und ihre Rontgendarstellung. Dtsch Zeitschr Chirur 1921; 162:168–97.

3. Seldinger SI. Catheter replacement of needle in percutaneous arteriography: new technique. Acta Radiol (Stockh) 1953; 39:368–76.

4. Weichel KL. Percutaneous transhepatic cholangiography: technique and application with studies of hepatic venous and biliary duct pressures, the chemical blood and bile and clinical results in a series of jaundiced patients. Acta Chir Scand 1964; Suppl. 330.

5. Molnar W, Stockum AE. Relief of obstructive jaundice through percutaneous transhepatic catheter – a new therapeutic method. Am J Roentgenol 1974; 122:356–67.

6. Ring EJ, Oleaga JA, Freiman DB, *et al.* Therapeutic applications of catheter cholangiography. Radiology 1978; 128:333–8.

7. Denning DA, Ellison EG, Carey BC. Preoperative percutaneous transhepatic biliary decompression lowers morbidity in patients with obstructive jaundice. Am J Surg 1981; 14:61–5.

8. Gobien RP, Stanley JM, Soucek CD, *et al.* Routine preoperative biliary drainage: effect on management of obstructive jaundice. Radiology 1984; 152:353–6.

9. Bonnell D, Ferucci JT, Mueller PR, *et al.* Surgical and radiological decompression in malignant biliary obstruction. A retrospective study using multivariated risk factor analysis. Radiology 1984; 152:347–51.

10. Nakayama T, Ikeda A, Okuda K. Percutaneous drainage of the biliary tract; technique and results in 104 cases. Gastroenterology 1978; 74:554–9.

11. Ishikawa Y, Oishi I, Miyai M, *et al.* Percutaneous transhepatic drainage; experience in 100 cases. J Clin Gastrenterol 1980; 2:305–14.

12. Berquist TH, May GR, Johnson CM, *et al.* Percutaneous biliary decompression: internal and external drainage in 50 patients. Am J Roentgenol 1981; 136:901–6.

13. Mueller PR, vanSonnenberg E, Ferrucci JT. Percutaneous biliary drainage; technical and catheter related problems in 200 procedures. Am J Roentgenol 1982; 138:17–23.

14. Carrasco CH, Zounoza J, Bechtel WJ. Malignant biliary obstruction; complications of percutaneous biliary drainage. Radiology 1984; 152:343–6.

15. Hamlin JA, Friedman M, Stein MG, Bray JF. Percutaneous biliary drainage: complications of 118 consecutive catheterizations. Radiology 1986; 158:199–202.

16. Gunther RW, Schild H, Thelen M. Review article: percutaneous transhepatic biliary drainage: experience with 311 procedures. Cardiovascular Intervent Radiol 1988; 11:65–71.

17. Venbrux AC, Osterman FC. Percutaneous transhepatic cholangiography and percutaneous biliary drainage: step by step. In LaBerge JM, Venbrux AC, eds. *Biliary interventions*. Fairfax, VA, SCVIR, 1995, 129–50.

18. Spies JB, Rosen RJ, Lebowitz AS. Antibiotic prophylaxis in vascular and interventional radiology: a rational approach. Radiology 1988; 166:381–7.

19. Spies JB, Abbruzzese MR. Use of antibiotics in interventional radiology. In *SCVIR 1994 Meeting Program*. Fairfax, VA, Society of Cardiovascular and Interventional Radiology, 1995, 190–4.

20. Weinger MB. General principles of conscious sedation. In *SCVIR 1994 Meeting Program*. Fairfax, VA, Society of Cardiovascular and Interventional Radiology, 1995, 66–72.

21. Savader SJ, Bourke DL, Venbrux AC, *et al.* Randomized double-blinded clinical trial of celiac plexus block for percutaneous biliary drainage. J Vasc Interv Radiol 1993; 4:539–42.

22. Rosenblatt M, Robalino J, Bergman A, *et al.* Pleural block: technique for regional anesthesia during percutaneous hepatobiliary drainage. Radiology 1989; 172:279–80.

23. Mueller PR, Ferrucci JT, vanSonnenberg E, *et al.* Obstruction of the left hepatic duct: diagnosis and treatment by selective fine-needle cholangiography and percutaneous biliary drainage. Radiology 1982; 145:297–302.

24. Russell E, Yrizzary JM, Montalvo BM, *et al.* Left hepatic duct anatomy: implications. Radiology 1990; 174:353–6.

25. Cope C. Improved anchoring of nephrostomy catheters: loop technique. Am J Roentgenol 1980; 135–402.

26. Muro A, Mueller PR, Ferrucci JT, *et al.* Bile cytology: a routine addition to percutaneous biliary drainage. Radiology 1983; 149:846–7.

27. Rabinovitz M, Zajko AB, Hassanein T, *et al.* Diagnostic value of brush cytology in the diagnosis of bile duct carcinoma: a study in 65 patients with bile duct strictures. Hepatology 1990; 12:747–52.

28. Yip CKY, Leung JWC, Chang MKM, *et al.* Scrape biopsy of malignant biliary structure through percutaneous transhepatic biliary drainage tracts. Am J Roentgenol 1989; 152:529–30.

29. Cope C, Marinelli DL, Weinstein JK. Transcatheter biopsy of lesions obstructing the bile ducts. Radiology 1988; 169:555–6.

30. Mladinich CR, Ackerman N, Berry CR, *et al.* Evaluation and comparison of automatic biopsy devices. Radiology 1992; 184:845–7.

31. Kim D, Porter DH, Siegel JB, *et al.* Common bile duct biopsy with the Simpson atherectomy catheter. Am J Roentgenol 1990; 154:1213–15.

32. Terasaki K, Wittich GR, Lycke E. Percutaneous transluminal biopsy of biliary strictures with a bioptome. Am J Roentgenol 1991; 156:77–8.

33. Herskovic A, Heaton D, Engler MJ, *et al.* Irradiation of biliary carcinoma. Radiology 1981; 139:219–22.

34. Conroy RM, Shahbazian AA, Edwards KC, *et al.* A new method for treating carcinomatous biliary obstruction with intracatheter radium. Cancer 1982; 49:1312–27.

35. Karani J, Fletcher M, Brinkley D, *et al.* Internal biliary drainage and local radiotherapy with iridium-192 wire in treatment of hilar cholangiocarcinoma. Clin Radiol 1985; 36:603–6.

36. Haffty BG, Mate TP, Greenwood LH, *et al.* Malignant biliary obstruction: intracavitary treatment with a high-dose rate remote after loading device. Radiology 1987; 164:574–6.

37. Fields JN, Emami B. Carcinoma of the extrahepatic biliary system: results of primary and adjuvant radiotherapy. Int J Radiat Oncol Biol Phys 1987; 13:331–8.

38. Hayes JK, Sapozink MD, Miller FJ. Definitive radiation therapy in bile duct carcinoma. Int J Radiat Oncol Biol Phys 1988; 15:734–44.

39. Pereiras RV, Owen JR, Hutson D, *et al.* Relief of malignant obstructive jaundice by percutaneous insertion of a permanent prosthesis in the biliary tree. Ann Intern Med 1978; 89:589–93.

40. Mueller PR, Ferucci JT Jr, Teplick SK, *et al.* Biliary stent endoprosthesis: analysis of complications in 113 patients. Radiology 1985; 156:637–9.

41. Lichtenstein DR, Carr-Locke DL. Endoscopic palliation for unresectable pancreatic carcinoma. Surg Clin North Am 1995; 75:969–87.

42. Adam AN. Biliary stent placement for malignancy. In *SCVIR 1995 Program*. Fairfax, VA, Society of Cardiovascular and Interventional Radiology, 1995, 89–90.

43. Davids PHP, Groen AK, Ruacos EAJ, *et al.* Randomized trial of self-expanding metal stents versus polyethylene stents for distal malignant biliary obstruction. Lancet 1992; 340:1488–92.

44. Wagner HMJ, Knyrim, Klose KJ. Controlled trial of plastic prostheses vs. metal stents in the treatment of malignant biliary obstruction. In *8th European Congress of Radiology abstracts book*, 1993, 182.

45. Hausegger KA, Wilding R, Flueckiger F, *et al.* Plastic versus expandable metal biliary endoprostheses: final

report of a randomized trial. Radiology 1993; 189:307.

46. Lammer J, Hausegger KA, Flueckiger F, *et al.* Common bile duct obstruction due to malignancy: treatment with plastic versus metal stents. Radiology 1996; 201:167–72.

47. Savader SJ, Trerotola SO, Merine DS, *et al.* Hemobilia after percutaneous transhepatic biliary drainage: treatment with transcatheter embolotherapy. J Vasc Interv Radiol 1992; 3:345–52.

Commentary (on Chapters 28 and 29)

SHARON WEBER AND LESLIE H BLUMGART

METASTATIC DISEASE

Palliation of jaundice in patients with malignant obstruction can be performed using surgical, endoscopic, or radiological techniques. The choice between these techniques is based on the overall condition of the patient and on the expected length of survival. In patients with a limited median survival due to metastatic disease, procedures performed in an outpatient setting, such as biliary intubation with endoscopic retrograde cholangiopancreatography (ERCP) or percutaneous transhepatic biliary drainage (PTBD), are preferred. The choice of approach is dependent upon the level of obstruction. Proximal obstruction due to cholangiocarcinoma or gallbladder carcinoma is almost never effectively palliated with ERCP-placed stents, although these stents are often successful for distal malignant obstruction. Clearly, patients with proximal obstruction have both an increased rate of failure with attempted stenting and an increased risk of recurrent cholangitis. Regardless, biliary stenting does result in symptomatic relief of jaundice and pruritus in the majority of patients. Compared to plastic stents, the placement of metallic stents is associated with a decreased rate of cholangitis and recurrent occlusion. In addition, Wall stents require no catheter care by the patient. Due to the risk of complications and often prolonged recovery time, surgical biliary bypass in patients with metastatic disease is rarely warranted.

LOCALLY ADVANCED DISEASE

Alternatively, in good-risk patients with locally advanced disease, surgical bypass can result in an improved quality of life due to a decreased risk of cholangitis and subsequent re-admission to the hospital. This is true for both distal and proximal malignant obstruction. Four prospective trials have compared surgical bypass to plastic stents for patients with distal bile duct obstruction.[1–4] Although surgical bypass resulted in greater early

morbidity and mortality, the long-term patency was improved and there was a lower incidence of recurrent jaundice and cholangitis. Of note, no prospective trial has compared surgical bypass to Wall stent.

In patients with locally advanced proximal obstruction, unresectable disease is often discovered at the time of open exploration. In this case, the patient has already undergone laparotomy and the added morbidity of surgical bypass is minimal. The alternative to surgical bypass is placement of a Wall stent. Although there is a near-90% 12-month patency rate after Wall stents are placed for distal biliary obstruction, the patency rate decreases to about 50% for proximal obstruction.[5] In these patients, segment III bypass can result in a patency rate of up to 80% at 1 year and is our preferred approach to biliary bypass in these patients.[6] Although less commonly used, the right hepatic duct can be approached at the base of the gallbladder fossa for biliary-enteric bypass. This approach is technically more difficult and results in a higher rate of late bypass failure.[6] Because many patients with locally advanced disease are found to be unresectable only after transection of the bile duct, biliary-enteric bypass with a Roux limb is required to restore continuity and can provide excellent palliation, even in the presence of microscopic disease at the bile duct margin.

RESECTABLE DISEASE

In patients with resectable disease, the goals of surgical management are both the eradication of tumor and the establishment of adequate biliary drainage. Complete surgical resection is the only potentially curative option in these patients. Distal obstruction from cholangiocarcinoma or pancreatic carcinoma is effectively treated with pancreaticoduodenectomy. Although bile duct tumors have historically been categorized based on their location in the proximal, mid, or distal duct, this classification has little clinical relevance because most of these patients will require hepatic and bile duct resection or pancreaticoduodenectomy. Very few patients will be amenable to bile duct excision alone. Therefore, it is of greater clinical value to separate these patients into two groups: those with obstruction at the proximal half or at the distal half of the bile duct.

Tumors of the biliary confluence are particularly difficult to treat because they are often discovered at an advanced stage when the lesion involves adjacent structures, including the portal vein or adjacent hepatic parenchyma. Complete resection, therefore, requires biliary and hepatic resection, occasionally with major vascular reconstruction. Both the incidence of curative resections and the outcome after resection have improved as the number of patients undergoing major hepatic resection has increased.[7]

PREOPERATIVE BILIARY DRAINAGE

Several investigators have proposed the routine use of preoperative biliary drainage in order to address several issues in patients with malignant obstruction. Hyperbilirubinemia results in significant physiologic disturbances, including renal dysfunction, bleeding diathesis, and friability of tissues that can make surgery hazardous. In addition, pruritus from jaundice is often extremely irritating for the patient. Because of both the need to establish a diagnosis and the potential palliative and physiological benefits of relieving jaundice, many patients undergo evaluation of the biliary tree with stent placement as an initial intervention. Unfortunately, it has become increasingly common for patients to be evaluated with ERCP and subsequent stent placement or PTBD before being evaluated by a surgeon. The increasing frequency of preoperative stent placement, whether plastic or Wall stents, can result in major difficulty at the time of surgery. After placement of a plastic stent, reactive edema and inflammation of the bile duct can make assessment of the extent of tumor exceedingly difficult, particularly for cholangiocarcinoma of the hepatic confluence or the mid-duct. In addition, referring physicians can considerably worsen the outcome by prematurely deeming patients unresectable and placing metallic Wall stents. These patients have often lost their only chance at curative resection, because removal of these stents is extremely difficult at any time and increases in difficulty the longer they are in place.

Although there is certainly a hypothetical advantage to preoperative biliary drainage, no benefit has been found in five separate, randomized, prospective trials evaluating the use of preoperative drainage in patients with pancreatic or peripancreatic tumors. Although the conclusions of these trials are hindered by the fact that most patients were unresectable and therefore underwent palliative biliary bypass only, none of these studies found any difference in postoperative mortality and only one showed a decrease in postoperative morbidity after preoperative drainage.[8] In this study, the only improvement in morbidity was a decrease in the rate of positive blood cultures; there was no difference in wound infection or intra-abdominal abscess rates. Again, all of these studies were limited by the fact that very few of the patients underwent resection; most patients underwent palliative bypass only.

Due to this problem, we retrospectively evaluated the postoperative outcome in a large number of patients undergoing resection. Of the 175 patients undergoing pancreaticoduodenectomy, the only factor associated with an increased risk of overall postoperative complications, infectious complications, intra-abdominal abscess, and death was the presence of a biliary drainage catheter.[9] In addition, we have performed a similar analysis on 71 patients with proximal cholangiocarcinoma, 41 of whom had preoperative biliary intubation. Although the preoperative bilirubin level was lower in stented patients, there was an increased risk of infectious complications in this group, including wound infection and intra-abdominal abscess.[10]

Although some authors have suggested that preoperative placement of bilateral biliary stents facilitates intraoperative dissection in patients with proximal obstruction, we have not found this to be true. In fact, preoperative drainage may increase the difficulty of dissection by increasing the amount of perihilar inflammation. Because of this, we do not routinely recommend biliary intubation in patients with malignant obstruction if they appear amenable to resection. There are three exceptions:

1 the occasional patient with cholangitis that is unresponsive to appropriate antibiotic therapy;
2 patients with severe pruritis who will experience a delay in surgical intervention;
3 patients undergoing neoadjuvant treatment.

Unfortunately, most patients presenting to tertiary referral centers have already undergone preoperative stenting by the time they are initially evaluated. In order to change this practice, surgeons must continue to stress the highly selective use of preoperative biliary stenting to their gastrointestinal and medical colleagues. By limiting the use of preoperative stents in patients with resectable disease, we may be able to improve postoperative morbidity and mortality.

REFERENCES

1. Bornman PC, Harries-Jones EP, Tobias R, VanSteigman G, Terblanche J. Prospective controlled trial of transhepatic biliary endoprosthesis versus biliary bypass surgery for incurable carcinoma of head of pancreas. Lancet 1986; 8472:69–71.

2. Shepard HA, Royle G, Ross APR, Diba A, Arthur M, Colin-Jones D. Endoscopic biliary endoprosthesis in the palliation of malignant obstruction of the distal common bile duct: a randomized trial. Br J Surg 1988; 75:1166–8.

3. Andersen JR, Sorenson SM, Kruse A, Rolckjaer M, Matzen P. Randomized trial of endoscopic endoprosthesis versus operative bypass in malignant obstructive jaundice. Gut 1989; 30:1132–5.

4. Dowsett JF, Russell RCG, Hatfield ARW, et al. Malignant obstructive jaundice: a prospective trial of bypass surgery versus endoscopic stenting. Gastroenterology 1989; 96:128A.

5. Becker CD, Glattli A, Maibach R, Baer HU. Percutaneous palliation of malignant obstructive jaundice with Wallstent endoprosthesis: follow-up and reintervention in patients with hilar and non-hilar obstruction. J Vasc Interv Radiol 1993; 4:767–72.

6. Jarnagin WR, Burke EC, Powers C, Fong Y, Blumgart LH. Intrahepatic biliary enteric bypass provides effective palliation in selected patients with malignant obstruction at the hepatic confluence. Am J Surg 1998; 175:453–60.

7. Chamberlain RS, Blumgart LH. Hilar cholangiocarcinoma: a review and commentary. Ann Surg Oncol 2000; 7(1):55–66.

8. Lygidakis NJ, vanderHeyde MN, Lubbers MJ. Evaluation of preoperative biliary drainage in the surgical management of pancreatic head carcinoma. Acta Chir Scand 1987; 153:665–8.

9. Povoski SP, Karpeh MS, Conlon KC, Blumgart LH, Brennan MF. Association of preoperative biliary drainage with postoperative outcome following pancreaticoduodenectomy. Ann Surg 1999; 230:131–42.

10. Hochwald SN, Burke EC, Jarnagin WR, Fong Y, Blumgart LH. Association of preoperative biliary stenting with increased postoperative infectious complications in proximal cholangiocarcinoma. Arch Surg 1999; 134:261–6.

Editors' selected abstracts (for Chapters 28 and 29)

Hilar cholangiocarcinoma: a review and commentary.

Chamberlain RS, Blumgart LH.

Department of Surgery, Montefiore Medical Center, Albert Einstein College of Medicine, Bronx, NY, USA.

Annals of Surgical Oncology 7(1):55–66, 2000, January–February.

Hilar cholangiocarcinoma is an uncommon cause of malignant biliary obstruction marked by local tumor spread for which surgery offers the only chance of cure. The diagnostic evaluation and surgical management of this disease continue to evolve. Although direct cholangiography and endoscopic biliary procedures have been used extensively to anatomically define the extent of tumor involvement, establish biliary decompression, and obtain histological confirmation of tumor, reliance on these invasive procedures is no longer necessary, and may be detrimental. Current noninvasive imaging technology permits accurate staging of the primary tumor and has improved patient selection for operative intervention without the need for invasive procedures. Overall survival has improved in accordance with an increasingly aggressive surgical approach. The propensity of this tumor for local invasion has led most experienced hepatobiliary centers to perform a partial hepatectomy in 50% to 100% of cases. Three-year survival rates of 35% to 50% can be achieved when negative histological margins are attained at the time of surgery. When resection is not feasible, either operative bilioenteric bypass or percutaneous transhepatic intubation can achieve significant palliation. There is no effective adjuvant therapy for this disease, and unless clear indications of unresectability exist, most patients should be considered for surgical exploration.

Triple-tissue sampling at ERCP in malignant biliary obstruction.

Jailwala J, Fogel EL, Sherman S, Gottlieb K, Flueckiger J, Bucksot LG, Lehman GA.

Indiana University Medical Center, Indianapolis, Indiana, USA.

Gastrointestinal Endoscopy 51(4):383–90, 2000, April.

Background: Procurement of cytologic samples by brushing is common practice at endoscopic retrograde cholangiopancreatography (ERCP) but has low sensitivity for cancer detection. Limited data are available on other techniques, including endoluminal fine-needle aspiration and forceps biopsy. This series reviews the yield of these three stricture sampling methods. Methods: In this prospective study, patients with biliary obstruction with a clinical suspicion of malignancy underwent triple-tissue sampling at one ERCP session. Final cancer diagnosis was based on all sampling methods plus surgery, autopsy, and clinical follow-up. Tissue specimens were reported as normal, atypia, or malignant. Results: A total of 133 patients were evaluated: 104 had cancer and 29 had benign strictures. Tissue sampling sensitivity varied according to the type of cancer; the highest yield was seen in ampullary cancers (62% to 85%). The cumulative sensitivity of triple-tissue sampling in the cancer patients was as follows: sensitivity was 52% if atypia was considered benign and 77% if it was considered malignant. The addition of a second or third technique increased sensitivity rates in most instances. No serious complications occurred from the tissue sampling methods. Conclusions: Tissue sampling sensitivity varied according to the type of cancer. Combining a second or third method increased sensitivity; general use of at least two sampling methods is therefore recommended.

Biliary dilatation: differentiation of benign from malignant causes – value of adding conventional MR imaging to MR cholangiopancreatography.

Kim MJ, Mitchell DG, Ito K, Outwater EK.

Department of Radiology, Thomas Jefferson University Hospital, Philadelphia, PA, USA.

Radiology 214(1):173–81, 2000, January.

Purpose: To determine the value of conventional T1- and T2-weighted images and gadolinium-enhanced dynamic magnetic resonance (MR) images as a supplement to MR cholangiopancreatographic (MRCP) images in differentiation of benign from malignant causes of biliary dilatation. *Materials and methods:* MR studies in 62 patients with biliary dilatation with proved causes included conventional T1- and less heavily T2-weighted images, as well as gadolinium-enhanced dynamic images and heavily T2-weighted MRCP images. Two radiologists reviewed MRCP images alone, MRCP images with nonenhanced T1- and T2-weighted MR images, and MRCP images with nonenhanced and gadolinium-enhanced dynamic images. *Results:* For differentiation of benign from malignant causes of biliary dilatation, the area under the receiver operating characteristic curve (A(z)) was significantly ($p < 0.05$) larger for MRCP images interpreted with T1- and T2-weighted images (0.9547 for reader 1, 0.8404 for reader 2) than for MRCP images alone (0.8144 for reader 1, 0.8122 for reader 2). The addition of gadolinium-enhanced dynamic MR images to MRCP images with nonenhanced T1- and T2-weighted images did not significantly increase accuracy (A(z) = 0.9554 for reader 1 and 0.8650 for reader 2), but the level of confidence was increased in 17%–24% of cases. *Conclusion:* Use of nonenhanced T1- and less heavily T2-weighted images with MRCP images significantly improved the diagnostic accuracy of MR examinations of pancreaticobiliary disease.

Extrahepatic biliary obstruction: magnetic resonance imaging compared with endoscopic ultrasonography.

Materne R, Van Beers BE, Gigot JF, Jamart J, Geubel A, Pringot J, Deprez P.

Dept of Radiology, Universite Catholique de Louvain, St-Luc University Hospital, Brussels, Belgium.

Endoscopy, 32(1):3–9, 2000, January.

Background and study aims: The aim of this study was to compare prospectively the diagnostic efficacy of magnetic resonance (MR) imaging and endoscopic ultrasonography (EUS) in extrahepatic biliary obstruction. *Patients and methods:* A total of 50 patients with suspected benign or malignant extrahepatic biliary obstruction underwent MR imaging, including MR cholangiopancreatography, and EUS, within a median time delay of 1 day. The final diagnosis was established by endoscopic retrograde cholangiopancreatography in 37 cases, intraoperative cholangiography in nine cases, and clinical and biochemical follow-up in four cases. *Results:* In total, 33 patients had extrahepatic biliary obstruction, of benign origin in 21 cases and of

malignant origin in 12 cases, whereas 17 had no evidence of obstruction. The sensitivity and specificity of MR imaging were 91% and 94%, respectively. There were one false-positive and three false-negative results, all related to choledochal sludge. The corresponding values for EUS were 97% and 88%. There were two false-positive results and one false-negative result. False-positive diagnoses were related to the presumed presence of biliary sludge and choledocholithiasis, whereas the false-negative diagnosis occurred in one patient with a final diagnosis of sludge. No significant difference in sensitivity and specificity was observed between the two imaging methods ($p > 0.05$). *Conclusion:* In our study MR imaging was as accurate as EUS in the diagnosis of extrahepatic biliary obstruction.

Palliation of hilar biliary obstruction from colorectal metastases by endoscopic stent insertion.

Valiozis I, Zekry A, Williams SJ, Hunt DR, Bourke MJ, Jorgensen JO, Morris DL, Craig PI.

Departments of Gastroenterology and Surgery, St. George and Westmead Hospitals, Sydney, Australia.

Gastrointestinal Endoscopy 51(4):412–7, 2000, April.

Background: In patients with hepatic metastases from colorectal carcinoma there is a distinct subgroup in whom jaundice is not due to hepatic replacement but rather biliary obstruction. We reviewed our experience with stent insertion in patients with malignant proximal biliary obstruction from metastatic colorectal carcinoma. *Methods:* Thirty-three patients were treated between July 1992 and December 1996. Placement of a single stent was attempted at initial endoscopic retrograde cholangiopancreatography. Hilar biliary obstruction was classified according to Bismuth's classification. *Results:* Successful stent placement was possible in 94% overall and at initial endoscopic retrograde cholangiopancreatography in 39% patients. Successful stent placement occurred significantly more often in patients with a type I stricture. Cholangitis was the principal complication occurring in 24% of patients. The 30-day mortality rate was 24%, with death occurring significantly less often in patients with a type I or II stricture. Overall, 45% of patients had a 30% fall in bilirubin at 1 week. The median survival was 81 days, with significantly longer survival seen in patients with a type I or II stricture. *Conclusions:* Endoscopic stent placement offers effective palliation in most patients with hilar obstruction from colorectal metastases. A subset of patients with type III stricture and greater than 3 intrahepatic metastases often do not benefit from stent insertion.

Performance characteristics of magnetic resonance cholangiography in the staging of malignant hilar strictures.

Zidi SH, Prat F, Le Guen O, Rondeau Y, Pelletier G.

Department of Gastroenterology, Bicetre Hospital, 94275 Le Kremlin Bicetre, France.

Gut 46(1):103–6, 2000, January.

Background: Magnetic resonance cholangiography (MRC) is currently under investigation for non-invasive biliary tract imaging. *Aim:* To compare MRC with endoscopic retrograde cholangiography (ERC) for pretreatment evaluation of malignant hilar obstruction. *Methods:* Twenty patients (11 men, nine women; median age 74 years) referred for endoscopic palliation of a hilar obstruction were included. The cause of the hilar obstruction was a cholangiocarcinoma in 15 patients and a hilar compression in five (one hepatocarcinoma, one metastatic breat cancer, one metastatic leiomyoblastoma, two metastatic colon cancers). MRC (T2 turbo spin echo sequences; Siemens Magnetomvision 1.5 T) was performed within 12 hours before ERC, which is considered to be the ideal imaging technique. Tumour location, extension, and type according to Bismuth's classification were determined by the radiologist and endoscopist. *Results:* MRC was of diagnostic quality in all but two patients (90%). At ERC, four patients (20%) had type I, seven (35%) had type II, seven (35%) and type III, and two (10%) had type IV strictures. MRC correctly classified 14/18 (78%) patients and underestimated tumour extension in four (22%). Successful endoscopic biliary drainage was achieved in 11/17 attempted stentings (65%), one of which was a combined procedure (endoscopic + percutaneous). One patient had a percutaneous external drain, one had a surgical bypass, and in a third a curative resection was attempted. Effective drainage was not achieved in six patients (30%). If management options had been based only on MRC, treatment choices would have been modified in a more appropriate way in 5/18 (28%) patients with satisfactory MRC. *Conclusion:* MRC should be considered for planning treatment of malignant hilar strictures. Accurate depiction of high grade strictures for which endoscopic drainage is not the option of choice can preclude unnecessary invasive imaging.

30

Management of soft tissue sarcomas of the extremity

JAMES F HUTH

INTRODUCTION

Soft tissue sarcomas are uncommon, representing less than 1% of all human malignancy. Approximately 6000 new cases are diagnosed in the USA per year. Most of these tumors originate in the extremity and the proximal thigh is the most common site. The incidence is equally distributed among all age groups and there is no significant difference in incidence based upon gender. The treatment of extremity sarcomas has changed dramatically in the past 50 years. Changes in treatment strategy have been directed toward improving outcomes in the three major areas of concern: (a) improving survival, (b) decreasing local recurrence rates, and (c) improving quality of life. However, before discussing strategies, it is important to understand issues regarding the epidemiology of this tumor, as well as issues regarding the clinical and pathologic staging of the disease.

ETIOLOGY

There are a number of factors known to increase risk for the development of sarcomas, but in the vast majority of patients there is no identifiable agent responsible for the development of the tumor. Exposure to radiation can result in the development of sarcomas, as evidenced by the increased incidence of this disease in individuals who had industrial exposure[1] or received radiation treatment for childhood and adult sarcomas.[2–4] It was initially hypothesized that orthovoltage (low kilovoltage) radiation of at least 2000 cGy was required to induce tumors, whereas megavoltage and high doses (greater than 4000 cGy) would decrease the rate of carcinogenesis. Children appear to be more prone to susceptibility and there appears to be a dose–response curve with a relative risk of 0.6 in those receiving < 1000 cGy (i.e., no

increased risk when compared to the general population) to 38.3 in those receiving > 6000 cGy.[5] Chemical agents have also been implicated: 3-methyl cholanthrene causes soft tissue sarcomas in laboratory animals, and Thorotrast and vinyl chloride have been implicated as causative agents in hepatic angiosarcoma in humans.[6] There are a multitude of inheritable genetic abnormalities that have recently been identified with various histologic subtypes of sarcoma. The *p53* gene has been associated with distinct familial cancer syndromes, including the Li–Fraumeni syndrome,[7] a rare inherited disorder characterized by high risk for the development of sarcomas of bone and soft tissue, breast, and other tumors. As the distribution of *p53* gene mutations becomes better understood, it is clear that this tumor suppressor gene is critical in cell regulation and its mutation is associated with a wide variety of human tumors.[8] Other genes with known association with sarcomas include the retinoblastoma (*Rb*) gene, and genes associated with neurofibromatosis (*NF-1* on chromosome 17, *NF-2* on chromosome 22).

STAGING

Clinical staging of soft tissue tumors of the extremity is critically important. The size of the primary tumor, extent of penetration into the surrounding tissues, histology and grade of the tumor, and metastatic spread are all important prognostic indicators which impact greatly upon treatment decisions. There is an excellent review of imaging of soft tissue tumors by Kransdorf *et al.* from the Armed Forces Institute of Pathology.[9] The development of computerized tomography (CT) and magnetic resonance imaging (MRI) has revolutionized the evaluation of these tumors. It is important to complete imaging studies prior to biopsy in patients suspected of having large malignant tumors of the extremity. The initial evaluation of a soft tissue mass should begin with a plain radiograph. This will reveal an underlying skeletal deformity or bony exostosis, which may be confused with a soft tissue mass. Plain radiographs show soft tissue calcifications that may be characteristic of specific diagnoses such as myositis osificans. They are also useful for assessing coexistent bony involvement such as remodeling, periosteal reaction, or bony destruction.

MRI is the preferred modality for imaging sarcomas. It provides superior soft tissue contrast, allows multiplanar imaging, and avoids the use of iodinated contrast agents. It is particularly useful for establishing the relationship between tumor and neurovascular structures. Although MRI, like any imaging modality, does not provide histologic information regarding whether a tumor is benign or malignant, certain diagnoses may be strongly suspected by MRI characteristics. These diagnoses include lipoma, liposarcoma, benign vascular lesions such as hemangioma, arteriovenous malformation, and pseudoaneurysm, hemosidern-laden lesions such as pigmented villonodular synovitis, fibromatosis, subacute hematomas, and ganglion cysts. The radiological evaluation of soft tissue tumors requires a close working relationship between the surgeon and radiologist in order to obtain the optimum MRI evaluation, including the appropriate use of T1-weighted, T2-weighted, stir image sequences, and a determination as to whether contrast agents such as gadolinium DTPA should be utilized. In addition to imaging at the local site, a chest CT scan is a useful screening tool to evaluate for pulmonary metastases.

A great deal of prognostic information can be gained by a thorough histopathologic evaluation of soft tissue tumors. A comprehensive review of classification schemes is beyond the scope of this chapter, but an excellent review has been presented by Hajdu and D'Ambrosia.[10] Regardless of the nature of the soft tissue lesion, pathologists may enhance the histopathologic diagnosis of soft tissue sarcomas by knowing the clinical presentation, size, and site of the tumor, and the age of the patient. There are three important components required for the accurate assessment of the malignant potential of a soft tissue sarcoma and these are used to determine its stage:

1 the histologic grade of the tumor,
2 the size of the tumor, i.e., whether the tumor is small (<5 cm) or large (>5 cm),
3 whether the tumor is superficial (above the superficial fascia) or deep (below the superficial fascia).

Grade is determined by several histologic criteria, which are outlined in Table 30.1.

Stage is determined by a combination of grading criteria as well as by the size and location of the tumor. There are currently two grading schemes used for soft tissue sarcomas, the system developed by the American Joint

Committee of Cancer (AJCC) (Tables 30.2 and 30.3) and the Memorial Sloan-Kettering Cancer Center (MSKCC) staging system (Table 30.4; Table 30.5). These systems combine the various tumor characteristics, which are then used to arrive at a stage, which is predictive of survival. Both systems are generally based on three criteria: tumor size, tumor grade, and the presence or absence of metastatic disease. The MSKCC system also considers the relationship of the tumor to the superficial fascia.

Table 30.1 *Grading of sarcomas*

Low-grade sarcomas	High-grade sarcomas
Good differentiation	Poor differentiation
Hypocellular	Hypercellular
Hypovascular	Hypervascular
Much stroma	Minimal stroma
Minimal necrosis	Much necrosis
<5 mitoses/high power field	>5 mitoses/high power field

Table 30.2 *AJCC staging parameters*

Stage or grade	Characteristics
Stage	
TX	Minimum requirements to assess primary tumor not metastasis
T0	No demonstrable tumor
T1	Tumor <5 cm
T2	Tumor >5 cm
T3	Destruction of cortical bone with invasion, invasion of major artery or nerve
N1	Histologically verified metastasis in regional lymph node
M1	Distant metastasis (clinical or radiologic evidence)
Grade	
G1	Well differentiated
G2	Moderately well differentiated
G3	Poorly differentiated

Table 30.3 *AJCC staging*

Stage	G	T	N	M
IA	1	1	0	0
IB	1	2	0	0
IIA	2	1	0	0
IIB	2	2	0	0
IIIA	3	1	0	0
IIIB	3	2	0	0
IIIC	1–3	1–2	1	0
IVA	1–3	3	0–1	0
IVB	1–3	1–3	0–1	1

Table 30.4 *MSKCC staging protocol*

Stage	Grade	Size (cm)	Depth
0	Low	<5	Superficial
I	Low	<5	Deep
	Low	>5	Superficial
	High	<5	Superficial
II	Low	>5	Deep
	High	<5	Deep
	High	<5	Deep
III	High	>5	Deep

Table 30.5 *Comparison of staging systems*

Stage	MSKCC signs	AJCC signs
0	3 favorable	
I	2 favorable	G1 T1 N0 M0
II	1 favorable	G2 T1 N0 M0
		G2 T2 N0 M0
III	0 favorable	G3 T1 N0 M0
		G3 T2 N0 M0
		G1–3 T1–2 N1 M0
IV	Distant metastases	T3 or distant metastases

SURGICAL THERAPY

Simple excision of soft tissue sarcomas has resulted in an unacceptably high rate of local recurrence, as high as 65%.[11] This resulted in amputation or compartment resection in an effort to obtain better local control rates, but local failure still occurred in 20–30% of cases.[12] Over the past two decades, significant advances have been made with respect to multimodality treatment of this disease, achieving local control rates of 95% and an amputation rate of less than 10%. These studies have combined either preoperative radiotherapy[13] or postoperative radiotherapy[14] with extremity-sparing surgery. Other investigators have included preoperative chemotherapy combined with radiation therapy in the treatment regimen, with excellent result.[15]

Brennan at the Memorial Sloan-Kettering Cancer Center in New York City has described the management strategy utilizing excision and postoperative brachytherapy.[16] The approach to high-grade, large tumors is wide local excision of the tumor with several centimeters of surrounding normal tissue if possible. This is followed by the intraoperative placement of iridium-192 sources directly into the tumor bed. This approach resulted in a decreased local recurrence rate in patients with high-grade tumors, but has not had an effect on local control in low-grade tumors. However, this approach was accompanied by an increase in wound complications at the operative site (22% in patients receiving brachytherapy compared to 3% in those receiving no therapy).

Eilber and colleagues at the University of California at Los Angeles have had extensive experience with neoadjuvant chemotherapy and radiation therapy in the treatment of extremity soft tissue sarcomas.[17] Encouraged by the improvements in outcome in the treatment of rhabdomyosarcoma in children when treated with multimodality therapy, they embarked upon a series of experiments to evaluate multimodality treatment of soft tissue sarcomas of the extremities. The concept was to give preoperative therapy before extensive surgical resection. The theoretical advantages of this approach were that:

1 chemotherapy and radiation are given to the tumor with undisturbed tissue planes and therefore better blood supply,
2 preoperative treatment provides an evaluation of the clinical response of the tumor to chemotherapy and radiation,
3 the reduction in tumor size and clarification of the tumor pseudocapsule allow for more adequate excision of the primary tumor.

Patients with high-grade tumors were treated with a neoadjuvant protocol. The primary tumor was resected 5 days to 2 weeks after preoperative therapy by wide local excision through normal tissue planes, with pathologic confirmation of tumor-free margins. No attempt was made to perform muscle group or compartment resections. For protocol 1 there was a minimum follow-up of 11 years in a group that consisted of 77 patients receiving preoperative intra-arterial adriamycin and 35 cGy to the extremity. Four patients required amputation (5.2%), two for primary disease, one for complications, and one for local recurrence. There were seven local recurrences (9%). Complications occurred in 27 patients (35%), and 12 required surgical correction of the complication. Pathologic necrosis in the tumor ranged from 10% to 100% (median 70%). There were nine complete pathologic responses (11.7%).

Because of the high local complication rate, the radiation dose was reduced in protocol 2 from 35 cGy to 17.5 cGy. Complications occurred in 35 (26%) of 137 patients, but only eight complications required reparation. However, the local recurrence rate increased to 15%. Ten amputations were required (7.3%), three for primary disease, five for local failure, and two for complications. The median necrosis rate dropped to 45% and there were only five complete responses to therapy (3.6%).

Protocol 3 evaluated the route of administration of chemotherapy, comparing intra-arterial doxorubicin to intravenous doxorubicin. Because of the results of protocol 2, the dose of radiation therapy was increased to 28 cGy in all 112 patients. There was a 9% local failure rate, equally distributed between the intra-arterial and intravenous chemotherapy groups. There were 26 wound complications (23%), which were also equally distributed between the intra-arterial and intravenous chemotherapy groups. Six patients required amputation (5.4%), one for primary tumor, three for local failure, and two for complications. The median tumor necrosis rate was 60%, with seven complete responses (6.3%). There were no differences in any of these parameters between the intra-arterial and intravenous arms of the protocol.

Because intra-arterial administration of chemotherapy appeared to offer no therapeutic advantage, protocol 4 consisted of intravenous doxorubicin combined with intravenous cisplatinum and the same radiation dose as protocol 3 (28 cGy). There were 46 patients enrolled in this trial. The complication rate was 18% (eight patients with four requiring operation.) Four amputations were required, one for primary tumor, two for recurrence and one for complications. The median tumor necrosis rate was 70%, with five complete responses (10.9%).

Protocol 5 added ifosfamide to the regimen given in protocol 4. Forty-four patients were treated. The complication rate was again 18% (eight patients with one requiring reparation). There was only one local failure and two (4.5%) amputations, both for primary tumor. The median tumor cell necrosis rate rose to 95% and 17 patients (39%) had complete responses.

Overall, for these five protocols there was a 10% local recurrence rate, a 27% complication rate, and a 5% amputation rate. Eilber and associates emphasize that the limb salvage rate in all of these protocols is extremely high (95%),[17] which is much better than rates for surgery alone, which range from 35–50% in various series. Most series with postoperative radiation therapy quote a limb salvage rate of 90%.

Barkley and associates from the University of Texas M.D. Anderson Cancer Center have reviewed their experience with the use of preoperative radiation therapy and conservative surgical resection in the treatment of soft tissue sarcomas.[18] The patients were selected for preoperative treatment because of large size of the tumor, or location that would require amputation if surgery were performed as the primary therapeutic modality. In the 110 patients who completed therapy, none required amputation and the wound complication rate was 14%. Ten patients developed a local recurrence with three of these being salvaged with amputation.

There would appear to be little dispute that multimodality therapy achieves improved results in the treatment of extremity sarcoma. However, there are vast differences among institutions regarding the timing and sequence of therapy as well as the choice of therapeutic modalities. Overall, the results from these institutions would appear to be similar with respect to local control and overall survival, regardless of the sequence of therapy. It should be noted, however, that all of these groups have dedicated groups of investigators working closely together to provide integrated multimodality treatment.

FUTURE CONSIDERATIONS

Currently, a great deal of investigation revolves around two issues: (1) the clinical significance of local failure, and (2) improving the overall survival. As discussed above, most series utilizing multimodality therapy quote a local failure rate of less than 10% in high-grade tumors. It is important to note that local control rates in low-grade sarcomas do not appear to be improved by either preoperative or postoperative radiation therapy. Furthermore, one might expect that patients with high-grade tumors who develop a local recurrence would have a worse overall survival than those who remained disease free at the local site, but this is not the case. The group at Memorial Sloan-Kettering Cancer Center[19] has studied this issue extensively and their results show that, despite a higher local recurrence rate in patients who did not receive radiation therapy (35% local recurrence versus 18% local recurrence in patients receiving brachytherapy), 5-year survival in these two groups was the same (80% for patients not receiving radiation versus 81% for those who did). In a series of 1041 patients treated at Memorial Sloan-Kettering Cancer Center, Pisters et al.[20] found that the presence of a microscopically positive surgical margin was an independent adverse prognostic factor for both local recurrence and disease-specific survival in these patients. A positive microscopic margin was associated with increasing size and depth of the primary tumor as well as large surgical blood loss and long duration of operation. Although, as stated above, radiation therapy will reduce the incidence of local recurrence in patients with microscopic positive surgical margins, this has no impact upon the development of distant metastases or overall survival in these patients. Thus, when a limb-sparing resection is carried out in experienced hands with a maximal extent of resection, the presence of a positive microscopic surgical margin is not necessarily an indication for amputation. This finding does provide important adverse prognostic information regarding the risk for future recurrence in these patients.

The quest for improved overall survival in this disease continues. To date, there have been few trials of systemic adjuvant chemotherapy for soft tissue sarcoma that have provided encouraging results. Baker and Zalupski[21] recently reviewed this issue. Adjuvant therapy trials are difficult because no one institution has enough patients fulfilling specific randomization categories to derive meaningful data. As pointed out by these authors, the demonstration of a significant increase in metastasis-free survival from 30% to 50% with adjuvant therapy requires 184 available patients. Of 11 trials that have attempted to evaluate adjuvant chemotherapy, only one has accrued this many patients. It is beyond the scope of this chapter on surgical strategies to review these trials, but the inclusion of local recurrences and disease-free survival statistics, as is done in many of these trials, interferes with an assessment of the *systemic* effects of adjuvant therapy. In addition, there are several differences of note among these trials that make comparison difficult, such as:

1 the percentage of high-grade tumors in each study varies considerably and tumor size is often not stated,
2 the dose intensity of doxorubicin varies nearly four-fold among the trials,
3 the duration of therapy ranged from 4 months to 2 years,
4 initiation of chemotherapy ranged from several weeks to several months.

Despite the difficulties enumerated above, there has been progress in the treatment of soft tissue sarcomas. The development of consistent methods of grading and staging tumors; the understanding of the prognostic significance of (1) staging systems, (2) local recurrence, and (3) response to preoperative chemotherapy; and the application of adjuvant trials based upon data derived from these prognostic factors provide methods that will aid greatly in the development of future multi-institutional trials.

REFERENCES

1. Martland HS, Humphries RE. Osteogenic sarcoma in dial painters using luminous paint. Arch Pathol 1929; 7:406–17.
2. Cahan WG, Woodard HQ, Higinbotham NL, *et al.* Sarcoma arising in irradiation: report of eleven cases. Cancer 1948; 1:3–29.
3. Davidson T, Westbury G, Harmer CL. Radiation induced soft-tissue carcinoma. Br J Surg 1981; 73:308–9.
4. Robinson E, Neugut AI, Wylie P. Review: clinical aspects of postirradiation sarcomas. J Natl Cancer Inst 1988; 80:233–40.
5. Tucker MA, D'Angio GJ, Boice JD, *et al.* For the Late Effects Study Group. Bone sarcomas linked to radiotherapy and chemotherapy in children. N Engl J Med 1987; 317:588–93.
6. Lloyd JW. Angiosarcoma of the liver of vinyl chloride/polyvinyl chloride production workers. J Occup Med 1975; 17:333–4.
7. Hartley AL, Birch JM, Blair V, *et al.* Patterns of cancer in the families of children with soft tissue sarcoma. Cancer 1992; 326:1301–8.
8. Toguchida J, Yamaguchi T, Dayton SH, *et al.* Prevalence and spectrum of germline mutations of the *p53* gene among patients with sarcoma. N Engl J Med 1992; 326:1350–2.
9. Kransdorf MJ, Jelinek JS, Moser RP. Imaging of soft tissue tumors. Radiat Clin North Am 1993; 31:359–72.
10. Hajdu SI, D'Ambosia FG. Histopathologic classification of limb sarcomas in relation to prognosis. Surg Clin North Am 1993; 2:509–35.
11. Alho A, Alvegard TA, Berlin O, *et al.* Surgical margin in soft tissue sarcoma: the Scandinavian Sarcoma Group experience. Acta Orthop Scand 1989; 60:687–92.
12. Rosenberg SA, Glatstein EJ. Perspectives on the role of surgery and radiation therapy in the treatment of soft tissue sarcomas of the extremities. Semin Oncol 1981; 8:190–200.
13. Suit HD, Poppe KH, Mankin HJ, Wood WC. Preoperative radiation therapy for sarcoma of soft tissue. Cancer 1981; 47:2269–74.
14. Lindberg RD, Martin RG, Romsdahl MD, Barkley HT. Conservative surgery and postoperative radiotherapy in 300 adults with soft tissue sarcomas. Cancer 1981; 47:2391–7.
15. Eilber FR, Morton DL, Eckardt J, Grant T, Weisenburger T. Limb salvage for skeletal and soft tissue sarcomas: multidisciplinary preoperative therapy. Cancer 1984; 53:2579–84.
16. Brennan MF. Management of extremity of soft-tissue sarcomas. Am J Surg 1989; 158:71–8.
17. Eilber FR, Eckardt GR, Yao SF, Seeger LL, Selch MT. Neoadjuvant chemotherapy and radiotherapy in the multidisciplinary management of soft tissue sarcomas of the extremity. Surg Oncol Clin North Am 1993; 2(6):511–620.
18. Barkley HT, Martin RG, Lindberg R, Zasars SK. Treatment of soft tissue sarcomas by preoperative irradiation and conservative surgical resection. Int J Radiat Oncol Biol Phys 1988; 14(4):653–9.
19. Harrison LB, Franzese F, Ganor JJ, Brennan MF. Long-term results of a prospective randomized trial of adjuvant brachytherapy in the management of completely resected soft tissue sarcomas of the extremity and superficial trunk. Int J Radiat Oncol Biol Phys 1993; 27:259–65.
20. Pisters PW, Leung DH, Woodruff J, Shi W, Brennan MF. Analysis of prognostic factors in 1,041 patients with localized soft tissue sarcomas of the extremities. J Clin Oncol 1996; 14(5):1679–89.
21. Baker LH, Zalupski M. Sarcoma: the role of adjuvant chemotherapy and a proposed new staging system. Monogr Pathol 1996; 38:240–51.

Author's note. The following articles, though not cited in the chapter, were used as references for it.

Rougraff B. The diagnosis and management of soft tissue sarcomas of the extremities in the adult. Curr Prob Cancer 1999; 23(1):1–50.

Pisters PWT. Combined modality treatment of extremity soft tissue sarcomas. Ann Surg Oncol 1998; 5(5):464–72.

Valle AA, Kraybill WG. Management of soft tissue sarcomas of the extremity in adults. J Surg Oncol 1966; 63:271–9.

Commentary 1

CHARLES FORSCHER

Dr Huth has provided a useful overview of the management of extremity soft tissue sarcomas. The summary of the current concepts of the etiology, staging, and surgical management of these tumors is concise and straightforward. Several points merit additional comment.

ETIOLOGY AND CLASSIFICATION

It is important to remember that there are many different types of soft tissue sarcomas which tend to be lumped together for purposes of management and analysis. We recognize differences in carcinomas based upon histology and site of origin but view adult sarcomas as one large category. Whereas patterns of failure tend to be similar for most sarcomas, hematogenous dissemination to the lung, for example, differences based on specific subtypes do exist. Myxoid liposarcomas of the extremity may present with metastasis to the retroperitoneum in addition to the lung – somewhat unique for sarcomas.[1] Although sarcomas are grouped together in part for the purpose of accrual to trials, it is clear that some tumors tend to be highly chemosensitive (e.g., synovial sarcoma) and others tend to be relatively chemoresistant (e.g., leiomyosarcoma, alveolar soft part sarcoma). The ability to delineate a useful therapy can be difficult in a setting in which sensitive and resistant sarcoma subtypes are mixed together.

Again, although we tend to view sarcomas as a single entity, there can be wide variation in clinical behavior within a single histologic subtype. Liposarcomas can range from relatively indolent tumors such as myxoid or well-differentiated liposarcomas with slow growth rates to round-cell or pleomorphic liposarcomas which are generally extremely high-grade tumors. Newer approaches, such as differentiation therapy, may be applicable to only certain subtypes of this disease.[2,3]

In the future, we should have improved knowledge of the genetic basis for different sarcomas. Synovial sarcomas demonstrate different fusion proteins: SYT-SSX1 and SYT-SSX-2 reflecting the product of the X:18 translocation observed in this disease. At present, the ability to detect these proteins holds promise as a diagnostic tool, and in the future may have prognostic and therapeutic applications.[4,5] Different fusion proteins in childhood rhabdomyosarcoma appear to have prognostic significance.[6]

STAGING

The revised American Joint Committee on Cancer (AJCC) staging system takes into account the observation from Memorial Sloan-Kettering Cancer Center (MSKCC) as to

Table 1. *Staging of sarcomas based on a tumor–node–metastasis–grade system*[7]

Tumor
  T1 tumors are ≤5 cm
    T1a – superficial to superficial fascia
    T1b – deep to superficial fascia
  T2 tumors are >5 cm
    T2a – superficial to superficial fascia
    T2b – deep to superficial fascia
Grade – either 1, 2, 3, or 4
  Grade 1 – well differentiated
  Grade 2 – moderately differentiated
  Grade 3 – poorly differentiated
  Grade 4 – undifferentiated
Regional lymph nodes
Distant metastases
Stage I
  Stage IA – G1, 2; T1a, b; N0; M0
  Stage IB – G1, 2; T2a; N0; M0
Stage II
  Stage IIA – G1, 2; T2b; N0; M0
  Stage IIB – G3, 4; T1a, b; N0; M0
  Stage IIC – G3, 4; T2a; N0; M0
Stage III – G3,4; T2b; N0; M0
Stage IV
  Stage IVA – any G; any T; N1; M0
  Stage IVB – any G; any T; any N; M1

T, tumor; G, grade; N, regional lymph nodes; M, distant metastases.

the importance of tumor depth as a prognostic factor. Now high-grade superficial tumors can be placed in an intermediate category reflecting their somewhat better prognosis compared to deep lesions of similar grade (Table 1).

One additional factor to bear in mind is that size is a continuous variable in the sarcomas. Tumors greater than 20 cm have a poorer prognosis than those whose size is between 10 cm and 20 cm, which is in turn worse than that of tumors which are between 5 cm and 10 cm.

SURGICAL AND COMBINED MODALITY MANAGEMENT

Dr Huth cogently summarizes the current surgical approaches at MSKCC, UCLA and MD Anderson. Interestingly, each institution has a slightly different approach:

MSKCC: surgery followed by postoperative brachytherapy.

UCLA: preoperative chemotherapy and radiation followed by surgery.

MD Anderson: preoperative radiation followed by surgery.

These diverse methods result in excellent local control rates, with local failure occurring in 10% or less of those treated. However, local control is only part of the picture. Survival and particularly disease-free survival are of paramount importance. In large, high-grade extremity sarcomas, data are emerging which point to the importance of chemotherapy in the management of these lesions.

A trial from the Italian Sarcoma Group compared the addition of chemotherapy with ifosfamide and epirubicin to surgery and radiation for large, high-grade extremity sarcomas.[8] Fifty-three patients received chemotherapy and 51 patients did not. The trial was stopped early as disease-free survival and overall survival were superior in the group who received chemotherapy. Further follow-up continues to show an advantage for the chemotherapy-treated group.[9,10]

A meta-analysis has been performed by the British Medical Research Council which analysed the use of adjuvant chemotherapy (primarily doxorubicin) in 1568 patients from multiple randomized trials. This study demonstrates a significant advantage for chemotherapy in local relapse-free interval, distant relapse-free interval, and a trend toward improvement in overall survival which did not reach statistical significance. This study included patients with trunk and abdominal sarcomas in addition to extremity lesions. When only extremity sarcomas are analysed, the benefit in overall survival with the use of chemotherapy is more pronounced.[11]

Data from separate studies at UCLA and Washington Cancer Institute suggest that the assessment of pathologic response to chemotherapy in soft tissue sarcomas may be an important factor, as it is in osteosarcoma of bone.[12] At UCLA, those with greater than 95% tumor necrosis in response to preoperative chemotherapy and radiation had a disease-free survival of 62% and an overall survival of 88%. Those with less than 95% necrosis had a disease-free survival of 47% and overall survival of 58% ($p = 0.001$ and $p = 0.003$). Several different regimens of chemotherapy and radiation have been used, including doxorubicin, cisplatin, and, more recently, incorporating ifosfamide. The addition of ifosfamide increased the percentage of patients achieving a good pathologic response (46% versus 13%). The Washington group utilized two different chemotherapy regimens including doxorubicin, intra-arterial cisplatin, and ifosfamide prior to surgery. Again disease-free survival and overall survival were superior in the group with ≥95% tumor necrosis (77% and 88%) versus the group with <95% necrosis (65% and 74%).

SUMMARY

Combined modality therapy with surgery, radiation, and chemotherapy, and a better understanding of the basic biology of soft tissue sarcomas should lead to techniques for better functional results and improved survival for our patients. It is hoped that the future will allow us to give more targeted (and ideally less toxic) treatments, with greater likelihood of benefit, and also to know which patients can be spared the toxic effects of treatment.

REFERENCES

1. Enzinger F, Weiss S (eds). In *Soft tissue tumors*, 3rd edn. Mosby, 1995, 462–3.
2. Demetri GD, Spiegelman B, Fletcher CDM, *et al.* Differentiation therapy for liposarcomas using troglitazone, a ligand for the PPAR-γ nuclear receptor: clinical translation of promising preclinical observations. ASCO Proc 1998; 17:517a.
3. Demetri GD, Spiegelman B, Fletcher CD, *et al.* Differentiation of liposarcomas in patients treated with the PPAR γ ligand troglitazone: documentation of biologic activity in myxoid/round cell and pleomorphic subtypes. ASCO Proc 1999; 18: Abstract 2064.
4. Kawai A, Woodruff J, Healey JH, *et al.* SYT–SSX gene fusion as a determinant of morphology and prognosis in synovial sarcoma. N Engl J Med 1998; 338(3):153–60.
5. Inagaki H, Nagasaka T, Otsuka T, *et al.* Association of SYT–SSX fusion types with proliferative activity and prognosis in synovial sarcoma. Mod Pathol 2000; 13(5):482–8.
6. Lynch JC, Triche TJ, Qualman SJ, *et al.* Prognostic significance of PAX3–FKHR and PAX7–FKHR gene fusions alveolar rhabdomyosarcoma. ASCO Proc 1999; 584a, Abstract 2299.
7. Fleming ID, Cooper JS, Henson DE, *et al.* (eds). Staging of sarcomas based on a tumor-node-metastasis-grade system. In *AJCC cancer staging manual*. Lippincott-Raven, 1992, 149–56.
8. Frustaci S, Gherlinzoni F, De Paoli A, *et al.* Preliminary results of an adjuvant randomized trial on high risk extremity soft tissue sarcomas (STS). The interim analyses. ASCO Proc 1997; 16:496a.
9. Frustaci S, Gherlinzoni F, De Paoli A, *et al.* Maintenance of efficacy of adjuvant chemotherapy (CT) in soft tissue sarcoma (STS) of the extremities: up-date of a randomized trial. ASCO Proc 1999; 18:546a.
10. Adjuvant chemotherapy for localized resectable soft-tissue sarcoma of adults: meta-analysis of individual data. Sarcoma Meta-analysis Collaboration. Lancet 1997; 350(9092):1647–54.
11. Henshaw RM, Priebat D, Perry D, *et al.* Induction chemotherapy for high grade extremity soft tissue sarcomas: histologic response and correlation of tumor necrosis to long term disease free and overall patient survival. ASCO Proc 2000; 19:553a, Abstract 2177.
12. Eilber FC, Rosen G, Eckardt J, *et al.* Treatment induced pathologic necrosis as a predictor of survival in patients receiving pre-operative therapy for extremity soft tissue sarcomas. Connective Tissue Oncology Society 5th Annual Meeting Abstracts. 1999, 11.

Commentary 2

ALLAN W SILBERMAN

Dr Huth has pointed out in his chapter on soft tissue sarcomas of the extremities that local control rates of 95% have been achieved with multimodality therapy. With high-grade tumors, this approach has a local failure rate of about 10%. The addition of either preoperative or postoperative radiation does not seem to improve upon the local failure rate of low-grade tumors. Although local control is still an important issue with extremity sarcomas originating from soft tissue, Dr Forscher points out that improving the disease-free survival and overall survival has become the paramount issue. The problem of

local control, however, remains the primary issue with soft tissues sarcomas arising from the retroperitoneum.

Retroperitoneal sarcomas are rare, insidious tumors, accounting for approximately 0.1% of all malignancies and < 15% of adult soft tissue sarcomas.[1] Like soft tissue sarcomas of the extremities, they are a varied group of malignancies arising from mesenchymal tissue. In an early series of 78 cases from Memorial Sloan-Kettering, the most common histology was liposarcoma (23/78), followed by leiomyosarcoma (14/78), and fibrosarcoma (12/78).[2] A recent report from the same institution

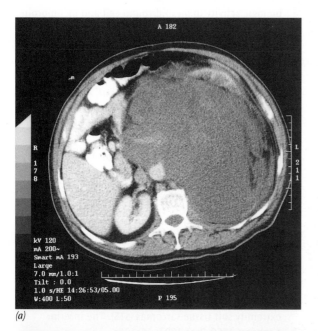

(a)

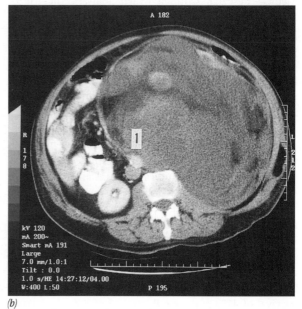

(b)

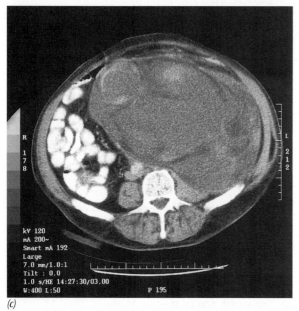

(c)

Figure 1 *CT scans of a massive left-sided retroperitoneal liposarcoma totally encompassing the left kidney and pushing the normal viscera, aorta, and inferior vena cava to the right (1). See also Plates 12 and 13.*

analysing 500 patients again showed liposarcoma (41%) and leiomyosarcoma (27%) to be the most common histologic subtypes.[3] The early symptoms of retroperitoneal sarcomas are usually vague, because the loose areolar tissue of the retroperitoneal space allows the tumor to expand relatively easily in several directions, except into the posterior musculature. Consequently, these tumors are often quite large when symptoms first occur and a diagnosis is established. The most frequent clinical presentations are weight loss and abdominal pain and/or a palpable abdominal or flank mass, but non-specific symptoms such as nausea, vomiting, and back pain are not unusual. More subtle presentations include neurologic symptoms from pressure or invasion of nerves such

as the femoral, genito-femoral or obturator nerves, or lower extremity swelling or edema from encroachment on the inferior vena cavae or iliac vein. These more subtle signs and symptoms often lead to delays in diagnosis because the medical evaluation is directed to neurologic or vascular studies, whereas the abdomen and retroperitoneum are not initially considered.

Computed tomography (CT) is the single most useful diagnostic procedure in the preoperative evaluation of patients with retroperitoneal masses. In addition to demonstrating the size and consistency of the tumor and its relationship to, and possible displacement of, adjacent retroperitoneal structures, CT-directed biopsies, either fine-needle aspirates or needle core biopsies, can lead

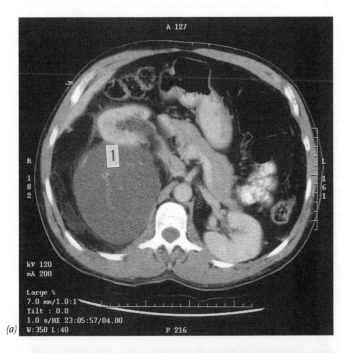

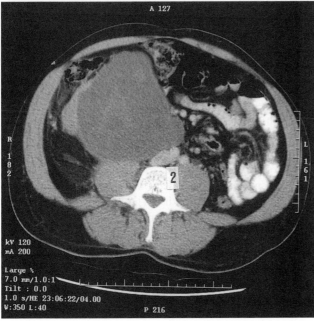

Figure 2 *(a) CT scan demonstrating right-sided retroperitoneal liposarcoma displacing the right kidney anteriorly (1). (b) Tumor mass pushing the inferior vena cava and iliac vessels to the left (2). Resection of the mass required partial non-anatomic right hepatic lobectomy, right hemicolectomy, and right uretero-nephrectomy, along with portions of retroperitoneal musculature.*

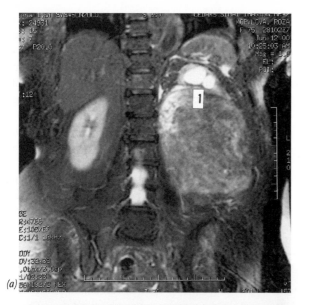

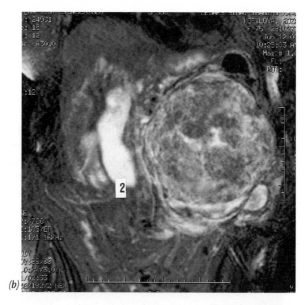

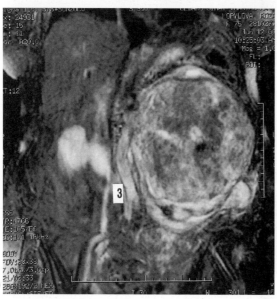

Figure 3 *(a) MRI scan demonstrating large, recurrent left-sided retroperitoneal liposarcoma displacing the left kidney and spleen superiorly (1). (b) Tumor causing obstruction of the proximal jejunum (2). (c) Tumor pushing the aorta to the right (3).*

to a tissue diagnosis which can be helpful in treatment planning and consideration of neoadjuvant therapy. Moreover, preoperative CT-guided biopsies will sometimes establish a diagnosis of a non-sarcomatous retroperitoneal malignancy, which may be more appropriately treated with non-surgical therapy, for example lymphomas or germ cell tumors. Magnetic resonance imaging (MRI) scans are increasingly being obtained preoperatively and can add additional information regarding tumor heterogeneity and vascular involvement; however, in this cost-cutting era, it is difficult to justify both CT and MRI unless a specific question, for example, patency of the portal vein or superior mesenteric vein, is being raised. Barium studies, intravenous pyelography, and arteriography, although still occasionally used in the preoperative evaluation of the patient with a retroperitoneal mass, have assumed much less importance since the introduction of CT and MRI.

The treatment of retroperitoneal sarcomas is simply stated, but often difficult to achieve: the complete removal of the tumor with clear surgical margins. As in other solid tumors, it is clear that the first surgical attempt at tumor removal is the best chance to cure the patient. In Lewis' analysis of 500 patients with retroperitoneal sarcomas, those presenting with primary disease had an 83% resection rate, with a median survival of 72 months. Those patients presenting with a local recurrence had a resection rate of 52%, with a median survival of 28 months.[3] The first surgical attempt for a left-sided retroperitoneal sarcoma may involve resection of diaphragm, stomach, pancreas, spleen, adrenal, kidney and ureter, small bowel, colon, pelvic organs, and vascular structures, with or without grafting (Figure 1, Plates 12 and 13). Removal of a right-sided retroperitoneal sarcoma may also involve resection of liver, biliary tract, and duodenum (Figure 2). These can be formidable, time-consuming operations and should be done at institutions where there is both experience and interest in the problem. The MRI scan shown in Figure 3 is from a patient presenting to our group who previously underwent two attempts at resection for a left-sided, well-differentiated liposarcoma for whom no organs were removed at either previous operation. Seventy percent distal pancreatectomy, splenectomy, adrenalectomy, uretero-nephrectomy, small-bowel resection, and left hemicolectomy were required to achieve complete resection. There can be no hesitation to resect involved organs; moreover, bowel and kidney will often approximate the tumor mass, but not be directly invaded. These organs should be resected to provide additional margin. Function of the contralateral kidney, of course, needs to be confirmed preoperatively.

Unlike patients with soft tissue sarcomas of the extremities for whom the cause of death is usually due to distant metastatic disease to the lungs, most patients with retroperitoneal sarcomas die of local recurrence. In Lewis' study, 75% of the patients with primary retroperitoneal disease died in the *absence* of distant disease.[3] This, of course, raises the question of adjuvant therapy delivered to the local area. Unfortunately, it is often not possible to deliver therapeutic radiation doses to the retroperitoneum for the control of microscopic/residual disease because of the inclusion of dose-limiting normal structures (spinal cord, bladder, bowel) in the radiation field.[4] In addition, no study has definitely shown that adjuvant chemotherapy, given either preoperatively or postoperatively, is effective treatment for retroperitoneal sarcomas. Newer approaches, such as intraoperative and/or postoperative intraperitoneal chemotherapy, neoadjuvant chemoembolization, or immunotherapy, need to be added to aggressive surgical resection in order to improve upon the current results in these often fatal diseases.

REFERENCES

1. Kinsella TJ, Sindelar WF, Lock E, Glatstein E, Rosenberg SA. Preliminary results of a randomized study of adjuvant radiation therapy in resectable adult retroperitoneal soft tissue sarcomas. J Clin Oncol 1988; 6:18–25.

2. Fortner JG, Martin S, Hajdus S, Turnbull A. Primary sarcoma of the retroperitoneum. Semin Oncol 1981; 8:180–4.

3. Lewis JJ, Leung D, Woodruff JM, Brennan MF. Retroperitoneal soft-tissue sarcoma: analysis of 500 patients treated and followed at a single institution. Ann Surg 1998; 228:355–65.

4. Singer S, Corson JM, Demetri GD, Healey EA, Marcus K, Eberlein TJ. Prognostic factors predictive of survival for truncal and retroperitoneal soft tissue sarcoma. Ann Surg 1995; 221:185–95.

Editors' selected abstracts

Predicators of functional outcomes following limb salvage surgery for lower-extremity soft tissue sarcoma.

Davis AM, Sennik S, Griffin AM, Wunder JS, O'Sullivan B, Catton CN, Bell RS.

University Musculoskeletal Oncology Unit, Mount Sinai Hospital and the University of Toronto, Toronto, Canada.

Journal of Surgical Oncology 73(4):206–11, 2000, April.

Background and objectives: Patient function has been conceptualized by clinical measures such as joint motion, muscle strength, disability, and general health status. The purpose of the current study was to evaluate tumor and treatment variables predictive of these conceptually different posttreatment functional outcomes in patients treated with limb preservation surgery for lower-extremity soft tissue sarcoma. *Methods:* One hundred seventy-two patients with minimum 1-year follow-up were evaluated using the following outcomes: impairment, measured by the 1987 and 1993 versions of the Musculoskeletal Tumor Society Rating Scale (MSTS); disability, measured by the Toronto Extremity Salvage Score (TESS); and general health status, using the Short Form-36 (SF-36). Tumor and treatment-related variables (age, gender, presenting disease status, anatomic site, tumor size, grade, depth, prior excision, irradiation, bone resection, motor nerve sacrifice, and complications) were extracted from the STS database. *Results:* Large tumor size, bone resection, motor nerve resection, and complications were predictive of lower MSTS 1987 and 1993 scores. Patients with large, high-grade tumors who required motor nerve resection were more disabled, as reflected by lower TESS scores. Only age and prior surgery were adverse predictors of SF-36 score. *Conclusions:* These results demonstrate that different factors are predictive of different patient outcomes, specifically, impairment, disability, and general health status. It is important to define function when counseling patients regarding their potential recovery based on tumor and treatment-related variables.

Extremity soft-tissue sarcomas selectively treated with surgery alone.

Fabrizio PL, Stafford SL, Pritchard DJ.

Division of Radiation Oncology, Mayo Clinic and Mayo Foundation, Rochester, MN, USA.

International Journal of Radiation Oncology, Biology, Physics 48(1):227–32, 2000, August 1.

Purpose: This study determined local control (LC), freedom from distant recurrence (FFDR), overall survival (OS), and potential prognostic factors in 34 adult patients with primary extremity or limb girdle soft-tissue sarcoma selectively managed with limb-conservation surgery alone. *Methods and materials:* The medical records of 34 patients who underwent surgery alone for localized soft-tissue sarcoma of the extremity were reviewed. Median duration of follow-up in survivors was 55 months (range, 24–143). There were 13 (38%) females. Eighteen (53%) of the tumors were low-grade, 15 (44%) were superficial, 15 (44%) were small (5 cm or less) and 16 (47%) involved the distal extremity. *Results:* Actuarial 5-year LC was 80%, FFDR was 86%, and OS was 82%. All recurrences (local and distant) were in patients with high-grade tumors; their 5-year LC was 60%, FFDR was 71%, and OS was 69%. In 2 patients, metastatic disease developed either concurrent with or after their local recurrence. Univariate analysis revealed better OS, FFDR, and LC for patients with low-grade tumors ($p < 0.05$). Female patients had significantly better FFDR and OS ($p < 0.05$). *Conclusion:* It is appropriate to consider withholding irradiation for selected patients with low-grade tumors resected with negative margins if, in the event of a local failure, a function-preserving surgical salvage is anticipated. For patients with high-grade sarcomas, the control of local and distant disease was not acceptable with limb-conservation surgery alone.

CT of recurrent retroperitoneal sarcomas.

Gupta AK, Cohan RH, Francis IR, Sondak VK, Korobkin M.

Department of Radiology, University of Michigan Hospitals, Ann Arbor, MI, USA.

American Journal of Roentgenology 174(4):1025–30, 2000, April.

Objective: We reviewed the medical records and CT scans of 33 patients with recurrent retroperitoneal sarcomas to determine the patterns of recurrent disease. *Materials and methods:* We reviewed the medical records and CT examinations obtained at the time the recurrence was diagnosed and tabulated data for all patients. Data for patients with high-grade malignancies were compared with those of patients with low-grade malignancies to determine whether there were differences in the interval between initial tumor resection and recurrence. We also compared CT appearances to determine patterns of recurrent disease. *Results:* Twenty-five of 33 recurrences were detected within 2 years of initial surgery. Only 16 patients had symptoms, and when present, most symptoms were nonspecific. In 28 (85%) patients, recurrent tumor was in the abdomen at the time of diagnosis. In nine patients, the largest detectable abdominal tumor was less than 5 cm in diameter. Interval to recurrence was similar for patients with low- and high-grade tumors. Although the CT appearance was similar for both grades, distant metastases were identified only in patients with high-grade malignancies. *Conclusion:* Primary retroperitoneal malignancies frequently recur within 2 years of initial surgical resection. For asymptomatic patients, diagnosis is typically made during routine follow-up CT. Most patients have abdominal recurrences that may be small when first detected.

Leiomyosarcoma of the inferior vena cava: prognosis and comparison with leiomyosarcoma of other anatomic sites.

Hines OJ, Nelson S, Quinones-Baldrich WJ, Eilber FR.

Department of Surgery, University of California–Los Angeles School of Medicine, Los Angeles, CA, USA.

Cancer 85(5):1077–83, 1999, March 1.

Background: Leiomyosarcoma of the inferior vena cava (IVC) is an uncommon tumor that many believe portends a poor prognosis compared with leiomyosarcoma with similar histology at other anatomic sites. Because of the limited international experience with this disease, the optimal management of these patients is unknown. *Methods:* From October 1978 to January 1997, 14 patients with leiomyosarcoma of the IVC were treated at the University of California–Los Angeles Medical Center. Wide resection was attempted in all patients. The characteristics of each patient were documented and compared with those of patients with leiomyosarcoma of the stomach ($n = 13$), small intestine ($n = 18$), retroperitoneum ($n = 19$), and uterus ($n = 10$) who were treated during the same time period. *Results:* Age, gender, tumor size, tumor grade, and lymph node status did not impact survival of patients with leiomyosarcoma of the IVC. Patients with positive surgical margins fared significantly worse ($p < 0.03$) compared with those who underwent complete resection. Radiation therapy diminished local recurrence and may improve median survival (6 months [$n = 2$] vs. 51 months [$n = 12$]) in this patient population. Patients who received combined chemotherapy and radiation lived longer than those who did not ($p < 0.05$). The 5-year cumulative survival rate (Kaplan–Meier method) was 53% for patients with leiomyosarcoma of the IVC, 47% for those with leiomyosarcoma of the stomach, 43% for those with leiomyosarcoma of the small intestine, 56% for those with leiomyosarcoma of the retroperitoneum, and 65% for those with leiomyosarcoma of the uterus. *Conclusions:* Despite having a tumor that originates from the IVC, patients with this tumor type can enjoy reasonably long term survival. It appears that these patients benefit from radiation therapy to control local disease. Survival of these patients is no worse than of patients with leiomyosarcomatous lesions of other origin. Aggressive surgical management combined with adjuvant therapy offers the best treatment for patients with leiomyosarcoma of the IVC.

Thoracoabdominal incisions and resection of upper retroperitoneal sarcomas.

Karakousis CP, Pourshahmir M.

State University of New York at Buffalo, Kaleida Health, Millard Fillmore Gates Hospital, Buffalo, NY, USA.

Journal of Surgical Oncology 72(3):150–5, 1999, November.

Background and objectives: There is a widespread impression among surgeons that a thoracoabdominal incision carries a substantially higher risk of morbidity and possible mortality over abdominal incisions. We decided therefore to critically review our experience of the last 4 years with these incisions. *Methods:* This is a retrospective review of all cases of retroperitoneal sarcomas of upper abdominal quadrants in the period May 1995 through February 1999. There were 33 consecutive patients and 34 thoracoabdominal incisions (1 patient had a second operation for recurrence). Their mean age was 54 years, with 13 >60 and 7 >70 years. *Results:* Eighteen patients were extubated immediately at the end of the procedure and the rest within 24 h. In the majority of instances (32 of 34 or 94%), the patients left the intensive care unit within 48 h. The most common postoperative complication was atelectasis (7 of 34, 21%). There was no postoperative death. The retroperitoneal tumor was resected in all 34 cases (100%). *Conclusions:* The thoracoabdominal incision for upper quadrant retroperitoneal sarcomas is tolerated well by the patients with a morbidity similar to that observed after routine abdominal incisions. It allows complete resection of the tumor in most (all in this series) cases.

Synovial sarcoma: a multivariate analysis of prognostic factors in 112 patients with primary localized tumors of the extremity.

Lewis JJ, Antonescu CR, Leung DH, Blumberg D, Healey JH, Woodruff JM, Brennan MF.

Departments of Surgery, Biostatistics, and Pathology, Memorial Sloan-Kettering Cancer Center, New York, NY, USA.

Journal of Clinical Oncology 18(10):2087–94, 2000, May.

Purpose: Synovial sarcoma is a high-grade tumor that is associated with poor prognosis. Previous studies analyzing prognostic factors are limited because of inclusion of heterogeneous cohorts of patients with nonextremity and recurrent tumors. The objective of this study was to determine independent prognostic factors of primary synovial sarcoma localized to the extremity. *Patients and methods:* Between July 1, 1982, and June 30, 1996, 112 patients underwent surgical resection for cure at our institution and then were followed-up prospectively. Clinical and pathologic factors examined for prognostic value included age, sex, tumor site and location, depth, size, microscopic status of surgical margins, invasion of bone or neurovascular structures, and monophasic or biphasic histology. The end points analyzed were the time to first local recurrence that was not preceded by a distant recurrence, time to any distant recurrence, and time to disease-related mortality. These end points were modeled using the method of Kaplan and Meier and analyzed by the log-rank test and Cox regression. *Results:* The median duration of follow-up among survivors in this cohort of 112 patients was 72 months. The 5-year local-recurrence, distant recurrence, and mortality rates were 12%, 39%, and 25%, respectively. Tumor size ≥ 5 cm ($p = 0.001$; relative risk [RR] = 2.7; 95% confidence interval [CI], 1.5 to 5.2) and the presence of bone or neurovascular invasion ($p = 0.04$, RR = 2.3; 95% CI, 1.0 to 5.3) were independent adverse predictors of distant recurrence. Tumor size ≥ 5 cm ($p = 0.003$; RR = 2.3; 95% CI, 1.4 to 6.3) and the presence of bone or neurovascular invasion ($p = 0.03$; RR = 2.7; 95% CI, 1.0 to 6.5) were also independent adverse predictors of mortality. *Conclusion:* The natural history of primary synovial sarcoma of the extremity is related to tumor size and invasion of bone and neurovascular structures.

Effect of reresection in extremity soft tissue sarcoma.

Lewis JJ, Leung D, Espat J, Woodruff JM, Brennan MF.

Departments of Surgery, Biostatistics, and Pathology, Memorial Sloan-Kettering Cancer Center, New York, NY, USA.

Annals of Surgery 231(5):655–63, 2000, May.

Objective: To determine whether reresection affects survival in patients with inadequately resected, primary extremity soft tissue sarcoma. This study correlates reresection with local recurrence-free survival, metastasis-free survival, and disease-free survival. *Summary background data:* Soft tissue sarcomas are rare neoplasms, with an incidence of approximately 6000 per year in the United States. Because these tumors are rare and benign soft tissue tumors are common, many are initially thought to be benign and are excised without wide margins. *Methods:* Patients who underwent treatment for primary tumors from July 1982 to June 1999 at a single institution were the subject of study. Two groups of patients were analyzed: those who underwent one definitive resection (one operation) and those whose tumors were previously resected and who were then referred for subsequent reresection (two operations). Patients were given adjuvant radiation or chemotherapy according to the standard of care. *Results:* Of 1092 patients with primary extremity soft tissue sarcoma who underwent resection, 685 underwent definitive radical resection and 407 underwent reresection after undergoing excisional resection elsewhere. Median follow-up was 4.8 years. The 5-year disease-free survival rate of the definitive resection (one operation) group was 70%; that of the reresection (two operations) group was 88%. On multivariate analysis, reresection was adjusted and controlled for age, grade, depth, size, histology, and margins. Reresection remained a significant predictor of improved disease-free survival, even after these adjustments. To determine whether this difference was stage- or referral-biased, the patient population was divided by AJCC stage. In all stages there was a trend toward improved outcome; this was most marked for those with stage III disease (> 5 cm, high-grade, and deep). *Conclusions:* Patients with extremity soft tissue sarcoma who undergo reresection with two 'primary' operations have an improved survival compared with those who undergo one operation. The most plausible explanation, referral and selection bias, is questionable given the significance of reresection as a variable after adjusting for stage and other risk factors. This suggests that where indicated and possible, reresection should be liberally applied in patients with primary extremity soft tissue sarcoma.

Influence of biologic factors and anatomic site in completely resected liposarcoma.

Linehan DC, Lewis JJ, Leung D, Brennan MF.

Departments of Surgery and Biostatistics, Memorial Sloan-Kettering Cancer Center, New York, NY, USA.

Journal of Clinical Oncology 18(8):1637–43, 2000, April.

Purpose: Soft tissue sarcoma (STS) encompasses a group of neoplasms that are anatomically and biologically diverse. Retroperitoneal/visceral (RP/V) tumors have a poorer prognosis than extremity/trunk (E/T) lesions, and this has been attributed to frequent presentation with tumors of large size and multiorgan involvement that precludes complete resection. The worse prognosis that is associated with RP/V tumors has also been thought to be histopathologically dependent and not necessarily related to anatomic site. The aim of this study was to determine the role of anatomic site and biologic features in prognosis and outcome in patients after complete resection by examining a large cohort of STS patients with a single histopathology, i.e., liposarcoma. *Methods:* All patients who were treated for liposarcoma from July 1, 1982, through July 1, 1998, were included. Univariate analyses were performed using log-rank test and Kaplan–Meier estimates, and multivariate analyses were performed using Cox regression. The three end points examined were local recurrence (LR), distant recurrence, and disease-specific survival (DSS). *Results:* Seven hundred twenty patients with liposarcoma were evaluated, and of these, 460 had completely resected primary or completely resected locally recurrent disease. Breakdown of anatomic site was 65% E/T ($n = 301$) and 35% RP/V ($n = 159$). The median follow-up period for patients who underwent complete resection was 42 months (range, 1 to 194 months). We found that RP/V site is a poor prognosticator that is independent of patient sex and age; tumor size, grade, and margin; and recurrent presentation. Sixty-nine percent of patients with RP/V tumors who died had local disease only and no distant metastasis at the time of death. *Conclusion:* In liposarcoma, tumor location exerts as strong an influence on prognosis as biology. In contrast to extremity liposarcoma, LR without distant metastasis often results in death for patients with RP/V tumors. For these patients, local control accomplished by complete surgical resection ± adjuvant radiation therapy should impact strongly on DSS.

A comparison of staging systems for localized extremity soft tissue sarcoma.

Wunder JS, Healey JH, Davis AM, Brennan MF.

University Musculoskeletal Oncology Unit, Mount Sinai Hospital, Department of Surgery, University of Toronto, Ontario, Canada.

Cancer 88(12):2721–30, 2000, June 15.

Background: Staging systems for soft tissue sarcoma (STS) are important to identify patients with similar systemic risk who might benefit from specific treatments. This study compared four commonly used staging systems for predicting systemic outcomes of patients with localized extremity STS, as proposed by the fourth and fifth editions of the American Joint Committee on Cancer/International Union Against Cancer (AJCC/UICC) staging system, the Memorial Sloan-Kettering Cancer Center (MSK) system, and the Surgical Staging System (SSS) of the Musculoskeletal Tumor Society. *Methods:* Three hundred consecutive adult patients with newly diagnosed nonmetastatic STS of the lower extremity were treated at Memorial Sloan-Kettering Cancer Center between 1982 and 1989. Metastasis-free survival was the end point of the study. The prognostic value of the four staging systems and their components were examined in univariate and multivariate analyses. The Akaike information criterion (AIC) was used to identify the system that best predicted the risk of systemic recurrence. *Results:* Compartment status, depth, grade, and size were all independent predictors of outcome within their respective staging systems. However, when compared with one another, only depth, grade, and size retained their prognostic significance. Of the four models, the AIC predicted that the MSK was the best predictor of systemic relapse, followed by the fifth edition of the AJCC/UICC staging system. *Conclusions:* Staging systems such as the MSK system or the fifth edition of the AJCC/UICC system, which include tumor depth, grade, and size as prognostic factors, are the most predictive of systemic relapse in patients presenting with localized extremity STS. Both of these systems identify the same group of patients at the highest risk who would be the most suitable for adjuvant chemotherapy trials.

31

Cryoablation of soft tissue sarcomas

LAWRENCE R MENENDEZ

INTRODUCTION

The treatment of soft tissue sarcomas remains controversial, but there is general agreement that local control of the tumor is essential in order to achieve a cure. The mainstay of treatment has therefore been wide surgical excision by means of a limb-sparing resection or amputation. In order to reduce the risk of local recurrence, radiation therapy has also been extensively utilized as a surgical adjuvant in the treatment of these tumors. The combination of surgery and radiation therapy has been generally effective in treating low-grade (stage IA and IB) sarcomas, but results have not been particularly impressive with high-grade (stage IIA and IIB) lesions.[1] More recently, patients with high-grade soft tissue sarcomas have also been treated with systemic chemotherapy in an attempt to improve local control and increase patient survival.

There are inherent problems with each of these treatment modalities. Wide surgical margins are sometimes difficult to achieve, especially when the tumor is adjacent to neurovascular structures, and many limb-sparing procedures result in major functional deficits and cosmetic deformities. Radiation therapy is also associated with significant risk and morbidity, including, for example, epidermolysis, fibrosis, stiffness, delayed wound healing, wound infection, radionecrosis of bone, degenerative arthritis, peripheral neuropathy, and the development of radiation-induced sarcomas. The morbidity of systemic chemotherapy in the treatment of cancer is well recognized and the efficacy of this modality in the treatment of soft tissue sarcomas is controversial.

In summary, the modalities currently used to achieve local control of soft tissue sarcomas are not completely effective and are associated with significant complications and morbidity. The search continues for another surgical adjuvant, which causes less morbidity than the current modalities and yet is as effective, or more so, in achieving local tumor control.

Cryosurgery is a therapeutic method of treating neoplastic tissue by freezing *in situ* in order to achieve devitalization.[2] The basic principles of cryosurgical techniques for the treatment of malignancies include rapid freezing, slow thawing, and the immediate repetition of the freezing and thawing cycle.[3,4] A tissue temperature of at least $-40\,^{\circ}\text{C}$ for at least 1 min is required to ensure cell necrosis.[2,5] The thawing process also disrupts cellular integrity by creating osmotic gradients and mechanical shearing forces.[6,7]

Cryoablation is now a recognized approach to the treatment of various malignant tumors occurring throughout the body.[2] The range of application of cryosurgical techniques to the treatment of cancer is widely diversified and is steadily increasing in scope. Cryosurgery is most useful in easily accessible areas of the body, but recent advances in technology now make it possible to treat tumors that are deep and relatively inaccessible. Cryoprobe transducers can provide a controllable and predictable area of necrosis, and their use is now the preferred method of cryosurgery in many situations. In addition, dramatic advances in imaging technology, especially the development of computer-enhanced, real-time intraoperative ultrasonography, have allowed the safe and precise monitoring of deep-seated visceral lesions that cannot be completely visualized. Malignancies in many parts of the body, including bone, have been treated with cryosurgical techniques. Until recently, soft tissue sarcomas had not been treated with this modality, even though these tumors are generally relatively accessible.

CRYOSURGERY OF SOFT TISSUE SARCOMAS: SAFETY AND FEASIBILITY

The results of a phase I study demonstrating the safety and feasibility of cryoablation of soft tissue extremity sarcomas have now been reported by Menendez and associates[8] at the University of Southern California (USC). Eligibility for entry into the USC study included: (1) biopsy-proven sarcoma; (2) absence of bone involvement; and (3) no prior treatment for the lesion. The evaluation and treatment of patients were planned in accordance with the schema shown in Figure 31.1. All

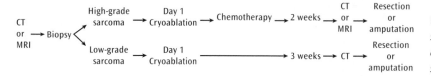

Figure 31.1 *Evaluation and treatment schema of phase I study of cryoablation of soft tissue extremity sarcomas.*

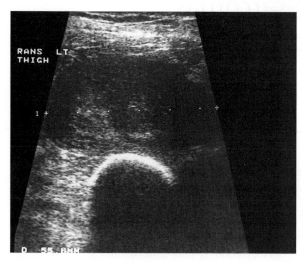

Figure 31.2 *Intraoperative ultrasonography of soft tissue sarcomas of the thigh using 7.5 MHz transducer. Note cursor used to measure tumor dimensions. Underlying femur appears as black hypoechoic mass surrounded by hyperechoic white rim.*

patients who met the eligibility criteria for this study underwent immediate cryoablation of the soft tissue sarcoma. The technique of cryoablation employed by Menendez *et al.* is as follows. The affected extremity is prepped and draped in the usual sterile fashion. Ultrasonography of the lesion is then performed utilizing 5.0 MHz or 7.5 MHz intraoperative transducers (BNK Medical Systems 3535 Ultrasound Scanning System). The dimensions of the tumor are measured and the volume to be cryoablated is calculated (Figure 31.2). A longitudinal incision is made over the sarcoma. Appropriate skin flaps or fascial cutaneous flaps are raised as needed. A cuff of normal tissue is left about the lesion except for a small strip along the more superficial area of the lesion. In this area, a small portion of the pseudocapsule of the tumor is visualized so that cryoprobes may be appropriately placed into the tumor. Any neurovascular structures not in direct continuity with the pseudocapsule are also mobilized and retracted. The skin flaps, fasciocutaneous flaps, and neurovascular structures are packed off with Gelfoam® (Upjohn Company, Kalamazoo, MI) and laparotomy pads. Ultrasonography is again performed and, once the lesion has been adequately visualized, one or more cryoprobes (Cryotech LCS 3000 Candela Laser Corporation, Wayland, MA; or CMS AccuProbe® 450 System Cryomedical Sciences, Inc., Rockville, MD) are strategically inserted into the lesion (Figure 31.3). Probes

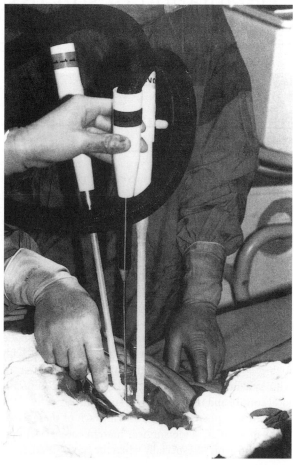

Figure 31.3 *Placement of three cryoprobes into sarcoma.*

of 3 mm, 8 mm, or 10 mm in diameter are inserted sequentially into the lesion at the discretion of the surgeon and depending on which cryoprobe system is employed. The probes are placed in such a manner as to insure a complete freeze of the tumor as well as a 5–10-mm cuff of normal tissue. Once the first cryoprobe reaches the appropriate position, which is documented with ultrasonography (Figure 31.4), it is secured in that position by passing liquid nitrogen into the probe and cooling it to approximately −100 °C so that it sticks to the surrounding tissue. Additional probes are inserted in an identical fashion as necessary. Once the probes are appropriately positioned and secured, liquid nitrogen is passed through these probes simultaneously in order to freeze the tumor. The freeze cycle is monitored with ultrasonography. The freezing interface is visualized as an advancing hyperechoic hemispheric rim with complete posterior or acoustic shadowing (Figure 31.5).

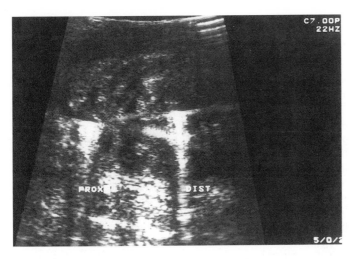

Figure 31.4 *The position of the cryoprobes is confirmed with intraoperative ultrasound.*

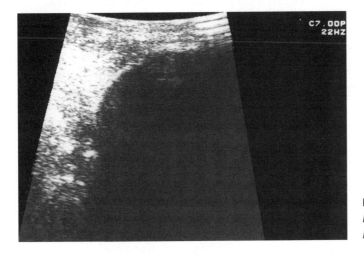

Figure 31.5 *Propagation of iceball viewed as hypoechoic mass surrounded by hyperechoic hemispheric rim.*

The iceball is extended beyond the tumor margin into normal tissue for a distance of 5–10 mm in an attempt to freeze satellite lesions that may be present in the reactive zone of the tumor. Once the iceball has reached the appropriate size, the flow of liquid nitrogen is halted and the iceball is allowed to thaw. Gaseous nitrogen is pumped through the probes to accelerate this process. When the probes reach a temperature of approximately 0 °C, a second freezing cycle is performed. The iceball is again monitored with the use of ultrasound and, once it has reached its appropriate size, gaseous nitrogen is again passed through the probes, allowing for another active thaw. Freezing temperatures, monitored with thermocouples located at the end of the probes, are maintained as close to −196 °C (the temperature of liquid nitrogen) as possible (see Plate 14). At the completion of the second thawing cycle, the probes are removed when the temperature at their tips reaches approximately 0 °C. The holes left by the cryoprobes are packed with Gelfoam®. The normal tissue over the strip of exposed pseudocapsule is approximated and the wound is irrigated. The fascia and skin are then closed in layers in routine fashion.

A suction drain is inserted prior to wound closure and compressive dressing is applied.

A total of 12 patients were entered into the USC trial. Patient data are summarized in Table 31.1. All of the sarcomas were resected after cryoablation. The resected specimens were examined histologically in order to determine the percentage of tumor necrosis and the adequacy of the surgical margins.

Cryoablation was successfully performed in all 12 patients. No cryosurgical ablation was considered suboptimal because of technical problems or considerations. No cryosurgical procedure had to be terminated because of intraoperative complications or technical considerations.

Complications are listed in Table 31.2. There were three cases each of peripheral nerve palsy and sterile serous wound drainage. There were no cases of wound infection, deep venous thrombosis, pulmonary embolism, nitrogen embolism, wound dehiscence, skin slough, or metabolic abnormalities. Postoperative pain was incisional only and no patients required prolonged or inordinate postoperative analgesic medication.

Table 31.1 *Patient data*

Patient	Sex	Age (years)	Diagnosis	Site	Stage
1	M	92	Malignant schwannoma	Right thigh	IIA
2	F	76	Malignant fibrous histiocytoma	Right thigh	IIA
3	F	49	Synovial cell sarcoma	Left buttock	IIB
4	M	46	Malignant schwannoma	Left leg	IIB
5	F	84	Malignant fibrous histiocytoma	Left thigh	IIB
6	M	45	Leiomyosarcoma	Right buttock	IA
7	M	66	Malignant fibrous histiocytoma	Left groin	IIIB
8	F	33	Malignant fibrous histiocytoma	Right buttock	IA
9	F	51	Malignant schwannoma	Right leg	IA
10	F	66	Fibrosarcoma	Left forearm	IIB
11	M	57	Malignant fibrous histiocytoma	Right arm	IIA
12	M	67	Malignant fibrous histiocytoma	Right shoulder	IB

Table 31.2 *Complications*

Patient	Complications
1	Neuropraxia
2	None
3	None
4	Sterile wound drainage and neuropraxia
5	None
6	None
7	Sterile wound drainage
8	None
9	Sterile wound drainage
10	None
11	Neuropraxia
12	None

All three cases of peripheral nerve palsy involved patients in whom a major peripheral nerve was frozen deliberately during the cryoablation procedure because of its proximity to the tumor (Figure 31.6). In these patients, it was felt to be hazardous to mobilize the nerve off the pseudocapsule of the tumor. All three instances demonstrated signs of recovery, two within 1 week of cryoablation and one within 4 months.

Of the three patients who developed serous wound drainage postoperatively, none became infected. The drainage subsided in time with conservative measures. No seromas needed to be evacuated surgically. All cases of wound drainage occurred in patients whose tumors were greater than 8 cm in diameter.

Subsequent surgical resection of the sarcoma was in no case adversely effected by the previous cryosurgical procedure. All sarcomas were resected with a wide margin.

There were three patients with low-grade lesions who did not receive chemotherapy prior to surgical resection. The percentages of tumor necrosis noted after resection were 75%, 75%, and 100%, respectively. There were three patients with high-grade sarcomas who did not receive chemotherapy prior to surgical resection. The percentages of tumor necrosis noted after resection in these patients were 99%, 100%, and 80%, respectively.

TREATMENT OF SOFT TISSUE SARCOMAS: GENERAL CONSIDERATIONS

The optimal treatment regimen for soft tissue sarcomas of the extremities has not yet been defined, and various strategies continue to evolve. To date, the fundamental pillar of treatment has been surgical excision by means of amputation or, more recently, by limb-sparing resection. The goal of surgical treatment is to achieve local control of the tumor. In order to accomplish this goal, the planned surgical margin is generally wide, i.e., the plane of resection is through normal tissue. This wide surgical margin theoretically eliminates any satellite lesions that may be in the reactive zone of the tumor. Significant functional and cosmetic defects may result from the sacrifice of normal tissue needed to obtain an en-bloc resection of the sarcoma. In addition, wide surgical margins are sometimes difficult to realize when the tumor is located in close proximity to major neurovascular structures. In limb salvage procedures especially, surgical margins are sometimes very narrow and the plane of resection between the tumor and the adjacent vital structures may be through the reactive zone of the tumor. The resulting 'marginal' margin may leave satellite lesions behind.

In order to reduce the risk of local recurrence, radiation therapy has been utilized extensively as a surgical adjuvant in the treatment of both low-grade and high-grade soft tissue sarcomas. This adjuvant radiation therapy has been administered both preoperatively and postoperatively via external-beam techniques. More recently, it has also been delivered by the technique of brachytherapy.

The combination of surgery and radiation therapy has been generally effective in the treatment of low-grade soft tissue sarcomas of the extremities. Overall survival in patients with stage IA and IB extremity sarcomas approaches 90% and local recurrence is generally in the range of 5–10%.[9] For high-grade (stage IIA and IIB) sarcomas, the results of surgery combined with radiation therapy are not as impressive. The overall survival rate

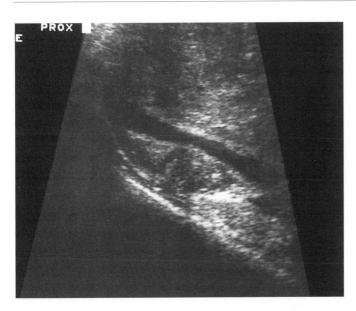

Figure 31.6 *Ultrasound examination demonstrating posterior tibial nerve surrounded by a malignant schwannoma. The nerve was deliberately frozen during cryoablation. The neuropraxia that followed was transient.*

for these patients is only about 60%, with local recurrence range as high as 20%.[9]

Radiation therapy in the treatment of soft tissue sarcomas is associated with potentially significant morbidity and risk. The ionizing radiation employed affects not only malignant tissue, but normal tissue as well. The common problems and complications associated with radiation therapy include:

1 burning and epidermolysis of skin,
2 fibrosis of muscle tendon and other connective tissue,
3 joint stiffness,
4 degenerative arthritis,
5 increased incidence and severity of wound infection,
6 increased risk of wound dehiscence and delayed wound healing,
7 radionecrosis of bone,
8 pathologic fracture,
9 development of radiation-induced sarcomas,
10 growth arrest in skeletally immature bones,
11 peripheral neuropathy secondary to direct radiation effect or to compression by scar and fibrotic tissue.

Additional surgical procedures are sometimes required to treat these complications. Because of the potential complications of radiation therapy and its limited effectiveness in producing cell necrosis and volume reduction of sarcomas, the search for another surgical adjuvant continues. Such an adjuvant should cause less morbidity than external-beam radiation therapy and yet be as effective, or even more so, in helping to achieve local control.

In order to improve local control and survival, most patients with high-grade soft tissue sarcomas are now treated with systemic chemotherapy as well as surgery and radiation. The addition of chemotherapy to the treatment schedule remains controversial, and the optimal choice and combination of drugs have not yet been elucidated. Indeed, there have not been consistent studies that demonstrate increased survival or decreased local recurrence when patients with soft tissue sarcomas are treated with systemic chemotherapy. Tumor necrosis in soft tissue sarcomas produced by chemotherapeutic effects is generally modest at best, with necrosis of 70% or less on average.[10] Nevertheless, many surgeons believe that the reactive fibrosis produced about the pseudocapsule of a sarcoma treated with systemic chemotherapy renders surgical excision easier and safer. In particular, mobilization of major neurovascular structures is particularly aided by this fibrosis. Thus, the majority of patients with soft tissue sarcomas are treated with systemic chemotherapy, although there may be no true scientific justification for this practice.

In summary, the present modalities employed to achieve local control in soft tissue extremity sarcomas are not completely effective and may be associated with significant complications and morbidity. The achievement of local control is essential in the successful treatment of soft tissue sarcomas. Without local control, all treatment regimens in patients with soft tissue sarcomas are doomed to failure and a cure will not be possible.

PRINCIPLES OF CRYOABLATION

Cryosurgical ablation is a therapeutic method of treating neoplastic tissue by freezing *in situ* in order to cause devitalization. Cryosurgery generally requires special instrumentation to produce freezing of tissue. Successful cryosurgery requires that the same volume of tissue must be frozen as would have been excised if the tumor had been treated surgically. For malignant tumors, an adequate amount of normal tissue around the lesion must also be frozen in order to achieve local control. In other words, a wide margin must be achieved with cryosurgical techniques just as it must be achieved with traditional surgery. The amount of tissue devitalized cryosurgically must extend past the reactive zone of a tumor and into surrounding normal tissue so that all satellite lesions are destroyed.

The basic principles of cryosurgical techniques for the treatment of malignancies include rapid freezing, slow thawing, and immediate repetition of the freezing and thawing, cycles.[3,4] The literature contains a wealth of reports detailing the development of this surgical specialty.[2] The use of freezing techniques in the treatment of malignancies began in the mid-nineteenth century when iced saline solutions were used to treat advanced carcinomas of the breast and cervix.[2] In the early twentieth century, cryosurgery was used to treat various skin diseases.[2] Modern cryosurgery made a significant breakthrough in 1961 with the development of an automated cryosurgical apparatus using liquid nitrogen.[11] In the decade that followed, scores of articles appeared detailing cryosurgical treatment of benign and malignant tumors.[12–32] Cryoablation is now a recognized approach to the treatment of various malignant tumors, including carcinoma of the skin,[33–35] tumors of the eye,[36–40] carcinomas of the oral cavity,[41–43] carcinoma of the liver, both primary and metastatic,[44–49] carcinoma of the vulva, vagina, and uterus,[50,51] carcinoma of the prostate,[16,52,53] metastatic carcinoma to bone,[15,54,55] malignant and aggressive primary bone tumors,[56–61] as well as others.

PATHOPHYSIOLOGY OF CRYOABLATION

The coldest temperature reached in tissue has been demonstrated to be the most important determinant in causing cell necrosis.[62] All living tissue subjected to a temperature of $-20\,°C$ or below for 1 min or longer will undergo necrosis.[5] Most authorities, however, recommend a treatment goal of at least $-40\,°C$ in all areas of tumor so as to minimize the risk of local recurrence.[2] The damaging effects on cellular integrity result from severe cold as well as from the process of freezing and thawing. Hypothermia deprives cells of the energy required to drive cellular processes, resulting in both metabolic uncoupling and compromised integrity of cell membranes and organelles. Tissue freezing results in both extracellular and intracellular propagation of pure water without electrolytes and proteins. The osmotic gradient which develops draws water from the intracellular spaces, leading to cell shrinkage and membrane damage.[6] Also, the shearing forces from the ice crystals are mechanically disruptive to organelles and cell membranes. Rapid freezing maximizes the cellular energy depletion.[2]

Thawing is also a damaging process, which subjects any remaining reactive cells to additional destructive forces. In early phases of warming, small ice crystals recrystallize into larger ones, which produce destructive shearing activity. As warming continues, melting occurs

and intact cells become exposed to a hypotonic environment. These new osmotic forces cause volume expansion and bursting of the cells. In contrast to the rate of freezing, a slow thaw is associated with optimal cellular damage.[2,7] Thrombosis and tissue obliteration of tissue microvasculature also occur throughout the entire cryodestructive process, and thus contribute to tissue anoxia and hypoxic cell death.[63]

The effects of freezing are non-selective; that is, normal as well as malignant tissue will be equally destroyed. An exception to this is the muscular wall of large arteries which has been shown to be relatively impervious to the effects of freezing.[64–67] Blood flow through these vessels acts like a heat sink and prevents freezing of the entire arterial wall. For this reason, a tourniquet should not be used when performing a cryosurgical ablation of an extremity sarcoma. Even after being frozen, these vessels will show no evidence of thrombosis or wall damage after thawing.

Another exception to the non-selective effects of freezing involves peripheral nerves. Marcove has documented peripheral nerve palsies after cryosurgical treatment of bone tumors.[57,68] Peripheral nerves that are frozen develop a neuropraxia and cease to function initially, but this has been found to resolve in about 3 months' time. Peripheral nerve palsies associated with cryosurgery appear to be transient, and there have been no reported cases of permanent nerve dysfunction.[69–72] Indeed, intraoperative intercostal nerve freezing has often been used to prevent post-thoracotomy pain. This surgically induced neuropraxia was also found to be transient.[73] This may be due to the unusual histology of peripheral nerves, which demonstrate long axons extending great distances from centrally located nuclei.

The probability of achieving total cell necrosis increases with two freeze–thaw cycles.[74] Although there is some debate as to the necessity of more than one freeze–thaw cycle in clinical practice, most surgeons performing cryoablation of malignant tumors perform two freeze–thaw cycles to assure maximal tissue destruction.[2,75,76] In many cases, the initial freeze is followed by a slow passive thaw, and the second freeze is followed by a relatively active thaw.

After cryoablation, necrotic, devitalized tissue is eliminated. The time required for slough of the necrotic tissue depends to some degree on the stroma. Cellular tissue sloughs quickly and is resorbed. Tissues with abundant fibrous stroma such as connective tissue are resistant to structural change, and the devitalized tissue requires a longer period of time for resorption.[2]

The basic feature of cryoablation is to devitalize neoplastic tissue by freezing in situ. In its simplest form, no tissue is excised except for the preliminary biopsy specimen. Necrotic tissue after freezing is merely allowed to slough and to be resorbed. When the goal is local control of a malignant tumor, care must be taken to use cryosurgery in a manner that produces a predictable area of necrosis that will encompass the tumor and an appropriate margin of normal tissue. This is the same care that must be taken when performing an en-bloc resection of a malignant tumor utilizing conventional means. The same principles of tumor surgery need to be followed for resection performed via cryoablation and for standard surgery.

Cryosurgical apparatus using liquid nitrogen is available in a variety of devices, ranging from expensive automated instruments to simple, hand-held devices that are nothing more than modified Thermos bottles or funnels. The type of apparatus chosen for use depends on the nature of the area of disease. Currently, the surgeon has the option to use liquid nitrogen in one of several ways. Liquid nitrogen can be poured or sprayed directly onto the tissues or it can be applied via a closed system with a cryoprobe so that the liquid nitrogen is never released on or into the tissue. The choice of technique depends on the site and size of the tumor. Cryosurgery for bone tumors, for example, has generally been undertaken utilizing a pour or spray technique. The major disadvantages of the spray or poured technique are related to the difficulty in controlling run-off of the liquid nitrogen onto normal tissues during treatment, as well as to the risk of insufflation of the tissue with associated nitrogen embolism if the sprayed technique is used. The cryoprobe technique provides a controllable and predictable area of necrosis, and is now the preferred method of cryosurgery in many situations, especially in large, bulky lesions in which a greater depth of freezing is required. There are several manufacturers, producing cryoprobes of different sizes, and each probe will create a freeze zone of different dimensions. It is important that the surgeon is familiar with the type of cryoprobe being utilized in order to rationally plan a safe and effective cryosurgical procedure. During the freezing process, the white, frosted appearance of the frozen tissue gradually extends away from the probe. When the freezing has encompassed a satisfactory volume of tissue, the process is stopped, the tissue is allowed to thaw, and the freeze–thaw cycle is repeated.

Ultrasound is routinely used during the cryoablation of hepatic and prostate tumors and other deep seated visceral lesions.[75] The freezing interfaces visualized as an advancing hyperechoic hemispheric rim with complete posterior or acoustic shadowing.[75] As the iceball expands, the hyperechoic rim increases in size, as does the area of acoustic shadowing. On the video monitor, the area of iceball appears as a black mass lined by a white rim. Ultrasound monitoring is important for reasons of both efficacy and safety. The temperature at the periphery of the cryolesion visualized on the ultrasound corresponds to 0 °C.[74] There is a 10–20 °C/mL decrease in the temperature from the outer rim of the iceball toward the center. Because a freezing temperature of −40 °C is required to assure tissue necrosis, there is a small rim of frozen tissue inward from the iceball's edge that may contain viable cells. Thus, as with traditional surgical resection, a margin of normal tissue surrounding the neoplasm is also

frozen in order to assure adequate treatment. Consequently, the surgeon should strive whenever possible to extend the iceball beyond the tumor margin into normal tissue for a distance of 5–10 mm.[75] Ultrasound monitoring of the freezing process can thus allow the surgeon to freeze the tumor while preventing undue freezing and necrosis of surrounding normal tissue. Freezing time varies, depending on the size of the tumor. It can range from 5 to 20 min or longer. The initial thawing period may also take 10–20 min or longer, depending on the size of the lesion. In a passive thaw, the iceball is allowed to defrost at room temperature. In an active thaw, heated gaseous nitrogen at approximately 60 °C is pumped into the probe to help accelerate the thawing process.

While performing cryoablation, care should be taken to isolate the tissue to be frozen from any surrounding vital structures if possible. Surgical packs and Gelfoam® can also be utilized to help with isolation. The outer portion of the probe and the delivery line should also be isolated from critical structures.

THE ROLE OF CRYOABLATION IN THE TREATMENT OF SOFT TISSUE SARCOMAS

Cryoablation is now a recognized approach to the treatment of malignant tumors. The range in application of cryosurgical techniques in the treatment of cancer is widely diversified and is steadily increasing in scope. Cryosurgery is most useful in easily accessible areas of the body, but recent advances in technology now make it possible to treat tumors that are deep and relatively inaccessible. Malignancies in many parts of the body, including bone, have been treated with cryosurgical techniques. Cryoablation is a technically feasible and safe technique in the treatment of soft tissue sarcomas of the extremity. Phase II studies are currently underway to evaluate the amount of tumor necrosis produced by this technique. Cryosurgical ablation of soft tissue sarcomas should be an effective method for treating these malignancies. No living tissue can withstand temperatures of −40 °C, especially when followed by a repeated freeze–thaw cycle. It is doubtful that soft tissue sarcomas will prove to be an exception.

The major complications associated with this technique are those involving the peripheral nerves. Although some patients do develop neuropraxia after direct exposure of the peripheral nerves to cryodestructive procedures, none has been permanent and the neuropraxia resulting from cryoablation is transient in nature.

No instances of thrombosis of major vessels in patients with cryoablation of extremity sarcomas have been reported. The major problem with vital structures is concern with peripheral nerves, blood vessels and, in certain instances, bone. Isolating these structures when possible can minimize the morbidity of the procedure. When the location of these structures in relationship to the tumor makes immobilization and isolation impossible, both peripheral nerves and blood vessels can be safely included in the freeze zone without sustaining permanent damage.

At present, there are several inherent problems with the cryoablation of soft tissue sarcomas. Of greatest concern is the quality of intraoperative imaging with ultrasound. If the tumor and propagating iceball are not adequately visualized, a portion of the tumor may not be adequately frozen. Lack of 100% tumor necrosis is secondary to inadequate freezing, which, in our experience, is the result of poor intraoperative imaging. Further technical advances with respect to ultrasound transducers need to be made in order to solve this problem. If imaging is satisfactory, complete tumor necrosis should be realized.

There are also concerns regarding the potential for local contamination when the cryoprobes are inserted. In order to minimize this risk, the tissues should be meticulously protected with surgical packing before the probes are inserted. The tracts created by the probes should also be plugged with Gelfoam® immediately upon their removal, while the tissue is still frozen and there is little or no bleeding.

In addition, there are some technical problems associated with the cryoprobe systems currently available. The commercially available probes were designed for the treatment of liver, prostate, and uterine tumors. They are long and somewhat unwieldy when applied to the treatment of extremity lesions. Also, the system can only accommodate a maximum of five probes simultaneously. When dealing with large, bulky sarcomas, five probes are sometimes inadequate. In such cases, the tumor must be frozen in sections. This can add considerable time to the procedure. The manufacturers of the cryoprobe systems are currently addressing these concerns.

SUMMARY

In summary, cryosurgical techniques can be applied safely to the treatment of soft tissue sarcomas of the extremity without causing serious morbidity. Additional phase II studies are necessary to evaluate the amount of necrosis produced by this technique and the effects of cryosurgery on local recurrence and patient survival. Only in this manner can the indications for the cryoablation of soft tissue sarcomas of the extremity be adequately elucidated. At present, cryosurgery is not meant to be used in lieu of conventional surgery in the treatment of soft tissue sarcomas, but rather in conjunction with standard surgical techniques. The idea is not to set cryosurgical ablation as a competing modality against surgical resection, but rather as a complementary modality. Only after careful study and evaluation should the role of this technique be expanded. In addition, cryosurgery can be used with systemic chemotherapy and radiation therapy when these modalities are indicated in the treatment of soft tissue sarcomas. Cryosurgery is a technically feasible and safe modality for the treatment of soft tissue extremity sarcomas.

REFERENCES

1. Enneking WF, Spanier SS, Goodman MA. A system for the surgical staging of musculoskeletal sarcomas. Clin Orthop 1980; 153:106–20.
2. Gage AA. Cryosurgery in the treatment of cancer. Surg Gynecol Obstet 1992; 174:73–92.
3. Gage AA. Probe cryosurgery. In Epstein E, Epstein E Jr, eds. *Skin surgery*, 6th edition. Philadelphia, WB Saunders, 1987; 465–79.
4. Gage AA, Torre D. Cryosurgery. In Webster J, ed. *Encyclopedia of medical devices and instrumentation*, Vol. 2. New York, John Wiley & Sons, 1988, 893–908.
5. Cooper IS. Cryosurgery for cancer. Fed Proc 1965; 24:5237–40.
6. Reite C. Mechanical forces as a cause of cellular damage by freezing and thawing. Biol Bull 1966; 131:197–203.
7. Mazur P. Physical chemical factors underlying cell injury in cryosurgical freezing. In Rand RW, Rinfret AP, Von Leder H, eds. *Cryosurgery*. Springfield, IL, Charles C Thomas, 1968; 32–51.
8. Menendez LR, Tan MS, Kiyabu MT, Chawla SP. Cryosurgical ablation of soft tissue sarcomas: a Phase I trial of feasibility and safety. Cancer 1999; 86:50–7.
9. Enneking WF. *Musculoskeletal tumor surgery*. New York, Churchill Livingstone, 1983, 141–84.
10. Kempf RA, Irwin LE, Menendez LR, *et al*. Limb salvage surgery for bone and soft tissue sarcoma. Cancer 1991; 68:738–43.
11. Cooper IS, Lee ASJ. Cryostatic congelation: a system for producing a limited, controlled region of cooling or freezing of biologic tissue. J Nerv Ment Dis 1961; 133:259–63.
12. Gonder MJ, Soanes WA, Smith V. Experimental prostate cryosurgery. Invest Urol 1964; 1:610–19.
13. Rand RW, Rashe AM, Paglia DE, *et al*. Sterotatic cryo-hypophysectomy. JAMA 1964; 189:255–9.
14. Gage AA, Keopf S, Wehrle D, Emmings F. Cryotherapy for cancer of the lip and oral cavity. Cancer 1965; 18:1649–51.
15. Zacarian S, Adham M. Cryotherapy of cutaneous malignancy. Cryobiology 1966; 2:212–18.
16. Gonder MJ, Soanes WA, Shulman S. Cryosurgical treatment of the prostate. Invest Urol 1966; 3:372–8.
17. Barton R. Cryosurgical treatment of nasopharyngeal neoplasms. Am Surg 1966; 32:744–7.

18. Hill C. Preliminary report on cryosurgery in otolaryngology. Laryngoscope 1966; 76:109–11.

19. Kaplan J, Kaplan I. Cryogenic electrocoagulation and spontaneous necrosis of a bladder neoplasm: a preliminary comparative study. J Urol 1966; 95:531–5.

20. Jordan W, Walker D, Miller G, Drylie D. Cryotherapy of benign and neoplastic tumors of the prostate. Surg Gynecol Obstet 1967; 25:1265–8.

21. Lincoff H, McLean J, Long R. The cryosurgical treatment of intraocular tumors. Am J Ophthalmol 1967; 63:389–99.

22. Crisp WE, Asadourian L, Ramberber W. Application of cryosurgery to gynecologic malignancy. Obstet Gynecol 1967; 30:668–73.

23. Blackwood J, Moore FT, Pace WG. Cryotherapy for malignant tumors. Cryobiology 1967; 4:33–8.

24. Ostergard D, Townsend DE. Malignant melanoma of the female urethra treated by cryotherapy with radical vulvectomy and anterior exenteration. Obstet Gynecol 1968; 31:75–82.

25. Dowd J, Flint L, Zinman L, Tripath V. Experiences with cryosurgery of the prostate in the poor-risk patient. Surg Clin North Am 1968; 48:627–32.

26. Gage AA. Cryotherapy for inoperable cancer. Dis Colon Rectum 1968; 2:36–44.

27. Torre D. Cutaneous cryosurgery. J Cryosurg 1968; 1:202–9.

28. Beggs JH. Cryotherapy as a palliative maneuver. JAMA 1968; 207:1570–2.

29. Marcove RC, Miller TR. Treatment of primary and metastatic bone tumors by cryosurgery. JAMA 1969; 207:1890–4.

30. Crisp WE. The use of cryosurgery in cancer of the uterine cervix. Int Surg 1969; 52:451–4.

31. Gage A. Cryosurgery for cancer – an evaluation. Cryobiology 1969; 5:241–9.

32. Miller D, Metzner D. Cryosurgery for tumors of the head and neck. Trans Am Acad Ophthalmol Otolaryngol 1969; 73:300–9.

33. Lubritz RR. Cryosurgery management of multiple skin carcinomas. J Dermatol Surg Oncol 1977; 3:414–16.

34. Kuflik EG. Cryosurgery for multiple basal-cell carcinomas on the nose: a case report. J Dermatol Surg Oncol 1984; 10:16–18.

35. Graham G, Clark L. Statistical analysis in cryosurgery of skin cancer. Clin Dermatol 1990; 8:101–107.

36. Abramson D, Lisman R. Cryopexy of a choroidal melanoma. Ann Ophthalmol 1979; 11:1418–21.

37. Fraunfelder FT, Boozman FW, Wilson RS, Thomas AH. No-touch technique for intraocular malignant melanomas. Arch Ophthalmol 1977; 95:1616–20.

38. Wilson RS, Fraunfelder FT. Circum-tumor cryoenucleation: a new no-touch technique for the prevention of metastatic seeding of intraocular cancer. Excerpta Medica International Congress Series 1979; 2:1870–3.

39. Lazar M, Geyer O, Rosen N, Godel V. A transconjunctival cryosurgical approach for intraorbital tumors. Aust NZJ Ophthalmol 1985; 13:417–20.

40. Hurwitz JJ, Mishkin SK. The value of cryoprobe-assisted removal of orbital tumors. Ophthalmic Surg 1988; 19:94–7.

41. Idem. Treatment of malignant soft tissue lesions of oral cavity pharynx, face and scalp. In Bradley P, ed. *Cryosurgery of the maxillofacial region*, Vol. 2. Boca Raton, FL, CRC Press, 1986, 1–30.

42. Weaver A, Smith D. Cryosurgery for head and neck cancer. Am J Surg 1974; 128:466–70.

43. Smith D, Weaver A. Cryosurgery for oral cancer – a six-year retrospective study. J Oral Surg 1976; 34:245–8.

44. Kuramoto S, Kamegai T. Cryosurgery for the liver tumor. Cryobiology 1978; 15:710.

45. Torigoshi Y, Ooke H, Kuramoto S, *et al*. Hepatic metastasis of rectum and colon cancer. Dig Dis Sci 1986; 31:125S.

46. Zhov XD, Tang ZY, Yu YQ, Ma ZC. Clinical evaluation of cryosurgery in the treatment of primary liver cancer. Report of 60 cases. Cancer 1988; 61:1889–92.

47. Ravikumar TS, Kane R, Cady B, *et al*. A 5 year study of cryosurgery in the treatment of liver tumors. Arch Surg 1991; 126:1520–4.

48. Polk W, Fong Y, Kerpeh M, Blumgart L. A technique for the use of cryosurgery to assist hepatic resection. J Am Coll Surg 1995; 180:171–6.

49. Steele G Jr. Cryoablation in hepatic surgery. Semin Liver Dis 1994; 14:120–5.

50. Wright VC, Davies EM. The conservative management of cervical intraepithelial neoplasia: the use of cryosurgery and the carbon dioxide laser. Br J Obstet Gynaecol 1981; 88:663–8.

51. Goncalves J. Cryovulvectomy – a new surgical technique for advanced cancer. Skin Cancer 1986; 1:17–31.

52. Bonney WW, Fallon B, Gerber WL. Cryosurgery in prostatic cancer: survival. Urology 1982; 19:37–42.

53. Bonney WW, Fallon B, Gerber WL, *et al*. Cryosurgery in prostatic cancer: elimination of local lesion. Urology 1983; 22:8–15.

54. Gursel E, Roberts M, Veenema R. Regression of prostatic cancer following sequential cryotherapy to the prostate. J Urol 1972; 108:928–32.

55. Eltahir K, Rietrich F. Clinical observations on tumor immunity in urologic cryosurgery. Z Urol Nephrol 1976; 69:135–40.

56. Gage A, Erickson R. Cryotherapy and curettage for bone tumors. J Cryosurg 1968; 1:60–6.

57. Marcove RC, Weis ID, Vaghaiwalla MR, *et al*. Cryosurgery in the treatment of giant cell tumors of bone. A report of 52 consecutive cases. Cancer 1978; 41:957–69.

58. Holland PS, Mellor WC. The conservative treatment of ameloblastoma, using diathreapy or cryosurgery. A 29-year review. Int J Oral Surg 1981; 10:32–6.

59. Jacobs PA, Clemency RE Jr. The closed cryosurgical treatment of giant cell tumor. Clin Orthop 1985; 192:149–58.

60. Marcove R, Stovel P, Huvos A, Bullough P. The use of cryosurgery in the treatment of low and medium chondrosarcoma. Clin Orthop 1977; 122:147–56.

61. Huvos A. Grading of bone tumors. Dev Oncol 1988; 55:14–17.

62. Gage A. What temperature is lethal for cells? J Dermatol Surg Oncol 1979; 5:459–61.

63. Pastena C, Reitmeier RJ, Moertel GG, Judd ES, Dockerty MB. The natural history of carcinoma of the colon and rectum. Am J Surg 1964; 108:826–9.

64. Cooper IS, Samma K, Wisniewska K. Effects of freezing in major arteries. Stroke 1971; 2:471–82.

65. Gage AM, Montes M, Gage AA. Freezing the canine thoracic aorta in situ. J Surg Res 1979; 27:331–40.

66. Bowers WD Jr, Hubbard RW, Daum RC, et al. Ultrastructural studies on muscle cells and vascular endothelium immediately after freeze–thaw injury. Cryobiology 1973; 10:9–12.

67. Giampapa VC, Oh C, Aufses AH. The vascular effect of cold injury. Cryobiology 1981; 1:49–54.

68. Marcove R. The surgery of tumors of bone and cartilage, 2nd edition. New York, Grove and Stratton Inc., 1984, 104–8.

69. Marcove RC, Lyden JP, Bullough P, Huvos AG. Giant cell tumors treated by cryosurgery: a review of 25 cases. J Bone Joint Surg 1973; 33:143.

70. Marcove RC, Weis LD, Vaghaiwalla MR, Person R. Cryosurgery in the treatment of giant cell tumors of bone. Clin Orthop 1978; 134:275.

71. Miles TS, Hribar D. Recovery of function after cryosurgical lesions of peripheral nerves in rats. Neurosci Lett 1981; 24:285–8.

72. Myers RR, Powell HC, Heckman HM, et al. Biophysical and pathological effects of cryogenic nerve lesion. Ann Neurol 1981; 10:478–85.

73. Nelson KM, Vincent RG, Bourke RS, et al. Intraoperative intercostal nerve freezing to prevent post-thoracotomy pain. Ann Thorac Surg 1974; 18:280–5.

74. Ravikumar TS, Steel G Jr, Kane R, King V. Experimental and clinical observations on hepatic cryosurgery for colorectal metastases. Cancer Res 1991; 51:6323–7.

75. Kane RA. Ultrasound-guided hepatic cryosurgery for tumor ablation. Semin Interv Radiol 1993; 10:132–42.

76. Steele G Jr. Cryoablation in hepatic surgery. Semin Liver Dis 1994; 14:120–5.

Commentary

KENNETH P RAMMING

Until the mid and late 1960s, amputation was virtually the only therapeutic option available for the management of extremity sarcomas. More recently, neoadjuvant regimens, including preoperative chemotherapy, initially adriamycin based, plus preoperative radiation therapy, were developed to enable oncologic surgeons to remove the cancer and still preserve the limb. Surgical techniques for such limb salvage surgery have gradually evolved, but the resected tumors inevitably approach a margin of resection, at least in some area of the specimen. An important benefit of this sequence of preoperative therapy followed by resection is that the operative specimen is available for pathologic examination so that the effectiveness of a given neoadjuvant regimen can be determined. For example, the degree of cellular necrosis induced by the preoperative treatment can be fairly well quantified. In only very rare cases to date has cell death approached 100%. Thus, a certain incidence of local recurrence, which can be as high 20–30% in some series, is almost inevitable.

In addition, preoperative radiation and chemotherapy are not without their complications. The marrow suppression and other side-effects of high-dose chemotherapy are well known. Significant toxicities and morbidity can also follow radiation therapy, including fibrosis, delayed wound healing, wound infection, radionecrosis of bone, degenerative arthritis, and epidermolysis. These toxicities can be progressive with time.

The use of cryotherapy prior to conventional limb salvage surgery is an innovative and quite possibly superior form of neoadjuvant preoperative therapy for sarcomas. Such lesions treated with intent to cure are generally readily accessible and, although they are usually large, the potential complications and the surgical difficulty in administering the cryosurgery appear to be much less than with the most commonly used form of cryotherapy, namely, treatment of inoperable malignancies in the liver. In the liver, the enormous blood flow through the organ is probably the major factor in cryoinduced systemic toxicity. The systemic and blood toxicities that are observed in hepatic cryotherapy do not appear to be present in cryotherapy of sarcomas, at least in Dr Menendez's series of 12 patients.

It is of interest that Dr Menendez made no particular effort to avoid freezing nerves when it was thought that this was necessary to provide an adequate margin. In three cases of neuropraxia, directly attributable to the cryosurgery, all nerves returned to normal function with time. This is of considerable interest to practitioners in the field of cryotherapy. For example, one of the putative advantages of cryotherapy in the treatment of prostatic cancer is that the degree of sexual dysfunction following cryosurgery is less than that following radical prostatectomy, presumably because the nerves regenerate. In contrast, this has also been an area of intense criticism of the cryotherapy method of treating prostate cancer, as critics have said that because sexual function returns, the nerves are not completely killed and, therefore, the destruction of the prostatic cancer must not be complete. Menendez suggests, however, that the fact that the neuropraxia is transient may be due to the unusual histology of peripheral nerves in which long axons extend great distances from centrally located nuclei. This is an interesting theoretical concept. Nonetheless, it is gratifying that in all cases the neuropraxia was temporary.

The fact that hypothermia has an adverse effect on solid malignancies has been known since the late 1800s. The first report is probably that of Dr James Arnott in 1893. He applied iced saline solutions directly to large ulcerating cancers and observed a reduction in size, odor, discharge, pain, and hemorrhage.[1] Through the decades, there have been a variety of delivery systems, most capable of somewhat slowing the growth of solid malignancies, but none capable of obliterating them completely. The first cryosurgical system capable of delivering liquid nitrogen utilizing trocar-type probes with an insulated shaft and metal tip was described by Cooper and Lee in 1961.[2] The capability of this device to produce an avascular cryolesion in the liver was demonstrated in animal models. During the following 20 years, cryosurgical treatment of tumors at various sites, such as the rectum, breast, skin, lung, brain, prostate, uterus, oral cavity, pancreas, and liver, was reported. However, it was not until the 1990s that two developments occurred which virtually revolutionized the delivery of extreme cold required for modern-day clinical cryotherapy. One was the development of commercially available, very reliable, delivery systems utilizing liquid nitrogen through hollow metal probes. The other, possibly more important, was the development of real-time intraoperative ultrasound. By this method, sterile sensors could be placed on the organs, usually the liver. As there is a phase change as the iceball in the tumor develops, reliable assessment of engulfment of the tumor by the tumor iceball, along with the normal margin or rim of the frozen normal tissue, could be accurately assessed.

The mechanism of tissue destruction by extreme cold has been fairly well elucidated. The more rapid the freeze, the more complete the cell destruction. As the freeze progresses, extracellular ice will form, causing an increase in the osmolarity of the extracellular fluid, creating an osmotic gradient, causing the cells to dehydrate. The

resulting changes in the intracellular milieu, such as changes in the pH, ionic concentration, and denaturation of cell proteins, can be lethal. When intracellular ice formation occurs, the cellular membranes and intracellular structures are incapacitated, and finally cell death will occur. Mechanical interactions between extracellular ice crystals and cells lead to the deformation of cells and rupture of cell membranes. In addition, the freezing causes complete disruption of the nutrient capillaries of the tumor. In biopsies of treated lesions 4–8 weeks after the treatment with cryotherapy, the cellular outline is completely obliterated, and what remains is only an amorphous mass. There is no evidence of vascularity in these residual tumors or tumor scars. Many investigators feel that the obliteration of the microvascular system of the tumor by cryotherapy is the most lethal cause of tumor cell death. Most practitioners in the field feel that it is essential to reach an intralesion temperature of at least −40 °C to obliterate tumor cells completely.

In liver cryotherapy sinusoidal congestion and hemorrhage and focal hepatocellular necrosis with pyknotic nuclei are present immediately after thawing. Electron microscopy reveals the degeneration of liver cell cytoplasm, a reduction in the amount of glycogen granules, and the degeneration and disappearance of mitochondria. During the following 24 h, progressive hepatocellular necrosis with the loss of nuclear detail, nuclear pyknosis and clumping of cytoplasm, as well as progressive congestion, are visible. At 12 h, an infiltrate of polymorphonuclear leukocytes and monocytes appears and, after 2–3 days, a cellular infiltrate of macrophages and fibroblasts surrounds the lesion. Disintegration of vessel walls and areas of eosinophilic necrosis are present within the lesion. During the following 2–8 weeks, the lesion is gradually replaced by fibrous tissue. No cellular detail is noted. Clinically, computerized axial tomography (CT scans) will initially show actual enlargement of the lesions. This has been a very deceptive observation for many radiologists, most whom are unfamiliar with changes after cryosurgical ablation of liver lesions. It has led to disturbing misdiagnoses of tumor progression when, in fact, the enlarged lesions simply reflect achievement of a proper margin of destroyed normal tissue around the tumor. In time, the body resorbs this tissue, and it is replaced by normal hepatic tissue. When patients are re-explored 1–2 years after cryosurgery, only slight dimpling of the Glisson's capsule is found, and in most instances there is virtually complete replacement of the ablated area by normal hepatic tissue.

Most of the clinical data on the use of cryosurgery for solid tumors have been in tumors of the liver, both metastatic and primary. Colorectal cancer is the third leading cause of cancer death in the USA, with more than 60 000 people dying of the disease annually. There are about 15 000 deaths from malignant hepatoma. Liver metastases are present in 15–25% of patients at the time of diagnosis of colorectal cancer. Almost 40% will develop metastases within a year of resection. The median survival time of patients with liver metastases from colorectal cancer who receive no treatment is less than a year. Unfortunately, though an enormous number of chemotherapy regimens and agents have been tried, the cure rate is probably less than 3%, at the cost of significant toxicity. These tumors are radiation insensitive, so there is no role whatsoever for radiation therapy.

Thus, almost the only cures with this disease have resulted from surgical resection of cancer of the colon metastatic but confined to the liver. Five-year survival rates of 20–50% have been reported from numerous centers. The techniques for liver surgery have been well established and are safe, and cures have been reported. Unfortunately, only about 20% of patients are candidates for liver resection. For patients with metastasis confined to the liver who are deemed *not* to be candidates for surgical resection, the reason is almost always the presence of multiple lesions too numerous to resect, or a large central lesion which, if resected, would disrupt the blood supply to the normal adjacent liver parenchyma. Thus, this is an unfortunate situation in which a very common tumor, and leading cause of death, has few therapeutic options. That is why there has been such an enormous effort to refine cryotherapy techniques in this widespread and lethal disease.

The criteria for cryosurgery are simple. By no means should cryosurgery be a replacement for conventional surgery. If conventional surgical techniques can result in complete excision of the tumor, they should be the treatment followed. Thus, the indications for cryosurgery are bilateral lesions, a central lesion not amenable to anatomic resection, contralateral nodules in a patient undergoing hepatic lobectomy, and, rarely, limited hepatic reserve such as cirrhosis and prior liver resection. The combination of conventional surgical resection and cryoablation is a very attractive one, and raises the number of patients who are candidates for liver resection. This most commonly occurs in patients who have a large but peripheral lesion in the right lobe, along with several nodules in the mid-left lobe. The right side can be resected and the left nodules easily treated with cryotherapy.

At the time of operation, the liver is completely mobilized. A biopsy is always taken, and the malignancy confirmed. Systematic mapping of the liver with ultrasound is made, with numerous prints being taken for the patient's record. Under ultrasonic guidance, the probes are placed into the lesion or lesions, and liquid nitrogen is flowed through the probes. Evaluation of the freeze is done both by palpation and, especially, by ultrasound evaluation. The progression of the iceball can easily be followed with intraoperative ultrasound. Though it was of great concern with pioneers, little regard is now given to whether or not large vessels are frozen because, as long as the blood supply is present in the hepatic artery or portal vein and/or aorta or vena cava, no permanent wall damage will occur. When freezing is complete with an adequate margin of normal hepatic parenchyma, heated nitrogen is flowed through the probes, and they are removed. The holes are packed with Gelfoam® or other hemostatic substances, such as platelet-enriched plasma gel. It is very important to stop the procedure at this time and observe the thaw. The most serious potential intraoperative complications are cracks, bleeding, or biliary fistula.

Cracks or fissures occur in the thaw phase. These are particularly frequent in large tumors where multiple probes have been used. They cannot be managed with conventional suture techniques, because the frozen tissue will not hold a stitch. They have to be treated with a combination of thrombogenic agents, usually Gelfoam® soaked in thrombin. The use of these agents, compression, and patience and time are the only way to handle these fissures.

Bleeding will usually occur in the presence of cracks. The use of the argon cautery and the conventional cautery, along with hemostatic agents, will eventually stop this. Any conventional causes of bleeding, such as a rent in a vessel, are simply treated with conventional suture and clamp techniques.

Bile leaks are infrequent, but the operative field should be vigorously inspected in every case, using irrigation and clean packs to make sure there is no evidence of bile leak. Should this occur, it is ideally treated with suture ligation and specific drainage to the area. On only rare occasions has it been necessary to put a T-tube into the main common duct and advance it up to the area of the leak.

Intraoperative hypothermia can occur. It is necessary to use warming blankets, ideally the Bair hugger. We use two of these in every case, and try to have the patient's temperature at normal or above normal by the time the cryotherapy phase of the operation is begun.

Complications from hepatic cryosurgery include those present with any major surgery, including wound breakdown, infection, pneumonia, and cardiac arrhythmias. However, there are some that can be specific to cryotherapy, as listed in Table 1.

In Dr Menendez's presentation of cryoablation of soft tissue sarcomas, his systemic complications were markedly few.

Table 1 *Complications of cryosurgery*

Major complications	Minor complications
Cryoshock phenomenon	Pleural effusions
Severe coagulopathy	Myoglobinuria
Hepatic hemorrhage	Fever
Biliary fistula	Increased thrombin time
Subphrenic or hepatic abscess	Transient increased LFTs
Cracks	Leukocytosis
Decreased platelets	Acute tubular necrosis

Occasionally, one can see a cryoshock phenomenon: a syndrome of multi-organ failure, severe coagulopathy and DIC, similar to septic shock but without evidence of any systemic sepsis. Most patients will have a degree of thrombocytopenia. This can be progressive over the postoperative 96 h, but rarely requires platelet infusion. Most patients will have significant changes in their clotting functions, occasionally with severe coagulopathy. Almost all patients require fresh frozen plasma during operation and postoperatively to correct this. Pleural effusions are common, but are rarely of any consequence. In any extensive cryotherapy against the diaphragm, we routinely place a chest tube at the time of surgery. Hepatic abscesses are rare. Acute tubular necrosis can occur, and its cause is obscure. Hydration and alkylation of the urine, along with the intraoperative administration of mannitol, have almost eliminated this problem. All patients will have very markedly elevated hepatic enzymes, but these return to normal, often by the time of discharge. Myoglobinuria is frequently present and seems to be of little clinical significance. The average stay in hospital is 5–6 days.

In 1998, Seifert et al.[3] presented a collective review of the world literature on hepatic cryotherapy. They gathered published results from almost 900 patients from 22 publications. I would estimate that the number of hepatic cryotherapies that have been done since then is at least double that. It is difficult to get an idea of survival from this compilation, although clearly there were some 5-year survivors reported. One of the great difficulties with evaluating any new anticancer modality is that it takes so long to get a large enough number of patients who have been observed for 5 years for significant survival data to be evaluated. Indeed, in 1997, Tandan et al.[4] tried to compare patients treated with cryosurgery and those treated with liver resection, and could come to no conclusions at all regarding survival.

In 1999, we reported our 6-year experience in 191 patients with liver metastases treated with cryosurgery (Table 2).[5] Between July 1992 and July 1998, 142 patients underwent cryotherapy, 61 females and 81 males, aged 30–76 (median age 60 years). Patients were evaluated preoperatively with spiral computerized tomography (CT scan) and intraoperatively with ultrasound. Lesions were frozen with liquid nitrogen delivered by steel probes for 15–30 min at $-190\,°C$. The iceball was monitored with real-time ultrasound. Multiple probes were used for lesions larger than 5 cm. One to 15 lesions were frozen (mean 3.4, median 3, mean size 3.1 cm). There was one operative death. Average intensive care unit and hospital stays were 1.5 and 6 days, respectively. The mean reduction in carcinoembryonic antigen (CEA) levels was 68%. The median follow-up from surgery was 13 months (1–58 months). The overall median survival was 35.1 months from the diagnosis of liver metastases and 30.2 months from the time of cryosurgery.

Table 2 *Survival after hepatic cryosurgery for unresectable metastatic colorectal cancer confined to the liver*

Year	Survival from date of cryosurgery (%)	Survival from date of diagnosis of liver metastases (%)
1	70	91
2	35	62
3	14	41
4	10	27

Virtually all of the patients referred to us with metastatic colorectal cancer confined to the liver were failures of conventional chemotherapy, usually 5-fluorouracil and leucovorin. As our program evolved, some patients were given chemotherapy postoperatively on a non-randomized basis. Twenty-three patients were treated with hepatic arterial 5-floxuridine (5FUDR), with an Infusaid pump placed at the time of surgery following cryosurgical ablation, that is, at the same operation. Thirty-five patients were treated with CPT-11. These patients were later in our series, because CPT-11 was not available when we started our cryosurgical program. In the evaluation of our data, somewhat to our surprise, we found that patients who received either hepatic artery 5FUDR or CPT-11 as post-surgical adjuvant therapy did significantly better than patients who received cryotherapy alone. We evaluated the data and found that age, comorbidity, hepatic dysfunction, size and number of lesions were equally matched between the postoperative adjuvant chemotherapy group and those receiving cryotherapy alone. The median survival after cryosurgery in the adjuvant intra-arterial FUDR and systemic CPT-11 groups was significantly higher ($p < 0.007$) than that for patients undergoing cryosurgery alone. Lesion size and number were not statistically significant prognostic indicators. Using unitary analysis, adjuvant chemotherapy, CEA levels of greater than 100 ng/ml, and a postoperative CEA reduction of less than 60% were significant prognostic indicators ($p < 0.05$). It is of great interest that even though virtually all these patients were chemotherapy failures preoperatively, there was a distinct therapeutic advantage to giving either intra-arterial 5FUDR or CPT-11 *after* cryotherapy treatment. Indeed, one of the advantages of cryotherapy is that it does not preclude the use of any other treatment, such as radiation therapy, chemotherapy, or immunotherapy. In the case of adjuvant chemotherapy in colorectal cancer, clearly from these data, a randomized trial comparing the modalities is needed.

Our results with cryosurgical ablation of hepatic metastases confined to the liver of non-colorectal origin are as follows:

Seventeen patients with unresectable *primary hepatocellular carcinoma* were treated with intraoperative cryotherapy; lesion size ranged from 4 cm to 18 cm.

Surgical mortality was 0%. Eight are currently alive. The median survival rates for these patients were:

All patients since diagnosis of metastasis	36 months (2–61)
All patients since cryosurgery	25 months (1–55)
Living patients since diagnosis of metastasis	34.5 months (7–61)
Living patient since cryosurgery	29.5 months (6–55)

Twelve patients with *metastatic breast cancer* confined to the liver underwent cryosurgical ablation. Surgical mortality was 0%. Twelve patients were available for follow-up; 7 are currently alive. The median survival rates for these patients were:

All patients since diagnosis of metastasis	47 months (7–120)
All patients since cryosurgery	23.5 months (3–56)
All living patients since diagnosis of metastasis	32 months (8–87)
All living patients since cryosurgery	23 months (3–56)

Twenty patients with *neuroendocrine carcinoma* confined to the liver underwent cryosurgical ablation. Nine patients are currently alive. The median survival rates for these patients were:

All patients since diagnosis of metastasis	35.5 months (8–118)
All patients since cryosurgery	19 months (0–47)
All living patients since diagnosis of metastasis	42 months (13–118)
All living patients since cryosurgery	26 months (13–47)

Thus, this rather large series from one institution includes 17 patients with hepatocellular carcinoma, 12 with metastatic breast cancer, and 20 with neuroendocrine carcinoma metastatic to the liver.

Our longest survivor was a man with colorectal cancer who was tumor free at 6 years after hepatic cryosurgery, and eventually died of metastatic cancer in the liver and other organs at 9 years. Why a patient who was tumor free at 6 years should eventually die of more colorectal cancer is not clear, but perhaps cryosurgery provided longer survival for a patient who would otherwise have been dead at a much earlier time, showing us significant changes in what we thought were patterns in the metastasis and biology of cancer and recurrences.

In summary, cryotherapy has been shown to be safe and therapeutic in other tumor systems and in other organ systems, particularly the liver. I applaud the pioneering use of this modality in Dr Menedez's presentation. There seems to be no reason why, in the hands of a competent sarcoma surgeon familiar with limb salvage, this form of adjuvant therapy, which surely has potential advantages over radiation therapy and chemotherapy, should not prove to be beneficial. The long-term results for these patients will indeed be of great interest.

REFERENCES

1. Bird HM. James Arnott, M.D. (Aberdeen), 1797–1883. A pioneer in refrigeration analgesia. Anesthesia 1949; 4:10–17.
2. Cooper IS, Lee ASJ. Cryostatic congelation: a system for producing a limited, controlled region of cooling or freezing of biologic tissue. J Nerv Ment Dis 1961; 133:259–63.
3. Seifert JK, Junginger T, Morris DL. A collective review of the world literature on hepatic cryosurgery. Royal College of Surgeons of Edinburgh. J R Coll Surg Edinb 1998; 43:141–54.
4. Tandan VR, Harmantas A, Gallinger S. Long-term survival after hepatic cryosurgery versus surgical resection for metastatis colorectal carcinoma, a critical review of the literature. Can J Surg 1997; 40:175–81.
5. Ramming KP, Saranton T, Adani K, et al. A six year institutional experience with hepatic cryosurgery for unresectable liver malignancies. Proceedings of the St. George Liver Oncology Group, Sydney, Australia, March 1999.

Editors' selected abstracts

Morbidity of adjuvant brachytherapy in soft tissue sarcoma of the extremity and superficial trunk.

Alektiar KM, Zelefsky MJ, Brennan MF.

Department of Radiation Oncology, Memorial Sloan-Kettering Cancer Center, New York, NY, USA.

International Journal of Radiation Oncology, Biology, Physics 47(5):1273–9, 2000, July 15.

Purpose: We have previously shown that adjuvant brachytherapy (BRT) improves local control in soft tissue sarcoma (STS) of the extremity and superficial trunk. A detailed assessment of the morbidity of this approach has not been examined. The purpose of this study was to evaluate the toxicity associated with adjuvant BRT in terms of wound complications, bone fracture, and peripheral nerve damage. *Methods and materials:* Between July 1982 and June 1992, 164 adult patients with STS of the extremity or superficial trunk were randomized intraoperatively to receive or not to receive BRT after complete resection. BRT was delivered with ^{192}Ir to a total dose of 42–45 Gy. The BRT and no-BRT arms were balanced with regard to age, sex, presentation (primary vs. recurrent), site, grade, size, and depth. Morbidity was assessed in terms of significant wound complication, bone fracture, and peripheral nerve damage (grade $\geqslant$3). The significant wound complications were defined as those wound problems requiring operative revision for coverage or threatened limb loss, persistent seroma requiring repeated aspirations and/or drainage, wound separation >2 cm, hematoma >25 ml, and/or purulent wound discharge. The median follow-up was 100 months. *Results:* The significant wound complication rate was 24% in the BRT group and 14% in the no-BRT group ($p = 0.13$). The rate of wound reoperation, however, was significantly higher in the BRT arm (10% vs. 0%; $p = 0.006$). Examination of other covariables that may have contributed to wound reoperation revealed the width of the excised skin (WES) to be a significant factor [1% (WES $\leqslant$4 cm) vs. 10% (WES >4 cm), $p = 0.02$]. Bone fracture only occurred in patients receiving BRT ($n = 3,4\%$), although this was not statistically significant ($p = 0.2$). The rate of peripheral nerve damage, however, was similar in both arms (7% vs. 7%). *Conclusion:* The overall morbidity associated with adjuvant BRT was not significantly higher than that with surgery alone. However, BRT and WES >4 cm were associated with significantly higher wound reoperation rate. This has significant implications for strategies designed to maximize wound coverage in patients who receive BRT.

Cryosurgery in the treatment of giant cell tumor. A long-term followup study.

Malawer MM, Bickels J, Meller I, Buch RG, Henshaw RM, Kollender Y.

Washington Cancer Institute, Washington Hospital Center, Washington, DC, USA.

Clinical Orthopaedics and Related Research (359): 176–88, 1999, February.

Between 1983 and 1993, 102 patients with giant cell tumor of bone were treated at three institutions. Sixteen patients (15.9%) presented with already having had local recurrence. All patients were treated with thorough curettage of the tumor, burr drilling of the tumor inner walls, and cryotherapy by direct pour technique using liquid nitrogen. The average followup was 6.5 years (range, 4–15 years). The rate of local recurrence in the 86 patients treated primarily with cryosurgery was 2.3% (two patients), and the overall recurrence rate was 7.9% (eight patients). Six of these patients were cured by cryosurgery and two underwent resection. Overall, 100 of 102 patients were cured with cryosurgery. Complications associated with cryosurgery included six (5.9%) pathologic fractures, three (2.9%) cases of partial skin necrosis, and two (1.9%) significant degenerative changes. Overall function was good to excellent in 94 patients (92.2%), moderate in seven patients (6.9%), and poor in one patient (0.9%). Cryosurgery has the advantages of joint preservation, excellent functional outcome, and low recurrence rate when compared with other joint preservation procedures. For these reasons, it is recommended as an adjuvant to curettage for most giant cell tumors of bone.

32

Pulmonary metastases

JOE B PUTNAM JR AND JACK A ROTH

INTRODUCTION

Systemic spread of metastases from primary neoplasms represents uncontrolled tumor and frequently heralds a rapid course of disease progression and eventual death. In contrast, isolated pulmonary metastases do not consistently represent a systemic or untreatable spread of a primary neoplasm. These patients, with metastases isolated only within the lungs, may have a unique biology, more amenable to local or systemic treatment options than patients with multi-organ metastases. Isolated pulmonary metastases should not be viewed as untreatable. Many patients who have complete resection of all metastases have associated longer survival than those patients who are unresectable. Long-term survival (greater than 5 years) may be expected in approximately one-third of all patients with resectable pulmonary metastases. Better survival awaits improvements in local control, systemic or regional chemotherapy, or modulation of tumor biology via bioimmunotherapy or gene transfer.

HISTORICAL PERSPECTIVE

Early attempts at resection of pulmonary metastases have been described.[1] A recent review by Martini *et al.* has chronicled the early attempts at resection of pulmonary metastases.[2] The first resections of pulmonary metastasis were reported in the mid-1980s while resecting primary chest wall tumors.[1] Divis[3] and Torek[4] described the first resection of a pulmonary metastasis as a separate procedure. Barney and Churchill[5] reported one of the first long-term survivors of pulmonary metastasectomy following resection of a metastasis from a patient with hypernephroma. After local control of the primary tumor and resection of the metastasis, the patient survived for 23 years and died from unrelated causes.

Alexander and Haight[6] reviewed the first large series (25 patients) of patients who had resection of metastases from carcinoma and sarcoma. Mannix in 1953 described for the first time resection of multiple pulmonary metastases from a patient with osteochondromas.[7] Few attempts were made at multiple resections for pulmonary metastases until Martini and coworkers in 1971 noted the value of multiple resections (multiple sequential operations) in the treatment of osteogenic sarcoma.[8] In the past 20 years, resections of solitary and multiple pulmonary metastases from numerous primary neoplasms have been performed, with good long-term survival in up to 40% of patients treated.

Autopsy studies have demonstrated that about one-third of patients with cancer will die with pulmonary metastases and a small percentage will die with metastases confined solely to the lungs. Metastases from osteogenic and soft tissue sarcomas commonly occur only in the lungs. Patients with other solid-organ neoplasms from melanoma, breast, or colon will have isolated pulmonary metastases less commonly, but these metastases may represent a favorable tumor biology and a treatable subset of such patients. In the absence of extrathoracic metastases, patients with isolated and resectable pulmonary metastases should undergo complete resection for treatment and possible cure of their disease.

PATHOLOGY

Neoplasms may metastasize in four ways: hematogenous, lymphogenic, direct invasion, and aerogenous. Underlying tumor biology and host resistance determine mechanisms of spread, location(s) of metastases, and extent of growth. Blood-borne metastases are most frequently found in the lung and liver. Clumps of tumor cells are filtered out in the lungs or may preferentially adhere to the underlying capillary endothelium. Tumor cells may travel by lymphatics and occupy a discrete position within the lung or may involve diffusely the entire lung, as is seen with lymphangitic spread of breast carcinoma or other metastatic adenocarcinomas. Rarely, metastases may metastasize to other organs; however, metastases can develop in draining pulmonary lobar, hilar, or mediastinal nodes, depending on the underlying histology. Direct invasion of metastases into other structures may occur as the metastasis grows. Aerogenous spread of tumor from one site within the bronchus to another site is rare, if it occurs at all.

SYMPTOMS

Symptoms rarely occur from pulmonary metastases; therefore, the diagnosis of metastases is routinely made on chest roentgenograms after primary tumor resection. Palliation for pain is rarely needed as the pleura is infrequently involved. Few ($< 5\%$) patients with metastases will present with symptoms of dyspnea, pain, cough, or hemoptysis.

DIAGNOSIS

Chest roentgenograms (CXRs) obtained after primary tumor resection may demonstrate pulmonary parenchymal changes consistent with metastases. Metastases may appear as solitary or multiple nodules, well-circumscribed or diffuse opacities, miliary or massive in appearance. Routine CXRs represent an effective means of screening patients for pulmonary metastases.

Patients without evidence of metastases on CXR rarely have metastases demonstrated by tomography. However, Lien et al.[9] showed that approximately half of patients with non-seminomatous testicular tumors have negative CXR but abnormalities identified on computed tomography (CT) scans. Chang and colleagues,[10] at the National Cancer Institute, prospectively evaluated linear tomograms and CT for pulmonary metastases. They found metastases in only 20% of nodules greater than 3 mm which were identified by CT and not by linear tomograms. CT provided a more sensitive but less specific examination than CXR for identifying metastatic lesions. CT of the chest provides a consistent anatomic reference for the resection of pulmonary metastases.

Patients with known metastases on CXR should undergo CT to identify other smaller metastases. CT of the chest will demonstrate nodules as small as 3 mm. When clinically correlated with the patient's age, prior history of malignancy, and prior treatment, a diagnosis of pulmonary metastases can be made. Dinkel et al.[11] stated that full lung linear tomograms (FLTs) may be 97% accurate in the diagnosis of pulmonary metastases, although without the sensitivity of high-resolution CT. Blickman and colleagues[12] studied 28 patients, comparing CT of the chest with whole-lung linear tomograms. They found no difference between the two studies in either sensitivity or specificity and concluded that the expense of CT was not justified. Feuerstein and associates[13] showed that magnetic resonance imaging (MRI) was as sensitive as CT scans for identifying pulmonary metastases but added little additional information. MRI is not routinely recommended for the evaluation of patients with pulmonary metastases confined to the pulmonary parenchyma; it may be of great value in planning the resection of pulmonary metastases involving other portions of the chest wall or adjacent thoracic organs.

One prospective study of 19 patients evaluated CT and FLTs to detect pulmonary metastases from osteogenic or soft tissue sarcomas. Pass and colleagues[14] noted that CT was significantly better than FLT in detecting metastatic nodules earlier (56 by CT versus 7 by FLT, $p = 0.001$) and smaller (7.6 mm by CT versus 13.2 mm by FLT, $p < 0.05$). They recommended that surgical decisions for the resection of pulmonary metastases be based on CT findings rather than on FLT.

Benign granulomatous diseases may mimic metastases; however, in patients with a prior diagnosis of malignancy, these nodules are probably metastases. Clinical stage I or II primary lung carcinoma may be indistinguishable from a solitary metastasis, particularly if the original tumor was squamous cell carcinoma or adenocarcinoma. For these two histologies specifically, thoracotomy and lobectomy would be the procedure of choice. Routine mediastinal lymph node dissection for solitary metastases from adenocarcinoma or squamous carcinoma would complete the staging. Fine-needle aspiration or thoracoscopic wedge excision may be helpful for the diagnosis or staging of pulmonary changes in high-risk patients. In patients with lymphangitic spread of cancer, biopsy may be required to differentiate neoplasm from infection.

TREATMENT OF PULMONARY METASTASES

The majority of patients with pulmonary metastases have multiple sites of metastases or unresectable pleural or pulmonary metastases. In these patients, treatment is directed to the palliation of symptoms. Although radiation therapy or chemotherapy is frequently used, little hope exists for cure. In patients with control of the primary tumor and metastases confined to the lungs, resection of all visualized or palpable metastases may be considered. Complete resection of pulmonary metastases is generally associated with improved patient survival, regardless of primary histology.

Chemotherapy

The value of chemotherapy for the treatment of pulmonary metastases that develop after treatment of the primary is controversial. The incidence of pulmonary metastases in patients with primary osteogenic sarcoma treated with surgical resection and adjuvant chemotherapy has dramatically declined compared to those patients treated with surgery alone, as described by Skinner et al.,[15] Goorin et al.,[16] Pastorino et al.,[17] and Yamaguchi et al.,[18] Bacci et al.[19] noted that in patients who receive adjuvant chemotherapy for primary osteogenic sarcoma, surgical resection of pulmonary metastases may be accomplished in a larger proportion (51%) than it can be in others who do not receive adjuvant chemotherapy (29%). Salvage chemotherapy with resection may be effective in prolonging survival in patients who develop pulmonary metastases from osteogenic sarcoma, as suggested by Marina et al.[20] and Pastorino et al.[21] however, Bacci et al.[22] and Al-Jilaihawi[23] and others have not seen a benefit. Bacci et al.[22] examined patients with osteogenic sarcoma of the extremity who presented with pulmonary metastases. Preoperat-ive chemotherapy (adriamycin, methotrexate, cisplatin), surgery, and postoperative chemotherapy (ifosphamide, VP-16) failed to provide disease-free or overall survival equivalent to that of patients without metastases at presentation. Seventy-three percent of patients with metastases at presentation experienced recurrence within 3.5 years compared to 27% of patients without metastases at presentation. Glasser and colleagues[24] showed that histologic response to chemotherapy (percentage necrosis) was the only independent predictor of enhanced survival in a study of 279 patients with stage II osteogenic sarcoma.

Completeness of resection after chemotherapy impacts significantly on subsequent survival. Kim and Louie[25] treated patients with metastatic renal cell carcinoma with interleukin-2 prior to surgical resection of residual tumor. Nine of 11 patients were alive and without evidence of disease at a median follow-up of 21 months. Lanza and associates[26] examined the response of soft tissue sarcoma metastases that were treated with chemotherapy prior to surgery. Patients were graded as having complete, partial, or no response/progression from the chemotherapy. Survival could not be predicted on the basis of response to chemotherapy alone. No prospective, randomized trial evaluating salvage chemotherapy followed by resection versus resection alone for pulmonary metastases for soft tissue sarcomas has been attempted.

Radiation therapy

Currently, radiation therapy is used for the palliation of symptoms of advanced metastases, e.g., extensive pleural involvement, bone metastases, etc. Radiation therapy is rarely used for the treatment of pulmonary metastases. Prophylactic lung radiation has been performed for osteogenic sarcoma. Burgers et al.[27] showed that patients with prophylactic lung radiation for primary osteogenic sarcoma had recurrence of pulmonary metastases similar to that of patients having adjuvant chemotherapy.

Surgery

In selected patients with resectable pulmonary metastases and absence of extrathoracic metastases, complete resection is generally associated with improved long-term survival, regardless of histology.

SELECTION OF PATIENTS FOR RESECTION

The criteria for the selection of patients with isolated pulmonary metastases for resection have been described by Takita et al.,[28] Morrow et al.,[29] McCormack and Martini,[30] and Mountain et al.[31] in an attempt to quantitate the tumor biology of the metastases and to identify patients who would benefit from surgical resection. Criteria have been proposed to identify and select patients who will benefit optimally from resection of their pulmonary metastases (Table 32.1).

Many patients with metastases will not benefit from surgery because of a biologically aggressive tumor characterized by extensive disease, a short disease-free interval between control of their primary tumor and identification of pulmonary metastases, or rapid metastatic growth. Tumor biology also differs with the same tumor histology based upon genetic factors and host (patient) resistance.

The surgeon has an obligation to consider complete resection for all patients who are potentially resectable. Resection does not change the natural history of pulmonary metastases: multiple, small nodules spread throughout all lobes may be unresectable for cure; however, in all patients, particularly in questionable cases, resectability or unresectability must be defined by a thoracic surgeon. Multiple wedge resections are commonly performed for the treatment of pulmonary metastases and, as well, segmentectomy or lobectomy. Pneumonectomy is rarely performed, although it may provide beneficial treatment in highly selected patients.[32]

Table 32.1 *Criteria for resection of pulmonary metastases*

Pulmonary nodules consistent with metastases
Control of primary tumor
All nodules potentially resectable with planned
  surgery/surgeries
Adequate postoperative pulmonary reserve anticipated
No extrathoracic metastases
Other indications for partial or complete resection of pulmonary metastases
Establish a diagnosis
Residual disease after chemotherapy
Obtain tissue for tumor markers or
  immunohistochemical studies
Decrease tumor burden

SURGICAL TECHNIQUES AND INCISIONS

Surgical procedures for resection include single thoracotomy, staged bilateral thoracotomies, median sternotomy, or the 'clam-shell' incision. These procedures have almost no mortality and minimal morbidity. Patients with bilateral metastases may be safely explored with either a median sternotomy or staged bilateral thoracotomies, as shown by Johnston[33] and Roth et al.[34] The incision(s) chosen does not influence patient survival if all metastases are resected; various advantages and disadvantages are unique to each approach (Table 32.2).

Patients with sarcomas and unilateral nodules often have multiple and bilateral metastases discovered during the operation. Johnston[33] and Roth et al.[34] discovered bilateral metastases in 38–60% of patients with preoperative unilateral sarcomatous metastasis. Post-resection survival rates after median sternotomy or bilateral staged thoracotomies and complete resection are similar.

A median sternotomy is recommended for patients with unilateral or bilateral nodules from osteogenic or soft tissue sarcomas. Median sternotomy should be considered the procedure of choice in patients with suspected bilateral metastases from any primary neoplasm. A thorough exploration for unilateral or bilateral nodules as well as resection of these sarcomatous nodules may be accomplished through a median sternotomy incision.

Prior to surgery, the patient is examined thoroughly for the extent of metastases and to assess whether an operation can be safely performed (Table 32.3). CXR and chest CT scans are reviewed and displayed prominently in the operating room. After bronchoscopy, a double-lumen endotracheal tube is placed. A median sternotomy incision is used and sequential deflation of each lung aids in the exposure and palpation of the pulmonary nodules. All nodules are resected with a margin of normal tissue. Nodules should not be 'shelled out' as viable tumor cells remain on the periphery of the resected area. Often, the decision of adequacy of margin is the surgeon's alone as lung parenchyma may become distorted around the nodule after resection, giving the illusion of a positive or close margin. Mediastinal lymph node metastases rarely occur from pulmonary metastases.[35,36]

Laser-assisted pulmonary resection using the neodymium–yttrium–aluminum garnet laser may provide a better means of resecting pulmonary metastases than the surgical stapler, as described by Kodama et al.,[37] Branscheid et al.,[38] Miyamoto et al.,[39] and Landreneau et al.[40] The disadvantages of laser resection may include longer operating time and a potential for prolonged postoperative air leaks; however, use of the laser may enhance the preservation of lung parenchyma, with less distortion. Bovie electrocautery may also spare lung parenchyma by removing the metastases with minimal distortion of the remaining lung. Air leaks, if they occur, can be sealed by oversewing the parenchymal defect or the use of fibrin glue.

Table 32.2 *Advantages and disadvantages of various surgical resections*

Median sternotomy	
Advantages	Bilateral thoracic explorations with one incision
	Less patient discomfort
Disadvantages	Resection of lesions posterior and medial (near the hila) may be difficult
	Difficult exposure to the left lower lobe in patients with obesity, congestive heart failure, or COPD (increased thoracic AP diameter)
Posterolateral thoracotomy	
Advantages	'Standard' approach
	Excellent exposure of the hemithorax
Disadvantages	Patient discomfort (*although minimized with thoracic epidural anesthesia*)
	Only one hemithorax may be explored at one operation
	A second operation is needed for bilateral metastases
Video-assisted thoracic surgery	
Advantages	Lobectomy potentially less immunosuppressive
	Excellent visualization
	Minimal morbidity and discomfort
	Excellent exposure for visceral pleural metastases
	May identify unresectable metastases, pleural studding, etc.
Disadvantages	Unable to fully evaluate metastases in the lung parenchyma
	Learning curve
	Length of procedure
	Potential for increased costs
	Potential for higher costs (staplers, disposable instruments)

COPD, chronic obstructive pulmonary disease.

Median sternotomy and 'clam-shell' incision

The patient is positioned supine, with the entire anterior thorax exposed from the neck to the umbilicus and laterally to each anterior axillary line. The sternum is divided. The pulmonary ligament is divided on each side to mobilize the lung completely. The lungs are sequentially deflated and palpated. Metastases are identified and resected, and then the deflated lung is reinflated. The

Table 32.3 *Preoperative evaluation prior to pulmonary metastasectomy*

Routine blood chemistries
Chest roentgenogram (PA and lateral)
Computed tomography (CT) of the chest (high resolution or spiral CT most sensitive)
Pulmonary function tests
Electrocardiogram
Optional (depending on symptoms and histology):
  CT abdomen
  CT brain
  CT of area of primary neoplasm
  Bone scan
  Other studies to exclude extrathoracic metastases

deflated right lung may be brought completely into the field, attached by only the hilar structures. Exposure of the left lower lobe may be more difficult than exposure of the other lobes because of the overlying heart. With appropriate gentle traction on the pericardium, the left lower lobe can be exposed quite readily and brought into the operative field. Various techniques to better visualize the lung may be employed, such as surgical packs behind the hilum of the deflated lung to elevate the parenchyma or technical aids such as an internal mammary artery retractor to exposure basilar tumors or posterior hilar left lower lobe masses.

The 'clam-shell' incision, as described by Bains *et al.*,[41] is a modification of the median sternotomy incision. Originally, this approach was developed from lung transplantation in order to enhance bilateral sequential single-lung transplantation. A curvilinear incision under the breasts/pectoral muscles is made and carried across the sternum at approximately the level of the fourth intercostal space. The sternum is divided transversely with a Gigli or oscillating saw, and the intercostal muscles are divided to open the chest anteriorly. Following placement of one or two chest retractors, the chest is opened, giving excellent exposure to hemithorax, bilateral hila, and mediastinum. The advantages of this approach include better exposure of the left hilum posteriorly and of the left lower lobe. The disadvantages include a large, painful incision and some difficulty with sternal reconstruction and stabilization.

Posterolateral thoracotomy

The posterolateral thoracotomy is a familiar and standard approach to pulmonary resection for carcinoma of the lung, although Urschel and Razzuk[42] have advocated median sternotomy for the resection of lung carcinoma. Posterolateral thoracotomy may provide better exposure for metastases located posteriorly near the hilum on the left side. In addition, for patients with bulky metastases, a posterolateral thoracotomy provides good access for

laser resection and optimal sparing of lung parenchyma; however, the surgeon is limited to operating in one hemithorax. Bilateral thoracotomies are rarely performed in the same patient at the same operation, although left thoracotomy following median sternotomy may be performed safely in selected patients.

Video-assisted thoracic surgery

Video-assisted thoracoscopic resection using high-resolution video imaging may be helpful for the diagnosis, staging, and resection of metastases, as suggested by Kodama *et al.*[37] and Miller *et al.*[43] However, its usefulness is limited as metastases can be identified only on the surface of the lung or the outer 10–20% (depending on size). Metastases within the lung parenchyma may be undetectable with this technique. Landreneau and associates[44] have described minimal morbidity and no mortality in 61 patients who underwent 85 thoracoscopic pulmonary resections. Lesions were small (<3 cm) and in the outer third of the lung parenchyma. Metastases in 18 patients were resected via thoracoscopy in this series. Video-assisted thoracic surgery (VATS) was the only procedure performed in these patients. At present, this approach can be advocated only for the diagnosis or staging of the extent of metastases. Complications of VATS may include failure to resect all metastases, positive margins, or pleural seeding with extraction of the metastasis.

The limitations of thoracoscopy continue to evolve as more experience with the technique is obtained and prospective studies mature. In an elegant study, McCormack and colleagues[45] considered a prospective study of VATS resection for the treatment of pulmonary metastases. After VATS, thoracotomy or median sternotomy was performed. They found that more nodules were found by thoracotomy and that VATS failed to identify all nodules. Limitations of the study were the inclusion as eligible patients those with two metastases, patients with prior sarcoma histology (frequently multiple and bilateral), and resolution limits with CT scans. VATS is not the standard approach for resection in patients with pulmonary metastases. However, it may be considered in patients with a solitary nodule and non-sarcomatous histology on high-resolution (spiral) chest CT scan.

Extended resection of pulmonary metastases

Pneumonectomy or other extended resection of pulmonary metastases may be performed safely in selected patients, with associated long-term disease-free survival. Less than 3% of all patients undergoing resection of pulmonary metastases will require an extended resection.

Pneumonectomy or en-bloc resection of pulmonary metastases with chest wall or other thoracic structures such as diaphragm, pericardium, and/or superior vena cava have been performed in a small number of patients with good results.[32] Nineteen patients had a pneumonectomy and 19 patients had other extended resection. The 5-year actuarial survival was 25%. Mortality was 5% and occurred in those patients having pneumonectomy, often after multiple prior wedge resections for metastases.

SELECTION OF INCISION AND CHOICE OF INITIAL PROCEDURE

The surgeon's choice of incision for resection of pulmonary metastases must reflect the goal of surgery: complete resection of the metastases with minimal morbidity. Resection of multiple, tiny, peripheral metastases may be possible; however, the biological impact of such an endeavor may be minimal. Patients with multiple metastases may undergo resection with good short-term results and the potential for long-term survival. Median sternotomy is well suited for resection of multiple peripheral metastases. For multiple or more centrally located metastases, staged bilateral thoracotomy may enhance the surgeon's ability to achieve complete resection and minimize pulmonary and other operative morbidity. Use of a lateral thoracotomy and the laser as a parenchymal-sparing modality may allow larger, more bulky metastases to be resected without the need for lobectomy. With median sternotomy, more centrally located tumors may require extensive or deep wedges, with significant diminution of pulmonary function in the residual lobar tissue. Transverse sternotomy or the 'clam-shell' incision may also be considered in lieu of bilateral staged thoracotomy. Use of the laser in contrast to the stapler minimizes compression and distortion of the lung (with resulting decrease in pulmonary function due to enfolding of the parenchyma). The laser maintains the 'topography' of the lung in a better manner.

Preoperative staging may suggest that a lobectomy or pneumonectomy may be required to resect all disease. In patients with solitary metastases, such resection may be associated with minimal morbidity and enhanced long-term survival. In patients with bilateral multiple metastases, incisions (median sternotomy versus bilateral staged thoracotomies with choice of side) must be planned with the goal of complete resection. In patients with potentially resectable metastases, I would recommend that the surgeon resect metastases from the least involved lung and then from the more involved lung. The rationale would be that, if the metastases within the least involved lung are unresectable, the patient is spared a second operation. If the metastases within the least involved lung are resectable, then the patient would have maximal parenchyma remaining when lobectomy is performed on the contralateral side, thereby enhancing patient safety and maximizing the opportunity for complete resection. This planning is particularly helpful in sarcomas, for which the metastases are frequently multiple and bilateral.

RESULTS OF RESECTION OF PULMONARY METASTASES

The results of resection for pulmonary metastasectomy require critical analysis of the factors that may potentially influence survival. Results should be based upon single primary histology (breast, colon, melanoma) or similar histology (e.g., soft tissue sarcomas) and sufficient numbers of patients. Prognostic indicators have been reviewed to assess their influence, singularly and in combination, on post-resection survival in patients with pulmonary metastases (Table 32.4) and to assist clinically in describing appropriate patients for resection. Age, gender, histology, grade, location, and stage of the primary tumor, disease-free survival, number of nodules on preoperative radiological studies, unilateral or bilateral metastases, tumor doubling time, and synchronous or metachronous metastases may be evaluated preoperatively. Postoperatively, the extent of resectability, the technique of resection, nodal spread, number of metastases and location, re-resection post-thoracotomy disease-free survival, and overall survival may also be examined.

Osteogenic sarcoma

Pulmonary metastases from osteogenic sarcoma may occur in up to 80% of patients who relapse after treatment for their primary neoplasm, whether or not they receive adjuvant chemotherapy.[16,46,47] Because these metastases are often isolated to the lungs, resection may render a significant number of patients disease free and may enhance long-term survival.[48] Five-year survival may range up to 40%.[49, 50]

Carter et al.,[51] Jaffe et al.,[52] Putnam et al.,[53] and Rosen et al.[54] have evaluated survival and prognostic factors in patients with pulmonary metastases from osteogenic sarcoma. In a series from the National Institutes of Health, Putnam et al.[53] evaluated 80 patients with osteogenic sarcoma of the extremity. Forty-three patients developed pulmonary metastases; 39 patients underwent one or more thoracic explorations for resection of their metastases. Five-year survival was 40%. Various prognostic factors were analysed. Fewer nodules (≤ three), longer disease-free interval, resectable metastases, and fewer metastases identified and resected were associated with longer post-thoracotomy survival. Resection was not possible if more than 16 nodules were identified on preoperative tomograms. A multivariate analysis did not find any combination of factors to be more predictive than the number of nodules identified on preoperative tomograms.

Table 32.4 *Prognostic indicators[a] associated with better post-resection survival for various tumor histologies*

Reference	Year	n	Stage of primary	Nodules CT FLT	METS resected	TDT (months)	Resect	DFI (months)	Median survival (months)	5-year survival (%)
Breast										
75	1992	33	NS	NS					58	36
74	1992	44	NS				+	>12	47[b]	50
114	1988	50	Neg nodes		NS			>18	13	12
Colorectal										
72	1992	139	NS		1[c]		+	NS	36	30.5
65	1988	66	NS		1[c]			>24[d]	42	38
115	1979	35	+		NS[c]			NS		22
68	1989	27	NS		NS[c]				27	9
69	1986	27	NS		NS[c]		+	>24	35	21
140	1985	62	NS		1[c]			NS	24	42
Osteogenic sarcoma										
21	1992	102					+			58
117	1985	38		≤4		NS	+	NS		
48	1987	39[e]		<4	<6		+	NS	20	38
53	1983	38		≤3	≤4	NS	+	>6	26	40
116	1988	27			1			>12	28	47 (at 3 years)
141	1984	32			NS		+	NS	24	32
50	1989	20					+	NS		37
Renal										
88	1992	23		NS	NS		+	NS	>49[b]	60
89	1988	39			NS[c]		+	NS	36	32.7
118	1983	44			NS		NS	>24	33	27
Soft tissue sarcomas										
83	1992	45			NS		+	NS		43
117	1985	67		≤4		>20 days	+	>12		
35	1984	67		≤4	<16	>20 days	+	>12	18	10
58	1989	63	NS	≤5 ≤3	NS	NS	+	>12	20.3	27
142	1989	28			NS			NS		35 (estimate)

Table 32.4 (Continued)

Reference	Year	n	Stage of primary	Nodules CT FLT	METS resected	TDT (months)	Resect	DFI (months)	Median survival (months)	5-year survival (%)
Ewing's sarcoma										
101	1987	19			≤4		+	NS	28[b]	15
Melanoma										
92	1992	98			+		+	+	22[b]	20
91	1991	56	NS	NS	NS	NS	+	NS	18	25
143	1990	29	NS		NS		+	NS	11[b]	4.5
90	1988	31	NS[f]	NS	NS		NS	NS	13	7 (estimate)
144	1988	47					+	NS	19	25
145	1985	17			NS			NS	16.5	11.1

CT, computed tomography; FLT, full lung linear tomograms; METS, metastases; Neg, negative; TDT, tumor doubling time; Resect, resectability; DFI, disease-free interval between control of primary tumor and identification of pulmonary metastases; NS, not significant.

[a]Age, sex, tumor grade, location of primary tumor are rarely prognostic indicators for either improved or poorer survival.
[b]Resectable patients only.
[c]Solitary versus multiple.
[d]Borderline significance ($p = 0.1$).
[e]Male gender was associated with improved survival.
[f]Nodal status was not significant.

Beattie and others[55] examined four of six survivors (>19 years) who had undergone multiple resections for multiple metastases. Surgical resectability was the only predictive factor associated with prolonged survival for recurrent osteogenic sarcoma. Chemotherapy had no effect on the post-thoracotomy survival following complete resection of pulmonary metastases from osteogenic sarcoma. However, it did prolong the disease-free interval between the surgical treatment of the primary and the appearance of pulmonary metastases. Belli et al.[50] suggest that chemotherapy may prevent or cure micrometastatic disease not amenable to surgery.

Soft tissue sarcomas

Soft tissue sarcomas comprise a family of non-ossifying malignant neoplasms arising from mesenchymal connective tissues. As with osteogenic sarcomas, Potter and colleagues[56] noted that local recurrence is common (20%) and metastases are predominantly to the lungs. Casson et al.[57] evaluated the determinants of 5-year survival in 58 patients who had complete resection and who were followed until death or for a minimum of 5 years. Absolute 5-year survival was 26% (15/58 patients). Favorable prognostic factors included tumor doubling time of greater than 40 days, unilateral disease, three nodules or fewer identified on preoperative tomograms, two metastases or fewer resected, and tumor histology (median survival 33 months for malignant fibrous histiocytoma versus 17 months for all others). Using multivariate analysis, the number of nodules (four or more) was the most significant prognostic indicator. The addition of tumor histology (malignant fibrous histiocytoma) improved the predictive ability of this model.

In patients with histologically documented pulmonary metastases from soft tissue sarcomas treated at the National Cancer Institute, Jablons et al.[58] and Putnam et al.[35] described significant preoperative predictors of enhanced survival. These included tumor doubling time (>20 days), number of metastases on preoperative tomograms (four or fewer nodules), and disease-free interval (>12 months). Predictive ability for better survival was improved when all three prognostic factors were combined. These patients represent those who will have the best response (i.e., prolonged post-resection survival) to pulmonary metastasectomy.

Resection of recurrent pulmonary metastases also improves post-resection survival.[59] Forty-three patients with two or more resections were recently reviewed by Pogrebniak et al.[60] In 31 resectable patients (31/43, 72%) median survival was 25 months, compared to unresectable patients with a median survival of only 10 months. A longer disease-free interval (≥18 months) was also associated with prolonged disease-free survival. Increased age and female gender were associated with an increased risk of death from disease in resected patients with recurrent pulmonary metastases, in contrast to initial isolated pulmonary metastases. In 39 patients with recurrent pulmonary metastases from adult soft tissue sarcomas, Casson et al.[61] noted that resectable patients and those with only one metastasis had the best post-resection survival. The results of chemotherapy for metastatic soft tissue sarcoma remain poor, with median survival ranging from 13 to 16 months.[62,63]

Colorectal neoplasms

Colorectal metastases commonly spread to local or regional nodes or are trapped in the liver through the portal venous drainage. Patients with prior colorectal neoplasms have had pulmonary metastases resected with prolonged post-resection survival. An absolute distinction cannot be made between a single carcinomatous metastasis and a primary bronchogenic carcinoma, except by direct visual comparison between the two neoplasms. Molecular determinants of origin are evolving.

As with other isolated pulmonary metastases, patients with pulmonary metastases from colorectal carcinoma may be resected safely, with low morbidity, mortality, and long-term survival. Recent reports[64–69] describe 5-year survival from 21% up to 50% following resection of pulmonary metastases from colon carcinoma. Differences in age, gender, location, grade and stage of the primary colorectal cancer are not associated with either improved or worsened survival after resection of these metastases. Patients with metachronous liver lesions excised for cure may also be candidates for resection of pulmonary metastases. Sauter et al.[70] evaluated 49 patients with isolated pulmonary metastases ($n = 18$) and hepatic metastases ($n = 31$). Patients with pulmonary metastases had a 47% 5-year survival, whereas patients with hepatic metastases had a 5-year survival of 19%. Pihl et al.[71] reviewed 1578 patients treated for colon and rectal cancer: 117 of 1013 patients with rectal carcinoma (11.5%) and 20 of 565 patients with colon cancer (3.5%) had recurrence in the lungs. Mansel et al.[69] evaluated 66 patients who underwent resection of pulmonary metastases from colorectal adenocarcinoma. Patients with solitary metastasis had a longer post-resection survival than others. The 5-year survival was 38% in both studies. In another study of 62 patients, Goya et al.[68] showed that only metastases <3 cm in diameter were associated with improved survival. Brister et al.[65] associated longer disease-free interval with prolonged post-thoracotomy resection.

In a large contemporary series from the Mayo Clinic, McAfee et al.[72] reported 139 patients who underwent resection of pulmonary metastases from colorectal carcinoma. The operative mortality was 1.4%, overall 5-year survival was 30.5%, and the median follow-up was 7 years. Patients with a solitary pulmonary metastasis and those with a preoperative carcinoembryonic antigen (CEA) level <4.0 ng/mL had a better post-thoracotomy than others. Longer disease-free interval and diameter of metastases <3 cm were not associated with improved survival.

Breast carcinoma

Patients with metastases from breast carcinoma usually do poorly as metastases occur in multiple sites. Patanaphan described 145 patients with metastatic breast carcinoma (145/558, 26%).[73] Bone (51%), lung (17%), brain (16%), and liver (6%) metastases occurred. The overall median survival was 12 months for patients with lung metastases mostly treated with palliative chemotherapy and/or irradiation. Lanza and associates[74] reviewed 44 women with a prior history of breast cancer

who underwent pulmonary resection for new pulmonary lesions. Seven patients who had benign nodules ($n = 3$) or unresectable metastases ($n = 4$) were excluded. In 37 resectable patients, the actuarial 5-year survival was 50% (Figure 32.1). Disease-free interval >12 months was associated with a longer median survival (82 months) and 5-year survival (57%) compared to patients with a disease-free interval of <12 months (15 months median, 0% 5-year survival; $p = 0.004$) (Figure 32.2). Estrogen receptor-positive status tended to be associated with a longer post-thoracotomy survival ($p = 0.098$).

Staren *et al.* evaluated 33 patients treated with surgical resection of pulmonary metastases from breast carcinoma and compared the results to those for 30 patients treated primarily with systemic chemotherapy and hormonal therapy.[75] Patients having complete resection of metastases had a better median survival than patients with medical therapy, particularly when single nodules

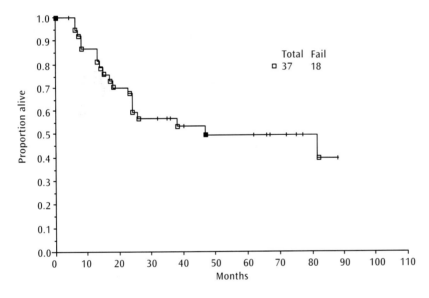

Figure 32.1 *Actuarial post-thoracotomy survival of 37 patients with history of breast cancer undergoing complete resection of malignant nodules (median survival, 47 ± 5.5 months). (From Lanza et al., 1992.[74])*

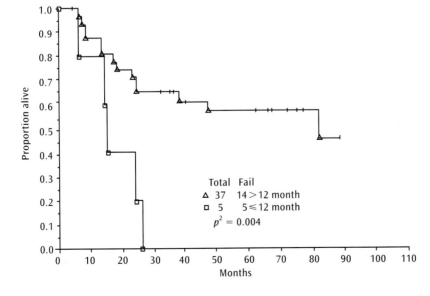

Figure 32.2 *Effect of initial disease-free interval after treatment for breast cancer. Preoperative disease-free interval is associated with prolonged post-thoracotomy survival (p = 0.004). (From Lanza et al., 1992.[74])*

were compared (58 months median survival versus 34 months, respectively). The 5-year survival amongst patients treated with some surgical resection was 36%, compared to 11% in those patients treated with other than surgical treatment.

Testicular neoplasms

Non-seminomatous testicular tumors can be diagnosed by the occurrence of new pulmonary nodules identified on CXR or by CT scan.[9,76] Metastatic testicular seminoma is usually identified as mediastinal nodal enlargement. Therefore, CT scan is more accurate in diagnosing of seminomatous metastases than plain CXRs.[77]

Cytoreductive surgery for disseminated non-seminomatous germ cell tumors of the testis may be performed after chemotherapy for removal of residual metastatic disease. The response to chemotherapy may be assessed when there is no further reduction in the size of the nodules. The majority of patients will require retroperitoneal lymph node dissections (69%), although thoracotomies may be required in 18% of patients.[78,79] Carsky and others evaluated 80 patients with germ cell tumors and lung metastases treated with chemotherapy and subsequent surgery.[80] Thirty-five percent ($n = 28$) achieved complete response after chemotherapy. Thirty-six patients with partial response underwent surgery for resection of metastases in the abdomen ($n = 17$), the lungs ($n = 15$), or both ($n = 4$); 27/36 patients achieved complete response after both chemotherapy and surgery. Carter et al.[81] noted that extensive pulmonary metastases (unresectable metastases) are a predictor of ultimate treatment failure.

Gynecological neoplasms

Fuller and colleagues,[82] from the Massachusetts General Hospital, reviewed a 40-year experience of treating 15 patients with pulmonary metastases from gynecologic cancer. Six patients had primary tumors involving the cervix, three the endometrium, two the ovary, two had uterine sarcomas, and two had choriocarcinomas. The 5-year survival was 36%. Lesions <4 cm in diameter and a disease-free interval of more than 36 months were associated with prolonged survival. Levenback et al.[83] reviewed 45 patients with pulmonary metastases from uterine sarcomas. Most patients (71%) had unilateral lesions and 51% had only one lesion. The 5-year survival was 43%. Unilateral metastases or fewer metastases were not significantly associated with prolonged survival.

Kumar reviewed 97 patients with metastatic gestational trophoblastic disease; chemotherapy was the treatment of choice.[84] Selective thoracotomy in patients with solitary lung metastases reduced the treatment time and the need for further aggressive chemotherapy. Overall, the 2-year survival after diagnosis was 65%. A disease-free

interval of less than 1 year was associated with poorer survival.

Barter et al.[85] studied 2116 patients with primary cervical malignancy between 1969 and 1984 and found 88 patients (4.2%) with pulmonary lesions consistent with metastases. The prognosis was poor with chemotherapy only (median survival 8 months; only 2/88 long-term survivors). Imachi et al.[86] identified 50 out of 817 patients (6.1%) treated for carcinoma of the uterine cervix who developed pulmonary metastases: 81% of patients had local recurrence or other metastases, and chemotherapy was given. The authors suggest that surgery may be considered for patients with pulmonary metastases without extrathoracic metastases.

Renal cell carcinoma

Various series have examined the value of resection of pulmonary metastases from renal cell carcinoma. Recent 5-year survival has ranged from 21%[87] to 60%.[88] Schott et al.[89] reviewed 938 patients undergoing nephrectomy for renal carcinoma. Thirty-nine patients (4.1%) underwent resection of pulmonary metastases. Patients with pulmonary metastases <2 cm in diameter and limited to one site had prolonged survival and disease-free interval compared to other patients. Dernevik and colleagues[87] resected 33 patients for pulmonary metastases, with a minimum follow-up period of 5 years or until death. Longer disease-free interval (>1 year) was associated with a longer overall survival than a shorter disease-free interval (<1 year). Pogrebniak and associates,[88] from the National Cancer Institute, reported on 23 patients who underwent resection of pulmonary metastases from renal cell carcinoma, of whom 18 had previous interleukin-2 based immunotherapy. Resectable patients (15/23, 65%) had a longer survival (mean 49 months; median not yet reached) compared to unresectable patients (median 16 months, $p = 0.02$). Post-resection survival did not depend on tomogram nodules, resected nodules, or the disease-free interval.

Melanoma

The overall biological behavior of melanoma cannot be predicted. Most commonly, pulmonary metastases occur in addition to metastases at other visceral sites and overall long-term survival is poor. In the rare patients who present with isolated pulmonary metastases, resection may be associated with long-term survival. Current 5-year survival ranges from 4.5% to 25%. Patients with multiple pulmonary metastases have poor long-term survival, as noted by Pogrebniak et al.[90]

Gorenstein and colleagues[91] evaluated 56 patients with histologically proven pulmonary metastases from melanoma. The overall post-resection survival was 25%

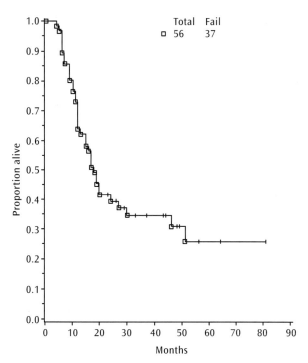

Figure 32.3 *Overall actuarial survival for patients with melanoma undergoing resection of pulmonary metastases. The median survival was 18 months. (From Gorenstein et al., 1991.[91])*

at 5 years (Figure 32.3). Patients with earlier primary stage melanoma, or patients with metastases to the lungs as the first site of metastases, had longer post-resection survival than other patients. Location of the primary tumor, histology, thickness, Clark level, nodal metastases, metastases doubling time, and type of resection of the primary tumor were not associated with improved post-resection survival.

Harpole et al.[92] evaluated pulmonary metastases in 945 patients with melanoma out of a population of 7564 melanoma patients. Bilateral as well as multiple metastases were present in the majority of these patients. Multivariate predictors of survival included complete resection, disease-free interval, chemotherapy, two or fewer metastases, negative lymph nodes, and histologic type. The overall 5-year survival for all patients was 4%, in contrast to 20% 5-year survival in patients with resection of pulmonary metastases.

Squamous cell carcinoma

Primary squamous cell carcinoma outside the lungs frequently metastasizes to the lungs. These lung neoplasms may be resected, with subsequent survival benefit. With solitary pulmonary lesions after the treatment of primary squamous cell carcinoma elsewhere in the body, the origin of the lesion is uncertain. The lesion may represent a solitary metastasis, a primary bronchogenic carcinoma, or a benign process. The recommended treatment for such a solitary lesion is bronchoscopy thoracic exploration,

and excisional biopsy. If a squamous cell carcinoma is identified, a lobectomy and mediastinal lymph node dissection should be performed as the patient should be treated as if the lesion were a second primary neoplasm. Less desirous would be a generous wedge excision and mediastinal lymph node dissection, as local control may be limited.

Finley *et al.*[93] described factors associated with improved survival in patients with squamous cell carcinoma metastases from head and neck cancers. These included complete resection, control of primary, early stage of the head and neck primary, one nodule on CXR, and longer disease-free interval (>2 years) from primary resection. Complete resection of all malignant disease was associated with 5-year survival of 29%. The number of nodules was not significantly associated with survival. In eight patients with more than one nodule, median survival was 2 years, and there were no 5-year survivors. Therefore, the benefits of resection of multiple pulmonary metastases from head and neck primary squamous cell carcinoma are not completely clear. In another study of 44 patients, the 5-year survival after pulmonary resection was 43%. Mazer *et al.*[94] noted that single nodules, primary tumor stage, or absence of locoregional recurrence were not associated with enhanced survival. The presence of mediastinal disease was associated with the worst outcome.

Lefor and colleagues[95] attempted to correlate primary carcinomas of the head and neck with subsequent development of pulmonary metastases or second primary lung carcinomas. An algorithm was used which considered the disease-free interval, histology, radiographic findings, and characteristics of the lung lesion, as well as the identification of mediastinal lymphadenopathy. The authors recommended that indeterminate lesions should be treated as primary lung carcinomas (e.g., lobectomy and mediastinal lymph node dissection), as this provides best local control of the disease as well as the potential for cure.

Childhood tumors

Primary tumors of childhood, such as hepatoma, neuroblastoma, hepatoblastoma, hepatoma, Ewing's sarcoma, and rhabdomyosarcoma, commonly spread to the lungs; however, other sites of metastasis are frequent, with the exception of osteogenic sarcoma. Chemotherapy remains the major treatment modality for metastases in multiple sites. Pulmonary resection for metastases may be required to document metastases in the lungs, to assess the tumor's response to chemotherapy or the viability of the remaining tumor, or to enhance post-resection survival in these children with resectable metastases.

Wilms' tumor

Patients with Wilms' tumor may present with pulmonary metastases at diagnosis or relapse after initial treatment.[96]

Early diagnosis using CT may identify metastases in up to 36% of patients, as shown by Wilimas et al.[97] Pulmonary metastases may be resected safely from children with Wilms' tumor, as recommended by de Kraker et al.[98] and Di Lorenzo and Collin.[99] In contrast, Green and others[100] evaluated 211 patients entered on the National Wilm's Tumor Study whose initial relapse was in the lungs. These patients failed to shown any survival advantage to resection of pulmonary metastases compared to treatment with chemotherapy and whole-lung irradiation.

Ewing's sarcoma

Ewing's sarcoma metastasizes preferentially to the lungs in children and may be resected. Patients with resectable pulmonary metastases from Ewing's sarcoma were examined by Lanza et al.,[101] and found to have prolonged survival (actuarial 5-year survival 15%, median survival 28 months) compared to those patients explored but found to have unresectable metastases (no survivors beyond 22 months, median survival 12 months; $p = 0.0047$). Patients with four nodules or fewer had better survival than patients with more than four nodules.

Osteogenic sarcoma

Osteogenic sarcoma metastasizes preferentially to the lungs. Resection of pulmonary metastases from osteogenic sarcoma is associated with prolonged post-resection survival, as noted by Beattie et al.,[55] Goorin et al.,[16] Pastorino et al.,[17] and Snyder et al.[49] Adjuvant therapy, such as chemotherapy[18,46] or lung irradiation,[26,100] may also be valuable, particularly for micrometastases. Post-resection survival may be as high as 39% at 5 years.[49]

INTERNATIONAL REGISTRY OF PULMONARY METASTASES

Pastorino and colleagues[103] have analysed over 5000 patients with pulmonary metastases in a multi-institutional, multinational, retrospective study. Multiple histologic groups were analysed. Favorable groups (e.g., improved survival) had complete resection and characteristics consisting of (1) solitary metastasis, (2) disease-free interval > 36 months, and (3) histology of germ cell neoplasm. Even in patients with 'unresectable disease,' some long-term (> 5 years) survival was noted.

RECURRENT PULMONARY METASTASES

If pulmonary metastases recur in the lungs, resection can again be accomplished safely, with prolonged post-thoracotomy survival. Patients are screened by the criteria in Table 32.1. Patients with pulmonary metastases may undergo multiple procedures for re-resection of metastases, with prolonged survival after complete resection. Several studies have reviewed the results of multiple resections for recurrent pulmonary metastases. Rizzoni and associates[59] described 29 patients with recurrent pulmonary metastases from soft tissue sarcomas with two or more resections. Patients with favorable tumor biology – resectable metastases, longer tumor doubling time, a small number of nodules (three or fewer), longer disease-free interval (> 6 months) – had longer overall survival. No operative mortality occurred and complications were 7.5%. The median survival was 14.5 months and overall 5-year survival was 22%. Resectable patients had a median survival of 24 months. These findings were confirmed by Casson and colleagues,[61] who described 39 patients with adult soft tissue sarcomas. Thirty-four patients were resectable (median survival 28 months; 5-year survival approximately 32%). Unresectable patients had a median survival of 7 months. The median survival following resection of a solitary recurrent metastasis was 65 months, compared to 14 months for patients with two or more nodules ($p = 0.01$).

METASTASIS OR PRIMARY BRONCHOGENIC CARCINOMA?

Pulmonary metastases from sarcomas or other distinctive non-pulmonary neoplasms are easy to diagnose. Solitary carcinomatous metastasis from breast or colon, or squamous cell carcinoma metastatic from head and neck primary tumors is difficult to distinguish from primary lung carcinoma. Patients with two or more pulmonary nodules can be considered to have metastases. In tumors without a propensity for bilaterality (e.g., non-sarcomatous histology), a solitary pulmonary nodule may be approached through a lateral thoracotomy incision. A generous wedge excision or lobectomy and mediastinal lymph node dissection should be performed. The final pathology may suggest a histology amenable to adjuvant therapy.

Traditionally, a comparison of the primary neoplasm and the lung nodule using light microscopy has been the only method for determining the origin of the lung nodule/neoplasm. Electron microscopy,[104] or specific molecular or genetic characteristics may identify more precisely the origin of these neoplasms. Ghoneim et al.[105] used monoclonal antibodies to assist in discriminating between primary bronchogenic adenocarcinoma and colon carcinoma metastatic to the lung. Slebos et al.[106] identified amplified K-ras oncogene expression in a pulmonary metastasis from colon adenocarcinoma which was also present in the primary tumor. Flint and Lloyd[107] used a monoclonal antibody to identify colorectal carcinoma in 46 patients. Cytology samples from patients with metastatic colon carcinoma and primary lung adenocarcinoma were examined. The monoclonal antibody was not sufficient to discriminate primary lung from metastatic adenocarcinoma. Flow cytometry and DNA analysis have been used by Nomori et al.,[108] Sauter et al.,[70] and Salvati et al.[109] to describe primary carcinomas of the lung and to distinguish them from metastases. Algorithms have been developed by Lefor et al.[95] for patients with squamous cell carcinomas of the head and neck who developed pulmonary nodules after treatment. The characteristics of metastases and of primary lung carcinoma were examined in an attempt to better direct subsequent therapy.

SURVIVAL ANALYSIS

Survival may be absolute or actuarial and is usually calculated from the time the surgical procedure is performed until death or until the date of last follow-up. For example: patients followed for a minimum of 5 years (survivors) or until death will provide an absolute 5-year survival rate (patients alive/all patients studied); patients followed for varying periods of time (e.g., 2–7 years) may be evaluated by using an actuarial survival curve. Actuarial survival and disease-free survival may be estimated using the method of Kaplan and Meier.[110] Patients, grouped into two or more populations, are defined as meeting or not meeting an objective criterion and compared to evaluate differences in survival. Univariate analysis (or comparisons between groups) may be made using the generalized Wilcoxon test of Gehan,[111] or log-rank test; if sample sizes are small, Thomas exact text[112] may be used. Cox's proportional hazards model[113] would be used to determine the relative effect of various prognostic indicators on survival. Univariate analysis will identify the most important prognostic indicators. Multivariate analysis evaluates the predictive ability of two or more prognostic indicators to provide additional prognostic value.

PROGNOSTIC INDICATORS

Predictors for improved survival have been studied retrospectively for various tumor types to identify selected patients who will benefit from pulmonary metastasectomy. These 'prognostic indicators' are clinical, biological, and molecular criteria which describe the biological interaction between the metastases and the patient and their association with prolonged survival. They may be used to identify those patients who are most likely to benefit after resection of pulmonary metastases.

The analyses of prognostic indicators in groups of patients with pulmonary metastases from heterogeneous tumors describe prolonged survival in patients with resectable metastases. Resectable patients, longer disease-free interval, longer tumor-doubling time, fewer metastases, and solitary metastasis are prognostic indicators generally associated with prolonged post-resection survival. Prognostic indicators should be studied in patients with the same primary tumor to define their association with post-resection survival. A wide variability exists in the characteristics of pulmonary metastases from different primary neoplasms and the subsequent survival of patients with these metastases. The study of prognostic indicators from the same primary neoplasm yields the most precise information on the association with post-resection survival.

Age and gender

Age or gender does not usually influence post-thoracotomy survival and, generally, these should not be considered as prognostic factors.

Location and stage of primary tumor

Post-resection survival is not usually influenced by the specific anatomic location of the primary tumor. Post-resection survival in patients with more advanced stage primary neoplasms does not usually differ from that of patients with earlier stage disease. However, initial or primary stage may suggest the biological aggressiveness of the tumor. Schlappack et al.[114] found that a negative nodal status predicted improved post-resection survival for patients with breast cancer. McCormack et al.[115] found better post-thoracotomy survival in patients with Dukes' stage A colorectal carcinoma (5-year survival 37.5%) compared to Dukes' C patients (5-year survival 15%), although this was not confirmed by others.[72]

Disease-free interval

The initial disease-free interval extends from resection of the primary tumor until pulmonary metastases or other metastases are detected. A short disease-free interval may indicate a more virulent tumor with a poor prognosis: metastases may be multiple and grow rapidly. A longer disease-free interval may represent a less biologically aggressive tumor and correlate with a longer post-resection survival. The disease-free interval may also be defined as the time between resection of the pulmonary metastases and recurrence of metastases in the lungs or elsewhere. Disease-free intervals of longer than 12 months are usually associated with improved survival in patients with breast carcinoma,[114] colorectal carcinoma,[65,69] osteogenic sarcoma,[116] soft tissue sarcomas,[35,117] and renal cell carcinoma.[118]

Number of nodules on preoperative imaging studies

CT has replaced linear tomograms as the examination of choice in patients with suspected pulmonary metastases. CT of the chest provides a study for patients with pulmonary metastases which is quite sensitive, but less specific than conventional linear tomography or CXR. Nodules may or may not represent metastases. Theoretically, earlier detection and treatment of metastases could improve survival. The laterality (unilateral or bilateral) of pulmonary metastases does not directly influence post-resection survival; the number of nodules is a more precise prognostic indicator.

Number of metastases resected

The physical appearance of nodules on preoperative roentgenograms usually corresponds to the number of metastatic nodules present; however, not all nodules are malignant.[90] Usually, the fewer the pulmonary metastases at the time of resection, the better the post-resection survival. Post-resection survival following complete resection of pulmonary metastases has been examined in patients with pulmonary metastases from multiple histologies to evaluate the influence of the number of metastases resected (see Table 32.2).

Tumor doubling time

Tumor doubling time is based on original observations by Collins et al.,[119] as calculated by Joseph et al.,[120,121] and has been analysed for multiple tumor types. It is calculated by measuring the same (growing) metastatic nodule on similar studies (for example serial CXRs) which are separated by a minimum of 10–14 days. The most rapidly growing nodule is selected. Tumor doubling time can be easily calculated by plotting changing diameters of pulmonary metastases on semilogarithmic paper; however, graphical error may be present. A mathematical formula may be used to calculate tumor doubling time precisely.

Tumor doubling time
$$= time^{a} \cdot [ln^{b} \, 2/3 \cdot ln(second \; diameter/first \; diameter)]$$
$$= 0.231 \cdot time/ln(second \; diameter/first \; diameter)$$

[a]Number of days between measurements.
[b]Natural logarithm.

Errors may occur in the calculation of tumor doubling time. All metastases do not grow at the same rate. In general, homogeneous metastases from the same primary neoplasm will grow at similar rates. Different growth rates of tumor nodules may reflect heterogeneity of metastases from the primary. The tumor doubling time may indirectly reveal the underlying biological nature of the metastases and, as such, influence the patient's post-resection survival.

Pulmonary metastases initially grow exponentially and, with increased size, the growth rate diminishes. Gompertz[122] described growth kinetics (expanded by Laird[123]) which considered a gradual diminution in tumor doubling time with time and increased size of the metastasis. Whether the growth rate is linear, exponential, or 'Gompertzian' may be difficult to evaluate as a CXR attempts to portray a three-dimensional structure in two dimensions. In addition, the growth rate measured over a few weeks represents only a brief period in the lifetime of the metastasis. Although this growth rate is presumed to be linear, this may not always be correct and tumor doubling time will only reflect growth during the interval measured. Rooser et al.[124] suggest that differences in tumor growth rates may be explained in part by tumor cell polyclonality.

Resectability

Complete resection consistently correlates with improved post-thoracotomy survival for patients with pulmonary metastases. If pulmonary metastases cannot be completely removed, the post-thoracotomy survival is shortened for patients with most tumors in comparison to those individuals completely resected.

Endobronchial or metastases

Involvement of mediastinal lymph nodes from pulmonary metastases is rare. Udelsman et al.[36] noted that patients with endobronchial metastases from adult soft tissue sarcomas have a short post-resection survival. Seven of 11 patients with endobronchial metastases lived 6 months or less. Jablons et al.[58] found that survival is poor (5 months) in patients with mediastinal lymph node involvement from soft tissue sarcomas compared to patients without nodal metastases (31 months).

Multivariate analysis of prognostic factors

The use of multivariate analysis may allow more accurate prediction of post-resection survival and better patient selection. Separate prognostic variables may be combined to enhance the predictive value for survival. Meyers et al.[125] found significant differences in post-resection survival in patients with pulmonary metastases from osteogenic sarcoma. Males with five or fewer nodules detected either radiologically or during surgery had a median survival of 560 days, compared to women with more than five nodules who had a median survival of only 128 days. Jablons et al.[58] noted the disease-free interval, gender, resectability, and truncal location in patients with pulmonary metastases from soft tissue sarcomas to be the best predictors of post-thoracotomy survival. Putnam *et al.*[35] noted that a disease-free survival > 12 months, tumor doubling time > 20 days, and four or fewer nodules on preoperative full lung tomograms as a single prognostic indicator was the best predictor of post-thoracotomy survival in patients with pulmonary metastases from soft tissue sarcomas. Roth *et al.*[117] compared prognostic indicators in patients with osteogenic sarcoma and soft tissue sarcoma. Tumor doubling time, number of metastases on preoperative FLTs, and disease-free interval when combined improved predictive ability over any single indicator or pair of indicators.

NOVEL TREATMENT STRATEGIES

Molecular events associated with pulmonary metastases have been identified in patients with osteogenic sarcoma. Amplification of the *MDM2* gene (the human homologue of a murine p53 binding protein) may regulate p53 protein function by inactivating the protein and deregulating/enhancing tumor growth. In one small study,[126] no detectable *MDM2* gene amplification in primary osteogenic sarcoma was found compared to 14% of metastases (3 PM, 1 local metastasis). Amplification of *MDM2* may be associated with metastases and tumor progression in osteogenic sarcoma.

In soft tissue sarcomas, alterations (mutations) of the *p53* gene (a tumor suppressor gene) may provide for uncontrolled cell growth. Restoration of normal *p53* ('wild-type') in soft tissue sarcomas may provide for more controlled cell growth or even programmed cell death (apoptosis). In one *in-vitro* study, transduction of wild-type *p53* into soft tissue sarcomas bearing mutated *p53* genes altered the malignant potential of the tumor. After transduction, transfected cells expressed wild-type *p53*, decreased cell proliferation, decreased colony formation in soft agar, and demonstrated decreased tumor formation in severe combined immunodeficient (SCID) mice *in vivo*. The ability to restore wild-type *p53* function in soft tissue sarcoma *in vitro* and in SCID mice may ultimately be considered as future therapy for patients with soft tissue sarcomas.[127] Other investigations have shown that pulmonary metastases from soft tissue sarcoma can develop from clonal expansion of primary tumor cells bearing *p53* mutations.[128] Examination of tissue specimens from osteogenic and soft tissue sarcomas demonstrated *p53* mutations in 25% of osteogenic sarcomas yet in only one of 16 metastases.[129]

The use of specific molecular markers may allow better selection of patients who will optimally benefit from surgery, chemotherapy, or other treatment modalities.

Other targets of gene therapy may include chemotherapy-resistant tumors or tumors with greater propensity for metastatic spread. Overexpression of the *MDR1* gene product P-glycoprotein is an important predictor of poor prognosis in osteosarcoma patients treated with chemotherapy. In these patients, the MDR phenotype is not *de novo* more aggressive (e.g., more metastatic); however, the poor outcome of patients with the MDR phenotype related to P-glycoprotein overexpression is related to the cells' failure to respond to cytotoxic drugs.[130] In another study,[131] 42% of patients with osteogenic sarcomas had metastases which expressed ErbB-2 and correlated with early development of pulmonary metastasis and poor survival. ErbB-2, therefore, may enhance tumor growth and promote metastases. These authors recommended that ErbB-2 might be considered as a prognostic factor for patients with osteosarcoma.

ErbB-2 protein is expressed in about 42% of osteosarcoma. It has been strongly correlated with early pulmonary metastasis and poor survival. It may enhance tumor aggressiveness and metastasis in osteosarcoma. As a marker, ErbB-2 may be useful as a prognostic indicator.[131]

A rodent model of osteogenic sarcoma has been developed with high propensity for pulmonary metastases. In this metastatic tumor model, matrix metalloproteinase (MMP)-2 activity is increased as is the expression of VEGF mRNA.[132]

Gene therapy strategies are being studied also. The systematic delivery of recombinant adenovirus (Ad) vector containing herpes simplex virus thymidine kinase (*TK*) gene (with an osteocalcin [OC] promoter [Ad-OC-TK]) supplemented with the prodrug acyclovir (ACV) may be an effective strategy for osteosarcoma metastases to the lungs.[133] Preclinical studies noted that following Ad-OC-beta-gal administration, specific beta-gal expression was found in tumor cells deposited in the lung. Induced rat osteogenic lung metastases in nude rats, followed by systemic Ad-OC-TK, and intraperitoneal ACV treatment were decreased (fewer tumor nodules) and had increased survival compared to controls. Ad-OC-TK/ACV may be a future treatment for pulmonary metastases from osteosarcoma. Other preclinical treatment methods may include nebulized interleukin-2 liposomes.[134]

Regional drug delivery to the lung (isolated lung perfusion)

Novel drug delivery systems may enhance chemotherapy treatment effects by increasing the drug concentration in lung tissues and minimizing the systemic effects of such treatment. In many patients, surgery has been used as salvage treatment after maximal chemotherapy response has been achieved. Systemic toxicity may limit the amount of chemotherapy given to an individual patient. Regional drug delivery to the lungs minimizes systemic drug delivery, preventing systemic toxicity; however, this technique dramatically increases the drug delivered to the lung over a short time period.

Recent preclinical studies in rodents with experimental pulmonary metastases from a methylcholanthrene-induced syngeneic sarcoma[135–137] have shown that chemotherapy may be delivered to pulmonary tissue in significantly higher concentrations than with systemic delivery. Minimal to no systemic toxicity was noted. In this model, isolated single-lung perfusion with adriamycin (doxorubicin) was safe and effective.[135] This simple microsurgical technique was performed in rats. Following left thoracotomy, the pulmonary artery and pulmonary vein were isolated and clamped. The lung was flushed prior to infusing doxorubicin. The infusion occurred over 10 min. Then the drug was flushed out, prior to removing the cannulas and restoring circulation. A perfusion concentration of 255 mg/L caused less general toxicity than a systemic dose equivalent to 75 mg/m^2, the extraction ratio was 58%, and the pulmonary tissue concentration of adriamycin was 25-fold higher than with the systemic dose. The technique was also effective: 9/10 animals treated at 320 mg/L had complete eradication of metastases from an implanted methylcholanthrene-induced sarcoma.[135]

Previous clinical studies of lung perfusion[138,139] have shown higher drug concentrations in pulmonary tissue, although clinical tumor response has been mixed. Johnston and colleagues described a continuous perfusion of the lungs with adriamycin (single lung, continuous perfusion) as a safe technique and subsequently applied their technique clinically, as recently reviewed.[139] Drug concentrations in normal lung and tumor generally increased with higher drug dosages. Two of eight patients had major complications: one patient developed pneumonia and sternal dehiscence, and one patient developed respiratory failure 4 days after lung perfusion. No objective responses occurred (0/4 patients with sarcomas). Although continuous perfusion with a pump circuit offers some theoretical advantages, the technique is cumbersome, equipment intensive, and time consuming, and has the inherent problem of the incompatibility of adriamycin and heparin. Pass *et al.*[138] examined isolated single-lung perfusion with tumor necrosis factor-alpha, interferon-gamma, and moderate hyperthermia for patients with unresectable pulmonary metastases. No hospital deaths occurred and a short-term (<6-month) decrease in nodule size was noted in three of 15 patients.

Phase I studies in patients with unresectable pulmonary metastases from soft tissue sarcomas are currently underway at The University of Texas MD Anderson Cancer Center in Houston. A paucity of effective treatment and the potential for high drug concentrations for pulmonary metastases by regional lung perfusion warrant further clinical study.

CONCLUSIONS

Isolated and resectable metastases to the lungs represent a unique biology amongst the host, the primary neoplasm, and the metastases. Patients may have long-term survival associated with complete resection of all pulmonary metastases. Is the associated long-term survival the result of surgery or the result of the unique biology of the tumor and its metastases? This question remains unanswered. Complete resection is the crucial characteristic associated with long-term survival – regardless of the primary tumor histology. Patients with resectable pulmonary metastases should undergo resection to render them disease free with the potential for long-term survival and cure. A suggested algorithm for the management of pulmonary metastases is presented in Table 32.5.

Various prognostic indicators may define the biological nature of the metastases, predict post-resection survival, and assist the clinician in selecting patients who will benefit from surgery. Prognostic factors are heterogeneous among different tumor histologies. Factors predictive of improved survival for one type of tumor may not be predictive for another. Various prognostic indicators used together may be better than any single prognostic indicator. Multivariate analyses of combinations of prognostic indicators in patients with osteogenic or soft tissue sarcomas may be helpful in deciding which patients would benefit from surgery. The use of prognostic indicators to deny patients the benefit of surgery remains inexact and should be used with additional clinical information. Nevertheless, careful use of prognostic indicators for a tumor type may facilitate the selection of patients for investigational therapies. Further and more detailed analyses of prognostic factors from larger populations of patients with single tumor histologies will better define the value of surgical resection in patients with pulmonary metastases and the value of prognostic indicators to select these patients. No single criterion in resectable patients consistently and reliably predicts which patients will have enhanced long-term survival following resection; however, unresectable patients do poorly despite adjuvant therapy. Bronchogenic carcinoma often cannot be excluded and solitary metastasis should be treated as a primary stage lung cancer. Current molecular biological techniques may best define the cell of origin of pulmonary metastasis and enable better adjuvant therapy for prolonged survival or cure.

Surgery for pulmonary metastases attempts to control mechanically the biological sequelae of primary malignancy. Surgical resection remains the best means of local control and the best way to render the patient disease free. Patients with complete resection of pulmonary metastases have associated long-term survival, in contrast to patients with unresectable metastases. However, surgery still remains unsuccessful in obtaining long-term or disease-free survival, or curing disease in 60–80% of patients with resectable metastases. The fundamental biology of the neoplastic and metastatic process is unchanged by surgery. Cure in these patients may require unique tumor biology, host–tumor interactions, and complete resection. The best results of the treatment of

Table 32.5 *Algorithm for the management of suspected pulmonary metastases*

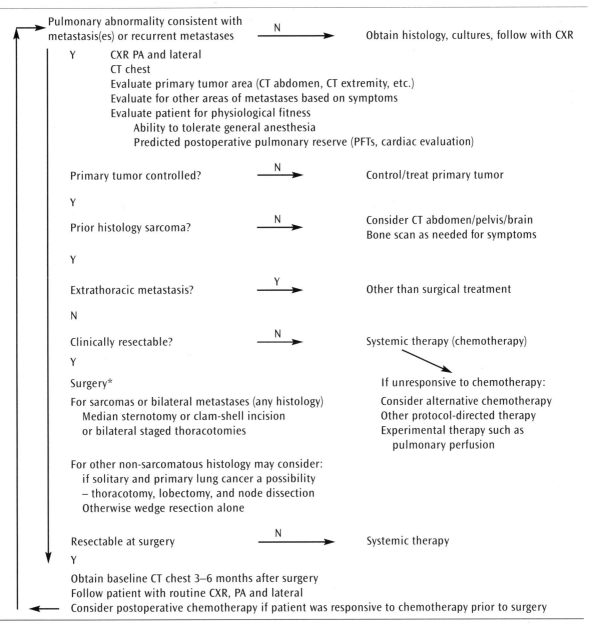

*The response to salvage chemotherapy after development of sarcomatous pulmonary metastases has not been shown to be associated with improved survival after resection compared to resection alone.

pulmonary metastases await improved adjuvant therapies or novel treatment strategies directed at biological and molecular events in the life cycle of the metastatic cell.

REFERENCES

1. Meade RH. *A history of thoracic surgery*. Springfield, IL, Charles C Thomas, 1961.
2. Martini N, McCormack PM. Evolution of the surgical management of pulmonary metastases. [Review] [33 refs]. Chest Surg Clin North Am 1998; 8(1):13–27.
3. Divis G. Ein Beitrag zur operativen Behandlung der Lungengeschwultse. Acta Chir Scand 1927; 62:329.
4. Torek F. Removal of metastatic carcinoma of the lung and mediastinum: suggestions as to technic. Arch Surg 1930; 21:1416–21.
5. Barney JD, Churchill EJ. Adenocarcinoma of the kidney with metastasis to the lung cured by nephrectomy and lobectomy. J Urol 1939; 42:269–76.
6. Alexander J, Haight C. Pulmonary resection for solitary metastatic sarcoma and carcinoma. Surg Gynecol Obstet 1947; 85:129–46.

7. Mannix EP. Resection of multiple pulmonary metastases fourteen years after amputation for osteochondroma of tibia. Apparent freedom from recurrence three years later. J Thorac Surg 1953; 26:544–9.

8. Martini N, Huvos AG, Mike V, Marcove RC, Beattie EJ Jr. Multiple pulmonary resections in the treatment of osteogenic sarcoma. Ann Thorac Surg 1971; 12(3):271–80.

9. Lien HH, Lindskold L, Fossa SD, Aass N. Computed tomography and conventional radiography in intrathoracic metastases from non-seminomatous testicular tumor. Acta Radiol 1988; 29:547–9.

10. Chang AE, Schaner EG, Conkle DM, Flye MW, Doppman JL, Rosenberg SA. Evaluation of computed tomography in the detection of pulmonary metastases: a prospective study. Cancer 1979; 43:913–16.

11. Dinkel E, Mundinger A, Schopp D, Grosser G, Hauenstein KH. Diagnostic imaging in metastatic lung disease. Lung 1990; 168(Suppl.):1129–36.

12. Blickman JG, Aarts JC, Oudkerk M, Simon M. Reconsideration of conventional tomography versus computerized tomography in the evaluation of lung metastases. Eur J Radiol 1986; 6:259–61.

13. Feuerstein IM, Jicha DL, Pass HI, et al. Pulmonary metastases: MR imaging with surgical correlation – a prospective study. Radiology 1992; 182:123–9.

14. Pass HI, Dwyer A, Makuch R, Roth JA. Detection of pulmonary metastases in patients with osteogenic and soft-tissue sarcomas: the superiority of CT scans compared with conventional linear tomograms using dynamic analysis. J Clin Oncol 1985; 3:1261–5.

15. Skinner KA, Eilber FR, Holmes EC, Eckardt J, Rosen G. Surgical treatment and chemotherapy for pulmonary metastases from osteosarcoma. Arch Surg 1992; 127:1065–70; discussion.

16. Goorin AM, Shuster JJ, Baker A, Horowitz ME, Meyer WH, Link MP. Changing pattern of pulmonary metastases with adjuvant chemotherapy in patients with osteosarcoma: results from the Multiinstitutional Osteosarcoma Study. J Clin Oncol 1991; 9:600–5.

17. Pastorino U, Gasparini M, Tavecchio L, et al. The contribution of salvage surgery to the management of childhood osteosarcoma. J Clin Oncol 1991; 9:1357–62.

18. Yamaguchi H, Nojima T, Yagi T, et al. The alteration in the pattern of pulmonary metastasis with adjuvant chemotherapy in osteosarcoma. Int Orthop 1988; 12:305–8.

19. Bacci G, Avella M, Picci P, Briccoli A, Dallari D, Campanacci M. Metastatic patterns in osteosarcoma. Tumori 1988; 74:421–7.

20. Marina NM, Pratt CB, Rao BN, Shema SJ, Meyer WH. Improved prognosis of children with osteosarcoma metastatic to the lung(s) at the time of diagnosis. Cancer 1992; 70:2722–7.

21. Pastorino U, Gasparini M, Valente M, et al. Primary childhood osteosarcoma: the role of salvage surgery. Ann Oncol 1992; 3(Suppl. 2):S43–6.

22. Bacci G, Picci P, Briccoli A, et al. Osteosarcoma of the extremity metastatic at presentation: results achieved in 26 patients treated with combined therapy (primary chemotherapy followed by simultaneous resection of the primary and metastatic lesions). Tumori 1992; 78:200–6.

23. Al-Jilaihawi AN, Bullimore J, Mott M, Wisheart JD. Combined chemotherapy and surgery for pulmonary metastases from osteogenic sarcoma. Results of 10 years' experience. Eur J Cardiothorac Surg 1998; 21:37–42.

24. Glasser DB, Lane JM, Huvos AG, Marcove RC, Rosen G. Survival, prognosis, and therapeutic response in osteogenic sarcoma. The Memorial Hospital experience. Cancer 1992; 69:698–708.

25. Kim B, Louie AC. Surgical resection following interleukin 2 therapy for metastatic renal cell carcinoma prolongs remission. Arch Surg 1992; 127:1343–9.

26. Lanza LA, Putnam JB Jr, Benjamin RS, Roth JA. Response to chemotherapy does not predict survival after resection of sarcomatous pulmonary metastases. Ann Thorac Surg 1991; 51:219–24.

27. Burgers JM, van Glabbeke M, Busson A, et al. Osteosarcoma of the limbs. Report of the EORTC-SIOP 03 trial 20781 investigating the value of adjuvant treatment with chemotherapy and/or prophylactic lung irradiation. Cancer 1988; 61:1024–31.

28. Takita H, Merrin C, Didolkar MS, et al. The surgical management of multiple lung metastases. Ann Thorac Surg 1992; 24:359–64.

29. Morrow CE, Vassilopoulos PP, Grage TB. Surgical resection for metastatic neoplasms of the lung: experience at the University of Minnesota Hospitals. Cancer 1980; 45:2981–5.

30. McCormack PM, Martini N. The changing role of surgery for pulmonary metastases. Ann Thorac Surg 1979; 28(2):139–45.

31. Mountain CF, McMurtrey MJ, Hermes KE. Surgery for pulmonary metastasis: a 20-year experience. Ann Thorac Surg 1984; 38:323–30.

32. Putnam JB Jr, Suell DM, Natarajan G, Roth JA. Extended resection of pulmonary metastases: is the risk justified? Ann Thorac Surg 1993; 55(6):1440–6.

33. Johnston MR. Median sternotomy for resection of pulmonary metastases. J Thorac Cardiovasc Surg 1983; 85:516–22.

34. Roth JA, Pass HI, Wesley MN, White D, Putnam JB, Seipp C. Comparison of median sternotomy and thoracotomy for resection of pulmonary metastases

in patients with adult soft-tissue sarcomas. Ann Thorac Surg 1986; 42:134–8.

35. Putnam JB Jr, Roth JA, Wesley MN, Johnston MR, Rosenberg SA. Analysis of prognostic factors in patients undergoing resection of pulmonary metastases from soft tissue sarcomas. J Thorac Cardiovasc Surg 1984; 87:260–7.

36. Udelsman R, Roth JA, Lees D, Jelenich SE, Pass HI. Endobronchial metastases from soft tissue sarcoma. J Surg Oncol 1986; 32:145–9.

37. Kodama K, Doi O, Higashiyama M, Tatsuta M, Iwanaga T. Surgical management of lung metastases. Usefulness of resection with the neodymium: yttrium–aluminum–garnet laser with median sternotomy. J Thorac Cardiovasc Surg 1991; 101:901–8.

38. Branscheid D, Krysa S, Wollkopf G, et al. Does ND-YAG laser extend the indications for resection of pulmonary metastases? Eur J Cardiothorac Surg 1992; 6:590–6; discussion.

39. Miyamoto H, Masaoka T, Hayakawa K, Hata E. Application of the Nd-YAG laser for surgical resection of pulmonary metastases. Kyobu Geka 1992; 45:56–9.

40. Landreneau RJ, Herlan DB, Johnson JA, Boley TM, Nawarawong W, Ferson PF. Thorascopic neodymium: yttrium–aluminum garnet laser-assisted pulmonary resection. Ann Thorac Surg 1991; 52:1176–8.

41. Bains MS, Ginsberg RJ, Jones WG, et al. The clamshell incision: an improved approach to bilateral pulmonary and mediastinal tumor. Ann Thorac Surg 1994; 58(1):30–2; discussion, 33.

42. Urschel HC Jr, Razzuk MA. Median sternotomy as a standard approach for pulmonary resection. Ann Thorac Surg 1986; 41:130–4.

43. Miller DL, Allen MS, Trastek VF, Deschamps C, Pairolero PC. Videothoracoscopic wedge excision of the lung. Ann Thorac Surg 1992; 54:410–13; discussion.

44. Landreneau RJ, Hazelrigg SR, Ferson PF, et al. Thoracoscopic resection of 85 pulmonary lesions. Ann Thorac Surg 1992; 54:415–19; discussion.

45. McCormack PM, Bains MS, Begg CB, et al. Role of video-assisted thoracic surgery in the treatment of pulmonary metastases: results of a prospective trial. Ann Thorac Surg 1996; 62(1):213–16.

46. Al-Jilaihawi AN, Bullimore J, Mott M, Wisheart JD. Combined chemotherapy and surgery for pulmonary metastases from osteogenic sarcoma. Results of 10 years' experience. Eur J Cardiothorac Surg 1988; 2:37–42.

47. Huth JF, Eilber FR. Patterns of recurrence after resection of osteosarcoma of the extremity. Arch Surg 1989; 124:122–6.

48. Meyer WH, Schell MJ, Kumar AP, et al. Thoracotomy for pulmonary metastatic osteosarcoma. An analysis of prognostic indicators of survival. Cancer 1987; 59:374–9.

49. Snyder CL, Saltzman DA, Ferrell KL, Thompson RC, Leonard AS. A new approach to the resection of pulmonary osteosarcoma metastases. Results of aggressive metastasectomy. Clin Orthop 1991; 270:247–53.

50. Belli L, Scholl S, Livartowski A, et al. Resection of pulmonary metastases in osteosarcoma. A retrospective analysis of 44 patients. Cancer 1989; 63:2546–50.

51. Carter SR, Grimer RJ, Sneath RS, Matthews HR. Results of thoracotomy in osteogenic sarcoma with pulmonary metastases. Thorax 1991; 46:727–31.

52. Jaffe N, Smith E, Abelson HT, Frei E. Osteogenic sarcoma: alterations in the pattern of pulmonary metastases with adjuvant chemotherapy. J Clin Oncol 1983; 1:251–4.

53. Putnam JBJ, Roth JA, Wesley MN, Johnston MR, Rosenberg SA. Survival following aggressive resection of pulmonary metastases from osteogenic sarcoma: analysis of prognostic factors. Ann Thorac Surg 1983; 38:516–23.

54. Rosen B, Huvos AG, Mosende C Jr, et al. Chemotherapy and thoracotomy for metastatic osteogenic sarcoma. Cancer 1978; 41:841–9.

55. Beattie EJ, Harvey JC, Marcove R, Martini N. Results of multiple pulmonary resections for metastatic osteogenic sarcoma after two decades. J Surg Oncol 1991; 46:154–5.

56. Potter DA, Glenn J, Kinsella T, et al. Patterns of recurrence in patients with high-grade soft-tissue sarcomas. J Clin Oncol 1985; 3:353–66.

57. Casson AG, Putnam JB, Natarajan G, et al. Five-year survival after pulmonary metastasectomy for adult soft tissue sarcoma. Cancer 1992; 69:662–8.

58. Jablons D, Steinberg SM, Roth J, Pittaluga S, Rosenberg SA, Pass HI. Metastasectomy for soft tissue sarcoma. Further evidence for efficacy and prognostic indicators. J Thorac Cardiovasc Surg 1989; 97:695–705.

59. Rizzoni WE, Pass HI, Wesley MN, Rosenberg SA, Roth JA. Resection of recurrent pulmonary metastases in patients with soft-tissue sarcomas. Arch Surg 1986; 121:1248–52.

60. Pogrebniak HW, Roth JA, Steinberg SM, Rosenberg SA, Pass HI. Reoperative pulmonary resection in patients with metastatic soft tissue sarcoma (see comments). Ann Thorac Surg 1991; 52:197–203.

61. Casson AG, Putnam JB, Natarajan G, et al. Efficacy of pulmonary metastasectomy for recurrent soft tissue sarcoma. J Surg Oncol 1991; 47:1–4.

62. Weh HJ, Zugel M, Wingberg D, et al. Chemotherapy of metastatic soft tissue sarcoma with a combination of adriamycin and DTIC or adriamycin and ifosfamide. Onkologie 1990; 13:448–52.

63. Elias A, Ryan L, Sulkes A, Collins J, Aisner J, Antman KH. Response to mesna, doxorubicin, ifosfamide, and dacarbazine in 108 patients with metastatic or unresectable sarcoma and no prior chemotherapy. J Clin Oncol 1989; 7:1208–16.

64. Murray KD. Excision of pulmonary metastasis of colorectal cancer. Semin Surg Oncol 1991; 7:157–61.

65. Brister SJ, de Varennes B, Gordon PH, Sheiner NM, Pym J. Contemporary operative management of pulmonary metastases of colorectal origin. Dis Colon Rectum 1988; 31:786–92.

66. Roberts DG, Lepore V, Cardillo G, et al. Long-term follow-up of operative treatment for pulmonary metastases. Eur J Cardiothorac Surg 1989; 3:292–6.

67. Scheele J, Altendorf Hofmann A, Stangl R, Gall FP. Pulmonary resection for metastatic colon and upper rectum cancer. Is it useful? Dis Colon Rectum 1990; 33:745–52.

68. Goya T, Miyazawa N, Kondo H, Tsuchiya R, Naruke T, Suemasu K. Surgical resection of pulmonary metastases from colorectal cancer: 10-year follow-up. Cancer 1989; 64:1418–21.

69. Mansel JK, Zinsmeister AR, Pairolero PC, Jett JR. Pulmonary resection of metastatic colorectal adenocarcinoma. A ten year experience. Chest 1986; 89:109–12.

70. Sauter ER, Bolton JS, Willis GW, Farr GH, Sardi A. Improved survival after pulmonary resection of metastatic colorectal carcinoma. J Surg Oncol 1990; 43:135–8.

71. Pihl E, Hughes ES, McDermott FT, Johnson WR, Katrivessis H. Lung recurrence after curative surgery for colorectal cancer. Dis Colon Rectum 1987; 30:417–19.

72. McAfee MK, Allen MS, Trastek VF, Ilstrup DM, Deschamps C, Pairolero PC. Colorectal lung metastases: results of surgical excision. Ann Thorac Surg 1992; 53:780–5; discussion.

73. Patanaphan V, Salazar OM, Risco R. Breast cancer: metastatic patterns and their prognosis. South Med J 1988; 81:1109–12.

74. Lanza LA, Natarajan G, Roth JA, Putnam JB Jr. Long-term survival after resection of pulmonary metastases from carcinoma of the breast. Ann Thorac Surg 1992; 54(2):244–7; discussion, 248.

75. Staren ED, Salerno C, Rongione A, Witt TR, Faber LP. Pulmonary resection for metastatic breast cancer. Arch Surg 1992; 127:1282–4.

76. Tesoro-Tess JD, Pizzocaro G, Zanoni F, et al. Reliability of diagnostic imaging after orchiectomy alone in follow-up of clinical stage I testicular carcinoma: excessive cost with potential risk. Lymphology 1987; 20:161–5.

77. Williams MP, Husband JE, Heron CW. Intrathoracic manifestations of metastatic testicular seminoma: a comparison of chest radiographic and CT findings. Am J Roentgenol 1987; 149:473–5.

78. Kulkarni RP, Reynolds KW, Newlands ES, et al. Cytoreductive surgery in disseminated non-seminomatous germ cell tumours of testis. Br J Surg 1991; 78:226–9.

79. Van Schil P, Vaneerdeweg W, Schoofs E, Van Oosterom A, Bourgeois N. Surgical excision of pulmonary metastases from primary testicular cancer – case reports. Acta Chir Belg 1989; 89:175–8.

80. Carsky S, Ondrus D, Schnorrer M, Majek M. Germ cell testicular tumours with lung metastases: chemotherapy and surgical treatment. Int Urol Nephrol 1992; 24:305–11.

81. Carter GE, Lieskovsky G, Skinner DG, Daniels JR. Reassessment of the role of adjunctive surgical therapy in the treatment of advanced germ cell tumors. J Urol 1987; 138:1397–401.

82. Fuller AF Jr, Scannell JG, Wilkins EW Jr. Pulmonary resection for metastases from gynecologic cancers: Massachusetts General Hospital experience, 1943–1982. Gynecol Oncol 1985; 22:174–80.

83. Levenback C, Rubin SC, McCormack PM, Hoskins WJ, Atkinson EN, Lewis JL Jr. Resection of pulmonary metastases from uterine sarcomas. Gynecol Oncol 1992; 45:202–5.

84. Kumar J, Ilancheran A, Ratnam SS. Pulmonary metastases in gestational trophoblastic disease: a review of 97 cases. Br J Obstet Gynecol 1988; 95:70–4.

85. Barter JF, Soong SJ, Hatch KD, Orr JW, Shingleton HM. Diagnosis and treatment of pulmonary metastases from cervical carcinoma. Gynecol Oncol 1990; 38:347–51.

86. Imachi M, Tsukamoto N, Matsuyama T, Nakano H. Pulmonary metastasis from carcinoma of the uterine cervix. Gynecol Oncol 1989; 33:189–92.

87. Dernevik L, Berggren H, Larsson S, Roberts D. Surgical removal of pulmonary metastases from renal cell carcinoma. Scand J Urol Nephrol 1985; 19:133–7.

88. Pogrebniak HW, Haas G, Linehan WM, Rosenberg SA, Pass HI. Renal cell carcinoma: resection of solitary and multiple metastases. Ann Thorac Surg 1992; 54:33–8.

89. Schott G, Weissmuller J, Vecera E. Methods and prognosis of the extirpation of pulmonary metastases following tumor nephrectomy. Urol Int 1988; 43:272–4.

90. Pogrebniak HW, Stovroff M, Roth JA, Pass HI. Resection of pulmonary metastases from malignant melanoma: results of a 16-year experience. Ann Thorac Surg 1988; 46:20–3.

91. Gorenstein LA, Putnam JB, Natarajan G, Balch CA, Roth JA. Improved survival after resection of pulmonary metastases from malignant melanoma (see comments). Ann Thorac Surg 1991; 52:204–10.

92. Harpole DH Jr, Johnson CM, Wolfe WG, George SL, Seigler HF. Analysis of 945 cases of pulmonary metastatic melanoma. J Thorac Cardiovasc Surg 1992; 103:743–8; discussion.

93. Finley RK 3, Verazin GT, Driscoll DL, *et al*. Results of surgical resection of pulmonary metastases of squamous cell carcinoma of the head and neck. Am J Surg 1992; 164(6):594–8.

94. Mazer TM, Robbins KT, McMurtrey MJ, Byers RM. Resection of pulmonary metastases from squamous carcinoma of the head and neck. Am J Surg 1988; 156:238–42.

95. Lefor AT, Bredenberg CE, Kellman RM, Aust JC. Multiple malignancies of the lung and head and neck. Second primary tumor or metastasis? Arch Surg 1986; 121:265–70.

96. Macklis RM, Oltikar A, Sallan SE. Wilms' tumor patients with pulmonary metastases. Int J Radiat Oncol Biol Phys 1991; 21:1187–93.

97. Wilimas JA, Douglass EC, Magill HL, Fitch S, Hustu HO. Significance of pulmonary computed tomography at diagnosis in Wilms' tumor. J Clin Oncol 1988; 6:1144–6.

98. de Kraker J, Lemerle J, Voute PA, Zucker JM, Tournade MF, Carli M. Wilm's tumor with pulmonary metastases at diagnosis: the significance of primary chemotherapy. International Society of Pediatric Oncology Nephroblastoma Trial and Study Committee. J Clin Oncol 1990; 8:1187–90.

99. Di Lorenzo M, Collin PP. Pulmonary metastases in children: results of surgical treatment. J Pediatr Surg 1988; 23:762–5.

100. Green DM, Breslow NE, Ii Y, *et al*. The role of surgical excision in the management of relapsed Wilms' tumor patients with pulmonary metastases: a report from the National Wilms' Tumor Study. J Pediatr Surg 1991; 26:728–33.

101. Lanza LA, Miser JS, Pass HI, Roth JA. The role of resection in the treatment of pulmonary metastases from Ewing's sarcoma. J Thorac Cardiovasc Surg 1987; 94:181–7.

102. Zaharia M, Caceres E, Valdivia S, Moran M, Tejada F. Postoperative whole lung irradiation with or without adriamycin in osteogenic sarcoma. Int J Radiat Oncol Biol Phys 1986; 12:907–10.

103. Pastorino U, Buyse M, Friedel G, *et al*. Long-term results of lung metastasectomy: prognostic analyses based on 5206 cases. J Thorac Cardiovasc Surg 1997; 113:37–49.

104. Herrera GA, Alexander CB, Jones JM. Ultrastructural characterization of pulmonary neoplasms. II. The role of electron microscopy in characterization of uncommon epithelial pulmonary neoplasms, metastatic neoplasms to and from lung, and other tumors, including mesenchymal neoplasms. Surv Synth Pathol Res 1985; 4:163–84.

105. Ghoneim AH, Brisson ML, Fuks A, Mobasher AA, Kreisman H. Monoclonal anti-CEA antibodies in the discrimination between primary pulmonary adenocarcinoma and colon carcinoma metastatic to the lung. Mod Pathol 1990; 3:613–18.

106. Slebos RJ, Habets GG, Evers SG, Mooi WJ, Rodenhuis S. Allele-specific detection of K-ras oncogene expression in human non-small-cell lung carcinomas. Int J Cancer 1991; 48:51–6.

107. Flint A, Lloyd RV. Colon carcinoma metastatic to the lung. Cytologic manifestations and distinction from primary pulmonary adenocarcinoma. Acta Cytol 1992; 36:230–5.

108. Nomori H, Hirohashi S, Noguchi M, Matsuno Y, Shimosato Y. Tumor cell heterogeneity and subpopulations with metastatic ability in differentiated adenocarcinoma of the lung. Histologic and cytofluorometric DNA analyses. Chest 1991; 99:934–40.

109. Salvati F, Teodori L, Gagliardi L, Signora M, Aquilini M, Storniello G. DNA flow cytometric studies of 66 human lung tumors analyzed before treatment. Prognostic implications. Chest 1989; 96:1092–8.

110. Kaplan EL, Meier P. Nonparametric estimation from incomplete observations. J Am Stat Assoc 1958; 53:457–81.

111. Gehan EA. A generalized Wilcoxon test for comparing arbitrarily singly-censored samples. Biometrika 1965; 522:203–23.

112. Thomas DG. Exact and asymptotic methods for the combination of 2×2 tables. Comput Biomed Res 1975; 8:423–46.

113. Cox DR. Regression models and life-tables. J R Stat Soc B 1972; 34:187–220.

114. Schlappack OK, Baur M, Steger G, Dittrich C, Moser K. The clinical course of lung metastases from breast cancer. Klin Wochenschr 1988; 66:790–5.

115. McCormack PM, Attiyeh FF. Resected pulmonary metastases from colorectal cancer. Dis Colon Rectum 1979; 22:553–6.

116. Pastorino U, Valente M, Gasparini M, *et al*. Lung resection as salvage treatment for metastatic osteosarcoma. Tumori 1988; 74:201–6.

117. Roth JA, Putnam JB, Wesley MN, Rosenberg SA. Differing determinants of prognosis following resection of pulmonary metastases from osteogenic and soft tissue sarcoma patients. Cancer 1985; 55:1361–6.

118. Jett JR, Hollinger CG, Zinsmeister AR, Pairolero PC. Pulmonary resection of metastatic renal cell carcinoma. Chest 1983; 84:442–5.

119. Collins VP, Loeffler RK, Tivey H. Observations on growth rates of human tumors. Am J Roentgenol 1956; 76:988–1000.

120. Joseph WL, Morton DL, Adkins PC. Prognostic significance of tumor doubling time in evaluating operability in pulmonary metastatic disease. J Thorac Cardiovasc Surg 1971; 61:23–32.

121. Joseph WL, Morton DL, Adkins PC. Variation in tumor doubling time in patients with pulmonary metastatic disease. J Surg Oncol 1971; 3:143–9.

122. Gompertz B. On the nature of the function expressive of the law of human mortality, and on a new mode of determining the value of life contingencies. Philos Trans 1825; 513–85.

123. Laird AK. Dynamics of tumor growth. Br J Cancer 1960; 18:490–502.

124. Rooser B, Pettersson H, Alvegard T. Growth rate of pulmonary metastases from soft tissue sarcoma. (Published erratum appears in Acta Oncol 1987; 26(6):496.) Acta Oncol 1987; 26:189–92.

125. Meyers PA, Heller G, Healey J, et al. Chemotherapy for nonmetastatic osteogenic sarcoma: the memorial Sloan-Kettering experience (see comments). J Clin Oncol 1992; 10:5–15.

126. Ladanyi M, Cha C, Lewis R, Jhanwar SC, Huvos AG, Healey JH. MDM2 gene amplification in metastatic osteosarcoma. Cancer Res 1993; 53:16–18.

127. Pollock R, Lang A, Ge T, Sun D, Tan M, Yu D. Wild-type p53 and a p53 temperature-sensitive mutant suppress human soft tissue sarcoma by enhancing cell cycle control. Clin Cancer Res 1998; 4(8):1985–94.

128. Pollock RE, Lang A, Luo J, El-Naggar AK, Yu D. Soft tissue sarcoma metastasis from clonal expansion of p53 mutated tumor cells. Oncogene 1997; 12:2035–9.

129. Mousses S, McAuley L, Bell RS, Kandel R, Andrulis IL. Molecular and immunohistochemical identification of p53 alterations in bone and soft tissue sarcomas. Mod Pathol 1996; 9(1):1–6.

130. Scotlandi K, Serra M, Nicoletti G, et al. Multidrug resistance and malignancy in human osteosarcoma. Cancer Res 1996; 56(10):2434–9.

131. Onda M, Matsuda S, Higaki S, et al. ErbB-2 expression is correlated with poor prognosis for patients with osteosarcoma. Cancer 1996; 77(1):71–8.

132. Asai T, Ueda T, Itoh K, et al. Establishment and characterization of a murine osteosarcoma cell line (LM8) with high metastatic potential to the lung. Int J Cancer 1998; 76(3):418–22.

133. Shirakawa T, Ko SC, Gardner TA, et al. In vivo suppression of osteosarcoma pulmonary metastasis with intravenous osteocalcin promoter-based toxic gene therapy. Cancer Gene Ther 1998; 5(5):274–80.

134. Khanna C, Anderson PM, Hasz DE, Katsanis E, Neville M, Klausner JS. Interleukin-2 liposome inhalation therapy is safe and effective for dogs with spontaneous pulmonary metastases. Cancer 1997; 79(7):1409–21.

135. Weksler B, Lenert J, Ng B, Burt M. Isolated single lung perfusion with doxorubicin is effective in eradicating soft tissue sarcoma lung metastases in a rat model. J Thorac Cardiovasc Surg 1994; 107(1):50–4.

136. Weksler B, Ng B, Lenert JT, Burt ME. Isolated single-lung perfusion with doxorubicin is pharmacokinetically superior to intravenous injection [see comments]. Ann Thorac Surg 1993; 56(2):209–14.

137. Weksler B, Schneider A, Ng B, Burt M. Isolated single lung perfusion in the rat: an experimental model. J Appl Physiol 1993; 74(6):2736–9.

138. Pass HI, Mew DJ, Kranda KC, Temeck BK, Donington JS, Rosenberg SA. Isolated lung perfusion with tumor necrosis factor for pulmonary metastases. Ann Thorac Surg 1996; 61(6):1609–17.

139. Johnston MR, Minchen RF, Dawson CA. Lung perfusion with chemotherapy in patients with unresectable metastatic sarcoma to the lung or diffuse bronchioloalveolar carcinoma. J Thorac Cardiovasc Surg 1995; 110(2):368–73.

140. Wilking N, Petrelli NJ, Herrera L, Regal AM, Mittelman A. Surgical resection of pulmonary metastases from colorectal adenocarcinoma. Dis Colon Rectum 1985; 28:562–4.

141. Goorin AM, Delorey MJ, Lack EE, et al. Prognostic significance of complete surgical resection of pulmonary metastases in patients with osteogenic sarcoma: analysis of 32 patients. J Clin Oncol 1984; 2:425–31.

142. Pastorino U, Valente M, Gasparini M, et al. Lung resection for metastatic sarcomas: total survival from primary treatment. J Surg Oncol 1989; 40:275–80.

143. Karp NS, Boyd A, DePan HJ, Harris MN, Roses DF. Thoracotomy for metastatic malignant melanoma of the lung. Surgery 1990; 107:256–61.

144. Wong JH, Euhus DM, Morton DL. Surgical resection for metastatic melanoma to the lung. Arch Surg 1988; 123:1091–5.

145. Thayer JO Jr, Overholt RH. Metastatic melanoma to the lung: long-term results of surgical excision. Am J Surg 1985; 149:558–62.

Commentary

STEVEN M GRUNBERG

Altered metabolism, loss of growth control, genetic instability, and variable response to therapy are all characteristics that define the neoplastic state. However, one of the most pathognomonic properties of a neoplasm is the ability to metastasize to distant organs. Although local treatment options may result in cure for early-stage neoplasms, the development of metastatic disease transforms the neoplasm from a localized to a systemic illness. Chemotherapy, hormonal therapy, immunotherapy, and now gene therapy are all modalities based on the premise that, in the setting of even one detectable site of distant disease, both macroscopic and microscopic metastatic disease must be addressed to regain the possibility of effective curative therapy.

However, despite the assumption by medical oncologists that cancer is by nature a systemic disease, surgery remains the modality responsible for the greatest number of cancer cures. This fact is the result of two basic premises of cancer therapy, one positive and one negative. On the positive side, although even the most indolent of cancers will become metastatic if allowed to grow for a long enough period without appropriate therapy, it is still possible to detect and treat a significant number of cancers early in their course. The appropriate time for aggressive local therapy may either be before the tumor has metastasized, when local therapy does remove all tumor, or at a time when micrometastatic disease is only moderately established and endogenous immune surveillance is still capable of controlling small amounts of residual disease after primary bulk disease has been resected. Even small-cell lung cancer, which is considered by most medical oncologists to be metastatic either macroscopically or microscopically in all cases at the time of presentation, can on occasion be cured by surgical resection after presentation as a solitary pulmonary nodule.[1] Thus, the TNM system, designed at a time when solid tumors were thought to follow a logical progression from the primary tumor site to nodal involvement and finally to distant metastatic disease, continues to serve as a valuable guide for predicting the probability of distant spread and for emphasizing the importance of local control.

On the negative side, the primary role of surgery in effecting cure of cancer is a reflection on the disappointing failure of systemic therapy to achieve cure in most cases of metastatic disease. This is not to say that there have not been significant and dramatic advances in the use of chemotherapy. Metastatic testicular cancer, previously an invariably fatal disease, is now often cured through the use of aggressive chemotherapeutic regimens.[2] Small-cell lung cancer, which previously had a median survival in the range of 2–3 months, now frequently has a median survival of a year or more.[3] Even increases in survival of non-small-cell lung cancer have been achieved through the addition of chemotherapy to multimodality regimens for regional disease[4] and the use of chemotherapy alone for advanced disease.[5] Adjuvant chemotherapy for diseases such as breast cancer is also commonly accepted.[6] However, most patients with metastatic disease will die of their cancer. Until this basic conclusion can be reversed through the development of more effective systemic treatments, attempts to palliate symptoms and extend survival through the control of locally detectable disease will continue to be made.

In their thorough review of the surgical treatment of pulmonary metastases, Putnam and Roth make the argument that surgical treatment is an important weapon in the overall therapeutic plan for such metastatic disease. Long-term survival rates of 20–30% for numerous tumor histologies after resection of pulmonary metastases are quoted. To place the role of the surgical resection of pulmonary metastases in perspective, one must carefully examine the underlying assumptions of the many case series that appear in the literature.

An important point is that the cases that appear in such surgical series are, and must be, highly selected. In many series, it is difficult to identify the overall denominator from which the cases for resection of pulmonary metastases have been selected. A smaller number of pulmonary metastases,[7] longer disease-free interval,[8] and longer doubling time[9] have been suggested as factors that increase the likelihood of successful outcome of pulmonary resection. However, these seem to be the characteristics that would also describe a tumor with a natural history of slow growth and late metastasis. The question therefore arises as to whether resection of pulmonary metastases increases long-term survival in some patients or whether the criteria for selecting patients for resection identify a group of patients with metastatic disease whose natural history would allow long-term survival with or without aggressive intervention. If the second possibility is to be considered, the medical oncologist would at least have to acknowledge that metastatic disease may not invariably lead to demise and that there exists a subset of patients for whom systemic therapy may also not be necessary.

Encouraging results have even been reported with multiple resections of pulmonary metastases. However, the natural history of a given tumor may change over time, and a long disease-free interval before first resection of pulmonary metastases does not necessarily imply that this characteristic of tumor growth will continue to apply.[10] Even in the setting of apparent success, the use of similar criteria to qualify patients for initial or repeated resection (e.g., small number of metastases, lack of extrathoracic disease, control of primary tumor) may simply continue to identify patients with a relatively benign natural history for whom the natural course of their tumor may be more important than the therapeutic interventions.[11]

One other important requirement for resection of pulmonary metastases is sufficient pulmonary reserve to retain good functional status after resection.[12] However, the presence of such a restriction for eligibility may select patients with a better baseline cardiovascular status that would be likely to lead to improved survival even if all other factors were ignored. Although not specifically mentioned in most series, the patient's overall performance status cannot help but be a factor in the surgeon's decision as to whether surgery is appropriate. Performance status is also commonly accepted as an excellent predictor of survival independent of any other therapeutic interventions.[13]

Although similar long-term survival rates may be noted with various tumor types after resection of pulmonary metastases, the natural history of the individual tumors must be taken into account. There is general acceptance, for example, that chemotherapy and surgery have important complementary roles in the management of metastatic germ cell tumor.[14] Although dramatic responses are often seen with chemotherapy for this disease, residual pulmonary nodules may still represent remaining neoplastic foci.[15,16] Of equal importance, residual parenchymal nodules may contain teratomatous foci that can undergo malignant degeneration and themselves metastasize at a later time.[17] In the treatment of soft tissue sarcomas, which are less sensitive to chemotherapy, the unique natural history in which pulmonary metastases are by far the dominant site of spread has led to the common use of repeated resection.[18] Squamous cell cancer of the head and neck represents a special case. These tumors seldom metastasize past the regional nodal basin. There is therefore a good possibility that a pulmonary nodule will represent an isolated metastatic site and that the patient would benefit from resection. In addition, the common risk factors for head and neck cancer and for lung cancer markedly increase the possibility that a pulmonary nodule in this setting represents a second tumor (primary bronchogenic carcinoma) that is indeed amenable to surgical cure.[19] In contrast, in diseases such as breast cancer[20] and melanoma,[21] which tend to disseminate early in their course to multiple organ systems, the relative risks and benefits of surgery must be more carefully considered.

The appropriate surgical approach for resection of pulmonary metastases has been a matter of discussion. In general, lateral thoracotomy or median sternotomy has been favored over video-assisted thoroscopic surgery (VATS) due to better exposure of the surgical field and the ability to locate and resect metastases that might not have been apparent through preoperative imaging.[22,23] However, the morbidity of a thorocotomy in terms of incisional pain and postoperative paresthesias is not always insignificant. If repeated surgical resection is feasible and anticipated, then identification of very small metastatic sites at the time of the first surgical procedure through wider exposure may be less essential because aggressive follow-up and intervention for newly identified lesions will then be undertaken.

As quality-of-life considerations become a more important component of therapeutic decision-making in oncology, questions concerning postoperative morbidity also become more important. If a procedure results in cure in the vast majority of cases, then a relatively high level of morbidity may be acceptable. However, at the present time, even among those cases carefully selected for surgical resection of pulmonary metastases, approximately 70–80% of patients will die of their cancer. One possible strategy to improve this situation would be the identification of prognostic factors accurate enough to select a subpopulation of patients with a very high chance of cure by pulmonary resection.[24] However, until such prognostic indicators are available, the effects of morbidity of treatment as compared to morbidity of tumor (often asymptomatic at the early stages of pulmonary metastases) as compared to possible alteration of the duration of survival through treatment must be considered. Methods to better determine patient preference and utility for various health states are presently under development and will prove valuable in making such decisions.

Dr Putnam and Dr Roth suggested that it is the responsibility of the thoracic surgeon to identify and propose resection of pulmonary metastases for appropriate patients. It is indeed the responsibility of the thoracic surgeon to identify patients for whom resection of pulmonary metastases is technically feasible. However, it is the responsibility of the entire multimodality team to identify therapeutic alternatives and to aid the patient in coming to an appropriate decision concerning treatment options. The answers to many of the questions raised above will not be soon forthcoming. The definitive clinical trial, randomizing patients who have been identified as having potentially resectable pulmonary metastases to resection or observation, is unlikely to be proposed or performed. Both physician and patient preference to actively pursue the most promising therapy in each individual case would make such a trial impossible. It is therefore reasonable to offer resection of pulmonary metastases as long as the strengths and limitations of the available literature are recognized and communicated. It is hoped that better multimodality therapy will lead to higher response and long-term survival rates that will then make the choice of optimal therapeutic options more clear cut.

REFERENCES

1. Lucchi M, Mussi A, Chella A, et al. Surgery in the management of small cell lung cancer. Eur J Cardiothorac Surg 1997; 12:689–93.

2. Hartmann JT, Kanz L, Bokemeyer C. Diagnosis and treatment of patients with testicular germ cell cancer. Drugs 1999; 58:257–81.

3. Bunn PA Jr, Carney DN. Overview of chemotherapy for small cell lung cancer. Semin Oncol 1997; 24 (2 Suppl. 7):S7-69–74.

4. Sause WT, Scott C, Taylor S, et al. Radiation Therapy Oncology Group (RTOG) 88-08 and Eastern Cooperative Oncology Group (ECOG) 4588: preliminary results of a phase III trial in regionally advanced, unresectable non-small-cell lung cancer. J Natl Cancer Inst 1995; 87:198–205.

5. Rapp E, Pater JL, Willan A, et al. Chemotherapy can prolong survival in patients with advanced non-small-cell lung cancer – report of a Canadian multicenter randomized trial. J Clin Oncol 1988; 6:633–41.

6. Esteva FJ, Hortobagyi GN. Adjuvant systemic therapy for primary breast cancer. Surg Clin North Am 1999; 79:1075–90.

7. Rizzoni WE, Pass HI, Wesley MN, Rosenberg SA, Roth JA. Resection of recurrent pulmonary metastases in patients with soft-tissue sarcomas. Arch Surg 1986; 121:1248–52.

8. Marincola FM, Mark JB. Selection factors resulting in improved survival after surgical resection of tumors metastatic to the lungs. Arch Surg 1990; 125:1387–92.

9. Ollila DW, Stern SL, Morton DL. Tumor doubling time: a selection factor for pulmonary resection of metastatic melanoma. J Surg Oncol 1998; 69:206–11.

10. Kamiyoshihara M, Hirai T, Kawashima O, Morishita Y. Resection of pulmonary metastases in six patients with disease-free interval greater than 10 years. Ann Thorac Surg 1998; 66:231–3.

11. Kandioler D, Kromer E, Tuchler H, et al. Long-term results after repeated surgical removal of pulmonary metastases. Ann Thorac Surg 1998; 65:909–12.

12. Dresler CM, Goldberg M. Surgical management of lung metastases: selection factors and results. Oncology 1996; 10:649–55.

13. Stanley KE. Prognostic factors for survival in patients with inoperable lung cancer. J Natl Cancer Inst 1980; 65:25–32.

14. Carter GE, Lieskovsky G, Skinner DG, Daniels JR. Reassessment of the role of adjunctive surgical therapy in the treatment of advanced germ cell tumors. J Urol 1987; 138:1397–401.

15. Liu D, Abolhoda A, Burt ME, et al. Pulmonary metastasectomy for testicular germ cell tumors: a 28-year experience. Ann Thorac Surg 1998; 66:1709–14.

16. Cagini L, Nicholson AG, Horwich A, Goldstraw P, Pastorino U. Thoracic metastasectomy for germ cell tumours: long term survival and prognostic factors. Ann Oncol 1998; 9:1185–91.

17. Ahmed T, Bosl GJ, Hajdu SI. Teratoma with malignant transformation in germ cell tumors in men. Cancer 1985; 56:860–3.

18. van Geel AN, Hoekstra HJ, van Coevorden F, Meyer S, Bruggink ED, Blankensteijn JD. Repeated resection of recurrent pulmonary metastatic soft tissue sarcoma. Eur J Surg Oncol 1994; 20:436–40.

19. Lefor AT, Bredenberg CE, Kellman RN, Aust JC. Multiple malignancies of the lung and head and neck. Second primary tumor or metastasis? Arch Surg 1986; 121:265–70.

20. McDonald ML, Deschamps C, Ilstrup DM, Allen MS, Trastek VF, Pairolero PC. Pulmonary resection in metastatic breast cancer. Ann Thorac Surg 1994; 58:1599–602.

21. Ollila DW, Morton DL. Surgical resection as the treatment of choice for melanoma metastatic to the lung. Chest Surg Clin North Am 1998; 8:183–96.

22. McCormack PM, Bains MS, Begg CB, et al. Role of video-assisted thoracic surgery in the treatment of pulmonary metastases: results of a prospective trial. Ann Thorac Surg 1996; 62:213–16.

23. Ferson PF, Keenan RJ, Luketich JD. The role of video-assisted thoracic surgery in pulmonary metastases. Chest Surg Clin North Am 1998; 8:59–76.

24. Pastorino U, McCormack PM, Ginsberg RJ. A new staging proposal for pulmonary metastases. Chest Surg Clin North Am 1998; 8:197–202.

Editors' selected abstracts

Metastasectomy as a cytoreductive strategy for treatment of isolated pulmonary and hepatic metastases from breast cancer.

Bathe OF, Kaklamanos IG, Moffat FL, Boggs J, Franceschi D, Livingstone AS.

Department of Surgery, University of Miami, FL, USA.

Surgical Oncology 8(1):35–42, 1999, July.

The authors sought to examine the utility of resection in conjunction with adjuvant chemotherapy for treatment of metastases from breast cancer isolated to the liver or lungs. Limitations of regional therapy were examined and potential agents for systemic therapy were reviewed. As resection of metastases is a controversial therapeutic approach, no clinical trials are available for review. Rather, evidence for a potential role for surgery rests on restrospective studies of small series of patients. Technical advances have rendered resection of liver and lung metastases safe. Long-term results as reported by other investigators support the role of metastasectomy in selected patients. The site of failure following ablation of liver metastases is usually in the liver. Following resection of lung metastases, nonpulmonary and disseminated recurrences are most common. Adjuvant therapy with docetaxel or any other agent or combination with significant activity against visceral metastases might potentiate long-term results.

Surgical treatment of pulmonary metastases.

Downey RJ.

Divisions of Thoracic Surgery and Critical Care Medicine, Memorial Sloan-Kettering Cancer Center, New York, NY, USA.

Surgical Oncology Clinics of North America 8(2):341, 1999, April.

Pulmonary metastatectomy has been widely adopted for the treatment of malignancies spread to the lungs. This article reviews the historical development of the procedure, pertinent anatomical background information, means of postoperative evaluation, and the conduct and results of surgery. [References: 72.]

Resection of lung metastases: Long-term results and prognostic analysis based on 5206 cases – the International Registry of Lung Metastases. [German]

Friedel G, Pastorino U, Buyse M, Ginsberg RJ, Girard P, Goldstraw P, Johnston M, McCormack P, Pass H, Putnam JB, Toomes H.

Abteilung fur Thoraxchirurgie, Zentrum fur Pneumologie und Thoraxchirurgie, Klinik Schillerhohe der LVA Wurttemberg, Stuttgart Gerlingen, Germany.

Zentralblatt fur Chirurgie 124(2):96–103, 1999.

The International Registry of Lung Metastases was established in 1991 to asses the long-term results of pulmonary metastasectomy. The Registry has accrued 5206 cases of lung metastasectomy, from 18 departments of thoracic surgery in Europe ($n = 13$), USA ($n = 4$) and Canada ($n = 1$). Of these patients 4572 (88%) underwent complete surgical resection. The primary tumor was epithelial in 2260 (43%), sarcoma in 2173 (42%), germ cell in 363 (7%), and melanoma in 328 (6%) patients. The disease-free interval was 0 to 11 months in 1729 (33%) cases, 12 to 35 months in 1857 (36%) and more than 36 months in 1620 (31%). Single metastases accounted for 2383 (46%) cases and multiple lesions for 2726 (52%). Mean follow up was 46 months. Analysis was performed by Kaplan–Meier estimates of survival, relative risk of death and multivariate Cox model. The actuarial survival after complete metastasectomy was 36% at 5 years, 26% at 10 years and 22% at 15 years (median 35 months); the corresponding values for incomplete resection were 13% at 5 years and 7% at 10 years (median 15 months). Among complete resections, the 5-year survival was 33% for patients with a disease-free interval of 0 to 11 months and 45% for those with a disease-free interval of more than

36 months; 43% for single lesions and 27 for four or more lesions. Multivariate analysis showed a better prognosis for patients with germ cell tumors, disease-free interval of 36 months and more and single metastases. These results confirm that lung metastasectomy is a safe and potentially curative procedure.

Surgery for pulmonary metastases from colorectal carcinoma.

Inoue M, Kotake Y, Nakagawa K, Fujiwara K, Fukuhara K, Yasumitsu T.

Department of Surgery, Osaka Prefectural Habikino Hospital, Habikino, Japan.

Annals of Thoracic Surgery 70(2):380–3, 2000, August.

Background: This study aims to clarify which patients would benefit by surgery for pulmonary metastases from colorectal carcinoma. *Methods:* A retrospective study was undertaken in 25 patients who had undergone complete resection. In all cases, prethoracotomy carcinoembryonic antigen (CEA) level was measured and mediastinal or hilar lymph nodes were histologically examined. *Results:* Overall 5-year survival was 39.2%. The 5-year survival rate for patients with a normal CEA level was 61.1%, as compared with 19.0% for patients with an elevated CEA level ($p = 0.0423$). The 5-year survival rate for patients without a lymph node metastasis was 49.5%, as compared with 14.3% for patients with a lymph node metastasis ($p = 0.0032$). No lymph node metastasis was a predictor of longer survival by univariate and multivariate analyses. The primary site, disease-free interval, and number and size of the metastasis were not significant prognostic factors. *Conclusions:* A resection for pulmonary metastasis from colorectal carcinoma is effective in patients with a normal CEA level and without a lymph node metastasis.

Pulmonary metastases of endocrine origin: The role of surgery.

Khan JH, McElhinney DB, Rahman SB, George TI, Clark OH, Merrick SH.

Division of Cardiac Surgery, University of California, San Francisco, CA, USA.

Chest 114(2):526–34, 1998, August.

Purpose: To determine the clinical course and outcome of patients undergoing pulmonary resection for metastatic endocrine tumors. *Methods:* Retrospective review of 47 patients with known endocrine tumors and pulmonary metastases who were evaluated for surgical resection between 1975 and 1996. *Results:* Tumors evaluated included the following: carcinoid (16), thyroid (12), pancreatic adenocarcinoma (10), adrenocortical carcinoma (6), pheochromocytoma (2), and parathyroid (1). Thirty-three patients were asymptomatic. Hormone secretion was noted in five patients. Twenty-five patients, who had isolated lung metastases, good control of the primary tumor, and no medical contraindication had surgical resection. The number of pulmonary nodules was not a limiting factor as long as all disease could be resected with adequate residual pulmonary function. CT was successful in directing resection in all patients. Twenty-six operations were performed in 25 patients and 22 patients were treated medically. Wedge resection was performed for lesions <2 cm (15), and lobectomy for larger or multiple nodules (10). Four patients had bilateral nodules resected. There was no operative mortality and no major complications. Actuarial 5-year survival was 61% for surgically treated patients. Independent predictors of poor survival included positive mediastinal lymph nodes at time of surgery ($p = 0.004$) and shorter disease-free interval ($p = 0.01$). At a median of 6.7 ± 1.2 years, six patients have developed radiographic appearance of a recurrence. A single patient with recurrent Hurthle cell cancer has had a successful reresection. The remaining patients have received chemotherapy. No patient with pancreatic carcinoma or adrenocortical carcinoma was a candidate for resection. All medically treated patients died within 6 months. *Conclusion:* Patients with endocrine tumors and pulmonary metastases are usually asymptomatic, their conditions are diagnosed accurately with CT, and they can achieve long-term survival comparable to other tumors (sarcoma) after pulmonary metastasectomy. *Clinical implications:* Patients with carcinoid, thyroid, pheochromocytoma, and parathyroid tumors with pulmonary metastases should undergo surgical resection if there is the following: (1) no evidence of extrathoracic disease; (2) good control of the primary tumor; (3) no medical contraindications for surgery; and (4) pulmonary function that can tolerate resection of all documented disease. The role of adjuvant chemotherapy in patients with positive lymph nodes needs further study.

Surgical treatment for both pulmonary and hepatic metastases from colorectal cancer.

Kobayashi K, Kawamura M, Ishihara T.

Metastatic Lung Tumor Study Group of Japan, Tokyo, Japan.

Journal of Thoracic & Cardiovascular Surgery 118(6):1090–6, 1999, December.

Objective: The role of surgery in the treatment of patients with pulmonary and hepatic metastases from colorectal cancer has not been delineated. *Methods:* Of the 351 patients enrolled in the Metastatic Lung Tumor Study Group of Japan between June 1988 and June 1996 who underwent thoracotomy for pulmonary metastases from colorectal cancer, 47 also underwent hepatic resection for metastatic tumors. The records of these patients were studied. *Results:* The 47 patients who underwent pulmonary and hepatic resection had a 3-year survival of $36\% \pm 8\%$, a 5-year survival of $31\% \pm 8\%$, and an 8-year survival of $23\% \pm 9\%$. The longest survival was 98 months. This patient was alive without recurrence. There was a significant difference in the cumulative survival of the patients with a solitary pulmonary metastasis and the patients with multiple pulmonary metastases ($p = 0.04$). Neither age, sex, location of the primary tumor, maximum diameter of the pulmonary metastases, method of pulmonary resection, number of hepatic metastases, nor method of hepatic resection was correlated with survival. However, 9 of 10 patients who survived 3 years or more after the initial thoracotomy had only one or two hepatic metastases. *Conclusion:* Surgical treatment of a solitary pulmonary metastasis concurrent with or after resection of hepatic metastases from colorectal cancer may be appropriate if the hepatic metastases are resectable for cure. Patients with a solitary pulmonary metastasis and a small number of hepatic metastases are good candidates for resection. Long-term survival can be expected.

The role of surgery in lung metastases.

Koodziejski L, Goralczyk J, Dyczek S, Duda K, Nabiaek T.

Centre of Oncology, Cracow, Poland.

European Journal of Surgical Oncology 25(4):410–17, 1999, August.

Aims: To evaluate the efficacy of pulmonary metastasectomy in 93 patients with lung metastases (LM) operated on from 1983 to 1997. *Methods:* We assessed: location and histological diagnosis of the primary tumor (PT); the extent of pulmonary resection; and disease-free interval (DFI). Survival analysis was undertaken using the Kaplan–Meier method. *Results:* Surgical complications occurred in eight (9%) patients; two (3%) died in hospital; seven (8%) were operated again because of further LM. In the whole patient group the average survival after metastasectomy was 40 months (median 22 months). The actuarial survival was 44% at 3 years and 35% at 5 years. With metastasectomy we achieved an overall survival after treatment of PT of 87 months (median 58 months). The actuarial survival was 58% at 5 years and 38% at 10 years. The average time between the treatment of PT and metastasectomy DFI was 4 years (median 41 months). Patients with a DFI of more than 2 years tended to live longer ($p = 0.086$). There were 23 patients with non-epithelial and 70 patients with epithelial tumours. Their DFIs were similar (mean 47, median 34 months for non-epithelial and mean 51, median 29 months for epithelial tumours). Of patients with non-epithelial tumours, 38% survived for 5 years and their survival curves were similar. In the group of tumours with the most frequent location, the results of metastasectomy did not differ considerably: 5 year survival rates of 20% for patients with kidney tumours, 28% for colorectal cancer, 30% for soft-tissue sarcoma, 28% for skin melanoma and 18% for breast cancer. *Conclusions:* Lung metastasectomy seems to be a safe and efficient method of treatment even for patients who show further metastases. According to our study it seems that, except for LM of breast carcinoma (which has a slightly worse prognosis), the results of surgical resection are not dependent on either the location or the histological pattern of the PT. For this reason patients indicated for operation can be selected according to similar criteria.

Lung metastases from melanoma: when is surgical treatment warranted?

Leo F, Cagini L, Rocmans P, Cappello M, Geel AN, Maggi G, Goldstraw P, Pastorino U.

Department of Thoracic Surgery, European Institute of Oncology, Via Ripamonti 435, Milan, 20141, Italy.

British Journal of Cancer 83(5):569–72, 2000, September.

Surgical treatment of lung metastases from melanoma is highly controversial as the expected outcome is much poorer than for other primary tumours and a reliable system for selecting patients is lacking. This study evaluated the long-term results of lung metastasectomy for melanoma, with the aim of defining a subset of patients with better prognosis. By reviewing the data of the International Registry of Lung Metastases (IRLM), we identified 328 patients who underwent lung metastasectomy for melanoma in the period 1945–1995. Survival was calculated by Kaplan–Meier estimate, using log-rank test and Cox regression model for statistical analysis. After complete pulmonary metastasectomy (282 patients) the 5- and 10-year survival was 22% and 16%, respectively. In this group of patients, a time to pulmonary metastases (TPM) shorter than 36 months or the presence of multiple metastases were independent unfavourable prognostic factors. There were no long-term survivors after incomplete resection (46 patients, $p < 0.01$). Using the IRLM grouping system, patients without risk factors (TPM >36 months and single lesion) experienced the best survival (29% at 5 years), followed by those with one risk factor only (20% at 5 years). On the other hand, those with two risk factors or incomplete resection showed a significantly poorer survival (7% and 0% at 5 years). Surgery plays an important role in carefully selected cases of pulmonary metastatic melanoma. The prognostic grouping system proposed by the International Registry of Lung Metastases provides a simple and effective method for improving the selection of surgical candidates.

Repeat resection of pulmonary metastases in patients with soft-tissue sarcoma.

Weiser MR, Downey RJ, Leung DH, Brennan MF.

Department of Surgery, Memorial Sloan-Kettering Cancer Center, New York, NY, USA.

Journal of the American College of Surgeons 191(2):184–90, 2000, August.

Background: Even after an apparent complete resection of sarcomatous pulmonary metastases, 40% to 80% of patients will re-recur in the lung. The benefit of subsequent re-resection is poorly defined. This study examines patient survival after repeat pulmonary exploration for re-recurrent metastatic sarcoma at a single institution. *Study design:* Between July 1982 and December 1997, data on 3,149 adult in-patients with soft tissue sarcoma were prospectively gathered. Of these, pulmonary metastases were present or developed in 719 patients and 248 underwent at least one resection. Of the patients relapsing in the lung after an apparently complete resection, 86 underwent reexploration. Disease-specific survival (DSS) after re-resection was the end point of the study. Time to death was modeled using the method of Kaplan and Meier. The association of factors to time-to-event end points was analyzed using the log-rank test for univariate analysis and the Cox proportional hazards model for multivariate analysis. Clinicopathologic factors were analyzed with the Pearson chi-square or Fisher's exact test when appropriate. *Results:* The median DSS after re-resection for all patients undergoing at least two pulmonary resections was 42.8 months with an estimated 5-year survival of 36%. The median DSS in patients with complete reresection was 51 months ($n = 68$) compared with 6 months in patients with an incomplete re-resection ($n = 16$, $p < 0.0001$). Patients with one or two nodules at re-resection ($n = 39$) had a median DSS of 51 months compared with 20 months in patients with three or more nodules ($n = 40$, $p = 0.003$). Patients in whom the largest metastasis re-resected was less than or equal to 2 cm ($n = 33$) had a median DSS of 44 months compared with 20 months in patients with metastasis greater than 2 cm ($n = 43$, $p = 0.033$). Patients with primary tumor high-grade histology ($n = 75$) had a median DSS of 32 months and patients with low-grade histology ($n = 11$) had a median DSS that was not reached ($p = 0.041$). Three independent prognostic factors associated with poor outcomes may be determined preoperatively: ≥ 3 nodules, largest metastases >2 cm, and high-grade primary tumor histology. Patients with either zero or one poor prognostic factor had a median DSS >65 months and patients with three poor prognostic factors had a median DSS of 10 months. *Conclusions:* Reexploration for recurrent sarcomatous pulmonary metastases appears beneficial for patients who can be completely re-resected. Outcomes are described by factors that may be determined preoperatively, including metastasis size, metastasis number, and primary tumor histologic grade. Patients who cannot be completely re-resected or those with numerous, large metastases and high-grade primary tumor pathology have poor outcomes and should be considered for investigational therapy.

Index